Vitamin D
Chemical, Biochemical
and Clinical Update

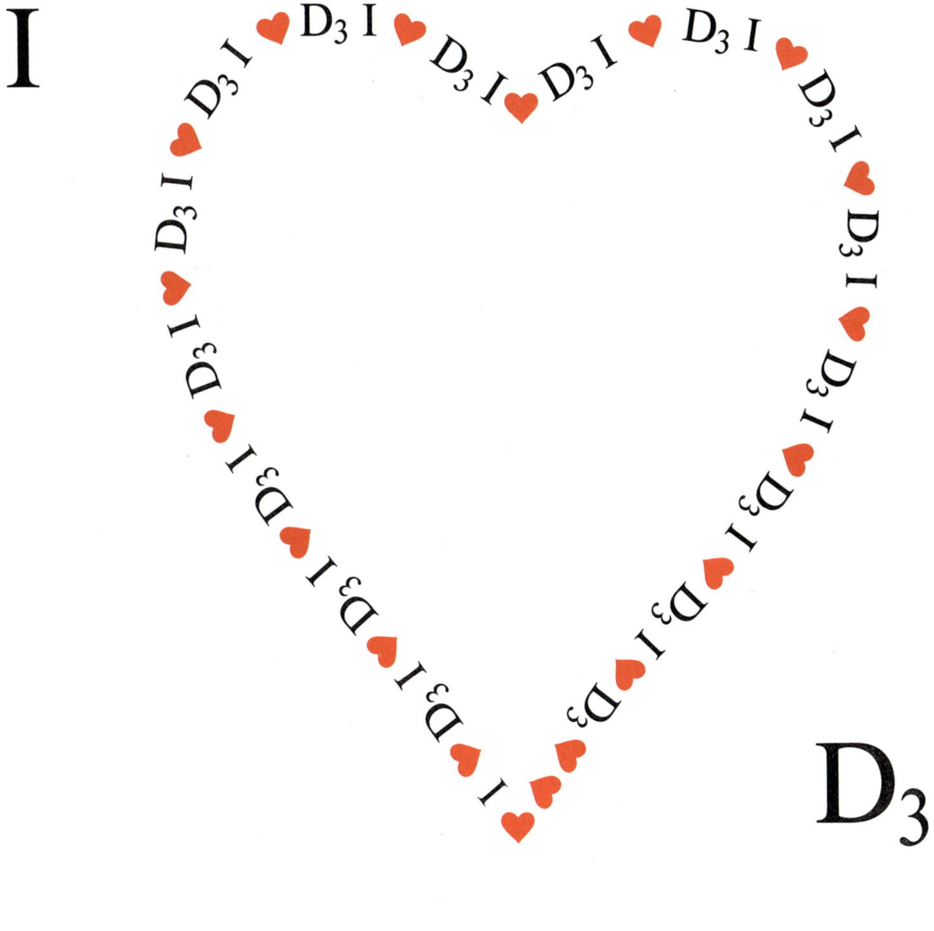

Vitamin D

Chemical, Biochemical and Clinical Update

Proceedings of the
Sixth Workshop on Vitamin D
Merano, Italy, March 1985

Editors
A. W. Norman · K. Schaefer
H.-G. Grigoleit · D. v. Herrath

W DE G

Walter de Gruyter · Berlin · New York 1985

Editors

A. W. Norman, Professor, Ph. D.
Department of Biochemistry
University of California
Riverside, CA 92521
USA

H.-G. Grigoleit, Dr.
Klinische Pharmakologie
Hoechst AG
D-6230 Frankfurt 80
Federal Republic of Germany

K. Schaefer, Professor, Dr.
St. Joseph-Krankenhaus I
D-1000 Berlin 42
Federal Republic of Germany

D. von Herrath, Dr.
St. Joseph-Krankenhaus I
1000 Berlin 42
Federal Republic of Germany

Library of Congress Cataloging in Publication Data

Workshop on Vitamin D (6th : 1985 : Merano, Italy)
Vitamin D : chemical, biological, and clinical update.
Includes bibliographies and indexes.
1. Vitamin D--Congresses. 2. Vitamin D--Metabolism--Congresses.
3. Vitamin D--Therapeutic use--Congresses.
I. Norman, A. W. (Anthony W.), 1938- . II. Title.
[DNLM: 1. Vitamin D--congresses. W3 WO512C 6th 1985 v / QU 173 W926 1985v]
QP772.V53W67 1985 612'.399 85-10403
ISBN 0-89925-066-1 (U.S.)

CIP-Kurztitelaufnahme der Deutschen Bibliothek

Vitamin D : proceedings of the ... Workshop on Vitamin D. –
Berlin ; New York : de Gruyter
Früher u. d. T.: Vitamin D and problems related to uremic bone disease
NE: Workshop on Vitamin D
6. Chemical, biochemical and clinical update : Merano, Italy, March 1985. – 1985.
ISBN 3-11-010181-5 (Berlin)
ISBN 0-89925-066-1 (New York)

ISBN 3 11 010181 5 Walter de Gruyter · Berlin · New York
ISBN 0-89925-066-1 Walter de Gruyter, Inc., New York

 Printing: Gerike GmbH, Berlin. Binding: Dieter Mikolai, Berlin. Printed in Germany.

Foreword

The Sixth Workshop on Vitamin D was held in the Centro Congressi of Merano, Italy, which is located in the northern Tyrol region of that country. The meeting was held from March 17–22, 1985. In attendance were 474 registered delegates from 27 countries. These include representatives from Algeria (2), Argentina (1), Australia (14), Austria (5), Belgium (12), Canada (15), Denmark (20), Federal Republic of Germany (24), Finland (6), France (37), German Democratic Republic (17, India (1), Israel (17), Italy (33), Japan (36), Norway (9), Poland (4), Saudi Arabia (2), South Afrika (2), Spain (7), Sweden (13), Switzerland (13), The Netherlands (25), Turkey (3), United Kingdom (36), United States (133) and Yugoslavia (2).

Interest and attendance at Vitamin D Workshops still continues to grow. Tabulated below are the dates and attendance as well as number of talks given at the six Vitamin D Workshops that have now been held. Since the time of the Fifth Workshop held in Williamsburg, Virginia in February of 1982, there has been a clear increase in attendance at the Workshop as well as in the number of submitted presentations. This reflects the continuing growth in research frontiers related to the vitamin D endocrine system.

Workshop Number	Date	Number of Delegates	Number of Countries Represented	Number of Presentations		Presentations per Delegate
				Talks	Posters	
I	October 1973	56	3	5	--	0.09
II	October 1974	221	22	84	--	0.39
III	January 1977	332	20	45	124	0.51
IV	February 1979	402	26	80	205	0.76
V	February 1982	455	25	95	298	0.86
VI	March 1985	474	27	77	380	0.96

The formal program of the Sixth Workshop on Vitamin D included 48 verbal presentations by invited speakers and 29 promoted free communications as well as 380 poster presentations. This program was conceived and put together by the Program Committee of the Sixth Workshop; members of this committee included R. Bouillon (Belgium), A. Caniggia (Italy), J. W. Coburn (USA), H. F. DeLuca (USA), S. Edelstein (Israel), J. A. Eisman (Australia), M. R. Haussler (USA), M. F. Holick

(USA), J. A. Kanis (United Kingdom), D. E. M. Lawson (United Kingdom), A. W. Norman (USA), J. L. H. O'Riordan (United Kingdom), W. H. Okamura (USA), B. L. Riggs (USA), T. Suda (Japan), M. Thomasset (France), M. Uskokovic (USA), R. H. Wasserman (USA). A major responsibility of the Program Committee was to review the 409 abstracts submitted as Free Communications and to individually „score" each abstract; from this group, 29 abstracts were selected by the Program Committee for inclusion on the verbal program of the meeting. In addition a special feature of the Sixth Workshop was a new component of the program entitled, „Late Breaking Events." A sub-committee of the Program Committee evaluated abstracts which were turned in at the time of the meeting in Merano; these presentations were to cover laboratory developments which occurred since the time of submission of abstracts in October 1984 and the occurrence of the meeting in March 1985. A total of 8 abstracts were received and 6 were programmed on the last day of the meeting as 7-minute presentations; the chapters for each of these „Late Breaking Events" are included in this volume.

Presented in this volume are papers prepared by the invited speakers as well as submittors of many of the Free Communications. The chapters in this book are grouped according to their general subject matter based on the classification made by the submitting authors, e. g. vitamin D chemistry, vitamin D metabolism and catabolism, receptors for $1,25(OH)_2D_3$, renal osteodystrophy, osteoporosis, etc.

Due to the large number of Free Communications (380) a major effort was made to allow adequate time for presentation and discussion of the many significant results that were presented by this mechanism. There were seven Poster Sessions scheduled throughout the meeting; during a 2–3 hour time interval the posters were „manned" by the submitting authors. Importantly, however, each poster was available for review for a minimum of 10–11 hours each day. Thus on each day approximately 100 posters were continuously presented throughout the day.

The highlights of the Sixth Workshop on Vitamin D were again amazing in terms of ther variety; undoubtedly this reflects the diverse interests of the chemists, biochemists, physiologists and clinicians who attended the meeting and who are actively conducting research in the various aspects of the vitamin D endocrine system. Clinical highlights included presentation of results of ongoing trials of $1,25(OH)_2D_3$ in the treatment of post-menopausal osteoporosis. There was uniformity of agreement in the four osteoporosis presentations that under appropriate circumstances $1,25(OH)_2D_3$ may make an important contribution to available treatment modalities. Also there was continuing status reports on the effectiveness of $1,25(OH)_2D_3$ in treatment of renal osteodystrophy. Several presentations focused on the application of $1,25(OH)_2D_3$ in the early onset of renal failure; again the utility of $1,25(OH)_2D_3$ was supported by the presentations given at the Workshop.

Several significant advances were also reported in terms of our basic understanding of the vitamin D endocrine system. Notable in this regard was the presentation of the molecular biological cloning of the mRNA for the D-binding protein; this resulted in the generation of the primary amino acid sequence for both the rat as well as human DBP. This important D-transport protein is apparently related to the protein families of albumin and α-feto protein. Also the amino acid sequence was reported, as derived from classical sequencing techniques, of the principle intestinal vitamin D induced 28,000 dalton calcium binding protein. An intriguing chemical observation was the sythesis of an analog of $1,25(OH)_2D_3$, namely $1,25S,26(OH)_3$-$\Delta 22$-D_3 which was highly active in mediating cell differentiation but had a diminished activity in terms of its hypercalcemic actions as compared to the parent $1,25(OH)_2D_3$. Clear and incisive evidence was presented that $1,25(OH)_2D_3$ could be produced at various extra-renal sites; in this regard it was intriguing to learn that γ-interferon could stimulate the production of $1,25(OH)_2D_3$ by pulmonary macrophages. Certainly the area of the program which attracted the largest submission of Free Communications was that relating to $1,25(OH)_2D_3$ receptors and their participation in cell differentiation. It is clear from these collective results that a micro/paracrine endocrine system exists for $1,25(OH)_2D_3$ in terms of mediating appropriate stem cell differentiation.

The Advisory Committee and the Program Committee would like to acknowledge the financial support of American Bio-Science Laboratories, Amersham International, Chugai Pharmaceutical Co. Ltd., Du Pont NEN Products Division, E. Merck, Fondazione Hoechst, Gambro Dialysatoren, Hoffmann-La Roche and Co. Ltd. (Basle), Hoffmann-La Roche (Nutley), Immuno Nuclear, Leo Pharmaceutical Products, Mead Johnson Nutritional Division, Nuclear Data, Inc., Roche S. P. A., Roussel Maestretti, Teijin Limited, and The Procter and Gamble Company. Without this generous governmental and multi-corporate financial support it would have been impossible to have a Vitamin D Workshop which included such a comprehensive program and world-wide attendance.

A special tribute is also due to the tireless efforts of the Workshop Conference Secretaries. Ms. Lean S. Gill and her colleagues in Riverside, Ms. June E. Bishop and Ms. Ann Hall were responsible for the bulk of the secretarial activities related to production of the abstract book and the advanced registration process. In addition Workshop Secretary, Ms. Pam Moore effectively and professionally handled the multitude of details concerned with the actual conduct of the meeting in Merano; in this capacity she was ably assisted by both Ms. June Bishop and Ms. Tieneka Hansson.

Anthony W. Norman, Riverside
Klaus Schaefer, Berlin
Dietrich von Herrath, Berlin
Hans-Günther Grigoleit, Frankfurt

March 1985

OFFICIAL SPONSORS
SIXTH WORKSHOP ON VITAMIN D

American Bio-Science Laboratories
USA

Amersham International plc
England

Chugai Pharmaceutical Co Ltd
Japan

Du Pont NEN Products Division
USA

E Merck
Fed Rep of Germany

Fondazione Hoechst
Italy

Gambro Dialysatoren (Munich)
Fed Rep Germany

Hoffmann-La Roche & Co Ltd (Basle)
Switzerland

Hoffman-La Roche (Nutley, New Jersey)
USA

Immuno Nuclear
USA

Leo Pharmaceutical Products
Denmark

Mead Johnson Nutritional Division
USA

Nuclear Data, Inc
(Molsgaard Medical A/S)

Roche S.P.A.
Italy

Roussel Maestretti
Italy

Teijin Limited
Japan

The Procter & Gamble Company
USA

Contents

Vitamin D

Metabolism and Catabolism

* Invited Presentation

Receptors for 1,25(OH)$_2$D$_3$

* Invited Presentation

Biological Actions for 24,25$(OH)_2D_3$

* Invited Presentation

Calcium Binding Proteins – Chemistry/Physiology/Molecular Biology

* Invited Presentation

Intestinal Ca and P Transport

Renal Actions of D Metabolites

* Invited Presentation

* Invited Presentation

Pregnancy/Neonatology

* Invited Presentation

D-Binding Proteins

* Invited Presentation

Photobiology

Evolutionary Aspects of Vitamin D

Chemistry of Vitamin D Seco-Steroids

* Invited Presentation

Assay Methodology: Vitamin D and Metabolites

* Invited Presentation

Pancreas/Diabetes and Vitamin D and Metabolites

* Invited Presentation

Cancer and Vitamin D (and Metabolites)

Renal Osteodystrophy

* Invited Presentation

* Invited Presentation

* Invited Presentation

Sarcoidosis

* Invited Presentation

Other Clinical Topics

Addendum

* Invited Presentation

* Invited Presentation

Vitamin D
Metabolism and
Catabolism

A COMPARISON OF VITAMIN D_2 AND D_3 IN MAN.

L. TJELLESEN, C. CHRISTIANSEN, L. HUMMER,
Department of Clinical Chemistry, Glostrup Hospital, Denmark.

INTRODUCTION

During the last 10 years extensive studies on vitamin D metabolism have demonstrated that vitamin D (cholecalciferol) is hydroxylated in the liver to 25-hydroxycholecalciferol ($25(OH)D_3$), which is further hydroxylated in the kidney either to 1,25-dihydroxycholecalciferol ($1,25(OH)_2D_3$) or to 25,26-dihydroxycholecalciferol ($25,26(OH)_2D_3$) or 24,25-dihydroxycholecalciferol ($24,25(OH)_2D_3$) (1). Furthermore, in the last few years a number of hydroxylated vitamin D analogues have been synthesized and it has become possible to measure the low levels of these compounds in serum (2). The 1α-hydroxylated compounds have particularly attracted clinical interest.

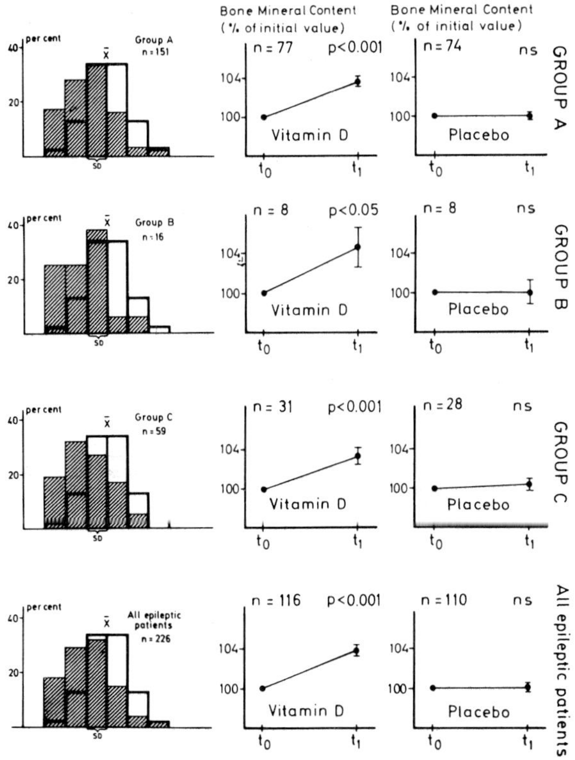

Fig. 1. An ideal normal histogram is superimposed with the percentage distribution of bone mineral content (BMC) in epileptics before vitamin D treatment (hatched areas).
The effect of three months' treatment with vitamin D_2 plus calcium and placebo plus calcium on BMC, expressed as per cent of initial value (right).

It is well documented that treatment of epileptic patients with phenytoin, phenobarbital and primidone produces disorders of bone and mineral metabolism (3,4,5). Recently, our group has demonstrated that epileptics on carbamazepine monotherapy do not develop pathophysiological changes in calcium and vitamin D metabolism (6,7). The features of this "antiepileptic drug induced osteomalacia" include hypocalcemia (3,4,5,8), raised serum alkaline phosphatase (3,5), a lower than normal bone mineral content (BMC) (fig. 1), hypomagnesaemia (9), bone biopsy findings characteristic of osteomalacia (10), and radiological findings of rickets in children (11, 12,13,14).

The two forms of vitamin D: ergocalciferol (D_2) and cholecalciferol (D_3) are thought to have equal effects in the treatment of osteomalacia, but some findings suggest that antiepileptic drug-induced osteomalacia is difficult to treat with vitamin D (15).

We have shown that vitamin D_2 in a dose of 2000 IU/day for three months increases BMC by 4% (3) (fig. 1), and that the effect of vitamin D_2 on BMC is dose dependent (16). In another study (17) we found that D_3 or $25(OH)D_3$ did not change the bone mineral content (fig. 2).

The aim of the present study was therefore to examine the serum concentration of vitamin D metabolites in epileptic patients <u>with</u> and <u>without</u> anticonvulsant osteomalacia compared to normals; and to examine the response of treatment with vitamin D_2 versus vitamin D_3 on vitamin D metabolites in epileptic patients <u>with</u> and <u>without</u> anticonvulsant osteomalacia compared to normals.

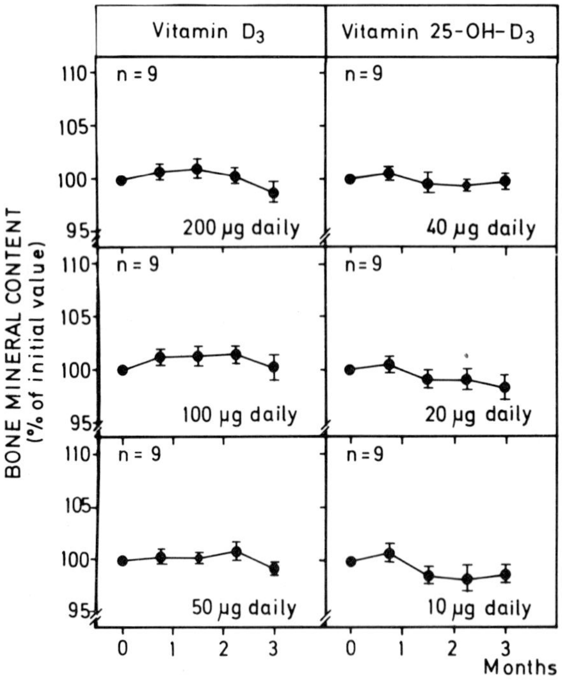

Fig. 2. Effect on bone mineral content of three different doses of vitamin D_3 and vitamin $25(OH)D_3$ as a function of time.

SUBJECTS

Three groups of subjects participated in the study:
Group 1 comprised twenty-two adult epileptic patients attending the epilepsy clinic at Glostrup Hospital as outpatients. All had received phenobarbitone for at least one year, and 13 were also receiving phenytoin. They had been treated for between 1 and 43 years (mean 21 years). The serum level of phenobarbitone ranged from 9 to 31 mg/l (mean 17 mg/l) and the serum level of phenytoin ranged from 4 to 18 mg/l (mean 14 mg/l). The trial was conducted as a double-blind investigation in the period from April to November 1983. The participants were allocated by random sampling numbers to two groups: oral treatment with either vitamin D_2 or vitamin D_3, 4000 IU/day for 24 weeks (table I). Moreover, all participants received 0.5 g calcium per day. Serum samples for determination of vitamin D metabolites were obtained before and after 24 weeks of vitamin D treatment.

Relevant clinical data in the three study populations.

Table I

	Number	Mean age (years)	Treatment group	Number	Mean age (years)
Epileptics on Phenytoin	22	51.2	D_2	12	48.6
			D_3	10	54.2
Epileptics on Carbamazepine	30	40.4	D_2	16	38.1
			D_3	14	43.1
Controls	19	33.4	D_2	9	31.8
			D_3	10	34.9

Group 2 comprised thirty adult epileptic patients attending the epilepsy clinic at Glostrup Hospital as outpatients. They had been treated with carbamazepine as the sole anticonvulsant therapy for between 1 and 10 years (mean 4 years) and the serum level ranged from 3 mg/l to 11 mg/l (mean 7 mg/l). The trial was conducted as a double-blind investigation in the period from May to December 1982.
The patients were allocated by random sampling numbers to two groups for oral treatment with either vitamin D_2 or vitamin D_3, 4000 IU/day for 24 weeks (table I). Serum samples for determination of vitamin D metabolites were obtained before and after 24 weeks of vitamin D treatment.
Group 3 comprised 19 normal subjects randomized to treatment with either vitamin D_2 or vitamin D_3 4000 IU/day (table I). Serum samples for determination of vitamin D metabolites were obtained before and after 8 weeks of vitamin D treatment.

METHODS

The serum samples were stored at -20°C until assayed, and all samples from the same participants were run in one assay to minimize the interassay variation. Five ml of serum was extracted by methanol/dichloromethane and the lipid extract was purified on Sephadex LH 20 according to the procedure described by Shepard et al. (18).

$25(OH)D_3$ / $25(OH)D_2$ assay

In the monohydroxylated fraction from the Sephadex LH 20 column, the serum concentration of 25(OH)D including $25(OH)D_3$ and $25(OH)D_2$ was measured by competitive protein binding assay (19), and the serum concentrations of $25(OH)D_3$ was measured by radioimmunoassay (20). Serum concentration of $25(OH)D_2$ was determined by the differences between the 25(OH)D and $25(OH)D_3$ result (19).

$24,25(OH)_2D$ / $24,25(OH)_2D_3$ / $25,26(OH)_2D$ assay

The fraction containing the dihydroxy metabolites was further chromotographed by a single step HPLC on a straight phase silica column (Lichrosorb Si 60) (18,21) and fractions eluting together with $24,25(OH)_2D_3$ and $25,26(OH)_2D_3$ standard preparation were collected for final assay. In the $24,25(OH)_2D$ fraction the $24,25(OH)_2D_3$ metabolite was measured by a selective radioimmunoassay (21) and $24,25(OH)_2D$ was measured by competitive protein binding assay (18). It has to be noted that the determination of $24,25(OH)_2D$ includes $24,25(OH)_2D_3$, $24,25(OH)_2D_2$, $25,26(OH)_2D_2$, and $25(OH)D_3$-26,23 lactone (22), whereas the radioimmunoassay of $24,25(OH)_2D_3$ is specific for $24,25(OH)_2D_3$ when applied to this fraction. The $25,26(OH)_2D_3$ is the only metabolite expected to be present in the $25,26(OH)_2D$ fraction (22).

$1,25(OH)_2D$

In the applied HPLC system $1,25(OH)_2D_2$ and $1,25(OH)_2D_3$ are almost coeluting and the elution volume containing both metabolites was collected. $1,25(OH)_2D$ was measured by competitive protein binding assay using cytosol from vitamin D deficient chick intestines, which equally recognizes $1,25(OH)_2D_2$ and $1,25(OH)_2D_3$ (23).

RESULTS

Initial values: Compared to the control group the 22 phenytoin treated patients (group 1) as a group had significant decreased serum 25(OH)D (14.5 ± 3.0 ng/ml versus 27.0 ± 2.5 ng/ml, $p < 0.01$), decreased serum $24,25(OH)_2D$ (1.2 ± 0.2 ng/ml versus 2.3 ± 0.5 ng/ml, $p < 0.05$), normal $25,26(OH)_2D_3$ (0.6 ± 0.1 ng/ml versus 0.9 ± 0.3 ng/ml, n.s.), and decreased $1,25(OH)_2D$ (18.9 ± 2.6 pg/ml versus 27.4 ± 2.1 pg/ml, $p < 0.01$).
The 30 carbamazepine patients as a group (group 2) had normal serum 25(OH)D (25.2 ± 1.8 ng/ml, n.s.) decreased serum $24,25(OH)_2D$ (1.2 ± 0.1 ng/ml, $p < 0.05$) normal $25,26(OH)_2D_3$ (0.9 ± 0.2 ng/ml, n.s.) and increased $1,25(OH)_2D$ (38.0 ± 3.1 pg/ml, $p < 0.05$).

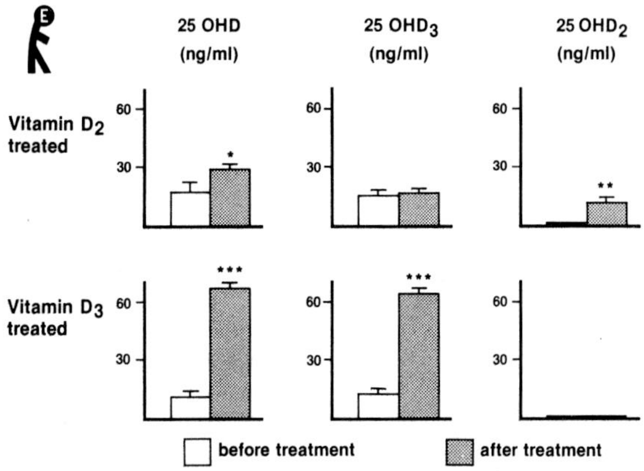

Fig. 3. Effect of treatment on serum 25(OH)D metabolites in epileptic patients in phenytoin therapy.

Effect of treatment

Group 1, phenytoin treated patients (fig. 3 and 4)

In the D_2 group there was no significant change in the serum vitamin D_3 metabolites ($25(OH)D_3$, $24,25(OH)_2D_3$ and $25,26(OH)_2D_3$), whereas serum $25(OH)D_2$ (and 25(OH)D) concentrations increased significantly. The rise in $24,25(OH)_2D$ together with the unchanged level of $24,25(OH)_2D_3$ during treatment with vitamin D_2, is caused by an increase in $24,25(OH)_2D_2$ and/or $25,26(OH)_2D_2$.
In the D_3 group a similar pattern was found, i.e. significant increases in the D_3 metabolites and unchanged levels of the D_2 metabolites. When comparing the response in the two vitamin D groups we found significant differences: treatment with vitamin D_3 produced a 2-4 fold higher increase in the corresponding metabolites than that of vitamin D_2.

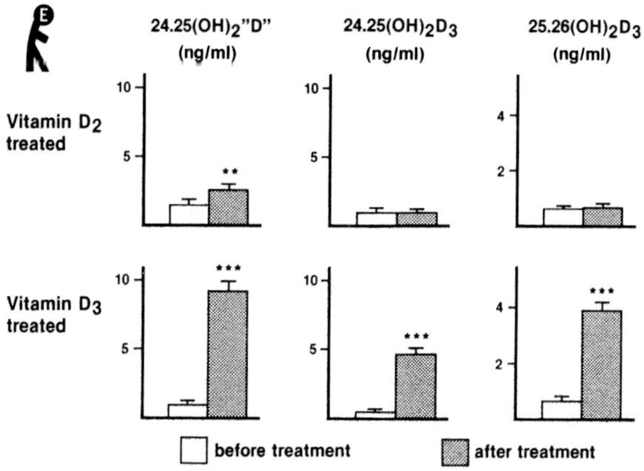

Fig. 4. Effect of treatment on serum levels of dihydroxy vitamin D metabolites in epileptic patients in phenytoin therapy.

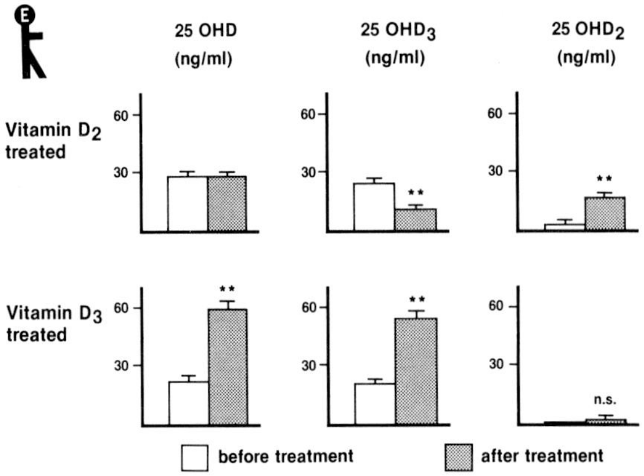

Fig. 5. Effect of treatment on serum 25(OH)D metabolites in epileptic patients in carbamazepine therapy.

Group 2, carbamazepine treated patients (fig. 5 and 6).

In the D_2 group, a significant increase in serum concentrations of $25(OH)D_2$ was found. However, the serum concentration of $25(OH)D_3$ decreased significantly. The serum concentrations of $24,25(OH)_2D_3$ and $25,26(OH)_2D_3$ decreased significantly, whereas the serum concentration of $24,25(OH)_2D$ was unchanged. In the D_3 group, serum concentrations of 25(OH)D, $25(OH)D_3$, and the dihydroxy metabolites $24,25(OH)_2D$, $24,25(OH)_2D_3$ and $25,26(OH)_2D_3$ all increased significantly during the trial. A comparison of the responses in the two vitamin D groups showed a difference in the changes during the treatment with vitamin D_2 and D_3. Treatment with vitamin D_2 did not increase serum concentrations of vitamin D metabolites due to a corresponding decrease in the vitamin D_3 metabolites, whereas vitamin D_3 treatment resulted in an increase in the serum concentrations of vitamin D metabolites caused by a 2-4 times increase in the vitamin D_3 metabolites.

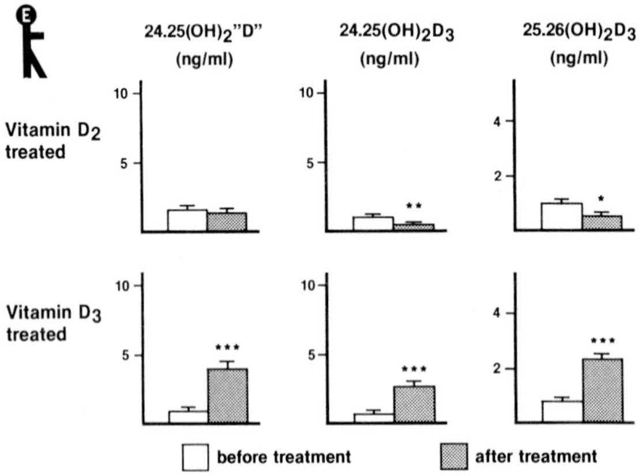

Fig. 6. Effect of treatment on serum levels of dihydroxy vitamin D metabolites in epileptic patients in carbamazepine therapy.

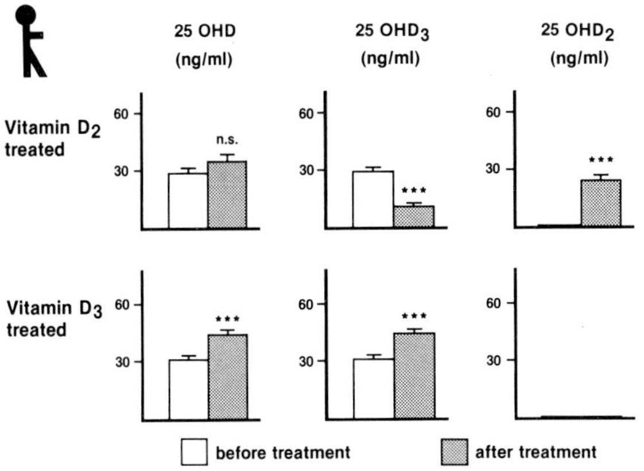

Fig. 7. Effect of treatment on serum 25(OH)D metabolites in normals.

Group 3, controls (fig. 7 and 8)

The response in the serum concentration of the 25-hydroxy vitamin D metabolites were similar to the findings in group 2, and so was the response in the vitamin D_3 treated group on the serum concentrations of $24,25(OH)_2D$, $24,25(OH)_2D_3$ and $25,26(OH)_2D_3$. In contrast the vitamin D_2 treated group showed a significant fall in the dihydroxy vitamin D metabolites.

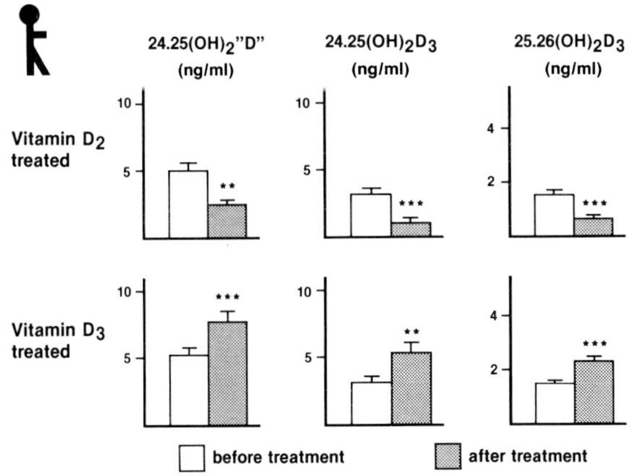

Fig. 8. Effect of treatment on serum levels of dihyd vitamin D metabolites in normals.

Effect of treatment on S-1,25(OH)$_2$D (fig. 9).

In all three groups there was no significant change in serum 1,25(OH)$_2$D during treatment with either vitamin D_2 or vitamin D_3.

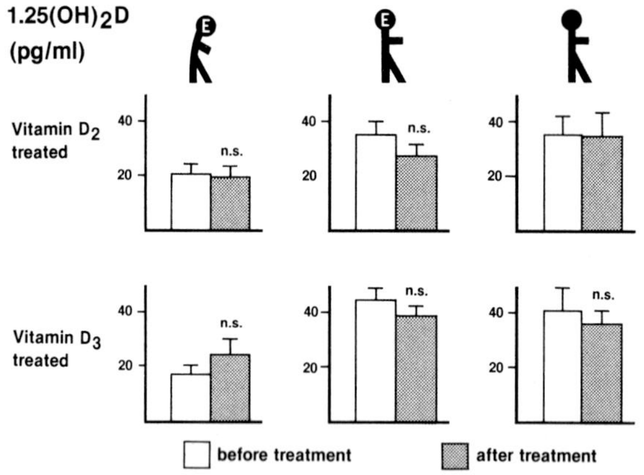

Fig. 9. Effect of treatment on serum 1,25(OH)$_2$D in the three groups (See text)

Effect of treatment on 24-h-U Ca/Cr (fig. 10).

In all three vitamin D_2 treated groups the 24-h urinary calcium excretion rate did not change during the treatment. In contrast the urinary calcium rose significantly in all three vitamin D_3 treated groups.

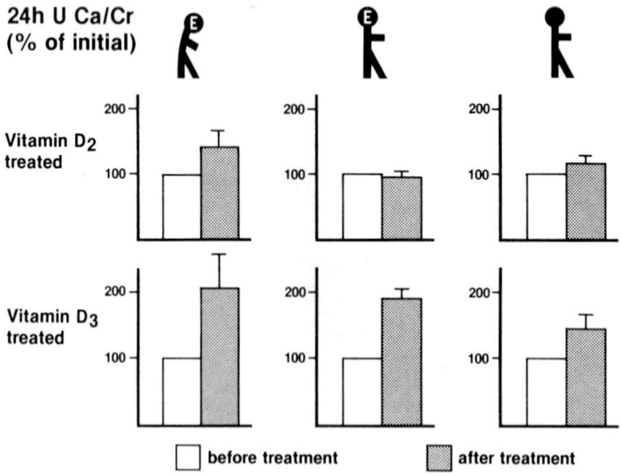

Fig. 10. Effect of treatment on 24-h urinary calcium excretion in the three groups (See text).

DISCUSSION

In 1975 we published the surprising finding that treatment of anticonvulsant osteomalacia with vitamin D_2 increased the bone mass whereas vitamin D_3 (or 25(OH)D_3) has no effect (3,17). These results disagree with the findings of Hahn and Halstead (24). At that time bone mass was measured by single photon absorptiometry on the distal part of the forearm (25), in an area corresponding to 1.2% of the total body calcium (26). Recently, we have demonstrated that this difference in the effect of vitamin D_2 and D_3 is of a generalized nature, since we found the same response when we used dual photon absorptiometry to measure the total body calcium (27).

During treatment with vitamin D_3 the carbamazepine treated patients (group 2) showed marked increases in all the vitamin D_3 metabolites. During treatment with vitamin D_2, the measured vitamin D_2 metabolites increased, but not to the same extent as did the D_3 metabolites during D_3 treatment. In contrast, the vitamin D_3 metabolites fell during the D_2 treatment so that the serum metabolites of D_2 and D_3 were constant during the treatment. In patients with anticonvulsant osteomalacia (i.e. group 1), who have low values of the vitamin D metabolites, we did not find this compensatory decrease in the serum D_3 metabolites during vitamin D_2 treatment, but the serum vitamin D metabolites were normalized. In contrast, vitamin D_3 treatment almost doubled the serum concentrations of vitamin D metabolites compared to the normal mean. These findings indicate that the two vitamins have both different quantitative and qualitative metabolic pathways in epileptic patients without anticonvulsant osteomalacia, whereas patients with anticonvulsant osteomalacia only show quantitative differences. Moreover, there may be some unknown regulatory mechanism between the hydroxylations of vitamin D_2 and D_3 in the liver, where the 25(OH)D metabolites are produced.

Our study cannot explain the different actions of vitamin D_2 and vitamin D_3 on bone mineral content in epileptic patients treated with phenobarbitone/phenytoin, but our present data proved a discrimination in the metabolism of orally dosed vitamin D_2 and vitamin D_3.

REFERENCES

1. Henry, H.L., Norman, A.W. (1984) Ann. Rev. Nutr., 4: 493-520.
2. Kumar, R. (1984) Physiol Rev. 64: 478-504.
3. Christiansen, C., Rødbro, P., Lund, M. (1973) Br. Med. J., 4: 695-701.
4. Hahn, T.J., Hendin, B.A., Scharp, C.R., Haddad, J. (1972) N. Engl. J. Med., 287: 900-904.
5. Richens, A., Rowe, D.J.F., (1970) Br. Med. J., 4: 73-76.
6. Tjellesen, L., Nilas, L., Christiansen, C. (1983) Acta Neurol. Scand. 68: 13-19.
7. Tjellesen, L., Gotfredsen, A., Christiansen, C. (1983) Acta Neurol. Scand. 68: 424-428.
8. Hunter, J., Maxwell, J.D., Stewart, D.A., Parsons, V., Williams, R. (1971) Br. Med. J., 4: 202-204.
9. Christiansen, C., Nielsen, S.P., Rødbro, P. (1974) Br. Med. J., 1: 198-199.

10. Dent, C.E., Richens, A., Rowe, D.J.F., Stamp, T.C.B. (1970) Br. Med. J. 4: 69-72.
11. Berger, G., Munde, B. (1970) Deutsche Gesundheitswesen, 15: 1549-1551.
12. Kruse, R. (1968) Monatsschr. Kinderheilkd., 116: 378-381.
13. Lifschitz, F., Maclaren, N.K. (1973) J. Pediatr., 83: 612-620.
14. Sotaniemi, E.A., Hakkarainen, H.K., Puranen, J.A., Lahti, R.O. (1972) Ann. Intern. Med., 77: 389-394.
15. Rowe, D.J.F., Stamp, T.C.B. (1974) Br. Med. J., 1: 392.
16. Christiansen, C., Rødbro, P. (1974) Acta Neurol. Scand., 50: 631-641.
17. Christiansen, C., Rødbro, P., Munck, P., Munck, O. (1975) Br. Med. J., 2: 363-365.
18. Shepard, R.M., Horst, R.L., Hamstra, A.J., DeLuca, H.F. (1979) Biochem. J., 182: 55-69.
19. Hummer, L., Tjellesen, L., Rickers, H., Christiansen, C. (1984) J. Clin. Lab. Invest. 44: 595-601.
20. Hummer, L., Nilas, L., Tjellesen, L., Christiansen, C. (1984) Scand. J. Clin. Lab. Invest., 44: 163-167.
21. Hummer, L., Christiansen, C. (1984) Clin. Endocrinol., 21: 71-79.
22. Horst, R.L., Littledike, E.T., Riley, J.L., Napoli, J.L. (1981) Anal. Biochem., 116: 189-203.
23. Hummer, L., Riis, B.J., Christiansen, C., Rickers, H. (1985) Scand. J. Clin. Lab. Invest., in press.
24. Hahn, T.J., Halstead, L.R. (1979) Calcif. Tissue. Int., 27: 13-18.
25. Christiansen, C., Rødbro, P., Jensen, H. (1975) Scand. J. Clin. Lab. Invest., 35: 323-330.
26. Christiansen, C., Rødbro, P. (1975) Scand. J. Clin. Lab. Invest., 35: 425-431.
27. Tjellesen, L., Gotfredsen, A., Christiansen, C. (1985) Calcif. Tissue Int., submitted.

METABOLISM OF 24R,25-DIHYDROXYVITAMIN D_3: AN APPROACH FROM SYNTHETIC STUDY.

S. Yamada,* E. Ino,* H. Takayama,* and T. Suda†
*Faculty of Pharmaceutical Sciences, Teikyo University, Sagamiko, Kanagawa 199-01, and † Department of Biochemistry, School of Dentistry, Showa University, Shinagawa, Tokyo 142, Japan

In vitamin D-supplemented state, 25-hydroxyvitamin D_3 is hydroxylated at the side chain to give 24R,25-dihydroxyvitamin D_3 [24R,25$(OH)_2D_3$] (1), 23S,25-dihydroxyvitamin D_3 (2), and 25,26-dihydroxyvitamin D_3 (3). Of these dihydroxylated metabolites, 24R,25$(OH)_2D_3$ has been received special attention. Because it is the major metabolite of vitamin D_3 whose plasma concentrations in most animals (4, 5) are at least ten-fold as high as those of the active metabolite, 1α,25-dihydroxyvitamin D_3. However, biological importance of 24R,25$(OH)_2D_3$ has still remained unclear. 24R,25$(OH)_2D_3$ was first considered to be an excretory metabolite, because of its low activity and rapid turnover in the birds (6). However, in the last seven years, evidence has been accumulated to suggest that 24R,25$(OH)_2D_3$ has its own specific biological activity (7, 8). To clarify the role of 24R,25$(OH)_2D_3$, we have been investigating the metabolism of 24R,25$(OH)_2D_3$. We have isolated and identified five new metabolites derived from 24R,25$(OH)_2D_3$ in vitamin D-supplemented state. We have synthesized all of those metabolites. This paper describes the metabolism of 24R,25$(OH)_2D_3$ in vitamin D-supplemented chicks and rats, and the syntheses of all of the metabolites derived from 24R,25$(OH)_2D_3$.

Metabolism of 24R,25$(OH)_2D_3$ in Vitamin D-Supplemented Chick Kidney. In 1978, Dr. Suda's group found a new in vitro metabolite which migrated prior to 25(OH)D_3 on a straight phase HPLC and designated the metabolite peak A (9). The metabolite is produced from either 24R,25$(OH)_2D_3$ or 25(OH)D_3 in the kidney from vitamin D-supplemented chicks.

The peak A metabolite was isolated in pure form by incubating 25(OH)D_3 with kidney homogenates from vitamin D-supplemented

Vitamin D. A Chemical, Biochemical and Clinical Update

chicks. The structure of the metabolite was determined to be 25-hydroxy-24-oxovitamin D_3 [25(OH)-24-oxo-D_3] on the basis of UV, mass, ^1H NMR, and IR spectra, as well as of some specific chemical reactions (10, 11). The structure of the metabolite was finally confirmed by chemical synthesis of this metabolite (12, 13).

25(OH)-24-oxo-D_3 was found to be metabolized to more polar compounds in vitamin D-supplemented chick kidney (Fig. 1). Panel A shows a Sephadex LH-20 chromatogram of the lipid extracts of the incubation mixture of 25(OH)-24-oxo-[^3H]D_3 with kidney homogenates from vitamin D-supplemented chicks. There are two metabolites peaks. These were separated into three peaks on a straight phase HPLC as shown in panel B. These were designated peak I, II, and IV in the order of increasing polarity (13).

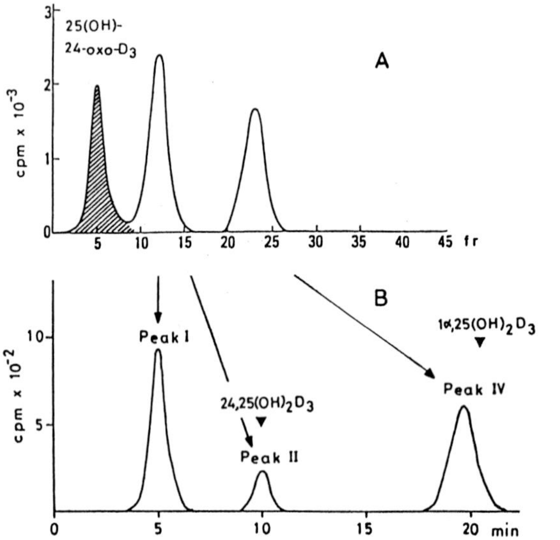

FIG. 1. Chromatographic profile of the metabolites of 25(OH)-24-oxo-[^3H]D_3 produced in vitamin D-supplemented chick kidney. A, Sephadex LH-20 chromatogram of lipid extracts of the kidney homogenates. The column was eluted with $CHCl_3$-hexane (75:25) and 5-ml fractions were collected. B, HPLC (Zorbax SIL, 0.46 x 25 cm, 2.5% methanol in CH_2Cl_2) profile of the fractions collected from Sephadex LH-20 column. Arrows show the elution position of authentic compounds.

All of these metabolites were isolated in pure form by incubating 50 µg of 25(OH)-24-oxo-D_3 with kidney homogenates from a total of 10 vitamin D-supplemented chicks. The yields of peak I, II, and IV were 2.6 µg, 3.0 µg, and 2.1 µg, respectively. The structure of the metabolites was determined on the basis of UV and mass spectra, and of some specific chemical reactions (14). The peak I was identified to be 23,25-dihydroxy-24-oxovitamin D_3 [23,25$(OH)_2$-24-oxo-D_3], the peak-II to be $24,25(OH)_2D_3$, and the peak IV to be 23,24,25-trihydroxyvitamin D_3 [$23,24,25(OH)_3D_3$]. The stereochemistry at C(24) of the isolated $24,25(OH)_2D_3$ was determined by comparing its trimethylsilyl ether with the trimethylsilyl ether of the authentic (24R)- and (24S)-$24,25(OH)_2D_3$ on a straight phase HPLC (Fig. 2). The trimethylsilyl ether of the isolated metabolite comigrated with the authentic compound with 24S-configuration. Thus the stereochemical configuration at C(24) in the $24,25(OH)_2D_3$ produced from 25(OH)-24-oxo-D_3 by metabolic reduction was determined to be not R, but S (15).

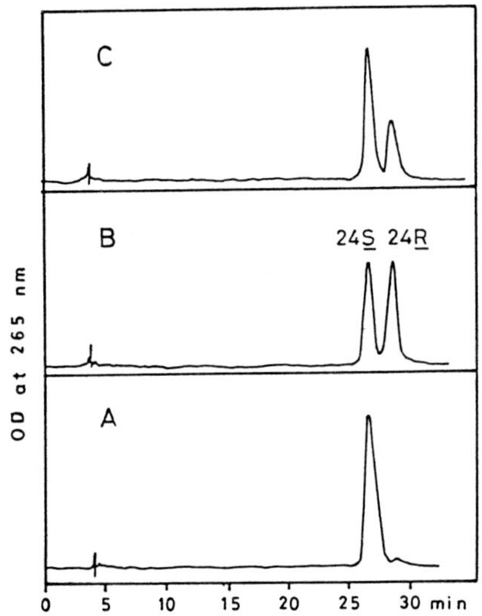

Fig. 2. Co-chromatography of tris(trimethylsilyl) ether of the $24,25(OH)_2D_3$ isolated from vitamin D-supplemented chick kidney incubated with 25(OH)-24-oxo-D_3 and tris(trimethylsilyl) ethers of the authentic (24R)- and (24S)-$24,25(OH)_2D_3$ on HPLC (Zorbax SIL, 0.46 x 25 cm, 2.5% $CHCl_3$ in hexane). A, Trimethylsilyl ether of the isolated metabolite; B, trimethylsilyl ethers of the authentic compounds; C, mixture of the silyl ethers of the isolated and the authentic two $24,25(OH)_2D_3$.

The metabolism of 24R,$25(OH)_2D_3$ in vitamin D-supplemented chick kidney is summarized as follows. 24-Hydroxyl group of 24R,$25(OH)_2D_3$ is first oxidized to ketone to give 25(OH)-24-oxo-D_3, which is then hydroxylated at the 23-position to give $23,25(OH)_2$-24-oxo-D_3. Reduction of the 24-oxo group of 25(OH)-24-oxo-D_3 also takes place to yield 24S,$25(OH)_2D_3$. It should be noted that the stereochemistry at C(24) of the $24,25(OH)_2D_3$ obtained from 25(OH)-24-oxo-D_3 by the reduction of the 24-oxo group is different from that in the $24,25(OH)D_3$ obtained from $25(OH)D_3$ by 24-hydroxylation. This suggests that the oxidation of the 24R-hydroxyl group and the reduction of the 24-oxo-group are catalyzed by two different enzymes. $23,24,25(OH)_3D_3$ is considered to be produced from $23,25(OH)_2$-

24-oxo-D_3 by the reduction of the 24-oxo group. Therefore the configuration at C(24) in this metabolite is supposed to be S. However, as an alternative pathway, 23-hydroxylation of 24S,25$(OH)_2D_3$ cannot be excluded. (Scheme 1)

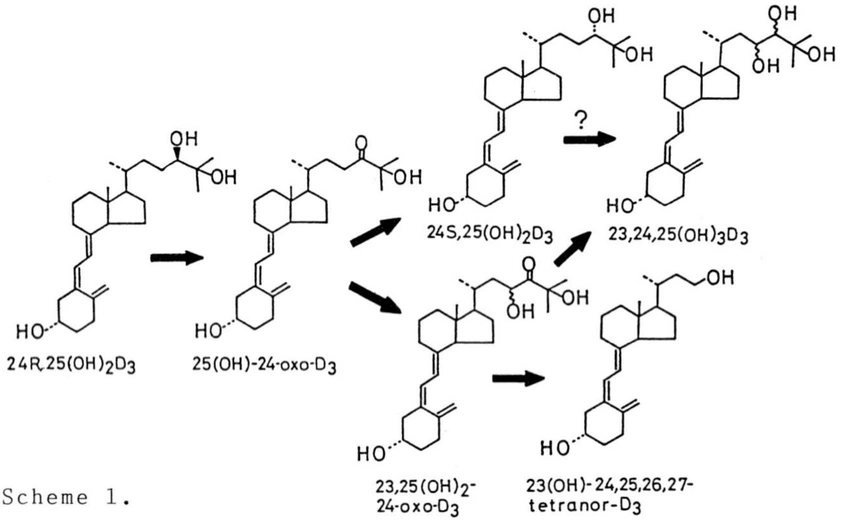

Scheme 1.

Metabolism of 24R,25$(OH)_2D_3$ in Vitamin D-Supplemented Rat Kidney. The metabolism of 24R,25$(OH)_2D_3$ in vitamin D-supplemented rats has been studied and a pathway similar to that in chicks was recognized (16, 17): 24R,25$(OH)_2D_3$ is oxidized at the 24-position to give 25(OH)-24-oxo-D_3 which is then hydroxylated at the 23-position to give 23,25$(OH)_2$-24-oxo-D_3. In addition to these metabolite, we, in collaboration with G. Jones's group, isolated and identified a new side chain cleavage metabolite, 23-hydroxy-24,25,26,27-tetranorvitamin D_3 [23(OH)-24,25,26,27-tetranor-D_3] from the perfused rat kidney incubated with 24R,25$(OH)_2D_3$ (16). 23(OH)-24,25,26,27-tetranor-D_3 was also obtained (1.6% yield) when 25(OH)-24-oxo-D_3 was incubated with kidney homogenates from rats predosed with 1α,25-dihydroxyvitamin D_3 (1.3 nmol/rat). In this experiment, the yield of 23,25$(OH)_2$-24-oxo-D_3 was as high as 18.5%. 23(OH)-24,25,26,27-tetranor-D_3 is considered to be produced by the cleavage of the bond between C(23) and C(24) in 23,25(OH)$_2$-24-oxo-D$_3$.

Syntheses of 24R,25(OH)$_2$D$_3$ and Its Metabolites. 24R,25(OH)$_2$D$_3$ and its metabolites were synthesized conveniently starting with two C(22) steroid synthons possessing provitamin D structure, phenylsulfone 3 and bromide 4, as summarized in Scheme 2. The phenylsulfone 3 is an especially useful nucleophilic C(22) steroid synthon from which 24R,25(OH)$_2$D$_3$, 25(OH)-24-oxo-D$_3$, 23,25(OH)$_2$-24-oxo-D$_3$, and 23,24,25(OH)$_3$D$_3$ were synthesized. The bromide 4 serves as electrophilic C(22) steroid synthon from which 23(OH)-24,25,26,27-tetranor-D$_3$ was synthesized. These two C(22) steroids can be readily obtained from ergosterol 1.

Scheme 2.

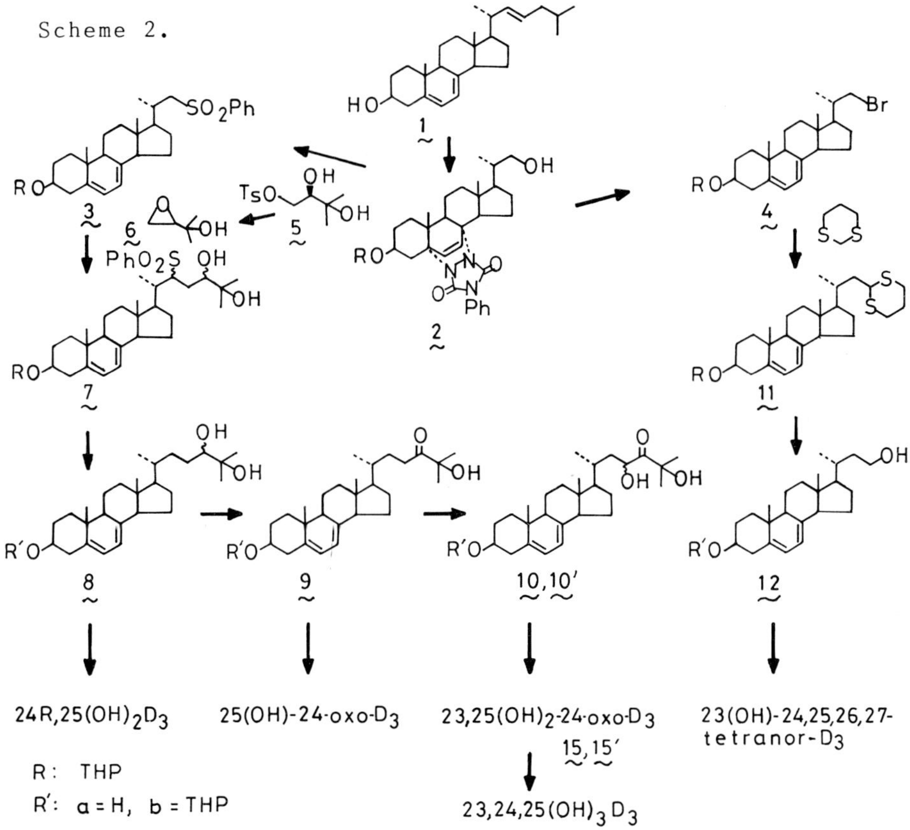

Syntheses of C(22) Steroid Synthons. After protection of the 5,7-diene part and the 3β-hydroxyl group, the side chain of ergosterol was cleaved by ozonolysis to give C(22) alcohol **2**. Deprotection of the 5,7-diene part was followed by tosylation and bromination to give the C(22) bromide **4**. The yield of the bromide **4** was about 25% from ergosterol. C(22) sulfone **3** was obtained from the alcohol **2** by tosylation, phenylsulfenylation, peracid oxidation, and deprotection of the 5,7-diene group. The overall yield of the sulfone **3** from ergosterol was about 28%.

Synthesis of 24R,25(OH)$_2$D$_3$. 24R,25(OH)$_2$D$_3$ was synthesized (18) conveniently and stereoselectively starting with the sulfone **3** and optically pure tosylate **5**. The reaction of the sulfone **3** with the chiral synthon **5** (LDA, THF, -20 °C) gave compound **7** (24R) in 86% yield. The tosylate **5** is considered to be converted to epoxyalcohol **R-6** under the reaction conditions before reacting with the sulfone **3**. The optically pure **5** was readily obtained from commercially available D-glyceraldehyde in 52% overall yield. Removal of the phenylsulfonyl group (Na-Hg, Na_2HPO_4, MeOH) and deprotection of the hydroxyl group gave the desired provitamin D **8a** (24R) (75%). The provitamin D was converted to 24R,25(OH)$_2$D$_3$ by UV irradiation followed by thermal isomerization.

Synthesis of 25(OH)-24-oxo-D$_3$. 25(OH)-24-oxo-D$_3$ was synthesized (12, 13) conveniently utilizing the intermediate of the synthesis of 24,25(OH)$_2$D$_3$, compound **8b**. In this case, however, racemic epoxyalcohol **6** was used as the side chain synthon. Oxidation (pyridine-SO_3, DMSO, Et_3N) of the 24-hydroxyl group followed by deprotection of the 3β-hydroxyl group gave the desired provitamin D **9a** (77%), which was converted to 25(OH)-24-oxo-D$_3$ in the usual manner.

Synthesis of 23,25(OH)$_2$-24-oxo-D$_3$. Synthesis of 23,25(OH)$_2$-24-oxo-D$_3$ started with compound **9b**, the intermediate of the synthesis of 25(OH)-24-oxo-D$_3$. Hydroxyl group at C(23) was introduced by peracid oxidation of its silyl enol ether. Treatment of **9b** with t-butyldimethylsilyl chloride in the presence of LDA (HMPA, THF, -20 °C) gave enolate **13** (84%) as a single isomer with regard to the enolate double bond. The 5,7-diene part of the enolate **13** was protected as a triazoline adduct (83%), and then the enolate was oxidized with m-chloroperbenzoic acid (CH_2Cl_2, 0 °C) to give the 23-hydroxylated derivative 14 (75%). The triazoline group was removed (K_2CO_3, DMSO, 60 °C, 51%) and the hydroxyl groups were deprotected (n-Bu_4NF, then MeOH, PPTS) to give the desired provitamin D as a mixture of two C(23) epimers, 10a and 10a' (3:7, 83%). The epimers were separated by HPLC on a reversed phase column. Each of the previtamin D (10a and 10a') was converted to the corresponding vitamin D, the minor and the less polar 15 and the major and the more polar 15', in the usual manner. The spectral properties of the two C(23) epimers of 23,25(OH)-24-oxo-D_3 synthesized are quite similar each other. Difference between the two epimers was found in their ^1H NMR spectra. The two epimers differ in the chemical shift of the proton at C(23): δ ($CDCl_3$) 15, 4.64 (m); 15', 4.72 (m). The ^1H NMR spectrum of the less polar isomer 15 was nearly identical with that of the natural metabolite reported by Dr. Norman's group (17): δ ($CDCl_3$) 4.65 (m, H-23). This suggests that the natural metabolite is identical with the less polar isomer of the two synthetic $23,25(OH)_2$-24-oxo-D_3. Single crystal X-ray analysis of the $23,25(OH)_2$-24-oxo-D_3 synthesized is progressing to determine the stereochemistry at C(23). Isolated and synthetic two $23,25(OH)_2$-24-oxo-D_3 were co-chromatographed on a reversed phase HPLC. As expected from the ^1H NMR spectra, both natural metabolites obtained from chicks and rats comigrated with the less polar isomer of the synthetic compound (Fig. 3). Thus the peak I metabolite was confirmed to be identical with the less polar isomer of the synthetic $23,25(OH)_2$-24-oxo-D_3.

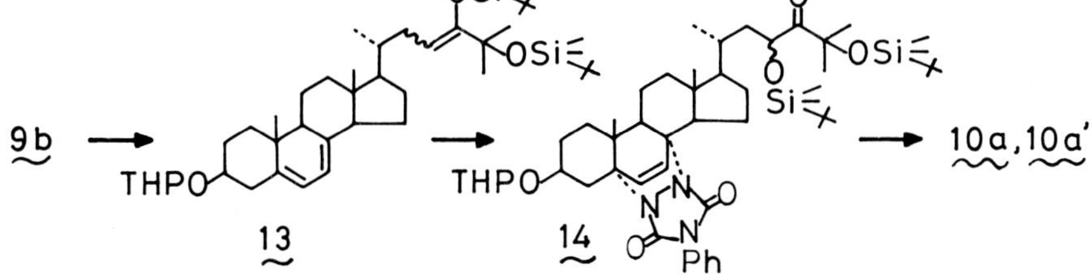

Scheme 3.

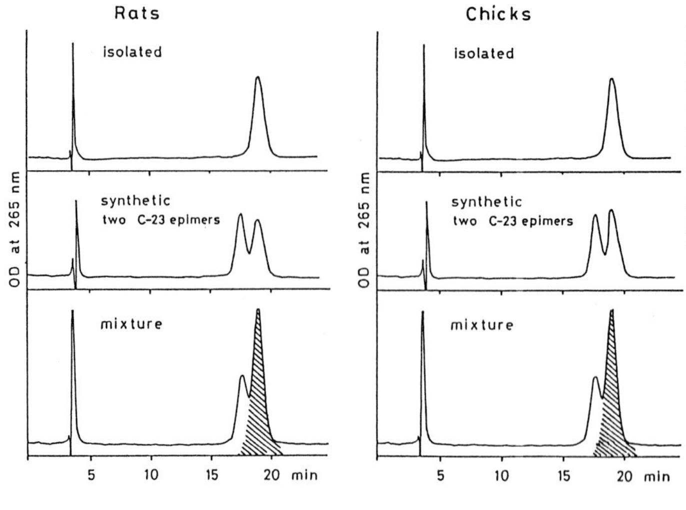

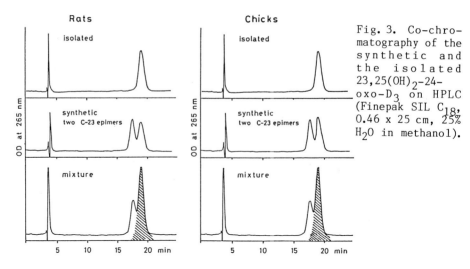

Fig. 3. Co-chromatography of the synthetic and the isolated $23,25(OH)_2$-24-oxo-D_3 on HPLC (Finepak SIL C_{18}, 0.46 x 25 cm, 25% H_2O in methanol).

Synthesis of $23,24,25(OH)_3D_3$. Since it was suggested that the stereochemistry at C(23) of the natural $23,24,25(OH)_3D_3$ is the same as that of the natural $23,25(OH)_2$-24-oxo-D_3, the less polar isomer of the synthetic $23,25(OH)_2$-24-oxo-D_3, which was determined to be identical with the natural metabolite, was reduced with $NaBH_4$ to obtain natural $23,24,25(OH)_3D_3$. The $23,24,25(OH)_3D_3$ thus obtained (75%) may be a mixture of the two C(24) epimers, but itself as well as its trimethylsilyl ether could not be separated chromatographycally. The synthetic $23,24,25(OH)_3D_3$ comigrated with the isolated metabolite on a straight phase (Zorbax SIL, 10% 2-PrOH in hexane) as well as on a reversed phase (Finepak SIL C_{18}, 30% H_2O in MeOH) HPLC. The mass spectra of the synthetic $23,24,25(OH)_3D_3$ and its trimethylsilyl ether are nearly identical with those of the natural metabolite and its trimethylsilyl ethers, respectively, to confirm the assigned structure (Fig. 4 and 5).

Synthesis of 23(OH)-24,25,26,27-tetranor-D_3. 23(OH)-24,25,26,27-tetranor-D_3 was synthesized starting with the C(22) bromide **4**. The reaction of the bromide **4** with lithio dithiane (THF, HMPA) gave the C(23) steroid **11** (95%). Hydrolysis of the dithio acetal group (HgO-BF_3, THF, 55%), reduction of the formyl group formed ($NaBH_4$, 90%), and deprotection of the 3β-hydroxyl group gave the desired provitamin

D 12, which was converted to 23(OH)-24,25,26,27-tetranor D_3 by the standard method. The tetranor D_3 thus synthesized comigrated with the natural metabolite on a straight as well as on a reversed phase HPLC. The mass spectra of the synthetic tetranor D_3 and its trimethylsilyl ether were nearly identical with those of the natural metabolite and its silyl ether, respectively, to confirm the proposed structure (16).

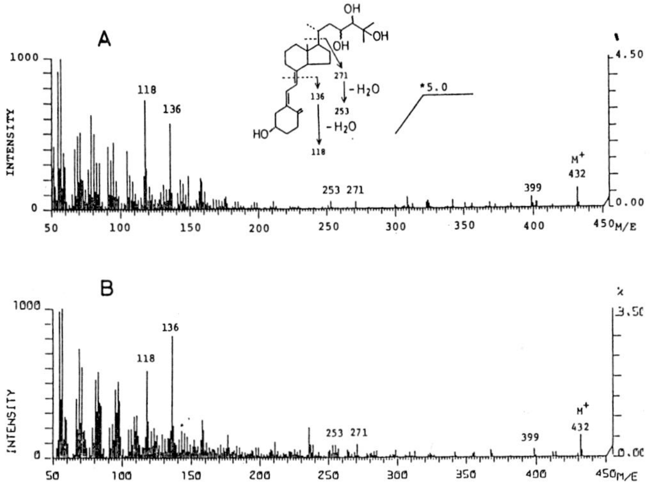

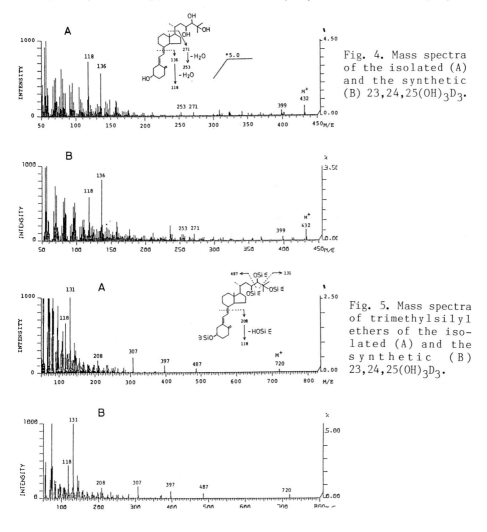

Fig. 4. Mass spectra of the isolated (A) and the synthetic (B) $23,24,25(OH)_3D_3$.

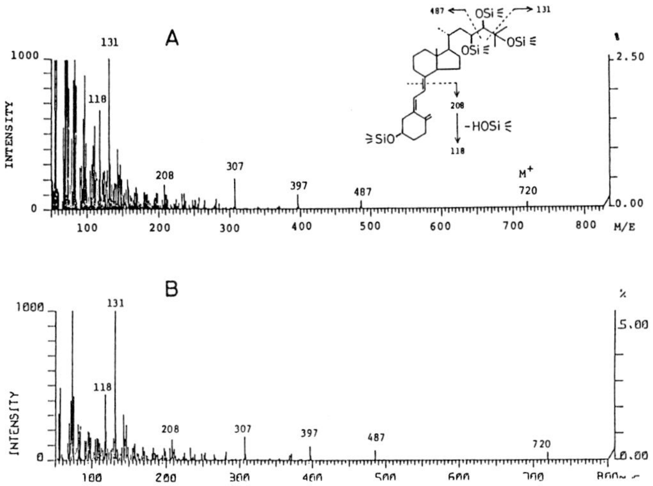

Fig. 5. Mass spectra of trimethylsilyl ethers of the isolated (A) and the synthetic (B) $23,24,25(OH)_3D_3$.

References

1. Holick, M. F., Schnoes, H. K., DeLuca, H. F., Gray, R. W., Boyle, I. T., and Suda, T. (1972) Biochemistry 11, 4251-4255
2. Tanaka, Y., Wichmann, J. K., Schnoes, H. K., and DeLuca, H. F. (1981) Biochemistry 20, 3875-3879
3. Suda, T., DeLuca, H. F., Tanaka, Y., and Holick, M. F. (1970) Biochemistry 9, 4776-4780
4. Shepard, R. M., Horst, R. L., Hamstra, A. J., and DeLuca, H. F. (1979) Biochem. J. 182, 55-69
5. Horst, R. L., Littledike, E. T., Riley, J. L., and Napoli, J. L. (1981) Anal. Biochem. 116, 189-203
6. Holick, M. F., Baxter, L. A., Schraufrogel, P. K., Tavela, T. E., and DeLuca, H. F. (1976) J. Biol. Chem. 251, 397-402
7. DeLuca, H. F. and Schnoes, H. K. (1983) Ann. Rev. Biochem. 52, 411-439
8. Edelstein, S., et al. (1982) in Vitamin D Chemical, Biochemical and Clinical Endocrinology of Calcium Metabolism (Norman, A. W., Schaefer, K., Herrath, D. v., and Grigoleit, H.-G., eds) pp 125-193, Walter de Gruyter, Berlin.New York
9. Takasaki, Y., Horiuchi, N., and Suda, T. (1978) Biochem. Biophys. Res. Commun. 85, 601-607
10. Takasaki, Y., Horiuchi, N., Takahashi, N., Abe, E., Shinki, T., Suda, T., Yamada, S., Takayama, H., Horikawa, H., Masumura, T., and Sugahara, M., (1980) Biochem. Biophys. Res. Commun. 95, 177-181
11. Takasaki, Y., Suda, T., Yamada, S., Takayama, H., and Nishii, Y., (1981) Biochemistry 20, 1681-1686
12. Yamada, S., Ohmori, M., Takayama, H., Suda, T., Takasaki, Y. (1981) Chem. Pharm. Bull. 29, 1187-1188
13. Takasaki, Y., Suda, T., Yamada, S., Ohmori, M., Takayama, H., and Nishii, Y., (1982) J. Biol. Chem. 257, 3732-3738
14. Yamada, S., Ohmori, M., Takayama, H., Takasaki, Y., and Suda, T. (1983) J. Biol. Chem., 258, 457-463
15. Yamada, S., Nakayama, K., Ohmori, M., Takayama, H., Shinki, T., Izumi, Y., and Suda, T. (1983) 26th Symposium on the Chemistry of Natural Products, Kyoto, pp 86-93
16. Jones, G., Kano, K., Yamada, S., Furusawa, T., Takayama, H., and Suda, T. (1984) Biochemistry 23, 3749-3754
17. Mayer, E., Reddy, G. S., Chandraratna, R. A. S., Okamura, W. H., Kruse, J. R., Popjak, G., Bishop, J. E., and Norman, A. W. (1983) Biochemistry 22, 1798-1805
18. Takayama, H., Ohmori, M., and Yamada, S. (1980) Tetrahedron Lett. 21, 5027-5028

EXTRA-RENAL PRODUCTION OF $1,25(OH)_2D_3$: THE METABOLISM OF VITAMIN D BY NON-TRADITIONAL TISSUES.

Rebecca S. Mason

Endocrine Unit, Royal North Shore Hospital, St. Leonards. NSW 2065, Australia.

Over recent years it has become apparent that the kidney can no longer be regarded as the unique site of biosynthesis (1) of 1,25 dihydroxyvitamin D_3 ($1,25(OH)_2D_3$). The extent and significance of this extra-renal synthesis of $1,25(OH)_2D_3$ in normal and pathological conditions has not yet been fully evaluated.

Whilst clear evidence for the existence and activity of extra-renal 25 hydroxyvitamin D- 24- and 26-hydroxylases has been obtained using in vitro (2,3,4) and in vivo (5,6) studies, the experiments relating to extra-renal 1α-hydroxylase activity have yielded somewhat conflicting results.

Problems with Experimental Systems

In order to try to evaluate the data obtained, it is worthwhile to distinguish between the types of subjects which have been used and to consider the limitations posed by different experimental methods. The difference between pregnant and non-pregnant subjects is clear. Much more blurred is the distinction between normal and pathological states. The nature of the problem requires the use of nephrectomized subjects. Whilst otherwise healthy, acutely-nephrectomized animals may be regarded as relatively "normal", this is not the case for anephric humans. Most of these patients, apart from other problems, have been on hemodialysis for some years. The occurrence of granulomatoid reactions to silicone from dialysis tubing (7) or other agents in such patients may be more widespread than is currently realized.

It has been known for some time that cells maintained in tissue culture may express characteristics which are different to those seen in the intact organism. Macrophages become activated during tissue culture (8). Tissue perfusion relationships are altered during cell culture, which may affect the ability of substrates such as 25OHD to enter the cells.

A second experimental problem relates to the identification of reaction products. Mass spectral analysis is not always able to be performed due to small quantities of sample. Lester et al. (9) have identified a 25 hydroxyvitamin D (25OHD) metabolite made by macrophages (10,11) and kidney cells which behaves like $1,25(OH)_2D_3$ during HPLC on silica with isopropanol:hexane (9:1 v/v). This compound has some affinity for the $1,25(OH)_2D_3$ calf thymus cytosol receptor (9) and presumably other binding proteins. This metabolite behaves quite differently to 1,25$(OH)_2D_3$ when methanol:methylene chloride solvent systems are used for HPLC (9,10,11). Those studies which rely on isopropanol/hexane separations and competitive protein binding assays require further clarification.

Many assays for 1,25$(OH)_2D$ in blood employ isopropanol/hexane HPLC and competitive protein binding analysis. In addition, assays for 1,25$(OH)_2D_3$ are imprecise and subject to non-specific interference, particularly at low concentrations of 1,25$(OH)_2D$ (12,13).

Pregnancy

There have been several studies which have demonstrated apparent synthesis of 1,25$(OH)_2D_3$ by homogenates of human (14,15) and rat (16) placenta, by human decidua in organ culture (17) and by chick chorio-allantoic membrane (18). Furthermore, nephrectomy of vitamin D-deficient pregnant rats has been reported to reduce but not abolish the production of putative $[^3H]$1,25$(OH)_2D_3$ from injected $[^3H]$25OHD_3 (19). On the evidence so far, the fetal kidney cannot be entirely excluded as a site of production of 1,25$(OH)_2D_3$ (20) in the in vivo studies. Moreover, in these studies the metabolite has been identified largely on the basis of co-chromatography of the compound with authentic 1,25$(OH)_2D_3$ on HPLC with isopropanol/hexane solvent mixtures.

"Normal" Subjects

The identity of putative 1,25$(OH)_2D_3$ synthesized in tissue culture by chick calvarial cells (21), normal human bone cells (22,23) and by chick intestinal cells (24) has been somewhat more conclusively established. In the case of chick calvarial cells, mass spectral identification of the metabolite has been reported (25). The metabolites co-chromatographed with authentic 1,25$(OH)_2D_3$ in a reverse phase system (22) and in a straight-phase system with methanol/methylene chloride (24). Pre-incubation of bone/calvarial cells with 1,25$(OH)_2D_3$ significantly diminished the activity of the 1α-hydroxylase enzyme (22).

There has been consistent failure, however, to detect $[^3H]$1,25$(OH)_2D_3$ from injected $[^3H]$25OHD_3 in serum, bone or intestinal tissue from non-pregnant anephric rats (1,5,26,27, 28) and human subjects (29,30) despite the use of high specific activity $[^3H]$25OHD_3 in more recent studies (5,27,28). Most workers have failed to detect 1,25$(OH)_2D_3$ in the serum of anephric human subjects using protein binding assay (31,32,33, 34,35,36,37), cytoreceptor assay (38), radioimmunoassay (39,40) and bioassay (41) techniques. The metabolite was also not detected in the serum of anephric sheep (12), chickens and rats (34). Low but detectable serum concentrations of 1,25$(OH)_2D_3$ have been occasionally reported in anephric human

human subjects (42,43). There have been three studies which suggest that a significant elevation in apparent 1,25$(OH)_2D_3$ may occur in anephric pigs (6) and humans (42,43) after vitamin D loading. Although similar findings have been reported in patients with minimal residual renal function (35,44), the compound assayed still has not been identified in more than one HPLC system.

Pathological Conditions: Malignancy

Two human melanoma cell lines (3) and one human osteosarcoma cell line (22) have been reported to synthesize putative 1,25$(OH)_2D_3$ in vitro. In each report the identity of the compound was determined in more than one HPLC system. Pre-incubation of the melanoma cells with 1,25$(OH)_2D_3$ resulted in inhibition of 1α-hydroxylase activity and induction of 24-hydroxylase activity (3).

Hypercalcemia in patients with melanoma is not common (45). Malignancy-associated hypercalcemia related to high serum concentrations of 1,25$(OH)_2D$ has been reported in 3 patients with non-Hodgkins lymphoma (46). At least two of these had a histiocytic component to their disease and it may be relevant to note the report by Sacher et al. (47) which emphasised the pathological gradations between histiocytic lymphoma, malignant histiocytosis and granulomatous disease.

Pathological Conditions: Granulomatous Diseases

Hypercalcemia associated with high serum concentrations of 1,25$(OH)_2D$ has now been described in patients with sarcoidosis (48,49,50,51), tuberculosis (52) and silicone-induced granulomas (53). Reports of the combination of hypercalcemia and high blood 1,25$(OH)_2D$ in an anephric sarcoid patient (54) and end stage renal failure patients with sarcoid or tuberculosis (52,55) suggest that significant extra-renal generation of 1,25$(OH)_2D_3$ may occur in these diseases.

Studies of sarcoid lymph node homogenate (4,56) and sarcoid macrophages in culture (57,58,59,60) have revealed that sarcoid tissue is apparently capable of generating 1,25$(OH)_2D_3$ from 25OHD_3. The product chromatographed with authentic standard on several HPLC systems (4,57,58), and partial mass spectral analysis was consistent with 1,25$(OH)_2D_3$ (J. Adams - personal communication).

The site of production of 1,25$(OH)_2D_3$ is probably abnormal in patients with sarcoidosis. Regulation of serum concentrations of this metabolite also seems to be abnormal in these patients. Under normal circumstances serum concentrations of 1,25$(OH)_2D$ are generally not related to levels of 25OHD (12,49,50). In patients with sarcoidosis, ingestion of vitamin D or exposure to sunlight (both of which raise serum 25OHD) results in elevated serum 1,25$(OH)_2D$ concentrations (48,49,50,51). Hypoparathyroid patients tend to be hypocalcemic and to have low levels of $1,25(OH)_2D$ (61). There are now two reports of hypoparathyroid patients who presented with hypercalcemia associated with high levels of $1,25(OH)_2D$ shortly after developing sarcoidosis (62,63). Both the patients, however, were receiving some form of vitamin D treatment (dihydrotachysterol and alphacalcidiol) at the time of study, which made the results difficult to interpret. A prostaglandin synthetase inhibitor (flurbiprofen) has been alleged to reduce blood $1,25(OH)_2D$ concentrations in recurrent stone formers (64) but had no significant effect on serum $1,25(OH)_2D_3$ in a patient with sarcoid-associated hypercalcemia (65). Thus there seem to be several differences between sarcoid and non-sarcoid patients in terms of their serum $1,25(OH)_2D$ response to various perturbations.

Features of $1,25(OH)_2D_3$ synthesis by kidney cells and by granuloma/sarcoid macrophages are compared in Table 1. It is possible that the inability of added $1,25(OH)_2D_3$ to suppress formation of putative $1,25(OH)_2D_3$ by sarcoid macrophages may contribute to the sensitivity of these patients to vitamin D.

TABLE 1

SYNTHESIS OF PUTATIVE $1,25(OH)_2D_3$ BY KIDNEY TISSUE OR GRANULOMAS/SARCOID MACROPHAGES[a]

	Kidney	Granulomas/Sarcoid Macrophages
Intracellular site	Mitochondria	Not Known
Km[b]	10-200 nM	100 nM
Production rates[b]	5-200 fmol/min/mg	83 fmol/min/mg
Inhibition by added $1,25(OH)_2D_3$	Yes	No
Distribution of newly formed $1,25(OH)_2D_3$	Less than 50% in medium	More than 90% in medium
Effect of prostaglandin synthetase inhibitor (aspirin)	Decrease	Not Known
24-Hydroxylase	Inducible by $1,25(OH)_2D_3$	Not inducible by $1,25(OH)_2D_3$

a - Data from Refs. 2,3,4,57,58,59,60,66,67. b - Variable.

In an attempt to determine the factors which may stimulate macrophages to express apparent 1α-hydroxylase activity (A. Norman, personal communication), human alveolar macrophages obtained during broncho-alveolar lavage from individuals without sarcoidosis were plated at a density of

0.5 x 10^6 cells/cm^2 in 24 well plates (Flow Laboratories, Sydney, Australia) in RPMI 1640 medium (Flow Laboratories, Sydney, Australia) with 5 μg/ml insulin (Sigma Chemical Co., Miss., U.S.A.), 30 μg/ml transferrin (Calbiochem-Behring, Sydney, Australia) and ethanolamine 2 x 10^{-5}M. The medium also contained 40 μg/ml gentamycin (David Bull Laboratory Ltd., Sydney, Australia), 120 μg/ml crystalline penicillin (Glaxo, Melbourne, Australia) and 10% (v/v) human serum. Medium was changed every 2 days. Cells were treated for 7 days with 50 μl of "macrophage acting factor". "MAF" consisted of the supernatant of white blood cells treated with phytohemagglutinin. This partially purified preparation contained interleukin-2 as well as γ-interferon (68). Control wells received medium only. At the end of the treatment period the cells were incubated with [^{3}H]25OHD for 16 hr at 37°C in serum free medium. In other experiments lipopolysaccharide preparations (10 μg/ml) and phorbol myristate acetate (10 ng/ml) were used to "stimulate" macrophage preparations (69). The results are seen in Table 2. Only the preparation containing γ-interferon was able to induce apparent 1α-hydroxylase activity.

TABLE 2

EFFECT OF VARIOUS AGENTS ON EXPRESSION OF "1α-HYDROXYLASE ACTIVITY" BY NON-SARCOID ALVEOLAR MACROPHAGES

		% Recovered Counts in $1,25(OH)_2D_3$ Fraction[a]	
Agent	Solvent[b] System	Untreated Cells	Treated Cells
Lipopolysaccharide	I/H	1.3 ± 0.8	1.2 ± 0.04
Phorbol ester	I/H	1.05 ± 0.5	1.3 ± 0.7
γ-Interferon (MAF)	I/H	2.5 ± 0.2	24 ± 6
γ-Interferon (MAF)	M/M	N.D.	18 ± 4

a - mean ± SEM. b - I/H = (isopropanol:hexane 9:1 v/v)
b - M/M = (methanol:methylene chloride 98:2 v/v)

There have been reports that 25OHD is metabolized by non-sarcoid mononuclear cells in culture to a compound which resembles authentic $1,25(OH)_2D_3$ (10,11). Table 3 compares the metabolism of 25OHD in normal mononuclear cells with that in sarcoid macrophages. These observations suggest that the metabolic activities of the cell types are different. The data in Table 2 suggests that γ-interferon may switch 25OHD metabolism in macrophages to a pathway which produces $1,25(OH)_2D_3$. γ-Interferon also has been reported to be the factor which primes macrophages for non-specific tumoricidal activity (70).

Table 3[a]

250HD METABOLISM BY MONONUCLEAR CELLS

	Normal	Sarcoid
Formation of "$1,25(OH)_2D_3$"	Yes (most samples)	Yes (less than 50% samples)
Co-chromatography with authentic $1,25(OH)_2D_3$ (methanol:methylene chloride)	No	Yes
Inhibition by added $1,25(OH)_2D_3$	No	No
Effect of phorbol-ester	Stimulation	No effect
Putative identity:	19nor - 10keto - $25OHD_3$	$1,25(OH)_2D_3$

a - Data from Refs. 9,10,11,58,59,60.

Conclusions

There is reasonable data to support the view that the synthesis of $1,25(OH)_2D_3$ can be demonstrated in certain normal cells in vitro. Except during pregnancy and possibly in anephric pigs given pharmacological doses of vitamin D, evidence that extra-renal synthesis of $1,25(OH)_2D_3$ occurs in vivo under normal circumstances, is lacking. It is not possible to determine whether small apparent increases in circulating $1,25(OH)_2D$ after vitamin D loading in anephric chronically-dialysed human subjects occur as a result of methodological artefact, the presence of granulomatoid abnormalities in some of these patients, or other factors.

Although synthesis of $1,25(OH)_2D_3$ by neoplastic cells has been described, the occurrence of malignancy-associated hypercalcemia together with apparently elevated serum $1,25(OH)_2D$ concentrations has so far been described in only a few reports. There is as yet little evidence to suggest that the $1,25(OH)_2D$ is synthesized at extra-renal sites.

The clearest evidence that significant extra-renal synthesis of $1,25(OH)_2D_3$ occurs, comes from in vivo and in vitro studies of patients with granulomatous disease. Abnormal regulation of this extra-renal synthesis may contribute to the propensity of such patients to develop hypercalciuria and hypercalcemia.

Acknowledgements

This work was supported by the National Health and Medical Research Council of Australia, the N.S.W. State Cancer Council, the University of Sydney Cancer Research Fund and the Coppleson Institute. Professor S. Posen made many valuable suggestions. Helen E. Thomas, Dianne Lissner, Angelika Trube and Deborah Reynolds gave valuable technical and secretarial assistance.

References

1. Frazer, D.R. and Kodicek, E. (1970) Nature 228, 764-766.
2. Chen, T.L., Hirst, M.A., Cone, C.M., Hochberg, Z., Tietze, H.U. and Feldman, D. (1984) J. Clin. Endocrinol. Metab. 59, 383-388.
3. Frankel, T.L., Mason, R.S., Hersey, P., Murray, E. and Posen, S. (1983) J. Clin. Endocrinol. Metab. 57, 627-631.
4. Mason, R.S., Frankel, T., Chan, Y.L., Lissner, D. and Posen, S. (1984) Ann. Int. Med. 100, 59-61.
5. Turner, R.T., Avioli, R.C. and Bell, N.H. (1984) Calc. Tiss. Int. 36, 274-278.
6. Littledike, E.T. and Horst, R.L. (1982) Endocrinology 111, 2008-2012.
7. Leong, A.S.Y., Disney, A.P.S. and Gove, D.W. (1982) N. Engl. J. Med. 306, 135-140.
8. Mosser, D.M. and Edelson, P.J. (1984) In: Macrophage Activation (D.O. Adams and M.G. Hanna Jnr, eds.) pp.87-91, Plenum Press, New York, London.
9. Lester, G.E., Horst, R.L. and Napoli, J.L. (1984) Biochem. Biophys. Res. Commun. 120, 919-925.
10. Gray, T.K., Maddux, F.W., Lester, G.E. and Williams, M.E. (1982) Biochem. Biophys. Res. Commun. 109, 723-729.
11. Cohen, M.S. and Gray, T.K. (1984) Proc. Natl. Acad. Sci. (USA) 81, 931-934.
12. Mason, R.S., Lissner, D., Grunstein, H.S. and Posen, S. (1980) Clin. Chem. 26, 444-450.
13. Mawer, E.B. (1982) In: Vitamin D, Chemical, Biochemical and Clinical Endocrinology of Calcium Metabolism (A.W. Norman, K. Schaefer, D.v. Herrath and H-G. Grigoleit, eds.) pp.623-628, Walter de Gruyter, Berlin, New York.
14. Whitsett, J.A., Ho, M., Tsang, R.C., Norman, E.J. and Adams, K.G. (1981) J. Clin. Endocrinol. Metab. 53, 484-488.
15. Savolainen, K.E., Kolonen, T. and Maenpaa, P.H. (1982) In: Vitamin D, Chemical, Biochemical and Clinical Endocrinology of Calcium Metabolism (A.W. Norman, K. Schaefer, D.v. Herrath and H.G. Grigoleit, eds.) pp.715-717, Walter de Gruyter, Berlin, New York.
16. Tanaka, Y., Halloran, B., Schnoes, H.K. and De Luca, H.F. (1979) Proc. Natl. Acad. Sci. USA 76, 5033-5035.
17. Weisman, Y., Harell, A., Edelstein, S., David, M., Spirer, Z. and Golander, A. (1979) Nature 281, 317-319.
18. Puzas, J.E., Turner, R.T., Forte, M. and Baylink, D.J. (1980) Gen. Comp. Endocrinol. 42, 116-122.
19. Gray, T.K., Lester, G.E. and Lorenc, R.S. (1979) Science 204, 1311-1313.

20. Sunaga, S., Horiuchi, N., Takahashi, N., Okuyama, K. and Suda, T. (1979) Biochem. Biophys. Res. Commun. 90, 948-955.
21. Turner, R.T., Puzas, J.E., Forte, M.D., Lester, G.E., Gray, T.K., Howard, G.A. and Baylink, D.J. (1980) Proc. Natl. Acad. Sci. (USA) 77, 5720-5724.
22. Howard, G.A., Turner, R.T., Sherrard, D.J. and Baylink, D.J. (1981) J. Biol. Chem. 256, 7738-7740.
23. Keck, E., Durdel, R., Schweikert, H.U., Kruck, F. and Kruskemper, H.L. (1981) Horm. Metab. Res. 13, 417.
24. Puzas, J.E., Turner, R.T., Howard, G.A. and Baylink, D.J. (1983) Endocrinology 112, 378-380.
25. Howard, G.A., Turner, R.T., Puzas, J.E., Knapp, D.R., Baylink, D.J. and Nichols, F. (1982) In: Vitamin D, Chemical, Biochemical and Clinical Endocrinology of Calcium Metabolism (A.W. Norman, K. Schaefer, D.v. Herrath and H.G. Grigoleit, eds.) pp. 3-5, Walter de Gruyter, Berlin, New York.
26. Gray, R., Boyle, I. and De Luca, H.F. (1971) Science 172, 1232-1234.
27. Reeve, L., Tanaka, Y. and De Luca, H.F. (1983) J. Biol. Chem. 258, 3615-3617.
28. Schultz, T.D., Fox, J., Heath, H.3rd and Kumar, R. (1983) Proc. Natl. Acad. Sci. (USA) 80, 1746-1750.
29. Mawer, E.W., Backhouse, J., Lumb, G.A. and Stanbury, S.W. (1971) Nature 232, 188-190.
30. Gray, R.W., Weber, H.P., Dominguez, J.H. and Lemann, J.Jnr. (1974) J. Clin. Endocrinol. Metab. 39, 1045-1056.
31. Brumbaugh, P.F., Haussler, D.H., Bursac, K.M. and Haussler, M.R. (1974) Biochemistry 13, 4091-4097.
32. Eisman, J.A., Hamstra, A.J., Kream, B.E. and De Luca, H.F. (1976) Arch. Biochem. Biophys. 176, 235-243.
33. Gray, R.W., Lemann, J.Jnr. and Adams, N.D. (1979) In: Vitamin D: Basic Research and Its Clinical Application (A.W. Norman, K. Schaefer, D.v. Herrath, H.G. Grigoleit, J. Coburn, H.F. De Luca, E.B. Mawer and T. Suda, eds.) pp.839-841, Walter de Gruyter, Berlin, New York.
34. Shepard, R.M., Horst, R.L., Hamstra, A.J. and De Luca, H.F. (1979) Biochem. J. 182, 55-69.
35. Lund, Bj., Clausen, E., Friedberg, M., Lund, Bi., Moszkowicz, M., Nielsen, S.P. and Sorensen, O.H. (1980) Nephron 25, 30-33.
36. Lambert, P.W., DeOreo, P.B., Hollis, B.W., Fu, I.Y., Ginsberg, D.J. and Roos, B.A. (1981) J. Lab. Clin. Med. 98, 536-548.
37. Reinhardt, T.A., Horst, R.L., Orf, J.W. and Hollis, B.W. (1984) J. Clin. Endocrinol. Metab. 58, 91-97.
38. Manolagas, S.C., Culler, F.L., Howard, J.E., Brickman, A.S. and Deftos, L.J. (1983) J. Clin. Endocrinol. Metab. 56, 751-760.
39. Clemens, T.L., Hendy, G.N., Graham, R.F., Baggiolini, E.G., Uskokovic, M.R. and O'Riordan, J.L.H. (1978) Clin. Sci. Mol. Med. 54, 329-332.

40. Gray, T.K., McAdoo, T., Pool, D., Lester, G.E., Williams, M.E. and Jones, G. (1981) Clin. Chem. 27, 458-463.
41. Stern, P.H., Hamstra, A.J., De Luca, H.F. and Bell, N.H. (1978) J. Clin. Endocrinol. Metab. 46, 891-896.
42. Lambert, P.W., Stern, P.H., Avioli, R.C., Brackett, N.C., Turner, R.T., Green, A., Fu, I.Y. and Bell, N.H. (1982) J. Clin. Invest. 69, 722-725.
43. Jongen, M.J.M., van der Vijgh, W.J.F., Lips, P., Netelenbos, J.C. (1984) Nephron 36, 230-234.
44. Halloran, B.P., Schaefer, P., Lifschitz, M., Levens, M. and Goldsmith, R.S. (1984) J. Clin. Endocrinol. Metab. 59, 1063-1069.
45. Burt, M.E. and Brennan, M.F. (1979) Am. J. Surg. 137, 790-794.
46. Breslau, N.A., McGuire, J.L., Zerwekh, J.E., Frenke, E.P. and Pak, C.Y.C. (1984) Ann. Int. Med. 100, 1-7.
47. Sacher, R.A., Jacobson, R.J., Lenes, B.A. and Rath, C.E. (1980) Am. J. Clin. Path. 74, 180-185.
48. Papapoulos, S.E., Fraher, L.J., Sandler, L.M., Clemens, T.L., Lewin, I.G. and O'Riordan, J.L.H. (1979) Lancet i, 627-630.
49. Bell, N.H., Stern, P.H., Pantzer, E., Sinha, T.K. and DeLuca, H.F. (1979) J. Clin. Invest 64, 218-225.
50. Stern, P.H., De Olazabal, J. and Bell, N.H. (1980) J. Clin. Invest. 66, 852-855.
51. Sandler, L.M., Winearls, C.G., Fraher, L.J., Clemens, T.L., Smith, R. and O'Riordan, J.L.H. (1984) Quart. J. Med. 53, 165-180.
52. Gkonos, P.J., London, R. and Hendler, E.D. (1984) N. Engl. J. Med. 311, 1683-1685.
53. Kozeny, G.A., Barbato, A.L., Bansal, V.K., Vertuno, L.L. and Hano, J.E. (1984) N. Engl. J. Med. 311, 1103-1105.
54. Barbour, G.L., Coburn, J.W., Slatopolsky, E., Norman, A.W. and Horst, R.L. (1981) N. Engl. J. Med. 305, 440-443.
55. Maesaka, J.K., Batuman, V., Pablo, N.C. and Shakamuri, S. (1982) Arch. Int. Med. 142, 1206-1207.
56. Van der Vijgh, W.J.F., Wijnberg, M., Netelenbos, J.C. and Lips, P. (1984) Calcif. Tiss. Int. 36(Suppl.2), S45.
57. Adams, J.S., Sharma, O.P., Gacad, M. and Singer, F.R. (1983) J. Clin. Invest. 72, 1856-1860.
58. Mason, R.S., Thomas, H.E., Lissner, D. and Posen, S. (1984) Calc. Tiss. Int. 36, 519.
59. Adams, J.S. and Gacad, M.A. (1985) This symposium.
60. Fraher, L.J., Flint, K.C., Hudspith, B.N., Johnson, N.McI. and O'Riordan, J.L.H. (1985) This symposium.
61. Lund, Bj., Sorensen, O.H., Lund, Bi., Bishop, J.E. and Norman, A.W. (1980) J. Clin. Endocrinol. Metab. 51, 606-610.
62. Mitchell, T.H., Stamp, T.C.B., Jenkins, M.V., Mawer, E.B. and Berry, J.L. (1983) Brit. Med. J. 286, 764-765.
63. Zimmerman, J., Holick, M.F. and Silver, J. (1983) Ann. Int. Med. 98, 338.
64. Buck, A.C., Brown, R.C., Davies, C.J., Sabur, R.Y.,

Murray, K. and Lucas, P.L. In: Proceedings of the 5th International Symposium on Urolithiasis and Related Clinical Research (Garmisch, April, 1984, in press).
65. Brown, R.C., Heyburn, P.J., Littlewood, T.J. and Beck, P. (1984) Lancet ii, 37.
66. Norman, A.W. (1979) Vitamin D: The Calcium Homeostatic Steroid Hormone. Academic Press, New York, London.
67. Wark, J.D., Larkins, R.G., Eisman, J.A. and Wilson, K.R. (1981) Clin. Sci. 61, 53-59.
68. Leibson, H.J., Gefter, M., Zlotnik, A., Marrack, P. and Kappler, J.W. (1984) Nature 309, 799-801.
69. Koretzky, G.A., Daniele, R.P. and Nowell, P.C. (1982) J. Immunol. 128, 1776-1780.
70. Schreiber, R.D. (1984) In: Macrophage Activation (D.O. Adams and M.G. Hanna, Jnr., eds.) pp.171-195, Plenum Press, New York, London.

REGULATION OF PRE-PROPARATHYROID HORMONE mRNA IN BOVINE PARATHYROID CELLS IN CULTURE BY VITAMIN D METABOLITES

Justin Silver, John Russell and Louis M. Sherwood

Hadassah University Hospital, Jerusalem, Israel, and Albert Einstein College of Medicine, New York, USA

Parathyroid hormone (PTH) is trophic to the renal synthesis of 1,25(OH)D_3, and both PTH and 1,25(OH)$_2D_3$ act to increase serum calcium. The resultant increase in serum calcium decreases PTH secretion and subsequently 1,25(OH)$_2D_3$ synthesis. What has not been well-documented is whether 1,25(OH)$_2$ D_3 itself has any direct effect on the synthesis and secretion of PTH. While some authors have suggested that vitamin D metabolites suppress PTH release other studies show either an increase or no effect (1-6). We have utilized molecular biology techniques to study the effects of vitamin D metabolites on preproPTH mRNA levels of bovine parathyroid cells in primary culture.

Materials and Methods

Isolated bovine parathyroid cells were prepared by collagenase digestion and plated in 16 mm tissue culture dishes (1 x 10^6 cells) in 1 ml of Dulbecco modified Eagle medium, containing 1.25 mM calcium, 10% fetal calf serum and 1% penicillin-streptomycin. After three days the medium was replaced by fresh medium and either vehicle alone (10 µl ethanol) or vitamin D metabolites in ethanol were added. At various time intervals, the medium was aspirated, the cells were removed and washed, and total cellular RNA was extracted with guanidine thiocyanate and guanidine hydrochloride followed by precipitation with alcohol (7). Concentrations of total RNA were calculated based on absorption at 260 nm, with 1 and 2 µg aliquots of RNA being spotted on nitrocellulose filters for dot blot hybridization (7). The filters were then hybridized with a cDNA probe that had been labelled with ^{32}P-nucleotides by nick translation. Following incubation, the filters were exposed to autoradiography and the resultant film scanned with a densitometer.

Results and Discussion

1,25(OH)$_2D_3$ (1 x 10^{-7}M) suppressed preproPTH mRNA by 15% at 24 hours, and 50% at 48-96 hours. When the effect of 1,25(OH)$_2D_3$ was tested at various concentrations, a significant effect was apparent at 10^{-11}M which increased progressively at higher concentrations up to a maximum at 10^{-6} - 10^{-7}M. 24,25-dihydroxyvitamin D_3 (24,25(OH)$_2D_3$ was approximately 10-fold less potent than 1,25(OH)$_2D_3$, while 25-hydroxyvitamin D_3 (25(OH)D_3) only showed a significant effect at 10^{-6}M. Vitamin D_3 itself had no effect, even at concentrations as high as 10^{-6}M. In order to be certain of the specificity of the effects, the cytoplasmic concentrations of mRNA for an unrelated protein alpha-actin, were studied, using a ^{32}P-labelled probe of chicken muscle alpha-actin. Cells cultured with 1,25(OH)$_2D_3$ in the medium at concentrations of 1 x 10^{-7}M for 48 hours showed no change in

Vitamin D. A Chemical, Biochemical and Clinical Update

alpha-actin mRNA despite a striking decrease in preproPTH mRNA. The effect of $1,25(OH)_2D_3$ (1×10^{-7}M) at 48 hours was largely reversible when the cells were then maintained in a $1,25(OH)_2D_3$-free medium for a further 48 hours.

These results show that $1,25(OH)_2D_3$ at physiologic concentration decreases steady-state levels of PTH mRNA, with greater potency than the less active vitamin D metabolites $24R,25(OH)_2D_3$ and $25(OH)D_3$, indicating that the parathyroid gland is a target organ for vitamin D. The sterol may exert a measure of control on total amount of hormone production by the gland, even if its effects on acute secretion are more questionable.

Acknowledgments

Supported in part by U.S. Public Health Service Grants AM 28556 and HD 15891.

References

1. Dietel, M., Dorn, G., Montz, R. and Altenahr, E. (1979) Endocrinology 105: 237-245.
2. Canterbury, J.M., Lerman, S., Claflin, A.J., Henry, H., Norman, A.W. and Reiss, E. (1978) J. Clin. Invest. 61: 1375-1383.
3. Chertow, B.S., Baylink, D.J., Wegedal, J.E., Su, M.H.H. and Norman, A.W. (1975) J. Clin. Invest.56: 668-678.
4. Oldham, S.B., Smith, R., Hartenbower, D.L., Henry, H.L., Norman, A.W. and Coburn, J.W. (1979) Endocrinology 104: 248-254.
5. Klahr, S. and Slatopolsky, E. (1980) Endocrinology 107: 602-607.
6. Slatopolsky, E., Weerts, C., Thielan, J., Horst, R., Harter, H. and Martin, K.J. (1984) J. Clin. Invest. 74: 2136-2143.
7. Russell, J., Lettieri, D. and Sherwood, L.M. (1983) J. Clin. Invest. 71: 1851-1855.

METABOLISM OF VITAMIN D IN PIGS WITH PSEUDO VITAMIN D DEFICIENCY RICKETS AFTER TREATMENT WITH HIGH DOSES OF VITAMIN D_3.

R. Kaune and J. Harmeyer*

Institute of Physiology, School of Vet. Med., 3000 Hannover, FRG

Introduction:

Besides classical vitamin D dependent rickets, there are other forms of rickets which are refractory to sunlight or dietary supply with vitamin D. One form is the pseudo vitamin D deficiency rickets, type I which is caused by the lack of the renal 25-OHD-1-hydroxylase (1). This inherited form of rickets has also been described in pigs (2).
Clinical, hematological and endocrinological features of the disease are similar to those of classical vitamin D deficiency rickets including hypocalcemia, increased activity of alkal. Pase, secondary hyperparathyreoidism, impaired mineralization, and enhanced mobilization of bone mineral. Plasma levels of vitamin D_3 are normal but 1,25-$(OH)_2D_3$ in plasma is unphysiologically low and 25-OHD_3 above normal. Piglets from this strain were used, to study why patients which suffer from this disease can effectively be treated with pharmacological doses of vitamin D_3.

Methods:

Rachitic piglets (4 to 6 weeks of age and 1.7 to 7.9 kg body weight) received a single i.m. injection of 0.25 to 1.25 mg vitamin D_3. Serial blood samples were taken over three weeks. Plasma concentrations of vitamin D_3 and its metabolites were analyzed as follows: 1. Lipid extraction with methanol/methylene-Cl. 2. Fractionation with different chloroform/n-hexane mixtures on Lipidex 5000 into three fractions: Vitamin D_3, 25-OHD_3, and the double hydroxylated metabolites. 3. Normal and reversed phase HPLC with UV-detection and radioimmunoassay for 1,25-$(OH)_2D_3$ (3).

Results:

Results are shown in the figure 1. Treatment with vitamin D_3 led to a transient increase in plasma Ca and the alkal. Pase which were seen for about one week after treatment. Clinical symptoms of rickets improved with pain relief from bone and an increased mobility. Three weeks after treatment rachitic symptoms redeveloped in association with severe hypocalcemia. Vitamin D_3 increased in plasma from 5.7 ± 3.1 to 140 ± 73 ng/ml in 2 to 3 days and declined to 13.6 ± 2.2 ng/ml within the following 10 to 14 days. 25-OHD_3 rose from 52.4 ± 18.5 during 7 days to 427 ± 64 ng/ml and declined slowly after that during the following 2 weeks with 25-OHD_3 concentrations still 4 times higher than before treatment.
Plasma 1,25-$(OH)_2D_3$ was elevated from 30.8 ± 10.4 to 117 ± 70 pg/ml in 2 to 3 days. This concentration is slightly above the physiological value of 71 ± 27 pg/ml from healthy control piglets. One week after treatment 1,25-$(OH)_2D_3$ concentrations had declined to 42 ± 14 pg/ml while 25-OHD_3 reached its maximum. 24,25-$(OH)_2D_3$ and 25,26-$(OH)_2D_3$ showed a slight increase after treatment, but the extent is varied in different animals.

Conclusions:

Piglets with pseudo vitamin D deficiency rickets type I produce large quantities of 25-OHD_3 when treated with high doses of vitamin D_3. They

* Supported by the Deutsche Forschungsgemeinschaft, Sonderforschungsbereich 146 "Versuchstierforschung".

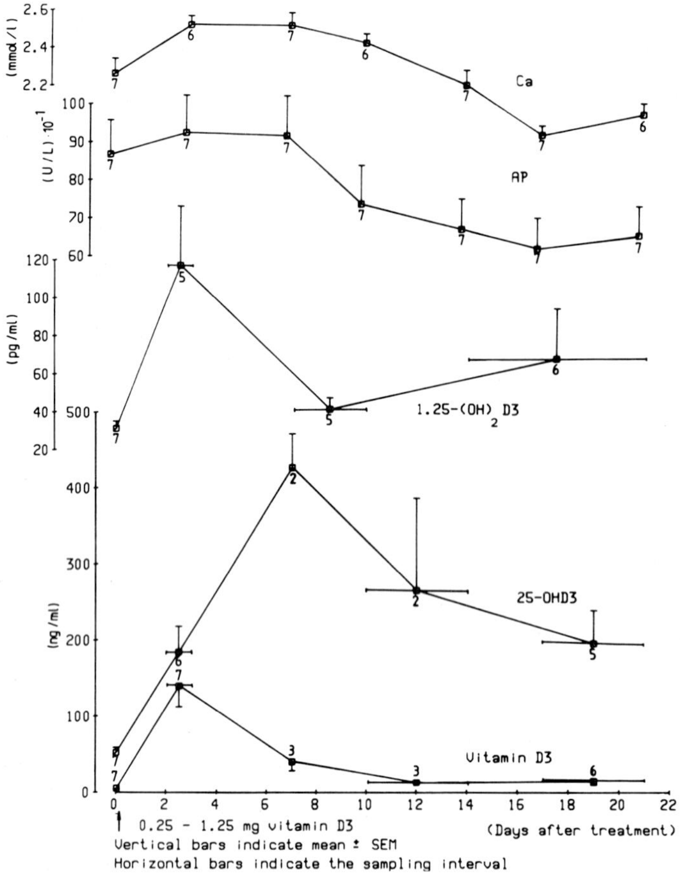

Fig. 1: Plasma concentrations of vitamin D_3, 25-OHD_3, 1,25$(OH)_2D_3$, alkal. Pase and Ca after treatment with vitamin D_3.

synthesize also significant amounts of 1,25-$(OH)_2D_3$. The transient healing of clinical symptoms which was seen after this treatment can be attributed to the short time normalization of plasma 1,25-$(OH)_2D_3$. Since the piglets have no renal 1-hydroxylase, extrarenal 1-hydroxylases with lower binding affinity may be responsible for elevation of 1,25-$(OH)_2D_3$ concentration (4).

References:

1. DeLuca, H.F. (1982) J. Am. Dietetic Ass. 80, 231-236.
2. Harmeyer, J., Grabe, C.v., Winkler, I. (1982) Expl. Biol. Med. 7, 117-125.
3. Lambert, P.W., Deoreo, T.B., Hollis, B.W., Fu, I.Y., Ginsberg, D.I., Roos, B.A. (1981) J. Lab. Clin. Med. 98, 536-548.
4. Littledike, E.T., Horst, R.L. (1982) Endocrinology 111, 2008-2013.

ISOLATION AND IDENTIFICATION OF 25-HYDROXYDIHYDROTACHYSTEROL$_2$, 1α,25-DIHYDROXYDIHYDROTACHYSTEROL$_2$ AND 1β,25-DIHYDROXYDIHYDROTACHYSTEROL$_2$.

R.BOSCH, C.VERSLUIS, J.K.TERLOUW, J.H.H.THIJSSEN AND S.A.DUURSMA.
Department of Internal Medicine, University Hospital, P.O.Box 16250, 3500 CG Utrecht, The Netherlands.

Dihydrotachysterol$_2$ (DHT$_2$) is succesfully used in the treatment of hypoparathyroidism and renal osteodystrophy. DHT$_2$ increases the calcium concentration in plasma by increasing intestinal calcium transport and mobilizing calcium from the skeleton. However, in contrast to dihydrotachysterol$_3$ no data are available concerning the metabolism of DHT$_2$. It is generally assumed that DHT$_2$ requires 25-hydroxylation before it can be effective. This assumption is supported by the finding that 25-hydroxydihydrotachysterol$_3$ is biologically more potent than dihydrotachysterol$_3$. It has been demonstrated that reconstituted mitochondrial cytochrome P-450 can carry out the 25-hydroxylation of DHT$_2$ when combined with ferredoxin and ferredoxin reductase. 1-Hydroxylation of DHT$_2$ which is equivalent to pseudo 3-hydroxylation is assumed to be most unlikely because, hitherto, there are no reports of the existence of (pseudo) 3-hydroxylases in animal systems.

In rats DHT$_2$ is rapidly metabolized to more polar forms. Two of these forms, preliminarily designated "c2" and "e" co-chromatograph with 25-hydroxydihydrotachysterol$_3$ and 1α,25-dihydroxyvitamin D$_3$ respectively. In view of the premises it was interesting to isolate and characterize these compounds. In order to conclusively prove the presence of DHT$_2$ in serum after oral administration, a compound, preliminarily designated "b", which co-chromatographs with authentic DHT$_2$, was isolated and identified as well.

Thirty, male Wistar rats (approx. 275 g) fed a diet adequate in Ca, P and vitamin D$_3$ were given 1.84 μmol of DHT$_2$ in 50 μl of ethanol by gastric tube. Ten h later, blood was collected by heart puncture yielding 128 ml of serum. Serum was extracted twice with 1 vol of ethyl acetate:cyclohexane (1:1, v/v) and once with 1.4 vol of methanol:ethyl acetate:water (4:5:5, by vol.). After drying the lipid extract was redissolved in n-hexane:propanol-2:water (85:15:0.05, by vol.) and applied to a Zorbax Sil 850 HPLC column (6.2x250 mm) which was developed with the solvent (1 ml/min). Crude "b" was eluted from 6-8 ml, crude "c2" from 8.5-11 ml and crude "e" from 18.5-24 ml.

Crude "e" was rechromatographed twice in the system described above. The fractions eluting at 19.5-21 ml were collected for further characterization. Crude "b" was further purified by using the same column with a solvent system of n-hexane:propanol2 (98.2:1.8, v/v); "b" eluted at 15-17 ml. Further purification of "c2" could be achieved by repeated chromatography in the HPLC system LichoSorb Si-60-5 (6.2x250 mm)/n-hexane:propanol-2:water (95:5:0.05, by vol.) In this sytem "c2" eluted at 23-25.5 ml. After drying "b", "c2" and "e" were redissolved in ethanol for UV spectroscopy. The UV spectrum of "b" corresponded to that of authentic DHT$_2$ showing peaks at 260.5, 251.2 (λ_{max}) and 242.8 nm; yield 5.05 μg. "c2" and "e" showed massive contamination by UV. However, when they were recorded against ethanolic solutions of their respective, preceeding HPLC fractions the spectra obtained were identical to that of DHT$_2$. The yield for both compounds was 1.3 μg. In view of the degree of purity of "c2" and "e" achieved mass spectrometric analyses were performed by GC/MS. Furthermore, the samples were trimethylsilylated to increase volatilities.

The mass spectrum of silylated "b" was identical to that of the trimethylsilyl ether of authentic DHT_2 showing peaks at m/z 470 ($M^{+\cdot}$), 380 ($M-(CH_3)_3SiOH(=TMSOH))^{+\cdot}$, 255 ($C_{17}-C_{20}$ cleavage; $(M-C_9H_{17}-TMSOH)^+$) and 121 (base peak; C_7-C_8 cleavage and concomitant H shift $(M-C_{19}H_{32}-TMSOH)^+$). The chromatographic, UV and mass spectral data demonstrated that DHT_2 is present in the circulation after oral administration.
Mass spectrometry of silylated "c2" showed a peak at m/z 121 (base peak), characteristic in the spectrum of silylated DHT_2, and a molecular ion at m/z 486 which was consistent with a monotrimethylsilyl ether of a monohydroxylated DHT_2 derivative. Ions at m/z 468 $(M-H_2O)^{+\cdot}$, 396 $(M-TMSOH)^{+\cdot}$ and 378 $(M-TMSOH-H_2O)^{+\cdot}$ confirmed the presence of a silylated and a free hydroxyl group in the compound. A fragment of m/z 255 ($(M-C_9H_{17}O-TMSOH)^+$; $C_{17}-C_{20}$ cleavage) established that the free, additional hydroxyl function was located in the side chain.
Additional evidence for structural assignment was obtained after prolonged silylation. Now, the mass spectrum of "c2" showed a molecular ion at m/z 558 which corresponds to a ditrimethylsilyl ether of monohydroxylated DHT_2. Fragments at m/z 255 and 131 (base peak; $(CH_3)_2C{=}O^+{-}Si(CH_3)_3$) indicated the presence of the additional hydroxyl group at C_{25}. Assuming a hydroxyl group at C_3, the mass spectral data together with the data of UV absorption and chromatography established the structure of "c2" as 25-hydroxydihydrotachysterol$_2$.
The total ion current chromatogram of silylated "e" demonstrated that this compound consisted of two components with almost identical mass spectra. Therefore, the following interpretation of the mass spectral data applies to both components. The molecular ion at m/z 646 suggested the incorporation of two additional hydroxyl groups into DHT_2. It is consistent with the molecular ion of a tritrimethylsilyl ether of dihydroxylated DHT_2. Fragments at m/z 343 $(M-C_{12}H_{25}OSi-TMSOH)^+$ and m/z 253 $(343-TMSOH)^+$ indicated the presence of one hydroxyl function in the side chain. A fragment at m/z 131 (base peak) established its location at C_{25}. The position of the second additional hydroxyl group was apparent from the ions at m/z 182 and 217. The fragment at m/z 182 could result from cleavage of the C_5-C_6 bond $(M-C_{24}H_{42}OSi-TMSOH)^+$ which suggested the presence of two hydroxyl groups in ring A. The ion at m/z 217 confirmed this interpretation since it could only be attributed to the fragment $(CH_3)_2SiO{-}CH{=}CH{-}CH{=}O^+Si(CH_3)_3$ arisen from cleavage of the C_3-C_4 and C_1-C_{10} bonds, with a hydroxyl group at C_1 and a hydroxyl group at C_3. These data defined the structure of the two epimers as the tritrimethylsilyl ether of 1-ambo,25-dihydroxydihydrotachysterol$_2$.
The tentative stereochemistry of the hydroxyl group at C_1 could be determined by comparison of the relative intensities of the ions at m/z 646 ($M^{+\cdot}$) and 556 $(M-TMSOH)^{+\cdot}$. The molecular ions of the epimers differed strongly in the rate of loss of TMSOH. An axial substituent in the A ring introduces non-bonded interactions into the ring and these will lower the stability of the molecular ion. Crowding of the trimethylsilyl ether functions at C_1 and C_3 will become maximal when both are in the axial orientation. As a result the molecular ion of the diaxial conformer will have a greater tendency to loose TMSOH compared with the equatorial(C_1)-axial(C_3) conformer. Thus, the structure of the epimer with the highest ratio $(M-TMSOH)^{+\cdot}/M^{+\cdot}$ could be tentatively identified as the tritrimethylsilyl ether of 1α,25-dihydroxydihydrotachysterol$_2$. Consequently, the other compound was the tritrimethylsilyl ether of 1β,25-dihydroxydihydrotachysterol$_2$.

STRESS TESTING OF CALCIUM REGULATORY HORMONES USING OUTPATIENT DIETARY CALCIUM DEPRIVATION

R.L. Prince, B.G. Hutchison, R.W. Retallack, J.C. Kent and G.N. Kent.

University Department of Medicine, Department of Renal Medicine and Department of Endocrinology and Diabetes, Sir Charles Gairdner Hospital, Nedlands, Western Australia.

Both parathyroid hormone (PTH) and 1,25 dihydroxyvitamin D (calcitriol) are important regulators of extracellular calcium homeostasis. The major regulator of PTH is serum calcium however the precise factors regulating calcitriol are still unclear. Nevertheless animal studies have shown consistent stimulation of calcitriol production by a low calcium diet (1). We have therefore developed a stress test of calcitriol secretory reserve using dietary calcium deprivation.

The test consisted of one week of dietary calcium deprivation. Subjects were provided with dietary guidelines in which dairy products and high calcium vegetables were excluded. This resulted in a dietary intake of approximately 4mmol calcium per day. The diet was supplemented with oral cellulose phosphate 5gms four times a day to further reduce calcium absorption. Magnesium chloride 1gm twice a day was given to prevent magnesium deficiency. Blood and urine samples were collected on days -4,0,2,4 and 7. Fasting two hour urine collections were used to assess parameters of renal phosphate and cAMP handling. 24 hour urine samples were collected to measure overall urine calcium excretion. The subjects consisted of 3 healthy males aged 31 to 35 and 3 healthy females aged 22 to 45.

Calcitriol was measured after extraction in an assay using either a rat osteogenic sarcoma cell line which carries a receptor for calcitriol or bovine thymus cytosol (2). PTH was measured by a 'mid-region' radioimmunoassay. Plasma and urine cAMP were measured in a radioimmunoassay. Urine and plasma phosphate, creatinine, calcium and albumin were measured by routine Technicon methods. Plasma adjusted calcium (Ca Adj) was calculated from the total plasma calcium and albumin concentrations. Statistical evaluation of results was by 2 tailed unpaired 't' tests using pooled basal values. Results are given as mean ± 1 standard deviation.

As there was no significant difference in results in males or females the results have been pooled. Results are shown in the table. There was a highly significant rise in calcitriol by day 2. This was associated with a significant fall in serum phosphate, plasma adjusted calcium and 24 hour urine calcium/creatinine ratio. Neither immunoreactive PTH nor nephrogenous cAMP altered however the renal tubular phosphate threshold

Vitamin D. A Chemical, Biochemical and Clinical Update

(Tmp) did fall significantly.

Days of calcium deprivation

	Day -4	Day 0	Day 2	Day 4	Day 7
Calcitriol (pg/ml)	39.4±11.9	48.5±15.0	70.2±16.4*	53.0±11.3	47.2±12.5
PTH (pM)	21.5±11.6	22.6±10.0	26.2±13.1	28.6±4.9	26.5±8.2
Ca Adj (mM)	2.30±0.09	2.26±0.05	2.22±0.04+	2.26±0.05	2.28±0.05
Serum phosphate (mM)	1.10±0.06	1.07±0.06	1.00±0.10+	1.00±0.04	1.02±0.10
Tmp (mM/1GF)	1.21±0.18	1.13±0.13	0.98±0.21	0.95±0.09+	0.97±0.12
Nephrogenous (nm/1GF)	6.5±6.0	9.6±8.2	10.5±3.7	7.3±8.5	10.3±7.4
24hr urine Ca/Cr ratio	0.30±0.15	0.31±0.01	0.13±0.4*	0.12±0.06	0.14±0.08

+p < 0.05 *p < 0.01 C.F. Day -4 and Day 0

These results show that dietary calcium deprivation in normal ambulant volunteers increases serum calcitriol levels. Previously this has only been shown for subjects admitted to hospital and consuming a liquid formula diet (3). The precise mechanism of calcitriol stimulation is not clear. In view of the fact that plasma calcium fell it is attractive to suggest that bioactive PTH levels rose, the fall in Tmp is consistent with this. However no change in immunoreactive PTH or nephrogenous cAMP was detected. Two important conditions in which deficiency of calcitriol has been suggested to be compensated for by a rise in circulating PTH levels are renal osteodystrophy and senile or type II osteoporosis. This test should prove useful in determining calcitriol reserve in these conditions. Should calcitriol reserve be deficient oral replacement of calcitriol may provide efficacious treatment.

(1) Omdahl, J.L., Gray, R.W., Boyle, I.T., Knutson, J. and DeLuca, H.F. (1972). Nature (New Biol) 237: 63-64.

(2) Nicholson, G.C., Kent, J.C., Gutteridge, D.H. and Retallack, R.W. (1985). Clin Endocrinol. (in press)

(3) Adams, N.D, Gray, R.W., and Lemann, J. Jr. (1979). J. Clin. Endocrinol. Metab, 48: 1008-1016

VITAMIN D METABOLISM AND GLUCOCORTICOID TREATMENT.

S. ADAMI, R. DORIZZI, D. TARTAROTTI, B. IMBIMBO and V. LO CASCIO.
Istituto di Semeiotica Medica. Policlinico, 37134 Verona, Italy.

Serum concentration of 1,25(OH)2D has been reported to decrease(1) or increase(2) after administration of glucocorticoids (GLS) in normal subjects, but GLS lower serum 1,25(OH)2D in hypercalcemic sarcoidosis(3) and they are rapidly effective in correcting hypercalcemia due to vitamin D intoxication. Here we present three separate observations which suggest that GLS therapy suppresses extra-renal 1-hydroxylase activity whenever occurring, whereas it has not direct effect on the renal enzyme activity.

EFFECT OF LONG TERM GLUCOCORTICOID TREATMENT

In 23 patients treated with prednisone or deflazacort(4) (Tab.1), serum phosphate significantly fell in both groups of patients and serum calcium increased only in prednisone patients. A statistically significant difference was found between the opposite changes in 1,25(OH)2D(5) observed in the two groups of patients. The rise in 1,25(OH)2D levels observed in deflazacort patients may be secondary to changes in phosphate metabolism but the stimulatory effect of hypophosphatemia may have been overriden in prednisone patients by the concomitant increase in serum calcium.

Tab.1: Serum calcium, phosphate, 25-OH-D and 1,25(OH)2D before and after long term treatment (3-6months) with prednisone or deflazacort (mean ± SE).

Serum calcium mg/dl		serum phosphate mg/dl		serum 25-OH-D ng/ml		serum 1,25(OH)D pg/ml	
Before	After	Before	After	Before	After	Before	After
Prednisone (10-25 mg/day;13 patients)							
9.1-0.1	9.3±0.1	3.8±0.1	3.6±0.1	13±3	12±2	38±3	30±4
Deflazacort(12-30 mg/day;10 patients)							
9.4±0.1	9.4±0.1	3.8±0.1	3.6±0.1	8±2	14±3	45±6	57±8

SERUM 1,25(OH)2D IN VITAMIN D INTOXICATION: EFFECT OF STEROID THERAPY.

Two patients with reumatoid arthritis were referred to us because of hypercalcemia discovered after 1-12 months of treatment with 10-0.25 mg of vitamin D2/day respectively (Tab.2). In both patients GLS treatment had been withdrawn for 2 months. Hypercalcemia was associated with raised levels of 1,25(OH)2D and administration of prednisone resulted in suppression of 1,25(OH)2D and reduction of calcium to within the normal range in both patients. In these two patients with reumatoid arthritis vitamin D intoxication seems to be due to high levels of 1,25(OH)2D since GLS,rapidly reducing serum 1,25(OH)2D, suppressed serum calcium to normal.

Tab.2: Serum calcium, 25-OH-D and 1,25(OH)2D in two patients with reumatoid arthritis and vitamin D2 intoxication before and after administration of prednisone (PN)(mean ± SD).

Vitamin D. A Chemical, Biochemical and Clinical Update

Pat. n.	age/sex	Serum calcium mg/dl		Serum 25-OH-D ng/ml		Serum 1,25(OH)2D pg/ml	
		before PN	After PN	Before PN	After PN	Before PN	After PN
1.	55/F	12.5±1.1	9.2±0.6	130±12	125±15	120±10	55±10
2.	52/F	13.4±0.9	9.0±0.8	225±25	212±14	132±14	40±12

EXTRA-RENAL PRODUCTION OF 1,25(OH)2D IN ANEPHRIC SUBJECTS: EFFECT OF STEROID THERAPY.

In two anephric subjects serum 1,25(OH)2D became detectable during treatment with 25-OH-D3, but 30 mg/day of prednisone suppressed 1,25(OH)2D back to undetectable values.(fig.1). These observations indicate that, if adequate substrate is available, an extra-renal, GLS-dependent, production of 1,25(OH)2D may occur.

CONCLUSIONS

1. Glucocorticoid therapy has not direct effect on renal production of 1,25(OH)2D but it suppresses extra-renal 1-hydroxylase activity.
2. Extra-renal production of 1,25(OH)2D may occur in anephric subjects and in reumatoid arthritis if adequate substrate (25-OH-D) is available.

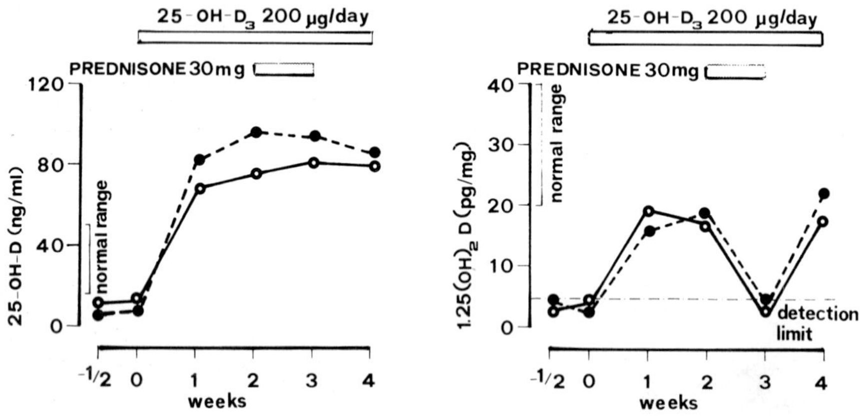

Fig.1 Serum 25-OH-D and 1,25(OH)2D in two anephric subjects during therapy with 25-OH-D3 and prednisone.

REFERENCES

1.Chesney RW, Mazess RB, Hamstra AJ, De Luca HF.(1978) Lancet 2:1123-1125.
2.Hahn TJ, Halster LR, Baran DT.(1978) J.Clin.Endocrinol.Metab.52:111-114.
3.Papapoulos SE,Clemens TL,Fraher LJ,O'Riordan JL.(1979) Lancet 1:672-630.
4.Lo Cascio V,Bonucci E,Imbimbo B,Ballanti P,Tartarotti D,Galvanini G,Adami S.(1984) Calcif. Tissue Intern.36:435-438.
5.Fraher L,Adami S,Clemens TL,Jones G., O'Riordan JLH. (1983) Clin. Endocrinol.19:157-165.

VITAMIN D-DEPENDENT RICKETS TYPE I IN PIGS

J. FOX, E.M.W. MAUNDER, A.D. CARE AND V.A. RANDALL

Departments of Animal Physiology & Nutrition and Biochemistry, University of Leeds, Leeds LS2 9JT, U.K.

Introduction

Two subclasses of hypocalcemic vitamin D-dependent rickets have been described in man. Type I is characterized by low circulating levels of 1,25-dihydroxyvitamin D (1,25-$(OH)_2D$), and is thought to be caused by a defective renal 1-hydroxylase enzyme (1). Type II is characterized by elevated 1,25-$(OH)_2D$ levels and is considered to be due to target-organ resistance (2). In 1962, pigs with inherited hypocalcemic rickets were described, the trait being transmitted by an autosomal-recessive mechanism (3). We have bred a strain of pigs with this condition to further elucidate its pathogenesis.

Methods

An approximately equal distribution of heterozygous (normocalcemic) and homozygous (hypocalcemic) piglets was produced by mating a homozygous boar, maintained clinically-normal by the administration of large doses of vitamin D_3, with heterozygous sows. The piglets were studied without vitamin D treatment at 7-9 weeks of age. Plasma N-terminal parathyroid hormone (iPTH), vitamin D metabolites and plasma and intestinal calcium-binding protein (CaBP) were measured by radioimmunoassays (4,5). iPTH levels are expressed as pmol-eq bPTH(1-84)/l. The metabolic clearance rate (MCR) and production rate (PR) of 1,25-$(OH)_2D$ was measured by infusing ^{3}H-1,25-$(OH)_2D_3$ to steady-state levels in plasma (4); values are expressed per kg metabolic bodysize (MBS; $kg^{0.75}$). Renal 25-$(OH)D_3$-1-and 24-hydroxylase enzyme activities were assessed by incubating 10% cortical homogenates with 100 pmol ^{3}H-25-$(OH)D_3$ for 15 min at 39°C. Duodenal cytosol, prepared in high-salt buffer was incubated with ^{3}H-1,25-$(OH)_2D_3$, layered on linear 4-20% sucrose gradients, and centrifuged at 225,000 x g for 18 h at 4°C. The gradient was fractionated and the elution of radioactivity compared with a 4.2S marker.

Results

Significant hypocalcemia was present in affected piglets at 3 weeks of age and became progressively more severe. By 8 weeks the prolonged hypocalcemia had induced a marked secondary hyperparathyroidism; hypophosphatemia and retarded growth were also significant features (Table 1). Plasma 1,25-$(OH)_2D$ levels were low or undetectable (<14 pmol/l) in the hypocalcemic animals; 24,25-$(OH)_2D_3$ levels were also significantly lower despite a 2.1-fold higher 25-$(OH)D_3$. The MCR of 1,25-$(OH)_2D_3$ was identical in both groups, resulting in an 8-fold difference in its PR. In incubations of renal homogenates, peaks of radioactivity coeluting with 24,25- and 1,25-$(OH)_2D_3$ on HPLC were clearly present in the normocalcemic piglets; there was no radioactivity other than unchanged 25-$(OH)D_3$ in homogenates from hypocalcemic animals. CaBP levels were significantly reduced in both plasma and intestine of hypocalcemic piglets, with the largest effect observed in the ileum. A similar degree of ^{3}H-1,25-$(OH)_2D_3$-binding was observed at a sedimentation coefficient of <4.2S in the duodenal cytosol of both normo- and hypocalcemic piglets. Binding was eliminated by a 100-fold molar excess of 1,25-$(OH)_2D_3$; a 10-fold excess of 25-$(OH)D_3$ was without effect. The hypocalcemia could be reversed by the administration of small doses of 1,25-$(OH)_2D_3$ or by pharmacologic doses of vitamin D_3.

Table 1. Plasma concentrations of relevant parameters, metabolic clearance rate (MCR) and production rate (PR) of 1,25-$(OH)_2D_3$, renal 25-$(OH)D_3$-hydroxylase enzyme activities, and intestinal CaBP levels in 7-9 week old normo- and hypocalcemic piglets (mean ± SEM).

Parameter	Normocalcemic(10)	Hypocalcemic(14)	P
Ca (mmol/l)	2.63 ± 0.04	1.44 ± 0.07	0.001
P (mmol/l)	2.71 ± 0.08	2.12 ± 0.07	0.001
iPTH (pmol/l)	< 23	120 ± 9	0.001
25-$(OH)D_3$ (nmol/l)	52 ± 5	111 ± 10	0.001
24,25-$(OH)_2D_3$ (nmol/l)	7.4 ± 0.7	5.0 ± 0.5	0.05
1,25-$(OH)_2D$ (pmol/l)	146 ± 23	22 ± 1	0.001
CaBP (nmol/l)	6.8 ± 0.6	4.9 ± 0.5	0.05
Weight (kg)	11.1 ± 1.2	7.0 ± 0.4	0.001
MCR of 1,25-$(OH)_2D_3$ (n = 4)			
ml/min per kg MBS	0.90 ± 0.02	0.90 ± 0.01	NS
PR of 1,25-$(OH)_2D$ (n = 4)			
fmol/min per kg MBS	177 ± 27	22 ± 1	0.001
Renal hydroxylase enzyme activities (pmol/min per g kidney cortex; n = 5)			
1-hydroxylase	3.1 ± 1.4	< 0.1	0.001
24-hydroxylase	0.8 ± 0.4	< 0.1	NS
Intestinal CaBP levels (nmol/g mucosa)			
Duodenum	58.5 ± 5.4	34.5 ± 3.0	0.001
Ileum	1.88 ± 0.22	0.59 ± 0.08	0.001

Discussion

The low circulating levels of 1,25-$(OH)_2D$ and absence of renal 1-hydroxylase enzyme activity, despite hypocalcemia, elevated iPTH and hypophosphatemia, the presence of apparently normal intestinal receptors for 1,25-$(OH)_2D_3$ and reversibility of the hypocalcemia by small doses of 1,25-$(OH)_2D_3$ all suggest that this condition is analogous to vitamin D-dependent rickets type I in man and distinguish it from type II. The similarity of the MCR of 1,25-$(OH)_2D_3$ in both groups confirms that the defect is caused solely by decreased 1,25-$(OH)_2D$ production, and demonstrates that the clearance of 1,25-$(OH)_2D$ is unaffected by a 7-8 fold difference in its plasma concentration. Further, it suggests that at physiologic levels, 1,25-$(OH_2D$ does not induce its own metabolism (6). The elevated 25-$(OH)D_3$ levels in affected piglets may represent a buildup of precursor since there was no 25-$(OH)D_3$ metabolism in renal homogenates, although the absence of 1,25-$(OH)_2D$-mediated inhibition of the 25-hydroxylase may also be a factor (7).

References

1. Fraser, D., Kooh, S.W., Kind, H.P., Holick, M.F. & DeLuca, H.F. (1975). N. Engl. J. Med. 289, 817-822.
2. Brooks, M.H., Bell, N.H., Love, L., Stern, P.H., Orfei, E., Queener, S.F., Hamstra, A.J. & DeLuca, H.F. (1978). N. Engl. J. Med. 298, 996-999.
3. Plonait, H. (1962). Deut. Tierarzkl. Woch. 69, 198-202.
4. Fox, J. & Ross, R. (1985). J. Endocrinol. - in press.
5. Murray, T.M., Arnold, B.M., Tam, W.H., Hitchman, A.J.W. & Harrison, J.E. (1974). Metabolism 23, 829-837.
6. Frolik, C.A. & DeLuca, H.F. (1972). J. Clin. Invest. 52 543-548.
7. Baran, D.T. & Milne, M.L. (1983). Calcif. Tiss. Int. 35, 461-464.

METABOLISM OF 25-OH-D_3 IN HUMAN PROMYELOCYTIC LEUKEMIA CELLS (HL-60). ISOLATION AND IDENTIFICATION OF 19-NOR-10-KETO-25-OH-D_3.

S. Ishizuka[1], T. Matsui[2], Y. Nakao[2], T. Fujita[2], T. Okabe[3] and A.W. Norman[4]

1) Teijin Institute for Bio-Medical Research, Tokyo, Japan, 2) Department of Medicine, University of Kobe, Kobe, Japan, 3) Faculty of Medicine, University of Tokyo, Tokyo, Japan, and 4) Department of Biochemistry, University of California, Riverside, CA 92521, U.S.A.

Recently it is demonstrated that the hormonal form of vitamin D_3, 1α,25-$(OH)_2D_3$, can induce in vitro differentiation of the murine myeloid leukemic cell line (M1 cell) and the human promyelocytic leukemia cell line (HL-60 cell) into monocyte-macrophages [1-4]. 25-OH-D_3 also can mediate induction of the differentiation of HL-60 cells into monocyte-macrophages when present at 250 time the concentrations of 1α,25-$(OH)_2D_3$ [5]. It is yet unclear whether induction of differentiation of HL-60 cells is by 25-OH-D_3 itself or by its metabolites. To solve this problem we investigated the metabolism of 25-OH-D_3 in HL-60 cells. In this report, we demonstrate that HL-60 cells metabolize 25-OH-D_3 to two unidentified metabolites during in vitro incubation. These two metabolites are identified as 5(Z)-19-nor-10-keto-25-OH-D_3 and 5(E)-19-nor-10-keto-25-OH-D_3.

Incubation of 25-OH-D_3 with HL-60 cells

The HL-60 cells (1 x 10^6 cells) were washed with serum-free RPMI-1640 medium and incubated with 1 µCi of [^{3}H]25-OH-D_3 (22 Ci/mmol) in 1 ml of serum-free RPMI-1640 medium for 1 min at 37°C in a humidified atmosphere of 5 % CO_2 in air. The reactions were terminated by adding two volumes of chloroform:methanol (1:1) to the cells and medium. To determine the structure of the metabolites of 25-OH-D_3, 550 µg of 25-OH-D_3 were incubated with HL-60 cells (3.6 x 10^9 cells) in 3 liters of serum-free RPMI-1640 medium at 37°C for 60 min, and then the metabolites were extracted with two volumes of chloroform:methanol (1:1).

Separation and purification of the metabolites by column chromatography

The chloroform phase was evaporated and the residue was dried by ethanol azeotrope. The chloroform extracts were chromatographed on a 1.5 x 25 cm Sephadex LH-20 column eluted with chloroform:n-hexane (50:50).
The 25-OH-D_3 (48 90 ml) and the 25-OH-D_3 metabolites (114-180 ml) fractions from the column were separatly pooled and concentrated.
The 25-OH-D_3 metabolite fractions from the Sephadex LH-20 column were then subjected to HPLC equipped with a 4.6 x 250 mm Zorbax Sil column, and eluted with 10 % isopropanol in n-hexane. The eluate was continuously monitored by ultraviolet absorption at 310 nm, and the ultraviolet absorbing metabolite 1 and metabolite 2 eluted between 25(S)26-$(OH)_2D_3$ and 1α,25-$(OH)_2D_3$ and eluted just before the elution position of 1α,25-$(OH)_2D_3$. The metabolite 1 and metabolite 2 were further purified by HPLC using a Zorbax Sil column eluted with 2.5 % methanol in dichloromethane.
The metabolite 1 was eluted at the same elution position as 24(R)25-$(OH)_2$ D_3 and the metabolite 2 was eluted between 24(R)25-$(OH)_2D_3$ and 25(S)26-$(OH)_2D_3$. According to these isolation and purification procedures, the total amount of 4.80 µg of metabolite 1 and 12.48 µg of metabolite 2 were

Vitamin D. A Chemical, Biochemical and Clinical Update

calculated, assuming an ε of 27,000 cm^{-1} [6].

Metabolism of [^{3}H]25-OH-D_3 in HL-60 cells

HL-60 cells metabolized [^{3}H]25-OH-D_3 to two new radioactive metabolites of 25-OH-D_3,metabolite 1 and metabolite 2 [7]. We investigated the time-course experiment of [^{3}H]25-OH-D_3 metabolism by HL-60 cells. Using 4.5 x 10^{-8} M of [^{3}H] 25-OH-D_3 as a substrate, the production of metabolite 1 and 2 reached the maximum level in 30 to 60 sec. and thereafter kept almost the same level for 60 min; this demonstrates that 25-OH-D_3 metabolism by HL-60 cells was remarkably rapid.

Identification of the two metabolites of 25-OH-D_3 by HL-60 cells

The structural confirmation of the two metabolites of 25-OH-D_3 was carried out as follows: (i) the isolated two metabolites comigrate with the authentic 5(Z)- and 5(E)-19-nor-10-keto-25-OH-D_3 on HPLC using two different solvent systems, respectively; (ii) the ultraviolet absorption spectra of the two metabolites display both the unique chromophore with λmax=310 nm; (iii) the mass spectral fragmentation patterns of the two isolated metabolites give both m/e 402, 384, 369, 359, 341, 315, 273, 177 and 133; (iv) the molecular weight of 402 and the loss of C_3H_7 fragments are mass spectral characteristics unique to 19-nor-10-keto-25-OH-D_3; (v) the FT-IR spectra of the two metabolites indicate both the very intense absorbance at 1678 cm^{-1}, which is indicative of a carbonyl group conjugated double bonds. From these results, the structure of the metabolite 1 and metabolite 2 was unequivocally determined to be 5(Z)-19-nor-10-keto-25-OH-D_3 and 5(E)-19-nor-10-keto-25-OH-D_3, respectively [6].

These unique metabolites, 5(Z)-19-nor-10-keto-25-OH-D_3 and 5(E)-19-nor-10-keto-25-OH-D_3, did not bind specifically to the chick intestinal 3.7 S receptor for 1α,25-$(OH)_2D_3$ [6,7]. It therefore appears that the 19-nor-10-keto-25-OH-D_3 is in a pathway of vitamin D_3 metabolic deactivation. However, Teitelbaum et al. recently reported that 19-nor-10-keto-25-OH-D_3 induces monocytic maturation of HL-60 cells in a manner similar to 1α,25-$(OH)_2D_3$ [8]. Hence, we are much interested in the biological and physiological functions of 19-nor-10-keto-25-OH-D_3.

REFERENCES

1. Abe, E., Miyaura, C., Sakagami, H., Takeda, M., Konno, K., Yamazaki, T., Yoshiki, S., and Suda, T.(1981) Proc. Natl. Acad. Sci. 78, 4990-4994
2. Tanaka,H., Abe, E., Miyaura, C., Shiina, Y., and Suda, T. (1983) Biochem. Biophys. Res. Commun. 117, 86-92
3. Matsui, T., Nakao, Y., Kobayashi, N., Kishihara, M., Ishizuka, S., Watanabe, S., and Fujita, T. (1984) Int. J. Cancer 33, 193-202
4. Yoshida, M., Ishizuka, S., and Hoshi, A. (1984) J. Pharm. Dyn.7, 962-968
5. Tanaka, H., Abe, E., Miyaura, C., Kuribayashi, T., Konno, K., Nishii, Y. and Suda, T. (1982) Biochem. J. 204, 713-719
6. Ishizuka, S., Norman, A.W., Matsui, T., Nakao, Y., Fujita, T., Okabe, T. Fujisawa, M., Watanabe, J., and Takaku, F. submitted
7. Okabe, T., Ishizuka, S., Fujisawa, M., Watanabe, J., and Takaku, F. (1985) Biochem. Biophys. Res. Commun. (in press)
8. Teitelbaum, S.L., Bar-Shavit, Z., Perry, III, H.M., Welgus, H.G., Kahn, A.J., Reitsma, P., Gray, R., and Horst, R. Sixth Workshop on Vitamin D (abstracts) p64

INFLUENCE OF CAFFEINE ON THE METABOLISM OF CALCIUM AND VITAMIN D IN YOUNG AND ADULT RATS.

J.K. Yeh and J.F. Aloia

Department of Medicine, Nassau Hospital, Mineola, N.Y. 11501

Introduction:

A negative calcium balance has been associated with caffeine intake in perimenopausal women (1). High caffeine intake has been found in an osteoporotic group as contrasted with age-matched controls (2). These observations suggest the possibility that caffeine intake may lead to a worsening of calcium balance. However, our laboratory observed an increase in calcium absorption in the intestine of the young rat after chronic administration of caffeine and the calcium balance of the rat was not decreased (3). The discrepancy between these two findings could be due to an age-related decline in the response of the renal production of 1,25-dihydroxyvitamin D ($1,25(OH)_2D$) to the hypercalciuric effect of caffeine. The current study was designed to investigate this hypothesis. The effect of caffeine administration on the metabolism of calcium and its regulating hormones in young and adult rats was studied.

Materials and Methods:

Male, Sprague-Dawley rats either after weanling (4 weeks old) or 12-13 months old were fed a diet containing 0.5% calcium and 0.54% phosphorus. After one week of adaption to the diet, caffeine was administered subcutaneously (10 $mg/(0.1Kg)^{3/4}$ metabolic body weight) daily for either 4 days or 14 days before the intestinal calcium absorption study (4). Control animals were injected with vehicle saline solution for 14 days. A 48 hour urine specimen was collected in a metabolic cage one day before the overnight fasting for the intestinal calcium absorption. Intestinal absorption was determined in the duodenum by the <u>in vivo</u> ligated loop technique (5). The solution injected into the loop had the following composition: 145mM NaCl, 2.0mM $CaCl_2$, 20mM glucose, 5mg% phenol red and 0.2uCi of ^{45}Ca per ml. The absorption period was 10 minutes and the animals were sacrificed by bleeding. Serum was collected for determination of calcium, $1,25(OH)_2D$, and iPTH (5,6).

Results:

Administration of caffeine to the young rat resulted in an increase in the urinary excretion of calcium after administration for 4 days. Serum $1,25(OH)_2D_3$ and iPTH levels did not increase until 14 days daily administration of caffeine. The increase in the intestinal calcium absorption was found in correspond to the change of serum PTH and $1,25(OH)_2D_3$. Serum calcium levels were decreased 4 days after caffeine adminstration but returned towards control levels after 14 days treatment. Administration of caffeine to the adult rat resulted in a consistent increase in the urinary excretion of calcium after 4 days treatment. However, the serum $1,25(OH)_2D_3$ and iPTH levels and intestinal calcium absorption were not changed throughout the 14 days administration of caffeine.

Vitamin D. A Chemical, Biochemical and Clinical Update

Discussion:

The current experiment supports the finding that caffeine intake is associated with a high urinary excretion of calcium (1,3). The increase in the intestinal calcium absorption in the young rat is the consequence of the calcitrol hormone regulation in response to the hypercalciuric effect of caffeine. However, these feedback changes in serum calcitrol hormone levels and intestinal calcium absorption after hypercalciuria was not apparent in the adult rat. It is believed that in the adult rat an age-related decline in the activity of the 1α-hydroxylase enzyme in the kidney leads to lower serum $1,25(OH)_2D$ levels and lower calcium absorption. Previous studies in rats and humans have demonstrated that there is an age-related decline in serum $1,25(OH)_2D$ and in calcium absorption by the intestine (7-9). The current finding of a consistent increase in the urinary excretion of calcium without a compensatory increase in intestinal calcium absorption in the adult rat may account for the negative calcium balance in association with caffeine intake in perimenopausal women (1).

Effect of the administration of caffeine on the serum $1,25(OH)_2D_3$, iPTH and the intestinal absorption and urinary excretion of calcium in the young and adult rats.

	Serum Ca (mg/dl)	$1,25(OH)_2D_3$ (pg/ml)	iPTH (ng/ml)	^{45}Ca Absorption (%)	Urinary Ca (mg/24hr)
YN	10.2±0.1	124±7.4	0.38±0.05	52.4±2.7	0.65±0.07
YC 4	9.5±0.2**	117±5.8	0.42±0.07	49.7±3.2	1.36±0.13**
YC 14	9.9±0.2	158±7.9**	0.85±0.10**	65.3±4.1*	1.83±0.20**
AN	9.6±0.1	48±3.4	0.87±0.04	28.2±1.4	1.25±0.07
AC 4	9.4±0.2	50±3.8	0.90±0.05	31.5±2.0	2.08±0.28**
AC 14	9.8±0.2	46±4.0	1.06±0.07*	25.7±2.1	3.05±0.40**

YN: Young normal; YC 4: Young rats + 4 days caffeine; YC 14: Young rats + 14 days caffeine; AN: Adult rats normal control; AC 4: Adult rats + 4 days caffeine: AC 14: Adult rats + 14 days caffeine. Values are mean ± S.E. of 7 observations. *;** Significantly different from the respective control ($p<0.05$; $p<0.01$)

References:

1. Heaney, R., Recker, R.R. (1982) J.Lab.Clin.Med.99:46-55.
2. Daniell, H.W. (1976) Arch. Intern Med.136:298-304.
3. Yeh, J.K., Aloia, J.F., Semla, H.M., Chen, S.Y.submitted - publication.
4. Kleiber, M.(1961) The Fire of Life, John Wiley and Sons, Inc.NY 177-216
5. Yeh, J.K., Aloia, J.F. (1984) Endocrinol 114:1711-1717.
6. Tenner, T.E., Buddingh, G., Yang, M.L., Pang, P., Patel, D., Savjani, G.(1985) in press.
7. Horst, R.L., DeLuca, H.F., Jorgensen, N.A. (1978) Metab.Bone Dis. Rel. Res. 1:29-33.
8. Armbrecht, H.J., Zenser, T.V., Gross, C.J., Davis, B.B. (1980) Am. J. Physiol. 239:E322-E327.
9. Avioli, L.V., McDonald, J.E., Lee, S.W. (1965) J. Clin. Invest. 44:1960-1967.

PHARMACOKINETICS OF 1,25-DIHYDROXYVITAMIN D IN THE RAT.

M.J.JONGEN, J.E.BISHOP, C.CADE and A.W.NORMAN.

Department of Biochemistry,University of California,Riverside,CA,USA.

Introduction: Despite intensive research in recent years on vitamin D metabolism there is relatively little information available on the pharmacokinetics of the physiologically active vitamin D metabolites and the factors that influence these pharmacokinetics. It was our aim to study the pharmacokinetics of 1,25-dihydroxyvitamin D (1,25(OH)$_2$D$_3$) under physiological conditions that are known to affect the production and/or degradation of this hormone. Dietary calcium and phosphate content and vitamin D deficiency are well known modulators of circulating 1,25(OH)$_2$D$_3$ concentrations. The effects of these physiological conditions were studied in the rat. Because vitamin D deficient rats have no endogenous 24,25-dihdyroxyvitamin D (24,25-(OH)$_2$D$_3$) they were also used as a model to study the effects of physiological doses of 24,25(OH)$_2$D$_3$ on the pharmacokinetics of 1,25-(OH)$_2$D$_3$.

Methods: Two to four months old male Holtzman rats were used in all experiments. They were fed a synthetic diet (0.73% Ca, 0.32% P, 2 IU D$_3$/g) from which virtually all calcium, phosphate and vitamin D could be omitted. Two types of experiments were done:

1. Vitamin D replete rats were equilibrated on the synthetic diet for several weeks. The rats were cannulated and kept on the same diet or put on a diet lacking either calcium or phosphate for 5 days, after which the pharmacokinetic experiment was done.
2. Rats were fed the vitamin D deficient diet for 6-8 weeks. Four or five days after cannulation the pharmacokinetic experiment was carried out. The effect of 24,25(OH)$_2$D$_3$ was studied by dosing the animals intravenously with 24,25(OH)$_2$D$_3$ approximately 14 hours before the experiment.

Experimental procedure: The rats were cannulated in the right jugular vein and allowed to recover for at least 4 days. On the day of the experiment they received a rapid intravenous dose of [^{3}H-26,27]-1,25-(OH)$_2$D$_3$ (Spec.act. 158 Ci/mmol). Blood samples (100-300µl) were taken from 5 minutes on with increasing time intervals during 3 days. Radioactivity was extracted from the blood with 5 ml hexane-isopropanol-n-butanol (93/3/4 v/v). The organic phase was separated and radioactivity measured after evaporation of the solvent. Two samples from each experiment were used to verify the identity of the radioactivity by HPLC using a silicic acid column with a gradient of isopropanol in hexane. Dpm per milliliter blood were calculated taking into account extraction efficiency and counting efficiency. After the experiment the rats were sacrificed and the blood taken for determination of plasma calcium, phosphate and vitamin D metabolites. Elimination half-lifes were determined with a computer program using nonlinear regression.

Results: Table 1 summarizes the results from all experiments. Short term phosphate or calcium deficiency did not effect the elimination half-life of 1,25(OH)$_2$D$_3$ in vitamin D replete rats. Vitamin D deficien-

Vitamin D. A Chemical, Biochemical and Clinical Update

cy approximately doubled the elimination half-life of 1,25$(OH)_2D_3$. In the vitamin D deficient rats physiological doses of 24,25$(OH)_2D_3$ did not result in a significant change of the elimination half-life of 1,25$(OH)_2D_3$. Figure 1 shows the results from vitamin D replete and vitamin D deficient rats.

Table 1: Results of pharmacokinetic experiments in vitamin D replete and vitamin D deficient rats (Mean and standard deviation).

Diet/treatment	$t_{1/2}$ elimin. (hours)	25(OH)D (nmol/l)	24,25D (nmol/l)	1,25D (pmol/l)
D replete:				
+Ca,+PO4 (n=6)	16.3±1.7	26.8±4.5	14.5±5.3	166±57*
-Ca,+PO4 (n=5)	18.6±1.0	21.0±7.7	12.1±3.7	447±116*
+Ca,-PO4 (n=6)	16.0±1.2	21.3±8.9	12.0±5.3	204±159*
D deficient:				
no 24,25D(n=7)	36.4±6.3	<10	<2	<45
2.5 ng/ml(n=3)	44.4±17.6	<10	<2	326,176,<45*
5.0 ng/ml(n=2)	42.1±5.7	<10	<2	<45
10 ng/ml (n=3)	37.3±6.8	<10	<2	<45
20 ng/ml (n=1)	27.6	<10	<2	<45

* Because of remaining ^{3}H-1,25$(OH)_2D_3$ in the samples only approximate values could be calculated.

Figure 1: Clearance of radioactivity from the blood in vitamin D replete (+D) and vitamin D deficient (-D) rats.

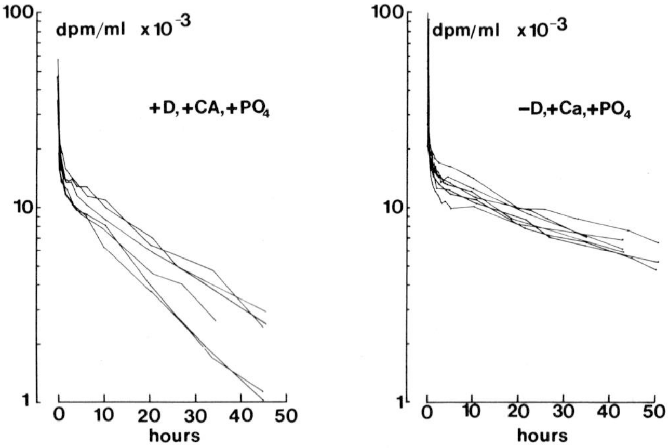

<u>Conclusions:</u> The elimination half-life of 1,25$(OH)_2D_3$ did not change with short term dietary phosphate or calcium depletion. This suggests that in vivo regulation of 1,25$(OH)_2D_3$ concentrations by dietary phosphate or calcium takes place at the production site of the hormone and not by changes in elimination rate. However, in vitamin D deficiency the elimination half-life is considerably increased which suggests that additional or different factors are involved in the regulation of 1,25$(OH)_2D_3$ concentrations. Our results also indicate that 24,25-$(OH)_2D_3$ is probably not the mediator of this change in elimination half-life.

EFFECT OF A RETINOID ON Ca AND VITAMIN D METABOLISM IN THYROPARATHYROIDECTOMIZED (TPTX) RATS

U. Trechsel and H. Fleisch
Department of Pathophysiology, University of Bern,
CH-3010 Bern, Switzerland

Vitamin A and its derivatives (retinoids) stimulate bone resorption by an unknown mechanism. We have studied the effect of a potent synthetic retinoid on Ca metabolism in thyroparathyroidectomized (TPTX) rats. Retinoid produced a decrease of intestinal Ca absorption and an increase of urinary Ca and plasma Ca. ^{45}Ca kinetics showed an increase of bone resorption but no change of bone formation. In order to investigate a possible role of $1,25(OH)_2D$ in the action of the retinoid on Ca metabolism, we have measured plasma $1,25(OH)_2D$ in retinoid treated TPTX rats.

The retinoid produced a dose-related decrease of plasma $1,25(OH)_2D$. This decrease of $1,25(OH)_2D$ was probably responsible for the observed impairment of intestinal Ca absorption. In contrast, the increased bone resorption was unlikely to be due to $1,25(OH)_2D$.

Since retinoid treatment produced a significant increase of plasma Ca it appeared possible that the decrease of plasma $1,25(OH)_2D$ was a consequence of the increase in extracellular Ca rather than a direct effect of the retinoid on the renal 1-hydroxylase. This hypothesis was supported by the finding of a good ($p < 0.001$) inverse correlation between plasma Ca and plasma $1,25(OH)_2D$. In order to corroborate it further, plasma $1,25(OH)_2D$ was measured in retinoid treated rats in which the increase of plasma Ca was prevented by blocking bone resorption with dichloromethylenebisphosphonate (Cl_2MBP). This compound is known to be a specific inhibitor of osteoclastic bone resorption. The results showed that preventing

Vitamin D. A Chemical, Biochemical and Clinical Update

the retinoid induced increase in plasma Ca with Cl_2MBP also abolished the decrease in plasma $1,25(OH)_2D$.

It is concluded that the retinoid increased bone resorption, probably by a $1,25(OH)_2D$ independent mechanism. A concomitant impairment of intestinal Ca absorption could be explained by a decrease of plasma $1,25(OH)_2D$. The inverse relationship between plasma $1,25(OH)_2D$ and plasma Ca suggests that the increase of plasma Ca observed in retinoid treated TPTX rats was involved in the inhibitory action of the retinoid on plasma $1,25(OH)_2D$.

We have previously demonstrated a Ca related modulation of plasma $1,25(OH)_2D$ in TPTX rats (1). The present study provides another example of a Ca-related, PTH independent modulation of plasma $1,25(OH)_2D$.

1. Trechsel, U., Eisman, J.A., Fischer, J.A., Bonjour, J.-P., Fleisch, H. (1980) Am. J. Physiol. 239:E119-E124.

FATTY ACID ESTERS OF CALCIOL AND ERCALCIOL IN HUMANS AND THEIR POSSIBLE METABOLIC FUNCTION

B. Zagalak, F. Neuheiser and H.-Ch. Curtius
University of Zurich, Department of Clinical Chemistry,
Institute of Pediatrics, 8032 Zurich, Switzerland

We have observed that about 15-25% of the total amount of calciol and ercalciol in serum or plasma of healthy adults (calciol 1-6 ng/ml serum) or children (calciol 5-15 ng/ml serum) are present in the form of lipophylic conjugates. These conjugates are also present in blood particles and in urine. They are easily hydrolized by cholesterol esterase from microorganisms (EC 3.1.1.13, Boehringer) or alkalines (5% KOH or 0.5 N sodium methylate in methanol) and the intact cis-vitamin D_3 and cis-vitamin D_2 can be essayed (1-3) in the hydrolysates as following:

Fig. 1 QUANTITATION OF FREE AND ESTERIFIED VITAMIN-D IN SERUM, PLASMA OR URINE (1)

SAMPLE + INTERNAL STANDARDS (vit. D_3-d_8, vit. D_2-d_3, vit. 25-OH-D_3-d_3)
↓ extraction x 2 (CH_2Cl_2: methanol, 2 : 1 v/v)
← 1. 5% KOH in methanol, reflux, 60 min., I.S.
   2. extraction mit CH_2Cl_2

ALUMINA COLUMN (4 g)
1. n-hexane (vit.-D fatty acid esters fraction) →
↓ 2. 3% ethanol in benzene (free vit.-D and β-sterols fraction)

DIGITONIN-CELITE-H_2O COLUMN
↓ n-hexane: ethyl acetate, 1 : 1 v/v

HPLC, LiChrosorb Si-60 Merck (4,6 x 250 mm)
↓ 3% methanol in CH_2Cl_2

HPLC, RP-18 COLUMN (4,6 x 250 mm)
↓ methanol

DERIVATIZATION (TMS-ETHER)
↓ TMCS: BSTFA, 1 : 4, R.T., 30 min.

GAS CHROMATOGRAPHY-MASS FRAGMENTOGRAPHY
↓ SE-30 capillary column (200°C - 300°C, 5°C/min.)

VITAMIN D_3: M^+, m/e 456 and m/e 464 (I.S.)
VITAMIN D_2: M^+, m/e 468 and m/e 471 (I.S.)
25-OH-VITAMIN-D_3: M^+-90, m/e 454 and m/e 457 (I.S.)

We attempted to isolate and then to identify these conjugates by chromatographic (LC, TLC, HPLC and GC, see Fig. 2) spectroscopic (UV and MS-EI- and MS-CI mode) and chemical (adducts with 4-phenyl-1,2,4-triazoline-3,5- dione) methods by comparison with synthetic references.
From 6 l of blood (Fig. 2) approx. 230 ng of pure cis-vitamin D_3 acetate and approx. 170 ng of other fatty acid esters of cis- vitamin D_3 as well as 66 ng of esterified vitamin D_2 were

Vitamin D. A Chemical, Biochemical and Clinical Update

isolated. The structure of isolated cis-vitamin D_3 acetate was confirmed by the above mentioned methods.

Fig. 2 FRACTIONATION OF FATTY ACID ESTERS OF VITAMIN $-D_3$ and $-D_2$ ISOLATED FROM HUMAN BLOOD (6 L).

n-Hexane Extract (23 gm. dry mass)

1. Silica gel-Kg-60-LC 5% E.A in n-Hexane

Vit.-D Long Chain Fatty Acid Esters

2. Silica gel-Kg-60-LC*
3. Silica gel-Kg-60-LC*
4. Silica gel-Kg-60-$AgNO_3$LC*

Fractions:	ml	Vit.D_3 ng	Vit.D_2 ng
C_{24}	300	49	14
C_{18}-C_{20}	100	42	18
C_{16}-C_{18}	100	79	34
C_{16}	100	-	-
C_3-C_4	100	-	-
C_3-C_4	100	-	-
C_2	100	10	10
C_2	100	10	10
C_2	500	10	10
Pyruvate	2200	-	-

Vit.-D Acetate

2. Silica gel-Kg-60-LC*
3. Silica gel Kg-60-HPLC*
4. RP-18-HPLC, MeOH
   Yield of Vit.D_3 Acetate: 200 ng totally
5. Gas Chromatography: Mass Spectrometry (SE-30)

* solvent: 2.5% ethyl acetate (E.A.) in n-Hexane

Similar results were obtained from urine extracts. We found that also approx. 50% of lipophylic conjugates of vitamin D_3 exist as calciol acetate and the rest in the form of long chain fatty acid esters.

An oral loading with 1 mg of calciol-d_3 of healthy adult control proved that the esterification of vitamin D_3 takes place in the body and showed that approx. 16% of deuterated calciol after 18 h was in the esterified form present in plasma and blood particles as following (calciol-d_3: calciol-d_3-esters in ng/1 ml blood): plasma 23.3:6.5, lymphocytes 8.1:7.0 granulocytes 0.32:0.6, erythrocytes 3.0:0.7.

We also observed an increase in the concentration of lipophylic conjugates by newborns.

We suggest that these esters could be a storage form of vitamin-D (4) and may be involved in the enzymatic regulation of the physiological level of calciol in humans.

In the pathway for biosynthesis and translocation of cutaneous calciol, proposed by Holick et al. (5), the concentration of vitamin D_3 depends principally on the photochemical processes. In contrast to this pathway, we therefore suggest that the physiological level of calciol in humans may be regulated by enzymatic (acyltransferases and esterases) rather than photochemical processes.

REFERENCES

1. B. Zagalak et al., (1984) Naturwissenschaften 71, 321.
2. B. Zagalak et al., (1983) Anal. Chem. Symp. Ser. 14, 347.
3. B. Zagalak et al., (1984) Spectroscopy, An International J. (Ottawa) 3 (in press).
4. D.R. Fraser (1969) Nutrition et Dieta 13, 17.
5. M.F. Holick et al., in: Vitamin D (A.W. Norman et al., eds.) de Gruyter, Berlin 1982, p. 1151.

DETECTION OF 1,24,25-TRIHYDROXYVITAMIN D_3 IN SOLANUM MALACOXYLON LEAF EXTRACTS INCUBATED WITH RUMINAL FLUID.

R.L. Boland[a], M.I. Skliar[a] and A.W. Norman[b]

[a]Departamento de Biologia, Universidad Nacional del Sur, 8000 Bahia Blanca, Argentina. [b]Department of Biochemistry, University of California, Riverside CA 92521, USA.

INTRODUCTION:

Leaves of Solanum malacoxylon contain a glycoside derivative of $1,25(OH)_2D_3$ (1). Incubation in vitro of S. malacoxylon leaf extracts with ruminal fluid potentiates their effects on intestinal calcium and phosphate transport. This has been related to the release of $1,25(OH)_2D_3$ from the corresponding glycoside and the production of more polar metabolites (2). The objective of this work was to identify vitamin D_3 metabolites produced by the action of rumen microbes on S. malacoxylon.

METHODS:

S. malacoxylon aqueous leaf extracts (1 vol) were incubated with sheep ruminal fluid (3 vol) at 38 °C for 72 h as previously described (2). Lipids were extracted with chloroform and chloroform-benzene (1:1, v/v) and purified by thin layer chromatography on silica gel G plates developed in chloroform-methanol (95:5, v/v). Bands comprised by Rf values of 0.20-0.50 were scrapped off and extracted with chloroform and methanol. The eluants were concentrated and chromatographed on Sephadex LH-20 columns (45 x 1.5 cm) equilibrated and eluted with methanol-petroleum ether (60:40, v/v). Two fractions which eluted at 60-100 ml and 100-130 ml evidenced biological activity (capacity to induce hypercalcemia in 15 day-old chick embryos). The first eluting bioactive fraction was evaporated and extracted with isopropanol-hexane (5:95, v/v) and used for HPLC analysis. Prior to HPLC the sample was spiked with tritiated vitamin D_3 metabolites. High pressure liquid chromatography was performed on a Waters Model LC-204 HPLC chromatograph using a Radial-Pak microporasil cartridge (10 microns, 8 mm x 10 cm). Isocratic and gradient elution were performed with isopropanol-hexane as specified in Results. Fractions of 2 ml were collected. Competitive protein binding assays using tritiated vitamin D metabolites as tracers were carried out as previously described (3).

RESULTS AND DISCUSSION:

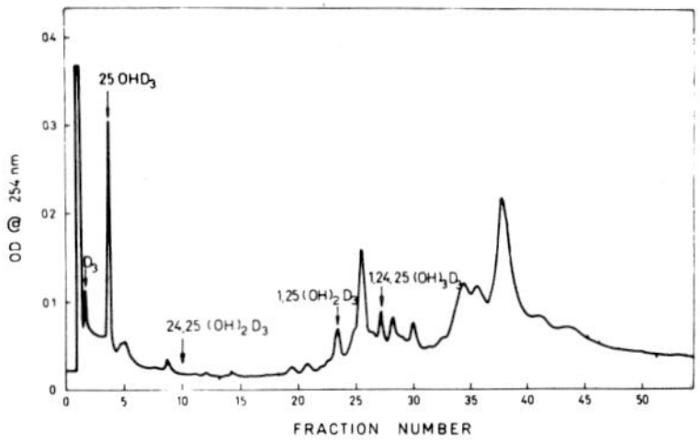

Fig. 1. HPLC profile of S. malacoxylon bioactive fraction isolated by Sephadex LH-20 chromatography. Elution: gradient of 4-60% isopropanol in hexane.

Vitamin D. A Chemical, Biochemical and Clinical Update

The biologically active fraction isolated by Sephadex LH-20 chromatography (60-100 ml) could be resolved in several fractions by gradient elution HPLC (Fig. 1). Fractions 2, 4, 24 and 28 had elution volumes similar to tritiated standards of vitamin D_3, 25OHD_3, 1,25$(OH)_2D_3$ and 1,24,25$(OH)_3D_3$, respectively. Fractions 2 and 4 produced a small displacement of ^{3}H-25OHD_3 from the serum vitamin D binding protein in the 25OHD_3 and 24,25$(OH)_2D_3$ assays (data not given), thereby indicating that only small amounts of vitamin D_3 and 25OHD_3 were contained in fractions 2 and 4, respectively. However, fractions 24 and 28, and to a smaller extent fraction 26, could effectively compete with ^{3}H-1,25$(OH)_2D_3$ for binding to the intestine cytosol receptor in 1,25$(OH)_2D_3$ binding assays (Fig. 2).

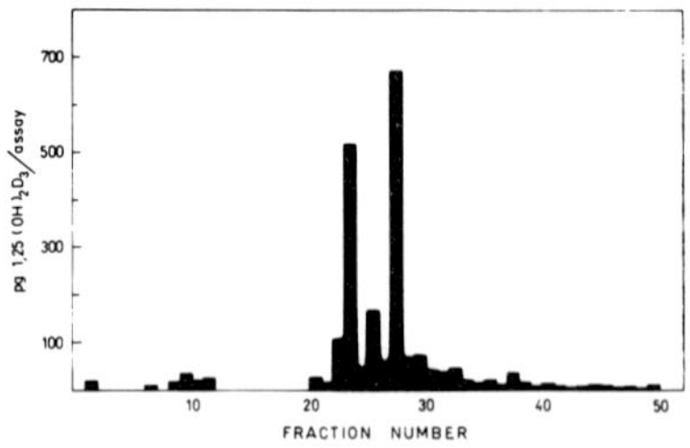

Fig. 2. 1,25$(OH)_2D_3$ competitive protein binding assays of <u>S. malacoxylon</u> fractions obtained by gradient elution HPLC.

Further chromatography of fractions 24 and 28 on HPLC columns eluted isocratically with isopropanol-hexane (8:92, v/v) and isopropanol-hexane (10:90, v/v), respectively, gave single UV absorbing peaks which had identical elution volumes as 1,25$(OH)_2D_3$ and 1,24,25$(OH)_3D_3$ standards, respectively. These peaks were effective to compete with ^{3}H-1,25$(OH)_2D_3$ in 1,25$(OH)_2D_3$ binding assays (data not given). Aplication of similar chromatographic isolation procedures coupled to competitive protein binding assays to <u>S. malacoxylon</u> extracts incubated with purified ß-glucosidase revealed the presence of only small amounts of fraction 28 in comparison with fraction 24 (data not shown). The results indicate that rumen microbes convert 1,25$(OH)_2$ D_3-glycoside of <u>Solanum malacoxylon</u> into free 1,25$(OH)_2D_3$ and a more polar metabolite. On the basis of its elution properties in various HPLC systems and its effectiveness to compete with ^{3}H-1,25$(OH)_2D_3$ for binding to the intestinal receptor it is suggested that this metabolite is 1,24,25$(OH)_3D_3$.

<u>REFERENCES</u>:

1. Haussler, M.R., Wasserman, R.H., Mc Cain, T.A., Peterlik, M., Bursac, K. M. and Hughes, M.R. (1976) Life Sciences <u>18</u>, 1049-1056.
2. Boland, A.R. de, Esparza, M., Gallego, S., Skliar, M. and Boland, R. (1978) Calcif. Tissue Res. <u>26</u>, 215-219.
3. Norman, A.W., Walters, M.R., Hunziker, W. and Bar, A. (1982) Adv. Exp. Med. Biol. <u>151</u>, 319-331.

THE PATHOGENESIS OF HYPERCALCAEMIA IN VITAMIN D POISONING.

M. DAVIES and E.B. MAWER
Department of Medicine, Royal Infirmary, Manchester M13 9WL, England.

INTRODUCTION

Early conceptions of the role of vitamin D imply that the formation of $1,25(OH)_2D$, was strictly regulated so that concentrations above normal would not be encountered (1). It is now recognised that increased serum concentrations of $1,25(OH)_2D$ are found in primary hyperparathyroidism and upon correcting vitamin D deficiency in which there is secondary hyperparathyroidism (2,3). An understanding of the underlying cause of vitamin D intoxication has been hampered by the small number of assays on serum of intoxicated patients and by conflicting results in such patients (4,5).

METHODS

Samples for assay of the hydroxylated metabolites of vitamin D_3 or vitamin D_2 were extracted with acetonitrile and applied to C18 silica sep-paks. Separation of the metabolites was effected by H.P.L.C. using automatic sample injector and programmable fraction collector.

$25(OH)D_2$ and $25(OH)D_3$ were assayed by UV absorbance on a second H.P.L.C. run, $24,25(OH)_2D$ was measured by competitive protein binding assay; $1,25(OH)_2D_2$ and $1,25(OH)_2D_3$ were assayed separately by RIA with antisera kindly donated by Professor J. O'Riordan. Calciferol was estimated by UV absorbance on H.P.L.C.

PATIENTS

8 subjects aged 15-78 yrs were studied. They had received 1.25mg - 5mg vitamin D_2 for between 5 months and 24 years. Serum was taken on admission and during recovery.

RESULTS

Serum calcium ranged from 3.01 - 4.05 mmol/l, creatinine 0.2 - 0.42 mmol/l, creatinine clearance in 6 patients 10 - 32 ml/min.

Serum $25(OH)D_2$ ranged from 583-1843 nmol/l and $1,25(OH)_2D$ mainly as $1,25(OH)_2D_2$ varied from 139 pmol/l - 313 pmol/l being raised in 7. In 4 patients $T\frac{1}{2}$ $25(OH)D$ varied from 25 - 68 days.

Significant relationships were found only between serum calcium and $25(OH)D_2$ ($p = 0.03$) and between serum $25(OH)D_2$ and calciferol.

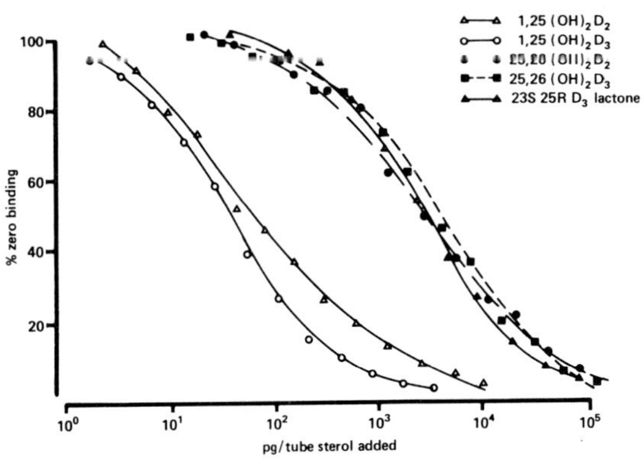

Fig 1.

No other metabolite was included in the assay for $1,25(OH)_2D_2$. The cross-reactivity was checked against all available vitamin D derivatives (Fig 1.) and $1,25(OH)_2D_3$ was excluded by H.P.L.C. Also the $1,25(OH)_2D_2$ fraction was rechromatographed on H.P.L.C. using dichloromethane: isopropanol (95:5) and no significant reduction in assayable activity for $1,25(OH)_2D_2$ was found.

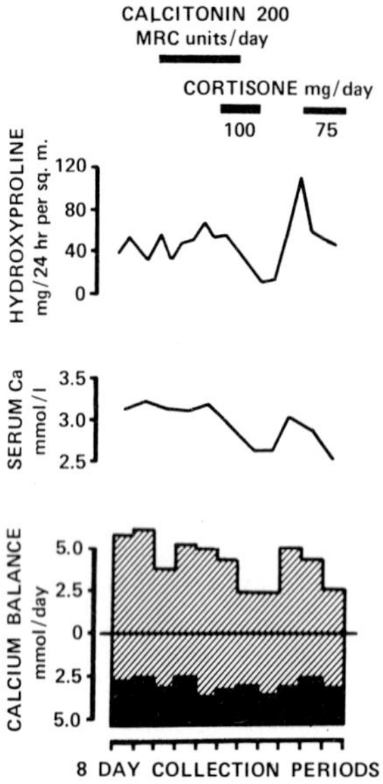

Fig 2 details the external calcium balance in one of the patients. There is negative calcium balance from urinary losses despite enhanced intestinal absorption. Steroids corrected hypercalcaemia without altering absorption. Hydroxyproline excretion fell and the evidence suggests that hypercalcaemia was corrected by reducing bone resorption.

CONCLUSIONS

High concentrations of both 25(OH)D and $1,25(OH)_2D$ occur in vitamin D poisoning. The high $1,25(OH)_2D$ occurs despite factors (such as hypercalcaemia) which favours suppression of synthesis. It seems that the increased $1,25(OH)_2D$ arises because of the increase in precursor 25(OH)D exerting a mass action effect on the renal 1 hydroxylase system. These high concentrations are such that both metabolites should produce increased bone resorption and enhanced intestinal calcium absorption. Hypercalcaemia is exacerbated by renal failure and by the possible effects of the vitamin D metabolites on the renal tubular reabsorption of calcium.

REFERENCES

1. Haussler, M.R. and McCain, T.A. (1977), New Engl. J. Med. 297, 974-983.
2. Brumbaugh, P.F., Haussler, D.H., Bressler, R. and Haussler, M.R. (1974) Science, 183, 1089-1091.
3. Stanbury, S.W., Taylor, C.M., Lumb, G.A., Mawer, E.B., Berry, J., Hann, J. and Wallace, J. (1981), Min. and Electrol. Metab. 5, 221-227.
4. Hughes, M.R., Baylink, D.J., Jones, P.G. and Haussler, M.R. (1976), J. Clin. Invest. 58, 61-70.
5. Mason, R.S., Lissner, D., Grunstein, J.S. and Posen, S. (1980), Clin. Chem. 26, 440-450.

VITAMIN D_3 UPTAKE BY THE ISOLATED PERFUSED LIVER IS DEPENDENT ON ITS TRANSPORT BY LIPOPROTEINS AND IS A SURFACE PHENOMENON

Justin Silver and Ehud Ziv

Hadassah University Hospital, Jerusalem, Israel

The liver is a major site of clearance and metabolism of vitamin D. After an intravenous injection of vitamin D to rats as much as 45% of the injected dose is retained by the liver at 1 hour (1,2). The mechanism of this hepatic uptake was not clear until it was shown that when added to an isolated liver perfusion on lipoproteins nearly 80% of the vitamin D was extracted by the liver at 1 hour as compared to about half the dose when added on vitamin D binding protein (DBP) (3). Lipoproteins play an important role in vitamin D transport because after intestinal absorption vitamin D is transported on chylomicrons (4), and after an intravenous injection vitamin D is initially bound to lipoproteins (5) before transferring to vitamin D binding protein (DBP) (6-8). We have now studied how the liver preferentially retains vitamin D from lipoproteins by comparing the uptake by the isolated perfused rat liver of vitamin D_3, cholesterol and triglycerides from different rat lipoproteins. The lipoprotein fractions studied were chylomicrons, very low density lipoprotein fraction (VLDL) and the high density lipoprotein fraction (HDL).

Materials and Methods (9)

Biosynthetically labelled lipoproteins were obtained from rats injected intravenously with either ($1-^{14}C$) palmitic acid or ($1,2(n)-^3H$) cholesterol 0.5 and 6 h respectively prior to exsanguination. The plasma was separated into individual lipoprotein fractions by sequential ultracentrifugation. Labelled chylomicrons were prepared with ^{14}C-palmitic acid, and all fractions were incubated with (^{14}C) or (^3H) vitamin D_3 for 16 h at 4^oC. The dialysed lipoprotein fractions (4 ml) were added to perfused rat livers (1) and aliquots sampled at timed intervals.

Results and Discussion

After ^3H-vitamin D_3 and ^{14}C-triglycerides (TG) were added to the perfusate of the isolated perfused rat liver on chylomicrons there was a much greater hepatic extraction of vitamin D_3 (mean=57% at 60 min) than TG (32%). When added on VLDL similar amounts of vitamin D_3 (63 ± 3%, n=6) and cholesterol (62 ± 2%, n=3) (p NS) were taken up by the liver at 60 min but much less TG (17 ± 4%, n=3) ($p<0.0005$). However from HDL, much more vitamin D_3 was taken up (60 ± 1%, n=5) than cholesterol (37 ± 4%, n=5) ($p<0.0005$).

VLDL cholesterol was largely unesterified (cholesterol : cholesterol ester = 8.8 : 1) and HDL cholesterol esterified (1 : 1.4). The unesterified cholesterol of VLDL is a lipoprotein surface component whilst the esterified cholesterol of HDL is a lipoprotein core component.

Vitamin D. A Chemical, Biochemical and Clinical Update

The hepatic retention of vitamin D was the same when added on either HDL or VLDL, despite the very different metabolism of these lipoprotein fractions. This suggests that the hepatic uptake of vitamin D is not dependent on the metabolism of lipoproteins, but is rather a surface phenomenon. The hepatic retention of vitamin D was similar to that of cholesterol in VLDL but more than cholesterol in HDL. VLDL cholesterol is mainly unesterified and situated more superficially in the lipoprotein, whilst HDL cholesterol is mainly esterified, situated in the lipoprotein core and not available for surface exchange. Thus the finding that the transfer of vitamin D to the liver was more than cholesterol from VLDL and not HDL, suggests that vitamin D is situated more superficially in the lipoprotein and therefore available for surface exchange. When compared to triglyceride uptake by the liver, vitamin D was taken up much faster from both VLDL and chylomicrons. This once again demonstrates that vitamin D uptake is not dependent on lipoprotein lipolysis and uptake.

All of the above data suggest that vitamin D is situated superficially in lipoproteins which facilitates its rapid transfer to the liver from lipoproteins. This should explain how vitamin D is preferentially accumulated by the liver after intestinal absorption and intravenous administration; when it would be bound by lipoproteins and not DBP.

Acknowledgment

This work was supported by a grant from the Israeli Ministry of Health and the Jonathan Beare Research Fund.

References

1. Olson, E.B., Knutson, J.C., Bhattacharyya, M.H. and De Luca, H.F. (1976) J. Clin. Invest. 57: 1213-1220.
2. Rojanasathit, S. and Haddad, J.G. (1976) BBA 421: 12-21.
3. Silver, J. and Berry, E. (1982) Min. & Electr. Metab. 7: 298-304.
4. Maislos, M., Silver, J. and Fainaru, M. (1981) Gastroenterology 80: 1528-1534.
5. Barragry, J.H., France, M.W., Boucher, B.J. and Cohen, R.D. (1979) Clin. Endocr. 11: 491-495.
6. Bouillon, R., van Baelen, H., Rombauts, W. and de Moor, P. (1976) Eur. J. Biochem. 66: 285-291.
7. Imawari, M., Kida, K. and Goodman De, W.S. (1976) J. Clin. Invest. 58: 514-523.
8. Haddad, J.G. and Walgate, J. (1976) J. Biol. Chem. 251: 4803-4809.
9. Ziv, E., Bar-On, H. and Silver, J. (1985) Eur. J. Clin. Invest. (in press).

EFFECTS OF LIPOPOLYSACCHARIDES ON CONVERSION OF 25-HYDROXYVITAMIN D_3 BY NORMAL HUMAN MACROPHAGES.

H. Reichel, *H. P. Koeffler, J. E. Bishop and A. W. Norman
Dept. Biochem., Univ. Calif., Riverside, CA 92521 and *Dept. Med., Univ. Calif., Los Angeles, CA 90024, USA.

Lipopolysaccharides (LPS) from the cell wall of gram-negative bacteria are known to have multiple effects on macrophages and other immunocompetent cells (I). When exposed to LPS macrophages from several tissues undergo activation and become more effective in host immune response. We studied the metabolism of $[^3H]$-25(OH)D_3 by normal human macrophages either in a resting or an activated state. Resting macrophages synthesized small amounts of a vitamin D metabolite behaving like 1,25$(OH)_2D_3$. In contrast, activation of macrophages resulted in a marked enhancement (5-100 fold) of the production of putative 1,25$(OH)_2D_3$.

Pulmonary alveolar macrophages (PAM) and monocytes were cultured in the presence of LPS under varying conditions. The cells were labeled with 10^{-7} M $[^3H]$-25(OH)D_3, 10.4 Ci/mmol. Lipid extracts of media or both media and cells were subjected to HPLC. Conversion of $[^3H]$-25(OH)D_3 was assessed by determining radioactivity of 1 min fractions. UV-absorbance of non-radioactive standards including 1,25$(OH)_2D_3$ served as a marker.

As shown in Fig. 1, the vitamin D metabolite produced by LPS-activated human PAM behaved like authentic 1,25$(OH)_2D_3$ on 4 different HPLC systems. These systems will separate all vitamin D metabolites presently known (2) including 19-nor-10-keto-25(OH)D_3. Synthesis of putative 1,25$(OH)_2D_3$ by LPS-stimulated macrophages was dose-dependent. The response and sensitivity varied between individuals. Fig. 2a depicts 1,25$(OH)_2D_3$-synthesis by PAM with increasing doses of LPS-B. Maximal 1,25$(OH)_2D_3$-production by PAM of this individual was noted at 100 µg LPS-B/10^6 cells. Fig. 2b shows the dose response of monocytes to LPS-RE, a subunit of LPS. Time course studies revealed a peak of 1,25$(OH)_2D_3$-synthesis by PAM after 2 days of exposure to LPS-B (Fig. 3). After a decrease, a new increase was noted at days 6-8. First effects of LPS on 1,25$(OH)_2D_3$-production could be seen after 12 hours.

In summary, significant production of the 1,25$(OH)_2D_3$-like metabolite _in vitro_ only occurred in macrophages, activated by LPS and similarly by γ-interferon (3). Assuming, the macrophage derived metabolite, is in fact, 1,25$(OH)_2D_3$, our observations might explain in part bone loss of periodontal disease. Abundance of gram-negative bacteria at sites of human periodontal disease (4) and occurrence of mononuclear phagocytes at sites of bone resorption in periodontosis (5) provide conditions _in vivo_, which correspond to the _in vitro_ conditions of our studies. However, no experimental data are available yet to support this hypothesis.

References

1. Morrison, D. C., and Ryan, J. L. (1979) Adv. Immunol. 28, 293-450.
2. Norman, A. W., Roth, J., and Orci, L. (1982) Endocr. Rev. 3, 331-366.

Vitamin D. A Chemical, Biochemical and Clinical Update

3. Koeffler, H. P., Reichel, H., Bishop, J. E., and Norman, A. W. (1985) Biochem. Biophys. Res. Commun., in press.
4. Newman, M. G., Socransky, S. S., Savitt, E. D., Propas, D. A., and Crawford, A. (1976) J. Periodontol. 47, 373-379.
5. Rifkin, B. R., and Heijl, L. (1979) J. Periodontol. 50, 636-640.

Work at UCLA was supported by USPHS grants CA-26038, CA-33936 and CA-3273 while work at UCR was supported by USPHS grant AM-14,750-013. HR was supported in part by the Deutsche Forschungsgemeinschaft.

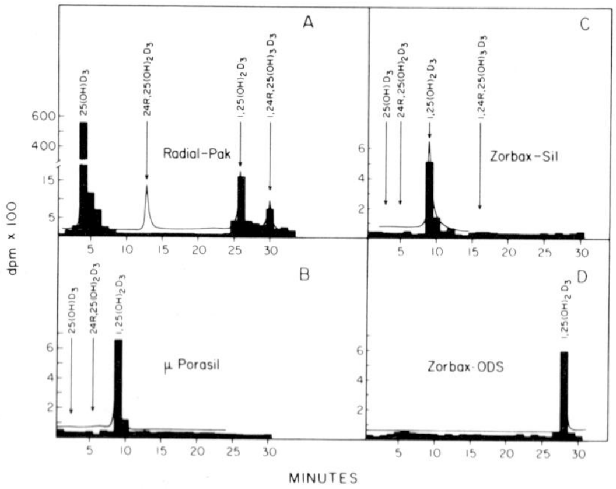

Fig. 1. Rechromatography on HPLC. Material comigrating with authentic $1,25(OH)_2D_3$ on the first column was collected, pooled and rechromatographed on three other systems. The HPLC systems were (a) Radial-Pak µPorasil cartridge, 4-60% isopropanol in hexane gradient, 2 ml/min, (b) µPorasil column, 10% isopropanol in hexane, 2 ml/min, (c) Zorbax Sil column, 10% isopropanol in dichloromethane, 1 ml/min, (d) Zorbax ODS column, reverse phase, 20% water in methanol, 1 ml/min.

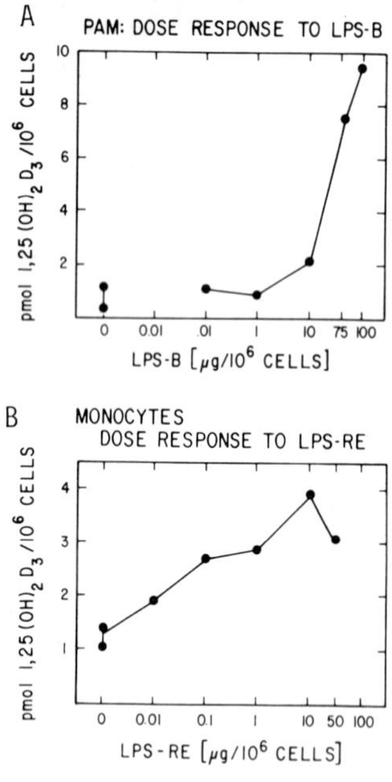

Fig. 2. Dose response LPS. Cells were cultured in the presence of different doses of LPS. A: PAM were exposed to LPS-B (= complete LPS molecule). B: monocytes were exposed to LPS-RE (= subunit of LPS: lipid A + ketodeoxyoctoanate).

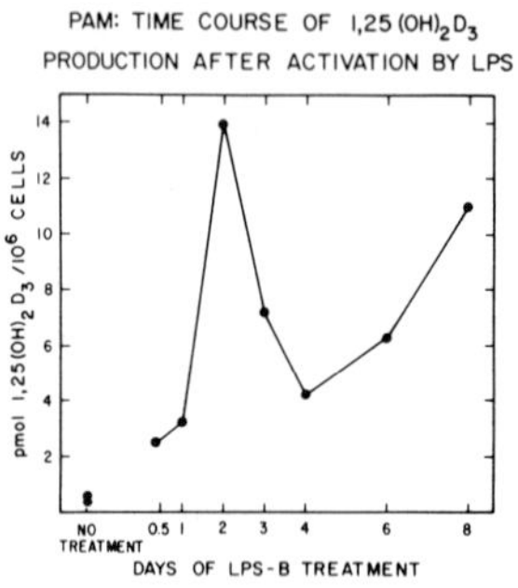

Fig. 3. Time course LPS. PAM were cultured in the presence of 7.5 µg LPS-B/10^6 cells over varying time periods.

CONTROL OF 1-HYDROXYLASE ACTIVITY IN PRIMARY HYPERPARATHYROID PATIENTS

V. LO CASCIO, S. ADAMI, R. DORIZZI, D. TARTAROTTI, G. SALVAGNO.
Istituto di Semeiotica Medica. Policlinico, 37134 Verona, Italy.

In primary hyperparathyroidism (PHPT) serum 1,25(OH)2D is frequently increased (1) and it is related to PTH serum levels (2). However we previously reported that when plasma calcium is very high it may override the PTH signal and suppress the 1-hydroxylase to produce a normal concentration (3). In this report we demonstrate that in PHPT patients serum 1,25(OH)2D concentrations are responsive to changes in serum calcium and are depending on the prevailing levels of its parent compound, 25-OH-D.

EFFECTS OF 25-OH-D TREATMENT

6 PHPT patients and 5 normal volunteers were given 50 ug/day of 25-OH-D3 for one month. In PHPT patients the consequent increase of serum 25-OH-D to supraphysiological levels were accompanied by parallel increase in serum 1,25(OH)2D (4) such that a significant positive correlation was found between the serum levels of the two vitamin D metabolites (fig.1). In the control subjects the 1,25(OH)2D concentrations did not change despite an increase of 25-OH-D comparable to that observed in PHPT patients. This should roule-out the possibility that the results observed in PHPT were due to interference of the parent compounds on our 1,25(OH)2D assay. In PHPT patients the increase in 1,25(OH)2D was accompanied by an increase in serum calcium and phosphate and by a fall in serum C-PTH (5) (fig.2). These observations indicate that in PHPT serum concentrations of 1,25(OH)2D may be a function of the blood levels of 25-OH-D.

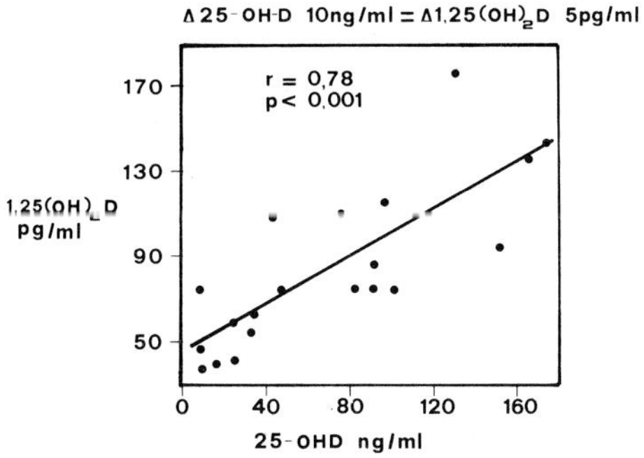

Fig.1 Correlation between serum concentrations of 25-OH-D and 1,25(OH)2D in 6 PHPT patients during treatment with 25-OH-D3.

EFFECTS OF AMINO-BUTANE DIPHOSPHONATE (ABDP).

In 9 patients with PHPT treatment with ABDP (5-25mg/day for 4-10 days), a powerful inhibitor of bone resorption, led to a transient significant fall in serum calcium and phosphate and to an increase in serum 1,25(OH)2D (fig.2). The decline in serum calcium was not accompanied by changes in PTH levels but it is possible that the unselected, predominantly C-terminal PTH assay used in this study was not sensitive enough to appreciate a small change in the secretion of biologically active hormone. Anyhow we have shown for the first time that in PHPT patients the 1,25(OH)2D levels are sensitive to changes in serum calcium and phosphate.

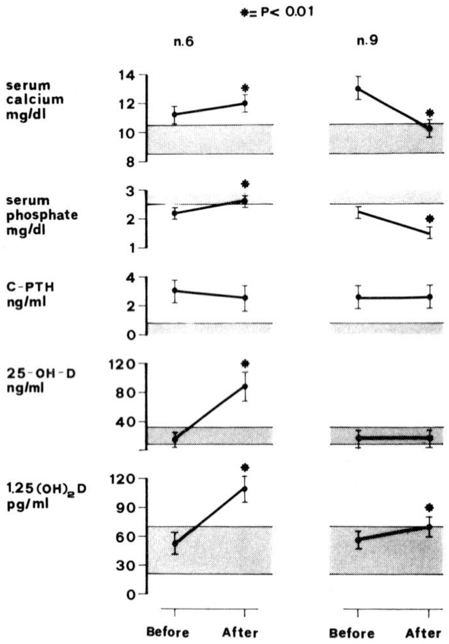

Fig.2 Changes in serum calcium, phosphate, C-PTH, 25-OH-D and 1,25(OH)2D before and after therapy with 25-OH-D (left pannel) and ABDP (right pannel)

REFERENCES

1. Kaplan R.A., Haussler M.R., Deftos L.J., Bone H., Pak C.Y.(1977). J.Clin. Invest. 59: 756-760.

2. Thakker R.V., Fraher L.J., Sudan H.L., Adami S. and O'Riordan JL.H. (1984). Calcif. Tissue Intern. 36 (suppl.2): s44.

3. Lo Cascio V., Adami S., Galvanini G., Cominacini L., Scuro L.A. (1984). Lancet 1: 755.

4. Tartarotti D., Adami S., Galvanini G., Dorizzi R., Piemonte G. and Lo Cascio V.(1984). J. Endocrinol. Invest. 6: 545-550.

5. Lo Cascio V., Vallaperta P., Adami S., Cominacini L., Galvanini G., Bianchi I., Ferrari M., Scuro L.A. (1978). Clin. Endocrinol. 8 : 349-356.

1,25 DIHYDROXY-VITAMIN D IN SERUM AFTER ORAL ADMINISTRATION OF VITAMIN D_3 IN HEALTHY SUBJECTS

S. Issa, B. Emde, H.v.Lilienfeld-Toal * and W. Burmeister
Department of Pediatrics, University Bonn, * Diabetes Hospital Bad Nauheim, F.R.G.

In vitamin D intoxication serum $1,25(OH)_2D$ is reported to be normal (1). In face of the high level of circulating precursor 25OHD this may be explained by hypercalcemia which is known to suppress the activity of renal 1-alpha-hydroxylase (2). We were interested if a large dose of vitamin D - as it is proposed for therapeutic use (3) - would increase serum $1,25(OH)_2D$ in healthy persons with normal serum calcium concentration.

We examined 25OHD and $1,25(OH)_2D$ in the serum of 1o healthy subjects after an oral administration of a bolus of 200.000 IU vitamin D_3. Determination of 25OHD and $1,25(OH)_2D$ was performed according to Reinhardt et al. (JCEM 58 91 1984): After extraction with acetonitrile from serum vitamin D metabolites have been purified using C18 sep-Pak and silica sep-Pak and were determined in binding assays using rat serum (4) and thymus cytosol as binding proteins (5, 6). In addition PTH, serum calcium, serum phosphate, cholesterol, alkaline phosphatase and 24hr urinary calcium excretion were determined in samples taken before, one day after and one, two, three, four, eight and twelve weeks following an oral gift of 200.000 IU vitamin D_3.

Results and discussion:
There was an immediate increase in serum $1,25(OH)_2D$ during the first day (fig 1). In contrast, peak concentration of serum 25OHD were after one week, when $1,25(OH)_2D$ showed already a tendency to decrease. All laboratory values concerning the calcium metabolism as listed above did not change in the samples taken during the period of observation.

Vitamin D. A Chemical, Biochemical and Clinical Update

According to these data a transient increase of the vitamin D metabolites 1,25$(OH)_2D$ and 25OHD in serum can be observed following an single oral administration of 200.000 IU D. In this situation the maximal concentration of serum 1,25$(OH)_2D$ preceeds that of 25OHD. This may be explained by the fact that renal tissue containing the 1-alpha-hydroxylase is exposed to an increasing extracellular concentration of 25OHD. The lack of further increase of 1,25$(OH)_2D$ concentration might reflect a product inhibition of 1-alpha-hydroxylase.
There was no clinical change exerted by the transient increase of serum 1,25$(OH)_2D$ in the subjects studied. Therefore, it does not seem to be of clinical importance.

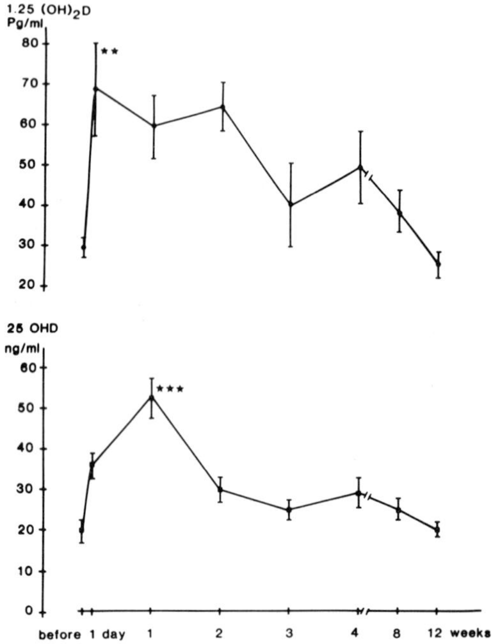

Fig. 1: Effect of oral administration of 200.000 IU vitamin D on serum 1,25$(OH)_2D$ and 25OHD in 1o healthy subjects ($M \pm SE$)
** $p < o,o1$ *** $p < o,oo1$

DIFFERENCES IN THE RATE OF METABOLISM OF VITAMIN D_2 AND VITAMIN D_3 IN MAMMALS.

I. HOLMBERG, T. BERLIN and I. BJÖRKHEM. Departments of Clinical Chemistry I and Urology, Huddinge Hospital, S-141 86 Huddinge, Sweden.

Introduction.

25-Hydroxylation is the first step in the metabolism of vitamin D (1). Chick liver homogenate has been reported to catalyze 25-hydroxylation of vitamin D_2 as effective as 25-hydroxylation of vitamin D_3 (2). Vitamin D_2 and vitamin D_3 have been considered to be metabolized equally effective also in mammals. However, in two recent *in vivo* studies results were obtained indicating differences in the metabolism of vitamin D_2 and vitamin D_3 (3,4).
The aim of the present work was to compare the 25-hydroxylation of vitamin D_2 and vitamin D_3 in mammalian liver *in vitro*, using the mitochondrial fraction from rat and human liver and a reconstitued system containing cytochrome P-450 from rat liver microsomes. The 25-hydroxylase in crude microsomes is very low due to the presence of inhibitor(s) in this fraction (5,6). Therefore purified microsomal cytochrome P-450 was used in the present study.

Methods.

The mitochondrial fraction was prepared from rat and human liver homogenate (5). Partly purified cytochrome P-450 from rat liver microsomes was obtained by octylamine sepharose chromatography and subsequent hydroxylapatite chromatography (6).
Incubations were performed as described previously (5,6).
25-Hydroxyvitamin D_2 and 25-hydroxyvitamin D_3 were analyzed by selected ion monitoring using deuteriumlabelled 25-hydroxyvitamin D_3 as internal standard (7). This standard was added to all incubations prior to the extraction and purification steps. Mass fragmentographic quantitation of 25-hydroxyvitamin D_3 was performed using the ion at m/e 586 (corresponding to the t-butyldimethylsilyl/trimethylsilyl derivative of 25-hydroxyvitamin D_3) and the ion at m/e 589 (corresponding to the t-butyldimethylsilyl/trimethylsilyl derivative of deuterium labelled 25-hydroxyvitamin D_3). 25-Hydroxyvitamin D_2 was quantitated using the ion at m/e 598 and the ion at m/e 589. The accuracy of the assay of 25-hydroxyvitamin D_2 was ascertained by addition of 29-226 pmol of 25-hydroxyvitamin D_2 to control incubation mixtures. The maximal error in these recovery experiments was about 25%.

Results.

Rat liver mitochondria catalyzed 25-hydroxylation of vitamin D_3 more efficiently than 25-hydroxylation of vitamin D_2 (Table 1). Also human liver mitochondria catalyzed 25-hydroxylation of vitamin D_3 (10 pmol/mg prot x min) more efficiently than 25-hydroxylation of vitamin D_2 (0.8 pmol/mg prot x min). There was a linear relationship between the rate of 25-hydroxylation of vitamin D_3 and the amount of mitochondrial protein. No such relationship could be obtained for incubation with vitamin D_2. A reconstituted system containing P-450 from rat liver microsomes catalyzed 25-hydroxylation of vitamin D_3. No significant amount of 25-hydroxyvitamin D_2 could be obtained in experiments with vitamin D_2 (Table 2).

Vitamin D. A Chemical, Biochemical and Clinical Update

Discussion.

No significant conversion into 25-hydroxyvitamin D_2 could be demonstrated in any of the experiments with microsomal cytochrome P-450. It should be pointed out, however, that the cytochrome P-450 fractions used were heterogenous and contained several isoenzymes of cytochrome P-450. It can not be completely excluded that there is a species of cytochrome P-450, specific for vitamin D_2 which is lost during the purification procedure.
The amount of product formed in incubations of vitamin D_2 with the mitochondrial fraction was very small and a final identifiction of the product as 25-hydroxyvitamin D_2 with a complete mass spectrum could not be performed.
The present results show a difference in the 25-hydroxylation of vitamin D_2 and vitamin D_3 in vitro. Vitamin D_3 has been reported to be more toxic than vitamin D_2 in several mammalian species (8-12). This might be due to a lower rate of 25-hydroxylation of vitamin D_2.

References.

1. DeLuca, H.F. (1979) Vitamin D. Metabolism and function. Monographs on endocrinology. Springer-Verlag, Berlin.
2. Jones, G., Schnoes, H.K. and DeLuca, H.F. (1976) J. Biol. Chem. 251, 24-28.
3. Horst, R.L., Napoli, J.L. and Littledike, E.T. (1982) Biochem. J. 204, 185-189.
4. Sommerfeldt, J.L., Napoli, J.L., Littledike, E.T., Beitz, D.C. and Horst, R.L. (1984) J. Nutr. 113, 2595-2600.
5. Björkhem, I. and Holmberg, I. J. Biol. Chem. (1979) 254, 9518-9524.
6. Andersson, S., Holmberg, I. and Wikvall, K. (1983) J. Biol. Chem. 258, 6777-6781.
7. Björkhem, I. and Holmberg, I. (1980) Methods Enzymol. 67, 385-393.
8. Hunt, R.D., Garcia, F.G., Felix, G. and Hegsted, D.M (1969) Am. J. Clin. Nutr. 22, 358-366.
9. Hunt, R.D., Garcia, G.G. and Walsh, J.R. (1972) J. Nutr. 102, 975-986.
10. Harrington, D.A. and Page, E.H. (1983) J. Am. Vet. Med. Assoc. 182, 1358-1369.
11. Roborgh, J.R. and De Man, Th.J. (1960) Biochem. Pharmacol. 3, 277-282.
12. Burgisser, H., Jacquier, C.I. and Leuenberger, M. (1964) Schweizer Archiv für Tierheilkunde 100, 714-718.

Table 1. 25-Hydroxylation of vit. D_2 and vit. D_3 by rat liver mitochondria.

Exper. No.	Formation of $25OHD_2$	Formation of $25OHD_3$
	pmol/mg mitochondrial prot. x min.	
1	< 0.7	1.0
2	1.3	2.5
3	< 0.7	1.6
4	< 0.7	2.5
5	0.7	1.7

Table 2. 25-Hydroxylation of vit. D_2 and vit. D_3 by cytochrome P-450 from rat liv liver microsomes.

Cytochr. P-450	Formation of $25OHD_2$	Formation of $25OHD_3$
	pmol/nmol cytochrome P-450 x min.	
Prep. 1	< 63	259
2	< 63	158
3	< 63	550
4	< 63	125
5	< 63	270

METABOLISM OF 1,25-DIHYDROXYERGOCALCIFEROL: Relation to the Biological Differences between Ergocalciferol and Cholecalciferol

Joseph L. Napoli and Ronald L. Horst, Department of Biochemistry, Un. Texas Health Science Ctr., Dallas, Texas and Department of Pathophysiology, Nat. Animal Disease Ctr., Ames, Iowa.

Studies with vitamin D_2 and vitamin D_3 have concluded that these two prohormones are equipotent in mammals (1). As a result, vitamin D_2 has been freely substituted for vitamin D_3 as a dietary supplement for humans and for most commercially important mammals. Precise recent measurements have shown that, in the rat, low doses of vitamin D_2 or vitamin D_3 produce the same degree of intestinal calcium transport, bone calcium mobilization, and calcification of rachitic cartilage (2). In contrast, high doses of vitamin D_2 have been reported to cause less hypercalcemia than high doses of vitamin D_3 (3). Moreover, recent work from our labs has demonstrated that vitamin D metabolism is species specific: when dosed with equimolar mixtures of vitamin D_2 and D_3, rats preferentially accumulate viramin D_2 metabolites, whereas pigs preferentially accumulate vitamin D_3 metabolites (4). [Discrimination against vitamin D_2 by chicken and new world monkeys had been known, but no previous example of discrimination against vitamin D_3 had been reported, and the discrimination against vitamin D_2 was presumed to be limited to the two examples cited.] At least one mechanism for this specificity is species-related affinity differences between vitamin D_2 and vitamin D_3 for the vitamin D serum carrier protein; these differences determine the relative amounts of each prohormone that is taken up by the liver and converted into the 25-hydroxylated forms, and thereby indirectly control the amount of dihydroxylated metabolites that are formed (5).

Another mechanism may lie in the nature of side chain metabolism. Recent work has shown that $1,25(OH)_2D_3$, in pharmacological and physiological levels, is converted, _in vivo_ and _in vitro_, into several side chain metabolites, which likely are responsible for modulating its action (6-8). These metabolites are: $1,24,25(OH)_3D_3$; 24-oxo-$1,25(OH)_2D_3$; 24-oxo-$1,23,24(OH)_3D_3$; and $1,25(OH)_2D_3$-26,25-lactone. Since the vitamin D_2 side chain has a C(24)-methyl group and a C(22)/C(23) double bond, formation of the latter 3 metabolites from $1,25(OH)_2D_2$ is improbable.

We report here the isolation, identification and biological assay of a new vitamin D_2 metabolite, $1,24,25(OH)_3D_2$. The new metabolite was obtained biologically from two different routes and two different precursors: $1,25(OH)_2D_2$ and $24,25(OH)_2D_2$. The products from each synthesis and isolation co-migrated on several HPLC systems capable of distinguishing all known $1,25(OH)_2D$ metabolites (9), and were chromatographically distinct from previously identified metabolites and synthetic standards. The structure was established by UV and mass spectral analysis of the metabolite, and its persilylated derivative, and by its periodate sensitivity.

Vitamin D. A Chemical, Biochemical and Clinical Update

$1,24,25(OH)_3D_2$ binds as well as $1,24,25(OH)_3D_3$ to the chick intestine and bovine thymus receptors, but has nearly twice the affinity for the rat intestine receptor (see Fig.), a result complimentary to our results discussed above; but has lower activity *in vivo* than $1,24,25(OH)_3D_3$ (see Table).

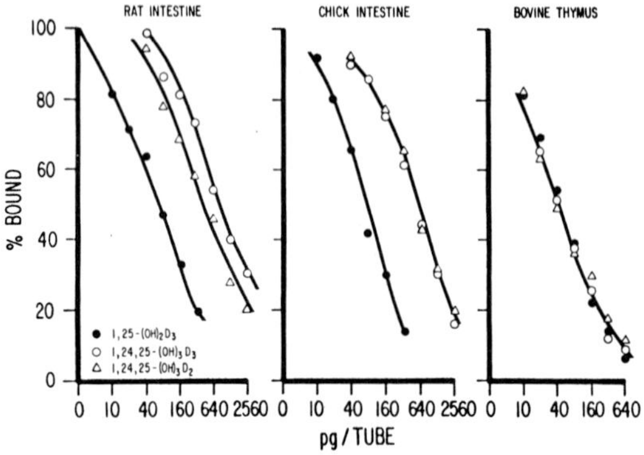

Activity of Vitamin D Metabolites in Rat (Mean ± SD, n = 6-7)

	Exp. 1		Exp. 2	
Metabolite (ng)	ICT	BCM	ICT	BCM
Control	1.5 ± 0.3	5.9 ± 0.3	1.7 ± 0.3	4.4 ± 0.3
$1,25(OH)_2D_2$ (12.5)	2.9 ± 0.4	6.5 ± 0.5	2.6 ± 0.5	5.4 ± 0.2
$1,24,25(OH)_3D_3$ (50)	3.0 ± 0.8	6.4 ± 0.6	----	----
$1,24,25(OH)_3D_2$ (800)	----	----	2.0 ± 0.4	4.4 ± 0.3

These data indicate that differences in the rates of metabolism of $1,24,25(OH)_3D_3$ and $1,25(OH)_3D_2$, and in the metabolites formed from them, rather than $1,24,25(OH)_3D_3$ or $_2$ themselves, are in part responsible for the biological differences between vitamins D_2 and D_3.

1. Bethke, R.M., Burroughs, W., Wilder, O.H.M., Edington, B.H. and Robison, W.L. (1946) Ohio Agric. Exp. Stn. Res. Bull. 667, 1-29
2. Napoli, J.L., Fivizzani, M.A., Schnoes, H.K., and DeLuca, H.F. (1979) Arch. Biochem. Biophys. 197, 119-125
3. Roborgh, J.R., and Deman, T.J. (1960) Biochem. Pharmacol. 3, 272-282
4. Horst, R.L., Napoli, J.L., and Littledike, E.T. (1982) Biochem. J. 204, 185-189
5. Reddy, G.S., Napoli, J.L., and Hollis, B.W. (1984) Calc. Tiss. Int. 36 (4), 524.
6. Napoli, J.L., Pramanik, B.C., Royal, P.M., Reinhardt, T.A., and Horst, R.L. (1983) J. Biol. Chem. 258, 9100-9107
7. Napoli, J.L., and Horst, R.L. (1983) Biochemistry 22, 5848-5853
8. Napoli, J.L., and Martin, C.A. (1984) Biochem. J. 219, 713-717
9. Napoli, J.L., and Horst, R.L. (1985) Methods in Enzymol., in press

SERUM 1,25-$(OH)_2D$ LEVELS INCREASE AFTER ORAL ADMINISTRATION OF THYROTROPIN-RELEASING HORMONE.

T.L. Storm, G. Thamsborg, S. Ladefoged, B. Lund and O.H. Sørensen.
Department of Medicine, Sundby Hospital, DK-2300,Copenhagen S, Denmark.

Introduction:
The serum levels of the vitamin D metabolite 1,25-dihydroxycholecalciferol (1,25-$(OH)_2D$) are increased in hypothyroidism and reduced in hyperthyroidism (1). These changes are thought to be secondary to an effect of the thyroid hormones on bone turnover. However, the direct influence of thyroid hormones on vitamin D metabolism is largely unknown. Prolonged stimulation with oral thyrotropin-releasing hormone (TRH) increases serum thyrotropin (TSH), 3,3',5-triiodothyronine (T_3) and thyroxine (T_4) in normal subjects (2). Therefore, a hyperthyroid state with increased levels of serum TSH can be achieved.

Aim of the study:
To investigate the effect of oral TRH on vitamin D metabolism.

Patients and methods:
Fifteen clinical euthyroid individuals (8 women and 7 men) were included in the study. None had any disease or received any medication known to interfere with bone or vitamin D metabolism.
Twenty mg of TRH was given orally at 08.00, 12.00, 16.00, 22.00 and at 08.00 the next morning (2). Blood samples for estimation of T_3-resin uptake, serum TSH, T_3, T_4, 1,25-$(OH)_2D$, calcium and phosphorus were drawn in the fasting state before and 28 hours after the first tablet was taken. Furthermore, 4 individuals were followed frequently throughout the test period by ionized calcium measurements. The free thyroid hormone indices (FT_3I and FT_4I) were calculated as the product of T_3-resin uptake and serum concentrations of T_3 and T_4, respectively. Student´s t test on paired differences was used for statistical evaluations.

Results: (n=15)	before TRH	after TRH	p-value
TSH (μU/ml)	1.0±1.1	4.2±7.9	< 0.01
FT_3I (arb. U)	167.5±50.0	289.0±47.9	< 0.01
FT_4I (arb. U)	8.1±2.0	11.9±2.3	< 0.01
1,25-$(OH)_2D$ (pg/ml)	35.8±5.5	40.9±8.5	< 0.02
24,25-$(OH)_2D$ (ng/ml)	2.9±3.0	3.5±2.4	ns
calcium (mmol/l)	1.23±0.03	1.24±0.03	ns
phosphorus (mmol/l)	1.06±0.16	1.15±0.19	< 0.01

Serum calcium did not change throughout the test period of 28 hours (n=4).

Vitamin D. A Chemical, Biochemical and Clinical Update

Discussion:

The increments of serum T_3 and T_4 to hyperthyroid levels were expected to increase the serum levels of calcium and phosphorus (3) thus depressing the formation of 1,25-$(OH)_2$D. However, in this study serum calcium was unchanged after 28 hours of oral TRH stimulation, but serum phosphorus increased significantly ($p<0.01$). Unexpectedly, serum 1,25-$(OH)_2$D increased from 35.8 to 40.9 pg/ml ($p<0.02$).
Intravenous administration of TRH has been shown to induce a significant decline in serum calcium within 20 minutes in healthy volunteers (4). Therefore, an acute (indirectly) stimulatory effect of TRH (or TSH) on 1,25-$(OH)_2$D production was possible. However, we were not able to show any hypocalcemic effect of oral TRH.
Since TRH is a potent stimulator of prolactin, the increment of serum 1,25-$(OH)_2$D could be due to increased serum levels of TRH stimulated prolactin, but further studies are needed to elucidate exactly why serum 1,25-$(OH)_2$D increase after oral TRH.

Conclusion:
The results indicate that orally administered TRH increases serum levels of phosphorus and 1,25-$(OH)_2$D. Whether TRH per se, or increased serum TSH and/or prolactin, or acute increase in T_3 and/or T_4, induce this effect remains to be elucidated.

References:
1. Bouillon R, Muls E, De Moor P. (1980), J Clin Endocrinol Metab 51, 793-797.
2. Kirkegaard C, Jørgensen PH, Friis T, Siersbæk-Nielsen K. (1982), Acta Med Scand 211, 477-480.
3. Mosekilde L, Melsen F, Bagger JP, Myhre-Jensen O, Sørensen NS. (1977), Acta Endocrinol (Kbh) 85, 515-525.
4. Röjdmark S, Andersson DEH, Edström E, Lamminpää K. (1983), Horm Metabol Res 15, 290-293.

VITAMIN D METABOLISM IN LIVER DISEASES

R. Morita, M. Fukunaga, N. Otsuka, T. Sone, S. Dokoh, Y. Fukuda, I. Yamamoto and K. Torizuka
Nuclear Medicine, Kawasaki Medical School, Kurashiki and Kyoto University, Kyoto, JAPAN

Introduction:

In patients with chronic liver diseases, an increase incidence of osteodystrophy has been described. Among the events which lead to the skeletal complications of the liver disease, the impaired hepatic hydroxylation of vitamin D_3 is being considered as a major factor rather than the intestinal malabsorption of vitamin D_3 (1)(2). We therefore determined plasma 25(OH)D and $1,25(OH)_2D$ levels as well as serum Ca, P, PTH and calcitonin levels in various liver diseases to study possible roles of deranged vitamin D metabolism in the development of skeletal complications.

Patients and Methods:

In total of 184 patients with various liver diseases were examined, the diagnosis of which was ascertained histologically except for fulminant and acute hepatitis. No patients with alcoholic liver injury was involved in this study. Plasma 25(OH)D levels were measured by CPBA after HPLC purification of the samples. Plasma $1,25(OH)_2D$ levels were measured by CPBA after the purification of $1,25(OH)_2D$ fraction by HPLC. Serum PTH levels were determined by a C-terminal specific RIA; using (65-84) human PTH as the standards, ^{125}I-tyr (65-84) human PTH as the tracer and anti-bovine PTH chicken anti-serum. The sensitivity of the assay was 160 pg/ml; (1-84) human PTH equivalent, and the mean normal value was 250±150 pg/ml. Plasma calcitonin levels were measured by the RIA using synthetic human calcitonin M, ^{125}I-[Asu 1,7] human calcitonin M and anti-human calcitonin rabbit anti-serum. The sensitivity of the assay was 25 pg/ml and the mean normal value was 30±40 pg/ml.

Results and Discussion:

In fulminant hepatitis (4 cases), serum Ca levels were significantly low, and the markedly elevated serum P, PTH and calcitonin levels were found (Fig. 1). The BUN levels were extremely high (136±66 mg/dl) in these patients and the abnormality was thought to be attributable to the renal excretory dysfunction associated with hepatic damage (hepato-renal syndrome). In acute hepatitis (49 cases), serum PTH and calcitonin levels were found elevated in the acute stage (49 cases). In the convalescent stage (19 cases), however, these values returned to normal and the values were closely correlated with those of the serum BUN levels ($r=0.88$, $p<0.001$ for C-PTH and $r=0.96$, $p<0.001$ for CT) suggesting the renal dysfunction as the major cause of the elevated PTH and calcitonin levels in acute liver diseases. Plasma $1,25(OH)_2D$ levels were distributed within the normal range in acute hepatitis and the damaged kidney was seemed to have ability to synthesize $1,25(OH)_2D_3$ at normal levels. Plasma 25(OH)D levels were found normal in patients with chronic hepatitis (42 cases), liver cirrhosis (55 cases) and primary biliary cirrhosis (PBC, 14 cases), and tended to low in hepatoma (20 cases)(Fig. 2). Plasma $1,25(OH)_2D$ levels were significantly low only in the patients with PBC among the other chronic liver diseases. These data indicate that the impairment of the hepatic and renal hydroxylation of vitamin D derivatives are minimum in the most cases with chronic hepatitis and liver cirrhosis, and that in patients with PBC, on the other hand, the major defect which leads to the skeletal complication might lay in the deficient renal hydroxylation of $25(OH)_2D_3$. The exact nature of the renal damage is unknown and should be elucidated.

Fig. 1

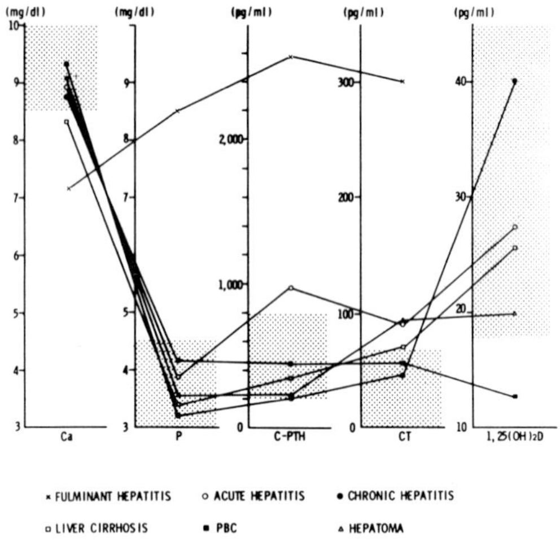

Fig. 2

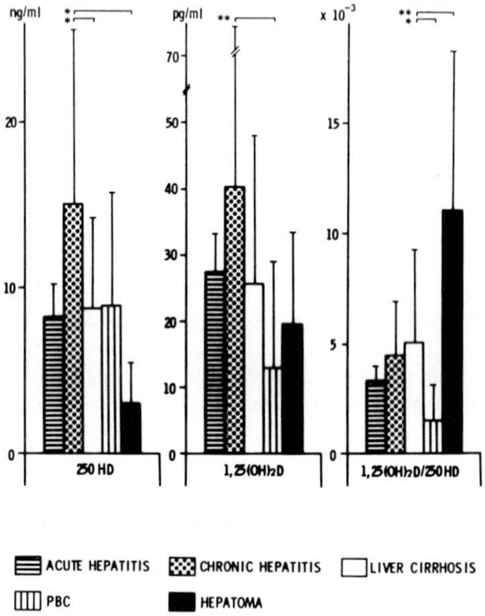

References:

1. Wagonfeeld, J.B., Nemchausky, B.A., Bolt, M., Horst, J.V., Boyer, J.L. and Rosenberg, I.H. (1976) Lancet 21, 391-394.
2. Sonnenberg, A., von Lilienfeld-Toal, Sonnenberg, G.E., Rohner, H.G. and Strohmeyer, G. (1977) Act. Hepato-Gastroent. 24, 256-258.

VITAMIN D METABOLISM: THE RENAL-PITUITARY AXIS.

R.W. GRAY AND J. LEMANN, JR.
Departments of Medicine and Biochemistry, MEDICAL COLLEGE OF WISCONSIN, Milwaukee, WI 53226 USA

Soon after 1,25-$(OH)_2$-vitamin D_3, produced in the kidney, was identified as the most rapidly acting and potent vitamin D metabolite stimulating Ca transport, studies were initiated to assess the regulation of renal synthesis of the hormone. The following paragraphs summarize current knowledge of the regulation of plasma 1,25-$(OH)_2$-D_3 concentrations and the renal synthesis of 1,25-$(OH)_2$-D_3 in response to dietary phosphate deprivation.

STUDIES IN LOWER MAMMALS

Table 1 summarizes the effects of PO_4-deprivation on plasma or serum levels and kidney production rates of 1,25-$(OH)_2$-D_3 in rats and mice. Tanaka and DeLuca were the first to demonstrate that dietary PO_4-deprivation in rats was accompanied by accelerated conversion of injected ^{3}H-25-OH-D_3 to ^{3}H-1,25-$(OH)_2$-D_3 in plasma, in approximate proportion to the degree of hypophosphatemia produced (1). Subsequent studies have shown that dietary PO_4-deprivation in vitamin D-replete rats results in striking elevations of serum 1,25-$(OH)_2$-D_3 concentrations within one to two days (2,3). This effect can be demonstrated in vitamin D replete, thyroxine replaced TPTX rats deprived of dietary phosphate (2). Thus, neither the availability of PTH nor CT mediates the effect of dietary PO_4-deprivation to raise serum 1,25-$(OH)_2$-D_3 concentrations. Subsequent studies have shown that kidney cortical slices, homogenates or kidney cortical mitochondria obtained from rats or mice previously deprived of dietary PO_4 in vivo produce greater quantities of 1,25-$(OH)_2$-D_3 when incubated in vitro with 25-OH-D_3 than do comparable tissues obtained from rats previously fed diets containing normal amounts of PO_4 (4-7). The product of such incubations has been isolated and identified as 1,25-$(OH)_2$-D_3 by mass spectroscopy (4). These studies provide firm support for the view that the rise in plasma 1,25-$(OH)_2$-D_3 concentrations that occur in response to PO_4-deprivation is the result of increased renal synthesis of the hormone and not accelerated tissue uptake or catabolism of 1,25-$(OH)_2$-D_3.

Gray and associates (8) have shown that the increase in renal synthe-

Vitamin D. A Chemical, Biochemical and Clinical Update

TABLE 1

Effects of PO_4 Deprivation on $1,25\text{-}(OH)_2\text{-}D_3$ in Rats and Mice

Ref.	Age of rats/mice	Sex	Diet P Content Control	Diet P Content Low P	Duration $-PO_4$	Effect
(1)	weanling rats	M	varies	0.1%	14 days	Accelerated conversion of injected $^3H\text{-}25\text{-}OH\text{-}D_3$ to $^3H\text{-}1,25\text{-}(OH)_2\text{-}D_3$ in plasma, in proportion to fall in plasma PO_4 regardless of acute PTX
(2)	weanling	M	0.6%	0.04%	14 days	Serum $1,25\text{-}(OH)_2\text{-}D$ in intact rats increased from 416 ± 34 SD pM (control) to 1980 ± 170 pM $(-PO_4)$, $p < 0.005$ and in thyroxine-replaced TPTX rats from 149 ± 50 pM (control) to 2190 ± 202 pM $(-PO_4)$, $p < 0.005$
						Plasma $1,25\text{-}(OH)_2\text{-}D$, pM: Control / $-PO_4$
(3)	rats, 6 wk	M	0.56%	0.02%	2-16 days	6 wk M: 228 ± 76 / 965 ± 360, $p < 0.001$
	6 wk	F				6 wk F: 146 ± 44 / 470 ± 200, $p < 0.001$
	22 wk	M				22 wk M: 105 ± 41 / 440 ± 230, $p < 0.001$
	22 wk	F				22 wk F: 101 ± 11 / 450 ± 130, $p < 0.001$
(5)	rats, 6 wk	M	0.56%	0.02%	4 days	$1,25\text{-}(OH)_2\text{-}D_3$ production by kidney cortical slices incubated with $25\text{-}OH\text{-}D_3$ increased from 17 ± 4 pmol/g wet wt/hour (control) to 128 ± 12 pmol/g wet wt/hour $(-PO_4)$; $p < 0.01$
(6)	mice, 4 wk	M/F	0.6%	0.02%	4-6 weeks	$1,25\text{-}(OH)_2\text{-}D_3$ production by kidney cortical homogenates incubated with $25\text{-}OH\text{-}D_3$ increased from 4.9 + 1.2 fmol/mg protein/min (control) to 17.0 ± 5.3 1983 fmol/mg protein/min $(-PO_4)$, $p < 0.001$
(7)	rats, 4 wk	M	0.6%	0.02%	4 days	$1,25\text{-}(OH)_2\text{-}D$ production by kidney cortical mitochondria incubated with $25\text{-}OH\text{-}D_3$ increased from 2.5 ± 0.8 fmol/mg protein/min (control) to 73 ± 23 fmol/mg protein/min $(-PO_4)$; $p < 0.005$

sis of 1,25-$(OH)_2$-D_3 in response to PO_4 deprivation cannot be accounted for by alterations, relative to controls, in either renal cortical content of total PO_4, acid-soluble PO_4 or the distribution of PO_4 as assessed by ^{31}P NMR spectrsocopy of perchloric extracts of kidney cortex. It is evident, however, that these studies would not detect a change in some small but critical phosphate pool that may be very important in determining the response to phosphate deprivation.

To determine whether a hormonal mechanism might mediate the augmentation of renal 1,25-$(OH)_2$-D_3 synthesis in response to PO_4-deprivation, classical endocrine ablation experiments were undertaken. Gray and associates observed that hypophysectomy completely prevented the rise in plasma 1,25-$(OH)_2$-D_3 in response to PO_4 deprivation (9). Moreover, hypophysectomy in rats previously deprived of PO_4 resulted in a rapid fall in plasma 1,25-$(OH)_2$-D_3 levels within 22 to 44 hours (5). By contrast, hypophysectomy did not blunt the rise in plasma 1,25-$(OH)_2$-D_3 levels or the increase in in vitro production of 1,25-$(OH)_2$-D_3 by kidney slices seen in response to dietary Ca-deprivation (5,9).

These observations naturally led to a series of hormonal replacement experiments. Only growth hormone (GH) but not PRL, TSH, ACTH or T_3 was shown to restore the rise in plasma 1,25-$(OH)_2$-D_3 concentrations or the augmentation of in vitro kidney slice 1,25-$(OH)_2$-D_3 synthesis in PO_4-deprived hypophysectomized rats (5,10). Other studies have shown that in intact rats, neither pituitary GH content (11) nor serum GH concentrations (5,10,11) are increased during dietary phosphate deprivation. Moreover, the administration of GH to hypophysectomized rats fed a diet containing normal amounts of PO_4 did not raise serum 1,25-$(OH)_2$-D_3 levels or in vitro production rates (5,10). These observations have led to the current view that augmentation of renal 1,25-$(OH)_2$-D_3 synthesis in response to dietary PO_4-deprivation is permissively dependent upon both an indirect effect of GH and on PO_4-deprivation.

The effects of GH on many tissues are mediated, at least in part, by somatomedins or insulin-like growth factors (12). The kidney, in comparison to other organs, has the highest content of somatomedin-C (SM-C) (13). Following hypophysectomy in rats, renal SM-C content falls to low levels and is restored to normal by in vivo administration of GH (13). In recent preliminary experiments, Gray and associates have prepared acid extracts of kidney using techniques identical to those employed for the extraction and radioimmunoassay of renal SM-C content (13). When such extracts were injected subcutaneously into PO_4-deprived hypophysectomized rats, plasma 1,25-$(OH)_2$-D_3 levels rose to 1520 ± 517 pM in comparison to 289 ± 91 pM in vehicle-injected animals ($p < 0.001$). Injection of the kidney extracts into hypophysectomized rats previously fed a normal PO_4 diet had no effect on plasma 1,25-$(OH)_2$-D_3 levels (192 ± 48 pM). These preliminary observations are analogous to the responses of hypophysectomized rats to GH and suggest that the augmentation of renal 1,25-$(OH)_2$-D_3 synthesis in response to dietary PO_4 deprivation is permissively dependent upon both an acid extractable factor, which may be SM-C, and upon PO_4-deprivation.

HUMAN BEINGS

Prior to the availability of techniques for the direct measurement of serum 1,25-$(OH)_2$-D concentrations, dietary PO_4-deprivation was observed to accelerate disappearance from plasma of injected ^{3}H-25-OH-D_3. Furthermore, restoration of PO_4 to the diet slowed disappearance of ^{3}H-25-OH-D_3 from the plasma. Those observations implied augmented conversion of 25-OH-D_3 to some further metabolite during PO_4 deprivation. This effect was independent of PTH since serum iPTH levels decreased during PO_4 deprivation (14). Moreover, the effect was apparently independent of serum PO_4 concentrations since serum PO_4 levels fell during PO_4 deprivation only among women but not among men whereas plasma ^{3}H-25-OH-D_3 disappearance was accelerated in both sexes (14).

Subsequently, as shown in Table 2, short term dietary PO_4 deprivation has been shown to raise serum 1,25-$(OH)_2$-D concentrations in healthy adults of both sexes (15,16,17) as well as in patients with hypoparathyroidism (18) and in children with moderately severe chronic kidney disease (19).

Other physiological circumstances affecting serum 1,25-$(OH)_2$-D concentrations may also be related to an alteration in PO_4 homeostasis. In a retrospective review of studies of healthy subjects fed various constant diets providing normal quantities of Ca, PO_4 and Mg, serum 1,25-$(OH)_2$-D levels were observed to be directly related to daily caloric

TABLE 2

Effects of PO_4-Deprivation in Human Beings

Ref.	Method of Achieving PO_4 Deprivation	Duration	Number of Subjects age, sex	Serum PO_4 mmol/liter Control	$-PO_4$	p	Serum $1,25-(OH)_2-D$ pmol/liter Control	$-PO_4$	p
(15)	Decreased diet PO_4 to 15 mmol/day + $Al(OH)_3$ 202 mmol/day	10 days	1 man, 3 women ages 48-50	1.13 ± 0.19 SD	0.77 ± 0.19	NS	101 ± 0	148 ± 9	< 0.025
(16)	Decrease in diet PO_4 to 16 mmol/day + $Al(OH)_3$ 308 mmol/day	4 days	6 men	1.0 ± 0.10	0.84 ± 0.06	< 0.05	118 ± 7	151 ± 14	< 0.05
(17)	Decrease in diet PO_4 from 52 to 29 mmol/day and oral $Al(OH)_3$, 155 mmol/day	18 days	7 healthy men ages 19-36	1.35 ± 0.20	1.33 ± 0.20	NS	80 ± 21	104 ± 26	< 0.001
(18)	Decrease in diet PO_4 to 16 mmol/day and $Al(OH)_3$	12-18 days	5 hypopara-thyroid adults	1.42 ± 0.22	0.77 ± 0.14	< 0.01	58 ± 14	161 ± 40	< 0.01
(19)	Decrease in diet PO_4 to 11 mmol/day and $Al(OH)_3$	5 days	7 children, moderate renal failure, GFR 25 to 50 ml/min/1.73 m^2	1.42 ± 0.17	1.35 ± 0.17	NS	62 ± 19	101 ± 13	< 0.005

intake/kg or individual average daily change in body weight as a reflection of energy balance as well as being inversely related to serum PO_4 concentrations (20). Serum 1,25-$(OH)_2$-D concentrations were not related to serum iPTH levels in these subjects. More recently a similar relationship between serum 1,25-$(OH)_2$-D and the average daily change in weight has been observed among men adapted to very low Ca diets (5 mmol/day) (7). Thus, some aspect of caloric intake or dietary composition in relation to PO_4 homeostasis, presumably acting via the pituitary-kidney axis, appears to be a determinant of serum 1,25-$(OH)_2$-D levels in healthy adults. In health, this regulating mechanism may be as important as the Ca-PTH axis.

Acknowledgements: Supported by USPHS AM22014, RR0058 and AM15089.

BIBLIOGRAPHY

1. Tanaka, Y., DeLuca, H.F. (1973) Arch. Biochem. Biophys. 154:566-574.
2. Hughes, M.R., Brumbaugh, P.F., Haussler, M.R., Wergedal, J.E., Baylink, D.J. (1975) Science 190:578-580.
3. Gray, R.W. (1981) Calcif. Tissue Int. 33:477-484.
4. Gray, R.W. and Napoli J.L. (1983) J. Biol. Chem. 258:1152-1155.
5. Gray, R.W. and Garthwaite, T.L. (1985) Endocrinol. 116:189-193.
6. Lobaugh, B. and Drezner, M.K. (1984) J. Clin. Invest. 71:400-403.
7. Gray, R.W. Unpublished.
8. Gray, R.W., Haasch, M.L., Brown, C.E. (1983) Calcif. Tissue Int. 35: 773-777.
9. Gray, R.W. (1981) Calcif. Tissue Int. 33:485-488.
10. Gray, R.W., Garthwaite, T.L. and Phillips, L.S. (1983) Calcif. Tissue Int. 35:100-106.
11. Lee, D.B.N., Brauthar, N., Walling, M.W., Silis, V., Carlson, H.E., Grindeland, R.W., Coburn, J.W. and Kleeman, C.R. (1980) Calcif. Tissue Int. 32:105-112.
12. Phillips, L.S., Vassilopoulou-Sellin, R. (1980) New Eng. J. Med. 302:371-380.
13. D'Ercole, A.J., Stiles, A.D. and Underwood, L.E. (1984) Proc. Nat'l. Acad. Sci. USA 81:935-939.
14. Dominguez, J.H., Gray, R.W. and Lemann, J. Jr. (1976) J. Clin. Endocrinol. Metab. 43:1056-1058.
15. Lufkin, E.G., Kumar, R. and Heath H., III. (1983) J. Clin. Endocrinol. Metab. 56:1319-1322, 1983.
16. Insogna, K.L., Broadus, A.E., Gertner, J.M. (1984) J. Clin. Invest. 71:1562-1569.
17. Maierhofer, W.J., Gray, R.W. and Lemann, J. Jr. (1984) Kidney Int: 25:571-575.
18. Wray, H.L., Mehlman, I., Kidd, G.S. and Cheatham, W.W. (1983) Calcif. Tissue Int. 35:706.
19. Portale, A.A., Booth, B.E., Halloran, B.P. and Morris, R.C., Jr. (1984) J. Clin. Invest. 73:1580-1589.
20. Lemann, J. Jr., Gray, R.W., Maierhofer, W.J. and Adams, N.D. (1984) Calcif. Tissue Int. 36:139-144.

Receptors for $1,25(OH)_2D_3$

FUNCTIONS AND MECHANISM OF ACTION OF THE 1,25-DIHYDROXYVITAMIN D_3 RECEPTOR

M.R. HAUSSLER, C.A. DONALDSON, M.A. KELLY, D.J. MANGELSDORF, S.L. MARION, and J.W. PIKE
Department of Biochemistry, College of Medicine, University of Arizona, Tucson, Arizona, USA

INTRODUCTION:

Within the past fifteen years the function of vitamin D has evolved into the vitamin D endocrine system (Fig. 1). The biochemical details of the metabolism of the vitamin to its $1,25(OH)_2D_3$ hormone and the exquisite physiologic regulation of the production of this hormone by the kidney are now well understood (1). Recent interest in the catabolism of $1,25(OH)_2D_3$ has led to the elucidation of a pathway involving C-24 oxidation and ultimate side-chain cleavage (2). We propose that this pathway is initiated by the $1,25(OH)_2D_3$ induced 24-hydroxylase (24-OHase) enzyme and that stimulation of this catabolic cascade is a major action of the hormone. In this fashion, $1,25(OH)_2D_3$ controls its own degradation. Thus, dynamically regulated levels of the hormone then participate in biological responses in the various $1,25(OH)_2D_3$ target tissues. As depicted in Fig. 1, these include the traditional mineral transporting organs and a variety of the other tissues. At the target cell level, $1,25(OH)_2D_3$ is thought to function as depicted in Fig. 2. The hormone associates with the unoccupied $1,25(OH)_2D_3$ receptor, which is in equilibrium between the cytoplasm and nucleus. This association strengthens the DNA binding capacity of the receptor. The complex then

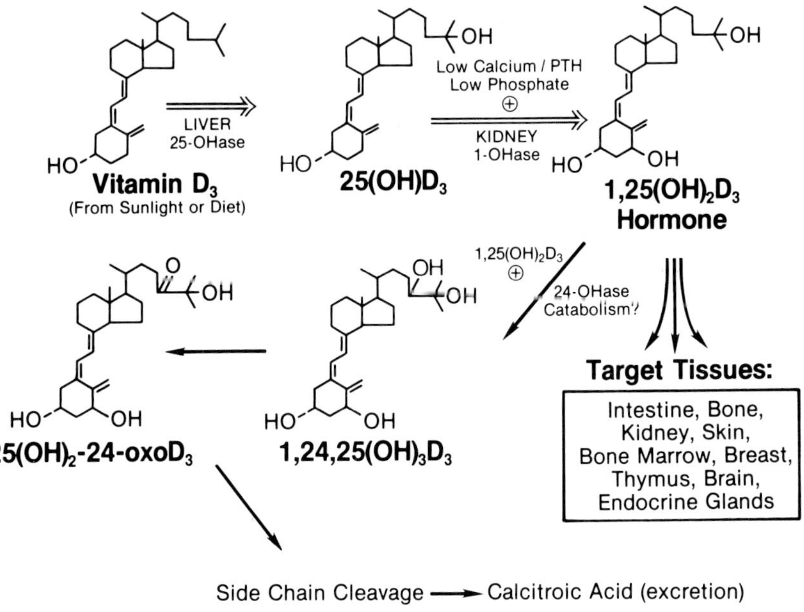

Figure 1. The vitamin D endocrine system.

Vitamin D. A Chemical, Biochemical and Clinical Update

activates genes coding for vitamin D induced bioactive proteins. These proteins are thought to carry out the biologic functions of the hormone in various target cells. These functions range from mineral homeostasis to cell differentiation, as depicted in Fig. 2. The current challenge is to define the mechanism whereby the 1,25(OH)$_2$D$_3$ receptor mediates the multitude of actions of this hormone and to characterize the biochemical function of 1,25(OH)$_2$D$_3$ in its plethora of target cells. Ultimately, the spectrum of bioresponses must be integrated into a composite picture defining the physiologic and pathophysiologic relevance of 1,25(OH)$_2$D$_3$ receptor action. The first step in this process is to dissect biochemically the 1,25(OH)$_2$D$_3$ receptor.

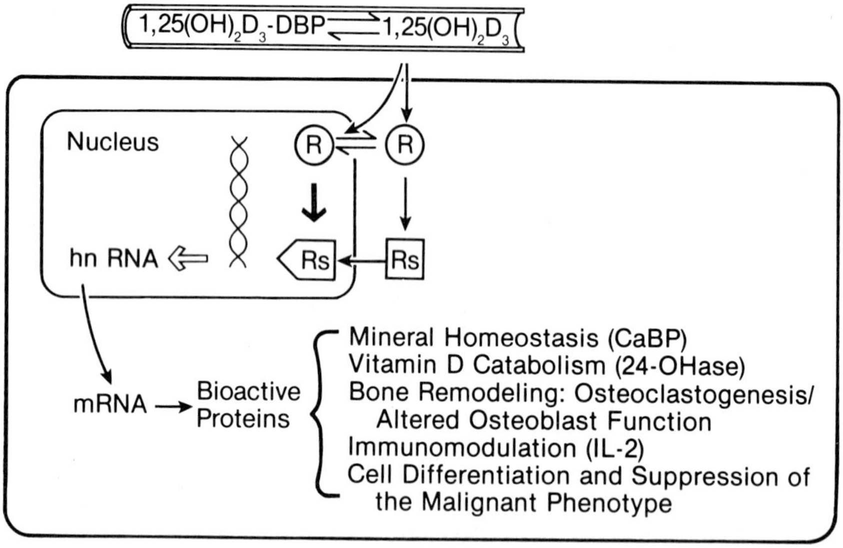

Figure 2. Mechanism of action of 1,25(OH)$_2$D$_3$ in target cells. Ⓡ = unoccupied receptor; [Rs] = occupied receptor; <[Rs] = activated occupied receptor.

THE 1,25(OH)$_2$D$_3$ RECEPTOR

Properties: The biochemical properties of the monomeric receptor as determined using crude or partially purified preparations from chick intestine and other target tissues are:

A. Protein of MW 50,000-60,000 daltons; Sedimentation Coefficient = 3.1-3.7S; $\leq$0.001% of soluble protein in target cells (3).
B. Isolated protein selectively binds 1,25(OH)$_2$D$_3$ with a K_d of 10^{-11}-10^{-10}M; Apparent affinity lowered but specificity enhanced in the presence of serum DBP (4,5).
C. Interacts with nuclei (K_d=10^{-10}M), chromatin and DNA; Association with nuclei is sensitive to nucleases (e.g., DNAse I) which cut transcriptionally active DNA (6).

D. Separate $1,25(OH)_2D_3$ and DNA binding domains; Extremely sensitive to proteolysis (7).
E. Evolutionarily conserved (in part) with immunocrossreactivity between fish, avian and mammalian $1,25(OH)_2D_3$ receptors (8).

Historical Account and Comparison with Other Receptors: The first insight that a biologically active vitamin D metabolite functions analogously to steroid hormones was obtained in 1968 when Haussler *et al.* (9) demonstrated that this metabolite was localized in target tissue nuclear chromatin in a saturable and specific manner after vitamin D administration, *in vivo*. It was next reported (10) in 1969 that the vitamin D metabolite could be extracted from chromatin by KCl, with 50% extraction occurring at 0.2 M KCl. Significantly, the metabolite remained bound to a receptor-like protein in the KCl extract as demonstrated by ammonium sulfate precipitation and CsCl ultracentrifugation. In fact, gel filtration suggested a MW of 50,000-70,000 daltons for the protease sensitive metabolite receptor (10). These data constitute the discovery of the vitamin D receptor and interestingly predate the identification of the active vitamin D metabolite as $1,25(OH)_2D_3$ (11). Tsai and Norman next showed that $1,25(OH)_2D_3$ association with chromatin in reconstituted systems was facilitated by a soluble factor (12). This factor was conclusively shown to be receptor-like by Brumbaugh and Haussler (13,14,15), who reported the following three critical characteristics of the macromolecule: i) binds vitamin D analogs in a rank order corresponding to their biologic potencies (13), ii) sediments at 3.0-3.5S in high salt sucrose gradients and iii) displays saturable high affinity binding, *in vitro* (15). These studies in 1973 and 1974 comprised the first pharmacological and biochemical identification of the receptor, *in vitro*. An important property of the receptor was revealed in 1979 when Pike and Haussler (3) observed that it is a DNA binding protein and the molecule was first purified utilizing DNA cellulose chromatography. Denaturing electrophoresis demonstrated that the purified chick intestinal $1,25(OH)_2D_3$ receptor consisted of several species of molecular weights 55,000-65,000 daltons (3). Biochemical work by Walters *et al.* (16) indicated that the unoccupied as well as occupied receptor was preferentially found in the target cell nucleus. In 1982, Pike *et al.* (17) developed monoclonal antibodies against the chicken $1,25(OH)_2D_3$ receptor which crossreacted with mammalian $1,25(OH)_2D_3$ receptors as well. These antibodies have recently been used to unequivocally identify the monomeric $1,25(OH)_2D_3$ receptor from chicken intestine as a doublet consisting of 60,000 and 58,000 molecular weight forms (Pike, this volume). Moreover, immunoblot detection of the mammalian $1,25(OH)_2D_3$ receptor indicates that it is a smaller protein of molecular weight 52,000-54,000. Recent unpublished immunocytochemical localization data using our antibody confirmed the suggestion of Walters *et al.* (16) that the receptor is predominately localized in the nucleus. Such immunocytochemical localization has been observed in human breast cancer tissue, mouse osteoblasts, mouse kidney, and rat hippocampus. These findings are consistent with recent results (18,19) suggesting that the estrogen receptor is also primarily a nuclear macromolecule. In fact, based upon its molecular size, DNA binding property, subcellular location, and capacity to induce new proteins, the $1,25(OH)_2D_3$ receptor bears a striking resemblance to the estrogen and thyroid hormone receptors and appears to belong in the super-family of steroid and thyroid hormone receptor proteins.

Distribution of the Receptor and Cell Culture Models: Table 1 lists the most significant tissues possessing the $1,25(OH)_2D_3$ receptor (via biochemical detection) as well as the specific cell type based upon autoradiographic localization of the hormone in nuclei as determined by Stumpf and coworkers (20). In order to study $1,25(OH)_2D_3$ action in this myriad of target cells, we and other groups have employed receptor-positive established cell lines representative of the $1,25(OH)_2D_3$ target cell types. These cell culture models are summarized in Table 1 and have been extremely valuable in probing both the mechanism and the wide ranging biologic function of the hormone.

TABLE 1. Relevant tissues and cells that possess the $1,25(OH)_2D_3$ receptor.

CATEGORY	TISSUES	SPECIFIC CELL TYPES	ESTABLISHED CELL LINES
	INTESTINE	ABSORPTIVE EPITHELIAL	INTESTINE - 407 (HUMAN)
CALCIUM CONTROL	BONE	OSTEOBLASTS	ROS 17/2.8 OSTEOSARCOMA (RAT)
	KIDNEY	DISTAL/PROXIMAL EPITHELIAL	$LLC-PK_1$ (PIG); $LLC-MK_2$ (MONKEY)
	PARATHYROID	CHIEF	----
	PANCREAS	β-CELLS	----
ENDOCRINE	PITUITARY	SOMATOMAMMOTROPH	GH_3 TUMOR (RAT)
	OVARY	?	CHINESE HAMSTER OVARY
	BREAST	EPITHELIAL	MCF-7 CARCINOMA (HUMAN)
	SKIN	EPIDERMAL	3T6 FIBROBLAST (MOUSE)
OTHER			G-361 MELANOMA (HUMAN)
	BONE MARROW	MONOCYTE	HL-60 LEUKEMIA (HUMAN)
			U-937 MONOBLAST (HUMAN)
	THYMUS	RETICULAR/T-LYMPHOCYTE	HSB-2 LYMPHOBLAST (HUMAN)
	BRAIN	SPECIFIC NEURONS	----

24-OHase Induction in Kidney Cell Lines: Two interesting models for evaluating receptor significance are the $LLC-PK_1$, and $LLC-MK_2$ renal cell lines, both of which contain a $1,25(OH)_2D_3$ inducible 24-hydroxylase. Chandler, et al. (21) previously reported that while $LLC-PK_1$ contained the classic $1,25(OH)_2D_3$ receptor, $LLC-MK_2$ possessed negligible amounts of high affinity receptor for $1,25(OH)_2D_3$. This suggested that $LLC-MK_2$ 24-OHase induction was either receptor-independent or that an atypical receptor was present in this cell line. Kelly et al. (22) have recently identified such a variant $1,25(OH)_2D_3$ receptor in LLC-MK_2. The variant receptor was detected by labeling intact cells with higher than normal levels of $1,25(OH)_2D_3$ followed by DNA cellulose chromatography. Combining these data with the fact that higher levels of $1,25(OH)_2D_3$ are required for optimum induction of 24-OHase in LLC-MK_2 compared to LLC-PK_1, we have proposed that the variant receptor in LLC-MK_2 is partially defective in binding the hormone. This hypothesis has been confirmed (Kelly, et al., unpublished) by demonstrating an immunoprecipitable variant receptor in LLC-MK_2 cells which binds $1,25(OH)_2D_3$ with a K_d that is approximately 10-fold higher than that in LLC-PK_1. This K_d variant is a model for one type of hormone receptor binding defect in vitamin D dependency rickets type II and provides additional proof of the obligatory role of the $1,25(OH)_2D_3$ receptor and its variants in the biologic action of the hormone.

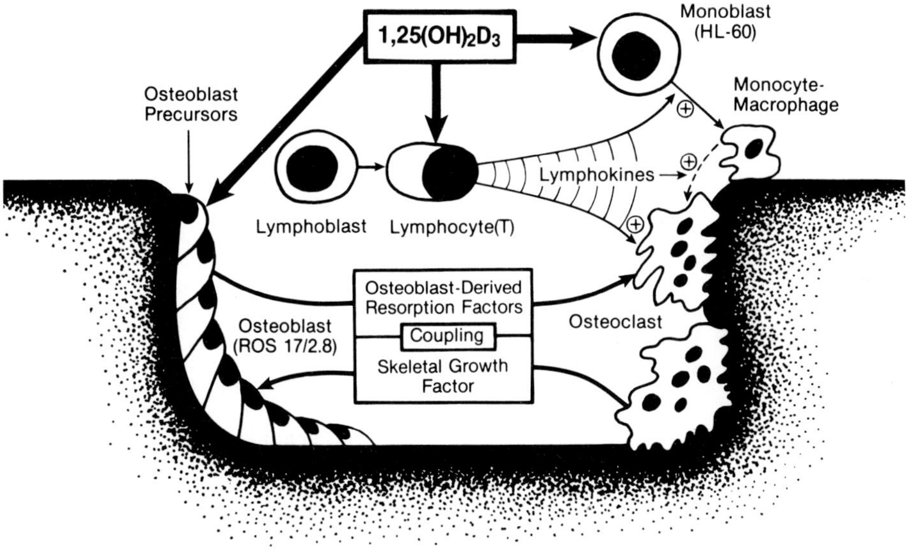

Figure 3. Proposed function of $1,25(OH)_2D_3$ and its receptor in bone remodeling and immunomodulation.

Differentiation of HL-60 Cells: An intensely studied model system for $1,25(OH)_2D_3$ induced differentiation is that of HL-60 cells. This leukemic cell line differentiates into macrophage-like cells when treated with $1,25(OH)_2D_3$ in culture (5,23). We have previously shown that saturation of the nuclear receptor by $1,25(OH)_2[^3H]D_3$ in complete culture medium correlates with the kinetics of $1,25(OH)_2D_3$ induced FMLP (chemotaxin) receptors (5). Thus, this expression of the differentiated phenotype, along with many others is mediated by the $1,25(OH)_2D_3$ receptor protein. One key effect of $1,25(OH)_2D_3$ in the HL-60 line is suppression of c-myc oncogene mRNA levels (24) which occurs rapidly and may reflect either the proliferation rate or more likely the triggering of the differentiation of

HL-60 cells. We have confirmed the results of Reitsma, et al. (24) that $1,25(OH)_2D_3$ dramatically attenuates c-myc mRNA levels in HL-60. Moreover, we have recently found that the receptor itself is modulated by the differentiation state of HL-60 cells. Treatment of HL-60 with the phorbol ester tumor promoter, TPA, for 72 hours elicits the production of macrophage-like cells which have an approximate 80 per cent suppression of the $1,25(OH)_2D_3$ receptor compared to untreated HL-60 cells. This finding may relate to the proposed role of monocytes and macrophages as osteoclast precursors (25). $1,25(OH)_2D_3$ increases osteoclast number, in vivo (26) and may (in part) mediate bone resorption by increasing the differentiation of osteoclast progenitors as illustrated in Fig. 3. Osteoclasts are thought not to possess $1,25(OH)_2D_3$ receptors and therefore it is their number but not their activity that is directly affected by $1,25(OH)_2D_3$. Our observation of dramatically reduced $1,25(OH)_2D_3$ receptor concentrations upon differentiation of HL-60 cells to macrophages could represent the first stage in the attenuation of receptor expression that is presumably complete upon fusion to multinucleate osteoclasts. As illustrated in Fig. 3 it is important to note that $1,25(OH)_2D_3$ indirectly augments the final stages of osteoclast differentiation through a newly recognized operation on T-lymphocytes. T-cells contain $1,25(OH)_2D_3$ receptors (27) and lymphokine production is modulated (28,29); at least one of these lymphokines has been shown to elicit macrophage-fusion to giant multinucleate osteoclast-like cells (29). Finally, $1,25(OH)_2D_3$ could cause bone resorption by binding to its well known receptors in osteoblasts (4) and bringing about the release of osteoblast-derived resorption factors as depicted in Fig. 3. Therefore, it is clear that, along with its mediating receptor, $1,25(OH)_2D_3$ accomplishes a complex yet elegant regulation of bone remodeling and bone remodeling cells. $1,25(OH)_2D_3$ responsive cells of the immune system appear to play a central role in the function of $1,25(OH)_2D_3$ on bone resorption but this may be only one facet of a more general action of the hormone as a novel immunomodulator.

Role of the $1,25(OH)_2D_3$ Receptor in Cell Proliferation and Differentiation: In addition to the above mentioned effects of $1,25(OH)_2D_3$ to induce 24-OHase activity in kidney cells and differentiation of HL-60 cells, $1,25(OH)_2D_3$ is known to elicit a number of other responses in cultured cells. These include inhibition of monolayer growth (4,30,31,32) and morphologic changes (4,31). Furthermore, in vivo studies indicate that $1,25(OH)_2D_3$ prolongs the survival time of nude mice inoculated with leukemia cells (33) and acts as an inhibitor of tumor promotion (34). Taken together, these data intimate that like vitamin A, $1,25(OH)_2D_3$ may be a natural antitumor agent. To further investigate this possibility, we have examined the influence of $1,25(OH)_2D_3$ on the colony forming ability of tumor cells in soft agar. Anchorage-independent growth in soft agar is a recognized assay for malignant transformation, since growth of cells in agar has been significantly correlated with tumorigenicity in immunologically suppressed host animals (35). Hamburger and Salmon have postulated that inhibition of colony formation in soft agar is an applicable means of determining the efficacy of potential anticancer drugs. Accordingly, we have studied the effects of $1,25(OH)_2D_3$ on the ability of a spectrum of malignant cell lines to form colonies in soft agar. We observed dramatic inhibition of anchorage-independent growth in a number of tumorigenic cell lines, all of which possessed significant quantities of the $1,25(OH)_2D_3$ receptor (Donaldson, et al., unpublished). To further delineate the rôle of the receptor in this process, we evaluated the action of a number of vitamin D analogs on the anchorage-independent growth of 3T6 cells (Fig. 4). $1,25(OH)_2D_3$ is a potent inhibitor of 3T6 colony formation in soft agar ($ID_{50} = 7 \times 10^{-10}$M). A longer acting fluorinated analogue, $24,24F_2$-$1,25(OH)_2D_3$, which binds equally well to the receptor (36) exhibits an inhibition four times more sensitive than $1,25(OH)_2D_3$. Trihydroxyvitamin D metabolites display intermediate potency in inhibiting 3T6 colony formation, with $1,24,25(OH)_3D_3$ being slightly less effective (75%) than $1,25(OH)_2D_3$ and $1,25,26(OH)_3D_3$ having one tenth the activity of the hormone. Of the monohydroxylated D vitamins, $1\alpha(OH)D_3$ shows the highest potency (1/250 that of $1,25(OH)_2D_3$). $24,25(OH)_2D_3$ exerts virtually no

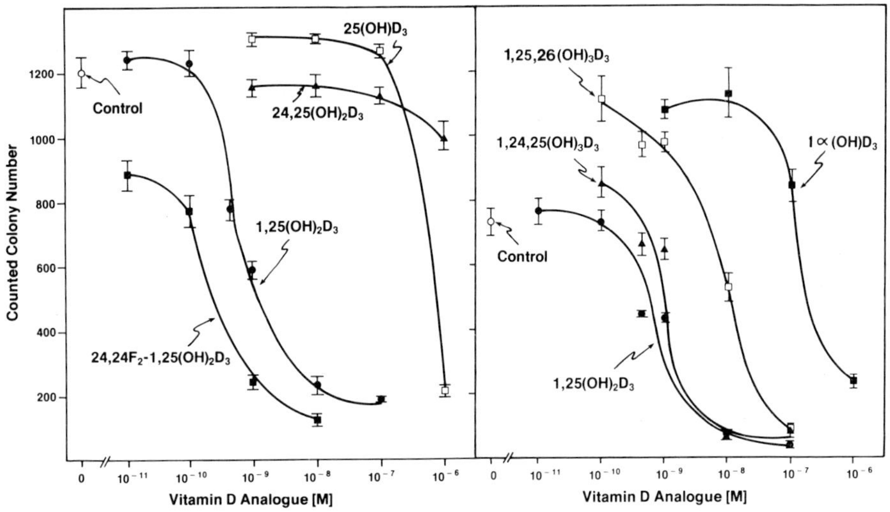

Figure 4. Influence of $1,25(OH)_2D_3$ and its analogues on colony formation by 3T6 cells in soft agar. Single cells were suspended in 0.3% agar in the appropriate cell culture medium containing 20% fetal bovine serum. Aliquots containing 10^4-10^5 cells were pipetted into each Petri dish onto a base layer containing 0.5% agar. Both lower and upper layers contained either the ethanol vehicle or vitamin D analogs at the appropriate concentration. Plates were incubated for approximately 2 weeks at 37°C, at which time the colonies were counted, utilizing an optical image analyzer. Colonies 50 μm or more in diameter (approximately 30 cells) were scored; data are depicted asthe mean of 3 to 5 plates ± SEM.

activity in this system, probably because of its high binding affinity for serum vitamin D binding protein combined with its low affinity for the intracellular $1,25(OH)_2D_3$ receptor (37,38). The pharmacologic profiles of the various vitamin D metabolites in these experiments correspond well with the rank order of these metabolites in binding to the receptor (37), verifying the assumption that the receptor mediates the inhibition of anchorage-independent growth.

PROPOSED BIOCHEMICAL MECHANISM AND BIOLOGICAL SIGNIFICANCE OF THE $1,25(OH)_2D_3$ RECEPTOR

The mechanism whereby $1,25(OH)_2D_3$ and its receptor suppress c-myc oncogene expression and inhibit anchorage-independent growth of tumor cells is unknown. However, these actions probably involve receptor binding to DNA, an event which alters transcription and may initiate the program for differentiation of transformed cells. Alternatively, since $1,25(OH)_2D_3$ is a calcium transport hormone, it may be an alteration of intracellular calcium that triggers cell differentiation and causes the apparent reversion of the malignant phenotype. Our current working model for the biochemical action of $1,25(OH)_2D_3$ is depicted in Fig. 5.

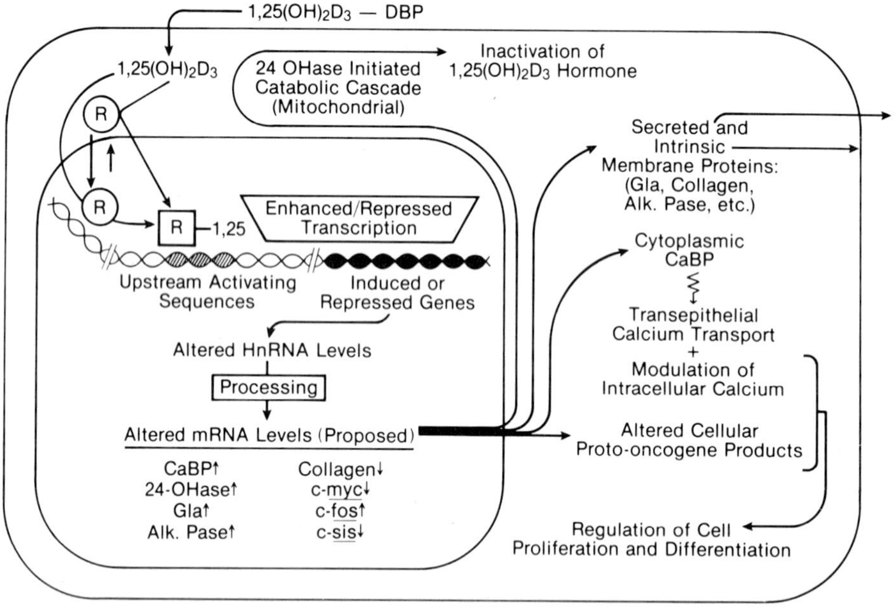

Figure 5. Working hypothesis for $1,25(OH)_2D_3$ mechanism - 1985.

In our integrated model we contend that a fraction of unoccupied receptor exists in the cytoplasm of target cells where it can complex with $1,25(OH)_2D_3$ prior to DNA binding. The majority of unoccupied receptor is apparently in the nucleus where it may be bound to DNA in regions of chromatin not modulated by the hormone. $1,25(OH)_2D_3$ binding is proposed to activate the receptor for "DNA walking" until it locates and binds to higher affinity upstream activating sequences of DNA that control vitamin D regulated genes. These upstream activating sequences are analogous to those found for other steroid hormone receptors (39-41). Altered DNA transcription then results in enhanced or repressed levels of various mRNA s. The altered mRNA levels pictured in Figure 5 are hypothetical except in the cases of CaBP, which has been shown to be increased (42), and c-myc and collagen which are decreased (24,43). The notion that the $1,25(OH)_2D_3$ receptor binds to regulatory/promoter sequences for each of the putative induced mRNA's is only one possible mechanism. Equally plausible is the concept that the 1,25$(OH)_2D_3$ receptor modulates transcription of a gene coding for a rapidly turned over protein that in turn regulates the expression of mRNA s for all vitamin D end-point proteins in a concerted fashion. Mechanisms incorporating altered stability and degradation rates of mRNA s must also be considered. Regardless of the exact sequence of events, there is little doubt that control of mRNA levels is the key manner in which 1,25$(OH)_2D_3$ ultimately orchestrates the concentration of its bioactive proteins. As illustrated in Fig. 5 one or more of the induced proteins then effects the altered function which is preprogrammed into the cell in terms of its responsiveness to the 1,25$(OH)_2D_3$ hormone. Thus, some target cells (i.e., kidney) may primarily inactivate 1,25$(OH)_2D_3$ and carry out transepithelial mineral transport. Bone cells respond by inducing an array of proteins required for the complex process of bone mineralization and remodeling. Finally, many cell types, including hematopoietic and transformed cells appear to respond to 1,25$(OH)_2D_3$ by differentiation and suppression of the embryonic or malignant phenotype. Astoundingly, what was traditionally a calcium absorption hormone has now been unveiled as a biological modifier capable of global maturation of target cells as well as alteration of specific cellular functions.

REFERENCES

1. Haussler, M.R. and McCain, T.A. (1977) N. Engl. J. Med. 297, 974-983 & 1041-1050.
2. Mayer, E., Bishop, J.E., Chandraratna, R.A.S., Okamura, W.H., Kruse, J.R., Popjak, G., Ohnuma, N. and Norman, A.W. (1983) J. Biol. Chem. 258, 13458-13465.
3. Pike, J.W. and Haussler, M.R. (1979) Proc. Natl. Acad. Sci. USA 76, 5485-5489.
4. Dokoh, S., Donaldson, C.A., and Haussler, M.R. (1984) Cancer Res. 44, 2103-2109.
5. Mangelsdorf, D.J., Koeffler, H.P., Donaldson, C.A., Pike, J.W., and Haussler, M.R. (1984) J. Cell Biol. 98, 391-398.
6. Pike, J.W. (1982) J. Biol. Chem. 257, 6766-6775.
7. Pike, J.W. (1981) Biochem. Biophys. Res. Commun. 100, 1713-1719.
8. Pike, J.W., Marion, S.L., Donaldson, C.A. and Haussler, M.R. (1983) J. Biol. Chem. 258, 1289-1296.
9. Haussler, M.R., Myrtle, J.F., and Norman, A.W. (1968) J. Biol. Chem. 243, 4055-4064.
10. Haussler, M.R. and Norman, A.W. (1969) Proc. Natl. Acad. Sci. 62, 155-162.
11. Holick, M.F., Schnoes, H.K., DeLuca, H.F., Suda, T. and Cousins, R.J. (1971) Biochemistry 10, 2799-2804.
12. Tsai, H.C. and Norman, A.W. (1973) J. Biol. Chem. 248, 5967-5975.
13. Brumbaugh, P.F. and Haussler, M.R. (1973) Life Sci. 13, 1737-1746.
14. Brumbaugh, P.F. and Haussler, M.R. (1974) J. Biol. Chem. 249, 1251-1257.
15. Brumbaugh, P.F. and Haussler, M.R. (1974) J. Biol. Chem. 249, 1258-1262.
16. Walters, M.R., Hunziker, W. and Norman, A.W. (1980) J. Biol. Chem. 255, 6799-6805.
17. Pike, J.W., Donaldson, C.A., Marion, S.L., and Haussler, M.R. (1982) Proc. Natl. Acad. Sci. 79, 7719-7723.

18. King, W.J. and Green, G.L. (1984) Nature 307, 745-747.
19. Welshons, W.V., Lieverman, M.E., and Gorski, J. (1984) Nature 307, 747-749.
20. Stumpf, W.E., Sar, M. and DeLuca, H.F. (1981) in Hormonal Control of Calcium Metabolism (Cohn, D.V., Talmage, R.V., and Matthews, J.L., eds.) 222-229, Excerpta Medica, Amsterdam.
21. Chandler, J.S., Chandler, S.K., Pike, J.W. and Haussler, M.R. (1984) J. Biol. Chem. 259, 2214-2221.
22. Kelly, M.A., Marion, S.L., Donaldson, C.A., Pike, J.W., and Haussler, M.R. (1985) J. Biol. Chem. 260, 1545-1549.
23. Bar-Shavit, Z., Teitelbaum, S.L., Reitsma, P., Hall, A., Pegg, L.E., Trial, J.A., and Kahn, A.J. (1983) Proc. Natl. Acad. Sci. USA 80, 5907-5911.
24. Reitsma, P.H., Rothberg, P.G., Astrin, S.M., Trial, J., Bar-Shavit, Z., Hall A., Teitelbaum, S.L. and Kahn, A.J. (1983) Nature 306, 492-494.
25. Ko, J.S. and Bernard, G.W. (1981) Am. J. Anat. 161, 415-425.
26. Holtrop, M.E., Karen, A.C., Clark, M.B., Holick, M., and Anast, C.S. (1981) Endocrinology 6, 2293-2301.
27. Provvedini, D.M., Tsoukas, C.D., Deftos, L.J., and Manolagas, S.C. (1983) Science 221, 1181-1183.
28. Tsoukas, C.D., Provvedini, D.M., and Manolagas, S.C. (1984) Science 224, 1438-1440.
29. Abe, E., Miyaura, C., Tanaka, H., Shiina, Y., Kuribayashi, T., Suda, S., Nishii, Y., DeLuca, H.F., and Suda, T. (1983) Proc. Natl. Acad. Sci. 80, 5583-5587.
30. Colston, K., Colston, M.J. and Feldman, D. (1981) Endocrinology 108, 1083-1086.
31. Frampton, R.J., Omond, S.A., and Eisman, J.A. (1983) Cancer Res. 43, 4443-4447.
32. Dokoh, S., Donaldson, C.A., Marion, S.L., Pike, J.W. and Haussler, M.R. (1983) Endocrinology 112, 200-206.
33. Honma, Y., Hozumi, M., Abe, E., Konno, K., Fukushima, M., Hata, S., Nishii, Y., DeLuca, H.F., and Suda, T. (1983) Proc. Natl. Acad. Sci. 80, 201-204.
34. Wood, A.W., Chang, R.L., Huang, M.T., Uskokovic, M., and Conney, A.H. (1983) Biochem. Biophys. Res. Commun. 116, 605-611.
35. Reid, L.C.M. (1979) Methods Enzymol. 58, 152-164.
36. Shina, Y., Abe, E., Miyaura, C., Tanaka, H., Yamada, S., Ohmori, M., Nakayama, K., Takayama, H., Matsunaga, I., Nishii, Y., DeLuca, H.F., and Suda, T. (1983) Arch. Biochem. Biophys. 220, 90-94.
37. Dokoh, S., Pike, J.W., Chandler, J.S., Mancini, J.M., and Haussler, M.R. (1981) Anal. Biochem. 116, 211-222.
38. Mallon, J.P., Matuszewski, D., and Sheppard, H. (1980) J. Steroid Biochem. 13, 409-413.
39. Renkawitz, R., Schutz, G., von der Ahe, D., and Beato, M. (1984) Cell 37, 503-510.
40. Dean, D.C., Gope, R., Knoll, B.J., Riser, M.E., and O'Malley, B.W. (1984) J. Biol. Chem. 259, 9967-9970.
41. Jost, J.-P., Seldran, M., and Geiser, M. (1984) Proc. Natl. Acad. Sci. 81, 429-433.
42. Hunziker, W., Siebert, P.D., King, M.W., Stucki, P., Dugaiczyk, A., and Norman, A.W. (1983) Proc. Natl. Acad. Sci. 80, 4228-4232.
43. Rowe, D.W. and Kream, B.E. (1982) J. Biol. Chem. 257, 8009-8015.

ULTRASTRUCTURAL-IMMUNOCYTOCHEMICAL LOCALIZATION OF 1,25-DIHYDROXYVITAMIN D_3 RECEPTORS IN OSTEOBLASTS AND OSTEOCYTES.

G. BOIVIN[1], P. MESGUICH[2], G. MOREL[2], J.W. PIKE[3], P.M. DUBOIS[2], P.J. MEUNIER[1] and M.R. HAUSSLER[3].
[1]INSERM U. 234, Faculté A. Carrel, 69008 Lyon, France ; [2]CNRS UA 559, Faculté Lyon-Sud, 69921 Oullins, France ; [3]Department of Biochemistry, University of Arizona, Tucson AZ 85724, U.S.A.

INTRODUCTION :

The osteoblast is an important site of action for the effect of 1,25-dihydroxyvitamin D_3 (1,25$(OH)_2D_3$) on bone formation (2,11). The receptors for 1,25 $(OH)_2D_3$ (1,25$(OH)_2D_3$-R) have been identified in numerous target organs (4,6) including bone tissue of chick, rat and mouse. 1,25$(OH)_2D_3$-R have been localized in the nucleus of target cells by both biochemical and autoradiographic methods (see review in 6). Furthermore, current evidence suggests that this protein mediates the biological action of 1,25 $(OH)_2D_3$ at the nuclear level (7). However, the cellular and subcellular locations of the receptor protein in bone tissue have not been established by histological methods.
Furthermore, there is current controversy over the cellular distribution of unoccupied steroid hormone receptors. According to the "two-step" hypothesis, these receptors are cytoplasmic proteins, but other data suggest that the receptors may reside in the nucleus and that cytosolic localization represents an artefact (12).
Recently, a combined method using immunocytochemistry on ultrathin sections obtained by cryoultramicrotomy (1,5) was developed, and made possible the ultrastructural localization of hormones and hormone-receptors normally extracted by conventional technique for electron microscopy.
The purpose of the present study is to applied immunocytochemistry after cryoultramicrotomy to bone tissue to established the ultrastructural localization of 1,25$(OH)_2D_3$-R in osteoblasts and osteocytes of neonatal mouse and rat calvaria.

MATERIAL AND METHODS :

The calvaria from 5 day-old mice and rats were fixed by immersion for one hour in 2.5 % glutaraldehyde in 0.1 M cacodylate buffer, pH 7.4 at 4°C. They were cut up into small pieces at the beginning of fixation. After washing in saccharose 0.2 M, tissues were post-fixed for one hour in 1 % buffered osmium tetroxide, and then washed again. Thereafter, tissues were incubated in 0.4 M sucrose as cryoprotectant. Freezing was performed in a cold gradient of fuming nitrogen (Biogel, CFPO, France) to -4°C before total immersion in liquid nitrogen (3).
The antibody used was a specific, high affinity (Kd = 1.8×10^{-11} M) monoclonal antibody (9A7Y) to chick intestinal receptor for 1,25$(OH)_2D_3$, obtained from confluent cultures of rat spleen/mouse myeloma hybrid SP2/0-9A7 (8,9,10). The antibody react with many 1,25$(OH)_2D_3$-R including those from rat and mouse tissues. Purified receptors were used in one of the controls of the immunocytochemical reaction.
Ultrathin sections were cut at -140°C on an ultrotome III (LKB, Stockholm, Sweden) fitted with a cryokit (3). The sections collected on collodion-coated nickel grids were incubated consecutively for ten min. periods with : a) monoclonal rat antibody directed against 1,25$(OH)_2D_3$-R (dilution from 2×10^{-4} to 2×10^{-8}) ; b) goat anti-rat γ-globulin

labeled with peroxidase ; c) 4-chloro-1-naphthol (ICN Pharmaceutical, Plainview N.Y., USA) solution in Tris buffered saline for three min..This solution was used with 0.01 % hydrogen-peroxide as enzymatic substrate ; d) 1 % phosphate buffered osmium tetroxide. After steps a and b, the grids were washed with 0.05 M Tris-HCl buffer, pH 7.6. After, steps c and d the grids were washed with distilled water. All washing steps were performed for ten min. The specificity of the immunocytochemical reaction was checked as follows : a) omitting the antibody serum ; b) using the antibody serum incubated overnight at 4°C with corresponding homologous antigen ; c) using the antibody serum incubated overnight at 4°C with heterologous antigens at 40 times greater concentration than homologous antigen.
Ultrathin sections were observed with a Siemens Elmiskop 101 electron microscope (P.M. Dubois's laboratory) and with a JEOL 1200 EX electron microscope (Centre de Microscopie Electronique et de Pathologie Ultrastructurale, Faculté A. Carrel, Lyon, France).

RESULTS :

After immunocytological reactions, the antigen-antibody complex appeared as small dense granules at least 30 nm in diameter. In the absence of anti-receptor serum, and when the antibody was incubated with homologous antigen, no immunocytological reaction was observed.
$1,25(OH)_2D_3$-R like immunoreactivity was detected in osteoblasts and osteocytes of mice and rats calvaria. The reaction products were mainly localized in the nucleus : at the nuclear membrane level, in the euchromatin and in the nucleolus. In the cytoplasm, the immunoreactivity was present in the cytoplasmic matrix but not in organelles, and it was never detected at the plasma membrane level.

CONCLUSIONS :

The application of immunocytochemistry after cryoultramicrotomy to bone tissue of neonatal mice and rats, provides ultrastructural evidence for the presence in osteoblasts and osteocytes of $1,25(OH)_2D_3$-R. The immunoreaction products were detected in the cytoplasm and mainly in the nucleus of these bone cells. These data imply that $1,25(OH)_2D_3$-R, as postulated for other steroid receptors (12), occur primarily in the nucleus.

REFERENCES :

1. Boivin, G., Morel, G., Meunier, P.J. and Dubois, P.M. (1983) Biol. Cell, 49, 227-230.
2. Canalis, E. (1983) Endocrine Rev. 4, 62-77.
3. Hemming, F.J., Mesguich, P., Morel, G. and Dubois, P.M. (1983) J. Microsc. 131, 25-34.
4. Henry, H.L. and Norman, A.W. (1984) Ann. Rev. Nutr. 4, 493-520.
5. Morel, G., Boivin, G., Dubois, P.M. and Meunier, P.J. (in press) Cell Tissue Res.
6. Norman, A.W., Roth, J. and Orci, L. (1982) Endocrine Rev. 3, 331-366.
7. Pike, J.W. (1982) J. Biol. Chem. 257, 6766-6775.
8. Pike, J.W. (1984) J. Biol. Chem. 259, 1167-1173.
9. Pike, J.W., Donaldson, C.A., Marion, S.L. and Haussler, M.R. (1982) Proc. Natl. Acad., Sci. USA, 79, 7719-7723.
10. Pike, J.W., Marion, S.L., Donaldson, C.A. and Haussler, M.R. (1983) J. Biol. Chem. 258, 1289-1296.
11. Raisz, L.G. and Kream, B.E. (1983) N. Engl. J. Med. 309, 29-35 and 83-89.
12. Schrader, W.T. (1984) Nature, 308, 17-18.

1,25-DIHYDROXYVITAMIN D RECEPTOR AND VITAMIN D-DEPENDENT CALCIUM-BINDING PROTEIN IN RAT BRAIN: COMPARATIVE IMMUNOCYTOCHEMICAL LOCALIZATION

T.L. Clemens, X.Y. Zhou, J.W. Pike, M.R. Haussler and R.S. Sloviter Regional Bone and Neurology Centers, Helen Hayes Hospital, West Haverstraw, N.Y. and Department of Biochemistry, University of Arizona, Tucson, AZ., USA

Introduction:
1,25-dihydroxyvitamin D_3 (1,25-$(OH)_2$-D_3) receptor activation in the intestine stimulates the synthesis of a calcium binding protein (CaBP) that may play a role in intestinal calcium transport. The finding that the brain contains large amounts of CaBP (1,2) along with the recent observation using autoradiography that some neurons bind 1,25-$(OH)_2$-D_3 suggest that certain brain cells are vitamin D responsive. These observations prompted us to visualize CaBP and 1,25-$(OH)_2$-D_3 receptors using immunocytochemistry to determine (i) the cellular and subcellular location of 1,25-$(OH)_2$-D_3 receptor and (ii) if all cells containing CaBP also contain the 1,25-$(OH)_2$-D_3 receptor.

Methods and Results: Brains from saline perfused rats were immersed-fixed in Bouin's fluid for 48 hrs. Adjacent Vibratome sections 50 um thick were incubated in 0.1 M Tris buffer containing either purified rat monoclonal antibody against the 1,25-$(OH)_2$-D_3 receptor (9A7, 0.3-1 ug/ml) (5) or polyclonal antibody (1,5000) raised against purified chick intestinal CaBP. Sections reacted with monoclonal antibody 9A7 were subsequently reacted with biotinylated rabbit-anti-rat, antibody. Antibodies were visualized using the Protein-A-avidin-biotin peroxidase technique (6). Immunologic controls included sections incubated with (i) Tris buffer, (ii) normal rat IgG (1 ug/ml), (iii) normal rabbit serum (1:1000) and (iv) monoclonal antibody 9A7 (0.3 ug/ml) preadsorbed with chick intestinal cytosol. 1,25-$(OH)_2$-D_3 receptor immunoreacitivity (IR) was present exclusively in cell nuclei and was widely distributed through the brain.

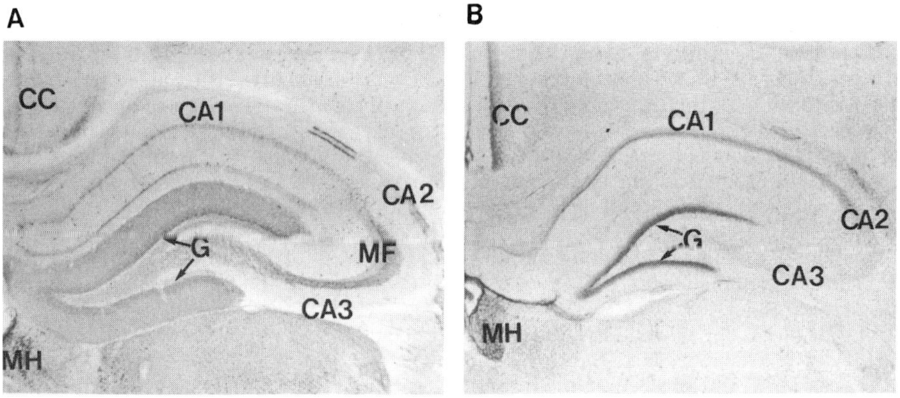

Figure 1: Localization of CaBP (A) and 1,25-$(OH)_2$-D_3 receptor (B) in the hippocampus of rat brain. CaBP staining was observed in cell bodies axons and dendrites of pyramidal cells (CA1 and CA2 but not CA3) granule cells, cells of medial habenula (MH) and cingulate cortex (CC). This pattern of staining was strikingly similar to that of the 1,25-$(OH)_2$-D_3 receptor (B).

Vitamin D. A Chemical, Biochemical and Clinical Update

A B

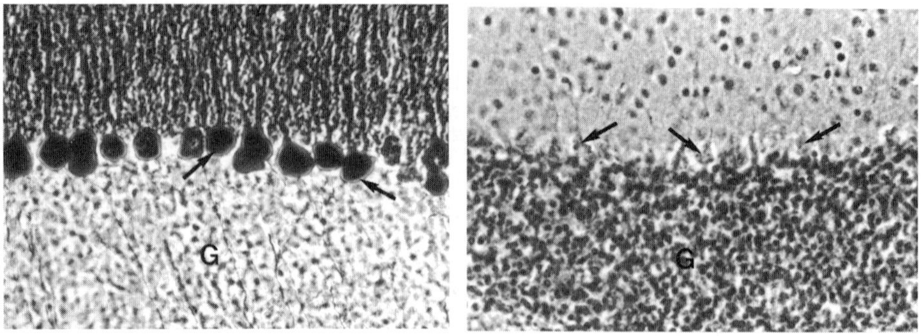

Figure 2: Immunocytochemical localization of CaBP (A) and the 1,25-$(OH)_2$-D_3 receptor (B) in rat cerebellum. High CaBP-like reactivity was observed in cell bodies (arrow), axons and dendrites of Purkinge cells but was low in the granule cell layer (G). By contrast, 1,25-$(OH)_2$-D_3 receptor immunoreactivity (B) was completely absent in Purkinje cells (arrows) but was found instead in the immediately adjacent granule cell nuclei.

Detailed comparisons of 1,25-$(OH)_2$-D_3 receptor IR and CaBP IR were made in hippocampus and cerebellum because the laminar distribution of cell types in these regions facilitated study and because both regions contain large amounts of CaBP (Figs. 1 and 2).

Discussion:

This study represents the first immunocytochemical demonstration of the 1,25-$(OH)_2$-D_3 receptor in brain. Its exclusive nuclear localization is consistent with previous biochemical studies showing that the 1,25-$(OH)_2$-D_3 binding activity was associated mainly with the nuclear compartment (7). The coexistence of CaBP and the 1,25-$(OH)_2$-D_3 receptor in hippocampal neurons supports the concept that vitamin D may affect these cells. However, the fact that cerebellar Purkinje cells, which are rich in CaBP but apparently lack the 1,25-$(OH)_2$-D_3 receptor, suggests that all CaBP-containing cells are not necessarily vitamin D responsive. This contention is further supported by results from our previous studies in which long-term vitamin D deficiency did not alter cerebellar CaBP concentrations (8). Further application of these immunocytochemical techniques to the mapping of the 1,25-$(OH)_2$-D_3 receptor and CaBP in other tissues are now underway and should lead to a better understanding of the mode of vitamin D action.

References:

1. Jande, S.S., Mater, L., Lawson, D.E.M., (1981), Nature (Lond). 2941, 765-767.
2. Thomasset, M., Parker, C.O., Cuisinier-Gleizes, P., (1982), Amer. J. Physiol. 243, E484-E488.
3. Feldman, S.C., Christakos, S., (1983), Endocrinology 113, 290-302.
4. Stumpf, W.E., Sar, M., Clark, S.A., DeLuca, H.F., (1982), Science 215, 1403-1405.
5. Pike, J.W., Marion, S.L., Donaldson, C.A., Haussler, M.R., (1983), J. Biol. Chem. 258, 1289-1296.
6. Hsu, S.M., Raine, L., Fanger, H., (1981), J. Histochem. Cytochem. 29, 577-580.
7. Walters, M.R., Hunziker, W., Norman, A.W., (1980), J. Biol. Chem. 255, 6799-6805.
8. Clemens, T.L., Christakos, S., Sloviter, R.S., (1984), Calc. Tiss. Intl. Program Abstract, Sixth Annual Meeting of the American Society for Bone and Mineral Research, A63.

NEW INSIGHTS INTO MEDIATORS OF VITAMIN D_3 ACTION.

J. WESLEY PIKE
Department of Biochemistry, University of Arizona Health Sciences Center, Tucson, Arizona USA 85724

Introduction:

Intracellular receptor proteins represent key elements in the mechanism of action of 1,25-dihydroxyvitamin D_3 (1,25(OH)$_2D_3$) (1). As DNA-binding proteins, their hypothetical function is to interact with regulatory regions of unique genes and thus alter the level of expression of biologically active proteins (2). Despite the central role receptors play in cellular responsiveness to hormone, however, these unique proteins have yielded reluctantly to investigation. This has been due primarily to their trace abundance in target cells and their extreme lability in cellular extracts. Recently, however, polyclonal and monoclonal antibodies raised against a number of steroid receptor proteins have made it possible to employ valuable immunologic methodology in their detection, characterization, and isolation (3,4). These antibodies have even proven useful in the molecular cloning of receptor genes (5,6). The purpose of this chapter is to describe the application of monoclonal antibodies which we have developed to the avian 1,25(OH)$_2D_3$ receptor (7-9) in the characterization of both avian and mammalian forms of this genomic regulating protein.

Characteristics of Monoclonal Antibodies to the Chick 1,25(OH)$_2D_3$ Receptor:

We raised antisera in Lewis rats against the partially purified 1,25(OH)$_2D_3$ receptor obtained from chick intestinal mucosa (8). Rat spleen cells were fused with a mouse myeloma (SP2/0-Ag 8) and the resulting hybridomas screened for the presence of anti-1,25(OH)$_2D_3$ receptor antibodies via immunoprecipitation. Three continuous lines, the SP2/0-9A7, SP2/0-4A5, and the SP2/0-8D3, were obtained which produce IgG2a, IgG2b, and IgM immunoglobulins, respectively, These antibodies proved unreactive to protein A, but displayed a very high affinity for the chick receptor of 1.8×10^{-11} M (9A7γ), 1×10^{-10} M (9A7γ), and 1×10^{-11} M (8D3μ) (10). Further, they exhibited extensive crossreactivity with all fish, amphibian, and mammalian receptors that we have tested, including the human. Importantly, the binding of antibody to the 1,25(OH)$_2D_3$ receptor does not alter the latter's affinity for 1,25(OH)$_2D_3$, but does qualitatively alter its *in vitro* binding to nuclei and DNA (10). Thus, these results suggest that the monoclonal antibodies we have obtained may recognize an antigenic determinant in or near the DNA binding domain of the chick 1,25(OH)$_2D_3$ receptor.

Immunologic Detection and Characterization of 1,25(OH)$_2D_3$ Receptors:

We developed a competitive radioligand immunoassay in order to detect and characterize certain properties of the native avian 1,25(OH)$_2D_3$ receptor (11). Application of this assay, in accord with hormone binding data (2), revealed that the receptor was a 3.3S macromolecule after sedimentation through a linear sucrose gradient and was a DNA binding protein which eluted from DNA cellulose at 0.22 M KCl. Separately, the immunoassay was also essential in evaluating the effects of administration of 1,25(OH)$_2D_3$ to chicks on the relative proportion of unoccupied and occupied 1,25(OH)$_2D_3$ receptors. While approximately 13% of receptor was occupied in the rachitic state, over 56% of this protein was endogenously occupied

Vitamin D. A Chemical, Biochemical and Clinical Update

with $1,25(OH)_2D_3$ following a 24 and 48 h treatment of 10 nmol $1,25(OH)_2D_3$. These findings are consistent with those of other studies utilizing radioligand exchange assays (12,13). However, despite these, as well as other applications of the radioligand immunoassay, certain imprecisions and limitations prevented its wide use in the measurement of $1,25(OH)_2D_3$ receptors.

We have recently adapted immunoblot methodology (14) to the characterization of both avian and mammalian receptors (15). In contrast to the radioimmunoassay, results obtained by this technique have been extremely insightful. Cells, tissue, or cellular extracts are denatured in 1% SDS and 2-mercaptoethanol at 100°C, and then electrophoresed by the method of Laemmli (15). Following electrophoretic transfer to nitrocellulose, the

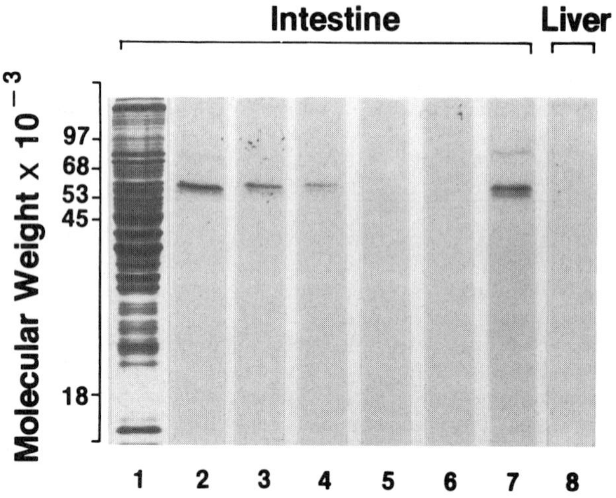

Fig. 1: Immunoblot detection of chick intestinal mucosal $1,25(OH)_2D_3$ receptor. Tissue extracts were prepared by homogenization in either 10 mM Tris-HCl, pH 7.4, 1 mM EDTA, 5 mM DTT, and 0.3 M KCl (cytosol) or the above buffer without KCl (nuclear) as described previously (15). The latter produced a nuclear fraction which was then extracted in the above buffer containing 0.3 M KCl. The samples were electrophoresed (16) and then either stained with Coomassie blue (Lane 1) or transferred to nitrocellulose (Lanes 2-8) and immunoblotted (15). Lane 2, 200 µg intestinal cytosol protein (2 ng receptor); lane 3, 100 µg intestinal cytosol protein (1 ng receptor); lane 4, 50 µg protein (0.5 ng receptor); and lane 5, 25µg protein (0.25 ng receptor) all probed with 4 µg/ml 9A7γ antibody. Lane 7, 200 µg of salt extracted nuclear protein (4 ng receptor) probed with 4 µg/ml 9A7γ. Lane 8, 200 µg of liver cytosol protein, probed with 4 µg/ml 9A7γ. Autoradiography was for 48 h at -70°C with a Cronex Hi-plus intensifying screen.

immobilized proteins are probed using monoclonal antibody, and then visualized using radioiodinated second antibody or protein A and autoradiography. Fig. 1 illustrates the detection of the chick $1,25(OH)_2D_3$ receptor after electrophoresis of crude intestinal mucosal extract prepared using either buffered 0.3 M KCl or from 0.3 M KCl extracts of the nuclear fraction (isolated after homogenization in low ionic strength buffer). Two antigenically-related species of 60,300 and 58,600 daltons are evident, particularly in the nuclear extract of mucosal tissue. These species are tissue specific (absent in liver), and detection is dependent upon tissue concentration and upon incubation with the specific 9A7γ (or 4A5γ, data not shown) antibody. Moreover, these species comigrate with two proteins detectable by Coomassie blue staining after extensive enrichment by previously described technique (2,8). It is unlikely that these two species represent different gene products and it is equally unclear at present whether form A is derived from B through a post-translational modification or whether form B is simply a proteolytic cleavage product of form A. These two species are not analogous, however, to the A and B forms of the avian progesterone receptor, since both forms of the $1,25(OH)_2D_3$ receptor bind to DNA. Interconversion of A and B is also evident _in vitro_, although immunoblot of mucosal tissue, solubilized directly in denaturing buffer to limit proteolysis, has revealed the equimolar presence of both of the $1,25(OH)_2D_3$ receptor forms (data not shown).

Table 1 represents a compilation of the molecular weights of occupied $1,25(OH)_2D_3$ receptors identified by immunoblot technique in cellular extracts obtained from a number of mammalian species. In contrast to the

Table 1. Comparison of the molecular weight of occupied $1,25(OH)_2D_3$ receptors derived from avian and mammalian sources.

Receptor Source[a]		Molecular Weight
Avian		
chick	intestine	60,300 (A) and 58,600 (B)
	kidney	60,300 (A) and 58,600 (B)
	parathyroid gld.	60,300 (A) and 58,600 (B)
Mammalian		
rat	intestine	53,500
	kidney	53,500
	bone (ROS 17/2.8)	53,500
mouse	fibroblast (3T6)	54,300
porcine	kidney ($LLC-PK_1$)	52,800
primate	kidney ($LLC-MK_2$)	52,800
human	fibroblast	52,300
	leukemic cell (HL-60)	52,300
	intestine (407)	52,300

[a]Parenthesis following source indicates the designated cultured cell line.

two avian forms, mammalian $1,25(OH)_2D_3$ receptors apparently exist as single species which exhibit a lesser molecular mass than that of the avian proteins. They are nonidentical in electrophoretic mobility with the murine receptors displaying molecular weights of 53,000-54,000 while the human protein migrates most rapidly, at 52,200. These polypeptides have been unequivocally identified as $1,25(OH)_2D_3$ receptors by virtue of their comigration with authentic $1,25(OH)_2D[^3H]D_3$-receptor complex on DNA cellulose. Furthermore, their subcellular distribution upon fractionation, as a function of $1,25(OH)_2D_3$ treatment, is consistent with that of previously identified biochemical data (17). Finally, while interspecies differences in the molecular weights of $1,25(OH)_2D_3$ receptors are evident, these proteins are apparently identical from tissue to tissue within a single species.

Functional Binding Domains on $1,25(OH)_2D_3$ Receptors:

We employed limited trypsin cleavage of intestinal cytosol proteins as a means of gaining insight into the molecular organization of the avian $1,25(OH)_2D_3$ receptor (18). Fragments which were generated were evaluated for charge (DEAE-HPLC), size (gel filtration, sedimentation), retention of $1,25(OH)_2[^3H]D_3$, DNA-binding activity and reactivity with monoclonal antibody. Two differentially trypsin-sensitive regions on the $1,25(OH)_2D_3$ receptor were identified under these conditions: cleavage within the most sensitive region of the receptor produced a large fragment of 53,000 daltons which retained complex with $1,25(OH)_2D_3$, lost predominant interaction with monoclonal antibody and failed to bind to DNA cellulose. These data support the interrelationship between the DNA binding domain and the epitope for monoclonal antibody (10), and suggest that while the DNA-binding domain is located at one end of the receptor molecule, the hormone-binding site is distal to that end and can be effectively separated enzymatically. We know, however, that one effect of the hormone-receptor interaction is to produce an increase in both avian and mammalian receptors' apparent affinity for DNA (17,19). Thus, while the molecular domains are separable, filling of the hormone-binding site is capable of functionally modifying the DNA binding region of the $1,25(OH)_2D_3$ receptor. The search for an intact DNA-binding domain produced by trypsin has relied upon its reactivity, and thus detectability, with monoclonal antibody and a small polypeptide of 16,000 daltons with weak DNA-binding activity has been identified. However, it is likely that cleavage by other proteolytic enzymes may be necessary in order to produce a unique $1,25(OH)_2D_3$ receptor fragment with DNA-binding activity equivalent to that of the native $1,25(OH)_2D_3$ receptor.

Isolation of $1,25(OH)_2D_3$ Receptors Utilizing Positive Immunoselection:

Purification of the $1,25(OH)_2D_3$ receptor from avian intestine has been accomplished utilizing a combination of techniques such as gel filtration, ion exchange chromatography, and group-selective affinity chromatography on such media as DNA cellulose and blue dextran- and heparin-Sepharose (2,8). While these techniques have produced analytical amounts of $1,25(OH)_2D_3$ receptor of varying degrees of purity, the yields of receptor are extremely poor and proteolysis is a major problem. Moreover, the laboriousness of the protocols suggest that this approach will be of limited usefulness in isolating sufficient receptor for chemical characterization. On the other hand, positive immunoselection of $1,25(OH)_2D_3$ receptor from cytosol or high salt nuclear extracts, utilizing immobilized anti-1,25(OH)$_2$D$_3$ receptor monoclonal antibodies is highly efficient, rapid, and yields a protein sample highly enriched for 1,25(OH)$_2$D$_3$ receptor. Fig. 2 depicts the results of such purification, employing Sepharose derivatized with either the 9A7γ or 4A5γ monoclonal antibody. As seen in the left panel, both the A and B forms of the avian intestinal receptor can be visualized by Coomassie blue staining after isolation from nuclear extracts by the immunoaffinity supports, and inspection of the staining patterns would suggest purity in the range of 20-50%. Immunoblot analysis of a small fraction of that which was stained, which, due to its stringency, would be expected to detect only high affinity interactions under denaturing conditions, reveal reactivity in each case with only the A and B forms, and these forms exactly comigrate with those identified in cytosolic extracts. Furthermore, components of this protein mixture (not yet

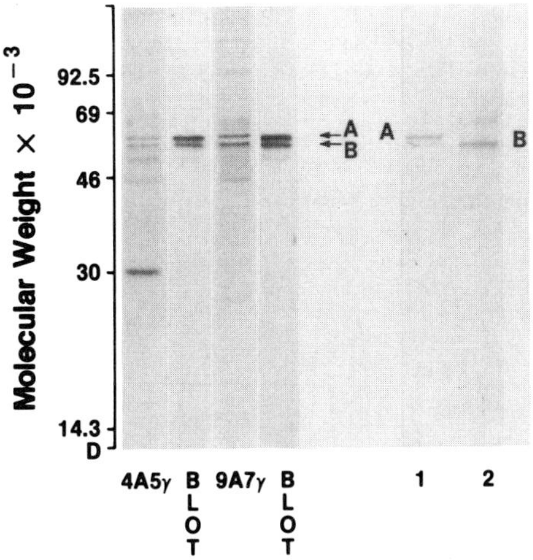

Fig. 2: Positive immunoselection of the chick 1,25(OH)$_2$D$_3$ receptor from 0.3 M KCl extracts of mucosal nuclei. Mucosa (6-8 grams) was homogenized in 10 mM of Tris-HCl, pH 7.5, 1 mM EDTA, and 5 mM DTT and the nuclear fraction collected by centrifugation. After two washes in the same buffer, the nuclear fraction was extracted in the above buffer containing KCl. Protein was shaken with either 9A7γ-Sepharose or 4A5γ-Sepharose (0.05 ml) overnight at 4°C, and the beads then collected and washed extensively in high salt containing 1.0% Triton X-100. Receptor was eluted with 3 M guanidine-HCl, precipitated and evaluated by SDS-PAGE. Left: "4A5γ" or "9A7γ" indicate resultant Coomassie stained proteins isolated by the monoclonal antibody derivatized to Sepharose and "Blot" indicates an immunoblot of a fraction of the sample. A and B indicate the two forms of the avian receptor. Right: Homogeneous isolation of A and B forms of the avian 1,25(OH)$_2$D$_3$ receptor (M_r = 60,300 and 58,600).

identified as A or B) have been shown to specifically bind $1,25(OH)_2[^3H]D_3$. As can be seen in the right panel of Fig. 2, both A and B can be isolated to homogeneity: polypeptide B is essentially pure, while form A is highly purified but often contaminated with a small portion of form B. This positive immunoselection procedure can also be utilized to isolate rat intestinal $1,25(OH)_2D_3$ receptors (data not shown), and promises to be extremely useful in the purification of preparative amounts of $1,25(OH)_2D_3$ receptor for chemical analyses.

Cellular Biology of the $1,25(OH)_2D_3$ Receptor:
The chick has been an excellent animal model from which great insight into $1,25(OH)_2D_3$ and its intracellular mechanism of action has been gained. Indeed, the $1,25(OH)_2D_3$ receptor was initially identified in the intestines of this species (20,21), and has been the receptor protein most extensively characterized. However, the identification of $1,25(OH)_2D_3$ receptors in a number of cultured mammalian cell lines has made it possible to study certain aspects of the cellular biology of the $1,25(OH)_2D_3$ receptor not possible in whole animal models. In this regard, we have pursued the mouse 3T6 fibroblast, which contains 15,000-20,000 molecules of receptor/ cell as a particular useful model system.

In suspense culture, 3T6 fibroblasts accumulate $1,25(OH)_2D_3$ with an internalization constant ($K_{int.}$) of approximately 6×10^{-10} M (17). The hormone

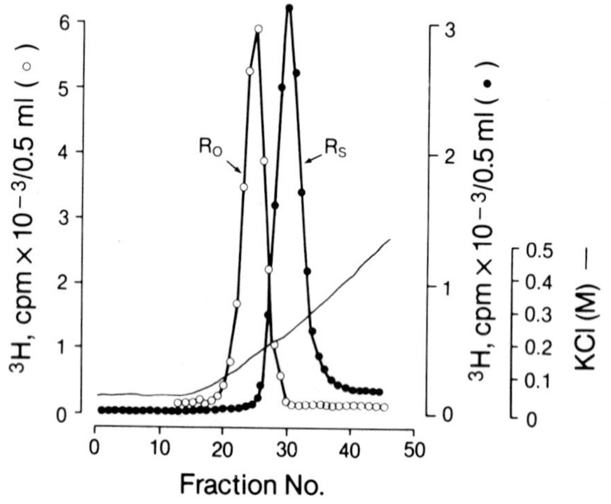

Fig. 3: Relative affinity of the 3T6 fibroblast $1,25(OH)_2D_3$ receptor for DNA. Unoccupied and in vivo occupied $1,25(OH)_2D_3$ receptors (17) were chromatographed on DNA cellulose and eluted during a linear gradient of KCl. Occupied receptor was estimated by direct radioactivity whereas unoccupied receptor was quantitated after incubation with $1,25(OH)_2[^3H]D_3$. R_o = unoccupied and R_s = occupied receptor.

can be identified associated with a protein which is bound to the nuclear fraction, sediments at 3.3S, and displays a molecular weight of 54,300 (Table 1). Its differential solubility (nuclear retention) as a function of occupancy by ligand, coupled with the observation that the unoccupied receptor elutes more readily than the $1,25(OH)_2[^3H]D_3$-receptor complex from DNA cellulose (Fig. 3), suggests that a primary effect of $1,25(OH)_2D_3$ on the macromolecule is to increase the protein's relative affinity for DNA. Employing immunoblot methodology, we have recently discovered that treatment of 3T6 cells in culture with 5 nM $1,25(OH)_2D_3$ causes not only increased receptor affinity for the subsequently isolated nuclear fraction, but that the in vivo occupied nuclear receptor has undergone covalant modification (22). Accordingly, the 3T6 receptor migrates electrophoretically under denaturing condition with an apparent molecular weight of 300-500 daltons greater than that of the unoccupied form. Incubation of monolayers of 3T6 cells with ^{35}S-methionine (in the presence or absence of $1,25(OH)_2D_3$) followed by immunoprecipitation of the internally labeled $1,25(OH)_2D_3$ receptor and then fluorography of the electrophoretically resolved precipitates also reveals an alteration in molecular mass as a function of $1,25(OH)_2D_3$. This modification is not apparent though in vitro formation of the $1,25(OH)_2D_3$ receptor complex, and is thus probably not a requirement for the receptor's increased affinity for DNA (the latter occurs regardless of the method by which receptors become occupied, i.e. in vivo or in vitro). The chemical nature of this modification remains unknown at present, although phosphorylation, acetylation, or nuclear ADP-ribosylation are viable possibilities, and can now be evaluated readily through the use of appropriately radiolabeled precursors and immunoprecipitation. It is likely that this modification of the 3T6 receptor may be an important key to its presently undefined function in the nucleus of target cells, although it could equally represent an inactivation signal.

Immunoblot methodology has also been utilized to examine the effect of $1,25(OH)_2D_3$ to autoregulate the concentration of its own receptor protein in 3T6 fibroblasts (23). Cells were treated in monolayer culture with 5nM $1,25(OH)_2D_3$ and the relative concentration of receptor in the nuclear fraction evaluated during the course of a 24 h exposure to hormone. Nuclear occupied receptor became evident within 1 h of $1,25(OH)_2D_3$ addition, and continued to increase substantially over the 24 h course of assay. This accumulation was not due to stabilization of nuclear receptor by $1,25(OH)_2D_3$ since cells treated with the protein synthesis inhibitor cycloheximide (20 μg/ml) revealed the appearance of nuclear receptor within 1 h of treatment, which reached a peak at 2 h and then began to slowly decline (nuclear inactivation?). Importantly, analogous results were obtained utilizing the transcriptional inhibitor actinomycin D (5 μM). While the details of this induction phenomenon need to be clarified, it seems likely that one biologic response of 3T6 fibroblasts to $1,25(OH)_2D_3$ appears to be the synthesis of increased receptor protein. Whether the $1,25(OH)_2D_3$ receptor complex directly regulates the expression of its own gene (autoregulation) or regulation is achieved through intermediate transcriptional events remains to be defined. Nevertheless, it is possible that in contrast to other factors which have been shown to regulate $1,25(OH)_2D_3$-binding activity, such as the glucocorticoids (24) or the retinoids (25), receptor regulation by $1,25(OH)_2D_3$ may represent an important facet of the molecular mechanism whereby $1,25(OH)_2D_3$ actually controls cellular biologic responses. Thus, increased receptor synthesis in the presence of $1,25(OH)_2D_3$ may serve to replenish receptors metabolically inactivated within the nucleus, and thereby maintain or enhance the response to $1,25(OH)_2D_3$.

These concepts are illustrated in Fig. 4, in which a model has been devised for the molecular mechanism of action of $1,25(OH)_2D_3$. The hormone diffuses into the cell and becomes bound to the $1,25(OH)_2D_3$ receptor, a protein which is either native to the nucleus or in equilibrium with that compartment. If the unoccupied receptor is bound to chromatin, then its interaction with the genome is modified and strengthened through hormonal ligand association by an as yet undefined molecular rearrangement which does not detectably alter its mass. Finally, prior to, because of, or during the course of specific DNA interaction, either as a functional modification or as an inactivation mechanism, the receptor becomes covalently altered. The biochemical result of these genome-receptor interactions is the altered synthesis of mRNAs which produce proteins active in cellular responsiveness. The concomitant induction of receptor mRNA, however, may serve to enhance or prolong the biologic action of

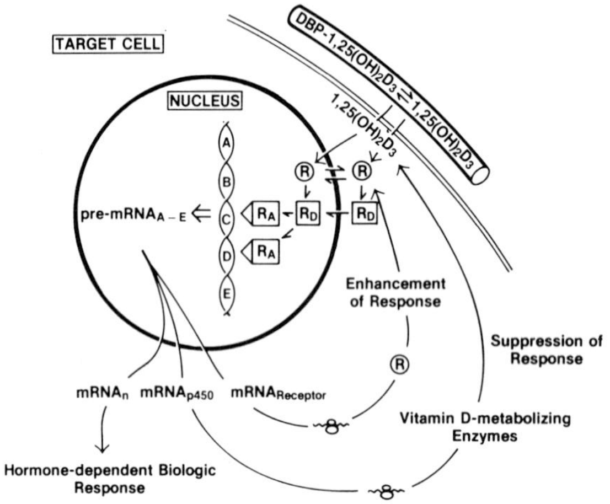

Fig. 4: Model for the mechanism of action of $1,25(OH)_2D_3$ in a typical mammalian target cell. R = $1,25(OH)_2D_3$ receptor; A-E = unique hormone-regulated genes.

$1,25(OH)_2D_3$ by acting as a positive feedback mechanism. Conversely, the $1,25(OH)_2D_3$-dependent induction of hormone-metabolizing enzymes common to many cells, such as the 25-hydroxyvitamin D_3-24-hydroxylase (26), may act as a compensatory mechanism to ultimately limit or suppress the effect of hormone on the cell.

Conclusions:
In conclusion, the immunologic approach to the study of $1,25(OH)_2D_3$ receptors, only several applications of which have been described in this chapter, holds promise in contributing to an eventual complete understanding of the mechanism of action of $1,25(OH)_2D_3$. Undoubtedly the most promising current avenues of research include elucidation of the chemical nature of pure $1,25(OH)_2D_3$ receptor, evaluation of the molecular arrangement of the polypeptide, an understanding of the receptor's biology, and the isolation of its natural gene. In all these ongoing pursuits, antibodies are proving essential as methodological reagents.

Acknowledgements:
This work is supported by National Institutes of Health grants AM-32313 and AM-34750 to JWP. I would like to also thank Ms. Noreen J. Sleator for technical assistance in several aspects of this work and Dr. M.R. Haussler for the use of laboratory facilities.

References:
1. Haussler,M.R.,McCain,T.A. (1977) N.Engl.J.Med.,297:974-983,1041-1050.
2. Pike,J.W.,Haussler,M.R. (1979) Proc.Natl.Acad.Sci.USA,76:5485-5489.
3. Greene,G.L.,Fitch,F.W.,Jensen,E.V. (1980) Proc.Natl.Acad.Sci.USA 77:157-161.
4. Edwards,D.P.,Weigel,N.L.,Schrader,W.T.,O'Malley,B.W.,McGuire,W.L. (1984) Biochemistry 23:4427-4435.
5. Zarucki-Schulz,T.,Kulomaa,M.S.,Headon,D.R.,Weigel,N.L.,Baez,M., Edwards,D.P.,McGuire,W.L., Schrader,W.T.,O'Malley,B.W. (1984) Proc. Natl.Acad.Sci.USA 81:6358-6362.
6. Meisfeld,R.,Okret,S.,Wikstrom,A.,Wrange,O.,Gustafsson,J-A,Yamamoto,K.R. (1984) Nature (London) 312:779-781.
7. Pike,J.W.,Donaldson,C.A.,Marion,S.L.,Haussler,M.R. (1982) Proc. Natl.Acad.Sci.USA 79:7719-7723.
8. Pike,J.W.,Marion,S.L.,Donaldson,C.A.,Haussler,M.R. (1983) J.Biol.Chem. 258:1289-1296.
9. Pike,J.W. (1983) J.Biol.Chem.259:1167-1173.
10. Pike,J.W.,Kelly,M.A.,Haussler,M.R. (1982) Biochem.Biophys.Res.Commun. 109:902-907.
11. Dokoh,S.,Haussler,M.R.,Pike,J.W. (1984) Biochem.J. 221:129-136.
12. Hunziker,W.,Walters,M.R.,Norman,A.W. (1980) J.Biol.Chem. 255:9534-9537.
13. Massaro,E.R.,Simpson,R.U.,DeLuca,H.F. (1983) Proc.Natl.Acad.Sci.USA 80:2549-2553.
14. Tobin,H.,Staehelin,T.,Gordon,H. (1979) Proc.Natl.Acad.Sci.USA 76:4350-4354.
15. Pike,J.W. (1985) J.Biol.Chem., under revision.
16. Laemmli,U.K. (1970) Nature (London) 227:680-685.
17. Pike,J.W.,Haussler,M.R. (1982) J.Biol.Chem. 258:8554-8560.

18. Allegretto,E.A.,Pike,J.W. (1985) J.Biol.Chem., under revision.
19. Hunziker,W.,Walters,M.R.,Bishop,J.E.,Norman,A.W. (1983) J.Biol.Chem. 258:8642-8648.
20. Haussler,M.R.,Norman,A.W. (1969) Proc.Nat.Acad.Sci.USA 62:155-162.
21. Brumbaugh,P.F.,Haussler,M.R. (1975) J.Biol.Chem. 250:1588-1594.
22. Pike,J.W. (1985) J.Biol.Chem., in preparation.
23. Pike,J.W. (1985) J.Biol.Chem., in preparation.
24. Chen,T.L.,Cone,C.M.,Morey-Holton,E.,Feldman,D. (1982) 257:13564-13569.
25. Petkovich,P.M.,Heersche,J.N.M.,Tinker,D.O.,Jones,G. (1984) J.Biol.Chem. 259:8274-8280.
26. Chandler,J.S.,Chandler,S.K.,Pike,J.W.,Haussler,M.R. (1984) J.Biol.Chem. 259:2214-2222.

RESISTANCE TO 1,25-DIHYDROXYCHOLECALCIFEROL IN MAN AND IN OTHER SPECIES

S.J. MARX, U.A LIBERMAN, C. EIL, D.A. DEGRANGE, AND M.M. BLIZIOTES

Mineral Metabolism Section, National Institute of Arthritis, Diabetes, and Digestive and Kidney Diseases, Bethesda, Md., U.S.A.

INTRODUCTION: GENERAL FEATURES OF THE $1,25(OH)_2D$ RESPONSE PATHWAY

$1,25(OH)_2D$ is a hormonally active seco-steroid with a mechanism of action analogous, in many if not all ways, to that of the true steroids. Through its interaction with nuclei of target cells, it controls a spectrum of responses. These responses can be divided into four categories (1): (1) transepithelial transport of minerals - this "classical" response to calciferols results in increased calcium flux into serum across intestinal mucosa, bone surface, and the renal tubules; (2) regulation of calciferol metabolism - $1,25(OH)_2D$ affects the concentrations (synthesis rate?) of 7-dehydrocholesterol in skin and of 25(OH)D, $1,25(OH)_2D$, and $24,25(OH)_2D$ in serum not to mention concentrations in serum for a host of additional oxidation products in this pathway; (3) regulation of peptide synthesis and secretion - effects on a small number of target peptides have been documented in vitro (collagen, osteocalcin, immunoglobulins, interleukin-2, and prolactin) but many others may be affected (insulin, etc); (4) inhibition of proliferation and stimulation of cell differentiation - this seems to be important in conversion of a macrophage-related stem cell to osteoclast or to other multinucleated giant cells and in maturation of skin and hair epithelium.

IN VIVO RESISTANCE TO $1,25(OH)_2D$: DEFINITION

We define resistance to $1,25(OH)_2D$ as a state where abnormally high concentrations of $1,25(OH)_2D$ are associated with a normal or even deficient response.

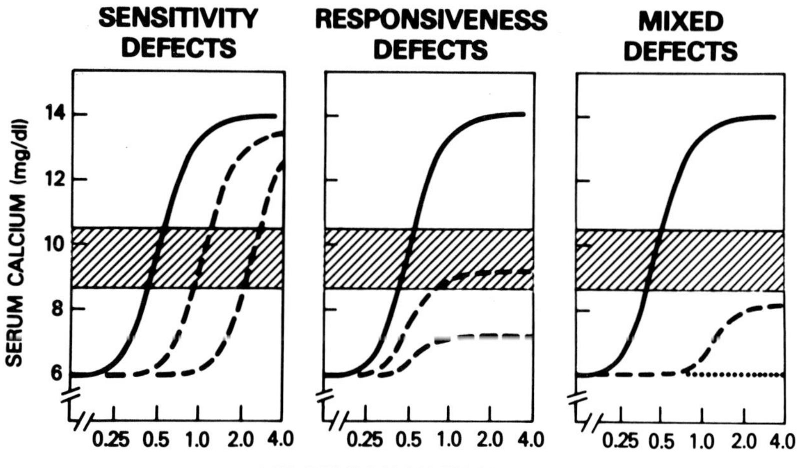

Figure 1. Variants in resistance of serum calcemic response to $1,25(OH)_2D_3$. Stippled zone indicates normal serum calcium; solid line is normal response (assuming baseline of $1,25(OH)_2D$ deficiency and constant calcium intake).

Though duodenal transport of calcium is a response of central importance in vivo, in clinical settings steady-state serum calcium and the simultaneous concentration of parathyroid hormone (PTH) are used as an index of this response. Resistance of serum calcium response to $1,25(OH)_2D$ can take several forms typefied by defects in maximal

Vitamin D. A Chemical, Biochemical and Clinical Update

response capacity, defects in response sensitivity, or mixed defects (this last includes lack of measurable response which cannot be assigned to the former two categories) (Figure 1) (1). Though the syndromes of hereditary resistance to $1,25(OH)_2D$ are diverse, they are all part of a single continuum; to date, there has not been evidence for selective resistance to single actions of $1,25(OH)_2D$.

ACQUIRED AND TEMPORARY RESISTANCE TO $1,25(OH)_2D$

Resistance caused by abnormal fluxes of calcium or phosphate to or from extracellular fluid: Our definition of resistance based upon the relation between calcium and $1,25(OH)_2D$ in serum incorporates several states in which serum concentrations of $1,25(OH)_2D$ rise to compensate or to attempt to compensate for large imbalances in fluxes of calcium (or even phosphate) (1). Examples of this include growing adolescents (such as the Bantu) with diets severely deficient in calcium, neonates (with rapidly mineralizing skeleton) who had been born prior to third trimester of gestation, and patients with renal wastage of calcium. Our definition also includes patients with selective wasting of phosphate by the kidney (2); these show hypophosphatemia, secondary elevation of $1,25(OH)_2D$, increased intestinal absorption of calcium, PTH suppression, and hypercalciuria. The secondary rise of $1,25(OH)_2D$ is in part maladaptive, and these patients, of course, benefit only from phosphate treatment; calciferols are not beneficial. All these groups are presumed to have normal target cell interactions in vivo with $1,25(OH)_2D$, and all but those with dietary calcium deficiency have normal response of intestinal calcium transport to $1,25(OH)_2D$; this highlights the problems inherent in our simplistic definition of resistance to $1,25(OH)_2D$ in vivo.

Acquired resistance to $1,25(OH)_2D$ in target cells: Cellular responsivity to $1,25(OH)_2D$ can be regulated in vivo. Tissue concentrations of $1,25(OH)_2D$ receptor are low in utero in the rat intestine but increase 2-3 weeks postpartum in association with development of $1,25(OH)_2D$-responsivity for intestinal transport of calcium (3). Glucocorticoids can regulate concentrations of $1,25(OH)_2D$ receptors; in the rat, glucocorticoids increase receptor concentrations, while in the mouse, glucocorticoids decrease them. In general $1,25(OH)_2D$ receptor concentrations are higher in dividing than in quiescent cells. It is highly probable that a host of factors will be shown to regulate responsivity to $1,25(OH)_2D$ at the level of the receptor and beyond it.

HEREDITARY RESISTANCE TO $1,25(OH)_2D$ IN MAN: CLINICAL SPECTRUM

The general features of resistance to $1,25(OH)_2D$ are rickets or osteomalacia, alopecia, hypocalcemia, secondary hyperparathyroidism, and high serum concentrations of $1,25(OH)_2D$ before or during treatment with calciferols. Each of these general features has shown a wide spectrum, but there are consistent correlations among all these features.

Serum calcium and calcemic response to calciferols: In the mildest forms of disease there is normocalcemia, mild secondary hyperparathyroidism, and mild elevation of $1,25(OH)_2D$ concentrations. Most reported cases, however, have had more severe dysfunction with hypocalcemia prior to treatment.

Approximately half of these cases have shown calcemic responses to high doses of calciferols (Figure 2); in some cases, even hypercalcemia has been provoked by vigorous therapy (Figure 2) (4). Some patients can respond satisfactorily to "natural" precursors of $1,25(OH)_2D$ (i.e. D_2 or $25(OH)D_3$), and serum $1,25(OH)_2D$ concentration as high as 19,000 pg/ml has been documented in a patient receiving 25(OH) D_3 (5). Other cases have remained hypocalcemic with high doses of calciferols (5); in some of these cases, patients have been judged to lack a calcemic response without having received sufficient therapeutic trials. An adequate trial must include (a) supplemental calcium by mouth, (b) a very high dose of a calciferol analog that insures maintenance of high serum concentrations of $1,25(OH)_2D$ (this can be accomplished by treatment with $1,25(OH)_2D_3$ or $1a(OH)D_3$ at doses in the range of 20-60 ug/day or by administering high doses of $1,25(OH)_2D$ precursors and documenting that repeated measurements of 1,25(OH)$_2$D are above 2000 pg/ml), and (c) a duration of therapy (about 3 months) sufficient to mineralize depleted bones and thus allow recovery from the hypocalcemia of "hungry bones". In patients without clear calcemic response to calciferols, some therapies remain promising. In cases with absent calcemic response to high doses of calciferols, provision of calcium alone (by oral administration of high dose - 2-4 grams elemental calcium per day) could ameliorate many disturbances.

Figure 2. Serum calcemic response as function of 1,25(OH)$_2$D dosage in patient 1B. Stippled zone indicates normal serum calcium; solid line is normal response (assuming baseline of 1,25(OH)$_2$D deficiency and constant calcium intake).

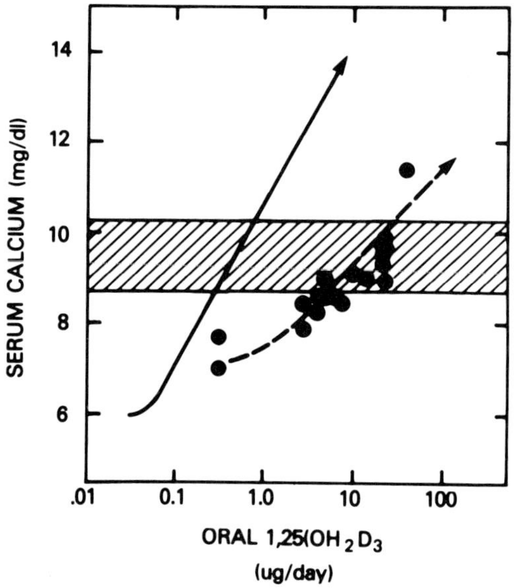

Several cases have shown suppression of secondary hyperparathyroidism, amelioration of hypophosphatemia, and improvement in radiographs despite continuation of hypocalcemia with high doses of calciferols (6). This could represent a direct action of calciferols on the kidney or the parathyroid gland independent of actions mediated through serum ionized calcium.

Age at presentation: The affected child appears normal at birth as fetal mineral homeostasis is determined largely by maternal concentrations of calcium and phosphate. It seems likely, however, that abnormalities in serum concentrations of 1,25(OH)$_2$D may be recognizable even in the first week of life. Most cases recognized to date have presented with rickets prior to age 3 years. When siblings have been followed prospectively, chemical disturbances have been evident prior to age 6 months. Some cases have not shown rickets, but have presented with osteomalacia as late as age 45 (7). All cases with late presentation have been normocalcemic, and they represent the mildest form of the disease.

Alopecia: Approximately half of reported cases have shown total alopecia or sparse hair. The alopecia can be present from birth, but typically hair is lost gradually between ages 3-6 months. Alopecia is a feature characteristic of the most severely affected patients; it is always associated with early age of presentation, and it is always present in patients with failure of calcemic response to calciferols. Conversely, all cases with apparently normal hair growth have shown satisfactory calcemic responses to calciferols (Figure 3B). Though some cases with alopecia have shown satisfactory calcemic responses to calciferols, none have shown improvement of hair growth. The clear association of alopecia with severe resistance to 1,25(OH)$_2$D indicates a role for this hormone in metabolism of the hair follicle.

Responses of calciferol metabolism enzymes: Concentrations of 25(OH)D or D in serum or 7-dehydrocholesterol in skin have not been analyzed closely in most cases. In one case there was an apparent deficiency of vitamin D 25-hydroxylase activity (8). Three types of abnormality have been documented in regulation of 1,25(OH) D (all presumably reflecting underlying abnormalities in 25(OH)D 1-alpha-hydroxylase activity). First, serum concentrations of 1,25(OH) D are generally high prior to and during therapy; this is attributable, only in part, to normal function of the parathyroid gland/1-hydroxylase axis. A second abnormality is that serum concentrations of 1,25(OH) D are usually disproportionally high considering the PTH concentration. This was most evident in a patient in remission during treatment with normal concentrations of calcium, phosphate, and PTH; brief administration of 25(OH)D resulted in endogenous generation of 1,25(OH) D concentrations of 2000 pg/ml (1). This suggested a deficiency of receptor mediated suppression of 1-hydroxylase activity. A third abnormality is that in some cases with all the usual activators of 1-hydroxylation functioning (i.e. high PTH and low phosphate in serum), serum concentrations of 1,25(OH) D have been normal or minimally elevated prior to therapy. While this phenomenon is not understood, it could result from the effects of severe hypocalcemia on the 1-hydroxylase system (9). One implication is that serum 1,25(OH) D prior to therapy is a poor predictor of the degree of underlying resistance to 1,25(OH) D (Figure 3A).

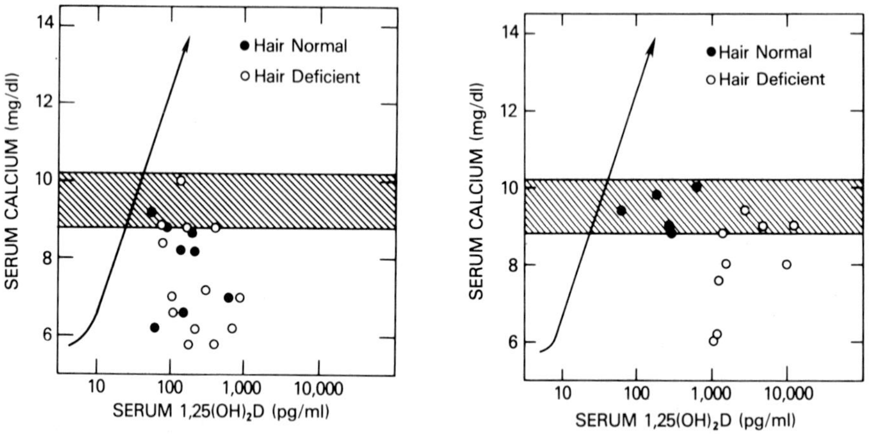

Figure 3. Serum calcium response as function of serum 1,25(OH) D. Stippled zone indicates normal serum calcium; solid line is normal response (assuming baseline of 1,25(OH) D deficiency and constant calcium intake). Each point represents one patient.
Left panel. Data obtained before administration of calciferol therapy.
Right panel. Data obtained during long-term administration of high doses of a calciferol. Plotted points represent maximal doses required without signs of toxicity.

Since 1,25(OH) D is a potent inducer of 25(OH)D 24-hydroxylase in vivo and in vitro, low serum concentrations of 24,25(OH) D might be predicted to arise from deficient function of 1,25(OH) D response mechanisms. Serum concentrations of 24,25(OH) D have generally been reported as normal. They have been low only in one case (10). However, low concentrations of 24,25(OH) D are, in fact, difficult to document as the techniques that have been applied to date have not insured that other cross-reacting metabolites had been eliminated completely.

Other possible target tissues: Hochberg and coworkers evaluated regulation of secretion of insulin, TSH, prolactin, growth hormone, and testosterone in six children with alopecia and resistance to $1,25(OH)_2D$ (11). They noted mild deficiencies in provoked secretion only of insulin and TSH, but these abnormalities were correctible by restoration of eucalcemia with calcium infusion.

Temporal variation in degree of resistance: With the indirect indices available, it is difficult to assess the possibility that general resistance may vary over time. For example, in several cases there has been striking radiographic improvement without therapy. We believe that the minimum criterion to support the possibility of a change in degree of resistance should be a clear change in the steady-state relation between $1,25(OH)_2D$ and calcium in serum without a causative change in calcium flux between serum and bone or between intestine and serum; thus a decrease of skeletal growth rate or an increase of oral calcium intake could easily result in confusion. Even with these caveats, at least one case has shown unexplained changes in degree of resistance to $1,25(OH)_2D$ (10). This patient, cited above as showing low concentrations of $24,25(OH)_2D$, showed a dramatic rise of serum calcium and a drop towards but not to normal of serum $1,25(OH)_2D$ concomitant with a period of therapy with $24,25(OH)_2D$.

PATTERNS OF CELLULAR DEFECTS WITH HEREDITARY RESISTANCE TO $1,25(OH)_2D$ IN MAN

Methodologic considerations: Hereditary defects in the $1,25(OH)_2D$ response pathway can be analyzed with cultured cells because of the near ubiquity of this response pathway. Cultured dermal fibroblasts can be used to assess most of the steps in hormone action from cellular uptake to induction of a bioresponse in cells. Below is a summary of the general techniques that have been applied.

a. Hormone uptake by intact cells. Intact cells in suspension are incubated with $[^3H]1,25(OH)_2D_3$ for 1 hour at 37 C, receptors are then extracted in a hypertonic lysing buffer, and bound and unbound hormone are then separated and measured (12).

b. Hormone binding with soluble extract. Cells are extracted with hypertonic KCl (0.3M); the supernate after centrifugation at 100,000 xg is termed soluble extract. On occasion, such soluble extracts have been called "cytosol"; this term is not accurate as the cellular location of unbound hormone receptors is not known and as hypertonic KCl can clearly extract receptors from all cell compartments including the nucleus. Soluble extract is incubated 15 hours at 4 C with graded concentrations of $[^3H]1,25(OH)_2D_3$; bound and unbound hormone are then separated and counted. The affinity and maximal capacity of hormone binding can then be derived (13).

c. Hormone localization to autologous nuclei. Dispersed cells are incubated at 37 C with $[^3H]1,25(OH)_2D_3$ for 45 minutes. The plasma membrane is dissolved with detergent and nucleus associated hormone is then measured. This assay is simultaneously an index of hormone binding to receptor, receptor sites for nuclear uptake, and cellular processes outside the receptor that help localize the receptor to the nucleus (14).

d. Receptor binding to nonspecific DNA. Occupied receptor is obtained by incubating soluble extract with $[^3H]1,25(OH)_2D_3$. This is then absorbed to DNA-cellulose and eluted with a linear gradient of KCl. Normal occupied receptors show high affinity for heterologous DNA (from calf thymus) and elute at approximately 0.22 M KCl (15).

e. $1,25(OH)_2D_3$ induction of $25(OH)D_3$ 24-hydroxylase activity (24-OHase). Cell monolayers are incubated with graded concentrations of $1,25(OH)_2D_3$ for 16 hours and then extensively washed; the wash procedure is critical because residual $1,25(OH)_2D_3$ at high concentration competes with $25(OH)D_3$ as an effective substrate for the 24-OHase enzyme. Cells are then dispersed or dispersed and homogenized and incubated with $[^3H]25(OH)D_3$. After brief incubation, $[^3H]24,25(OH)_2D_3$ is isolated and measured (16-18). The normal maximal response to $1,25(OH)_2D_3$ is at least 40-fold over baseline.

Heterogenous intracellular steps for defects in $1,25(OH)_2D_3$ interaction with cultured skin fibroblasts: There has been a striking heterogeneity in the cellular defects associated with hereditary resistance to $1,25(OH)_2D$ (Figure 4). We shall review published and unpublished studies; in many cases, not all relevant assays have been performed, while in others additional specialized techniques have been applied (ex: analysis of immunoreactive receptor in hormone binding negative cases).

1. Hormone binding negative. The commonest abnormality documented has been absence of detectable hormone binding with soluble extract. When nuclear localization of hormone has been tested, it too has been unmeasurable in these kindreds. With cell extracts from three of these kindreds, receptor was measured by immunoassay and cross-reacting protein was found in normal amounts; furthermore, the protein showed normal sedimentation in sucrose density gradient (19). This suggests that most, if not all, hormone binding negative mutants represent focal abnormalities in the hormone binding domain of the receptor and not receptor deletions.

2. Deficient hormone binding capacity. We have observed a binding capacity 10 percent of normal in two kindreds. In both there was a normal binding affinity. In one kindred, an identical deficiency in capacity for nuclear localization of hormone was documented (13).

3. Deficient hormone binding affinity. Two kindreds have shown 20- to 30-fold reductions in hormone binding affinity but a normal binding capacity with soluble extract (20).

4. Unmeasurable nucleus localization of hormone. With cells from two kindreds hormone binding to soluble extract was normal or near normal yet there was no detectable hormonal localization to the nucleus of intact cells. An identical defect was demonstrated with dermal fibroblasts and osteoblast-like cells cultured from bone of one patient (21).

5. Normal or nearly normal hormone localization to the nucleus. Four kindreds have shown this pattern (15, 16, 18). In three (two unpublished), receptor elution from DNA-cellulose was abnormal suggesting that the mutation involved the structure of a DNA binding domain of the receptor (15).

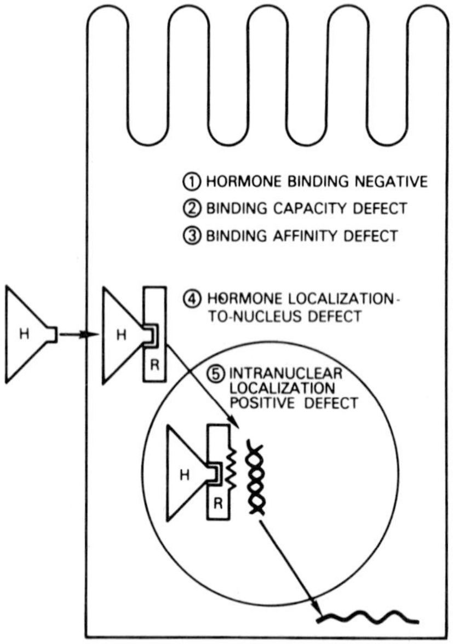

Figure 4. Five classes of defect in cellular interactions with $1,25(OH)_2D_3$ associated with hereditary resistance to $1,25(OH)_2D$. This is a pictorial formulation not intended to prejudge the issue over the normal location of unoccupied receptors and the question of whether some or all the mutations affect structure of the receptor.

<u>Relation of intracellular defect site to features in vivo</u>: The type of defect detected with fibroblasts has provided no uniform correlation with clinical features. For example, at least one patient with unmeasurable hormone binding to soluble extract showed a transient calcemic response to calciferols in vivo (we have speculated that a severe defect in affinity could account for these findings) (5). For another example, two kindreds showed

unmeasurable hormone localization to nucleus; however, both showed calcemic responses to high doses of calciferols (1). Lastly, normal or near normal hormone localization to the nucleus was associated with alopecia and no response to calciferols in two kindreds but with a calcemic response and no alopecia in another (16, 18). It seems likely that each type of defect can produce a spectrum of severity of clinical features. This leads to the prediction that some parameters showing incomplete deficiencies, such as hormone binding capacity or hormone binding affinity, should correlate with degrees of clinical abnormality. The number of cases evaluated has been too few to evaluate this. In one kindred a 90 percent deficiency in binding capacity was associated with failure of the calcemic response to calciferols; in another kindred a 20-fold decrease in binding affinity was associated with alopecia and a calcemic response to high doses of calciferols (5, 20).

Assessment of responses to calciferols in vitro: A wide spectrum of human cells is amenable to sampling for assessment of calciferol responsivity; it includes epidermal keratinocytes, circulating monocytes (differentiation and multinucleation response), B-lymphocytes (inhibition of proliferation and of immunoglobulin secretion), and T-lymphocytes (inhibition of proliferation and of interleukin-2 secretion). However, only dermal fibroblasts have been tested extensively.

The peak response of 24-hydroxylase in dermal fibroblasts (18) occurs after exposure to 10^{-7} M $1,25(OH)_2D_3$ (Figure 5); the half-maximal response occurs after exposure to 3×10^{-9} M

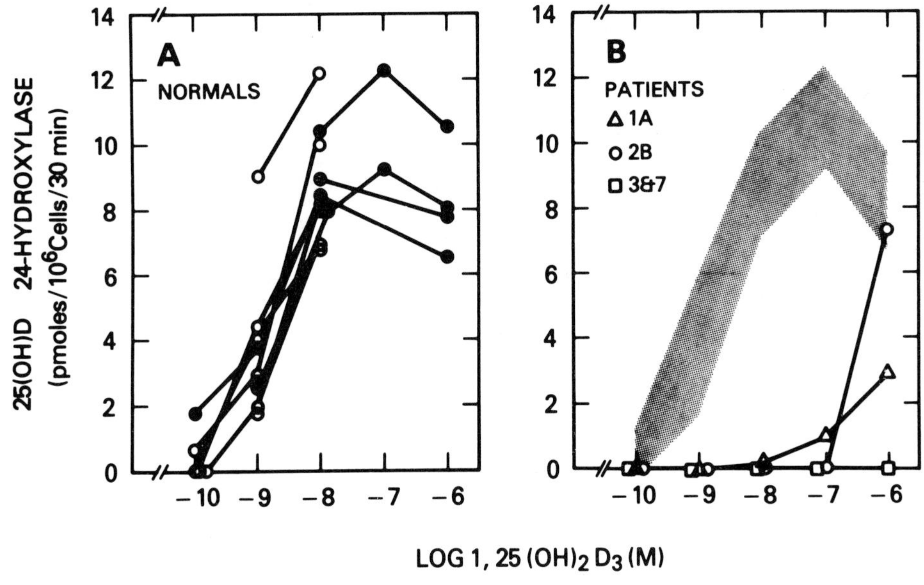

Figure 5. $25(OH)D_3$ 24-hydroxylase response to $1,25(OH)_2D_3$ in cultured dermal fibroblasts. Patients 1A and 2B both show normal hormone binding to soluble extract but unmeasurable hormone localization to nucleus. Both showed calcemic responses to high doses of $1,25(OH)_2D_3$ in vivo. Patients 3 and 7 both show normal hormone binding to soluble extract and 30-50% of normal hormone localization to nucleus. Neither showed a calcemic response to high doses of calciferols (18).

$1,25(OH)_2D_3$; and the minimal dose for a detectable response is 3×10^{-10}M. 24-hydroxylase induction by $1,25(OH)_2D_3$ has been abnormal in cells from every case of hereditary resistance to $1,25(OH)_2D$ tested to date. Our own studies have shown unmeasurable induction even at

10^{-6} M 1,25$(OH)_2D_3$ in two kindreds; in both kindreds there was no calcemic response to high doses of calciferols. We have found measurable induction in two other kindreds but at doses of 1,25$(OH)_2D_3$ 100-fold or higher than normal (Figure 5); in both of these kindreds, there were also calcemic responses to high doses of 1,25$(OH)_2D_3$ in vivo. Studies from other laboratories have confirmed this overall pattern with two kindreds showing responses in vivo and in vitro and four kindreds lacking responses in vivo and in vitro.

Hormonal inhibition of proliferation has also been tested as an index of bioresponse in cultured dermal fibroblasts (22). While, deficient response was documented in the one kindred tested, the normal response was too small for wide application.

TRANSMISSION AND GEOGRAPHY OF HEREDITARY RESISTANCE TO 1,25$(OH)_2$D IN MAN

In about half the kindreds reported to date, parental consanquinity has strongly suggested autosomal recessive inheritance. And no kindred data have been inconsistent with this mechanism. Parents have been reported as normal, but detailed studies have not been done. In several cases, subtle abnormalities have been suggested from analyses of skin fibroblasts from parents (17).

There has been a striking clustering of cases close to the Mediterranean (Figure 6). This clustering is true for kindreds showing all types of cellular defect; therefore, it is not simply a clustering of one mutation.

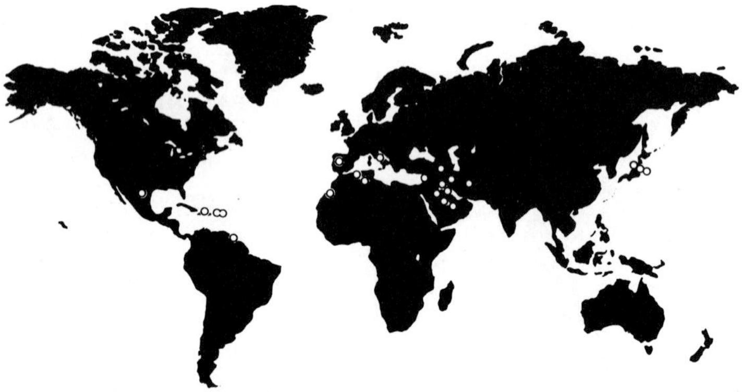

Figure 6. Geographic distribution of 22 kindreds with resistance to 1,25$(OH)_2$D based on published and unpublished data. Clustering about Mediterranean is evident; 3 kindreds from Puerto Rico and Mexico are Hispanic in origin.

The geographic clustering plus the suggestion of detectable changes with fibroblasts from heterozygotes suggest that the heterozygous state might confer some advantage to persons.

RESISTANCE TO 1,25$(OH)_2$D IN NEW WORLD PRIMATES

Osteomalacia associated with high concentrations of 1,25$(OH)_2$D has been reported in marmosets and tamarins (23), two closely related species of New World monkey. Furthermore, serum concentrations of 1,25(OH) D were found to be high in all members of the same species without osteomalacia (mean serum concentration in marmoset approximately 10-fold the human mean). Unusual features in metabolism of the true steroids have previously been studied among New World primates as compared to Old World primates, of which man is a member (24). The New World primates show higher serum concentrations of cortisol (by 20-fold for total hormone and by 100-fold for free hormone), aldosterone (by 2-fold), peak luteal phase progesterone (by 10-fold), and peak preovulatory estradiol (by 5-fold). This resistance has been associated with abnormalities in transport proteins and target receptors for these steroids. Whereas "resistance" to any one of these hormones has deleterious consequences or is undocumented (presumably lethal) in man, it is normal for these animals. With soluble extracts from B-lymphocytes transformed by Epstein-Barr virus, we have noted an 8-fold lower affinity for $1,25(OH)_2D_3$ in marmoset (Saguinus oedipus) than human (25); at the same time the marmoset cells also showed a 50% decrease in binding capacity for $1,25(OH)_2D_3$. To date there has been no satisfactory answer to the fascinating question of what beneficial role steroid or seco-steroid hormone resistance might have in natural selection of these animals. Resistance to $1,25(OH)_2D$ could cause tolerance or even dependence upon dietary components rich in bioactive calciferols; the recent recognition of glycosides of $1,25(OH)_2D$ in certain plants points to one potential source.

RESISTANCE TO $1,25(OH)_2D$ IN MUTANT CELL LINES

Kuribayashi et al have developed variant strains from HL-60 human promyelocytic leukemia cells (26). Cells from the parental strain show a dramatic differentiation towards mature macrophages after incubation with $1,25(OH)_2D_3$. As a component of this response, $1,25(OH)_2D_3$ also inhibits proliferation of these cells, and this feature has been used to select for cells not inhibited by $1,25(OH)_2D_3$ in cultures. Two variant cell strains were described. In each case $1,25(OH)_2D_3$ binding with soluble extract showed normal affinity but decreased capacity. In the parental strain, several classes of agents induce a similar program of differentiation; one variant strain showed selective deficiency of response to $1,25(OH)_2D_3$ while another showed global deficiency of response to all classes of inducer.

Kelley et al have documented a receptor variant in LLC-MK2 cells, derived from kidney of the rhesus (Macacca mulatta), an Old World monkey (27). In these cells, 24 hydroxylase induction showed the hormonal specificity expected for mediation by a $1,25(OH)_2D$ receptor but all analogs were required at 100-fold the doses required in control cells. While receptor could not be detected with standard radioligand techniques, it was demonstrable after purification with DNA-cellulose. Presumably, this is a low-affinity receptor. Our own studies of hormone binding with soluble extract from virus transformed B-lymphocytes of the stump-tailed macaque (Macacca arctoides), another Old World monkey, have shown normal (i.e., similar to human) affinity and capacity for $1,25(OH)_2D_3$, indicating that $1,25(OH)_2D_3$ binding in the LLC-MK2 strain is not representative of all non-human Old World primates (25).

CONCLUSIONS

Hereditary resistance to $1,25(OH)_2D$ in man shows a spectrum of features. The variable features including serum calcium (from severe hypocalcemia to normocalcemia), bone status (from infantile rickets to late onset osteomalacia), and hair growth (from absent to apparently normal) form a continuum with direct correlation among these features.

Analyses of cultured dermal fibroblasts allow recognition of intracellular steps in which genes determining 1,25(OH) D interactions are abnormal. At least five classes of mutation have been identified. Each might reflect modification of a separate functional domain of the receptor for $1,25(OH)_2D$. However, some could result from mutations outside the receptor gene. There are good correlations between deficiencies in responsivity to high doses of calciferols in vivo versus in vitro (measured by induction of $25(OH)D_3$ 24-hydroxylase). The features in vivo and in cultured fibroblasts suggest that the defective gene(s) determine the $1,25(OH)_2D$ effector pathway similarly in all target tissues.

"Resistance" to $1,25(OH)_2D$ is a feature of normal marmosets and is associated with abnormal hormone binding to the 1,25(OH) D receptor. Since these animals also show resistance to the true steroids, some events during evolution favored a coordinated modification of effector pathways for these structurally related hormones. The geographic clustering about the Mediterranean for all classes of mutation causing resistance to 1,25(OH) D in man also suggests some evolutionary advantage for the heterozygote.

REFERENCES

1. Marx S.J., Liberman U.A., Eil C., Gamblin G.T., deGrange D.A., Balsan S. (1984) Rec. Prog. Horm. Res. 40: 589-615.
2. Tieder M., Modai D., Samuel R., Arie R., Halabe A., Bab I., Gabizon D., Liberman U.A. (1985) N. Eng. J. Med. 312: 611-616.
3. Halloran B.P., DeLuca H.F. (1981) J. Biol. Chem. 256: 7338-7342.
4. Marx S.J., Swart E.G., Hamstra A.J., DeLuca H.F. (1980) J. Clin. Endocrinol. Metab. 51: 1138-1142.
5. Balsan S., Garabedian M., Liberman U.A., Eil C., Bourdeau A., Guilloza H., Grimberg R., LeDeunff M.J., Lieberherr M., Guimbaud P., Broyer M., Marx S.J. (1983) J. Clin. Endocrinol. Metab. 57: 803-811.
6. Hochberg Z., Benderli A., Levy J., Vardi P., Weisman Y., Chen T., Feldman D. (1984) Am. J. Med. 77: 805-811.
7. Fujita T., Nomura M., Okajima S., Furuya H. (1980) 50: 927-931.
8. Zerwekh J.E., Glass K., Jowsey J., Pak C.Y.C. (1979) J. Clin. Endocrinol. Metab. 49: 171-175.
9. Tanaka Y., DeLuca H.F. (1983) Biochem. J. 214: 893-897.
10. Liberman U.A., Samuel R., Halabe A., Kauli R., Edelstein S., Weisman Y., Papapoulos S.E. Clemens T.L., Fraher L.J., O'Riordan J.L.H. (1980) Lancet I: 504-507.
11. Hochberg Z., Borochowitz Z., Benderli A., Vardi P., Oren S., Spirer Z., Heyman I., Weisman Y. (1985) J. Clin. Endocrinol. Metab. 60: 57-61.
12. Adams J.S., Gacad M.A., Singer F.R. (1984) J. Clin. Endocrinol. Metab. 59: 556-560.
13. Liberman U.A., Eil C., Marx S.J. (1983) J. Clin. Investig. 71: 192-200.
14. Eil C., Marx S.J. (1981) Proc. Nat. Acad. Sci. 78: 2562-2566.
15. Hirst M., Hochman H., Feldman D. (1985) J. Clin. Endocrinol. Metab. 60: 490-495.
16. Griffin J.E., Zerwekh, J.E. (1983) J. Clin. Invest. 72: 1190-1199.
17. Chen T.L., Hirst M.A., Cone C.M., Hochberg Z., Tietze H.U., Feldman D. (1984) J. Clin. Endocrinol. Metab. 59: 383-388.
18. Gamblin G.T., Liberman U.A., Eil C., Downs R.W. Jr., deGrange D.A., Marx S.J. (1985) J. Clin. Invest. In press.
19. Pike J.W., Dokoh S., Haussler M.R., Liberman U.A., Marx S.J., Eil C. (1984) Science 224: 879-891.
20. Castells S., Greig F., Fusi M., Finberg L., Yasumura S., Liberman U.A., Eil C., Marx S. (1984) Pediat. Res. 18: 291E.
21. Liberman U.A., Eil C., Holst P., Rosen J.F., Marx S.J. (1983) J. Clin. Endocrinol. Metab. 57: 958-961.
22. Clemens T.L., Adams J.S., Horiuchi N., Gilchrist B.A., Cho H., Tsuchiya Y., Matsuo N., Suda T., Holick M.F. (1983) J. Clin. Endocrinol. Metab. 56: 824-830.
23. Shinki T., Shiina Y., Takahashi N., Tanioka Y., Koizumi H., Suda T. (1983) Biochem. Biophys. Res. Comm. 114: 452-457.
24. Lipsett M.B., Chrousos G.P., Tomita M., Brandon D.D., Loriaux D.L. (1985) Rec. Prog. Horm. Res. In press.
25. Liberman U.A., deGrange D.A., Marx S.J. (1985) FEBS Lett In press.
26. Kuribayashi T., Tanaka H., Abe E., Suda T. (1983) Endocrinol. 113: 1992-1998.
27. Kelly M.A., Marion S.L., Donaldson C.A., Pike J.W., Haussler M.R. (1985) J. Biol. Chem. 260: 1545-1549.

ADMINISTRATION OF 1,25DIHYDROXYVITAMIN D_3 RESULTS IN INCREASED CHOLINE ACETYLTRANSFERASE ACTIVITY IN SPECIFIC BRAIN NUCLEI

J. SONNENBERG†, V. N. LUINE, L. KREY and S. CHRISTAKOS†

Department of Biochemistry, UMDNJ-New Jersey Medical School, Newark, NJ and Department of Neuroendocrinology, The Rockefeller University, New York, NY USA

Introduction

Gonadal and adrenal steroid hormones at specific brain target sites, have been shown to alter a number of neural proteins, including choline acetyltransferase (CAT) and monamine oxidase (MAO). It has been suggested that these hormone dependent enzyme changes alter neurotransmitter levels and turnover. In a recent autoradiographic study, receptors for 1,25dihydroxyvitamin D_3 (1,25$(OH)_2D_3$) have been localized in discrete brain nuclei (Stumpf and DeLuca (1982) Science 215, 1403). In this study, we have considered whether 1,25$(OH)_2D_3$ might also effect levels of specific brain proteins.

Results

The nuclei sampled were those in which receptors for 1,25$(OH)_2D_3$ and/or vitamin D dependent calcium binding protein have been localized (Fig. 1).

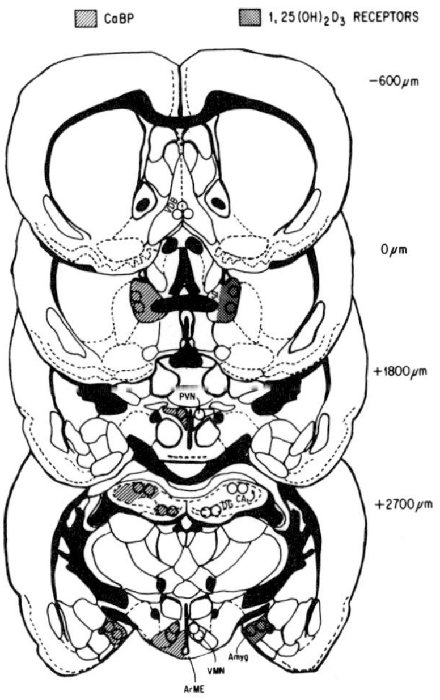

Fig. 1. Localization of nuclei samples. All nuclei were reported to possess receptors for 1,25$(OH)_2D_3$ and/or CaBP. Abbreviations are as follows: A-ME, arcuate nucleus and median eminence; Amyg, medial amygdaloid nucleus; CA_1, CA of the hippocampus; DG, dentate gyrus; PVN, paraventricular nucleus; St, bed nucleus of the stria terminalis.

Vitamin D. A Chemical, Biochemical and Clinical Update

In vitamin D replete male rats, significant elevations in CAT were observed in the bed nucleus of the stria terminalis (St), which has the strongest nuclear concentration of $1,25(OH)_2D_3$ binding, and in the arcuate median eminence (A-ME) which receives projections from the bed nucleus. Rats were made vitamin D replete by 8 daily intraperitoneal injections of 100 or 200 ng $1,25(OH)_2D_3$ as well as by constant intraventricular infusion (i.v.i.) by ALZET minipump of 25 ng $1,25(OH)_2D_3$ for 7 days. The percent increase ranged from 12-45% and was related to the i.p. dose administered (Fig. 2).

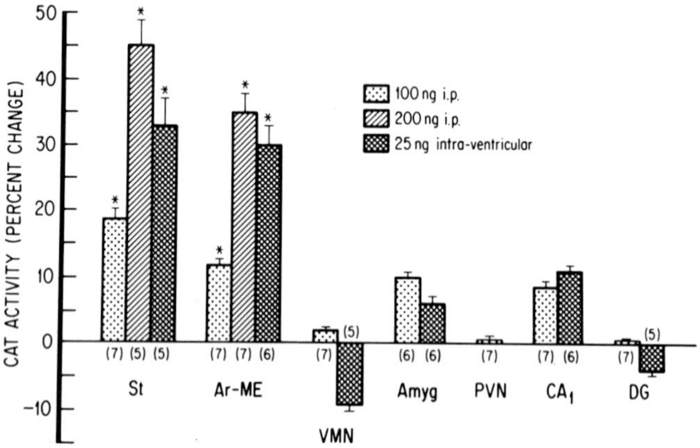

Fig. 2. Effect of $1,25(OH)_2D_3$ administration on CAT activity in discrete brain nuclei. Activity is expressed as the percent change in the $1,25(OH)_2D_3$ treated rats compared to vitamin D deficient controls. Data are presented as mean ± SE. The numbers in parentheses represent the number of determinations. Data was analyzed by student's t test where $p < 0.05$.

Constant i.v.i. of 2 mM Ca^{++} or 125 ng $25(OH)D_3$/day for 7 days did not alter CAT activity (data not shown). No significant changes in MAO were observed with vitamin D repletion. Since the A-ME of the hypothalamus is an important regulatory site in the neuroendocrine axis, serum testosterone was measured by RIA. Serum testosterone was significantly increased 2-5 fold ($p < 0.05$) in rats made vitamin D replete by constant i.v.i. of 25 ng $1,25(OH)_2D_3$ or by i.p. injection of 100 or 200 ng $1,25(OH)_2D_3$. Administration of testosterone to gonadectomized male rats does not similarly alter CAT activity in these nuclei (Muth et al. (1980) Neuroendo. 30, 329). Our results suggest for the first time, that $1,25(OH)_2D_3$ may effect cholinergic activity in discrete brain regions and that $1,25(OH)_2D_3$ may play a role in the regulation of certain neurohormones.

COMPARISON OF CELLULAR AND SUBCELLULAR DISTRIBUTION OF VITAMIN D METABOLITES [1,25(OH)$_2$ VITAMIN D$_3$, 24,25(OH)$_2$ VITAMIN D$_3$, 25(OH) VITAMIN D$_3$] IN TARGET TISSUES.

W.E. Stumpf, S.A. Clark, Y.S. Kim and H.F. DeLuca
Departments of Anatomy and Pharmacology, University of North Carolina, Chapel Hill, NC 27514 and Department of Biochemistry, University of Wisconsin, Madison, WI 53706, USA.

Introduction

The question, whether or not 25(OH) vitamin D$_3$ and 24,25(OH)$_2$ vitamin D$_3$ are steroid hormones similar to 1,25 (OH)$_2$ vitamin D$_3$ can be studied by autoradiography with radiolabeled compounds and competition with unlabeled compounds. Autoradiography, as developed in our laboratory, has been used as a probe to identify and characterize target cells with nuclear concentration and retention of ^{3}H 1,25 (OH)$_2$ vitamin D$_3$, including B cells of pancreatic islets, thyrotropes and pituicytes in the pituitary, certain neurons in defined brain regions, pyloric muscle, parenchymal cells of the parathyroid, epithelial cells of mammary glands, cells in the placenta and yolk sack, osteoblasts, stomach endocrine cells, cells in the epidermis and hair shaft, dental pulp cells, certain fibroblasts, epithelium of esophagus, podocytes in the kidney, and others (1-12). Many of these newly discovered cell types have since been confirmed to contain nuclear receptors, although biochemical confirmation is still lacking for tissues which are difficult to isolate. The advantage of the sensitivity and resolution of autoradiography, which leaves the tissue structure relatively intact, has been utilized in order to answer the question about the presence or absence of nuclear target sites for these metabolites of vitamin D$_3$.

Methods

Sprague Dawley rats young adult male and female, pregnant rats at day 18 and 20, neonatal rats 9-hour, 2½-day, and 6-day old, were kept under conditions of vitamin D-deficient diet, injected intraperitoneally with 0.1 to 0.5 ug/100g bw of ^{3}H 1,25(OH)$_2$ vitamin D$_3$, ^{3}H 25(OH) vitamin D$_3$ or ^{3}H 24,25(OH)$_2$ vitamin D$_3$ (spec. act. 160 Ci/mM), and sacrificed 2-4 hours afterwards. In addition, unlabeled metabolites, identical to or different from the labeled compound, were injected in excess prior to the labeled compound, in order to obtain evidence for or against specificity. The labeled compounds were purified and provided by the laboratory of Dr. DeLuca (Madison, WI). Autoradiograms were prepared by our thaw-mount autoradiographic procedure, which excludes or minimized diffusion and redistribution of tissue constitutents.

Results

Autoradiograms with ^{3}H 1,25 (OH)$_2$ vitamin D$_3$ showed typical nuclear concentration in the target tissues listed. This nuclear concentration was blocked, when unlabeled 1,25 (OH)$_2$ vitamin D$_3$ was injected in excess prior to the labeled hormone. No such effect was seen with unlabeled 25 (OH) vitamin D$_3$ or 24,25 (OH)$_2$ vitamin D$_3$. Autoradiograms with ^{3}H 25(OH) vitamin D$_3$ or with ^{3}H 24,25 (OH)$_2$ vitamin D$_3$ did not show nuclear concentration

Vitamin D. A Chemical, Biochemical and Clinical Update

in the tissues studied, which include fetal and neonatal bone, cartilage, intestine, skin, oral epithelium, teeth and kidney. With ^3H 25 (OH) vitamin D_3 as well as with ^3H 24,25 $(OH)_2$ vitamin D_3, accumulation of radioactivity was seen, however, in the apical cytoplasm of epithelial cells of kidney proximal tubules. Pretreatment with excess unlabeled metabolite, 25(OH) vitamin D_3 or 24,25 $(OH)_2$ vitamin D_3, did not prevent this cytoplasmic uptake of radioactivity.

Conclusions

The autoadiographic data obtained indicate the presence of nuclear receptors for 1,25 $(OH)_2$ vitamin D_3, but absence of nuclear binding for 25 (OH) vitamin D_3 and 24,25 (OH) vitamin D_3 in tissues identified as genomic target tissues for 1,25 $(OH)_2$ vitamin D_3.

References

1. Stumpf, W.E., Sar, M., Reid, F.A., Tanaka, Y. and DeLuca, H.F. (1979) Science 206: 1188-1190.
2. Stumpf, W.E., Sar, M., Narbaitz, R., Reid, F.A., Deluca, H.F. and Tanaka, Y. (1980) PNAS 77: 1149-1153.
3. Sar, M., Stumpf, W.E. and DeLuca, H.F. (1980) Cell Tiss. Res. 209: 161-166.
4. Narbaitz, R., Stumpf, W.E., Sar, M., DeLuca, H.F. and Tanaka, Y. (1980) Gen. Comp. Endocrin. 42: 283-289.
5. Stumpf, W.E., Sar, M., Clark, S.A., Lieth, E. and DeLuca, H.F. (1980) Neuroendocrin. Lett. 2: 297-301.
6. Esvelt, R.P., DeLuca, H.F., Wichmann, J.K., Yoshizawa, S., Zurcher, J., Sar, M. and Stumpf, W.E. (1980) Biochemistry 19: 6158-6161.
7. Clark, S.A., Stumpf, W.E., Sar, M., DeLuca, H.F. and Tanaka, Y. (1980) Cell Tiss. Res. 209: 515-520.
8. Narbaitz, R., Stumpf, W.E. and Sar, M. (1981) J. Histochem. Cytochem. 29: 91-100.
9. Stumpf, W.E., Sar, M. and DeLuca, H.F. (1981) in Hormonal Control of Calcium Metabolism, Eds. D.V. Cohn, R.V. Talmage and J.L. Matthews Jr., pp. 222-229, Excerpta Medica, Amsterdam.
10. Sar, M., Miller, W.L. and Stumpf, W.E. (1981) Physiologist 24: 70.
11. Clark, S.A., Stumpf, W.E. and Sar, M. (1981) Diabetes 30: 382-386.
12. Chertow, B.S., Clark, S.A., Baranetsky, N.G., Sivitz, W.I., Stumpf, W.E. and Waite, A.T. (1981) Clin. Res. 29: 402A.
13. Stumpf, W.E., Sar, M., Reid, F.A., Huang, S., Narbaitz, R. and DeLuca, H.F. (1981) Cell Tiss. Res. 221: 333-338.
14. Narbaitz, R., Sar, M., Stumpf, W.E., Huang, S. and DeLuca, H.F. (1981) Horm. Res. 15: 263-270.
15. Narbaitz, R., Stumpf, W.E., Sar, M. and DeLuca, H.F. (1982) Acta Anatomica 112: 208-217.
16. Stumpf, W.E., Sar, M., Clark, S.A. and DeLuca, H.F. (1982) Science 215: 1403-1405.
17. Kim, Y.S., Stumpf, W.E., Clark, S.A., Sar, M. and DeLuca, H.F. (1983) J. Dent. Res. 62: 58-59.
18. Narbaitz, R., Stumpf, W.E., Sar, M., Huang, S. and DeLuca, H.F. (1983) Calcif. Tiss. Int. 35: 177-182.

EFFECT OF VITAMIN D DEFICIENCY AND SUPPLEMENT ON PTH DEGRADATION BY THE KIDNEY

T. FUJITA, H. BABA, M. FUKASE, M. SASE, M. FUKUSHIMA AND Y. NISHII.

Third Division, Department of Medicine, Kobe University School of Medicine, Kobe and Chugai Research Institute, Tokyo, Japan.

INTRODUCTION:

Parathyroid hormone (PTH), the main physiological controlling agent for renal 1α-hydroxylation of 25(OH) vitamin D_3, is known to be degraded by at least 5 different enzymes[1-5] including cathepsin B and D[6] and ATP-activated membrane bound enzyme reported by Botti et al.[7]. Since PTH and vitamin D form a close functional circuit, it is quite possible that vitamin D status of the organism influences PTH degradation as well as its secretion. Since new enzymes with activity of limited hydrolysis of PTH were found in the supernatant fractions of rat kidney[8], attempts were made to define the effect of vitamin D deficiency and supplements on PTHase activities in the kidney supernatant.

MATERIALS AND METHODS:

Rat renal cortex was minced and homogenized in 8 volumes of 0.45M sucrose containing 0.68mM EDTA pH 7.0, centrifuged at 3000 r.p.m. for 10 minutes, followed by recentrifugation of the supernatant at 40,000 r.p.m. (100,000 × g) for 60 minutes. PTHase activity was measured by incubating 0.4 ml 0.1 M Tris-HCl (pH 6-10), 0.5 ml H_2O and 50 μl sample or buffer with 0.5 μg TCA PTH at 37°C for 10 minutes. At the end of the incubation, 1 ml 10 % TCA and 50 μl 10 % BSA was added. After centrifugation for 10 minutes at 3000 r.p.m. the supernatant was treated with ether and the aqueous layer was subjected to radioimmunoassay for PTH using Sorin Kit. Since original intact PTH was completely precipitated by 10 % TCA, PTH-like immunoreactivity in the TCA-supernatant indicating the amount of fragments as the product of limited hydrolysis of PTH could be used as the index for PTHase activity. PTHase activity with optimal pH at 4.0, 7.3 and 9.0 was found. Vitamin D deficient Spraque-Dawley rats were placed on normal calcium vitamin D deficient diet from the 4th to 9th week after birth, and divided into 4 groups. In the first group, low calcium, vitamin D dificient diet alone was given in the 9th week, with addition of 1α(OH)VD_3 in the 2nd 1α25$(OH)_2VD_3$ in the 3rd group, 4th normal control group received ordinary diet throughout.

RESULTS:

As shown in Fig. 1, PTHase activity at pH 7.3 rose significantly in vitamin D deficiency. Supplement with 0.25 μg/kg 1α(OH) vitamin D_3 did not decrease the PTHase activity but the same dose of 1α25$(OH)_2$vitamin D_3 tended to decrease it towards the control level. PTHase activity at pH 4.5 and 9.0 did not change.

SUMMARY AND CONCLUSION:

PTHase activity at pH 7.3 in the 100,000 × g supernatant of rat kidney increased significantly in vitamin D deficient

Vitamin D. A Chemical, Biochemical and Clinical Update

rat and was restored towards normal by $1\alpha25(OH)_2$ VD_3 supplement, but PTHase activities at pH 4.5 and 9.0 did not change. PTHase with pH optimum at 7.3 might be involved in the functional control of PTH-$1\alpha25(OH)_2$VD-axis. Although nothing is known about the physiological significance of this enzyme, the PTHase could be facilitating PTH action by activation instead of inhibiting it by degradation, since its activity is augmented on the need of more PTH activity.

REFERENCES:

1. Orimo, H., Fujita, T., Morii, H., Nakao, K. (1965) Endocrinology 76:255-258.
2. Orimo, H., Fujita, T., Yoshikawa, M., Morii, H., Nakao, K. (1965) Endocrinology 77:428-432.
3. Fujita, T., Ohata, M., Orimo, H., Yoshikawa, M., Maruyama, M. (1969) Endocrinologia Japonica 16:383-389.
4. Fujita, T., Orimo, H., Ohata, M., Yoshikawa, M., Maruyama, M. (1970) Endocrinoly 86:42-49.
5. Maruyama, M., Fujita, T., Ohata, M. (1970) Archives of Biochemistry and Biophysics 38:245-253.
6. Hamilton, J.W., Jilka, R.L., MacGregor, R.R. (1983) Endocrinology 113:285-292.
7. Botti, R.E., Heath, E., Frelinger, A.L., Chuang, J., Roos, B.A., Zull, J.E. (1981) J. Biol. Chem. 256:11483-11488.
8. Fujita, T., Baba, H., Yoshimoto, Y., Fukase, M., Kishihara, M., Tomon, M., Fukami, T., Imai, Y., Nishii, Y., Fukushima, M. (1984) Endocrine Control of Bone and Calcium Metabolism p238-241.

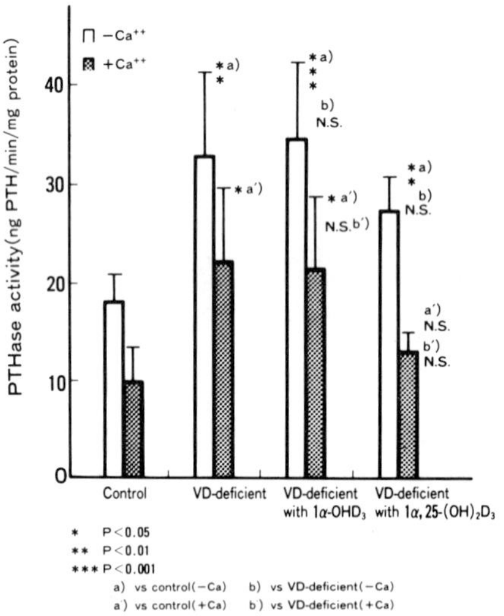

Figure 1. Effect of vitamin D deplention and repletion on PTHase activity at pH 7.3 in rat kidney supernatant fraction.

IN VITRO STABILITY OF THE CALF THYMUS 1,25-DIHYDROXYVITAMIN D_3 RECEPTOR

T. Koskinen and M. Hahl, Department of Clinical Sciences, University of Tampere, P.O. Box 607, SF-33101 Tampere, Finland

Although receptors for $1,25(OH)_2D_3$ have been demonstrated almost ubiquitously in tissues, the biochemical properties of only that from chick intestine have been studied in detail. This is mainly due to the low levels of the receptor in most tissues, as well as to its instability in vitro. Reinhardt et al. (1) have shown that calf thymus contains significant amounts of a $1,25(OH)_2D_3$ receptor. The good availability of thymus tissue suggests several possibilities for the use of this receptor in further studies. The purpose of the present study was to characterize its stability in various in vitro conditions.

Materials and methods

Ammonium sulfate-precipitated receptor pellets were prepared (1) from the thymus tissue of 6-week-old calves. The homogenization buffer contained 50 mM Tris-HCl, 500 mM KCl, 5 mM DTT, 10 mM Na_2MoO_4 and 1.5 mM EDTA, pH 7.5 (TKEDMo buffer). The pellets were redissolved (0.8-3 mg protein/ml); a) in TKEDMo buffer, and incubated at various temperatures; b) in TKEDMo buffer, pH 4.5-12.7, and incubated at +25°C for 1 h; c) in modified TKEDMo buffer (KCl 0-500 mM, DTT 0-5 mM, Na_2MoO_4 0-10 mM), and preincubated for 1 h at +25°C. In a) and b), the incubation mixture contained labeled $1,25(OH)_2D_3$ with and without excess nonradioactive $1,25(OH)_2D_3$; in c) the ligands were added after the preincubation followed by further incubation at +25°C for 1 h. Bound and free sterols were separated with dextran-coated charcoal. The precentage of specific binding from total was calculated.

Results and discussion

The calf thymus $1,25(OH)_2D_3$ receptor was found to be very stable at 0°C and +4°C: no loss of specific binding occurred between 2 h and 48 h (Fig. 1). At +25°C the binding activity declined between 7 to 24 h, while it was rapidly lost at +37°C. The pH optimum of the receptor was at pH 7.7, and good stability was observed at the pH range 7-10 (Fig. 2). Outside this range the specific binding was quickly destroyed.

Vitamin D. A Chemical, Biochemical and Clinical Update

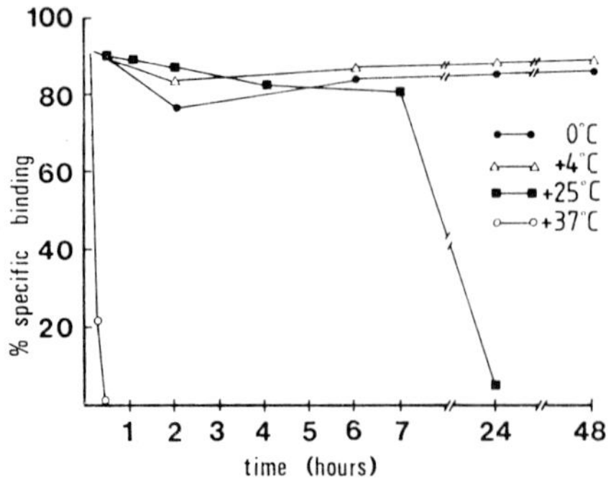

Fig. 1. The effect of temperature and duration of incubation on $1,25(OH)_2D_3$ specific binding.

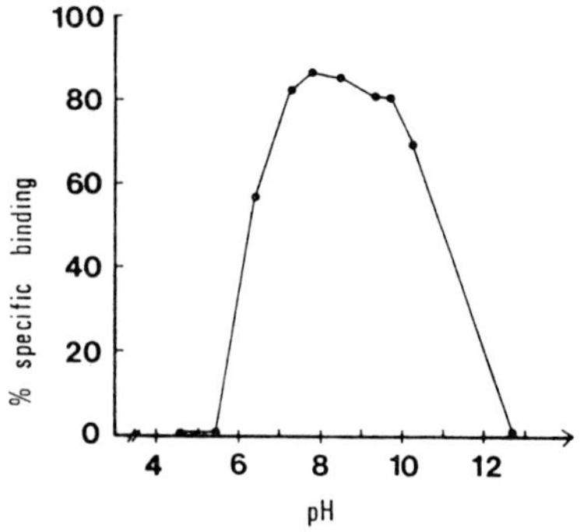

Fig. 2. The effect of pH on $1,25(OH)_2D_3$ specific binding.

There were no dramatic changes in the stability of the receptor caused by various KCl, molybdate or DTT concentrations (data not shown). The specific binding was about 88 % even without DTT in preincubation buffer, which indicates that a sulfhydryl moiety may not be very crucial in the stability of the thymus receptor.

The receptor was quite stable in conditions which could be used in its purification. Neither is its stability a problem in the recently described assay of serum $1,25(OH)_2D$ (2). The properties of the calf thymus receptor contrast with those reported for the chick intestinal receptor, which appears to be easily denatured (3).

References

1. Reinhardt, T.A., Horst, R.L., Littledike, E.T. and Beitz, D.C. (1982) Biochem. Biophys. Res. Commun. 106, 1012-1018.
2. Reinhardt, T.A., Horst, R.L., Orf, J.W. and Hollis, B.W. (1984) J. Clin. Endocrinol. Metab. 58, 91-98.
3. Mellon, W.S., Franceschi, R.T. and DeLuca, H.F. (1980) Arch. Biochem. Biophys. 202, 83-92.

$1,25(OH)_2D_3$ RECEPTORS IN SERTOLI CELLS AND SEMINIFEROUS TUBULES IN MOUSE AND RAT

J. Merke, U. Hügel, E. Ritz
Department Medicine, University of Heidelberg, 69 Heidelberg (FRG)

$1,25(OH)_2D_3$ receptors have recently been demonstrated in whole testis (1, 2, 3). It has not been delineated whether such receptors are present on endocrine or exocrine testicular structures. This problem was examined in the present study.

Material and Methods:

Non-rachitic adult male SD rats (8 weeks, 250 g) and NMRI mice (7 weeks, 40 g) were raised on standard diet. Whole testis, Leydig cells, separated from seminiferous tubuli by Percoll density gradient (0-90%) after Schumacher; Sertoli cell preparation after Dorrington (collagenase dispersion); spermatogonia as germinal cell enriched fraction according to Tung. Viability by trypan-blue exclusion (≥ 95%) of cells; identification of cells by NADH indicator (NBT) to characterize Leydig cells; cAMP stimulation with HCG or LH (25 U/ml) in vitro.
As described previously (Merke, 1983) (1) receptor characterization in cytosol and nuclear extracts by sucrose density gradient analysis; Scatchard plot; binding kinetics; degradation studies with proteases/nucleases; DNA cellulose affinity chromatography.

Results:

In whole testis of rats and mice we confirmed our previous findings of specific receptors in rat (in this study: mouse testis N_{max} 95 fmol/mg protein; K_D 1.6×10^{-10}M). In pure (≥ 95%) Leydig cell preparations, no significant binding could be detected using an assay which reproducibly detected ≥ 2 fmol/mg protein specific binding of $1,25(OH)_2D_3$ in intestinal mucosa of rat and mouse. In seminiferous tubules of rat and mouse, specific binding of $1,25(OH)_2D_3$ could be demonstrated both in cytosolic and nuclear fractions (for mouse: K_D 1×10^{-10} M; N_{max} 80 fmol/mg protein; for rat: K_D 3.0×10^{-10}M; N_{max} 52 fmol/mg protein). Binding was reversible (i.e. abolished by 100-fold molar excess of $1,25(OH)_2D_3$) and not abolished by 100-fold molar excess of $25(OH)D_3$. Separate analysis of Sertoli cells and spermatogonia fractions respectively showed specific binding exclusively in Sertoli cells (72 fmol/mg protein).
The $[^3H]$-$1,25(OH)_2D_3$ nuclear receptor complex of seminiferous tubules or Sertoli cells associated with DNA under conditions of low ionic strength (0.1 M KCl) and could be eluted as single peak at 0.25 M KCl. Incubation of the nuclear fractions with 100-fold molar excess of $1,25(OH)_2D_3$ completely obliterated the radioactive peak on DNA cellulose chromatogram, demonstrating specificity for the receptor macromolecule.

Discussion:

The present study shows typical $1,25(OH)_2D_3$ receptors in cytosolic and nuclear fractions of seminiferous tubules and Sertoli cells, but not Leydig cells of rat and mouse testis. The

Vitamin D. A Chemical, Biochemical and Clinical Update

3.5 S binding macromolecule could be easily differentiated from the 4 S serum binding protein (DBP) and the 6 S tissue binding protein complex for $25(OH)D_3$. Scatchard analysis revealed presence of a single class of non interacting binding sites with high binding selectivity ($1,25(OH)_2D_3 > 25(OH)D_3 > 1\alpha(OH)D_3 > 24\ R,25(OH)_2D_3$), low binding capacity and high binding affinity (K_D). Circulating $1,25(OH)_2D_3$ levels in rodents are in the range of measured K_D. Partial receptor occupancy in vivo is suggested by the finding that $1,25(OH)_2D_3$ receptor recovery was twice as high in cytosolic fractions of testis prepared at high as opposed to low ionic strength.
Absence of receptors on Leydig cells is particularly surprising since earlier studies of our laboratory documented $1,25(OH)_2D_3$ actions in vivo on LH-stimulated cAMP generation of uremic rat testis (2). We cannot exclude that such $1,25(OH)_2D_3$ actions are mediated by non-genomic, e.g. liponomic, mechanisms.
The presence of $1,25(OH)_2D_3$ receptor in Sertoli cells but not spermatogonia, is of note since in rodents whole testis $1,25(OH)_2D_3$ receptor concentration was shown to increase during puberty in parallel with spermatogenesis (3). Further studies must clarify whether possible actions of $1,25(OH)_2D_3$ on spermatogenesis are mediated indirectly via $1,25(OH)_2D_3$ receptor bearing Sertoli cells.

Literature:

1. Merke, J., Kreusser, W., Bier, B., Ritz, E. (1983) Europ.J. Biochem. 130, 303-308
2. Merke, J., Kreusser, W., Ritz, E. (1982) J. Steroid Biochem. 17: CXI
3. Walters, M. (1984) Endocrinology 114,2167-2174

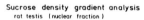

Sucrose density gradient analysis
rat testis (nuclear fraction)

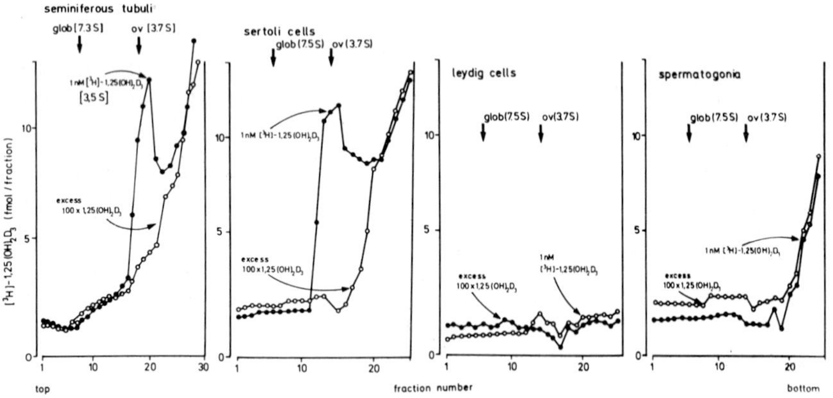

$1,25(OH)_2D_3$ RECEPTOR IN PULMONARY ALVEOLAR MACROPHAGES

J. E. Bishop, H. Reichel, H. P. Koeffler and A. W. Norman. Dept. Biochem., Univ. Calif., Riverside, CA 92521 and Dept. Med., Univ. Calif., Los Angeles, CA 90024, USA.

Introduction: Recent evidence of several laboratories has demonstrated that the vitamin D endocrine system extends to hematolymphopoietic tissue. Although primarily produced in the kidney, $1,25(OH)_2D_3$ has also been shown to be produced in vitro, among other tissues, in placenta (1), in bone cells (2), in sarcoid lymph nodes (3) and in human pulmonary alveolar macrophages (PAM) (4,5). Receptors for $1,25(OH)_2D_3$ have been demonstrated in human monocytes, in activated B and T lymphocytes (6) and in several malignant cell lines of myeloid (7) and lymphoid lineages (6). We were prompted to look for $1,25(OH)_2D_3$ receptors in PAM because (a) monocytes as direct precursors of PAM express $1,25(OH)_2D_3$-receptors and (b) interactions between $1,25(OH)_2D_3$ and PAM have been reported recently. Here we summarize preliminary results of our studies using rat and rabbit PAM.

Methods: PAM were obtained by bronchoalveolar lavage and were washed with α-medium with or without 10% FCS or phosphate-buffered saline (PBS). Rabbits yielded 0.3-2.6 X 10^7 PAM each (assayed for receptor individually) and 0.8-1.2 X 10^6 PAM were obtained from each rat (assayed in groups of 6-10). More than 95% of the cells isolated were identified as macrophages by their morphology and by staining with α-naphthyl acetate esterase. Viability was determined by trypan blue exclusion. Cells were homogenized in a high ionic strength buffer (KTED) and centrifuged. Aliquots of the 103,000 X g supernatant were incubated with $[^3H]$-$1,25(OH)_2D_3$ in the presence or absence of excess unlabelled $1,25(OH)_2D_3$ or $25(OH)D_3$. 5-to-20% sucrose gradients were prepared in KTED with 300 μM PMSF, and the incubation mixtures were applied. After centrifugation, fractions were collected from the bottom of the tube and counted to determine radioactivity. ^{14}C-labelled bovine serum albumin and ovalbumin were used as marker proteins.

Results: Rabbit PAM and rat PAM, collected and washed in PBS before homogenization yielded a radioactive peak migrating at approximately 3.7S on a 5-20% sucrose density gradient. Binding to this receptor macromolecule was competible with excess unlabelled $1,25(OH)_2D_3$ but not with $25(OH)D_3$ (Fig. 1).

Appearance of the $1,25(OH)_2D_3$ receptor in macrophages was dependent on an experimental procedure avoiding contact of macrophages with serum. In control experiments trace amounts of fetal calf serum (FCS) were found to bind $[^3H]$-$1,25(OH)_2D_3$ significantly as determined by the presence of a 4.0S-4.1S radioactive peak in sucrose density gradients. Thus, interference of the vitamin D binding protein in serum masked the $1,25(OH)_2D_3$ receptor peak in macrophages washed repeatedly in culture medium containing 10% FCS.

The total binding of $[^3H]$-$1,25(OH)_2D_3$ to the receptor varied between different cell preparations of PAM of the same species, and, as

Vitamin D. A Chemical, Biochemical and Clinical Update

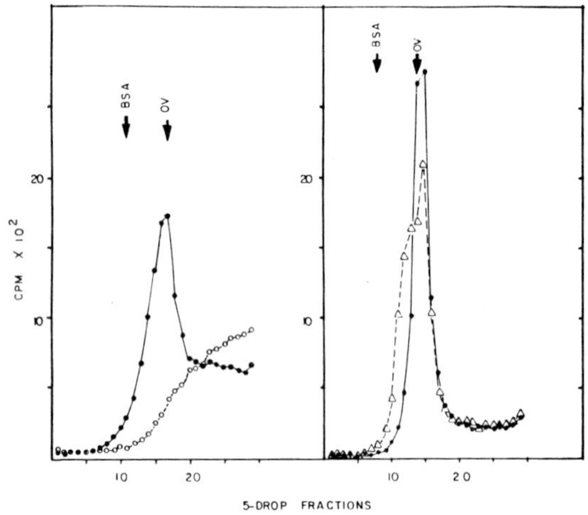

Fig. 1. Sucrose density gradients of rabbit PAM $1,25(OH)_2D_3$ receptor. ● = $[^3H]$-$1,25(OH)_2D_3$, O = plus excess $1,25(OH)_2D_3$, Δ = plus excess $25(OH)D_3$.

expected, higher binding occurred with an increasing number of macrophages obtained by bronchial lavage. Studies to further characterize this receptor are currently underway in our laboratories.

Our preliminary findings provide further evidence for involvement of $1,25(OH)_2D_3$ in the function of hematopoietic cells. The presence of a receptor molecule for $1,25(OH)_2D_3$ could be demonstrated in pulmonary alveolar macrophages. There are no data available at this point on expression of $1,25(OH)_2D_3$ receptors in other macrophage populations.

References:

1. Gray, T. K., Lester, G. E., and Lorence, R. S. (1979) Science 204, 1311-1313.
2. Howard, G. A., Turner, R. T., Sherrard, D. J., and Baylink, D. J. (1981) J. Biol. Chem 256, 7738-7740.
3. Mason, R., Frankel, T., Chan, Y. L., Lissner, D., and Posen, S. (1984) Ann. Intern. Med. 100, 59-61.
4. Adams, J. S., Sharma, O. P., Gacad, M. A., and Singer, F. R. (1983) J. Clin. Invest. 72, 1856-1860.
5. Koeffler, H. P., Reichel, H., Bishop, J. E., and Norman, A. W. (1985) Biochem. Biophys. Res. Commun. (in press).
6. Provvedini, P. M., Tsoukas, C. D., Deftos, L. J., and Manolagas, S. C. (1983) Science 221, 1181-1183.
7. Mangelsdorf, D. J., Koeffler, H. P., Donaldson, C. A., Pike, J. W., and Haussler, M. R. (1984) J. Cell Biol. 98, 391-398.

$24R,25(OH)_2D_3$: AN ALLOSTERIC EFFECTOR OF $1,25(OH)_2D_3$ BINDING TO ITS CHICK INTESTINAL RECEPTOR.

F. Wilhelm, F. P. Ross and A. W. Norman
Dept. Biochem., University of California, Riverside, CA 92521, U.S.A.

To date there has been no report of a direct effect of $24R(OH)_2D_3$ on $1,25(OH)_2D_3$ binding to its chick intestinal receptor. We report here an allosteric inhibitory effect of $24R,25(OH)_2D_3$ on $1,25(OH)_2D_3$ binding to its receptor. This effect is expressed at a physiological molar ratio (1) of 10:1, $24R,25(OH)_2D_3$: $1,25(OH)_2D_3$, through modulation of the positive cooperativity of $1,25(OH)_2D_3$ binding we have previously described (2). Intestinal chromatin was prepared from normal 4 week old chicks, in the presence of PMSF, and assayed for specific $[^3H]$-$1,25(OH)_2D_3$ binding in the presence or absence of 10-fold excess 24R,25-$(OH)_2D_3$. $[^3H]$-$24R,25(OH)_2D_3$ binding was likewise assessed by hydroxylapatite assay (3). Data were plotted via Scatchard and Hill plots. A Hill coefficient (n_H) less than one indicates negative cooperativity and greater than one, positive cooperativity (4).

Both $1,25(OH)_2D_3$ and $24R,25(OH)_2D_3$ showed positive cooperativity in binding to chick intestinal chromatin (Fig. 1, Table 1). $1,25(OH)_2D_3$ had a higher affinity and a greater number of binding sites than 24R,25-$(OH)_2D_3$.

TABLE 1

METABOLITE	K_d (nM)	n_H	B_{max} (fmol/mg protein)
$24R,25(OH)_2D_3$ (n=6)	34.0 ± 6.4	1.40 ± 0.13	47 ± 8
$1,25(OH)_2D_3$ (n=6)	1.86 ± 0.08	1.39 ± 0.07	170 ± 14

In the presence of a 10-fold physiological molar excess of 24R,25-$(OH)_2D_3$, the $1,25(OH)_2D_3$ saturation binding curved showed a significant shift to the right (Fig. 2) and reduction in affinity and cooperativity without a change in binding capacity (Table 2).

TABLE 2

	K_d (nM)	n_H	B_{max} (fmol/mg protein)
Control	0.97 ± 0.09	1.49 ± 0.06	200 ± 9
$+24R,25(OH)_2D_3$	1.36 ± 0.04	1.26 ± 0.06	189 ± 11
	($p < 0.1$)	($p < 0.03$)	(N.S.)

Vitamin D. A Chemical, Biochemical and Clinical Update

These results collectively suggest that 24R,25(OH$_2$D$_3$ is a physiological allosteric effector of 1,25(OH)$_2$D$_3$ binding to its chick intestinal receptor. The effect is expressed at a 10-fold molar ratio over 1,25-(OH)$_2$D$_3$. The reduction in affinity and cooperativity is independent of competition with 1,25(OH)$_2$D$_3$. The chick intestinal receptor for 1,25(OH)$_2$D$_3$ appears to be an allosteric protein regulated by 24R,25-(OH)$_2$D$_3$.

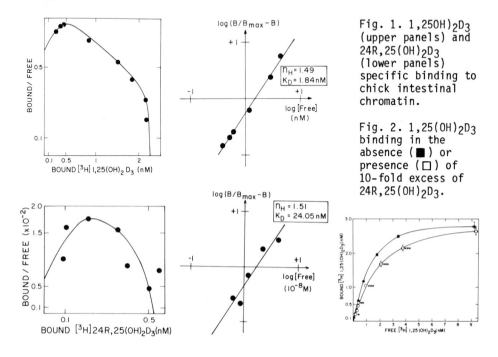

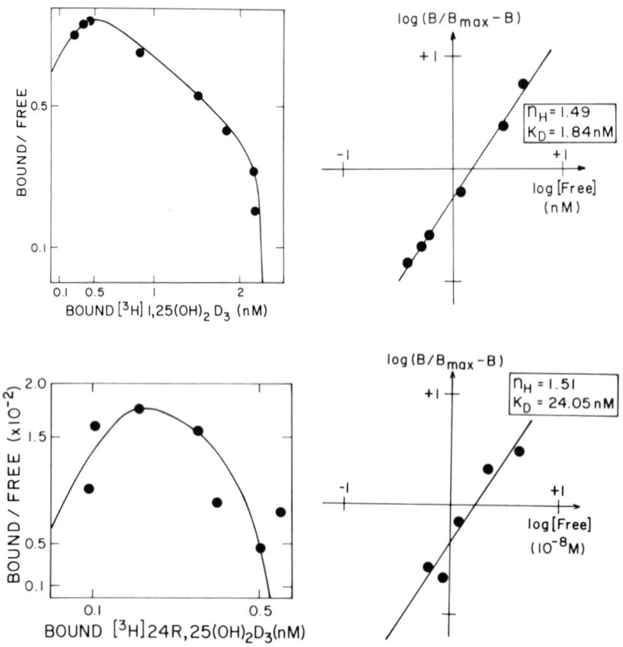

Fig. 1. 1,250H)$_2$D$_3$ (upper panels) and 24R,25(OH)$_2$D$_3$ (lower panels) specific binding to chick intestinal chromatin.

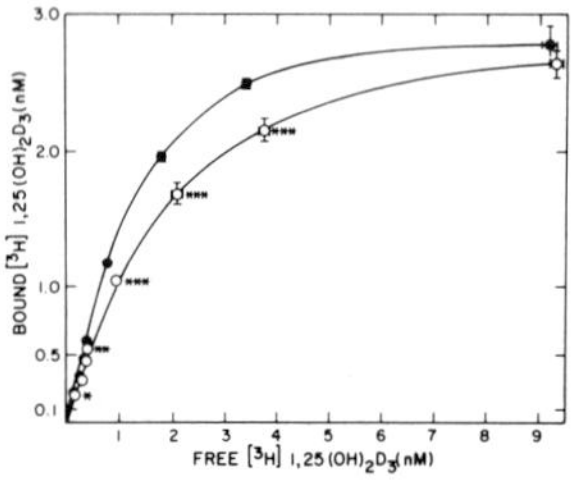

Fig. 2. 1,25(OH)$_2$D$_3$ binding in the absence (■) or presence (□) of 10-fold excess of 24R,25(OH)$_2$D$_3$.

References:

1. Bouillon, R. and Van Baelen, H. (1981) Calcif. Tiss. Int. 33, 451-453.
2. Wilhelm F. and Norman, A. W. (1984) FEBS Letters 170, 239-242.
3. Wecksler, W. R. and Norman, A. W. (1979) Anal. Biochem. 22, 314-323.
4. Hill, A. V. (1910) J. Physiol. 40, 4-7.

EFFECT OF CALCIUM AND PHOSPHATE ON 1,25(OH)2D RECEPTOR IN OSTEOGENIC SARCOMA CELL LINE (UMR 106)

M. Nakada, M. Fukase, Y. Imai, Y. Kinoshita and T. Fujita
Third Division, Department of Medicine, Kobe University, Kobe, 650, JAPAN

It is well known that rat osteogenic sarcoma cell(UMR 106) established by T.J. Martin et al. is responsive to PTH, but not responsive to CT, and has 1.25(OH)$_2$D(1,25-D) receptor(1). In addition, UMR 106 cell has high levels of alkaline phosphatase(Al-P) activity. However, since no direct evidence for the local regulator of vitamin D receptor has been reported, we examined the effect of varying concentrations of calcium(Ca) and phosphate(P) on 1,25-D receptor and the nuclear uptake of 1,25-D in the cell.

METHOD

When UMR 106 cells reached 70-80% confluency, medium was replaced with serum-free medium (Ham's F 12) containing varying concentrations of Ca and P, and the cells were maintained for another 24 hrs.. Then cells were washed with PBS, and homogenized with a Teflon Pestel. Cytosol was prepared by centrifugation at 105,000 x g for 60 min at 0-4 C. Equilibrium binding assay was carried out by the method of Mellon et al.(2). For the nuclear uptake of 1,25-D, intact monolayer cells in serum-free medium were incubated with tritiated 1,25-D for 1 hr. at 37 C, and then washed with either PBS or physiologic saline for phosphate experiments. Cells were suspended with ice cold lysing buffer(0.25 M Sucrose, 20 mM Tris, 1.1 mM $MgCl_2$, 0.5% Triton X-100, pH 7.85), centrifuged 3,000 rpm twice, and then radioactivity associated with nuclei (pellet) was counted (3). Al-P activity in the cells was determined by using p-nitrophenyl-phosphate as the substrate (4).

RESULTS

1,25-D binding to cytosol preparations of cells in the presence of 0.3, 1.2, or 2.5 mM Ca was examined individually. Scatchard analysis gave an apparent dissociation constant of 6.7×10^{-11} M for 0.3 mM Ca, 6.1×10^{-11} M for 1.2 mM Ca and 6.0×10^{-11} M for 2.5 mM Ca, and showed no difference of affinity in varying Ca concentrations, while maximum binding capacity/mg protein was 52 fmol, 39.5 fmol, 31.6 fmol for the respective Ca concentration.

The nuclear uptake of 1,25-D in the intact monolayer cells was decreased depending on the increasing concentrations of Ca and P as described in table 1.

Table 1

	Ca (mM) (P 1.0 mM)					P (mM) (Ca 1.2 mM)			
Nuclear uptake	0.3#	1.2	1.6	2.1	2.5	0.3##	1.0	2.0	3.0
	100	61	48	31	28	100	69	67	53

(#,## Each value was expressed as the percentage of specific nuclear uptake of 1,25-D at 0.3 mM Ca and P)

These data indicate that in hypercalcemic condition both of the receptor number and the nuclear uptake of 1,25-D are higher than those in hypocalcemic condition without any alteration of affinity.

Vitamin D. A Chemical, Biochemical and Clinical Update

Next, changes of Al-P activity in these cells were also examined in different Ca and P conditions. The results demonstrated that Al-P activity was increased depending on the increasing concentrations of Ca and P in the medium. (Table 2)

Table 2

	Ca (mM)				P (mM)			
Al-P#	0.3	1.2	1.8	3.0	0.3	1.0	2.0	3.0
	1.47	1.67	1.67	1.78	1.01	1.08	1.16	1.29

(#μ mole PNP/min/mg protein)

In addition, verapamil and nicardipine, a calcium antagonist, which is postulated to decrease Al-P activity, did suppress the enzyme activity. (Table 3)

Table 3

	control	verapamil, 10^{-6} M	micardipine, 10^{-6} M
Al-P#	1.82	1.55	1.49

(#μ mole PNP/min/mg protein)

Furthermore, Al-P activity in UMR 106 cells was actually induced by 1,25-D on dose depending fashion (10^{-11}–10^{-9}) as described in Table 4.

Table 4

	control	10^{-11}M	10^{-10}M	10^{-9}M	10^{-8}M	10^{-7}M	(1,25-D)
Al-P#	1.51	1.50	1.67	1.88##	1.71##	1.85##	

(#μ mole PNP/min/mg protein)

(## significant difference, $P < 0.05$)

In summary, 1) In UMR 106 cells low calcium ion increased the maximum binding capacity of 1,25-D receptor directly without any alteration of affinity, while high calcium ion decreased. 2) Calcium and phosphate concentration had negative correlation with the content of nuclear upatake of 1,25-D. 3) Alkaline phosphatase activity was increased depending on calcium and phosphate concentration. 4) 1,25-D induced alkaline phosphatase activity. From these results it will be concluded that 1) Calcium and phosphate ions are important factors for the regulation of 1,25-D action and 2) Environmental calcium and phosphate concentration may give an important signal for bone turnover.

REFERENCE

1. Partridge, N.C., Frampton, R.J., Eiseman, J.A., Michelangeli, V.P., Elms, E., Bradley, T.R. and Martin, T.J.(1980) FEBS LETTERS 115, 139-138
2. Mellon, W.S., Franceschi, R.T. and Deluca, H.F. (1980) Arch. Biochem. Biophys., 202, 83-87
3. Eil, C. and Marx, S.J. (1981) Proc. Natl. Acad. Sci. USA. 78, 2562-2565
4. Manolagas, S.C., Burton, D.W. and Deftos, L.J. (1981) J. Biol. Chem., 256, 7115-7117.

TEMPORAL RELATIONSHIP OF 1,25-DIHYDROXYCHOLECALCIFEROL RECEPTOR EXPRESSION AND EFFECTS ON ACTIVATED LYMPHOCYTES.

D.M.Provvedini, C.D.Tsoukas[ϕ], L.J.Deftos, and S.C.Manolagas,
Division of Endocrinology/Metabolism, University of California, San Diego, and VAMC, La Jolla, CA 92161;ϕDepartment of Basic and Clinical Research, Scripps Clinic and Research Foundation, La Jolla, CA 92037, USA.

INTRODUCTION :

We have previously shown that human peripheral blood lymphocytes express receptors for 1,25-dihydroxycholecalciferol {$1,25(OH)_2D_3$}upon activation (1) and that the hormone acts as a potent inhibitor of interleukin 2 (IL-2) and cell proliferation (2). In order to elucidate the temporal relationship of these events, we have studied the time course of the $1,25(OH)_2D_3$ receptor expression, IL-2 production and proliferation of lymphocytes for 3 days following activation with phytohemagglutinin (PHA). In addition, we examined the effect of $1,25(OH)_2D_3$ on the cell cycle of the PHA-activated cells.

MATERIALS AND METHODS :

Peripheral lymphocytes from healthy subjects were isolated on Ficoll and cultured in RPMI medium in the presence of 1 μg/ml of PHA. Cell proliferation, blast transformation, IL-2 activity, stage of cell cycle and 1,25-$(OH)_2D_3$ receptor concentration were determined by previously described methods (2-4).

RESULTS :

TABLE I : TIME COURSE OF LYMPHOCYTE ACTIVATION IN VITRO (PHA)

DAYS IN CULTURE :	0	1	2	3
PARAMETER TESTED :				
1) CELLS IN CULTURE (percent compared to day zero)	100%	58%	75%	158%
2) BLAST CELLS (percent of total cells)	0	0.3%	53%	82%
3) PROTEIN DETERMINATION ($ug/10^6$ cells)	27	30	51	98
4) [3H]THYMIDINE INCORPORATION ($cpm/10^6$ viable cells)	3,600	5,700	173,135	289,977
5) CELL CYCLE :				
% in G0	93%	69%	22%	10%
% in G1a	1.3%	26%	27%	16%
% in G1b	0	0.3%	23%	34%
% in S	0	0.2%	18%	28%
% in G2/M	0.1%	1%	8%	12%
6) INTERLEUKIN-2 ACTIVITY (units)	0	10	8	5
7) $1,25(OH)_2D_3$ BINDING				
- $K_d (x10^{-10}$ M)	-	1.6	2.1	1.8
- N_{max}(fmoles bound/10^6 viable cells)	-	9.1	29.5	14.5
- N_{max}(fmoles bound/mg protein)	-	282	511	126
- Binding sites/cell	-	5,470	17,759	8,729

Vitamin D. A Chemical, Biochemical and Clinical Update

Table I shows the time course of lymphocyte activation. After 1 day following the addition of PHA, 26% of cells entered the G1a phase. At this time IL-2 activity in the culture supernatant was maximal, while 1,25 - $(OH)_2D_3$ receptors were present and DNA synthesis was insignificant. At day 2 IL-2 declined from its peak value, $1,25(OH)_2D_3$ receptor concentration reached its peak and DNA synthesis was present. At day 3 both IL-2 activity and $1,25(OH)_2D_3$ receptor concentration declined, while DNA synthesis kept rising. When $1,25(OH)_2D_3$ was added simultaneously with PHA ($1x10^{-12}$ - $1x10^{-8}$ M and 1 μg/ml, respectively) the percentage of cells in the culture blocked at G1a phase increased progressively from 48 hours and up to 4 days in a dose dependent fashion (Table II).

TABLE II : EFFECTS OF $1,25(OH)_2D_3$ ON CELL CYCLE OF ACTIVATED LYMPHOCYTES (PHA)

	G_0	G_{1a}	G_{1b}	S	G_2M
DAY ZERO	94%	1.2	0	0	0
DAY 1					
-control	78.3%	17.2%	0.3%	0.3%	0.4%
- 1,25 (10^{-12})	74.1%	21.6%	0.1%	0.3%	0.4%
- (10^{-10})	73.6%	20.2%	0.1%	0.2%	0.7%
- (10^{-8})	74.4%	19.4%	0.1%	0.1%	0.6%
DAY 2					
-control	31.3%	19.9%	15.2%	15.9%	12.0%
- 1,25 (10^{-12})	32.6%	21.4%	13.8%	14.9%	11.5%
- (10^{-10})	32.0%	21.1%	16.9%	13.8%	10.3%
- (10^{-8})	36.2%	24.2%	14.6%	12.2%	9.3%
DAY 3					
-control	17.1%	14.0%	31.5%	20.5%	14.7%
- 1,25 (10^{-12})	14.9%	16.2%	33.3%	22.8%	10.7%
- (10^{-10})	13.3%	14.0%	35.7%	21.6%	11.3%
- (10^{-8})	20.2%	32.0%	18.0%	16.1%	13.8%
DAY 4					
-control	8.3%	27.3%	26.8%	23.9%	11.2%
- 1,25 (10^{-12})	13.8%	46.9%	14.1%	14.7%	9.4%
- (10^{-10})	15.6%	49.3%	10.6%	12.0%	7.8%
- (10^{-8})	18.0%	55.0%	7.7%	9.4%	7.6%

CONCLUSIONS :

These rsults indicate that $1,25(OH)_2D_3$ receptor expression is an early event associated with activated (G1a-G1b) and not necessarily proliferating ($S-G_2M$) lymphocytes. The anti-proliferative effect of $1,25(OH)_2D_3$ on activated lymphocytes is exerted by blocking cells in the G1a phase.

REFERENCES :

1. Provvedini,D.M.,Tsoukas,C.D.,Deftos,L.J.,and Manolagas,S.C. (1983) Science 221, 1181-1183.
2. Tsoukas,C.D.,Provvedini,D.M.,and Manolagas,S.C. (1984) Science 224, 1438-1440.
3. Darzynkiewicz,Z.,Traganos,F.,Sharpless,T.,and Melamed,M.R. (1976) Proc. Natl. Acad. Sci. USA 73, 2881-2884.
4. Manolagas,S.C.,and Deftos, L.J. (1980) Biochem. Biophys. Res. Commun. 95, 596-602.

IS LIGAND OVERESTIMATION RESPONSIBLE FOR THE OBSERVED COOPERATIVITY IN THE BINDING OF 1,25-DIHYDROXYVITAMIN D_3 TO CHICK INTESTINAL CHROMATIN

F. P. ROSS, F. E. WILHELM and A. W. NORMAN
Department of Biochemistry, University of California-Riverside.

Introduction:

Several mechanisms can influence the effects of hormones on cells. These include: a) downregulation of receptor number, e.g. the β-adrenergic receptor (1); b) modulation of receptor responsiveness by mechanisms such as i) receptor phosphorylation, e.g. the androgen receptor (2) ii) receptor autophosphorylation, e.g. the insulin receptor (3) iii) action of various cellular effectors such as Ca^{2+}, cAMP on the receptor (4).

Recently, the estrogen receptor has been shown to exhibit positive cooperativity for the natural ligand (5), a phenomenon which is modulated by an estrogen metabolite, estriol (6). We have reported that the receptor for $1,25(OH)_2D_3$ exhibits an analogous co-operativity (7). We were concerned that our result was an artifact caused by binding of radio-labelled hormone to the assay tubes. If this binding was saturable and of low capacity it would yield erroneous results mainly at low ligand concentrations. The reduced free ligand levels could manifest in Hill plot analysis as positive co-operativity.

Methods:

Intestinal chromatin was isolated from 3 week old vitamin D deficient chicks by homogenization in TED buffer (10 mM Tris, 1,5 mM EDTA, 1 mM DTT, pH 7, 4) followed by washing the pellet 3 times with TED-0.5% Triton. Duplicate experiments were set up in which aliquots (100µl) of the resuspended (49%) chromatin in TED were incubated in triplicate with 0.2 - 10 nM $[^3H]$-$1,25(OH)_2D_3$ (10µl, 17 Ci/mmol, Amersham) in the presence or absence of 200x excess of nonradioactive $1,25(OH)_2D_3$.

One set of tubes was treated in the standard fashion (8) with a suspension of hydroxylapatite (HAP) in TED to determine free (A) and bound (B). The contents of the second set were transfered totally with Pasteur pipettes to counting vials for measurement of total radioactivity (C). The incubation tubes in this set were extracted with 1 ml ethanol and the extracts were dried and counted (D). Subtraction of (B+D) from (C) allowed determination of total "free" ligand. The data from both experiments were analysed by Scatchard and Hill plot analysis.

Results:

Over the entire range of ligand concentration used 9.0 ± 0.6% of the ligand was bound. Computation showed that the corrected values still exhibited non-linear Scatchard plots typical of co-operativity (Fig 1A o = corrected, o = uncorrected). This was confirmed by the Hill plots (Fig 1B o = corrected, o = uncorrected) in which the n_H value is unchanged at 1.60. The K_d value obtained from the corrected data (0.68 nM) was significantly ($p > 0,05$) lower than in the original analysis (1,16 nM).

Vitamin D. A Chemical, Biochemical and Clinical Update

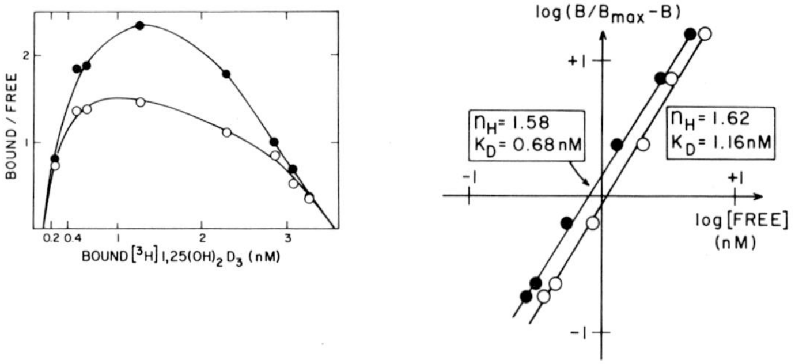

Figure 1. Scatchard (1A) and Hill (1B) plots of binding of 3H 1,25-dihydroxy vitamin D to chick intestinal receptor. The results are shown with (o) and without (o) correction for non-specific binding to the incubation tube.

Conclusion:

These results show the absence of an experimental artifact in our previous experiments and confirm our understanding that the chick intestinal chromatin receptor for $1,25(OH)_2D_3$ does manifest positive co-operativity with respect to its ligand.

References:

1. Davies, A. O. and Lefkowitz, R. J. (1981) in Receptors and Recognition (R. Lefkowitz, ed) Vol 13, pp. 83-121, London, Chapman α Hall.
2. Goueli, S.A., Holtzman, J. L. and Ahmed, K. (1984) Biochem. Biophys. Res. Comm. 123, 778-784.
3. Zick, Y., Kasuga, M., Kahn, C.R. and Roth, J. (1983) J. Biol. Chem. 258, 75-80.
4. Rasmussen, H. and Barrett, P.Q. (1984) Physiol. Revs. 64, 938-984.
5. Notides, A. C., Lerner, N. and Hamilton, D. E. (1981) Proc. Natl. Acad. Sci. U.S.A. 18, 4926-4930.
6. Sasson, S. and Notides, A. C. (1984) J. Steroid Biochem. 20, 1021-1026.
7. Wilhelm, F. E. and Norman, A. W. (1984) FEBS Lett. 170, 239-242.

ACCUMULATING EVIDENCE FOR A PHYSIOLOGICAL ROLE FOR 1,25-DIHYDROXYVITAMIN D_3 IN NEW TARGETS: TESTIS AND HEART.

M.R. WALTERS, B.C. OSMUNDSEN, R.M. CARTER, P. C. RIGGLE, AND J.R. JETER*
Departments of Physiology and Anatomy,* Tulane Medical School, New Orleans, LA 70112

Within the past few years, the range of possible 1,25-dihydroxyvitamin D_3 [1,25$(OH)_2D_3$] target tissues has expanded considerably from those involved in the classical function of extracellular calcium homeostasis -- gut, bone, and kidney (1-3). As previously discussed in detail (4,5), the tissues which have now become candidates for consideration as authentic 1,25$(OH)_2D_3$ target tissues have been defined by the presence of 1,25$(OH)_2D_3$ receptors and/or the vitamin D-related calcium binding proteins (CaBP's). Attempts have been made to categorize these tissues (4,5) according to putative 1,25$(OH)_2D_3$ function therein or general uniformity of tissue/organ function. However, since these new putative targets participate in a myriad of physiological functions within the body, developing a uniform hypothesis of 1,25$(OH)_2D_3$ function therein at the tissue/organ level has been difficult. As a result, our laboratory has developed the working hypothesis (4) that 1,25$(OH)_2D_3$ receptors regulate very basic cellular events involved in/regulated by cellular Ca^{++} and its receptors (Fig. 1). However, the important question of whether 1,25$(OH)_2D_3$ receptors in these new tissues are physiologically relevant, i.e. functional, generally remains to be answered. Possible exceptions include the pancreas (5,7), blood cells/precursors (8-12), and pituitary (13). However, in many of these studies the effects ascribed to 1,25$(OH)_2D_3$ may be indirect -- i.e. secondary to plasma calcium regulation (14-16). In fact, this caveat plagues many ongoing studies of 1,25$(OH)_2D_3$ function in possible new targets and seriously complicates experimental design.

As detailed below, this laboratory has pioneered definition of the uterus, testis, and heart as possible new 1,25$(OH)_2D_3$ targets. These studies are being pursued to investigate possible 1,25$(OH)_2D_3$ functions therein by a series of physiological and biochemical procedures as described.

Authentic 1,25$(OH)_2D_3$ Receptors in Heart, Testis, and Uterus

Sucrose gradient and Scatchard analyses previously provided evidence for the presence of authentic 1,25$(OH)_2D_3$ receptors in rat heart (17), testis (18), and uterus (19) using the criteria of chromatin localization in low salt buffers (20,21), sedimentation coefficient, steroid specificity, and the Scatchard parameters of saturability and high affinity. Confirmatory reports on testis (22) and uterine (23) receptors have also appeared.

No 1,25$(OH)_2D_3$ Receptors in *P. polycephalum*

Recognizing that phylogenetic distribution can provide clues to evolving function in biochemical systems and stimulated by recent evidence of steroid hormone receptor-like systems in several species of fungi (24-26), the possible presence of 1,25$(OH)_2D_3$ receptors in the slime mold *Physarum polycephalum* was examined during life cycle stages (27). These sucrose gradient analyses of KCL-extracted chromatin preparations (17-19) provided

Vitamin D. A Chemical, Biochemical and Clinical Update

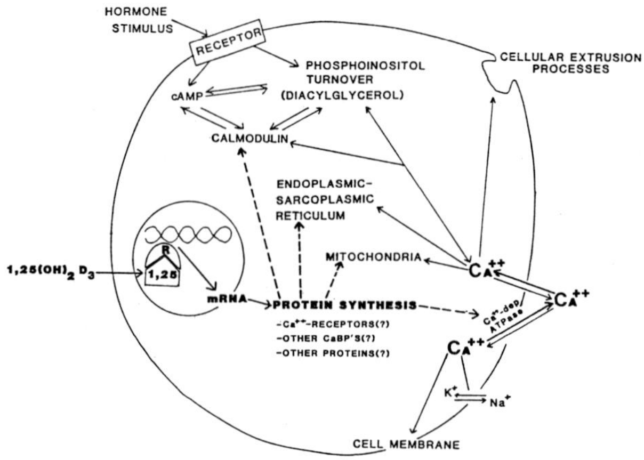

Fig. 1. A working model of possible $1,25(OH)_2D_3$ effects on intracellular Ca^{++} homeostatis in new target tissues. Bold-faced symbols represent well-known phenomena in the vitamin D endocrine system. Other symbols: solid lines, sites of known effects of intracellular Ca^{++}; dashed lines, undocumented steps through which $1,25(OH)_2D_3$ might affect Ca^{++} homeostasis within the cell.

Fig. 2. Sucrose gradient analysis of ^3H-$1,25(OH)_2D_3$ binding components in KCl-chromatin extracts of the slime mold Physarum polycephalum. Samples were taken from both the log growth phase of the microplasmodia (A) and the surface plasmodia (B) life cycle stages. These tissues were homogenized in TED buffer (10 mM Tris, 1.5 mM EDTA, 1.0 mM dithiothreitol, pH 7.4) with Trasylol and PMSF prior to chromatin preparation by three washes of the 6000 rpm pellet. The KTEDMo (TED + 0.3 M KCl and 10 mM Na_2MoO_4) + Trasylol-resuspended chromatin was incubated (4°C, 1h) with 1.0 nM ^3H-$1,25(OH)_2D_3$ in the absence (○) or presence (●) of 1.0 uM $1,25(OH)_2D_3$ prior to loading onto 5-20% sucrose gradients. Following ultracentrifugation and fractionation (4 drops), excess ^3H-$1,25(OH)_2D_3$ was removed by the HAP assay (18). Symbols: ●——, ^3H-$1,25(OH)_2D_3$; ○, ^3H-$1,25(OH)_2D_3$ + excess $1,25(OH)_2D_3$; arrow = 3.6S.

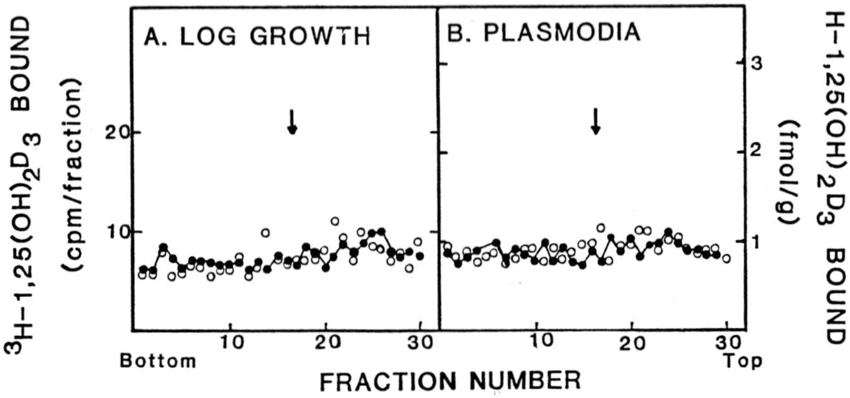

no evidence for $1,25(OH)_2D_3$ receptors either during the log growth phase of the microplasmodia (Fig. 2A) or when differentiated into surface plasmodia (Fig. 2B). Thus, at the present level of sensitivity of the detection methods used, there is no evidence for specific ^3H-$1,25(OH)_2D_3$ binding proteins in the slime mold Physarum polycephalum during these two very different life cycle stages.

Cellular Localization of $1,25(OH)_2D_3$ Receptors in Rat Testis

In addressing the question of the physiological relevance of $1,25(OH)_2D_3$ receptors in unexpected tissues, the possibility that the presence of low levels of the receptor simply represent "leaky" gene expression must be considered (4). One approach to this problem is to ask whether this protein is restricted to selected cell types or evenly distributed throughout the organ. $1,25(OH)_2D_3$ receptor cellular localization in the testis was first investigated by teasing apart the interstitial tissue and seminiferous tubules (18). Under these conditions, $1,25(OH)_2D_3$ receptors were selectively localized (>90%) in the seminiferous tubules as compared to the interstitial tissue, including the steroidogenic Leydig cells (18). More recent studies to localize the receptors have included comparision of testicular $1,25(OH)_2D_3$ receptor levels after cryptorchidism or busulfan treatment. When germ cell function was disrupted by these procedures, there was no change in $1,25(OH)_2D_3$ receptor levels. Conversely, when Sertoli cells were also damaged by long-term cryptorchidism, there was a substantial reduction (63.2 %, $P<0.001$) in $1,25(OH)_2D_3$ receptor levels. Although further studies are necessary to unequivocally establish the cellular localization of testis $1,25(OH)_2D_3$ receptors, these observations seem to suggest their localization in the Sertoli cells.

Physiological Regulation of $1,25(OH)_2D_3$ Receptor Levels

Another criterion which can provide evidence for the functional relevance of $1,25(OH)_2D_3$ receptors is whether receptor levels change with changing physiological function of the respective tissue. Such correlation of $1,25(OH)_2D_3$ receptor levels to physiological state has been established in both uterus and testis. In uterus, $1,25(OH)_2D_3$ receptor levels parallel the degree of estrogen-stimulation (19,22), which is well known to increase uterine growth and function therein. In the testis (but not mucosa) the level of $1,25(OH)_2D_3$ receptors increased approximately two-fold at the time of puberty (18), correlating temporally with the onset of spermatogenesis and mature function of this organ.

Testis $1,25(OH)_2D_3$ Receptors And Aging

Importantly, Scatchard analyses also indicate that testis $1,25(OH)_2D_3$ receptor levels and affinity do not change appreciably after puberty/maturity during the normal rat life span (Table 1), indicating that the testis receptors are stable throughout the aging process in this species.

Presence of Vitamin D-Responsive Proteins in New Targets?

An ultimate criterion which must be fulfilled before concluding that $1,25(OH)_2D_3$ receptors function in a new putative target tissue is the

TABLE 1: SIMILARITY OF TESTIS $1,25(OH)_2D_3$ RECEPTORS IN MATURE AND IN AGED RATS: SCATCHARD ANALYSES

AGE (MONTHS)	$1,25(OH)_2D_3$ RECEPTORS N (fmol/g)	K_D (nM)	N†
3	99.7 ±9.7	0.33 ±.08	4
19*	102.3 ±6.4	0.33 ±.06	2

*Near the end of their normal life span as judged by the deaths of the remaining rats of this age group.

†Each observation represents data from testes pooled from 2-3 individual rats.

direct correlation of hormonal stimulus with a concrete physiological/biochemical response. As discussed previously, there are reports of CaBP and/or its mRNA in both testis (18) and heart (17). However, these reports are often incomplete with respect to vitamin D regulation or conflicting with respect to the possible identity (28 k vs 10 k dalton) of the CaBP's therein. In order to resolve these issues and in recognition that $1,25(OH)_2D_3$ function in these tissues may involve other (not usually considered vitamin D-regulated) CaBPs, a study of the entire CaBP profile in these tissues was initiated by ^{45}Ca binding to nitrocellulose membrane transblots from SDS-PAGE gels according to a modification of the procedure of Maruyama (28). By using 15% polyacrylamide concentrations, the molecular weight range of 10-40,000 daltons was selectively studied in these experiments.

As summarized in Table 2, there was no major difference in the number or molecular weights of the CaBP's observed in all tissues studied to date (rat intestinal mucosa, kidney, testis, and heart). Thus in addition to both the "small" mucosal and the "big" renal CaBP, there was evidence for ^{45}Ca-binding to proteins co-migrating with ("like") parvalbumin and calmodulin in all these tissues. However, there were important differences in the apparent quantity (reflected by autoradiographic band intensity and frequency) of these proteins and their regulation by $1,25(OH)_2D_3$. As expected, neither the parvalbumin-like nor the calmodulin-like proteins seem to be $1,25(OH)_2D_3$ regulated in any tissue. Interestingly, these experiments also seem to indicate that the "big" 28k CaBP is not $1,25(OH)_2D_3$ regulated in the testis. However, these preliminary data suggest that further study and amplication of the technique may demonstrate that the "small" 13 K CaBP is $1,25(OH)_2D_3$-regulated in both the heart and testis. Thus, these studies provide strong impetus and a useful technique for pursuing the question of $1,25(OH)_2D_3$ function in new putative target tissues.

TABLE 2. SUMMARY OF THE CALCIUM BINDING PROTEINS (CaBP)[1] DETECTED BY ^{45}Ca-BINDING TO NITROCELLULOSE TRANSBLOTS FROM SDS-PAGE PROFILES OF TISSUE CYTOSOLS[2]

TISSUE	SMALL CaBP 13,000 ±500	PARVALBUMIN-LIKE 15,500 ±200	CALMODULIN-LIKE[6] 17,000 ±500	19,600 ±600	BIG CaBP 28,500 ±1000
MUCOSA					
INTENSITY[3]	++++	++	+	++	++
(FREQ)[4]	(13/14)	(8/15)	(8/15)	(9/15)	(8/15)
D-REGULATED[5]	**	θ	θ	θ	*
(FREQ)	(7/7)	(0/7)	(0/7)	(0/7)	(3/7)
KIDNEY					
INTENSITY	++	++	+	++	+++
(FREQ)	(7/15)	(7/15)	(7/15)	(11/15)	(14/15)
D-REGULATED	*	θ	θ	θ	**
(FREQ)	(5/7)	(0/7)	(0/7)	(0/7)	(10/10)
TESTIS					
INTENSITY	+	+	+	+	+
(FREQ)	(5/11)	(4/14)	(9/14)	(11/14)	(12/14)
D-REGULATED	*	θ	θ	θ	θ
(FREQ)	(3/5)	(0/5)	(0/5)	(0/5)	(0/5)
HEART					
INTENSITY	+	++	+	++	+
(FREQ)	(4/6)	(5/7)	(4/8)	(8/8)	(6/8)
D-REGULATED	*	θ	θ	θ	N.D.
(FREQ)	(2/4)	(0/4)	(0/4)	(0/4)	

[1]MOLECULAR WEIGHTS (DALTONS) WERE TAKEN FROM THE ABOVE TISSUE WHERE IT IS MOST PROMINENT.

[2]CYTOSOLS WERE PREPARED IN TED BUFFER (10 mM TRIS, 1.5 mM EDTA, 1.0 mM DITHIOTHREITOL, pH 7.4) CONTAINING TRASYLOL AND PMSF.

[3]++++(VERY INTENSE); +++(BRIGHT); ++(AVERAGE INTENSITY); + (DIMLY VISIBLE); - (NOT SEEN)

[4]FREQUENCY = NUMBER OF TIMES VISUALISED/NUMBER OF EXPERIMENTS.

[5]REGULATION BY $1,25(OH)_2$VITAMIN D_3: ** (YES); * (MAYBE); θ (NOT REGULATED); N.D. (NO DATA)

[6]CALMODULIN-LIKE CaBP'S SOMETIMES SEEMED TO APPEAR AS A DOUBLET.

References

1. Norman, A.W. (1979) Vitamin D: The Calcium Homeostatic Hormone, Academic Press, New York.
2. Haussler, M.R. and McCain, T. (1977) New Engl. J. Med. 297, 974-983, 1041-1050.
3. DeLuca, H.F. and Schnoes, H.K. (1983) Ann. Rev. Biochem. 52, 411-39.
4. Walters, M.R., Cuneo, D.L. and Jamison, A.P. (1983) J. Steroid Biochem. 19, 913-920.
5. Norman, A.W., Roth, J., and Orci, L. (1982) Endoc. Rev. 3, 331-366.
6. Kadowaki, S. and Norman, A.W. (1984) J. Clin. Invest. 73, 759-766.
7. Seino, Y., Sierra, R.I., Sonn, Y.M., Jafari, A., Birge, S.J. and Alvioli, L.V. (1983) Endocrinology 113, 1721-1725.
8. Abe, E., Shina, Y., Miyaura, C., Tanaka, H., Hayashi, T., Kanegasaki, S., Saito, M., Nishii, Y., DeLuca, H.F., and Suda, T. (1984) Proc. Natl. Acad. Sci. USA 81, 7112-7116.
9. Bar-Shivat, Z., Teitelbaum, S.L., Reitsma, P., Hall, A., Pegg, L.E., Trial, J., and Kahn, A.J. (1983) Proc. Natl. Acad. Sci. U.S.A. 80, 5907-5911.
10. Mangelsdorf, D.J., Koeffler, H.P., Donaldson, C.A., Pike, J.W., and Haussler, M.R. (1984) J. Cell. Biol. 98, 391-398.
11. Suda, D., Enomoto, S., Abe, E., and Suda, T. (1984) Biochem. Biophys. Res. Comm. 119, 807-813.
12. Tsoukas, C.D., Provvedini, D.M., and Manoaogas, S.C. (1984) Science 224, 1438-1440.
13. Wark, J.D. and Tashjian, A.H. (1983) J. Biol. Chem. 258, 12118-12121.
14. Miyaura, C., Abe, E., and Suda, T. (1984) Endocrinology 115, 1891-1896.
15. Tanaka, Y., Seino, Y., Ishida, M., Yamaoka, K., Satomura, K., Yabuuchi, H., Ishida, H., Seino, Y. nd Imura, H. (1984) Proceedings Intl. Congr. Endocrinology 8, 1380A.
16. Hochberg, Z., Borochowitz, Z., Benderli, A. Vardi, P., Oren, S., Spirer, Z., Heyman, I., and Weisman, Y. (1985) J. Clin. Endocrinol. Metab. 60, 57-61.
17. Walters, M.R., Wicker, D.C., and Riggle, P.C. (1985) J. Molec. Cell Cardiol. (In Press).
18. Walters, M.R. (1984) Endocrinology 114, 2167-2174.
19. Walters, M.R. (1981) Biochem. Biohys. Res. Comm. 103, 721-726.
20. Walters, M.R., Hunziker, W., and Norman, A.W. (1980) J. Biol. Chem. 255, 6799-6805.
21. Walters, M.R., Hunziker, W., and Norman, A.W. (1982). J. Steroid. Biochem. 15, 491-495.
22. Merke, J., Kreusser, W., bier, B., and Ritz, E. (1983) Eur. J. J. Biochem. 130, 303-310.
23. Levy, J., Zuili, I., Yankowitz, N., and Shany, S. (1984) J. Endocr. 100, 265-269.
24. Burshell, A., Stathis, P.A., Do, Y., Miller, S.C., and Feldmn, D. (1983) J. Biol. Chem. 259, 3450-3456.
25. Loose, D.S., Stover, E.P., Restrepo, A., Stevens, D.A., and Feldman, D. (1983) Proc. Natl. Acad. Sci. U.S.A. 80, 7659-7663.
26. Riehl, R.M. and Toft, D.O. (1984) J. Biol. Chem. 259, 15324-15330.
27. Jeter, J.R., Cameron, I.L., Smith, N.K.R., Steffens, W.L., and Wille, J.J. (1982) Cytobios 35, 47-62.
28. Maruyama, K., Mikawa, T., Ebashi, S. (1984) J. Biochem. 95, 511-519.

CHEMICAL SYNTHESIS AND BIOLOGICAL EVALUATION OF PHOTOAFFINITY - LABELLED DERIVATIVES OF VITAMIN D_3, 25-HYDROXYVITAMIN D_3, AND 1,25-DIHYDROXYVITAMIN D_3

R. Ray, S.D. Rose, S.A. Holick, and M.F. Holick,
Department of Nutrition & Food Sciences, Massachusetts Institute of Technology, Cambridge, Ma 02139, U.S.A.

Introduction

Photoaffinity labelling of peptide and steroid hormone receptors has been effectively used for probing ligand binding sites (1). However, this powerful tool has not been used to investigate ligand-receptor interactions for vitamin D_3 and its biologically important metabolites. We, hereby, report chemical synthesis and biological evaluation of photolabile derivatives of vitamin D_3 (PL-D_3), 25-hydroxyvitamin D_3 (PL-25-OH-D_3) and 1,25-dihydroxyvitamin D_3 (PL-1,25-$(OH)_2$-D_3.

Methods & Results

Synthesis: PL-D_3 and PL-25-OH-D_3 were synthesized by DCC-coupling of vitamin D_3 and 25-OH-D_3 with N-(4-azido-2-nitrophenyl) glycine (2). For PL-1,25-$(OH)_2$-D_3, 1-tert butyldimethylsilyloxy —25-hydroxyvitamin D_3 was coupled with the glycine derivative followed by desilylation with 5% HF (figure 1).

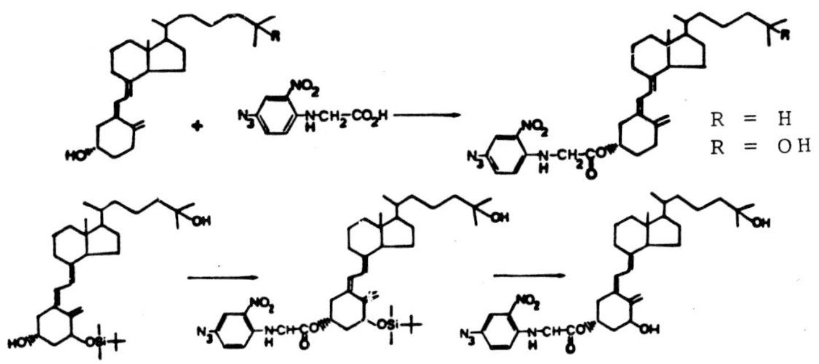

Figure 1

Biological Assay for PL-1,25-$(OH)_2$-D_3, in vivo: Weanling Holtzman rats, fed on a vitamin D-deficient, calcium-supplemented diet, were given intravenous doses of one of the following: 95% ethanol (control), 0.125 g of vitamin D_3, and 1.0 g of PL-1,25-$(OH)_2$-D_3. Rats were sacrificed after 24 hours. Serum Ca and intestinal Ca transport were determined by standard methods (3). Animals given 1.0 g PL-1,25-$(OH)_2$-D_3 showed increased intestinal Ca transport (S/M=3.8$\pm$0.1, compared to 1.9$\pm$0.1 for the control) and elevated serum Ca level (8.1$\pm$0.1, compared to 4.6$\pm$0.1 for the control)(3).

Competitive Binding Assays of PL-25-OH-D_3 & PL-1,25-$(OH)_2$-D_3
These assays were performed according to previously published procedures. Results are shown in figure 2 and figure 3. PL-25-OH-D_3 was approximately 100-fold less active than 25-OH-D_3 in displacing 50% Of the maximally bound [^{3}H]25-OH-D_3 (figure 2). PL-1,25-$(OH)_2$-D_3 was approximately 20-fold less active than 1,25-$(OH)_2$-D_3 (figure 3).

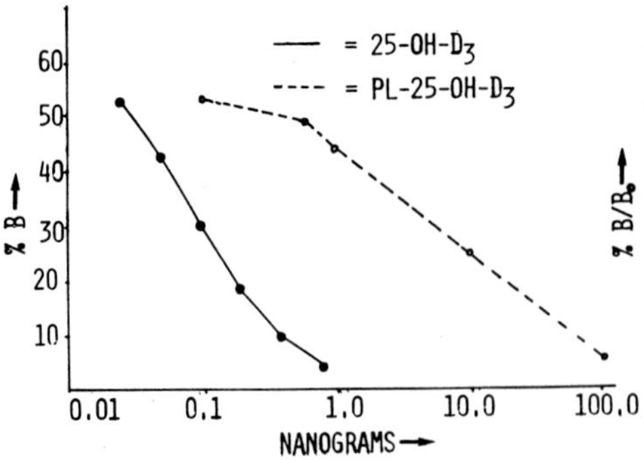

Figure 2: Competitive Binding Assay for PL-25-OH-D_3

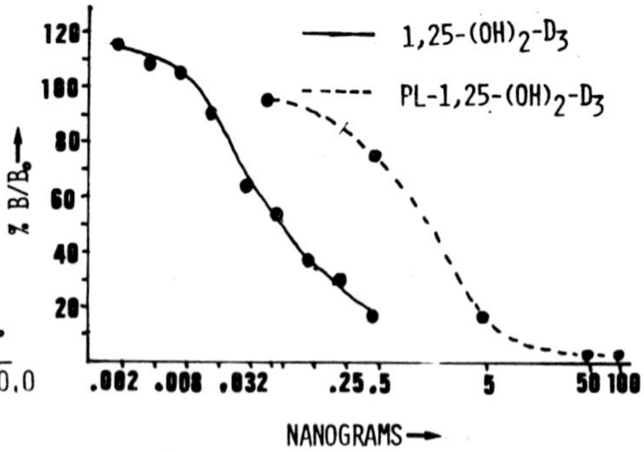

Figure 3: Competitive Binding Assay for PL-1,25-$(OH)_2$-D_3

Assay for the Receptor-Blockade by Irradiated PL-1,25-$(OH)_2$-D_3. Sucrose Density Gradient Sedimentation Analysis

Two quartz tubes containning PL-1,25-$(OH)_2$-D_3 were incubated at room temperature followed by irradiation of one (+UV). [^{3}H]1,25-$(OH)_2$-D_3 was added to each tube followed by incubation and charcoal-treatment. The supernatents were analyzed by sucrose density gradient sedimentation procedure. Results are shown in figure-4. A single peak of radioactivity (approximately 3.7S) was observed in both the samples indicating specific binding of PL-1,25-$(OH)_2$-D_3 to the receptor for 1,25-$(OH)_2$-D_3. Moreover, when the sample was irradiated prior to incubation with [^{3}H]1,25-$(OH)_2$-D_3, the amplitude of the 3.7S peak was significantly diminished.

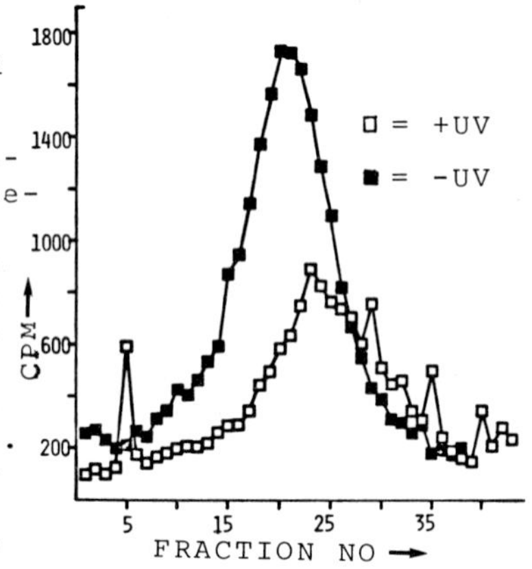

Figure 4: Sucrose Density Gradient Sedimentation Analysis with chick intestinal cytosol & PL-1,25-$(OH)_2$-D_3 (+UV & -UV).

Discussion

Both PL-25-OH-D_3 and PL-1,25-$(OH)_2$-D_3 stimulated intestinal Ca transport and bone calcium mobilization. These synthetic analogs competed for the binding sites (of rat plasma binding protein and chick intestinal cytosol respectively) with the normal substrates. Furthermore, PL-1,25-$(OH)_2$-D_3, upon irradiation, was covalently and specifically bound to the receptor.

References

1. Das,M., Fox,C.F., Ann. Rev. Biophys. Bioeng., (1979) 8: 165-193.
2. Levy,D., Biochem. Biophys. Acta, (1973) 322: 329-336.
3. Schacter,D., Kimber,V., Schenker,H., Am. J. Physiol., (1961) 200: 1263-1271.
4. This work was supported in part by NIH grants AM 27334 and AM 32324.

MULTIPLE FORMS OF CHICKEN INTESTINAL NUCLEAR 1,25-DIHYDROXYVITAMIN D_3 (1,25$(OH)_2D_3$) RECEPTORS. W.S. Mellon and S. Radparvar, School of Pharmacy, University of Wisconsin, Madison, WI 53706

Introduction. The biological function of 1,25$(OH)_2D_3$ as a calcemic and phosphatemic hormone presumably is mediated through an intracellular receptor system. At least for the chick intestine, the 1,25$(OH)_2D_3$ receptor has been purified as an apparent homogeneous protein with a molecular weight of 65-67,000 (1, 2). However, Hunziker *et al*., (3) have presented results that demonstrate biochemical heterogeneity in the 1,25$(OH)_2D_3$ receptor system which may represent distinct multiple forms. The present study was initiated to investigate physical/chemical properties of occupied and unoccupied nuclear 1,25$(OH)_2D_3$ receptors.

Methods. Nuclear 1,25$(OH)_2D_3$ receptors were obtained from purified intestinal nuclei of 3-5 week-old white Leghorn cockerels which were fed a vitamin D-deficient diet. In some instances, chicks were injected with 30 nmol 1,25$(OH)_2D_3$ I.V. 2 h prior to sacrifice. Receptor extraction was carried out at 0-4°C using Tris-HCl (50 mM), $MgCl_2$ (5 mM), DTT (5 mM), and KCl (300 mM), pH 7.5 (TMDK-0.3). Receptor labeling was accomplished by incubation with 1,25$(OH)_2[^3H]D_3$ directly (unoccupied) or using an exchange assay (total) as previously described (4). Linear 4-20% sucrose density gradient analysis was employed to monitor 1,25$(OH)_2D_3$ receptor form(s) (5). Additionally, receptor was purified and monitored for heterogeneity using Fast Protein Liquid Chromatography (FPLC). Generally, receptor was applied to a strong anion exchange column (Mono Q), washed with 10 ml TMDK-0.03 and finally eluted with a linear KCl gradient at a flow rate of 1.0 ml/min.

Results. Depending upon the volume of high ionic strength buffer (TMDK-0.3) utilized to extract nuclei (1:4 to 1:0.1, w/v), the receptor complexes, formed upon incubation with 1,25$(OH)_2[^3H]D_3$, sedimented on sucrose density gradients with a range of sedimentation coefficients (Fig. 1). The S value of the species observed was dependent upon the receptor concentration. With receptor concentrations $\leq$ 0.3 nM, receptor complexes sedimented as 3.7 S macromolecules (designated as monomers); within the range of 0.4 to 1.6 nM, migration as 4.5 to 6.9 S macromolecules (designated as oligomers) was observed. Similar findings also were observed with *in vivo* occupied receptors. When oligomeric forms were diluted with TMDK-0.3 to a receptor concentration $\leq$ 0.3 nM, receptors sedimented as 3.7 S macromolecule. Likewise, the monomer when subjected to concentration by lyophilization or filtration, sedimented as oligomers. Monomeric receptor treated with trypsin (0.1 mg/ml) or heated to 25°C for 2-4 hr lost its ability to aggregate. Contrariwise, the oligomeric forms are stable to warming at 25°C for at least 6 hr. Receptor complexes treated with RNase, DNase, β-glucuronidase, or lipase, were able to aggregate. Furthermore, monomeric receptors (0.21 nM) concentrated 6-fold using either BSA, ovalbumin, or chick liver cytosol, sedimentated as 3.7 S macromolecules. In contrast, monomers concentrated with receptor heated to 37°C could still aggregate. Both monomers and oligomers have similar ionic properties as demonstrated by anion exchange chromatography (FPLC). Both receptor forms are capable of being resolved into two components upon rechromatography of the

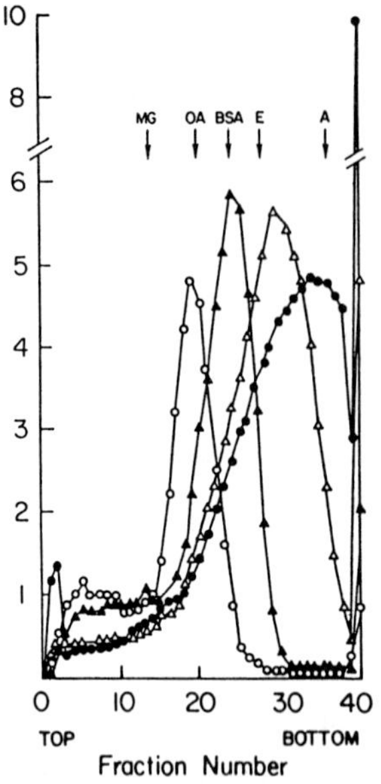

Figure 1. Sedimentation behavior of 1,25 $(OH)_2[^3H]D_3$ nuclear receptor at various receptor concentrations.

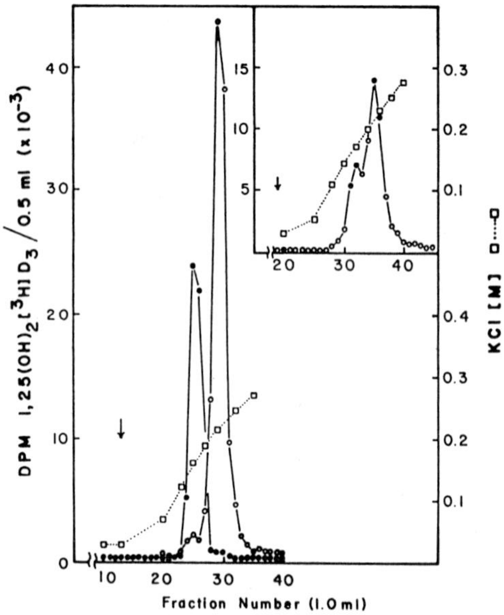

Figure 2. Separation of two $1{,}25(OH)_2[^3H]D_3$ receptor species by FPLC using a strong anion exchanger.

original peaks (see inset, Fig. 2); peak I eluting at 160 mM KCl and Peak II eluting at 215 mM KCl (Fig. 2). Preliminary results indicate that both peak I and II sediment as 3.7 S macromolecules on sucrose density gradients. Upon 5-fold concentration, neither Peak I nor Peak II aggregated. In contrast, equal portions of concentrated Peak I and II did form a 4.5 S oligomer.

In summary, these findings suggest that oligomer formation may result from multiple receptor subunit interactions. Moreover, two distinct monomer forms of nuclear receptor, as seen on FPLC, may be responsible for this aggregatory phenomenon. However, it is possible that binding of receptor to an accessory protein was responsible for oligomer formation.

References.

1. Pike, J.W., and Haussler, M. (1979) Proc. Natl. Acad. Sci. U.S.A. 76, 5485-5489.
2. Simpson, R.U., and DeLuca, H.F. (1982) Proc. Natl. Acad. Sci. U.S.A. 79, 16-20.
3. Hunziker, W., Walters, M.R., Bishop, J.E., and Norman, A.W. (1983) J. Biol. Chem. 258, 8642-8648.
4. Radparvar, S., and Mellon, W.S. (1984) J. Steroid Biochem. 20, 807-815.
5. Mellon, W.S. (1985) Endocrinology, in press.

DEFECTIVE BINDING AND FUNCTION OF 1,25-DIHYDROXY VITAMIN D_3 ($1,25(OH)_2D_3$) RECEPTORS IN PERIPHERAL MONONUCLEAR CELLS OF PATIENTS WITH END ORGAN RESISTANCE TO $1,25(OH)_2D$.

R. KOREN, A. RAVID, Z. HOCHBERG, Y. WEISMAN, A. NOVOGRODSKY and U.A. LIBERMAN,
Beilinson Medical Center, Rambam Medical Center, Ichilov Medical Center, Israel.

Fibroblasts cultured from human skin biopsies are an accepted and available model for vitamin D action in target organs. Fibroblasts obtained from patients with the syndrome of end organ resistance to $1,25(OH)_2D$ (vitamin D dependent rickets type II-DDII) exhibited defects in the intracellular $1,25(OH)_2D$ effector system. These defects were revealed by assays of equilibrium binding of ^3H-$1,25(OH)_2D_3$ with high salt cell extracts ("cytosol"), nuclear uptake of the hormone by intact cells and induction of 25-hydroxy vitamin D 24 hydroxylase. However fibroblast cultures are expensive and time consuming. This study is an attempt to provide an alternative model for vitamin D target organs using peripheral blood mononuclear cells.

Human T lymphocytes acquire receptors for $1,25(OH)_2D_3$ upon mitogenic stimulation and mitogen-induced lymphocyte proliferation is inhibited ((40-60)% n=24) by physiological concentrations (10^{-10}-10^{-9})M of $1,25(OH)_2D_3$. Mononuclear cells were obtained from 20 ml blood samples and cultured for 72 hours in presence of 10 μg/ml concanavalin A or 1 μg/ml phytohemagglutinin and increasing concentrations of $1,25(OH)_2D_3$. ^3H-thymidine incorporation into DNA was assayed in intact cells and binding of ^3H-$1,25(OH)_2D_3$ was measured in "cytosol". We found that lymphocytes from a group of 5 patients from 3 different kindreds with DDII do not acquire receptors for $1,25(OH)_2D_3$ upon mitogenic stimulation. However, the stimulation of these lymphocytes is refractory to inhibition by $1,25(OH)_2D_3$. The mitogenic stimulation of lymphocytes from a sixth patient from an additional kindred were not inhibited by $1,25(OH)_2D_3$, although the cells acquired a normal number of cytosolic receptors upon mitogenic stimulation. These results are similar to those obtained previously with skin fibroblasts from the same patients.

Vitamin D. A Chemical, Biochemical and Clinical Update

We conclude: a: A functional receptor for 1,25$(OH)_2D_3$ is essential for the action of the hormone in mononuclear cells. b: These receptors are probably controled genetically by the same mechanism as the expression of receptors in "classical" target organs. Therefore mononuclear cells can serve in a fast bioassay for the presence of functional receptors for 1,25$(OH)_2D$ in human subjects.

TRYPTIC CLEAVAGE OF CHICK 1,25-DIHYDROXYVITAMIN D_3 RECEPTOR

E.A. ALLEGRETTO and J.W. PIKE
Department of Biochemistry, Arizona Health Sciences Center, University of Arizona, Tucson, AZ 85724

The receptor for 1,25-dihydroxyvitamin D_3 (1,25$(OH)_2D_3$) is a cytosoluble, 60 kilodalton (K) protein that specifically binds the active form of the vitamin and mediates its action in target cell nuclei (1,2). Like other steroid hormone receptors, the 1,25$(OH)_2D_3$ receptor is thought to regulate gene expression via its capacity to bind to DNA (3,4). While the physiological effects of 1,25$(OH)_2D_3$ are well known, there is a paucity of physical information on the receptor itself. This deficiency of data is mainly due to the fact that the receptor is a proteolytically sensitive protein of trace abundance (<0.001% of the total cell protein) within target cells. We have attempted to gain insight into the structure-function relationship of the 1,25$(OH)_2D_3$ receptor by subjecting chick intestinal cytosol to trypsin (30', 10°C). Physical characterization of the resulting trypsin-derived polypeptide fragments was achieved through sedimentation analysis, gel filtration chromatography, and DEAE anion-exchange HPLC. Intactness of functional ligand-binding domains was evaluated by assessing macromolecular retention of 1,25$(OH)_2D_3$ as well as by determining reactivity to DNA and monoclonal antibody (5). Action at site I (~2.0 μg trypsin/200 μl 10% chick intestinal cytosol) resulted in the formation of a 50 K fragment which retained hormone and partial monoclonal antibody reactivity, but had lost DNA binding activity (see table below). Immunoblot methodology revealed the disappearance of the 60 K

CHARACTERISTICS OF 1,25$(OH)_2D_3$ RECEPTOR - TRYPTIC FRAGMENTS

	STRUCTURAL				FUNCTIONAL		
	MOLECULAR WEIGHT (K)		S	CHARGE(M)*	DNA	McAb[γ]	1,25$(OH)_2D_3$
	Gel Filtration	Immunoblot	SDG	DEAE-HPLC			
INTACT	62.5	60.3	3.0-3.6	0.25	+	+	+
		58.5			+	+	
SITE I	53	50	2.4-3.0	0.25	-	±	+
		20			±	+	-
SITE II	44	-	2.4-3.0	0.20	-	-	+

*Concentration of KCl in eluant.
[γ]McAb; Monoclonal Antibody, assessed by immunoblot or SDG.

receptor and the appearance of a 50 K and ~20 K band upon trypsin treatment at this concentration. Preliminary DNA-cellulose chromatography experiments indicate that the 20 K fragment is a low affinity DNA-binder. Higher trypsin concentrations (site II) resulted in the formation of a 44 K fragment which bound 1,25$(OH)_2D_3$, but not antibody or DNA. An immunoblot of this material showed that the epitope for monoclonal antibody was destroyed with high trypsin concentrations. The model below schematically illustrates the effects of trypsin on the 1,25$(OH)_2D_3$ receptor. The monomeric cytosolic receptor (left top) which has reactive sulfhydryl

Vitamin D. A Chemical, Biochemical and Clinical Update

groups in or near the binding domains for both $1,25(OH)_2D_3$ (6) and DNA (7), is shown to co-exist with receptor aggregates (right top). 60% of the 50 K hormone-binding fragments that are generated with low concentrations of trypsin, bind antibody (middle right) whereas ~40% do not (middle left). Trypsin treatment of DNA cellulose purified $1,25(OH)_2D_3$ receptor confirmed the results obtained with crude cytosolic preparations. Our findings suggest that while the steroid-binding site of the $1,25(OH)_2D_3$ receptor is remarkably stable to limited trypsin digestion, the determinant for monoclonal antibody and the domain for DNA-binding are readily inactivated and are thus highly vulnerable to attack by trypsin. The observations summarized in the table and the model are consistent with the hypothesis that the functional domains for $1,25(OH)_2D_3$ and DNA are distinct and therefore potentially separable from each other for further study to gain insight into the topology functionality of the $1,25(OH)_2D_3$ receptor.

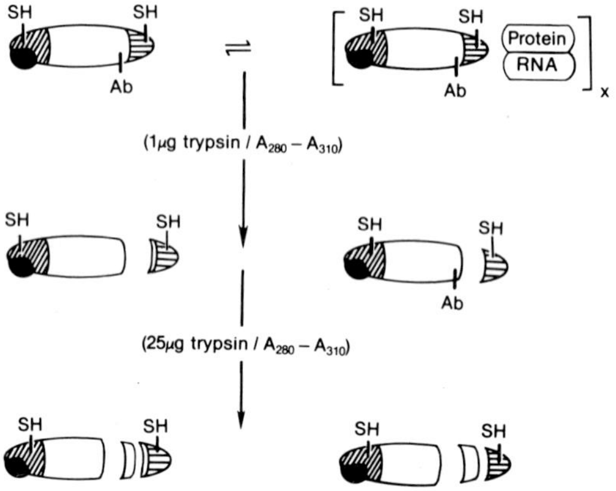

Proposed model for the effects of trypsin on the chick cytosol $1,25(OH)_2D_3$ receptor. -SH, cysteine residue; -Ab, monoclonal antibody binding site; $[\,]_x$, receptor-protein/nucleic acid low salt aggregates; diagonal slash, $1,25(OH)_2D_3$ binding domain; horizontal slash, DNA-binding domain; solid area, $1,25(OH)_2D_3$ ligand, 1 μg trypsin/A_{280}-A_{310} = 2.0 μg trypsin/200 μl cytosol.

References:

1. Haussler, M.R. and Brickman, A.S. (1982) in Disorders of Mineral Metabolism (Coburn, J.W., ed.) Academic Press, Inc., New York, Vol. II, 359-431.
2. DeLuca, H.F. and Schnoes, H.K. (1976) Annu. Rev. Biochem. 45, 631-666.
3. Pike, J.W. and Haussler, M.R. (1979) Proc. Natl. Acad. Sci. USA 76, 5485-5489.
4. Pike, J.W. (1982) J. Biol. Chem. 257, 6766-6775.
5. Pike, J.W. (1984) J. Biol. Chem. 259, 1167-1173.
6. Wecksler, W.R., Ross, F.P., and Norman, A.W. (1979) J. Biol. Chem. 254, 9488-9491.
7. Pike, J.W. (1981) Biochem. Biophys. Res. Commun. 100, 1713-1719.

TESTICULAR CALCITRIOL RECEPTORS; APPEARANCE DURING DEVELOPMENT AND PRESENCE IN ADULT TESTICULAR CELL CULTURES.

F.O. Levy, L. Eikvar, A. Frøysa, J. Cervenka, T. Yoganathan and V. Hansson
Institutes of Medical Biochemistry and Pathology, University of Oslo, Norway.

The rat testis contains a receptor for calcitriol (1,25-dihydroxy-vitamin D_3) (1,2,3,4). Earlier, we have shown that this receptor is present both in seminiferous tubules and interstitial tissue of adult rats, but not in cultured Sertoli cells or peritubular (myoid) cells isolated from immature (19-day-old) rats (3). It is not known whether this lack of calcitriol receptors in cultured cells from immature rats is due to the culture conditions or to the age of the animals.

The aim of this study was to examine whether there are developmental changes in the concentration of calcitriol receptors in the rat testis, and to elucidate which of the testicular cell types contain such receptors. Some of the results have been presented in a preliminary report (5).

MATERIALS AND METHODS.

Animals. Male Sprague Dawley rats were raised on a standard laboratory diet and kept on a 12 h light/12 h dark cycle.

Cytosol preparation. Whole testis cytosol was prepared from decapsulated testes which were rinsed in ice-cold phosphate-buffered saline (PBS). The testes were then homogenized at 0^oC in 5 volumes of high-salt buffer containing 10 mM Tris-HCl, 300 mM KCl, 1.5 mM EDTA, 1 mM DTT and 10 mM Na_2MoO_4 (KTEDMo buffer, pH 7.4 at 23^oC) in a Dounce all glass homogenizer. The homogenates were left at 0^oC for 30 to 60 min to extract nuclear receptors before preparation of a 105,000 g supernatant (cytosol).

Differential displacement of $[^3H]$-calcitriol binding to the serum vitamin D binding protein (DBP). $[^3H]$-calcitriol binding to DBP was eliminated by the following procedure: First, cytosol was labelled to equilibrium at 0^oC with $[^3H]$-calcitriol (0.3-0.5 nM) with and without excess unlabelled calcitriol. After labelling, an excess of unlabelled calcidiol (25-OH-D_3) (1.0 µM) was added, and the incubation was continued for 1 h at 0^oC. Due to the rapid dissociation of $[^3H]$-calcitriol from the DBP ($t_{1/2}$ < 5 min) and the very slow dissociation from the receptor ($t_{1/2}$ >> 48 h) (3), this procedure completely eliminated binding of $[^3H]$-calcitriol to the DBP without reducing the binding to the receptor (Fig. 1, right panel). After the 1 h incubation with unlabelled calcidiol, bound and free steroids were separated by hydroxylapatite assay or sucrose gradient centrifugation as described in (3).

RESULTS AND CONCLUSIONS.

Receptors for calcitriol can be detected in whole testis cytosol using either a hydroxylapatite batch assay or sucrose gradient centrifugation after "differential displacement" of binding to the contaminating DBP with cold calcidiol (25-OH-D_3) (Fig. 1).

Vitamin D. A Chemical, Biochemical and Clinical Update

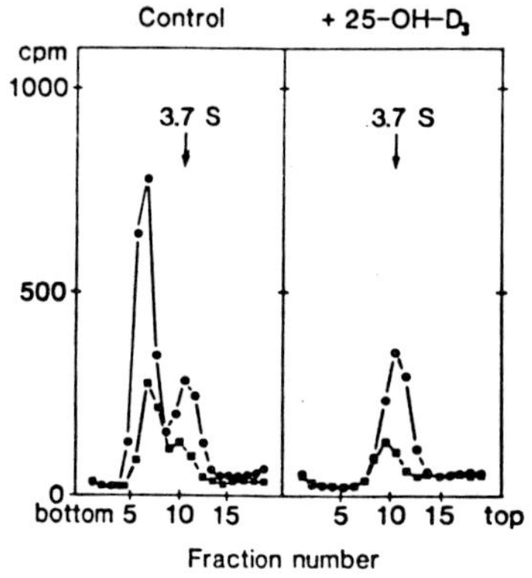

Figure 1. Sucrose gradient analysis of [^{3}H]-calcitriol binding in cytosol from whole testis of adult rats, before (left) and after (right) "differential displacement" of bound [^{3}H]-calcitriol from the contaminating DBP with an excess of unlabelled calcidiol.

The testicular calcitriol receptors were undetectable before day 24, and the concentration of receptors increased during development to reach adult levels (6-8 fmol/mg protein) around day 50-60.

The lack of receptors in the immature rat testis is not due to degrading enzymes; cytosol from pooled equal volumes of testis homogenates of immature and adult rats had binding levels exactly half of "adult controls".

The increase in specific [^{3}H]-calcitriol binding during development is due to an increase in the number of receptors, and is not due to a change in binding affinity ($K_d \approx 1 \times 10^{-11}$ M at 0^oC).

Receptors for calcitriol can be detected in adult testicular cell cultures, containing a mixture of Sertoli cells and peritubular (myoid) cells. Calcitriol receptors were not detected in testicular germ cells (pachytene spermatocytes and round spermatids) from 32-day old rats. The final answer to which of the cell types in the seminiferous tubules that contain these receptors must await better procedures for isolation of pure cells from adult testicular tissue.

REFERENCES.

(1) Walters, M.R., Cuneo, D.L. and Jamison, A.P. (1983) J. steroid Biochem. 19, 913-920.
(2) Merke, J., Kreusser, W., Bier, B. and Ritz, E. (1983) Eur. J. Biochem. 130, 303-308.
(3) Levy, F.O., Eikvar, L., Jutte, N.H.P.M., Frøysa, A., Tvermyr, S.M. and Hansson, V. (1985) J. steroid Biochem. 22 (4).
(4) Walters, M.R. (1984) Endocrinology 114, 2167-2174.
(5) Levy, F.O., Eikvar, L., Jutte, N.H.P.M. and Hansson, V. Program, Third European Workshop on Molecular and Cellular Endocrinology of the Testis, Lyon (L'Arbresle), France, April 26-28, 1984 (Abstract).

1,25DIHYDROXYVITAMIN D_3 RECEPTORS AND ACTIVITIES IN SKELETAL AND HEART MUSCLE

R.U. SIMPSON, G.A. THOMAS, and A.J. ARNOLD,
Dept. of Pharmacology, Univ. of Michigan, Ann Arbor, MI 48109 U.S.A.

INTRODUCTION:

A recognized function of vitamin D_3 is to promote growth and development of muscle (1). Muscle myopathy is a prominent feature of vitamin D deficiency or disturbance of vitamin D metabolism. It has been suggested that the action of 1,25$(OH)_2D_3$ on muscle is secondary to its action to regulate blood calcium (2). Others, however, have shown that 1,25-$(OH)_2D_3$ has direct effects on muscle metabolism and contractile processes (3). We here report that two established heart and skeletal myoblast lines, and excised muscle cells possess 1,25$(OH)_2D_3$ receptors. We demonstrate that proliferation of the myoblasts is inhibited by 1,25$(OH)_2D_3$ and that receptor concentration in the cells is decreased when cells were differentiated to fused myotubes.

MATERIALS AND METHODS:

Cell culture: Heart (H9c2), skeletal myoblast (G-8) lines and isolated heart cells were cultured in Dulbecco's media (DMEM) with 10% fetal calf and 10% horse sera. Differentiation of lines was induced by "differentiation media" as described by Rowin *et al.* (4). All cells were kept at 37°C in 5% CO_2.

Cell preparations: Cells were removed from flask with 10 mM EDTA in phosphate buffered saline, rinsed, resuspended in 2 volumes of TKED buffer and cytosols were prepared as previously described (5). Muscle cells were isolated using enzyme digestion by the technique of Jacobson (6).

Binding studies: 1,25$(OH)_2$-[^3H]D_3 (AMERSHAM) in ethanol was added in the presence or absence of 10-100 fold excess nonradioactive calciferols. Bound hormone was separated from free and sucrose gradient (TKED buffer) analysis was as previously described (5). Equilibrium binding data was analyzed by the method of Scatchard.

Cell proliferation and DNA synthesis: Cells were incubated with 1.0 µCi/ml [^3H]thymidine at 37°C for 1 hr, harvested and counted in a Coulter counter (Zf) or lysed and DNA was TCA precipitated.

RESULTS:

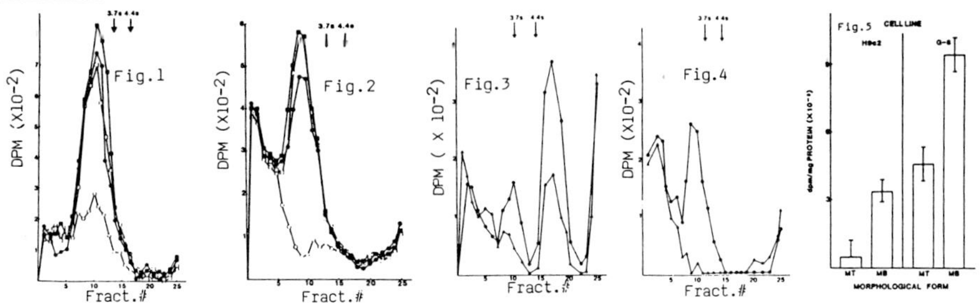

Figure 1-5. Sucrose density gradient analysis of 1,25$(OH)_2$[^3H]D_3 binding in G-8 skeletal myoblasts (Fig. 1), H9c2 heart myoblast (Fig. 2), isolated heart cells (Fig. 3), and primary culture of heart cells (Fig. 4). Effect of low-serum induced differentiation on 1,25$(OH)_2D_3$ receptor concentration in H9c2 and G-8 cells (Fig. 5)(MB myoblasts; MT myotubes).

Vitamin D. A Chemical, Biochemical and Clinical Update

Figures 1 and 2 show gradient profiles of 1,25(OH)$_2$[^{3}H]D$_3$ binding in skeletal G-8 (1) and heart H9c2 (2) myoblast lines. For analysis cytosol was incubated with 1.0 nM 1,25(OH)$_2$[^{3}H]D$_3$ alone (■) or with 10 nM cold 1,25(OH)$_2$D$_3$ (○), 24,25(OH)$_2$D$_3$ (□) or 25(OH)D$_3$ (●). The data show that a 3.2s sedimenting 1,25(OH)$_2$D$_3$ receptor exists in both myoblast cell lines. Furthermore, figure 3 shows that enzyme isolated heart muscle cells possess 2 binding species: a 3.2-3.4s and a 6.0s binding macromolecule. Figure 4 is a sucrose gradient profile of a primary culture of beating rat heart cell cytosol; only the 3.2-3.4s 1,25(OH)$_2$D$_3$ receptor is present. Scatchard analysis of 1,25(OH)$_2$D$_3$ binding in myoblast cell cytosols were performed (data not shown). The Kd was 8.4 x 10^{-11}M with 25.9 fmol/mg protein sites for the H9c2 myoblasts and the Kd was 3.8 x 10^{-11}M with 62.4 fmol/mg sites for G-8 cells. Incubating the H9c2 and G-8 lines in "differentiation media" the myoblasts differentiated to fused myotube form (data not shown). Figure 5 shows that G-8 and H9c2 cells differentiated to myotubes possessed less 1,25(OH)$_2$D$_3$ receptor than myoblast cells. We examined the possibility that 1,25(OH)$_2$D$_3$ may affect the proliferation of the myoblasts. Figure 6 shows a dose-dependent inhibition of cell proliferation of the G-8 cells by 1,25(OH)$_2$D$_3$. Figure 7 shows that 1,25(OH)$_2$D$_3$ dose dependently inhibited DNA synthesis in the G-8 myoblast line. For both experiments, cells were cultured for 48 hrs, dosed and 48 hrs later cell number and DNA synthesis was assayed.

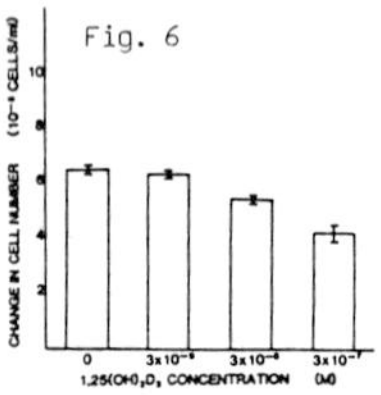

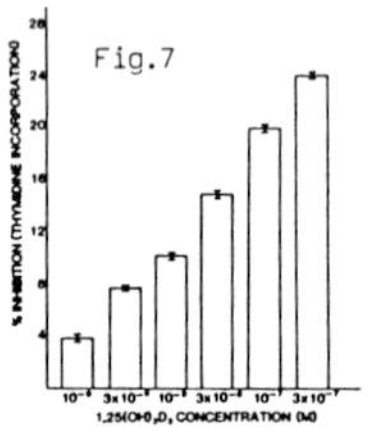

Figure 6. Action of 1,25(OH)$_2$D$_3$ on G-8 myoblast proliferation.
Figure 7. Action of 1,25(OH)$_2$D$_3$ on G-8 myoblast DNA synthesis.

DISCUSSION:

It has long been recognized that vitamin D affects muscle (1). Our data suggest that skeletal and heart muscle possesses 1,25(OH)$_2$D$_3$ receptors and are target tissues for 1,25(OH)$_2$D$_3$. Our data also suggest that 1,25(OH)$_2$D$_3$ may induce terminal differentiation of myoblasts. Further studies of the action of 1,25(OH)$_2$D$_3$ on muscle are required and should yield important new information.

Selected References:

1. Steenbock, H. and Herting, D.C. (1955) J. Nutr. 57, 449-468.
2. Wassner, S.J., Li, J.B., Sperduto, A. and Norman, M.E. (1983) J. Clin. Invest. 72, 102-112.
3. Guiliani, D.L. and Boland, R. (1984) Cal. Tis. Int. 36, 200.
4. Rowin, K.S. and Nadal-Ginard, B. (1983) Proc. Natl. Acad. Sci. (USA) 80, 6390-6394.
5. Simpson, R.U. and DeLuca, H.F. (1980) Proc. Natl. Acad. Sci. (USA) 77, 5822-5824.
6. Jacobson, S.L. (1977) Cell Struct. Funct. 2, 1-9.

IMPACT OF MICROCOMPUTERS ON VITAMIN D RESEARCH

Organiser: Glenville Jones
Departments of Biochemistry and Medicine
Queen's University, Kingston, Ontario, Canada K7L 3N6

INTRODUCTION

No area of academic pursuit is immune to the effects of computers - not even vitamin D research. Though many of us dislike the invasion of these intruders into our laboratories and offices, few of us can deny that computers save us time and perform tedious repetitive tasks effortlessly. Whether we use this "saved" time sensibly is debatable. Computer power has been at the fingertips of scientists for some time, but costly hardware and complicated software limited its application to the vitamin D field. At the last two Workshops on Vitamin D there were few reports involving computer applications.

With the advent of the microcomputer the cost and complexity of computing has been much reduced. This has resulted in widespread software development in scientific fields and in the integration of this technology into scientific instrumentation in the form of microchips. Thus today's instruments have an improved electronic stability and increased automation over yesterday's models.

The purpose of this discussion is not to advertise today's instruments or to extol the virtues of this computer or that but rather to explore the areas of vitamin D research which have benefitted in the past or will benefit in the future from the use of microcomputers.

Microcomputers can be used in:-

1) Quantitation and identification of vitamin D during chromatography.
2) Radio ligand binding assays and Scatchard analysis.
3) Screen and plotter graphics of vitamin D.

These will be each examined in some detail.

QUANTITATION AND IDENTIFICATION OF VITAMIN D DURING HPLC

HPLC of vitamin D is now a decade old (Matthews *et al.*, 1974; Jones and DeLuca, 1975; Ikekawa and Koizumi, 1976) and since then assays for 25-OH-D, vitamin D and 24,25-$(OH)_2D_3$ have been developed (Jones, 1977; Shepard *et al.*, 1977; Dreyer and Goodman, 1981). These assays were based upon the UV absorption spectrum of vitamin D with the characteristic λ_{max} = 265 nm, λ_{min} = 228 nm and ε_{265} = 18,300. Most methods utilize a mercury lamp detector with a strong mercury line at 254 nm. The technique is sensitive. As little as 1 nanogram of vitamin D in an HPLC peak can be detected using a 254nm

Vitamin D. A Chemical, Biochemical and Clinical Update

detector. However accurate quantitation is dependent upon other UV containing contaminants being absent from the peak. Since the two criteria for identification of the vitamin D by this technique are:-

a) its absorbance at 254 nm, and
b) its retention time,.

the method is subject to frequent interference by contaminants.

Quantitation of peaks in HPLC is performed by measuring the area under peaks and comparison to a standard. Traditionally this was done manually with a planimeter or automatically using an integrator. Integrators are dedicated instruments equipped with complex algorithms and designed for the purposes of accurately measuring peak areas and allocating the area under a fused set of peaks.

Recently microcomputer-based integration has been introduced by many companies (Nelson Analytical; Adalabs; Waters) which take existing microcomputers (HP or IBM; Apple; Dec 350) and combine them with new software to perform the same tasks as integrators. Usually these systems have advantages over integrators:-

1) Much more data can be stored in the disk-drives of the microcomputer so that raw data from an HPLC run can be saved and not just the processed data as in most integrators. This permits repeated reprocessing of raw data until the operator is satisfied.

2) Manual reintegration (Fig. 1) becomes feasible as a result where the operator can decide where peaks start and end and where baselines should be. This is particularly useful to the vitamin D area where we are usually pushing

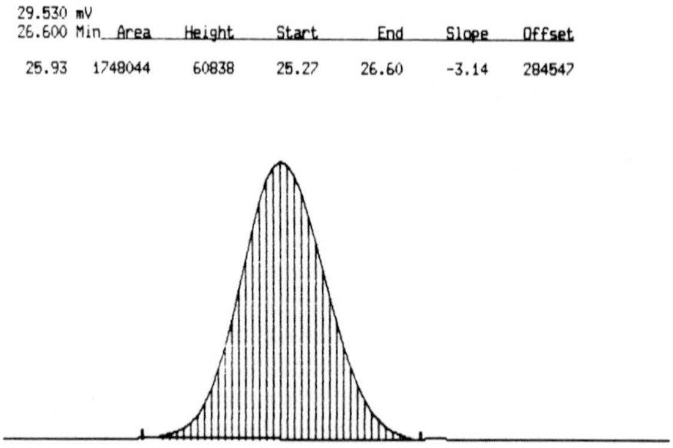
29.530 mV
26.600 Min Area Height Start End Slope Offset
25.93 1748044 60838 25.27 26.60 -3.14 284547

Figure 1. Use of Scanner program from Waters Expert software to integrate area under peak. The computer used is a DEC 350. (with permission of Waters)

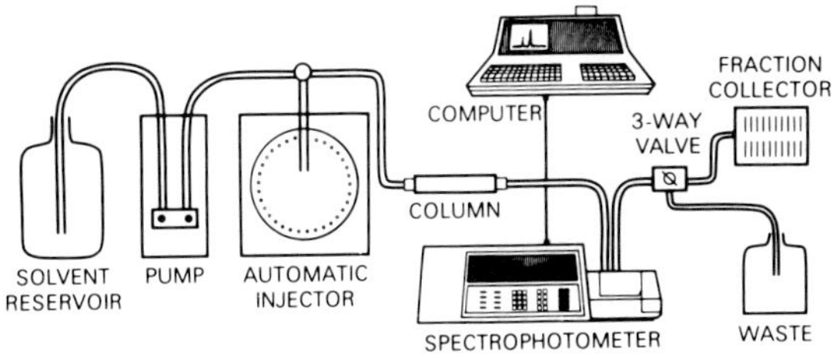

Figure 2. (A) Diode-array spectrophotometer in an HPLC set-up

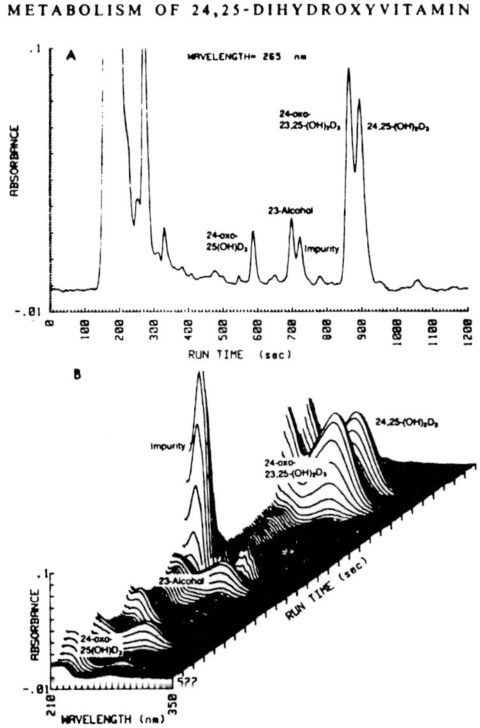

Figure 2. (B) Results of 2- and 3-dimensional HPLC using diode array spectrophotometer (reproduced from Jones et al., 1984).

et al., 1983; Jones et al., 1984; Jones, 1985). The technique allows scanning of the complete UV (and VIS) spectrum every 1-3 seconds during an HPLC run. One obtains a 3-dimensional rather than a 2-dimensional chromatogram (Fig. 2). Our data was obtained using a combination of the HP 8450 spectrophotometer and a HP 9816 microcomputer. The software was written by Tat Ying Wong in my laboratory and is available to anyone who can use it (software free; $25 cost to cover disk and sensitivity limits to their maximum and integration based upon algorithms falls down.

3) The microcomputer can perform other tasks such as instrument control, data manipulation at the same time as it is acquiring new data.

4) The software can be improved and changed with minimal modification to the chromatograph.

During the late 1980's we will see more shifts in this direction because of economics. Using the microcomputer the instrument companies need to develop only the software and not the hardware - the microcomputer. With this switch to microcomputer quantitation has also come the possibility of customising data output to suit the operator's needs:
further data analysis using operator designed software;
customised data reports;
graphs "camera-ready" for publication in whatever format and size is needed.

In the field of vitamin D these general improvements have helped but further changes just around the corner will have an even bigger impact. Newer high sensitivity detectors are being designed which can transmit several UV signals simultaneously to the microcomputer (eg. Waters 490 Multiwavelength detector). This takes advantage of the microcomputer's well recognised power to "crunch" data extremely quickly. From the standpoint of vitamin D quantitation, the ability to simultaneously monitor 4 or more wavelengths allows for greater specificity. By simultaneously quantitating vitamin D peaks at 228 nm, 254 nm, 265 nm and 285 nm, the operator is in a position to recognise the existence of contaminating peaks and remove them by arithmetical means. Microcomputer software again allows this manipulation to be performed with the minimum of inconvenience.

Other less-sensitive detectors are now available based upon diode-array spectrophotometry. This technique uses a deuterium lamp and rather than selecting a specific wavelength of light, uses 200 diodes to measure about 200 separate wavelengths simultaneously. This technique generates 200 times as much data, but sampling intervals are usually lengthened over standard UV detectors in order not to saturate the computer with data. Models include Hewlett Packard 8450 or 8451 spectrophotometers fitted with a flow cell; Hewlett Packard HP1040A, HPLC detector; and LKB Model 2140 Spectral Detector with IBM computer.

Though it is doubtful that present diode-array spectrophotometric detectors are sensitive enough to allow for the measurement of 25-OH-D_3 in normal plasma, they certainly provide excellent selectivity where sensitivity is not a critical factor. We recently published two or three papers on the use of computerised diode-array spectrophotometry in the study of vitamin D metabolism in the perfused kidney (Jones mailing). Software of this type can be made quite specific for vitamin D - to recognise the unique features of vitamin D and display them visually.

RADIO-RECEPTOR ASSAYS AND SCATCHARD ANALYSIS

Radio-receptor assays, whether competitive binding assays or radioimmunoassays, have become established technique in the measurement of plasma vitamin D metabolite concentrations. Commercially available kits (Yamasa; Amersham; Immunonuclear) and simplified chromatography have made these assays feasible even for routine biochemistry laboratories. Data analysis from such assays has been computerised for a decade or more. Mainly through the work of David Rodbard, NIH (Rodbard and Lewald, 1970) we now have several mathematical treatments of radio-receptor assay curves (eg. LOGIT vs LOG DOSE; SPLINE FIT; and 4 PARAMETER LOGISTIC) that permit accurate weighting and interpolation of data. Many of these treatments have been incorporated into computer programs and are available from Biomedical Computing Technology Information Center (BCTIC) at the Vanderbilt Medical Centre for no cost. Some have been adapted for microcomputers (eg. BASIC programs RIA001 and RIA004, BCTIC). Several useful handbooks have been produced on this subject (see references).

BCTIC also distributes programs based upon Scatchard analysis (Scatchard, 1949) but these are usually for larger computers and are written in FORTRAN. Mr. Tat-Ying Wong and I have also written a radioimmunoassay program for the Hewlett-Packard HP85 incorporating logit vs log dose treatment, interpolation of plasma vitamin D data and a section for directly transferring the results to printed sheets for transmission to the physician. This program is presently being adapted for the IBM-PC. Listing is available on request. Sample output is shown below (Fig. 3).

SCREEN AND PLOTTER GRAPHICS OF VITAMIN D

This technique is in its infancy. 2-dimensional representations of the vitamin D molecule are relatively easy to develop and are based upon establishing an X-Y template for the vitamin D structure. Analogs of vitamin D can be readily made by simple modifications to this basic structure eg. additions of -OH groups in 1,25-$(OH)_2D_3$. Using an HP85 computer scaling is easy to change and a molecule which filled the screen can now be put into the left-upper quandrant of the screen. See example shown below (Fig. 4).

Convenience of computer graphics tends to be highly dependent not only on the model of computer but also on the peripherals (printer or plotter) used. Often the quality of screen graphics is poor compared to the resolution one can obtain on a good plotter. Thus there is often little desire to copy screen graphics on to the printed page and with some combinations of computer and printer/plotter this is difficult.

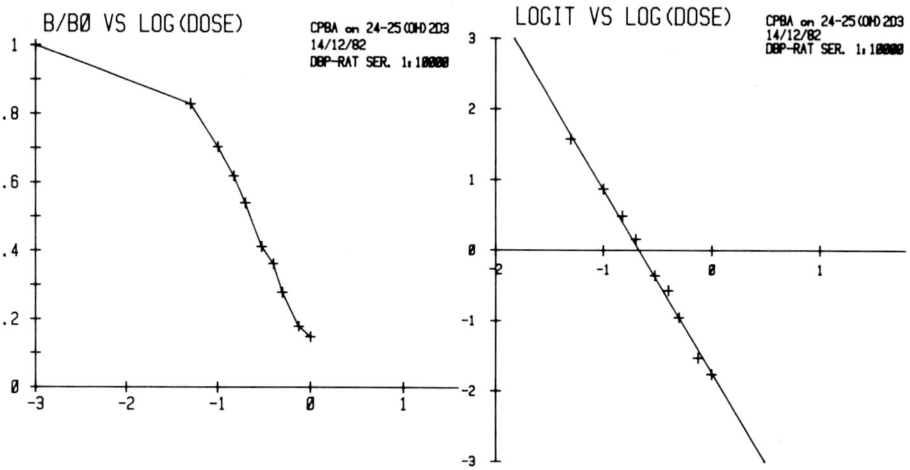

Figure 3. Two computer outputs of B/Bo vs LOG(DOSE) and LOGIT vs LOG(DOSE) for a 24,25-$(OH)_2D_3$ binding assay using a Hewlett-Packard HP85 computer program.

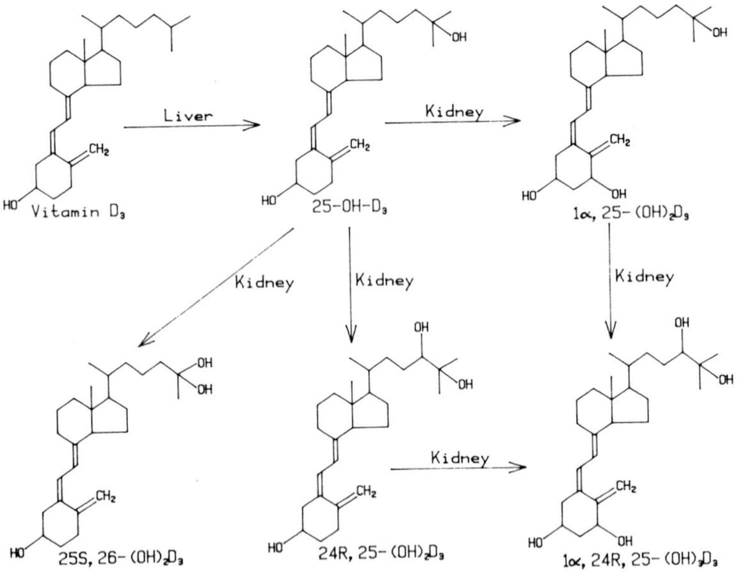

Fig. 4. Plotter graphics produced with an HP85 computer and HP 7225 plotter.

However, recently screen graphics has improved (eg. Macintosh) and the need to exactly "screen-dump" onto a plotter/printer becomes advantageous. Printer/plotters based upon inkjet or laser technology (eg. Hewlett Packard Thinkjet or Laser Jet Printers) are able to reproduce very accurately a complex vitamin D representation (Fig. 5). This type of graphics can be quite useful in documentation writing when coupled with a program such as Lotus 1,2,3 (Lotus Development Corp.).

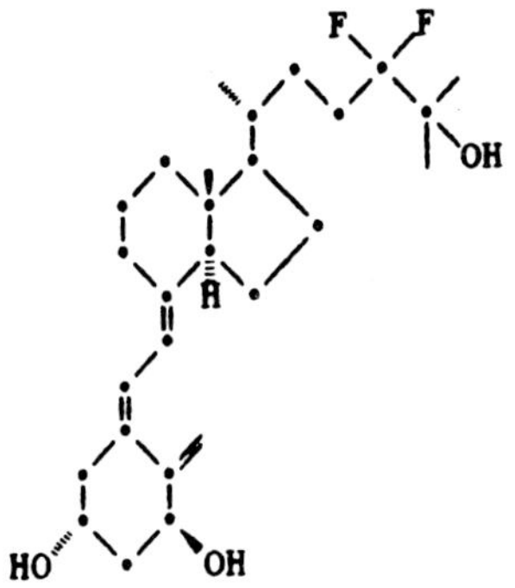

$1,25(OH)_2$-$24F_2$-D_3
Ro 22-9343

Figure 5. Vitamin D structure produced on a jet printer.

CAUTION:

Commercially available software is subject to copyright protection and the reproduction of such software is ILLEGAL. The author recommends strict adherence to the copyright laws. Similarly, the privately written non-copyright programs referred to in this chapter, are not guaranteed in any way. Such programs may contain "bugs" or simply will not work on other computer systems. They are provided with the proviso that the recipient does not hold the program owner responsible for damage or law suits which might arise out of use of the programs.

DISCUSSION

Owen Parkes (University of British Columbia) introduced a number of applications of microcomputers for group discussion. These included:

1) Information and reference storage and retrieval

A data base management program has been developed by O. Parkes for information manipulation based upon free field entry and compatible with Wordstar.
Dr. H. Makin (London) reported his experience with the fixed field data management system - SCI Mate. The CPM based software was very slow when loaded with over 1000 references and was asked to retrieve specific individual references.

2) Wordprocessing, particularly as related to manuscript preparation. How long before electronic mail in papers?
O. Parkes also recommended the generation of a biyearly newsletter advertising programmes that are available and user reports on commercially available programs. G. Jones agreed to mail such a list of programs to all present at the session and to all those who later requested it. O. Parkes recommended a subscription to "Byte" magazine as an aid to all those entering the computer field.
It was pointed out by E. Kaptein (University of Southern California) that the present use of microcomputers was a passing phase and that the future would likely bring a return to mainframe computers by use of microcomputers as terminals. This development she felt would reduce the opportunity to develop "personalised" software. She also reported her own use and modification of Rodbard programs.
A great interest was expressed by T. Freund (Fairleigh Dickinson University) in the need for modelling programs that could be used to predict changes in calcium homeostatic pools following perturbations of a single parameter.
G. Jones pointed out that many microcomputer word processing systems and associated printers are not designed for such complex typing problems as the formula - $^3H\ 1,25(OH)_2D_3$.
Similarly graphic and statistical software available rarely contains error-bars and makes it necessary to use artist modification of computer printer/plotter graphics. One impressive piece of software written for DEC series computers (VAX, DEC 350, PDP 11 Series) is the RS-1 of Bolt, Berenek and Newman. Though expensive it accepts ASCII files generated by many other programs and privides comprehensive statistical analysis.

REFERENCES:

1. Matthews, et.al. (1984), FEBS Letters 48, 122
2. Jones, G., and DeLuca, H.F. (1975), J. Lipid Res. 16, 448
3. Ikekawa, N. and Koizumi (1976)

4. Jones, G. (1977) in: Vitamin D, Biochemical, Chemical and Clinical Aspects related to Calcium Metabolism, Eds. Norman, A.W. et al, 491
5. Shepard (1979) Biochem.J. 182, 55-69
6. Dreyer, B. and Goodman, D. (1981), Analyt.Biochem. 114, 37-41
7. Jones, G., Kung, M., and Kano, K. (1983), J.Biol.Chem.
8. Jones, G., et.al. (1984), Biochemistry 23, 3749-3754
9. Jones, G. (1985) Methods in Enzymology Vitamins and Enzymes, in press.
10. Rodbard, D. and Lewald, (1970), Acta Endocr. 64, Suppl. 147, 79-103
11. Scatchard, (1949)
12. BCTIC, Room 1302, Vanderbilt Medical Centre, Nashville, Tennesee 37232, USA
13. Computers in Endocrinology (Serono Symposia Publications from Raven Press Vol. 14), Rodbard, D. and Forte, G., eds. Raven Press, New York, 1984.

Cell Differentiation and Vitamin D (+ Metabolites)

1,25-DIHYDROXYVITAMIN D_3 AND THE HEMATOPOIETIC SYSTEM

Helmut Reichel*, H. Phillip Koeffler+, Richard Barbers+, Reinhold Munker+ and Anthony W. Norman*, *Dept. Biochem., Univ. Calif., Riverside, CA 92521 and +Dept. Med., Univ. Calif., Los Angeles, CA 90024.

Introduction: In the last few years interactions between the vitamin D endocrine system and the hematopoietic system have been observed *in vivo* and *in vitro*.

An increased frequency of bacterial infections (1), along with impaired reaction to non-specific inflammatory stimuli (2) and decreased leukocyte chemotaxis and phagocytosis (3) were demonstrated in vitamin D deficient children. Rachitic children were found to have anemia and extramedullary hematopoiesis (4), with improved hematologic findings after treatment with vitamin D_3.

The recent demonstration of specific receptors for $1,25(OH)_2D_3$ in a number of normal and malignant human hematopoietic cells suggested a biological role for $1,25(OH)_2D_3$ extending its established properties in mineral and bone metabolism (5). $1,25(OH)_2D_3$ was found to bind specifically to human monocytes and to activated, but not to resting B- and T-lymphocytes (6,7). A number of malignant cells from the lymphoid (6,8) and myeloid (9,10) lineage also express specific receptors for $1,25(OH)_2D_3$.

Human myeloid leukemic cell lines have been used extensively in recent years to study the role of $1,25(OH)_2D_3$ in the differentiation of hematopoietic stem cells. Figure 1 provides a flow chart of stem cell differentiation, showing widely used myeloid cell lines at their stage of differentiation.

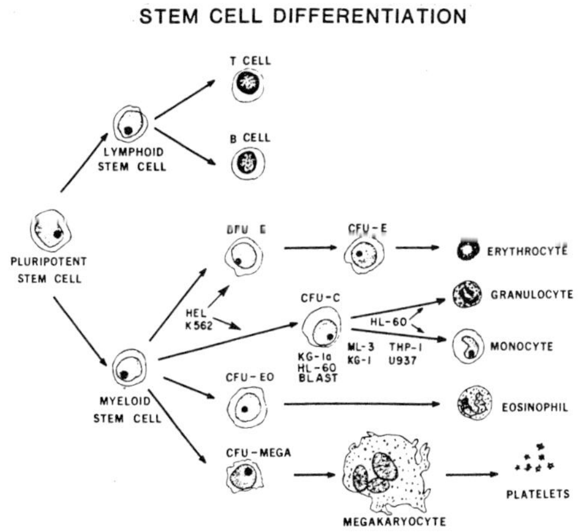

Fig. 1: Flow chart of stem cell differentiation. Cell lines shown at stage of differentiation. Arrows indicate differentiation potential.

Vitamin D. A Chemical, Biochemical and Clinical Update

In this report we will outline some effects of $1,25(OH)_2D_3$ on the differentiation and clonal growth of human myeloid cells, refer to the effects of $1,25(OH)_2D_3$ on patients with the myelodysplastic syndrome and then focus on our most recent work on the role of human macrophages in the metabolism of the vitamin D endocrine system.

$1,25(OH)_2D_3$ and Myeloid Differentiation:

In 1981 it was reported for the first time that $1,25(OH)_2D_3$ could induce differentiation of the mouse myeloid cell line MI (11) and the human promyelocytic cell line HL-60 (12). Furthermore, when $1,25(OH)_2D_3$ was administered *in vivo* to mice inoculated with M1 leukemic cells, survival of the mice was prolonged significantly (13).

It became clear that $1,25(OH)_2D_3$ differentiated HL-60 cells towards macrophages and not toward granulocytes (10,14) at dose levels as low as 10^{-10}M. HL-60 cells, exposed to $1,25(OH)_2D_3$ become adherent to plastic, increase phagocytic activity, reduce nitroblue tetrazolium, express non-specific acid-esterase and express receptors for the FMLP chemoattractant (10). Other alterations induced in HL-60 cells by $1,25(OH)_2D_3$ comprise C3-rosette formation (15), expression of monocyte-macrophage-specific surface antigens (14,16) and the capacity to resorb bone (17).

Another study was carried out to determine whether $1,25(OH)_2D_3$ also can induce differentiation of normal human myeloid stem cells (GM-GFC) (18). Bone marrow cells from normal donors were plated in soft agar with a source of colony-stimulating factor (CSF) and incubated with different concentrations of $1,25(OH)_2D_3$. As shown in Table 1, $1,25(OH)_2D_3$ stimulated formation of monocyte/macrophage colonies (MMC) in a dose-dependent fashion. Exposure of GM-GFC to 10^{-7}M $1,25(OH)_2D_3$ resulted both in an increase of the absolute number of macrophage-colonies and in an increase of the relative number of MMC compared to granulocyte colonies. Control incubations were carried out in the presence of CSF but not $1,25(OH)_2D_3$.

Similarly, $1,25(OH)_2D_3$ affected colony formation of monocytes/macrophages in peripheral blood cells, obtained from patients with chronic myelogenous leukemia and acute nonlymphocytic leukemia (18). Since only supraphysiological doses of $1,25(OH)_2D_3$ ($\geq 10^{-9}$M) were effective, there is still no evidence, if $1,25(OH)_2D_3$ also induces monocyte/macrophage differentiation of GM-GFC *in vivo*. The *in vitro* results suggest that $1,25(OH)_2D_3$ may enhance differentiation of myeloid progenitor cells predominantly towards mononuclear phagocytes. Since monocytes are probable precursors of osteoclasts (19), bone metabolism might thus be influenced by $1,25(OH)_2D_3$.

$1,25(OH)_2D_3$ and the Clonal Growth of Leukemic Cells

Further studies were related to *in vitro* effects of $1,25(OH)_2D_3$ on clonal growth of leukemic cells (20). Either cells from established myelogenous leukemia cell lines or cells freshly obtained from patients with myelo-

Table 1

Differentiation and Proliferation of Norman Human Myeloid Colony Forming Cells: Effects of $1,25(OH)_2D_3$

$1,25(OH)_2D_3$ (M)	Number of Colonies (% of control)	Neutrophilic Colonies (%)	Neutrophil-Macrophage Mixed Colonies (%)	Macrophage Colonies (%)	Absolute Number of Macrophage Colonies
0	100	56 ± 8*	10 ± 1	34 ± 4	31
10^{-10}	102 ± 6	58 ± 5	6 ± 1	36 ± 3	33
10^{-9}	120 ± 5	39 ± 4	5 ± 1	56 ± 4	61
10^{-8}	110 ± 6	29 ± 5	6 ± 1	65 ± 4	65
10^{-7}	91 ± 8	12 ± 3	3 ± 1	85 ± 6	71

Table 1: Nonadherent mononuclear cells from the bone marrow of 8 normal volunteers were cultured in the presence of 2.5% T-lymphocyte conditioned medium and different concentrations of $1,25(OH)_2D_3$. On day 10 of culture colonies were counted. Morphology of colonies was determined by dual esterase and luxol fast blue staining.

* Mean ± SE

genous leukemia were cultured in soft agar in the presence of $1,25(OH)_2D_3$ in different concentrations.

$1,25(OH)_2D_3$ (10^{-11} - 8x 10^{-8}M) inhibited clonal growth of myelogenous cell lines blocked at more mature stages of differentiation while it had no effect on clonal growth of less mature myelogenous cell lines (Table 2A). Clonal growth of leukemic cells was inhibited by $1,25(OH)_2D_3$ in cells obtained from 6 out of 9 patients with acute myelogenous leukemia and of 3 out of 4 patients with chronic myelogenous leukemia (Table 2B). In contrast, bone marrow cells taken from 11 patients with treated leukemia in remission showed no suppression of colony-formation, when exposed to $1,25(OH)_2D_3$.

Table 2A

Myeloid Leukemia Cell Lines: Inhibition of Clonal Growth by $1,25(OH)_2D_3$

CELL LINE	DESCRIPTION	ED-50++ (M)
HL-60+	Promyelocytes	1 x 10^{-11}
U937 +	Monoblast	2 x 10^{-9}
THP-1+	Monoblast	9 x 10^{-9}
M-1+*	Myeloblast	1 x 10^{-8}
HEL	Myelomonoblast/Erythoblast	2 x 10^{-8}
KG-1	Myeloblast	No inhibition
KG-1a	Early Myeloblast	No inhibition
HL-60 Blast	Early Myeloblast	No inhibition
K562	Early Myeloblast/Erythroblast	No inhibition

+Induction of differentiation by $1,25(OH)_2D_3$.
++ED-50: Concentration of $1,25(OH)_2D_3$ producing a 50% inhibition of cloonal growth.
*M-1: Is a murine cell line; all other lines are human.

$1,25(OH)_2D_3$ and Myelodysplasia

Hematopoiesis in myelodysplasia is characterized by the preponderance of a defective leukemic stem cell clone which may progress to malignancy. The ineffective hematopoiesis frequently results in anemia, thrombocytopenia, leukopenia and an increased number of bone marrow blast cells.

Table 2B

Myeloid Leukemia Cells Freshly Obtained from Patients: Inhibition of Clonal Growth by $1,25(OH)_2D_3$

PT. NO.	DIAGNOSIS*	CELL SOURCE**	ED-50+ (M)
1	AML	BM	5×10^{-11}
2	AML	BM	5×10^{-11}
3	AML	PB	2×10^{-9}
4	AMML	BM	4×10^{-9}
5	CML (Ph^-)	PB	4×10^{-9}
6	CML (Ph^+)	PB	5×10^{-9}
7	CML (ph^+)	BM	8×10^{-9}
8	AMML	BM	2×10^{-8}
9	CML (ph^+)	PB	1×10^{-7}
10	AML	BM	5×10^{-7}
11	AML	BM	No inhibition
12	AML	PB	No inhibition
13	CML (Ph^+)	PB	No inhibition
14	AML	BM	Stimulation°

*Diagnosis: AML, acute myelogenous leukemia; AMML, acute myelomonocytic leukemia; CML, chronic myelogenous leukemia with (+) or without (-) the Philadelphia chromosome (Ph).

**Cell Source: BM, bone marrow; PB, peripheral blood.

+ED-50: Concentration of $1.?5(OH)_2D_3$ producing a 50% inhibition of clonal growth.

°Colony formation was five fold increased in the presence of 5×10^{-8}M $1,25(OH)_2D_3$ and colony stimulating factor (CSF) as compared to plates containing CSF alone.

A trial of administering $1,25(OH)_2D_3$ (2 µg/day p.o.) to patients with the myelodysplastic syndrome was initated to evaluate in vivo effects of $1,25(OH)_2D_3$ on induction of differentiation and on inhibition of clonal proliferation (21). As shown in Table 3, hematologic findings had not improved significantly by the end of the treatment period in the 19 patients studied. The majority of patients developed hypercalcemia during the study and 6 of the 19 patients had progressed to acute myelogenous leukemia.

1,25(OH)2D3 and the Macrophage

Recently, further evidence for the involvement of Vitamin D metabolites with hematopoietic tissue has been provided by reports on interactions between macrophages and the vitamin D endocrine system.

Vitamin D-deficient mouse peritoneal macrophages and bone marrow polymorphonuclear leukocytes were shown to have defective chemotaxis and impaired phagocytic ability (22). The latter function could be restored in vivo by incubating the macrophages with $1,25(OH)_2D_3$. Vitamin D-replete mice had normal inflammatory and phagocytic response. In addition, reduced attachment of macrophages to bone was reported to occur in vitamin D-deficient rats (23) due both to defective bone matrix and to impaired capacity of the macrophages, per se, to attach to bone.

A possible role of $1,25(OH)_2D_3$ in the activation of macrophages was suggested by Abe, et al. (24). $1,25(OH)_2D_3$ ($\geq 10^{-10}$ M) could directly induce fusion of murine alveolar macrophages in vitro. Indirectly, this effect occured after incubation of macrophages with conditioned media

Table 3

Treatment of Preleukemia Patients with $1,25(OH)_2D_3$*

	Median	Range	p-Value**
Granulocytes (μl blood)			
start***	2300	180-11520	
peak	3750	486-29820	.0014
end	3110	96-24480	.0694
Macrophages (μl blood)			
start	50	3-8435	
peak	300	43-16900	.004
end	80	3-10200	.03156
Platelets (10^3/μl blood)			
start	58	12-300	
peak	105	23-610	.0006
end	65	4-360	1.0000
Marrow blasts (%)			
start	10	3-20	
end	15	4-70	.0136
Serum Calcium (μg/dl)			
start	8.9	8.2-10.4	
peak	10.8	9.7-17.8	.0004
end	10.3	9.6-12.4	.0004

* Results represent data from 18 preleukemic patients.

** Represents Wilcoxon signed rank test p-values (adjusted). Values are compared to base-line (starting) values and $p \leq 0.05$ is significant.

*** Start, initial value before therapy; peak, highest value during therapy; end, value on last day of therapy.

from T-cell or spleen-cell cultures, treated with $1,25(OH)_2D_3$. Follow-up studies indicated that the direct effect of $1,25(OH)_2D_3$ on fusion of macrophages involved RNA and protein-synthesis, but not DNA-synthesis (25). $1,25(OH)_2D_3$ enhanced glucose consumption, induced cytotoxity and increased expression of Fc receptors in mouse alveolar macrophages (26).

Metabolism of $25(OH)_2D_3$ in macrophages was studied by Gray, et al. Rodent peritoneal macrophages converted $[^3H]$-$25(OH)_2D_3$ to a more polar metabolite in vitro (27). This metabolite could not be identified since its elution position was different from those of known vitamin D metabolites. Incubations of human neutrophils and monocytes and resident rat peritoneal macrophages with $[^3H]$-$25(OH)_2D_3$ yielded three peaks (28). The peaks were designated as a lactone-derivative of $25(OH)_2D_3$, as putative $24,25(OH)_2D_3$ and as a novel metabolite.

Several lines of evidence indicate that macrophages and $1,25(OH)_2D_3$ are involved in the pathophysiology of abnormal calcium metabolism found in 20-30% of patients with sarcoidosis. Subjects with sarcoidosis were shown to have elevated $1,25(OH)_2D_3$ serum levels during episodes of hypercalcemia (29,30). The demonstration of increased serum $1,25(OH)_2D_3$ in a nephrectomized patient with sarcoidosis (31) led to the suggestion, that in sarcoidosis extrarenal cells can produce clinically significant amounts of $1,25(OH)_2D_3$. Macrophages from lung and granulomatous tissue have been identified as possible sources of $1,25(OH)_2D_3$ in sarcoidosis.

Adams, *et al.* (32) showed that pulmonary alveolar macrophages (PAM) from five out of seven patients with sarcoidosis could convert [^{3}H]-25(OH)D_3 to 1,25(OH)$_2D_3$ *in vitro*. The identity of the 1,25(OH)$_2D_3$-like metabolite produced by PAM was assessed by comigration with authentic 1,25(OH)$_2D_3$ on different HPLC-systems and by binding of the metabolite to the chick intestinal receptor for 1,25(OH)$_2D_3$. In contrast, PAM, from two patients with idiopathic pulmonary fibrosis could not metabolize [^{3}H]-25(OH)D_3. Mason *et al.* incubated homogenates of granulomatous tissue, obtained from lymph nodes of patients with sarcoidosis with [^{3}H]-25(OH)D_3. 25(OH)D_3 was converted to 1,25(OH)$_2D_3$ (33). Lymph node homogenates obtained from normal subjects did not metabolize. [^{3}H]-25(OH)D_3. However a recent study investigating metabolism of [^{3}H]-25(OH)D_3 by sarcoid granulomatous tissue (34) yielded different results. 25(OH)D_3 was converted to a vitamin D metabolite behaving chromatographically like 19-nor-10-keto-25(OH)D_3.

Recent work in our laboratories was undertaken to assess a possible role of normal human macrophages from lung alveoli, peripheral blood and bone marrow in the metabolism of vitamin D_3 and 25(OH)D_3. In an extension of previously published studies we compared the [^{3}H]-25(OH)D_3 metabolizing capacity of resting and of activated macrophages. We found that resting macrophages synthesized and secreted at most only very small amounts of a metabolite, behaving in several regards like 1,25(OH)$_2D_3$. However, activation of the macrophages by γ-interferon (γ-IFN) induced a marked enhancement (5 to 100 fold) of the production of the putative 1,25(OH)$_2D_3$ *in vitro* (35).

Pulmonary alveolar macrophages (PAM) obtained by bronchial lavage, bone-marrow macrophages obtained by iliac crest biopsy and monocytes were plated into culture dishes. Non-adherent cells were removed by several washes. Over 99% of the remaining adherent cells had the morphology of macrophages and stained for macrophage-specific α-naphtyl-esterase activity. After incubation with γ-IFN under varying conditions, cells were labelled with [^{3}H]-25(OH)D_3. Metabolism of [^{3}H]-25(OH)D_3 by the macrophages was examined by applying lipid extracts of cells, supernatants or both to high performance liquid chromatography (HPLC). Chemically synthesized authentic vitamin D metabolites, including 1,25(OH)$_2D_3$ were added to each sample. UV-absorbance of the standards served as marker for tritium peaks representing vitamin D metabolites which were synthesized by macrophages. The radioactivity was determined in 1 min/2 ml fractions by liquid scintillation measurements.

In order to evaluate the identity of the 1,25(OH)$_2D_3$-like product of activated macrophages, peak fractions, comigrating with authentic 1,25(OH)$_2D_3$ on the first HPLC-system, were collected, pooled and subsequently rechromatographed on three different HPLC-systems. The systems were: (a) Radial-pak cartridge, 4-60% isopropanol in hexane gradient; (b) Zorbax-Sil column, 10% isopropanol in dichloromethane, isocratic; (c) μ-Porasil column, 10% isopropanol in hexane, isocratic; (d) Zorbax ODS 20% water in methanol, reverse phase. The metabolite, produced by γ-IFN activated pulmonary macrophages exactly comigrated with authentic 1,25(OH)$_2D_3$ on each of the four systems.

In addition, we assessed binding of the putative $1,25(OH)_2D_3$ from activated PAM to the chick intestinal $1,25(OH)_2D_3$ receptor. We also tested the macrophage-derived vitamin D metabolite in a bioassay involving induction of calcium absorption from intestine and calcium mobilization from bone. In both experiments, the metabolite from PAM behaved like authentic $1,25(OH)_2D_3$. (HR, HPK, AWN manuscript in preparation).

Synthesis of putative $1,25(OH)_2D_3$ by γ-IFN stimulated PAM occured in a dose- and time-dependent fashion. First effects of increased $1,25(OH)_2D_3$ synthesis by PAM were noted at 100 to 200 units of γ-IFN/10^6 cells (Fig. 2A). $1,25(OH)_2D_3$ production further increased with higher γ-IFN doses. As shown in Fig. 2B, maximal stimulation of PAM to produce $1,25(OH)_2D_3$ was seen after 1 day of incubation with 500 units γ-IFN. The plateau level was sustained for 6 days. Inactivation of γ-IFN by acid-degradation abolished the stimulatory effect of γ-IFN on $1,25(OH)_2D_3$ synthesis by PAM.

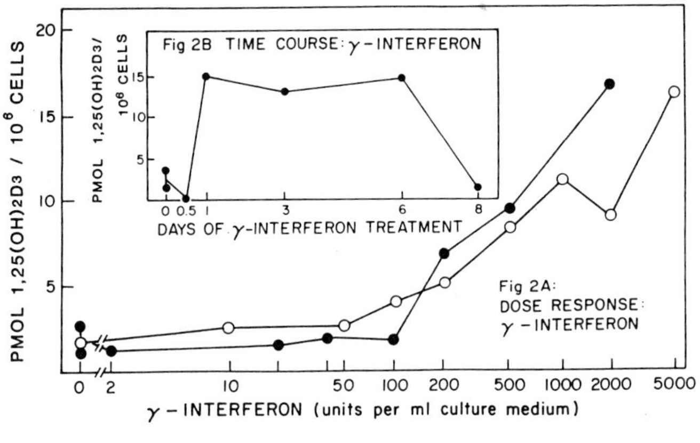

Fig. 2. Exposure of human pulmonary macrophages (PAM) to recombinant human γ-interferon. Appearance of $1,25(OH)_2D_3$ after treatment: (A) with different doses of γ-IFN; (B) with 500 U of γ-IFN over different periods of time.

We also studied the effects of bacterial lipopolysaccharides (LPS) on metabolism of $[^3\text{-H}]\text{-}25(OH)D_3$ by human macrophages from different tissues. Lipopolysaccharides present in the cell wall of gram-negative bacteria, are known to have various effects on macrophages, B-lymphocytes and possibly T-lymphocytes (36). Macrophages from peritoneum, lung, blood and bone marrow undergo activation when exposed to LPS. In summary, we found that LPS, like γ-IFN, markedly enhanced $1,25(OH)_2D_3$ synthesis by human macrophages. This effect was mediated by the lipid moiety (lipid A) of LPS and could be overcome by adding polymyxin B to the cultures. In contrast, polymyxin B had no effect on the γ-IFN stimulated increase in $1,25(OH)_2D_3$ synthesis by macrophages. (HR, HPK, AWN manuscript in preparation).

Table 4 summarizes the results of our studies of vitamin D metabolism in macrophages and other hematopoietic cells from normal individuals. $1,25(OH)_2D_3$-synthesis in a given cell type varied quantitatively within a wide range in cells from different individuals. Pulmonary alveolar macrophages had, on average, the highest production of $1,25(OH)_2D_3$ compared to macrophages from other tissues. Lymphocytes and neutrophils exposed to γ-IFN, LPS or phorbol-myristate-acetate did not generate a $1,25(OH)_2D_3$-like metabolite.

Although all available evidence suggests that the vitamin D metabolite, produced by macrophages, in fact is $1,25(OH)_2D_3$, it has to be emphasized that definite proof only can be obtained by analytical techniques like mass spectrometry. The necessary material has not yet been collected. However, none of the known vitamin D metabolites, except $1,25(OH)_2D_3$ would behave like $1,25(OH)_2D_3$ on the four employed HPLC-systems, the binding to chick intestinal $1,25(OH)_2D_3$-receptors and the induction of calcium absorption from intestine and calcium resorption from bone in chickens.

Table 4

Synthesis of Putative $1,25(OH)_2D_3$ by Hematopoietic Cells and Skin Fibroblasts exposed to γ-IFN or Lipopolysaccharides

Cell Type	N	Maximal observed activity of $1,25(OH)_2D_3$ production in fmol/30 min/10^6 Cells					
Pulmonary alveolar macrophages	16	(1)	520	(9)	802		
		(2)	508	(10)	115		
		(3)	1045	(11)	487		
		(4)	67	(12)	90		
		(5)	145	(13)	0		
		(6)	510	(14a)	583 +	b)	339ˣ
		(7)	1390	(15a)	212 +	b)	65ˣ
		(8)	700	(16a)	55 +	b)	67ˣ
Peripheral blood monocytes	7	(1)	41,5	(5)	108		
		(2)	0	(6)	227		
		(3)	30,8	(7)	0		
		(4)	62,9				
Bone marrow macrophages	5	(1)	14,2	(4)	0		
		(2)	0	(5)	16		
		(3)	6,0				
Lymphocytes	2	(1)	0	(2)			
Neutrophils	2	(1)	0	(2)	0		
Skin fibroblasts	1	(1)	0				

N: Number of individuals studied

ˣActivity for a) LPS and b) γ-IFN stimulation

(Cells were cultured in the presence of different doses of γ-IFN (1000-5000 units/10^6 cells) or LPS (10-100μg/10^6 cells). Rates of $1,25(OH)_2D_3$ production are expressed as fmoles of $1,25(OH)_2D_3$ generated by 10^6 cells in 30 minutes.).

Therefore, our findings imply that macrophages from different populations have the ability to synthesize and secrete $1,25(OH)_2D_3$ and that significant $1,25(OH)_2D_3$ production is dependent on an activated state of macrophages. Necessary activation can be induced at least by γ-interferon and lipopolysaccharides.

Our in vitro observations of macrophages as a possible extrarenal source of $1,25(OH)_2D_3$ have been preceded by a number of reports on extrarenal $1,25(OH)_2D_3$ production by other tissues. Human bone (37) and human placenta and decidua (38,39) among other tissues, were shown to have 1α-$25(OH)D_3$ hydroxylase activity in vitro. In contrast, no $1,25(OH)_2D_3$ could be detected in nephrectomized rats (40) when blood, intestine and bone were examined. However, it is difficult to conclude from the last study, that a possible $1,25(OH)_2D_3$ synthesis by macrophages does not occur in vivo, since the small amounts of $1,25(OH)_2D_3$ secreted by resting macrophages certainly would not be detectable in serum and since a possible release of $1,25(OH)_2D_3$ by macrophages might be important only for microenvironmental processes.

Elevated serum levels of $1,25(OH)_2D_3$ (29), observed occasionally in patients with sarcoidosis, might be explained in part by our findings. Accumulation of activated T lymphocytes at sites of alveolitis in pulmonary sarcoidosis (41) results in locally high levels of γ-IFN which will stimulate macrophages to release $1,25(OH)_2D_3$. Thus granulomatous disease possibly provides a paradigm demonstrating in vivo relevance of our observations.

What remains to be shown is whether the in vitro interactions between the hematopoietic system and the vitamin D endocrine system reported by others as well as by our laboratories play a role in health and disease in man.

References:

1. Stroeder, T. (1975) In: Norman, A.W., Schaefer, K., Grigoleit, H.-G., Herrath, D.von and Ritz, E.[eds], Vitamin D and Problems Related to Uremic Bone Disease. DeGruyter, Berlin, 675-687.
2. Lorente, F., Fontan, G., Jara, P., Casa C., Garcia-Rodriguez, M.C. and Ojeda, J.A. (1976) Acta Paediatr. Scand. 65, 695-699.
3. Stroeder, J., and Kasal, P. (1970) Acta Paediatr. Scand. 65, 288-292.
4. Yetgin, S., and Ozsoylu, S. (1982) Scand. J. Haematol. 28, 180-185.
5. Norman, A.W., Roth, J., and Orci, L. (1982), Endocrine Reviews 3, 331-336.
6. Provvedini, D.M., Tsoukas, K.D., Deftos, L.J., and Manolagas, S.C. (1983) Science 221, 1181-1183.
7. Bhalla, A.K., Amento, E.P., Clemens, T.L., Holick, M.F., and Krane, S.M. (1983) J. Clin. Endocrinol. Metab. 57, 1308-1310.
8. Walter, R.M., Freake, H.C., Iwasaki, J., Lynn, J., and MacIntyre, I. (1984) Metabolism 33, 240-243.
9. Peacock, M., Jones, S., Clemens, T.L., Amento, E.P., Kurnick, J., Krane, S.M., and Holick, M.F. (1982) In: Norman, A.W., Schaefer, K., Herrath, D.von, Grigoleit, H.-G. [eds], Vitamin D, Chemical, Biochemical and Clinical Endocrinology of Calcium Metabolism. De Gruyter, Berlin, 83-85.
10. Mangelsdorf, D.J., Koeffler, H.P., Donaldson, C.A., Pike, J.W., and Haussler, M.R. (1984) J. Cell Biol., 98, 391-398.
11. Abe, E., Miyaura, C., Sakagami, H., Takeda, M., Konno, K., Yamazaki, T., Yoshiki, S., and Suda, T. (1981) Proc. Natl. Acad. Sci. USA 78, 4990-4994.
12. Miyaura, C., Abe, E., Kuribayashi, T., Tanaka, H., Konno, K., Nishii, Y., and Suda, T. (1981) Biochem. Biophys. Res. Commun. 102, 937-943.
13. Honma, Y. Hozumi, M., Abe, E. Konno, K. Fukushima, M., Hata, S., Nishii, Y., DeLuca, H.F., and Suda, T. (1983) Proc. Natl. Acad. Sci. USA 80, 201-204.
14. Tanaka, H., Abe, E., Miyaura, C. Shiina, Y., and Suda T. (1983) Biochem. Biophys. Res. Commun. 117, 86-92.
15. Tanaka, H., Abe, E., Miyaura, C., Kuribayashi, T., Konno, K., Nishii, Y., and Suda, T. (1982) Biochem. J. 204, 713-719.
16. McCarthy, D.M., San Miguel, J.F., Freake, H.C., Green, P.M., Zola, M., Catovsky, D., and Goldman, J.M. (1983) Leuk. Res. 7, 51-55.
17. Bar-Shavit, Z., Teitelbaum, S.L., Reitsma, P., Hall, A., Pegg, L.E., Trial, J., and Kahn, A.J. (1983) Proc. Natl. Acad. Sci. USA 80, 5907-5911.
18. Koeffler, H.P., Armatruda, T., Ikekawa, N., Kobayashi, Y., and DeLuca, H.F. (1984) Cancer Res. 44, 5624-5628.
19. Burger, E.H., van der Meer, J.W.M., van de Gevel, J.S., Gribnau, J.C., Thesingh, C.W., and van Furth, R. (1982) J. Exp. Med. 156, 1604-1614.
20. Munker, R., Norman, A. W., and Koeffler, H. P. Effect of vitamin D metabolites on clonal growth and differentiation of human myeloid cells. (submitted).

21. Koeffler, H. P., Hirji, K., and Itri, L. Southern California Leukemia Group. Cancer Chemotherapy Reports (in press).
22. Bar-Shavit, Z., Noff, D., Edelstein, S., Meyer, M., Shibolet, S., and Goldman, R. (1981) Calcif. Tissue Int. 33, 673-676.
23. Bar-Shavit, Z., Kahn, A. J., and Teitelbaum, S. L. (1983) J. Clin. Invest. 72, 526-534.
24. Abe, E., Miyaura, C., Tanaka, H., Shiina, Y., Kuribayashi, T., Suda, S., Nishii, Y., DeLuca, H. F. and Suda, T. (1983) Proc. Natl. Acad. Sci. USA 80, 5583-5587.
25. Tanaka, H., Hayashi, T., Shiina, Y., Miyaura, C., Abe, E., and Suda, T. (1984) FEBS Letters 174, 61-65.
26. Abe, E., Shiina, Y., Miyaura, C., Tanaka, H., Hayashi, T., Kanegasaki, S., Saito, M., Nishii, Y., DeLuca, H. F., and Suda, T. (1984) Proc. Natl. Acad. Sci. USA 81, 7112-7116.
27. Gray, T. K., Maddux, F. W., Lester, G. E., and Williams, M. E. (1982) Biochem. Biophys. Res. Commun. 109, 723-729.
28. Cohen, M. S., and Gray, T. K. (1984) Proc Natl. Acad. Sci. USA 81, 931-934.
29. Bell, N. H., Stern, P. H., Pantzer, E., Sinha, T. K., and DeLuca, H. F. (1979) J. Clin. Invest. 64, 218-225.
30. Papadopoulos, S. E., Clemens, T. L., Fraher, L. J., Lewin, J. G., Sandler, L. M., and O'Riordan, J. L. H. (1979) Lancet 1, 627-629.
31. Barbour, G. L., Coburn, J. W., Slatopolsky, E., Norman, A. W., and Horst, R. L. (1981) N. Engl. J. Med. 305, 440-443.
32. Adams, J. S., Sharma, O. P., Gacad, M. A., and Singer, F. R. (1983) J. Clin. Invest. 72, 1856-1860.
33. Mason, R., Frankel, T., Chan, Y. L., Lissner, D. and Posen, S. (1984) Ann. Intern. Med. 100, 59-61.
34. Okabe, T., Ishizuka, S., Fujisawa, M., Watanabe, J., and Takaku, F. (1984) Biochem. Biophys. Res. Commun. 123, 822-830.
35. Koeffler, H. P., Reichel, H., Bishop, J. E., and Norman, A. W. (1985) Biochem. Biophys. Res. Commun. (in press).
36. Morrison, D. C. and Ryan, J. L. (1979) Adv. Immunol. 28, 293-450.
37. Howard, G. A., Turner, R. T., Sherrard, D. J., and Baylink, D. J. (1981) J. Biol. Chem. 256, 7738-7740.
38. Whitsett, J. A., Ho, M., Tsang, R. C., Norman, E. J., and Adams, K. G (1981) J. Clin. Endocrinol. Metab. 53, 484-488.
39. Weisman, Y., Harell, A., Edelstein, S., David, M., Spirer, Z., and Golander, A. (1979) Nature 281, 317-319.
40. Shultz, T. D., Fox, J., Heath, H. III., and Kumar, R. (1983) Proc. Natl. Acad. Sci. USA 80, 1746-1750.
41. Crystal, R. G., Roberts, W. C., Hunninghake, G. W., Gadek, J. E., Fulmer, J. D., and Line, . R. (1981) Ann. Intern. Med. 94, 73-94.

Work at UCLA (HPK) was supported by USPHS grants CA-26038, CA-33936 and CA-3273 while work at UCR (AWN) was supported by USPHS grant AM-14, 750-013. HPK is a scholar of the Leukemia Society and has a Career Development Award from the USPHS. HR and RM were supported by the Deutsche Forschungsgemeinschaft.

VITAMIN D AND MACROPHAGE DIFFERENTIATION

Steven L. Teitelbaum, Zvi Bar-Shavit, Pieter H. Reitsma, Howard G. Welgus, and Arnold J. Kahn

Washington University Medical Center, St. Louis, Missouri, U.S.A.

INTRODUCTION

1,25-dihydroxyvitamin D ($1,25(OH)_2D$ is generally viewed as a hormone which functions to maintain calcium homeostasis. Indeed it has only recently been appreciated that $1,25(OH)_2D$ may affect tissues other than intestine and bone. The realization that the steroid may have more global effects is derivative of recent documentation that specific $1,25(OH)_2D$ receptors exist in a variety of tissues many of which, by first approximation, do not seem to impact on calcium metabolism. Thus, the skin fibroblast is a rich source of such receptors (1), and the magnitude of ligand binding by this cell is altered in genetic diseases of bone (2).

Despite the fact that extraskeletal and extraintestinal $1,25(OH)_2D$ receptors have been recognized for some years, their significance in most circumstances remains enigmatic. On the other hand, this steroid has been shown to have effects which initially appear not to be primarily calcium-related but do offer insight into the biology of its ubiquitous receptor. To date, these "extra-calcitropic" effects appear by and large to primarily entail cell growth and differentiation (3,4). While it has become increasingly apparent that the steroid may play a role in promoting differentiation of a variety of cells, our laboratory has focused on the hematopoietic effects of $1,25(OH)_2D$, and in particular, the manner in which it influences monocytic differentiation.

Monocytes and Bone Resorption

Our interest in the effects of $1,25(OH)_2D$ on monocyte differentiation stems from early studies involving hormonal control of bone resorption. In these experiments we determined that the in vitro addition of $1,25(OH)_2D$ does not alter the resorptive activity of fully differentiated macrophages, while in contrast, pretreatment of vitamin D-deficient mice with the steroid enhances the capacity of their mononuclear phagocytes to resorb bone in culture (5). These observations suggested to us that $1,25(OH)_2D$ may stimulate bone resorption via enhanced differentiation of osteoclast precursors which are members of the monocyte-macrophage family. This hypothesis prompted us to embark on a series of experiments aimed at examining the effects of $1,25(OH)_2D$ on monocyte differentiation. These studies utilized a human promyelocytic leukemia cell line HL-60 which has the capacity to differentiate, under the influence of various stimuli, along either granulocytic or monocytic pathways (4).

Consistent with our hypothesis, physiological concentrations of $1,25(OH)_2D$ induce HL-60 to differentiate along a monocytic pathway as judged by lysozyme production and secretion and the acquisition of monocyte-specific esterase activity and surface antigens (4). In addition, HL-60 cells treated with $1,25(OH)_2D$, acquire the capacity to attach to and resorb bone (4)

Vitamin D. A Chemical, Biochemical and Clinical Update

(Fig. 1) and metabolize arachadonic acid in a manner similar to authentic monocytes (6). Clearly then, $1,25(OH)_2D$ induces monocytic differentiation of HL-60, and recent observations in our laboratory suggest the same pertains to human bone marrow-derived macrophage precursors.

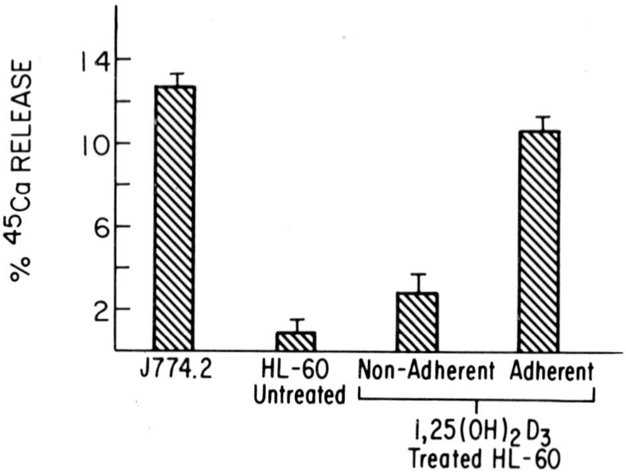

Figure 1. $1,25(OH)_2D_3$ induction of bone resorption by HL-60. Cells were cocultured with ^{45}Ca-labeled, devitalized rat bone, and resorption monitored as a function of cell-mediated mobilization of the bone isotope. Note that untreated HL-60 cells and those exposed to $10^{-8}M$ $1,25(OH)_2D$ but do not acquire the capacity to adhere to plastic fail to substantially resorb bone. In contrast, those HL-60 cells which become plastic-adherent under the influence of $1,25(OH)_2D_3$ (approximately 50% of total cells) degrade bone as effectively as the mature macrophage-like cell line J774.2 (from Bar-Shavit, et al., Proc Natl Acad Sci USA 80:5907-5911, 1983, with permission of editor).

Oncogene Expression and $1,25(OH)_2D$

When HL-60 is exposed to $1,25(OH)_2D$, a fall in the proportion of cells in S-phase of the replicative cycle ensues, leading to a profound decline in proliferative rate (4). As expression of specific oncogenes such as c-myc has been shown to reflect, or perhaps induce, alterations of cell replication (7), we assessed transcription of c-myc by HL-60 under the influence of $1,25(OH)_2D$ (8). These "dot-blot" experiments which involved hybridization of a cDNA probe to c-myc mRNA documented that transcription of this oncogene by HL-60 falls dramatically and rapidly following $1,25(OH)_2D$ exposure (Fig. 2). The rapidity of this change is such that it precedes all other phenotypic effects of the steroid on HL-60 and hence, suggests that altered c-myc transcription may in some way be causally related to $1,25(OH)_2D$-induced differentiation.

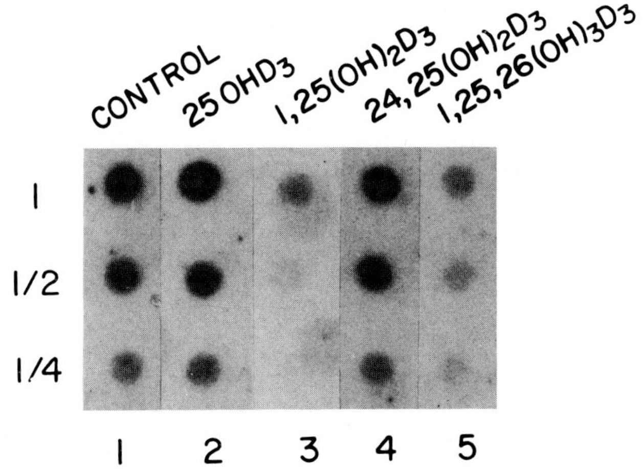

Figure 2. RNA "dot-blots" from HL-60 cells following exposure to $1,25(OH)_2D_3$. In this type of experiment, cells are collected after 4-72 h incubation with the vitamin D_3 metabolite, total RNA is extracted and then aliquoted onto nitrocellulose filters with and without further dilution (1/2, 1/4). After baking, the filters are hybridized overnight at 42°C with nick-translated DNA probes ($4x10^6$ c.p.m. ml^{-1}), and the unbound fraction is removed by extensive washing. The filters are then autoradiographed for various periods of time at -70°C. The myc probe is a 1.7 kilobase ClaI-EcoRI fragment covering most of the 3' exon of the normal human myc gene. The reduction in myc mRNA levels is specific for metabolites hydroxylated at carbon 1. $1,25(OH)_2D_3$ is effective in suppressing myc gene expression between 10^{-9} and 10^{-7}M (values that coincide with the minimal doses necessary to affect other phenotypic changes in HL-60). (From Reitsma, et al., Nature 306:492-494, 1983, with permission of editor).

Reversibility of $1,25(OH)_2D$-Induced Monocytic Differentiation

In recent years a body of information has accumulated indicating that $1,25(OH)_2D$ has the capacity to promote in vitro maturation of a variety of tumor cell lines, including HL-60 (4,9). Consequently, there is now considerable interest in the possible involvement of this metabolite in regulating normal cell differentiation as well as in its possible utility as an anti-neoplastic agent. Hence, it is of particular importance to document whether vitamin exposure evokes terminal or irreversible differentiation of transformed cells. We found, in fact, that withdrawal of $1,25(OH)_2D$ from mononuclear HL-60 leads to loss of features of differentiation in a sequence which mirrors their appearance when the cells mature under the influence of the steroid (Fig. 3). The reversion to a less mature phenotype begins chronologically with the reappearance of abundant myc mRNA followed by disappearance of the monocyte-specific antigen 63D3 and finally renewed proliferative activity. These revertants also re-acquire the capacity to respond to 1,25(OH)$_2$D in a manner similar to virgin HL-60 cells.

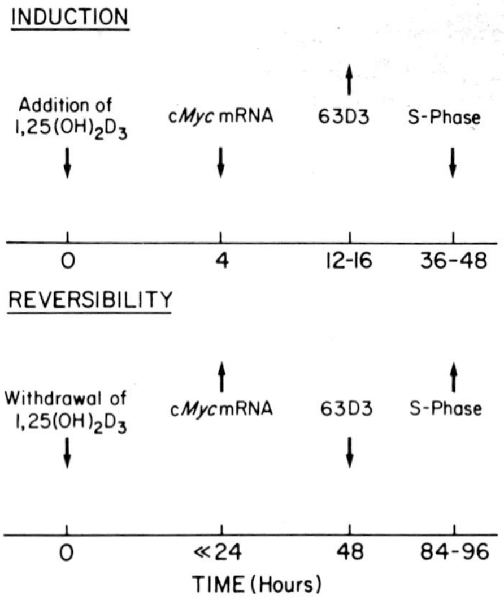

Figure 3. Kinetic patterns of induction of monocytic differentiation of HL-60 by 1,25(OH)$_2$D$_3$ and reversibility of maturation following withdrawal of the metabolite. Note that both events mirror each other with alterations of expression of the oncogene, c-myc, occurring first, followed by changes in the monocyte-specific membrane antigen, 63D3. Finally, the cell cycle is modified.

The exception to the "rule" of reversion is the multinucleated HL-60 cells which appear in large numbers in cultures exposed to 1,25(OH)$_2$D (4). In contrast to their cocultured mononuclear counterparts, these polykaryons do not dedifferentiate to a more immature condition following vitamin withdrawal but remain viable and 63D3 antigen-positive. How the multinucleated cells manage to stabilize cell phenotype is not known, but the phenomenon almost certainly has to do with achieving developmental commitment, perhaps even prior to cell fusion. In this regard, it is instructive to note that glucocorticoids, which are potent inhibitors of macrophage differentiation (10,11), also block giant cell formation.

Monocytic Maturation and Collagen Remodeling

Macrophages and their multinucleated derivatives have been implicated in connective tissue remodeling and clearly have the capacity to degrade collagen (12). We have recently documented, however, that human pulmonary alveolar macrophages also secrete collagenase inhibitor (CI), a protein of M_r 28,500, which stoichiometrically blocks the action of collagenase (13). Because 1,25(OH)$_2$D induces monocytic maturation in HL-60, we studied the production of CI under the influence of the steroid with the specific goal of determining if synthesis of the protein is developmentally associated. We found that while untreated HL-60 cells release no CI, when the cells are exposed to either 1,25(OH)$_2$D or phorbol ester which also promotes their monocytic differentiation (4), they release immunoreactive CI in a dose-dependent fashion. This CI is immunologically and functionally identical to its counterpart produced by native human macrophages, and as reflected by immunoprecipitation of administered ^{35}S-cysteine, the secreted CI represented new protein synthesis.

SUMMARY

These studies and those from other laboratories give credence to the hypothesis that 1,25(OH)$_2$D promotes monocytic differentiation. Because monocytes and osteoclasts derive from similar precursors (14), there is a probable relationship between the maturational effect of the vitamin on monocytes and skeletal homeostasis. On the other hand, one must consider the likelihood that the skeletal manifestations of vitamin D are perhaps the most recognized of a host of biological effects of this steroid. The possibility exists, for example, that 1,25(OH)$_2$D has a more global effect on cell differentiation than its putative influence on osteoclast maturation. Thus, 1,25(OH)$_2$D-induced enhancement of absorption of calcium may conceivably reflect trophic effect on development of intestinal cells. Analogous scenarios may also pertain to possible effects of 1,25(OH)$_2$D on the immune system. In any event, 1,25(OH)$_2$D can no longer be considered solely as a calcitrophic hormone, but an agent with the capacity to regulate differentiation and function of a variety of cells.

REFERENCES

1. Feldman, D., Chen, T., Hirst, M., Colston, K., Karasek, M., and Cone, C. (1980) J. Clin. Endocrinol. Metab. 51, 1463-1465.

2. Pike, J.W., Dokoh, S., Haussler, M.R., Liberman, U.A., Marx, S.J., and Eil, C. (1984) Science 224, 879-881.

3. Chen, T.L., Hirst, M.A., Cone, C.M., Hochberg, Z., Tietze, H-U., and Feldman,D. (1984) J. Clin. Endocrinol. Metab. 59, 383-388.

4. Bar-Shavit, Z., Teitelbaum, S.L., Reitsma, P., Hall, A., Pegg, L.E., Trial, J., and Kahn, A.J. (1983) Proc. Natl. Acad. Sci. USA 80, 5907-5911.

5. Kahn, A.J., Malone, J.D., and Teitelbaum, S.L. (1980) In: Hormonal Control of Calcium Metabolism, Eds. D.V. Cohn, R.V. Talmage, and J.L. Matthews, Excerpta Medica, Amsterdam, pp. 182-189.

6. Stenson, W.F., Teitelbaum, S.L., and Bar-Shavit, Z. (1985) Abstracted in Proceedings from the 7th Annual Meeting of the American Society for Bone and Mineral Research.

7. Kelly, K., Cochran, B.H., Stiles, C.D., and Leder, P. (1983) Cell 35, 603-610.

8. Reitsma, P.H., Rothberg, P.G., Astrin, S.M., Trial, J., Bar-Shavit, Z., Hall, A., Teitelbaum, S.L., and Kahn, A.J. (1983) Nature 306, 492-494.

9. Amento, E.P., Bhalia, A.K., Kurnick, J.T., Kradin, R.L., Clemens, T.L., Holick, S.A., Holick, M.F., and Krane, S.M. (1984) J. Clin. Invest. 73, 731-739.

10. Thompson, J., and van Furth, R. (1970) J. Exp. Med. 131, 429-442.

11. Zalman, F., Maloney, M.A., and Patt, H.M. (1979) J. Exp. Med. 149, 67-72.

12. Teitelbaum, S.L., Stewart, C.C., and Kahn, A.J. (1979) Calcif. Tissue Int. 27, 255-261.

13. Welgus, H.G., Campbell, E.J., Bar-Shavit, Z., Senior, R.M., and Teitelbaum, S.L. (1985) J. Clin. Invest. - in press.

14. Teitelbaum, S.L., and Kahn, A.J. (1980) Min. Electrolyte Metab. 3, 2-9.

ACKNOWLEGMENTS

This work was supported by NIH grants DE05413, AM32788 (Teitelbaum), DE04629 (Kahn), AM35805, AM01525 (Welgus), American Cancer Society grant IN36 (Reitsma). Drs. Bar-Shavit and Reitsma are recipients of Arthritis Investigator Awards.

SIMILARITY OF THE EFFECTS OF 1,25$(OH)_2D_3$ AND RETINOIC ACID ON INTERLEUKIN (IL) 1, 2 AND 3 PRODUCTION.

U. Trechsel, V. Evêquoz, B. Hodler and H. Fleisch
Department of Pathophysiology, University of Bern,
CH-3010 Bern, Switzerland

INTRODUCTION

Previous studies from this and other laboratories have shown that physiological concentrations of 1,25$(OH)_2D_3$ increase the production of IL 1 and decrease that of IL 2 in vitro. Moreover, we have found 1,25$(OH)_2D_3$ to increase the release of IL 3 by the murine myelomonocytic cell line WEHI-3. Since IL 1 and IL 3 might be involved in the local regulation of bone metabolism, it is conceivable that the stimulatory effect of 1,25$(OH)_2D_3$ on bone resorption might partly be mediated by IL 1 and/or IL 3.

Retinoids are another class of compounds which stimulate bone resorption in vitro and resorption as well as formation in vivo. We have studied the effect of retinoid acid on the production of IL 1,2 and 3 in the same model systems that had been used to study 1,25$(OH)_2D_3$ and have found a striking similarity of the effects of the two compounds on lymphokine production.

METHODS

Models for the production of interleukins were the release of IL 1 by the murine macrophage cell line P388D_1 and by human peripheral blood mononuclear cells (PBL), of IL 2 by rat spleen cells, and of IL 3 by the murine WEHI-3 cell line. Interleukin assays were the stimulation of collagenase by chondrocytes for IL 1, proliferation of the IL 2 dependent cell line CTLL for IL 2 and that of the IL 3 dependent cell line DCL 32 for IL 3.

Vitamin D. A Chemical, Biochemical and Clinical Update

RESULTS

Retinoic acid stimulated IL 1 release by P388D$_1$ cells in a dose-related fashion, starting at 10^{-9}M and maximally at 10^{-8}-10^{-6}M. With PBL a maximal stimulation of IL 1 release was observed with 10^{-7}M retinoic acid. IL 2 production by rat spleen cells stimulated with Concanavalin A was decreased by retinoic acid between 10^{-9}M and 10^{-6}M in two experiments, but unaffected in a third. IL 3 release by WEHI-3 cells was stimulated by retinoic acid in a dose-related fashion. The maximal response varied between 10^{-10}M and 10^{-8}M in different experiments.

DISCUSSION

These results demonstrate that retinoic acid affects the production of the interleukins 1,2 and 3 in a very similar fashion as does 1,25$(OH)_2D_3$. It is tempting to speculate that both compounds might stimulate bone resorption through a stimulation of IL 1 and/or IL 3 production. IL 1 has already been shown to stimulate bone resorption in organ culture in vitro. In contrast, an effect of IL 3 on bone has not yet been reported. However, IL 3 is thought to act as a multi-colonystimulating factor in the differentiation of bone marrow cells and seems to be identical with the mast cell growth factor. On the basis of these multiple activities it is conceivable that IL 3 might not only influence bone resorption, possibly through an effect on mast cells, but also bone formation.

SYNERGISTIC REGULATION OF 1,25-DIHYDROXYVITAMIN D_3 AND γ-INTERFERON IN c-myc ONCOGENE EXPRESSION ON HUMAN PROMYELOCYTE, HL-60.

T. MATSUI, Y. NAKAO, T. NAKAGAWA, T. KOIZUMI, Y. KATAKAMI, T.SUGIYAMA and T. FUJITA.
Third Division, Department of Medicine, and Department of Pathology, Kobe University School of Medicine, Kobe Japan.

INTRODUCTION:

The human promyelocytic leukemia cell line, HL-60, cells can be induced to differentiation into morphologically and functionally mature granulocytes or macrophage-like cells by compounds such as dimethylsulfoxide, retinoic acid, 1,25-$(OH)_2D_3$, lymphocyte-conditioned medium and phorbol esters. Differentiation of HL-60 cells is accompanied by growth inhibition and decreased levels of expression of the proto-oncogene c-myc, homologous to the transforming gene of avian myelocytomatosis virus (MC29). Recent studies on c-myc expression suggest its importance in the control of the growth and differentiation of normal cell, although the mechanisms regulating c-myc expression remain unknown. It therefore appeares worth while to investigate the regulation of c-myc expression by phisiological bioactive molecules. However, not all of these differentiation-inducing agents act under phisiological conditions. In addition, the factors in the lymphocyte-conditioned medium involved in the differentiation have not been completely identified. Recently, interferon-γ, a lymphokine derived from the culture medium, has been suggested to infuluence cell differentiation along the monocytic pathway. A great deal of attention has been focused on the immunomodulatory role of IFN-γ with respects to its ability to activate macrophages, but its precise role in monocyte-differentiation and oncogene-expression has not been clarified. Some recent reports, on the other hand, have shown an immunoregulatory effects of 1,25-$(OH)_2D_3$ as well as IFN-γ apart from their differentiation-inducing effects. The present study was undertaken to determine the differences between the effects of recombinant human IFN-γ and 1,25-$(OH)_2D_3$ on the differentiation of HL-60 cells and oncogene-expression, and to investigate the biologic interaction between IFN-γ and 1,25-$(OH)_2D_3$ in producing these effects. Because co-existence of these substances is quite conceivable in the phisiologic environment, we also examined the potential significance of such combination.

MATERIALS AND METHODS:

HL-60 cells were cultured in the presence or absence of IFN-γ or 1,25-$(OH)_2D_3$. To assess the qualitative and quantitative cell surface phenotypic changes in HL-60 cells, monoclonal anti human-monocyte antibodies, Mo2, 63D3, OKM1, OKM5 and OKT9 were used in flowcytometric analysis, as previously reported (1). Functional differentiation was assessed by the capacities of phagocytosis and NBT-reduction. To evaluate the levels of c-myc expression, Northern blot hybridization analysis was carried out.

Vitamin D. A Chemical, Biochemical and Clinical Update

RESULTS:

After 4 day culture with IFN-γ, the monocyte-specific cell surface antigens, Mo2 and OKM1, increased in a dose-dependent manner. 1,25-$(OH)_2D_3$ alone induced phenotypic changes but the potency of 1,25-$(OH)_2D_3$ was quite low at a physiological concentration of human serum, 0.1nM. The addition of both 0.1 nM 1,25-$(OH)_2D_3$ and IFN-γ induced synergistic changes in cell surface antigens. In functional differentiation, the effects of 1,25-$(OH)_2D_3$ and IFN-γ were cooperative, and dramatic morphological changes were also induced by the combination of these agents. Another monocyte-specific antigen 63D3 was increased by IFN-γ as well as by 1,25-$(OH)_2D_3$. On the other hand, OKM5, adherent monocyte-specific antigen, appeared on HL-60 cells treated with IFN-γ but not on those treated with 1,25 $(OH)_2D_3$. However, synergistic enhancement of OKM5 expression was seen under the combined treatment. In contrast, transferrin receptors recognized by the monoclonal antibody, OKT9 were synergistically decreased by IFN-γ and 1,25-$(OH)_2D_3$. Some difference was also found in the time-courses of OKM1 expression between IFN-γ and 1,25-$(OH)_2D_3$-treatment. OKM1 expression by IFN-γ occured about 24 hr after that caused by 1,25-$(OH)_2D_3$ (2).

The amount of c-myc mRNA was reduced by either IFN-γ or 1,25-$(OH)_2D_3$. The amount of action mRNA was not reduced in these differentiated cells. These findings demonstrate the selective reduction in c-myc mRNA transcription. A synergistic reduction of c-myc expression was seen in the combined treatment with IFN-γ and 1,25-$(OH)_2D_3$. This was confirmed by densitometic analysis as described blow.

Treatment	Relative density (%)
Control	42
IFN-γ	24
1,25-(OH)-$_2D_3$	30
IFN-γ and 1,25-$(OH)_2D_3$	4

These results indicate that human recombinant IFN-γ induces a monocytie phenotype in the HL-60 cells via a mechanism different from the action of 1,25-$(OH)_2D_3$.

The interaction of the two phisiological bioactive molecules may play an important role not only in normal cell differentiation, but also in the function of cell-mediated immunity.

REFERENCES:

1. Matusi, T., Nakao, Y., Kobayashi, N., Kishihara, M., Ishizuka, S., Watanabe, S. and Fujita, T. (1984) Int. J. Cancer, 23:193-202.
2. Matsui, T., Nakao, Y., Kobayashi, N., Koizumi, T., Nakagawa, T., Kishihara, M. and Fujita, T. (1985) Cancer Res. 45:311-316.

MODULATION OF CELL DIFFERENTIATION AND TUMOR PROMOTION BY 1α,25-DIHYDROXYVITAMIN D_3 [$1\alpha,25(OH)_2D_3$]

T. SUDA, E. ABE, C. MIYAURA, H. TANAKA, Y. SHIINA, T. HAYASHI, H. NAGASAWA, K. CHIDA*, H. HASHIBA*, M. FUKUSHIMA**, Y. NISHII**, and T. KUROKI*

Department of Biochemistry, School of Dentistry, Showa University, 1-5-8 Hatanodai, Shinagawa-ku, Tokyo 142, *Department of Cancer Cell Research, Institute of Medical Science, University of Tokyo, Tokyo 108, and **Research Laboratories of Chugai Pharmaceutical Company, Tokyo 171, JAPAN

For a long time, the only known function of $1\alpha,25(OH)_2D_3$ was a regulator of the extracellular calcium homeostasis by enhancing intestinal calcium transport and bone mineral mobilization. However, a specific cytosol/nuclear receptor for $1\alpha,25(OH)_2D_3$ was recently found in almost all tissues except the liver and skeletal muscle, and this raised the question of whether $1\alpha,25(OH)_2D_3$ has more subtle functions in a wide variety of tissues and cells besides the known target tissues of vitamin D such as bone and intestine.

A break through was made by the independent studies of Colston et al. (1) and Abe et al. (2). The former group (1) reported that $1\alpha,25(OH)_2D_3$ inhibits growth of human malignant melanoma cells (Hs 695T), and the latter (2) clearly demonstrated that the vitamin not only inhibits proliferation of mouse myeloid leukemia cells (M1), but also induces differentiation of M1 cells into monocyte-macrophages. We extended this original observation to other types of cells, in particular focussing on hematopoietic cells and skin-derived cells. We also found that $1\alpha,25(OH)_2D_3$ is involved in tumor promotion in a mouse skin chemical carcinogenesis system.

Table 1 summarizes the effect of $1\alpha,25(OH)_2D_3$ on modulation of cell differentiation and tumor promotion in hematopoietic cells and skin-derived cells so far reported. A wide variety of the effects of $1\alpha,25(OH)_2D_3$ (1 - 17) indicates that the vitamin is not only a calcium-regulating hormone, but also an immuno-modulator. We review here our recent findings on modulation of cell differentiation and tumor promotion by $1\alpha,25(OH)_2D_3$.

1. Fusion and Activation induced by $1\alpha,25(OH)_2D_3$ and their relation in alveolar macrophages

In 1983, Bar-Shavit et al. (14) and Abe et al. (4) independently reported that $1\alpha,25(OH)_2D_3$ induces fusion of macrophages to form multinucleated giant cells. It is believed that cells of the macrophage-monocyte series may be precursors of multinucleated osteoclasts. The former group (14) demonstrated that the multinucleated giant cells induced from HL-60

Vitamin D. A Chemical, Biochemical and Clinical Update

Table 1. The differentiating action of $1\alpha,25(OH)_2D_3$ in hematopoietic cells and skin-derived cells

Cells	Origin	Action	References
Hematopoietic cells			
M1	mouse myeloid leukemia	Cell growth ↓ Differentiation into monocyte-macrophages ↑	(2)
HL-60	human myeloid leukemia	Cell growth ↓ Differentiation into monocyte-macrophages ↑	(3-5)
U937	human histiocytic lymphoma	Cell growth ↓ Differentiation into monocyte-macrophages ↑	(5-7)
$P388D_1$	mouse macrophage-like lymphoma	Cell growth ↓ Differentiation into monocyte-macrophages ↑	(8)
Friend	mouse erythro-leukemia	DMSO-induced differentiation into erythrocytes ↓	(9)
Activated T-lymphocytes	human and mouse T-cells	Production of IL-2 ↓	(10,11)
Monocyte-macrophages	mature U937 cells	Production of monokines ↑	(12)
B-lymphocytes	human peripheral B-cells	Production of immunoglobulin ↓	(13)
Alveolar macrophages	ddy mouse lung	Fusion ↑ Activation ↑	(15-17)
HL-60 (long culture)	human myeloid leukemia	Fusion ↑ Bone-resorbing activity ↑	(14)
Skin-derived cells			
Hs 695T	human melanoma	Cell growth ↓	(1)
Epidermal cells	C57BL mouse skin	Terminal differentiation ↑	(22)
	SENCAR mouse skin	TPA-induced ODC activity ↓	(25)
	CD-1 mouse skin	DMBA- and TPA-induced papilloma formation ↓	(26)
B16	mouse melanoma	Melanin synthesis ↑	(23)

↑ stimulation, ↓ inhibition

cells by $1\alpha,25(OH)_2D_3$ exhibit a marked increase in the ability to bind and degrade bone matrix, the functional characteristics of bone-resorbing cells.

On the other hand, we used alveolar macrophages (15). Spleen cells obtained from 6- to 8-week-old male mice, ddy strain, were cultured with either 15 μg/ml of phytohemagglutinin (PHA) or concanavalin A (Con A), or 12 nM $1\alpha,25(OH)_2D_3$. After culture for 3 days, spleen cells were removed by centrifugation and conditioned media were obtained. Alveolar macrophages from mice of the same strain were cultured for 3 days in modified MEM containing 5% human serum either with conditioned media of spleen cell cultures, or directly with PHA, Con A or $1\alpha,25(OH)_2D_3$. Fusion rate of macrophages was expressed as percentages of total number of nuclei within giant cells containing at least 3 nuclei in a cell to total number of nuclei counted (Fig. 1). Figure 2 shows the time course of

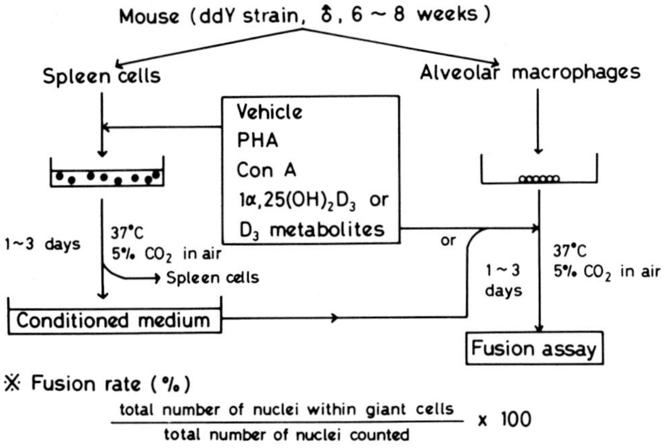

Fig. 1 The assay procedure for measuring fusion rate of alveolar macrophages treated with mitogens or $1\alpha,25(OH)_2D_3$ directly, or with conditioned media from stimulated spleen cell cultures.

change in fusion of alveolar macrophages directly induced by the vitamin or by a spleen cell-mediated indirect mechanism. About 80% of the macrophages fused to form multinucleated giant cells on day 3, similarly with each of the three conditioned media from spleen cell cultures (Fig. 2, left) (15). Conditioned media from stimulated spleen cell cultures contain both mitogens or $1\alpha,25(OH)_2D_3$ and a fusion factor produced by spleen cells. Thus, the question remains whether the stimulating effect of conditioned media on fusion of macrophages is due to a direct action of PHA, Con A or $1\alpha,25(OH)_2D_3$, or to an indirect action involving a fusion factor released from stimulated spleen cell cultures. $1\alpha,25(OH)_2D_3$ added to the macrophages directly induced fusion of about 35% of the cells on day 3. Neither PHA nor Con A induced fusion (Fig. 2, right)

(15).

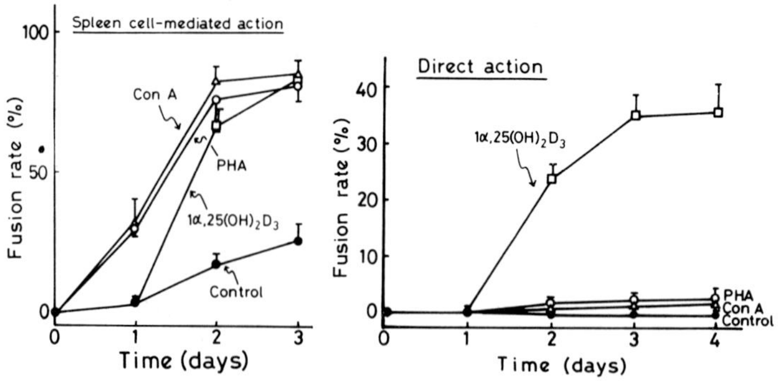

Fig. 2 Time course of change in fusion of alveolar macrophages induced by PHA, Con A or 1α,25(OH)$_2$D$_3$ directly, or by a spleen cell-mediated indirect mechanism (15).

To confirm the direct action of the vitamin, the preparation of alveolar macrophages were pretreated with anti-Thy 1.2 antibody and complement to eliminate lymphocytes which might have contaminated the macrophage preparation. The concentrations of anti-Thy 1.2 antibody and complement used were enough to suppress the Con A-induced enhancement of DNA synthesis by spleen cells (Fig. 3, right) (16). Alveolar macrophages pretreated with or without anti-Thy 1.2 antibody and complement fused similarly when they were incubated with 1α,25(OH)$_2$D$_3$ (Fig. 3, left) (16). Thus, it is concluded that 1α,25(OH)$_2$D$_3$ is capable of inducing fusion of mouse alveolar macrophages

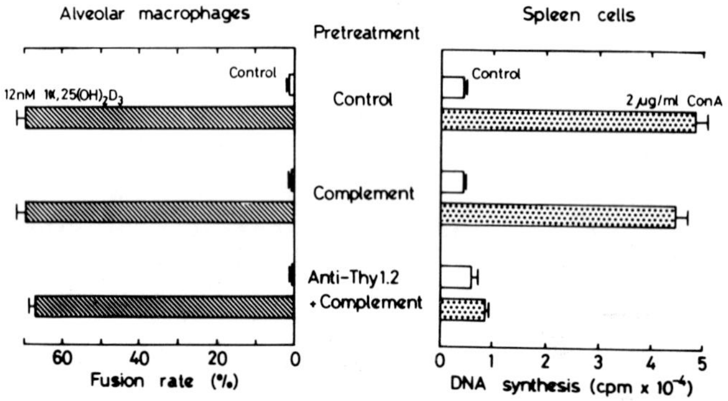

Fig. 3 Effects of pretreatment with anti-Thy 1.2 antibody and/or complement on fusion of alveolar macrophages (left) and DNA synthesis of spleen cells (right). DNA synthesis was determined by incorporating 1 μCi/ml of [^{3}H]-thymidine into DNA for the last 24 hours of the 72 hours' culture period in the presence or absence of 2 μg/ml of Con A. Alveolar macrophages were incubated for 3 days with or without 12 nM 1α,25(OH)$_2$D$_3$ (16).

by a direct mechanism (15, 16) and also by an indirect mechanism, the latter mediated by spleen cells (15). PHA and Con A also induce production of a lymphokine which exhibits macrophage fusion activity (MFF). Conditioned media of spleen cell cultures treated with PHA or Con A contain these mitogens which per se do not induce fusion directly (15). However, the conditioned medium of spleen cells treated with $1\alpha,25(OH)_2D_3$ contains the vitamin which does induce fusion directly (15, 16). Thus, the indirect action of the vitamin is complicated. The isolation of MFF and the relation between MFF and $1\alpha,25\text{-}(OH)_2D_3$ in inducing fusion of macrophages are being explored in our laboratory.

We next examined the possibility whether multinucleated giant cells formed from alveolar macrophages exhibit bone-resorbing activity. The activity was assessed using ^{45}Ca-labelled dead bone particles. Macrophages treated with 0.005-5 ng/ml of $1\alpha,25(OH)_2D_3$ exhibited bone-resorbing activity in parallel with the increase of fusion rate of macrophages. It is of great interest that the bone-resorbing activity was significantly enhanced without forming multinucleated giant cells when alveolar macrophages were treated with 0.05 ng/ml of $1\alpha,25(OH)_2D_3$. These results indicate that not only multinucleated giant cells formed from alveolar macrophages but also mononuclear macrophages treated with $1\alpha,25(OH)_2D_3$ exhibit bone-resorbing activity, though the activity increases in parallel with the increase of fusion rate of the macrophages. These results are in accord with those obtained by Bar-Shavit et al. (14) using HL-60 cells.

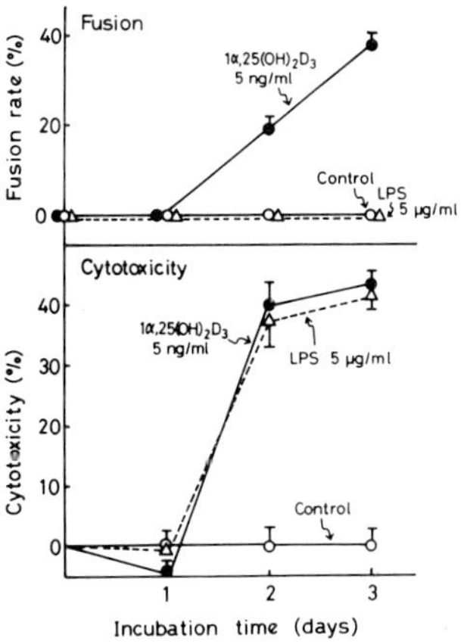

Fig. 4 Time course of change in the fusion and cytotoxicity of alveolar macrophages treated with 5 ng/ml of $1\alpha,25(OH)_2D_3$ or 5 μg/ml of LPS. B16 melanoma cells were the target cells used to examine cytotoxicity (17).

The most important role of macrophages is in the host defense mechanism against bacterial infection and growth of tumor cells. It is known that macrophages are activated by lipopolysaccharides (LPS), muramyldipeptides (MDP), or lymphokines. Activation of macrophages can be detected by morphological changes, increase in glucose consumption, phagocytic activity and cytotoxicity, and production of interleukin 1 (IL-1). We examined whether $1\alpha,25(OH)_2D_3$ activates alveolar macrophages. Figure 4 shows the relation between fusion and cytotoxicity of alveolar macrophages. Cytotoxicity was measured against B16 melanoma cells after alveolar macrophages were treated with either 5 ng/ml of $1\alpha,25(OH)_2D_3$ or

5 μg/ml of LPS. Like LPS, $1\alpha,25(OH)_2D_3$ induced cytotoxicity with a 1,000-fold difference in the effective dose levels of the two compounds. The cytotoxicity induced by the vitamin attained a similar maximal level on day 2 (Fig. 4, bottom) (17). In contrast, unlike $1\alpha,25(OH)_2D_3$, LPS did not stimulate fusion of macrophages at all (Fig. 4, top) (17). Therefore, it is concluded that $1\alpha,25(OH)_2D_3$ induces both fusion and activation, whereas LPS elicits activation only (17).

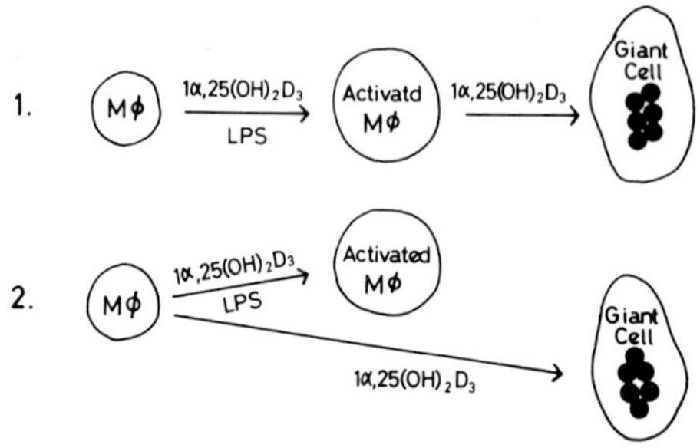

Fig. 5 Two hypothetical relations between fusion and activation of alveolar macrophages.

The relation between activation and fusion of alveolar macrophages is most interesting. There are two possible processes in this relation. The first hypothesis is that the activation of macrophages is prerequisite to the fusion, and the second one is that the fusion and activation occur independently (Fig. 5). At the present time, it is difficult to conclude which possibility is more plausible. In either case, it is clear that the vitamin induces fusion and activation whereas LPS elicits activation only. It is reported that macrophages treated with LPS produce IL-1 (18). This monokine not only stimulates proliferation and differentiation of lymphocytes (19), but also induces collagenase and proteoglycanase activity of chondrocytes (20) as well as bone-resorbing activity (21). Therefore it may be possible that the activated mononuclear macrophages induced by the vitamin exhibit cytotoxicity and also production of monokines which may lead to bone resorption.

2. Inhibition of Tumor Promotion in Mouse Skin by $1\alpha,25(OH)_2D_3$

During the studies on cell differentiation by $1\alpha,25(OH)_2D_3$, we found some similarities in the actions of $1\alpha,25(OH)_2D_3$ and tumor promoters such as 12-0-tetradecanoylphorbol-13-acetate (TPA). Like TPA, $1\alpha,25(OH)_2D_3$ stimulated differentiation of myeloid leukemia cells (Ml, HL-60, U937) into macrophages (2-7), blocked DMSO-induced differentiation of Friend erythroleukemia cells (9), and stimulated terminal differentiation of skin epidermal cells (22). This prompted us to examine whether $1\alpha,25(OH)_2D_3$ also exhibits a promoting activity.

One of the most widely used systems to study the sequential development of cancer is the initiation-promotion model on mouse skin. In this model, a low subthreshold dose of a complete carcinogen such as 7,12-dimethylbenz[a]anthracene (DMBA) is applied only once to the mouse skin to initiate the carcinogenic process. One week later, this treatment is followed by repeated applications of non-carcinogenic tumor promoters such as TPA or teleocidin B for 20-30 weeks. This consecutive treatment causes papilloma formation on mouse skin. This system is useful not only in examining tumor-initiating and tumor-promoting activities of a given compound, but also in finding anti-promoting activity of a compound if the agent is given concurrently with a known promoter. However, it takes 20-30 weeks to obtain either positive or negative results in this chemical carcinogenesis system.

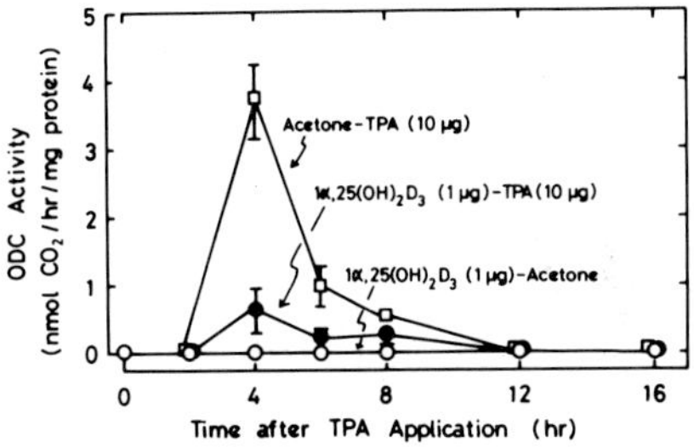

Fig. 6 Time course of change in inhibition of TPA-induced ODC activity in mouse skin by 1α,25-$(OH)_2D_3$ (25).

It is known that some early occurring changes are well correlated with tumor promotion. They include induction of dark cells (primitive skin stem cells) and induction of ornithine decarboxylase (ODC) activity (24). Since ODC induction occurs as early as 4 hours after application of TPA, we first examined the effect of 1α,$25(OH)_2D_3$ on ODC induction. Topical application of 10 μg of TPA greatly induced ODC activity (25). The activity attained a maximum 4 hours after TPA application and it rapidly decreased thereafter (Fig. 6). Concomitant topical application of 1 μg of 1α,$25(OH)_2D_3$ 30 minutes before TPA application markedly inhibited the TPA-induced ODC activity. The vitamin alone did not induce ODC activity at all, suggesting that 1α,$25(OH)_2D_3$ is an anti-promoter but not a promoter in mouse skin carcinogenesis (25). The dose required for 50% inhibition was 0.063 μg or 0.15 nmol, which was about half that of retinoic acid (25).

While this study was in progress, Wood <u>et al</u>. (26) reported that the topical application of 1α,$25(OH)_2D_3$ in the promotion phase suppressed papilloma formation. After a single topical application of 20 nmol of DMBA, CD-1 mice were given 16 nmol of TPA twice a week for 15 weeks. The animals were concomitantly given either acetone or 0.5 or 2 nmol of 1α,$25(OH)_2D_3$ twice a week 1 hour prior to TPA application. The 1α,$25(OH)_2D_3$ treatment inhibited tumor formation in a dose-dependent manner. Application of 0.5 and 2 μg of 1α,25-$(OH)_2D_3$ reduced the percentage of tumor-bearing mice from 88% to 59 and 18%, respectively. The same amounts of the vitamin also reduced the number of tumors per mouse from 8.6 to 3.4 and 0.8, respectively (26). We also confirmed the anti-promoting activity of 1α,$25(OH)_2D_3$ in SENCAR mice (unpublished results).

In the course of further examining the anti-promoting action of 1α,$25(OH)_2D_3$, we were interested in the unique bio-

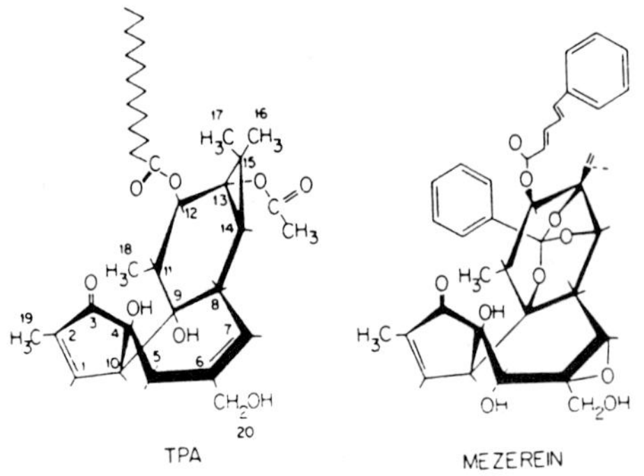

Fig. 7 Comparison of the structures of TPA and mezerein.

logical activity of a newly isolated tumor promoter, mezerein. Mezerein is a diterpene and its basic structure is similar to TPA (Fig. 7). Mezerein is a weak promoter, and its overall promoting activity is less than 2% of that of TPA (24). The activity of mezerein in inducing dark cells is only one-tenth that of TPA, but mezerein is as potent or even more potent than TPA in inducing ODC activity and DNA synthesis (Table 2) (24). Based upon these experimental results, Slaga (24) classified the promotion phase into two stages: Stage I involves induction of dark cells and Stage II induction of ODC activity. TPA induces both Stage I and Stage II promotion. In contrast, mezerein is involved only in Stage II promotion.

Table 2 Comparison of cellular and biochemical responses to TPA and mezerein in tumor promotion.

	Specific for	Relative response	
		TPA	Mezerein
Tumor promotion		100	< 2
Induction of dark cells	Stage I	100	<10
ODC	Stage II	80	100
epidermal cell proliferation	Stage II	50	100
DNA synthesis	Stage II	50	100

Slaga et al. Carcinogenesis 7:19 (1982)

Using this two-stage promotion protocol, we further examined the anti-promoting activity of 1α,25-$(OH)_2D_3$. First, 10 nmol of DMBA was topically applied as an initiator to all SENCAR mice one week before promotion. Then, 5 μg of TPA as a Stage I promoter only once and subsequently 5 μg of mezerein as a Stage II promoter once a week for 19 weeks were applied. 1α,25$(OH)_2D_3$ (1 μg) was applied to mouse skin 30 minutes before treatment with either Stage I promoter or Stage II promoter, or both Stage I and II promoters. Application of both mezerein and 1α,25$(OH)_2D_3$ was stopped at 20 weeks, but the experiment was continued up to 30 weeks. When 1α,25$(OH)_2D_3$ was applied to either Stages I and II or Stage II alone, tumor formation was markedly suppressed and only 17-25% of the animals had tumors at 20 weeks, indicating about 70-80% inhibition compared with the control to which 1α,25$(OH)_2D_3$ was not applied. Although tumors developed gradually after discontinuance of 1α,25$(OH)_2D_3$ and mezerein application, a significant inhibition by about 50% was still observed at 30 weeks [10 weeks after discontinuance of 1α,25-$(OH)_2D_3$ and mezerein application]. Application of 1α,25$(OH)_2$-D_3 to Stage I alone, however, did not suppress tumor formation. Similarly, inhibitory effect of the vitamin was observed in the number of tumors formed: only 0.3-0.4 tumors per mouse were formed at 20 weeks when $1\alpha,25(OH)_2D_3$ was applied to either Stage II alone or Stages I and II. Control animals formed 3.0 tumors per mouse.

Figure 8 summarizes the various stages of skin carcinogenesis and a site where $1\alpha,25(OH)_2D_3$ inhibits tumor promotion. One of the most important events in Stage I promotion involves induction of dark basal keratinocytes, which is specifically inhibited by a protease inhibitor (tosylphenylalanine chloromethyl ketone, TPCK) or an anti-inflammatory steroid (fluocinolone acetonide, FA). In contrast, induction of ODC activity and epidermal cell proliferation are involved in Stage II promotion. Therefore, it is likely that $1\alpha,25(OH)_2D_3$ inhibits tumor promotion, especially Stage II promotion in the two-stage promotion system.

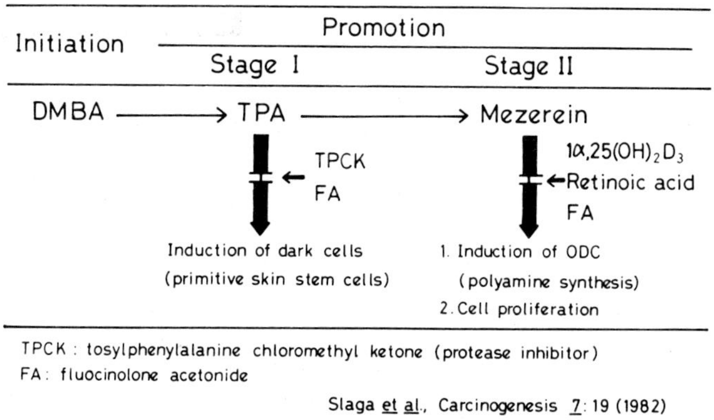

Fig. 8 Various stages of skin carcinogenesis and a site where $1\alpha,25(OH)_2D_3$ inhibits tumor promotion.

A series of the studies from our laboratory and other laboratories have suggested that $1\alpha,25(OH)_2D_3$ is a natural important modulator of cell growth, cell differentiation, tumor promotion and immune response. This hypothesis is now in more detail under investigation in our laboratory.

REFERENCES

1. Colston, K., Colston, M. J. and Feldman, D. (1981) Endocrinology 108, 1083-1086.
2. Abe, E., Miyaura, C., Sakagami, H., Takeda, M., Konno, K., Yamazaki, T., Yoshiki, S. and Suda, T. (1981) Proc. Natl. Acad. Sci. USA 78, 4990-4994.
3. Miyaura, C., Abe, E., Kuribayashi, T., Tanaka, H., Konno, K., Nishii, Y. and Suda, T. (1981) Biochem. Biophys. Res. Commun. 102, 937-943.

4. McCarthy, D. M., San Miguel, J. F., Freake, H. C., Green, P. M., Zola, H., Catovsky, D. and Goldman, J. M. (1983) Leukemia Res. 7, 51-55.
5. Tanaka, H., Abe, E., Miyaura, C., Shiina, Y. and Suda, T. (1983) Biochem. Biophys. Res. Commun. 117, 86-92.
6. Dodd, R. C., Cohen, M. S., Newman, S. L. and Gray, T. K. (1983) Proc. Natl. Acad. Sci. USA 80, 7538-7541.
7. Olsson, I., Gullberg, U., Ivhed, I. and Nilsson, K. (1983) Cancer Res. 43, 5862-5867.
8. Goldman, R. (1984) Cancer Res. 44, 11-19.
9. Suda, S., Enomoto, S., Abe, E. and Suda, T. (1984) Biochem. Biophys. Res. Commun. 119, 807-813.
10. Tsoukas, C. D., Provvedini, D. M. and Manolagas, S. C. (1984) Science 224, 1438-1440.
11. Bhalla, A. K., Amento, E. P., Serog, B. and Glimcher, L. H. (1984) J. Immunol. 133, 1748-1754.
12. Amento, E. P., Bhalla, A. K., Kurnick, J. T., Kradin, R. J., Clemens, T. L., Holick, S. A., Holick, M. F. and Krane, S. M. (1984) J. Clin. Invest. 73, 731-739.
13. Lemire, J. M., Adams, J. S., Sakai, R. and Jordan, S. C. (1984) J. Clin. Invest. 74, 657-661.
14. Bar-Shavit, Z., Teitelbaum, S. L., Reitsma, P., Hall, A., Pegg, L. E., Trial, J. and Kahn, A. J. (1983) Proc. Natl. Acad. Sci. USA 80, 5907-5911.
15. Abe, E., Miyaura, C., Tanaka, H., Shiina, Y., Kuribayashi, T., Suda, S., Nishii, Y., DeLuca, H. F. and Suda, T. (1983) Proc. Natl. Acad. Sci. USA 80, 5583-5587.
16. Tanaka, H., Hayashi, T., Shiina, Y., Miyaura, C., Abe, E. and Suda, T. (1984) FEBS Letters 174, 61-65.
17. Abe, E., Shiina, Y., Miyaura, C., Tanaka, H., Hayashi, T., Kanegasaki, S., Saito, M., Nishii, Y., DeLuca, H. F. and Suda, T. (1984) Proc. Natl. Acad. Sci. USA 81, 7112-7116.
18. Gery, I. and Waksman, B. H. (1972) J. Exp. Med. 136, 143-155.
19. Farrar, J. J., Mizel, S. B., Fuller-Farrar, J., Farrar, W. L. and Hilfiker, M. L. (1980) J. Immunol. 125, 793-806.
20. Gowen, M., Wood, D. D., Ihrie, E. J., Meats, J. E. and Russell, G. G. (1984) Biochem. Biophys. Acta 797, 186-193.
21. Gowen, M., Wood, D. D., Ihrie, E. J., McGuire, M. K. B. and Russell, G. G. (1983) Nature (London) 306, 378-380.
22. Hosomi, J., Hosoi, J., Abe, E., Suda, T. and Kuroki, T. (1983) Endocrinology 113, 1950-1957.
23. Hosoi, J., Abe, E., Suda, T. and Kuroki, T. (1985) Cancer Res. 45, in press.
24. Slaga, T. J., Fischer, S. M., Weeks, C. E., Nelson, K., Mamrack, M. and Klein-Szanto, A. J. P. (1982) Carcinogenesis 7, 19-34.
25. Chida, K., Hashiba, H., Suda, T. and Kuroki, T. (1984) Cancer Res. 44, 1387-1391.
26. Wood, A. W., Chang, R. L., Huang, M. T., Uskokovìc, M. and Conney, A. H. (1983) Biochem. Biophys. Res. Commun. 116, 605-611.

HUMAN "OSTEOBLAST-LIKE" CELLS IN CULTURE : RESPONSIVENESS TO 1,25-$(OH)_2D_3$

M.F. Harmand, L. Bordenave, R. Duphil, M. Thomasset*, D. Ducassou.

INSERM SC 31, Université de Bordeaux II, F.33076 Bordeaux Cédex.
*INSERM U.120, 44 Chemin de Ronde - F78110 Le Vésinet.

Human "osteoblast-like" cells are derived without proteolytic digestion from explants (4 - 5 mm^3 - washed free of marrow) of trabecular, cortical or alveolar bone of children. Medium (DMEM) is supplemented with 10 % FCS and 10 μg/ml ascorbic acid. As early as the third day for trabecular bone, much later (3 - 4 weeks) for both alveolar or cortical bone, cells grow out of the explants. They exhibit a typical flattened multipolar appearance with long cytoplasmic extensions and a centrally located nucleus with numerous nucleoli. As soon as confluency is reached, subcultures are achieved. Cells are subcultured up to 6 times. The doubling time is 10, 6 and 3 days respectively for cortical, trabecular and alveolar bone cells, arising from pre-pubertal children of 5 years old. After prolonged culture (2 months) in the same passage, cells form a multilayered system with localized macroscopic structures showing small deposits which contain high levels of Ca and P as detected by electron probe X-ray analysis.

Biochemical characterization of cells :

An optimal cell density (0.5×10^4 - 2×10^4 cells/cm^2) was found which permits the best phenotype expression as defined with the three following parameters :

- pure collagen type I synthesis is checked by an immunoperoxydase study using specific antibodies (kindley donated by Institut Pasteur - Lyon - France) against human collagen type I and III.
- specific non-collagenous protein synthesis is studied, after ^{3}H-Serine and ^{32}P incorporation, in both medium and cell compartment i.e. proteoglycans, phosphophorins, osteocalcin (Sephadex - G100 chromatography ; DEAE ion exchange chromatography ; electrophoresis ; hexuronic acid and protein assay).
- High alkaline phosphatase (AP) activity : 375 n mol Pi/min/μg DNA at 2×10^4 cells/cm^2.

These 3 culture models derived from various kinds of human bone express several osteoblast-like characteristics even after extended serial passages.

Responsiveness to 1,25-$(OH)_2D_3$

Cells from the 2nd subculture (alveolar and trabecular bone) are platted at 4×10^3 cells per well in plastic multiwell dishes (1.5 cm diameter wells) and allowed to attach for 24 hours at 37°C in a humidified atmosphere containing 5 % CO_2 . The experiment is initiated by adding medium supplemented with 5 % of "charcoal-stripped" FCS (1) over 24 hours. Thereafter fresh medium containing 1,25-$(OH)_2D_3$ (10^{-13} to 10^{-7} M) and 5 % "charcoal-stripped" FCS is added and changed every 3 days.

No change in morphology, nor in collagen type is noted.

Low concentrations of 1,25-$(OH)_2D_3$ stimulate slightly (+ 19 % $P < 0.01$

Vitamin D. A Chemical, Biochemical and Clinical Update

- 10^{-12} M) at early stages of incubation (12 h), whereas higher doses result in a marked and progressive inhibitory effect on growth. This effect is maximum at 10^{-8} M : 54 % of control value are reached after a 6 days incubation period.

These opposite effects are difficult to explain, but could be modulated by cell density, the former appearing at low cell density (2.5 x 10^3 cells/cm^2), the latter at higher cell density (1 x 10^4 cells/cm^2).

On the other hand AP activity is submitted by 1,25-$(OH)_2D_3$ treatment to a bimodal variation.
A first acute mode appears as early as the first hour of incubation with the vitamin D metabolite : 137 % of the control value is measured at 10^{-8}M in cell compartment. Thereafter AP levels appear rather reduced in treated cultures when compared to control ones after incubation periods of 3 and 6 hours.
A second mode is observed starting after a 12 hours incubation period, with also increasing AP activity : 200 % and 237 % of the control values were measured respectively in the medium and the cells after a 6 days incubation period, at 10^{-8}M (maximum effect).
Furthermore this double effect, maximum for the same metabolite concentration (10^{-8}M), which should be divided into acute and chronic, is difficult to explain. Could it be the translation of some kind of cell population heterogeneity ?

1,25-$(OH)_2D_3$ seems to promote cell differentiation expression by slowing growth and increasing the AP specialized function. This was observed by other authors on mouse "osteoblast-like" cells (2) or osteogenic sarcoma cells (3) (4), and could suggest a general action of 1,25-$(OH)_2D_3$ on target cells in stimulation of phenotype expression or modulation of maturation (1).

A second function related to 1,25-$(OH)_2D_3$ was investigated : total RNA extracted from trabecular bone "osteoblast-like" cells was assayed for CaBP 9 kDA by dot-blot hydridization using the specific ^{32}P cDNA probe. Autoradiograms of cDNA hybridized filters reveal the presence of detectable CaBP 9 kDa mRNA. Thus, this "osteoblast-like" strain could be a useful model to study the control of the expression of CaBP 9 kDa gene by 1,25-$(OH)_2D_3$.

Conclusion

These first results indicate that these three bone-cell culture models arising from humans are suitable experimental systems to study further the role of 1,25-$(OH)_2D_3$ in bone formation and metabolism.

References

1 - Harmand, M.F., Thomasset M., Rouais, F., Ducassou D. (1984) - J. Cell Physiol. 119, 359-365.
2 - Chen, T.I., Cone, C.M., Feldman, D. (1983) - Calcif. Tissue Int., 35, 806-811.
3 - Majeska, R.J., Rodan, G.S. (1982) - J. Biol. Chem., 257, 3362-3365.
4 - Mulkins, M.A., Manolagas, S.C., Deftos, L.J., Sussman, H.H. (1983) - J. Biol. Chem., 258, 6219-6225.

ROLE OF 1,25 DIHYDROXYVITAMIN D_3 IN THE IMMUNE SYSTEM

Stavros C. Manolagas

Department of Medicine, Division of Endocrinology/Metabolism
University of California at San Diego and VA Medical Center
La Jolla, CA 92161

Important interactions between the endocrine and the immune systems have been long appreciated (1,2). Moreover, hormones such as glucocorticoids have assumed a major role in the treatment of immune disorders. In this article, I review a series of recent discoveries which indicate that the hormonal form of vitamin D_3, namely $1,25(OH)_2D_3$, also interacts with the immune system and might play a biologically important role in the regulation of the immune response.

Receptors for $1,25(OH)_2D_3$ in cells of the immune system

That $1,25(OH)_2D_3$ might interact with cells of the immune system was initially suggested by the discovery of receptors for $1,25(OH)_2D_3$ in such cells. Several studies have demonstrated that monocytic cell lines, macrophages as well as peripheral monocytes from humans possess receptor proteins that bind $1,25(OH)_2D_3$ with high affinity ($Kd=10^{-10}$ M), and specificity (3,4). The receptor - $1,25(OH)_2D_3$ complexes from immune cells bind to DNA in a manner similar to that described in the classical target tissues of the hormone (4).

In contrast to monocytes/macrophages peripheral resting T and B lymphocytes do not possess $1,25(OH)_2D_3$ receptors. However, in-vitro activation of lymphocytes with mitogenic lectins such as phytohemagglutinin and concanavalin A causes the expression of $1,25(OH)_2D_3$ receptor proteins (4,5). Expression of $1,25(OH)_2D_3$ receptors upon in-vitro activation occurs also in normal human B-lymphocytes transformed with Epstein-Barr virus as well as in normal lymphocytes activated in-vitro by co-culture with lymphocytes from histoincompatible individuals. The evidence for the expression of the $1,25(OH)_2D_3$ receptor upon activation of lymphocytes

Vitamin D. A Chemical, Biochemical and Clinical Update

along with the finding of $1,25(OH)_2D_3$ receptor proteins in established malignant lymphocytic-lines (4) suggest an association between stage of activation and/or differentiation of cells of the lymphoid lineage and this receptor. This suggestion is supported by studies in rat and mouse thymic lymphocytes. Lymphocytes of the T lineage co-exist in the thymus at different stages of maturation and mitotic activity. Large and medium size cells located mainly in the subcapsular and medullary regions undergo a rapid series of mitotic divisions and give rise to small mitotically inert cells which are located almost exclusively in the thymic cortex (6). Provvedini et al. have detected $1,25(OH)_2D_3$ receptor macromolecules in the large cells but found no specifically bound radioactivity in the small cells (7). In agreement with these findings, Ravid et al. detected $1,25(OH)_2D_3$ receptors in medullary immunoincompetent mouse thymocytes, but found them absent from cortical immature cells (8).

Recent studies from our laboratory indicate that expression of $1,25(OH)_2D_3$ receptor in activated lymphocytes is a phenomenon that takes place in vivo. We have detected $1,25(OH)_2D_3$ receptor proteins in activated lymphocytes present in thymus and tonsils of normal children (9). In addition we have obtained evidence that unlike circulating lymphocytes from normals, circulating lymphocytes from over 80% of patients with rheumatoid arthritis express $1,25(OH)_2D_3$ receptors (10); it is established that in rheumatoid arthritis and other autoimmune disorders peripheral lymphocytes are activated and are involved in the disease process (11).

Effects of $1,25(OH)_2D_3$ on the immune function of monocytes

Using established monocytic cell lines it has been demonstrated that $1,25(OH)_2D_3$ promotes in-vitro the differentiation of monocytes towards the macrophage phenotype (12-19). Using normal peripheral human monocytes, we have found that $1,25(OH)_2D_3$ induces morphological changes as well as changes in lysosomal hydrolases consistent also with a hormone dependent promotion of the differentiation of these cells toward the macrophage phenotype (4).

Two observations raise the possibility that $1,25(OH)_2D_3$ might be also involved in specialized immune functions mediated by monocytic cells. Amento et al. found that $1,25(OH)_2D_3$ in combination with a factor from human T lymphocytes augmented the production of interleukin-1 in the U-937 cell line (20). Using the myelo monocytic cell line Wehi-3, we have obtained evidence that $1,25(OH)_2D_3$ enhances by 2 - 3 fold the gamma-interferon (γ-IFN)-induced expression of the Class II major histocompatibility complex antigens (Ia molecules), which mediate antigen presentation to lymphocytes (21). This enhancement leads to increased capacity of the Wehi-3 cells to stimulate antigen-specific Ia-restricted activation (details of these findings are given in the chapter by Morel et al. in this book). The $1,25(OH)_2D_3$ modulation of γ-IFN induction of Ia antigens suggests that the hormone might promote monocytes to function more efficiently as antigen-presenting cells. The relationship, if any, of the two observations to the prodifferentiation action of $1,25(OH)_2D_3$ on monocytes are at this stage unknown. However, in view of suggestions that the two main functions of monocytic cells, namely phagocytosis and antigen presentation could be expressions of two different cell types(22), it is feasible that the $1,25(OH)_2D_3$ effects on antigen presentation and differentiation are exerted on two distinct monocytic cell types.

Effects of $1,25(OH)_2D_3$ on thymocytes

The receptor data discussed above suggest that certain thymic cells are targets for $1,25(OH)_2D_3$ actions. We have examined in our laboratory the effects of $1,25(OH)_2D_3$ on primary culture of rat thymocytes. In cultures maintained in the absence of the hormone the number of viable cells decreased progressively. This phenomenon has been demonstrated by others both in vitro as well as in-vivo and it is thought to reflect natural death or suppression of lymphocytic clones (23). The addition of $1,25(OH)_2D_3$ in our cultures exerted a partially protective dose dependent effect against the spontaneous lytic involution of the thymic cells (24). In addition to this evidence Ravid et al. (8) have observed that $1,25(OH)_2D_3$ inhibited the response of medullary mouse thymocytes to phytohemagglutinin and IL-2 but had no effect on the cortical subpopulation, which did not contain the $1,25(OH)_2D_3$ receptor protein.

The significance of the presence of $1,25(OH)_2D_3$ receptor at certain stages of differentiation of thymic cells and of the evidence for an effect of the hormone on certain thymic cells is not clear at this stage. In view of the evidence for the prodifferentiation actions of $1,25(OH)_2D_3$ on monocytes, however, it is likely that the hormone is also involved in intrathymic differentiation of T-cells.

Effects of $1,25(OH)_2D_3$ on activated lymphocytes

Activation of lymphocytes by either mitogenic lectins or antigens triggers the release of lymphokines including interleukin-2 (IL-2) (25). Under the influence of IL-2 the T-cells reactive to the initial antigen proliferate and differentiate to cells that mediate effector functions (26). Such functions include cytotoxicity and either help or suppression of antibody production. Prompted by the evidence for the expression of the $1,25(OH)_2D_3$ receptor in activated lymphocytes, we examined the effect of the hormone on IL-2 (27). We have found that the media from PHA activated human lymphocytes grown in the presence of $1,25(OH)_2D_3$ exhibited reduced IL-2 activity. This effect was dependent on the concentration of $1,25(OH)_2D_3$. Fifty percent reduction of IL-2 activity in the medium as compared to media from control cultures that were maintained in the absence of $1,25(OH)_2D_3$ occurred at $2x10^{-12}$ - $10x10^{-12}$ M. The order of potency of other metabolites of vitamin D_3 on IL-2 suppression corresponded closely to their respective order of affinity for the specific $1,25(OH)_2D_3$ receptor and to their order of potency in other biological effects. This indicates that the inhibition of IL-2 by $1,25(OH)_2D_3$ is probably mediated via the specific receptor. In view of the lymphocyte growth-promoting properties of IL-2, we expected that $1,25(OH)_2D_3$ would have an effect on cellular proliferation. In fact, $1,25(OH)_2D_3$ mediated significant inhibition (50%) of PHA stimulated lymphocytes with total concentration as low as 10^{-11} to 10^{-10} M. This anti-proliferation effect, however, had later time kinetics than the effect on IL-2. After 2 days of culture the inhibitory effect of the hormone on cellular proliferation was less potent than its inhibitory effect on IL-2. However, significant inhibition of proliferation was seen after 3 days. Since the appearance of the $1,25(OH)_2D_3$ receptors in lymphocytes requires hours after mitogenic activation, it seems conceivable that the difference in time kinetics could be due to the time interval during which the cells were unresponsive to the effects of the hormone, but sensitive to the effects of the mitogen.

Rigby et al., independently, confirmed the potent inhibitory effect of $1,25(OH)_2D_3$ on IL-2 and on proliferation (28). In addition, they demonstrated that the inhibition of proliferation by $1,25(OH)_2D_3$ could be only partially restored by addition of exogenous IL-2. Thus, $1,25(OH)_2D_3$ might inhibit proliferation of activated lymphocytes through other mechanisms in addition to interferring with IL-2.

We have also examined in our laboratory the combined effect of $1,25(OH)_2D_3$ and of the potent synthetic glucocorticoid triamcinolone acetonide on IL-2 in PHA activated human lymphocytes. Glucocorticoids have been known to inhibit IL-2 production by animal and human lymphocytes in-vitro (1,25). We found that over a range of concentrations of $1,25(OH)_2D_3$ [10^{-12} to 10^{-8} M] and triamcinolone the combination of two steroids potentiated each other's effect in inhibiting IL-2.

In addition to the profound effects of $1,25(OH)_2D_3$ on IL-2 production and lymphocyte proliferation the hormone has potent immunoregulatory properties on the effector phases of the immune response. We have determined that $1,25(OH)_2D_3$ inhibits the generation of cytotoxic lymphocytes during a mixed lymphocytic reaction. Reduction of the cytotoxic response to one half of maximal in our experiments was mediated at $8x10^{-10}$ M concentrations of the hormone. Lemire et al. on the other hand have shown that $1,25(OH)_2D_3$ inhibits immunoglobulin production induced by activation with pokeweed mitogen (23). We have confirmed their findings and further observed that $1,25(OH)_2D_3$ can inhibit the production of polyclonal immunoglobulins M or G induced by the Epstein-Barr virus. Fifty percent inhibition of the IgM response was effected by $10x10^{-10}$ M concentration of $1,25(OH)_2D_3$ while similar inhibition of IgG required 10 times higher concentrations of the hormone. Since the pokeweed mitogen driven antibody response depends on the presence of T cells, it is of interest that additions of exogenous IL-2 in our studies did not reverse the inhibitory effect of $1,25(OH)_2D_3$. This observation along with the fact that

$1,25(OH)_2D_3$ inhibits the Epstein-Barr virus induced antibody, (a T cell independent response) supports the contention that the immunoregulatory effects of $1,25(OH)_2D_3$ may be mediated through other mechanisms in addition to interferring with IL-2.

Summary of Evidence

The evidence indicating that the hormonal form of vitamin D, $1,25(OH)_2D_3$, is involved in the regulation of the immune system can be summarized as follows:

1. Cells of the monocyte/macrophage series contain receptors for $1,25(OH)_2D_3$ regardless of their activation stage. Cells of the lymphoid series express also $1,25(OH)_2D_3$ receptor but only at certain stages of their differentiation pathway and upon activation.

2. $1,25(OH)_2D_3$ promotes the differentiation of monocytes towards the macrophage phenotype and enhances the function of macrophages in non-specific immune processes such as phagocytosis. In addition, $1,25(OH)_2D_3$ might enhance the function of monocytes in antigen-presentation.

3. $1,25(OH)_2D_3$ is a potent inhibitor of interleukin-2 produced by activated lymphocytes and exerts suppressive effects on the effector function of both T and B lymphocytes. In addition, $1,25(OH)_2D_3$ might be involved in the intrathymic differentiation of T-lymphocytes.

Goals of Future Research

The experimental evidence for the involvement of $1,25(OH)_2D_3$ in immunoregulation raises issues of basic as well as of clinical importance. The major effects of $1,25(OH)_2D_3$ on its classical target tissues involve calcium translocation. On the other hand, alteration of calcium pools or an increase in cytoplasmic ionized calcium along with protein kinase C activation appear to be of major importance in lymphocyte activation/proliferation and the subsequent immune response (30,31,32). It should be noted that in addition to the $1,25(OH)_2D_3$ receptors, lymphocytes possess receptors for other calcium regulating hormones such as parathyroid hormone and calcitonin (33,34). Both these peptide hormones that act through cAMP have been shown to influence the proliferation of lymphocytes. Thus, it will be of interest to determine whether the role of $1,25(OH)_2D_3$ and of other calcitropic hormones on lymphocytes is linked to calcium regulation. I expect that $1,25(OH)_2D_3$ and its receptor will be useful tools in studies aiming to elucidate the molecular details of the lymphocyte activation/proliferation process vis-a-vis intracellular calcium, cAMP and protein kinases.

Future studies will be also needed to determine the relevance of the immunoregulatory properties of $1,25(OH)_2D_3$ to the immune response in-vivo. Available evidence from in-vivo studies appears consistent with a stimulatory influence of $1,25(OH)_2D_3$ on the non-specific component of the immune response, which is mediated by monocytes/macrophages. Indeed, vitamin D-deficient rickets in humans is frequently associated with recurrent infections (35). Investigation of defects in the defense mechanisms of such patients has revealed an impaired ability to respond to non-specific inflammatory stimuli (36) and decreased mobility and impaired capacity of their leukocytes to phagocytize (37). Bar-Shavit and colleagues have further shown that macrophages from vitamin-D_3 deficient mice function abnormally and that this can be corrected in-vitro as well as in-vivo with the addition of $1,25(OH)_2D_3$.

Very little, if any, is known on the other hand at the present vis-a-vis the relevance of the suppressive influence of $1,25(OH)_2D_3$ to the lymphocyte mediated (antigen dependent or specific) immune response in-vivo (39,40). Considering the evidence that $1,25(OH)_2D_3$ might potentiate monocyte/macrophage function in antigen presentation, while on the other hand might suppress activated lymphocyte function I speculate that the overall influence of the hormone on immunity in-vivo will depend upon the balance of such positive and negative feedbacks. In turn such balance would probably depend a) on the accumulation of the hormone in the different cells of the immune system and b) on the ability of lymphocytes to respond to the signals of the hormone by expressing receptor proteins. Through inhibition of proliferation and its suppressive influence on the effector function of activated lymphocytes $1,25(OH)_2D_3$ could act as the brake of an undesirably excessive immune response or an inappropriate proliferation of lymphocytes. In this context, it is of interest to note that abnormally proliferating lymphoid tissues such as lymphomas and

and sarcoid are capable themselves of synthesizing 1,25$(OH)_2D_3$ from its precursor 25$(OH)D_3$ (41,42).

The preliminary evidence for the potentiation of the 1,25$(OH)_2D_3$ effects on IL-2 by glucocorticoids raises the possibility that 1,25$(OH_2D_3$ or newer analogs with lesser hypercalcemic properties might have a place in the therapeutic manipulation of immune disorders.

Acknowledgements

The author wishes to acknowledge C.D. Tsoukas, D.M. Provvedini and L.J. Deftos for their collaboration in these studies and M.E. Hornbeck and D. Curran for technical assistance. Supported by the National Institute of Health(AI 21761)and the Veterans Administration.

REFERENCES

1. Cupps, T.R., and Fauci, A.S. (1982) Immunological Reviews 65:133-155.

2. Grossman, C.J. (1985) Science 227:257-261.

3. Peacock, M., Jones, S., Clemens, T.L., Amento, E.P., Kurnick, J.T., Krane, S.M., and Holick, M.F. (1982) In: Vitamin D: Chemical, Biochemical and Clinical Endocrinology of Calcium Metabolism. Eds.: A.W. Norman, K. Schaefer, D.V. Herrath, and H-G. Grigoleit (Walter De Gruyter, Berlin) pp.83-85.

4. Provvedini, D.M., Tsoukas, C.D., Deftos, L.J., and Manolagas, S.C. (1983) Science 221:1181-1183.

5. Bhalla, A.K., Amento, E.P., Clemens, T.L., Holick, H.F., and Krane, S.M. (1983) Journal of Clinical Endocrinology and Metabolism 57:1308-1310.

6. Droege, D.L., and Zucker, R. (1975) Transplantation Reviews 25:3-25.

7. Provvedini, D.M., Deftos, L.J., and Manolagas, S.C. (1984) Biochemical and Biophysical Research Communications 121:277-283.

8. Ravid, A., Koren, R., Novogrodsky, A., and Liberman, U. (1984) Biochemical and Biophysical Research Communications 123:163-169.

9. Provvedini, D.M., Sobol, R.E., Rulot, C., Deftos, L.J., and Manolagas, S.C. (1985) In: Proceedings of the 7th Annual Meeting of the American Society for Bone and Mineral Research, in press.

10. Werntz, D.A., Tsoukas, C.D., Provvedini, D.M., Vaughan, J.H., Deftos, L.J., and Manolagas, S.C. (1984) Calcified Tissue International 36:528.

11. Winchester, R.J., and Kunkel, H.G. (1979) Advances in Immunology 28:221-229.

12. Miyaura, C., Abe, E., Kuribayashi, T., Tanaka, H., Konno, K., Nishii, Y., and Suda, T. (1981) Biochemical and Biophysical Research Communications 102:937-943.

13. Tanaka, H., Abe, E., Miyaura, C., Shiina, Y., and Suda, T. (1983) Biochemical and Biophysical Research Communications 117:86-92.

14. Mangelsdorf, D.J., Koeffler, H.P., Donaldson, C.A., Pike, J.W., and Haussler, M.R. (1984) Journal of Cell Biology 93:391-398.

15. Matsui, T., Nakao, Y., Kobayashi, N., Kishihara, M., Ishizuka, S., Watanabe, S., and Fujita, T. (1984) International Journal of Cancer 33:193-202.

16. Reitsma, P.H., Rothberg, P.G., Astrin, S.M., Trial, J., Bar-Shavit, Z., Hall, A., Teitelbaum, S.L., and Kahn, A.J. (1983) Nature 306:492 -494.

17. Abe, E., Miyaura, C., Sakagami, H., Takeda, M., Konno, K., Yamazaki, T., Yoshiki, S., and Suda, T. (1981) Proceedings of the National Academy of Sciences USA 78:4990-4994.

18. Dodd, R.C., Cohen, M.S., Newman, S.L., and Gray, T.K. (1983) Proceedings of the National Academy of Sciences USA 80:7538-7541.

19. Olsson, I., Gullberg, U., Ivhed, I., and Nilsson, K. (1983) Cancer Research 43:5862-5867.

20. Amento, E.P., Bhalla, A.K., Kurnick, J.T., Kradin, R.L., Clemens, T.L., Holick, S.A., Holick, M.F., and Krane, S.M. (1984) Journal of Clinical Investigation 73:731-739.

21. Morel, P.A., Wegmann, D.R., Provvedini, D.M., Manolagas, S.C., and Chiller, J.M. (1985) Proceedings of the Symposium "Leukemia 1985", Keystone, Colorado, Jan 27-Feb 2, 1985.

22. Sun, D., and Lohmann-Matthes, M.L. (1982) European Journal of Immunology 12:134-140.

23. McPhee, D., Pye, J., and Shortman, K. (1979) Thymus 1:151-162.

24. Provvedini, D.M., Miller, M.M., Werntz, D.A., Deftos, L.J., and Manolagas, S.C. (1984) Calcified Tissue International 36:523.

25. Smith, K.A. (1980) Immunological Reviews 51:337-357.

26. Ruscetti, F.W., and Gallo, R.C. (1981) 57:379-394.

27. Tsoukas, C.D., Provvedini, D.M., Manolagas, S.C. (1984) Science 224:1438-1448.

28. Rigby, W.F.C., Stacy, T., and Fanger, M.W. (1984) Journal of Clinical Investigation 74:1451-1455.

29. Lemire, J.M., Adams, J.S., Sakai, R., and Jordan, S.C. (1984) Journal of Clinical Investigation 74:657-661.

30. Lichtman, A.H., Segel, G.B., and Lichtman, M.A. (1983) Blood 61:413-422.

31. Weiss, M.J., Daley, J.F., Hodgdon, J.C., and Reinherz, E.L. (1984) Proceedings of the National Academy of Sciences USA 81:6836-6840.

32. Truneh, A., Albert F., Golstein, P., and Schmitt-Verlust, A. (1985) Nature 313:318-320.

33. Marx, S.J., Aurbach, G.D., Gavin, III, J.R., and Buell, D.W. (1974) Journal of Biological Chemistry 249:6812-6816.

34. Yamamoto, I., Potts, J.T., Jr., and Segre, G.V. (1983) Journal of Clinical Investigation 71:404-407.

35. Stroder, J. (1975) In: Vitamin D and Problems Related to Uremic Bone Disease. Ed: A.W. Norman (Walter De Gruyter, Berlin) pp.679-687.

36. Lorente, F., Fontan, G., Jara, P., Casa, C., Garcia-Rodriguez, M.C., and Ojeda, J.A. (1976) Acta Paediatrica Scandinavica 65:695-699.

37. Stroder, J., and Kasal, P. (1970) Acta Paediatrica Scandinavica 65:288-292.

38. Bar-Shavit, Z., Noff, D., Edelstein, S., Meyer, M., Shibolet, S., and Goldman, R. (1981) Calcified Tissue International 33:673-676.

39. Miyakoshi, H., Aoki, T., and Hirasawa, Y. (1981) Clinical Nephrology 16:119-125.

40. Fujita, T., Matsui, T., Nakao, Y., and Watanabe, S. (1984) Mineral and Electrolyte Metabolism 10:375-378.

41. Breslau, N.A., McGuire, J.L., Zerwekh, J.E., Frenkel, E.P., and Pak, C.V.C. (1984) Annals of Internal Medicine 100:1-7.

42. Mason, R.S., Frankel, T., Chan, Y.L., Lissner, D., and Posen, S. (1984) Annals of Internal Medicine 100:59-61.

EFFECT OF 1α-HYDROXYVITAMIN D_3 ON THE IMMUNE RESPONSE

Y. Ohsugi,* T. Nakano,* T. Komori,* K. Ueno,* Y. Sugawara,* M. Fukushima,* T. Yamamoto,* Y. Nishii,* T. Masuda,** M. Matsuno**

* Research Laboratories, Chugai Pharmaceutical Co., Ltd., 41-8, Takada 3 chome, Toshima-ku, Tokyo 171,
** Department of Orthopedic Surgery, Hokkaido University, Kita-15, Nishi-7, Kita-ku, Sapporo 060, JAPAN

Restoration of Thymic Involution and the Depressed Lymphocyte Proliferation by 1α-Hydroxyvitamin D_3 in Renal Osteodystrophy rats

We have previously reported that a single injection of homologous glycopeptide causes renal osteodystrophy with severe hyperparathyroidism in rats (1) and also shown clinical effectiveness of an active form of vitamin D_3 in curing bone damage observed in this new experimental model (2). In that study, 30 rats were divided into 5 groups on the 280th day after the injection of glycopeptide. Various doses of vitamin D_3 derivatives (10 µg/kg D_3, 2 µg/kg 25-hydroxyvitamin D_3 ($25OHD_3$), 0.1 µg/kg 1α,25-dihydroxy-vitamin D_3 ($1\alpha,25(OH)_2D_3$), and 0.2 µg/kg 1α-hydroxyvitamin D_3 ($1\alpha OHD_3$) were daily administered orally to the nephritic rats for 23 days before sacrifice. Table 1 shows that oral administration of $1\alpha OHD_3$ and $1\alpha,25(OH)_2D_3$ prevented the thymic involution occurred in these nephritic rats. There is a correlation between the clinical efficacy on the renal osteodystrophy and wet weight of the thymus; i.e. $25OHD_3$ and D_3 which were ineffective in curing renal damage, did not prevent the thymic involution. In contrast, both $1\alpha OHD_3$ and $1\alpha,25(OH)_2D_3$ were much more potent than the others in curing diseases and prevented the thymic involution.

Furthermore, nephritic control rats had a lower responsiveness of the peripheral lymphocytes to mitogens such as phytohemagglutinin (PHA) and concanavalin A (Con A). $1\alpha OHD_3$ and $1\alpha,25(OH)_2D_3$, but not D_3 and $25OHD_3$ showed an augmenting effect on the lymphocyte reactivity (Data not shown).

Among the tested derivatives, $1\alpha,25(OH)_2D_3$ and $1\alpha OHD_3$ were the most potent in augmenting the depressed immune response and in preventing the thymic involution. Daily administration of $1\alpha OHD_3$ at a dose level of 0.1 µg/kg caused a marked improvement of the immunological defect. However, doses of vitamin D_3 100 times higher were not enough to cure these abnormalities. This strikingly contrasts with the relative potency of vitamin D_3 and its derivatives in preventing rickets in vitamin D-deficient

Vitamin D. A Chemical, Biochemical and Clinical Update

Table 1. Effect of Daily Administration of Each Vitamin D_3 Derivatives for 23 Days on Thymus Weight of Nephritic Rats

	Drugs	Thymus weight (mg/100 g B.W.)	Therapeutic effect on renal osteodystrophy
Normal	Vehicle	18.6 ± 2.4[a)]	-
Nephritic rats	Vehicle	11.9 ± 1.2	-
	$1\alpha OHD_3$	20.2 ± 1.0[a)]	Remarkable
	$1\alpha,25(OH)_2D_3$	16.9 ± 1.6[a)]	Remarkable
	D_3	13.2 ± 2.4	Moderate
	$25OHD_3$	14.5 ± 2.5	Moderate

Various doses of vitamin D derivatives (10 µg/kg D3, 2 µg/kg $25OHD_3$, 0.1 µg/kg $1\alpha,25(OH)_2D_3$, and 0.2 µg/kg $1\alpha OHD_3$) were administered orally for 23 days before sacrifice. Values are means ± S.E. of 6 rats.

a) $P<0.05$ vs nephritic rats given vehicle (medium chain triglyceride).

animals. It has been reported that the antirachitic effectiveness of $1\alpha OHD_3$ was only 2-6 times higher than vitamin D_3 in vitamin D-deficient animals (3-5). The critical factor in this discrepancy is, most likely, the impaired conversion of $25OHD_3$ to $1\alpha,25(OH)_2D_3$ in the nephritic rats. In vitamin D deficiency, renal biosynthesis of $1\alpha,25(OH)_2D_3$ is not disturbed. It has been reported that $1\alpha OHD_3$ is quickly converted to $1\alpha,25(OH)_2D_3$ in the liver (6,7). In the mean time, it was reported that physiological concentrations of $1\alpha,25(OH)_2D_3$ induced differentiation of murine (8) and human (9) myeloid leukemic cells. Provvedini et al. (10) reported that the receptors for $1\alpha,25(OH)_2D_3$ were present on human monocytes, and also on T and B lymphocytes activated in vitro by mitogenic lectin or Epstein-Barr virus, respectively; these receptors were not present in resting lymphocytes. Tsoukas et al. (11) also reported that physiological concentration of $1\alpha,25(OH)_2D_3$ suppressed the release of interleukin-2 in vitro. These lines of evidence together with the present findings suggest that active vitamin D_3 might play some role in the differentiation of bone marrow precursor cells and might be involved in the regulation of immune response.

Immunoregulation by 1αOHD$_3$ in Mice

The following experiments were performed in mice to clarify the point described above. First, the influence of 1αOHD$_3$ on the primary immune response against sheep red blood cells (SRBC) was examined. Balb/c mice were intravenously immunized with SRBC. Two or three days after SRBC injection, spleens were removed for the determination of direct plaque-forming cells (PFC). 1αOHD$_3$ dissolved in medium chain triglyceride (MCT), was orally given at doses of 0.05, 0.1, or 0.2 μg/kg body weight.

As shown in Fig. 1, 1αOHD$_3$ enhanced the primary anti-SRBC PFC response in mice immunized with $1x10^7$ SRBC. PFC number of MCT-treated control mice was 351±62/spleen and 3.76± 0.75/10^6 spleen cells, when PFC assay was done 2 days after immunization (Fig. 1-A). In contrast, PFC numbers/spleen of mice orally given 1αOHD$_3$ immediately after SRBC immunization were 484±79 and 571±104 at doses of 0.05 and 0.2 μg/kg, respectively (38 and 63% increases in mean value). Slight increases in PFC/10^6 cells were observed at doses of 0.05 and 0.2 μg/kg of 1αOHD$_3$ (24 and 39% increases in mean value, respectively). The enhancing effect of 1αOHD$_3$ was more obvious 3 days after immunization (Fig. 1-B). The groups given 1αOHD$_3$ in doses of 0.05 and 0.2 μg/kg recorded 54% ($p<0.05$) and 111% ($p<0.001$) increases in mean values of PFC/spleen in comparison with 3122±495 PFC/spleen of the control group. A significant increase in the number of PFC/10^6 cells ($p<0.001$; 90% increase in mean value) was also detected at a dose of 0.2 μg/kg compared with 28.4±4.2 PFC/10^6 cells of the control group. 1αOHD$_3$, on the other hand, did not influence the PFC response induced by immunization with $5x10^8$ SRBC (optimal dose of antigen) (Fig. 1-B). The number of PFC/spleen of MCT-treated control group was 27000±1411, and those of 1αOHD$_3$-administered groups were 31488±1546 and 24000±2337 at doses of 0.1 and 0.2 μg/kg, respectively. No differences were also observed in numbers of PFC/10^6 cells. Reproducibility of the results was confirmed in the repeated experiment.

These results indicated that 1αOHD$_3$ had no effect on the antibody formation induced by immunization with $5x10^8$ SRBC. When the dose of antigen was reduced to 1/50 of the optimal, the immune response was markedly lowered. In such conditions 1αOHD$_3$ significantly augmented the anti-SRBC PFC response. This suggests that 1αOHD$_3$ potentiated the suboptimal immune response by accelerating the helper T cell-function and/or B cell proliferation and differentiation to catch up with the optimal immune response. Thus, augmentation by 1αOHD$_3$ is dependent on the magnitude of PFC response.

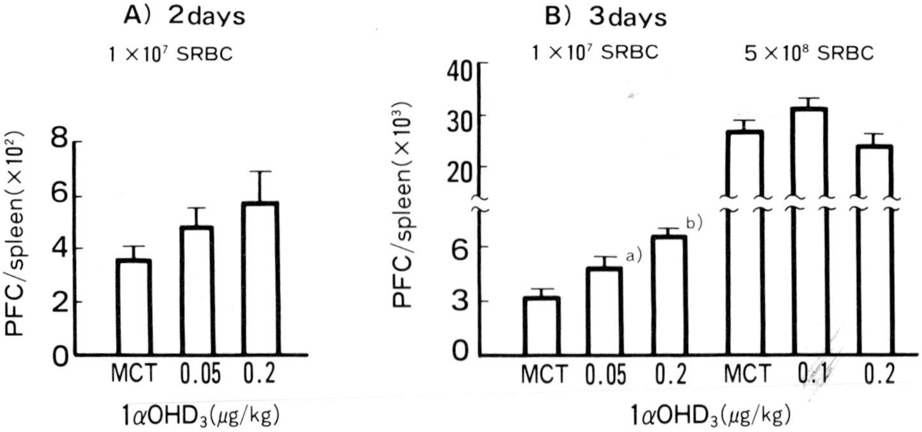

Fig. 1. Effect of $1\alpha OHD_3$ on the Primary Anti-SRBC PFC Response.

A) Balb/c mice were intravenously injected with 1×10^7 SRBC and $1\alpha OHD_3$ was orally administered immediately after immunization. Mice were sacrificed two days after immunization and their spleens were used for the anti-SRBC direct PFC assay. PFC assay was performed as described by Cunningham and Szenberg.
B) Balb/c mice were intravenously injected with 1×10^7 or 5×10^8 SRBC and $i\alpha OHD_3$ was oraliy administered immediately after, and again 24hrs after, immunization. Mice were sacrificed three days after immunization and their spleens were used for the anti-SRBC direct PFC assay. Values are means±S.E. obtained from 7-10 mice. a)$p<0.05$, b)$p<0.001$. Significantly different from the MCT-administered group.

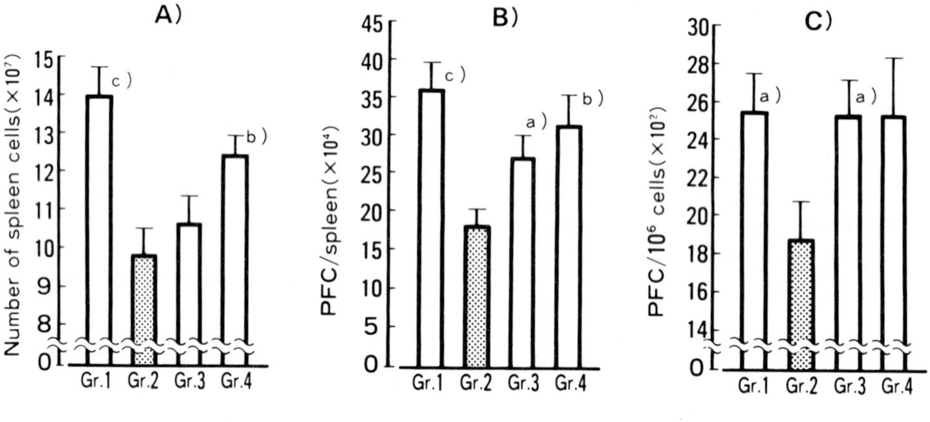

Fig. 2. Effect of $1\alpha OHD_3$ on Suppressed Immunity Caused by Restraint-Stress.

Gr. 1. Non-stress and MCT. Gr. 2. Stress and MCT. Gr. 3. Stress and $1\alpha OHD_3$ (0.1μg/kg).
Gr. 4. Stress and $1\alpha OHD_3$ (0.2μg/kg).
BDF_1 mice were subjected to restraint-stress for 2 days (12 hours a day, from 8:30 to 20:30) and were intravenously immunized with 5×10^8 SRBC 13 hours after release from the second day's restraint. $1\alpha OHD_3$ or MCT was orally administered immediately after, and again 24 hours after, immunization. Mice were sacrificed 4 days after immunization and their spleens were used for the anti-SRBC direct PFC assay. Bars and vertical lines represent mean values±S.E. obtained from 7-9 mice. Closed bars indicate the control group.
a)$p<0.05$, b)$p<0.02$, c)$p<0.01$. Significantly different from the stressed control group (Gr. 2).

To confirm this immunoregulatory activity of 1αOHD$_3$ another experimental assay system established by Okimura and Yamamoto (13) was used. They reported that restraint-stress caused the depression of helper T cell function and decreased anti-SRBC PFC response, while B cell function was not impaired. BDF$_1$ mice (male, 6-7 wks old) were restrained in small wire cages in which they could hardly move, for 2 days (12 hours a day, from 8:30 to 20:30). Non-stressed control mice were kept without food and water. These animals were immunized with 5x10^8 SRBC 13 hours after release from the second day's restraint. Splenic PFC assay was performed 4 days after immunization.

It was repeatedly confirmed that restraint-stress remarkably reduced the number of spleen cells and the anti-SRBC PFC response. In all 5 experiments the mean numbers of spleen cells and PFC/spleen decreased by over 30% and over 50%, respectively. Fig. 2 clearly shows that the oral administration of 1αOHD$_3$, at doses of 0.1 and 0.2 μg/kg body weight, resulted in recovery from the reduced numbers of spleen cells, PFC/spleen and PFC/10^6 cells. In particular, at a dose of 0.2 μg/kg, significant increases in the number of spleen cells ($p<0.02$) and the number of PFC/spleen ($p<0.05$) were observed compared with the stressed control group. The mean value of PFC/10^6 cells also completely recovered to the level of the nonstressed group, though there was no statistically significant difference (Fig. 2-C). Fasting did not influence antibody formation in this experimental system (data not shown).

These results clearly show that 1αOHD$_3$ significantly restores the stress-induced immunosuppression to near the normal level. It is likely that this immunoregulatory effect of 1αOHD$_3$ is due to the increase in the depressed helper T cell function.

Finally, experiment was performed to examine whether 1αOHD$_3$ would have a suppressive effect on the enhanced immune response. Colchicine is known to enhance antibody formation, inactivating suppressor cell activity (14,15). DNP-KLH (100 μg) and colchicine (1 mg/kg body weight) were intraperitoneally injected into Balb/c mice. MCT or 1αOHD$_3$ was orally administered immediately after, and again 24 hours after, immunization. Mice were sacrificed 6 days after immunization and their spleens were used for the anti-DNP direct PFC assay. DNP-coated SRBC was prepared using $CrCl_3$ by the method of Gronowicz et al (16) and used for PFC assay. As shown in Fig. 3, 1αOHD$_3$ significantly suppressed the anti-DNP PFC response which was enhanced over 4-fold by colchicine; especially at a dose of 0.1 μg/kg. The numbers of PFC/spleen and PFC/10^6 cells were decreased by 77% and 80% ($p<0.05$ and $p<0.01$, respectively).

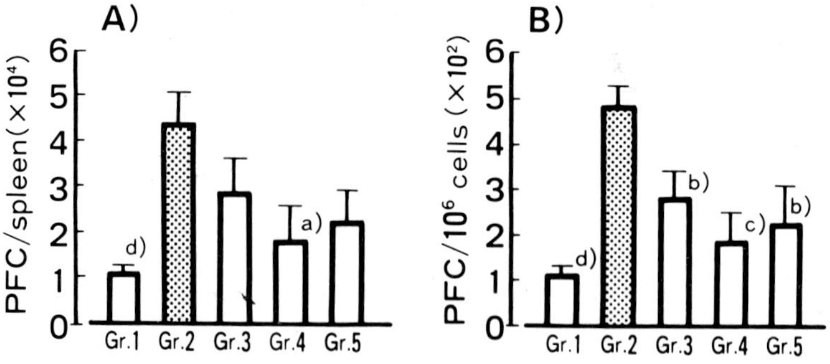

Fig. 3. Suppressive Effect of 1αOHD$_3$ on the Anti-DNP PFC Response Augmented by Colchicine

Gr. 1. MCT alone, Gr. 2. Colchicine and MCT(control), Gr. 3. Colchicine and 1αOHD$_3$ (0.05μg/kg), Gr. 4. Colchicine and 1αOHD$_3$(0.1μg/kg), Gr. 5. Colchicine and 1αOHD$_3$(0.2μg/kg).

DNP-KLH (100μg) and colchicine (1 mg/kg body weight) were intraperitoneally injected into Balb/c mice. MCT or 1αOHD$_3$ was orally administered immediately after, and again 24 hours after, immunization. Mice were sacrificed 6 days after immunization and their spleens were used for the anti-DNP direct PFC assay. Bars and vertical lines represent mean values±S.E. obtained from 5-6 mice. Closed bars indicate the control group. a)$p<0.05$, b)$p<0.02$, c)$p<0.01$. Significantly different from the MCT control group (Gr. 2).

These findings indicate that 1αOHD$_3$ has the ability to suppress the hyperimmune response induced by colchicine, which is known to increase the antibody formation at doses of 1-1.5 mg/kg in mice, when injected simultaneously with antigens. This enhancing effect is attributed to the inhibition of mitotic division which is necessary for the suppressor T cells to obtain their activity. Thus, 1αOHD$_3$ seemed to stimulate the proliferation and differentiation of the suppressor T cells when the induction of these cells was inhibited by colchicine.

It is noteworthy that 1αOHD$_3$ obviously increased the number of spleen cells reduced by restraint-stress (Fig. 2-A), and also slightly increased the number of spleen cells in experiments of anti-SRBC PFC response performed repeatedly (data not shown). Tsoukas et al. (11) and Lemire et al. (17) reported that 1α,25(OH)$_2$D$_3$ suppressed DNA synthesis and immunoglobulin produced by normal human peripheral blood lymphocytes activated in vitro by PHA or pokeweed mitogen. We suppose that these discrepancies might result from a difference in experimental conditions (in vitro vs in vivo), and a difference in the magnitude of stimulation.

In conclusion, $1\alpha OHD_3$ was shown to enhance immune response which has been lowered by reducing antigen dosage, or by restraint-stress. $1\alpha OHD_3$ also suppressed the hyperimmune response induced by colchicine. It should be noted that $1\alpha OHD_3$ never enhanced or suppressed immune responses beyond the normal level. Further studies are needed to clarify the mechanisms of the effect of $1\alpha OHD_3$ on these immune responses.

Effect of $1\alpha OHD_3$ Treatment on the Development of Autoimmune Diseases in NZB/NZW F_1 Hybrid Mice

It has been reported that some immunoregulatory drugs such as levamisole (18) and lobenzarit disodium (CCA) (19-21) prevent the spontaneous development of autoimmune diseases in NZB/NZW F_1 hybrid (B/W F_1) mice. These lines of evidence together with the findings showing immunoregulatory effect of $1\alpha OHD_3$ prompted us to examine whether $1\alpha OHD_3$ could prevent the development of autoimmunity in these mice. Female B/W F_1 mice were divided into 3 groups at 7 weeks of age. A group of 6 to 7 mice were given $1\alpha OHD_3$ every day except for Sunday at a daily dose of 0.05 or 0.2 μg/kg. Control mice were given vehicle only. Mice were sacrificed at 8 months of age and their spleens were used for the measurement of Con A-induced suppressor cells. Suppressor T cell activity was determined as described in our previous paper (21). As shown in Table 2, splenic suppressor T cell activity from vehicle-treated control mice is lower than that from young mice. Treatment with $1\alpha OHD_3$ in a dose of 0.2 μg/kg prevented the age-related loss of suppressor T cell activity. Lower dose of $1\alpha OHD_3$, however, was ineffective.

Naturally occurring thymocytotoxic autoantibody (NTA) in the serum was titrated at 8 months of age according to the method previously described (21). As shown in Fig. 4, larger dose of $1\alpha OHD_3$ insignificantly lowered the serum NTA titer, but lower dose did not. NTA is known to be cytotoxic against the murine thymocytes in vitro in the presence of complement, and recently it was found that NTA preferentially attacked the suppressor T cells (22), playing the crucial role in the regulation of the immune responses. Thus, it is very likely that the preservation of suppressor T cell activity by $1\alpha OHD_3$ is attributed to the inhibition of NTA production. Furthermore, autoantibody against ssDNA was also quantitated using enzyme linked immunosorbent assay. However, $1\alpha OHD_3$ failed to suppress the appearance of this antibody at that time. Moreover $1\alpha OHD_3$ had no beneficial effect on the development of proteinuria and life span (data not shown).

Table 2. Preservation of the Age-related Decline of Splenic Con A-induced Suppressor T Cell Activity by the Treatment with $1\alpha OHD_3$ in Female NZB/NZW F_1 Hybrid Mice

Group	Suppression (%)
MCT Control	39.7 ± 10.0
$1\alpha OHD_3$ 0.05 µg/kg	25.6 ± 6.6
$1\alpha OHD_3$ 0.02 µg/kg	72.3 ± 6.8[a)]
Young Control[b)]	80.1 ± 2.9[a)]

A group of 6-7 female NZB/NZW F_1 hybrid mice were given $1\alpha OHD_3$ every day except for Sunday from 7 weeks to 8 months of age. Mice were sacrificed 2 days after the last drug administration. Suppressor T cell activity was assayed by the suppression of splenic anti-SRBC PFC response (see ref. #16). The percent of suppression was determined by following formula:

$$100 - \frac{\text{PFC number of cultures with suppressor cells}}{\text{PFC number of cultures without suppressor cells}} \times 100$$

a) $P<0.05$ compared with MCT control by Student's t-test
b) 2 month-old NZB/NZW F_1 hybrid mice

These findings indicate that $1\alpha OHD_3$ was unable to suppress the development of autoimmunity, despite of its restoring effect on the depressed suppressor T cell activity. It might be possible that the ability of $1\alpha OHD_3$ to potentiate suppressor T cell was not high enough to improve autoimmunity. Alternative explanation is that $1\alpha OHD_3$ act on not only T cells, but also B cells. This undesirable action might cause the acceleration of autoantibody production.

Disappearance of Anti-DNA Autoantibody in the Old Patients with Osteoporosis following $1\alpha OHD_3$ Treatment

Some of the old patients with osteoporosis develop anti-DNA autoantibody in their serum. Anti-DNA-positive patients were treated with $1\alpha OHD_3$ (1 µg/day) for 1 to 3 months. As shown in Fig. 5, anti-DNA antibody titer decreased to the normal range within 1 month after the beginning of the treatment.

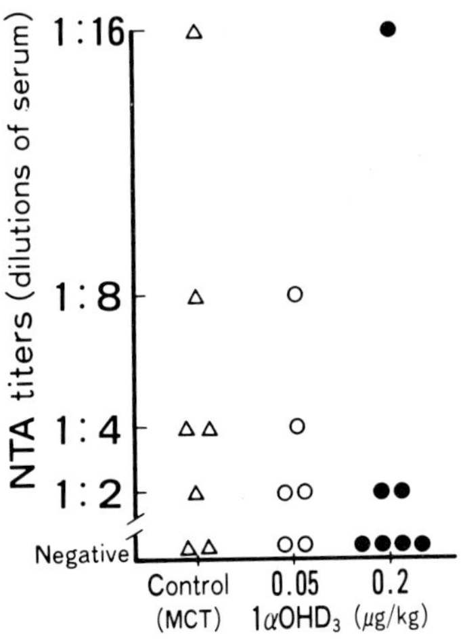

Fig. 4. Serum NTA Titers in 8-month-old 1αOHD$_3$-treated and Control NZB/NZW F$_1$ Hybrid Mice.

Female NZB/NZW F$_1$ hybrid mice were treated with 1αOHD$_3$ as described in Table 2.

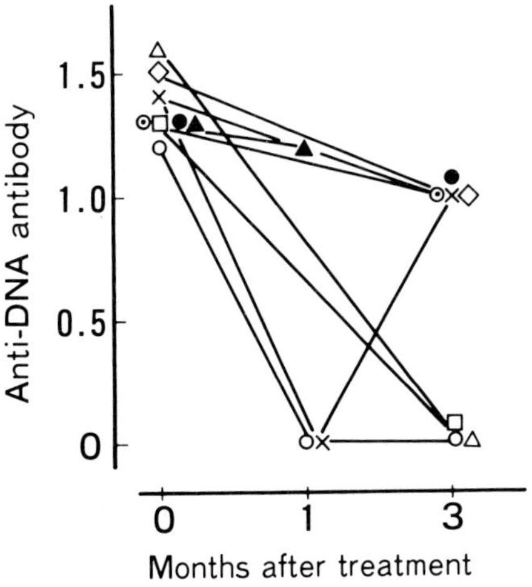

Fig. 5. Disappearance of Anti-DNA Antibody in the Old Patients with Osteoporosis following 1αOHD$_3$ Treatmant.

Patients were treated with an oral dose of 1αOHD$_3$(1μg/day). Anti-DNA antibody was tested by using assay test kit.

Further studies will be needed to clarify whether the inhibition of anti-DNA production by 1αOHD$_3$ is attributed to its activating effect on suppressor T cells.

Summary

It was found that 1αOHD$_3$ played some role in the regulation of the immune response in animals as well as humans.

References

(1) Nishii, Y., Ono, M., Fukushima, M., Shimizu, T., Niki, R., Ohkawa, H., Takagaki, Y., Okano, K. and Suda, T. (1980) Endocrinology 107, 319-327.

(2) Fukushima, M., Niki, R., Ohkawa, H., Shimizu, T., Matsunaga, I., Nakano, H., Takagaki, Y., Nishii, Y., Okano, K. and Suda, T. (1980) Endocrinology 107, 328-333.

(3) Cork, D. J., Haussler, M. R., Pitt, M. J., Rizzardo, E., Hesse, R. H., Pechet, M. M. (1974) Endocrinology 94, 1337-1345.
(4) Boris, A., Hurley, J. F., Trmal, T. (1977) In Vitamin D: Chemical and Clinical Aspects Related to Calcium Metabolism (Norman, A. W. et al), pp. 553. Walter de Gruyter, Berlin and New York
(5) Holick, M. F., Kasten-Schraufrogel, P., Tavela, T., DeLuca, H. F. (1975) Arch. Biochem. Biophys. 166, 63-66.
(6) Fukushima, M., Suzuki, Y., Tohira, Y., Matsunaga, I., Ochi, K., Nagano, H., Nishii, Y., Suda, T. (1975) Biochem. Biophys. Res. Commun. 66, 632-638.
(7) Holick, M. F., Tavela, T. E., Holick, S. A., Schnoes, H. K., DeLuca, H. F., Gallagher, B. M. (1976) J. Biol. Chem. 251, 1020-1024.
(8) Abe, E., Miyaura, C., Sakagami, H., Takeda, M., Konno, K., Yamazaki, T., Yoshiki, S., Suda, T. (1981) Proc. Natl. Acad. Sci. USA., 78, 4990-4994.
(9) Miyaura, C., Abe, E., Kuribayashi, T., Tanaka, H., Konno, K., Nishii, Y., Suda, T. (1981) Biochem. Biophys. Res. Commun. 102, 937-943.
(10) Provvedini, D. M., Tsoukas, C. D., Deftos, L. J., Manolagas, S. C. (1983) Science 221, 1181-1183.
(11) Tsoukas, C. D., Provvedini, D. M., Manolagas, S. C. (1984) Science 224, 1438-1440.
(12) Cunningham, A. J., Szenberg, A. (1968) Immunology 14, 599-600.
(13) Okimura, T., Yamamoto, I. (1977) Proc. Jap. Soc. Immunol., 12, 766-767.
(14) Shek, PN, Coons, A. H. (1977) J. Exp. Med. 147, 1213-1227.
(15) Shek, P. N., Waltenbaugh, C., Coons, A. H. (1977) J. Exp. Med. 147, 1228-1235.
(16) Gronowicz, E., Coutinho, A., Melchers, F. (1976) Eur. J. Immunol. 6, 588-590.
(17) Lemire, J. M., Adams, J. S., Sakai, R., Jordan, S. C. (1984) J. Clin. Invest. 74, 657-661.
(18) Vogler, C. (1977) Clin. Res. 25, 637.
(19) Ohsugi, Y., Nakano, T., Hata, S., Niki, R., Matsuno, T., Nishii, Y., Takagaki, Y. (1978) J. Pharm. Pharmac. 30, 126-128.
(20) Ohsugi, Y. (1985) Immunotherapy (In press)
(21) Nakano, T., Yamashita, Y., Ohsugi, Y., Sugawara, Y., Hata, S., Takagaki, Y. (1983) Immunopharmacology 5, 293-302.
(22) Shirai, T., Hayakawa, K., Okumura, K., Tada, T. (1978) J. Immunol. 120, 1924-1929.

VITAMIN D PHOTOBIOLOGY: RECENT ADVANCES IN THE BIOCHEMISTRY AND SOME CLINICAL APPLICATIONS.

M.F. Holick
Vitamin D Laboratory, Endocrine Unit, Massachusetts General Hospital and Harvard Medical School, Boston, MA and Department of Applied Biological Sciences, Massachusetts Institute of Technology, Cambridge, MA, 02139, USA

INTRODUCTION

In the 19th century Sniadecki (1) and Palm (2) independently concluded from their own clinical observations that the sunless environment that children were raised in the polluted cities in Poland and Great Britian was in some way responsible for the development of the bone deforming disease, rickets. It was not until 1919 when Huldschinsky (3) unequivically demonstrated that he could cure rickets in children by exposing them to radiation from a mercury-arc lamp that prompted a serious investigation to determine whether exposure to sunlight alone could cure this crippling disease. Finally, in 1921 Hess and Unger (4) reported that they cured rickets in 8 children by doing nothing more than exposing them to sunlight several times a week for a few months on the roof of their hospital. These pioneering studies unveiled a truely unique association between the absolute dependence of many mammals, including humans, on exposure to sunlight for the maintenance of calcium metabolism and bone mineralization.

PHOTOBIOLOGY OF VITAMIN D IN HUMAN SKIN

It is now established that when adult human skin is exposed to sunlight the radiation between 290 and 315 nm penetrates into the epidermis to photolyze provitamin D_3 (7-dehydrocholestrol) to previtamin D_3 (5, 6). Greater than 90% of the epidermal provitamin D content is in the actively growing layers (namely the stratum spinosum and stratum basale) and therefore most of the cutaneous previtamin D_3 that is made is in these layers. Because very little of this high energy ultraviolet radiation penetrates into the dermis, very little previtamin D_3 is

Vitamin D. A Chemical, Biochemical and Clinical Update

synthesized in this tissue and usually accounts for less than 10% of the total cutaneous content.

Previtamin D_3 is thermally labile and spontaneously isomerizes to vitamin D_3 at room temperature. In warm blooded mammals including humans, it takes about 24 hours for approximately 50% of the previtamin D_3 to isomerize to the thermally more stable vitamin D_3. After 3 days essentially all of the previtamin has equilibrated to vitamin D_3 (Fig. 1)). Once vitamin D_3 is formed, it is translocated into the circulation by the vitamin D-binding protein for transport to the liver for its first hydroxylation. Because the vitamin D-binding protein has little affinity for provitamin D_3, previtamin D_3, lumisterol, or tachysterol it is believed that these products remain in the epidermis and are degraded as the epidermal cells differentiate and die (7).

REGULATION OF CUTANEOUS PREVITAMIN D_3 PHOTOSYNTHESIS

Melanin is an effective ultraviolet radiation absorber and competes with provitamin D_3 for UV-B photons thus limiting previtamin D_3 formation. However, it is unlikely that melanin evolved for the sole purpose of preventing vitamin D intoxication in the populations that lived at or near the equator as has been suggested (8). Previtamin D_3 is a photolabile isomer that readily isomerizes to lumisterol and tachysterol. It has now been demonstrated that during the initial exposure to sunlight, provitamin D_3 is efficiently converted to previtamin D_3. However, Once about 10 to 15% of the provitamin D_3 is converted to previtamin D_3, a photoequilibrium begins to form whereby further irradiation leads to the formation of lumisterol and tachysterol (Fig. 1). Because of the spectral composition of sunlight the major photoisomer that is formed is the biologically inert lumisterol (6). Therefore, it is unlikely that an intoxicating amount of vitamin D_3 is ever generated in the skin as a result of a single excessive exposure to sunlight because the solar irradiation limits the amount of previtamin D_3 that is actually formed.

PHOTOSYNTHESIS OF 24-DEHYDROPREVITAMIN D_3 IN MAMMALIAN SKIN

It has been assumed that mammalian skin has the capacity to produce only one vitamin D, vitamin D_3. A reverse-phase HPLC analysis of a lipid extract from skins of 14-day-old rats has revealed that there is an

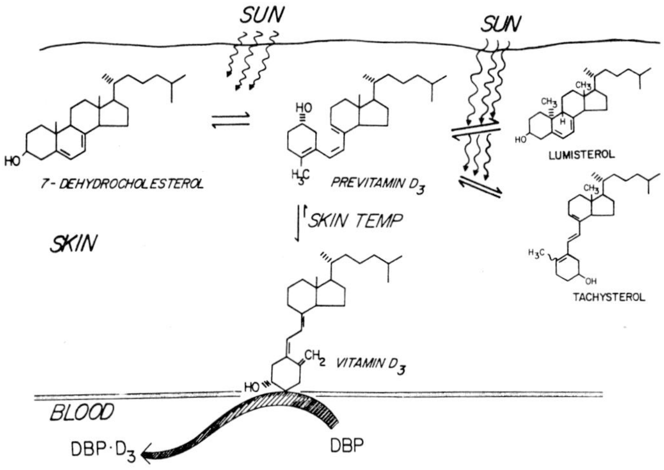

Fig. 1. Schema for the steps in the formation of previtamin D3, which then is subject to thermal isomerization to vitamin D3. Once formed, vitamin D3 is specifically translocated into the circulation by the vitamin D binding protein (DBP). During continual exposure to sunlight, previtamin D3 undergoes photoisomerization to form the biologically intert photoproducts, lumisterol and tachysterol. (with permission)

additional provitamin D that can be separated from provitamin D3. This provitamin D was isolated and purified for spectroscopic analysis. Its ultraviolet absorption spectrum demonstrated maxima at 295, 282, and 271 nm which are characteristic of a conjugated 5,7-diene. A mass spectrum revealed a molecular ion at m/z 382 indicating that it was two mass units less than provitamin D3. To be certain that this new sterol was a provitamin D, it was exposed to UV-radiation. The major photoproduct was found to have an ultraviolet absorption spectrum with a maximum at 260 nm and a minimum at 230 nm which are characteristic of the 6,7-cis-triene system for previtamin D. A mass spectral analysis of this photoproduct showed a molecular ion at m/z 382 (21.5%) and major fragments at m/z 349 (22.5%); 323 (9%); 271 (9%); 253 (12%); 176 (14%); 158 (42%); 136 (40%); 118 (46.5%); 81 (58.5%); 69 (100%). The peaks at m/z 271 and m/z 253 arise from the loss of the side chain and the loss of the side chain minus water, respectively, indicating that structure of the A,B,C, and D rings are the same as for provitamin D3 and that the unsaturation was in the the side chain. The base peak at m/z 69 that arose from the allylic cleavage of the 22-23 bond indicated that the unsaturation was between

C-24 and C-25. Confirmation of the Δ^{24} unsaturation was provided by the 270-MHz ^1H NMR spectrum. When compared with the spectrum of provitamin D_3 there was an additional signal in the olefin region that was a psuedo triplet at 5.09 ppm integrating for one proton. In addition, the C-26 and C-27 methyl groups were displayed at 1.68 and 1.60 ppm that are typical for allylic methyl protons. Thus, the compelling spectroscopic data unequivically identified this new cutaneous provitamin D as cholesta-5,7,24-trien-3β-ol (24-dehydroprovitamin D_3) (Fig. 2). To be certain that this new cutaneous provitamin D is photolyzed in the skin similar to provitamin D_3, skin from 14-day-old rats was exposed to simulated sunlight or kept in a UV-free environment. Lipid extracts of the skin were made and chromatographed on a straight-phase HPLC system (6). The previtamin D region was recovered and chromatographed on a C-18-reverse phase HPLC in methanol. Two major peaks were observed and only found in the extracts obtained from the irradiated skin. Both peaks had an ultraviolet maximum at 260 nm and a minimum at 230 nm characteristic of previtamin D. The earlier migrating peak (rt = 10.02

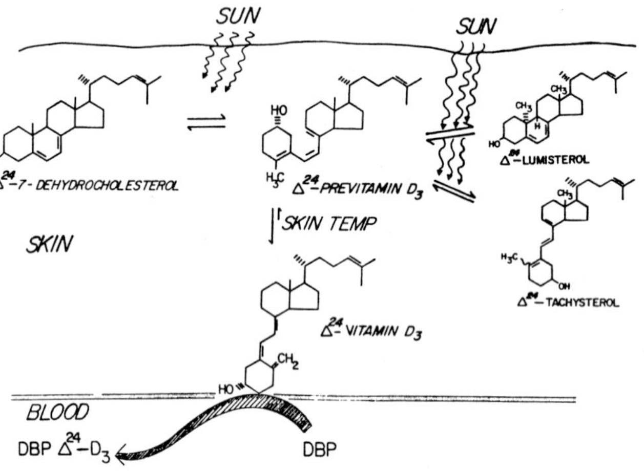

Fig. 2. Schema for the steps in the formation of Δ^{24}-previtamin D_3, which then is subject to thermal isomerization to Δ^{24}-vitamin D_3. Once formed, Δ^{24}-vitamin D_3 is specifically translocated into the circulation by the vitamin D binding protein (DBP). During continual exposure to sunlight, Δ^{24}previtamin D_3 undergoes photoisomerization to form the biologically intert photoproducts, Δ^{24}-lumisterol and Δ^{24}-tachysterol.

min) was identified as 24-dehydroprevitamin D_3 and the peak with a rt = 11.64 min was provitamin D_3.

The physiologic role of this new mammalian vitamin D remains to be determined. What is known is that in 14-day-old rats this new provitamin accounts for 20 to 25% of the total provitamin D content in the skin. Furthermore 24-dehydroprovitamin D_3 has been detected in human skin.

EFFECT OF AGING ON CUTANEOUS PROVITAMIN D STORES.

In Europe, where the fortification of foods with vitamin D is not practiced, vitamin D nutrition principally occurs as a result of exposure to sunlight. It is well recognized that in the United Kingdom between 20 and 40% of women and men with fractures of the proximal femur suffer from vitamin D deficiency and osteomalacia (9-13). Recently, it has been demonstrated that vitamin D deficiency and osteomalacia is also common amoung patients with hip fractures in the midwestern and northeastern United States (14,15).

To determine whether aging affected the capacity of the skin to produce vitamin D_3, we analyzed the epidermal and dermal concentrations of 7-dehydrocholesterol in surgically obtained skin samples from individuals between the ages of 8 and 92 years. As shown in Figure 3,

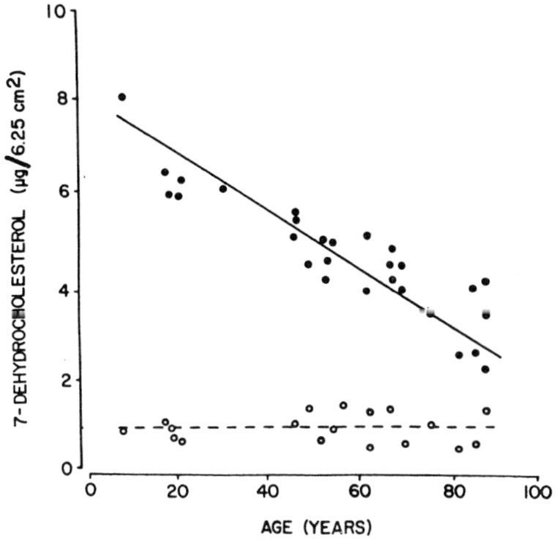

Fig. 3. Effect of aging on 7-dehydrocholesterol concentrations in human epidermis and dermis. Concentrations of 7-dehydrocholesterol (provitamin D_3) per unit area of human epidermis (-●-), and dermis (-o-) obtained from surgical specimens from donors of various ages.

there is an age- related decrease in the concentration of provitamin D3 in the epidermis. The dermal concentrations of the vitamin D_3 precusor appear to remain relatively constant throughout life. To determine what impact the age-related decrease in epidermal stores of provitamin D_3 might have, selected skin samples were exposed to simulated sunlight and the previtamin D_3 concentrations were determined in the epidermis and dermis. Greater than 85% of the cutaneous previtamin D_3 resided in the epidermis. A comparison of the amount of previtamin D_3 produced in the skin from the 77 and 82-year-old subjects was less than 50% of that produced in the skin from the 8 and 18-year-old subjects. These observations suggest that aging significantly decreases the capacity of human skin to produce vitamin D_3. Recognition of this may be very important for the elderly who infrequently go outdoors and depend on solar irradiation for their vitamin D nutrition.

EFFECT OF 1,25-$(OH)_2$-D_3 ON EPIDERMAL DIFFERENTIATION

It is now recognized that a variety of tissues and circulating cells that are not directly involved in regulating calcium homeostatis such as The ovary, stomach, pituitary, pancrease, lymphocytes, and monocytes have cytosolic and nuclear receptors for 1,25-$(OH)_2$-D_3 (16-22). In addition, it has been shown that the dermal fibroblasts and epidermal keratinocytes also have high-affinity, low-capacity receptors for the hormone (19-21). In culture, dermal fibroblasts that have receptors for 1,25-$(OH)_2$-D_3 respond to this hormone by increasing cell generation time in a dose-dependent manner (23). We have found this response to be exquisitively sensitive to the concentration of the hormone and has been valuable in evaluating the potential biologic activity of vitamin D metabolites and analogs.

To determine whether the effect of 1,25-$(OH)_2$-D_3 on the growth of fibroblasts was a physiologic rather than a non-specific response, fibroblasts from a patient with vitamin D-dependent rickets, type II, that lacked receptor activity for the hormone were evaluated. Whereas a 30 to 50% inhibition in fibroblast cell division was observed in normal cultures incubated with 10^{-8}M of 1,25-$(OH)_2$-D_3 there was no inhibition of

DDR-II fibroblast cell division time at concentrations up to 10^{-6}M of the hormone (23).

Cultured human and mouse keratinocytes also possess receptors for 1,25-$(OH)_2$-D_3 (23-25). In culture, 1,25-$(OH)_2$-D_3 causes a dose-dependent increase in the epidermal differentiation of human and mouse keratinocytes (23-25). The number of attached human basal cells decreased when exposed to 10^{-8}M of 1,25-$(OH)_2$-D_3 while the number of attached squamous cells, terminally differentiated cells floating in the medium and cornified envelopes increased concurrently and there was a shift to lighter cellular density. Transglutaminase, an enzyme responsible for the formation of the cornified envelope, has served as a good biological marker of epidermal differentiation. Analysis of homogenates of epidermal cells that had been exposed to 1,25-$(OH)_2$-D_3 has revealed that the activity of this calcium dependent enzyme is enhanced when compared to homogenates of cells not exposed to 1,25-$(OH)_2$-D_3 (20). Thus, it appears that 1,25-$(OH)_2$-D_3 has the potential of regulating epidermal differentiation.

PSORIASIS AND 1,25-$(OH)_2$-D_3

Psoriasis is a disfiguring disorder of the skin that affects at least 1% of the population. Because this disease is characterized by the hyperproliferation of the epidermis, most investigators have believed that the etiology of this disease is due to a defect in the differentiation of basal cells. Because 1,25-$(OH)_2$-D_3 is a potent differentiator of cultured mouse (19) and human keratinocytes (20) and that the response of 1,25-$(OH)_2$-D_3 receptor positive dermal fibroblasts to 1,25-$(OH)_2$-D_3 is a predictor of this response, we investigated the biologic responsiveness of cultured dermal fibroblasts from psoriatic patients to this hormone. To our surprise, we found that 1,25-$(OH)_2$-D_3 at 10^{-8}M and 10^{-6}M had no effect on the cell generation time of cultured dermal fibroblasts obtained from non-lesion areas of psoriatic patients whereas 10^{-5} and 10^{-4}M of 1,25-$(OH)_2$-D_3 did. Cultured dermal fibroblasts from normal volunteers showed the expected 30%, 59%, 72%, and 92% increase in cell generation time when incubated with 1,25-$(OH)_2$-D_3 at 10^{-8}, 10^{-6}, 10^{-5}, and 10^{-4}, respectively. Therefore, it appears that psoriatic fibroblasts have a partial but not absolute resistance to the action of $1,25-(OH)_2-D_3$. To determine whether this partial resistance was due to a decrease in the number of $1,25-(OH)_2-D_3$ receptors or a defect in the cytosolic or nuclear binding of this hormone, sucrose density gradient, DNA cellulose chromatography and Scatchard analysis were performed on normal and psoriatic fibroblasts. Psoriatic dermal fibroblasts were found to have cytoplasmic and nuclear receptors for $1,25-(OH)_2-D_3$ with physical chemical properties identicle to those of normal fibroblasts i.e. the same k_d, B_{max} and sedimentation coefficient (26).

Therefore, our data suggest that psoriatic dermal fibroblasts have a defect in the expression of $1,25-(OH)_2-D_3$ action on cell growth. These observations may provide the basis for a diagnostic test for this disorder as well as a treatment since pharmacologic concentrations (1000 to 10000-fold higher concentrations) of $1,25-(OH)_2-D_3$ are able to overcome this resistance. In addition, these data clearly demonstrate for the first time a biochemical disorder that is present in the dermis of unaffected areas of psoriatic patients. These observations suggest that psoriasis is not just a localized disease of the epidermis, but rather a disease that affects all of the epidermis and dermis.

CONCLUSION

For reasons not yet understood, exposure of skin to sunlight was essential for the development of the mineralized skeleton for terrestrial vertebrates. It has been established that mammalian skin is the site for the photosynthesis of one vitamin D, vitamin D_3. Recent observations from our laboratory suggest that the skin is capable of making at least two vitamin Ds, vitamin D_3 and 24-dehydrovitamin D_3. Furthermore, the skin is not only a synthetic organ for vitamin D but it is a target organ for its 1,25-dihydroxy metabolite. The new revelations that $1,25-(OH)_2-D_3$ can induce morphologic and biochemical differentiation of cultured human keratinocytes, coupled with the observation that psoriatic dermal fibroblasts have a partial resistance to the action of this hormone may herald an exciting new role for $1,25-(OH)_2-D_3$

endocrine system for the diagnosis and treatment of this hyperproliferative disorder.

REFERENCES

1. Sniadecki, J., 1840 (Cited by W. Mozolowski): Jedrzej Sniadecki (1768-1883). (1939) Nature 143, 21.
2. Palm, T.A. (1890) Practitioner 45, 270-279, 321-342.
3. Huldschinsky, K. (1919) Dtsch. Med. Wochenschr. 45, 712-713.
4. Hess, A.F. and Unger, L.J. (1921) J. Am. Med. Assoc. 77, 39.
5. Holick, M.F, MacLaughlin, J.A., Clark, M.B., Holick, S.A., Potts, J.T., Jr., Anderson, R.R., Blank, I.H. and Parrish, J.A. (1980) Science 210, 203-205.
6. MacLaughlin, J.A., Anderson, R.R., and Holick, M.F. (1982) Science 216, 1001-1003.
7. Holick, M.F., MacLaughlin, J.A., and Doppelt, S.H. (1981) Science 211, 590-593.
8. Loomis, F. (1967) Science 157, 501-506.
9. Nordin, B.E.C., Peacock, M., and Aaron, J. (1980) Clinics. Endocrinol. Metab. 9, 177.
10. Exton-Smith, A.N., Hodkinson, H.M., and Stanton, B.R. (1966) Lancet ii, 999-1001.
11. Chalmers, J., Conacher, D.H., Gardner, D.L., and Scott, P.J. (1967) J. Bone Jt. Surg. 49B, 403-423.
12. Jenkins, D.H.R., Robert, J.G., Webster, D., and Williams, E.O. (1973) J. Bone Jt. Surg. 55B, 575-580.
13. Aaron, J.E. Gallagher, J.C., and Anderson J. (1974) Lancet i, 7851.
14. Sokoloff, L. (1978) Am. J. Surg. Path. 2, 21-30.
15. Doppelt. S.H., Neer, R.M., Daly, M., Bourret, L., Schiller,A. and Holick, M.F. (1983) Orthop. Trans. 7;3, 512-513.
16. Stumpf, W.E., Sar, M., Reid, F.A., Tanaka, Y., and DeLuca, H.F. (1979) Science 206, 1188-1190.
17. Franceschi, R.T., Simpson, R.V., and DeLuca, H.F. (1979) Biochem. Biophy. 210, 1-13.

18. Abe, E., Miyaura, C., Sakagami, H., Takeda, M., Konno, K., Yamazaki, T., Yoshiki, S., and Suda, T. (1981) Proc. Natl. Acad. Sci. USA 78, 4990.
19. Simpson, R.U., and DeLuca, H.F. (1980) Proc. Natl. Acad. Sci. USA 77, 5822.
20. Colston, K., Horst, M. and Feldman, D. (1980) Endocrinology 107, 1916.
21. Clemens, T.L. Horiuchi, N., Nguyen, M. and Holick, M.F. (1981) FEBS Lett. 134, 203-206.
22. Provvendini, D.M., Tsoukas, C.D., Deftos, L.J., and Manologous, S.C. (1983) Science 221, 1183.
23. Clemens, T.L. Adams, J.S., Horiuchi, N., gilchrest, B.A., Cho, H., Tsuchiya, Y., Matsuo, N., Suda, T., and Holick, M.F. (1983) J. Clin. Endocrinol. Metab. 56, 824-830.
24. Hosomi, J., Hosoi, J., Etsuko, A., Suda, T., and Kuroki, T. (1983) Endocrinology 113, 1950.
25. Smith, E., and Holick, M.F. (1985) Proceedings of the Sixth Workshop on Vitamin D, Merano, Italy, March, 1985, Walter de Gruyter (in press).
26. MacLaughlin, J., and Holick, M.F. (1985) Proceedings of the Sixth Workshop on Vitamin D, Merano, Italy, March, 1985, Walter de Gruyter (in press).
27. This work was supported by NIH grants AM27334, AG04616, and AG04390.

INTERACTION OF 1,25(OH)$_2$D WITH THE CAMP CLASS OF BIOLOGICAL SIGNALS.

BD Catherwood and JE Rubin, Department of Medicine, University of California and VA Medical Center, San Diego, CA.

Many tissues have receptors for both steroid hormones and agents which activate adenylate cyclase (AC). For example, osteoblasts have intracellular receptors for 1,25(OH)$_2$D and membrane receptors for PTH and prostaglandin E (PGE); PTH and 1,25(OH)$_2$D also have some similar effects on osteoblast function (1). However, little is known about ways in which steroid hormones and AC agonists interact at specific target tissues.

We are studying the effect of 1,25(OH)$_2$D on the AC in various cell types. We have shown an attenuative effect of treatment with 1,25(OH)$_2$D on cAMP response to hormonal challenge in whole cells as well as a similar effect on AC activity in membrane preparations of these cells. In rat osteosarcoma cells we have demonstrated opposing regulatory effects of 1,25(OH)$_2$D and glucocorticosteroids. Detailed study of this interaction dissociated two 1,25(OH)$_2$D effects: direct attenuation of activation of the guanine nucleotide-binding regulatory protein via the PTH receptor and interference with the as yet undefined mechanism(s) of glucocorticosteroid augmentation of AC (2). In the U937 human monoblastic cell line the cAMP response of whole cells to isoproterenol and prostaglandin is also attenuated after culturing with 1,25(OH)$_2$D (3). In normal human lymphocytes, cAMP production in response to forskolin, an agent which presumably works near the catalytic subunit, and to prostaglandin is augmented during activation by lectins and significantly decreased by 1,25(OH)$_2$D. Finally, the adenylate cyclase of T84 human colon carcinoma cells, which is activated by vasoactive intestinal polypeptide (VIP), shows a similar attenuated response when exposed to 1,25(OH)$_2$D in culture (Table).

TABLE: 1,25(OH)$_2$D attenuation of T84 cell cAMP production (Exp 1-3; pmol cAMP/10^6cells/10min) and adenylate cyclase activity (Exp.4; pmol/mg/min).

EXP.	ACTIVATOR	CELL TREATMENT (48hr)	
		None	1,25(OH)$_2$D(10^{-8}M)
1	VIP (10^{-8}M)	186 ± 21	81 ± 10
2	VIP (10^{-8}M)	509 + 62	236 ± 22
3	VIP (10^{-8}M)	194 ± 14	70 ± 9
4	Gpp(NH)p (25uM)	8 ± 1.5	3 ± 0.2
	VIP (10^{-6}M) + Gpp(NH)p (25uM)	33 ± 3	20 ± 3
	VIP (10^{-6}M) + GTP (25uM)	19 ± 1	9 ± 1

In these various cells types the 1,25(OH)$_2$D attenuation occurs with EC_{50}'s of $7x10^{-11}$ to 10^{-9} M and specificity (24,25(OH)$_2$D and 25(OH)D are less than 1/100 as potent) appropriate for mediation by a receptor dependent system. This 1,25(OH)$_2$D action appears after a 12 hour delay in rat osteosarcoma cells, and has a similar delay in the other cell types. This evidence, in diverse endocrine responsive cells including a normal human type cell, may point to a general mechanism of 1,25(OH)$_2$D action on adenylate cyclase activity(2).

Vitamin D. A Chemical, Biochemical and Clinical Update

$1,25(OH)_2D$ may also modulate subsequent effects of adenylate cyclase agonists on cell function. This is suggested by our data in the U937 cell line that $1,25(OH)_2D$ and cAMP agonists act in synergy to cause cell differentiation. As a marker for differentiation we have measured C5a receptor induction; C5a is a complement derived chemotactic factor present in a subset of human monocytes and inducible in the remainder. The U937 cell carried in culture has less than 2000 C5a receptors per cell; when incubated with dibutyryl cAMP the C5a receptor is induced to more than 150,000 per cell. Neither $1,25(OH)_2D$ alone, nor cAMP agonists alone (prostaglandin, isoproterenol, forskolin) change the baseline C5a receptor number. However, we have shown that when physiologic concentrations of AC agonists are combined with phosphodiesterase inhibitor and $1,25(OH)_2D$ for 3 - 4 days in cell culture, receptors are induced to levels nearly as high as those achieved with pharmacologic doses of dBcAMP. The effects of $1,25(OH)_2D$ and the cAMP agonists are dose dependent. The induced receptors have high affinity for C5a (Kd ca. 1nM). $24,25(OH)_2D$ and 25(OH)D do not facilitate the cAMP agonist to induce receptors. Butyrate alone does not cause receptor induction, but, when combined with cAMP agonists, can substitute for $1,25(OH)_2D$. We would like to speculate that C5a receptor induction, and possible other differentiated cell functions, are dependent on cAMP signals, but these may require a facilatory effect in the cAMP pathway brought about by $1,25(OH)_2D$ action on the genome.

We have thus demonstrated two seemingly opposite interactions of $1,25(OH)_2D$ with cAMP agonists in the U937 cell. On the one hand $1,25(OH)_2D$ is required to facilitate cAMP action at the same time $1,25(OH)_2D$ diminishes the ability of the cell to generate cAMP in response to a hormone stimulus. The site of synergistic interaction must be located at or beyond the cAMP dependent protein kinase; we plan to investigate its location.

The action of $1,25(OH)_2D$ to attenuate cAMP hormone agonist effects may serve an integrative function in cells besides the osteoblast. For instance, the attenuative effect of $1,25(OH)_2D$ on the amount of cAMP produced endogenously would limit the cAMP signal to U937 differentiation. The same type of control is suggested by our studies in activated lymphocytes. PGE and $1,25(OH)_2D$ both inhibit IL-2 secretion in these cells (4,5). PGE presumably causes this effect through a cAMP dependent mechanism. $1,25(OH)_2D$ then, while itself limiting IL-2 production, could protect the cell against excessive IL-2 inhibition by limiting the cAMP generated by PGE.

The adenylate cyclase complex is ubiquitous as a second messenger system. Since $1,25(OH)_2D$ receptors are now known to be widespread, the ability to modulate cAMP signals could endow $1,25(OH)_2D$ with a role in diverse cellular function and a mechanism for integration with other classes of hormones.

1. Wong G, Luben RA, and Cohn DV (1977) Science 197:663-665.
2. Catherwood BD (1985) J.Biol.Chem. 260:736-743.
3. Rubin JE and Catherwood BD (1984) Biochem.Biophys.Res.Comm. 123:210.
4. Goodwin JS, Kaszubowski PA and Williams RC (1979) J.Exp.Med. 150:1260-1264.
5. Tsoukas C, Provvedini DM and Manolagas SC (1984). Science 224:1438-1440.

THE EFFECT OF CALMODULIN ANTAGONISTS AND CYTOCHALASIN ON PROLIFERATION AND 1,25-$(OH)_2D_3$-INDUCED DIFFERENTIATION OF HUMAN PROMYELOCYTE.

T. MATSUI, Y. NAKAO, T. NAKAGAWA, T. KOIZUMI, M. KISHIHARA and T. FUJITA.
Third Division, Department of Medicine, Kobe University School of Medicine, Kobe, Japan.

INTRODUCTION:

Calcium ion are speculated to regulate a broad spectrum of cellular functions, including cell mitosis, exocytosis, cell motility and metabolic activity. Regulation of biological processes by calcium ions involves an interaction with high affinity calcium-binding protein. Calmodulin, a ubiquitous Ca^{2+}-binding protein, is a component of a number of Ca^{2+} dependent enzyme systems and may mediate the effect of Ca^{2+} on a wide variety of cellular functions. In particular, calmodulin-Ca^{2+} may be an important intermediate in the Ca^{2+}-regulating microfilament-related motility in a variety of cells. Recently, 1,25-$(OH)_2D_3$ has been suggested to modulate calmodulin-system of duodenum in Ca^{2+} transport. Thus we examined the calmodulin and microfilaments systems in human leukemic cells, which are inducible to mature monocyte by 1,25-$(OH)_2D_3$, using calmodulin antagonists and microfilament-disrupting agent.

MATERIALS AND METHODS:

The human promyelocytic leukemia, HL-60, cells were cultured with or without various chemicals, such as 1,25-$(OH)_2D_3$, trifluoperazine dihydrochloride(TRIF), W5, W7, W12, W13, cytochalasin B and D. The ability to reduce NBT, the activity of phagocytosis and cell surface antigenic changes were determined as reported previously (1).

RESULTS:

Phagocytic capacity can be induced in HL-60 cells cultured with active vitamin D_3 analogues as reported previously (1). To eveluate the specific effect of W7 and W13 as calmodulin antagonists on HL-60, phagocytic activity of the cells preincubated with 1,25-$(OH)_2D_3$ for 48hr was assayed in the presence of W5, W7, W12 or W13. W7 and W13 inhibited phagocytosis in a dose dependent manner. On the other hand, W5 and W12, which interact more weakly with calmodulin and inhibit the activation of Ca^{2+}-calmodulin-dependent enzymes to a lesser extent than W7 and W13, respectively, did not inhibit phagocytosis even at 40μM.

W7 supressed the cell proliferation significantly, compared with control or W5. Treatment with W13 reduced cell growth in a dose-dependent manner, and there was a significant difference in antiproliferative effect between W12 and W13. TRIF was a potent inhibitor of HL-60 cell proliferation.

Incubation of HL-60 cells treated with 1,25-$(OH)_2D_3$ in the presence of W7 or W13 did not suppress the induction of matu-

Vitamin D. A Chemical, Biochemical and Clinical Update

re myeloid phenotypic changes. The increases in the percentage of NBT-positive and OKM1-binding cells after 10nM 1,25-$(OH)_2D_3$ treatment were not inhibited but enhanced slightly by W7 and W13. TRIF did not inhibit the OKM1 expression induced by 1,25-$(OH)_2D_3$ as did W7 and W13.

The induction of phagocytosis by 1,25-$(OH)_2D_3$ in the presence of W7 or W13 was inhibited to 40% until 48hr. However, this inhibitory effect disappeared when these antagonists were washed out just before the assay of phagocytosis. The induction of optimal differentiation required the continuous exposure to 1,25-$(OH)_2D_3$ until 96hr (1). These results indicate that calmodulin antagonists inhibit phagocytosis, but not the induction of phagocytic capacity by 1,25-$(OH)_2D_3$ in HL-60 cells.

Cytochalasin B and D, which disrupt microfilaments, reduced cell proliferation of HL-60, and induced polynucleation. In contrast, the increase in percentage of NBT-positive cells and the decrease in percentage of transferrin receptor-positive cells induced by 1,25-$(OH)_2D_3$ were enhanced by cytochalasins B and D. Monocyte-associated antigen was also induced by 1,25-$(OH)_2D_3$ in the presence of cytochalasins. 1,25-$(OH)_2D_3$ did not reduce the formation of polynuclear cells by cytochalasin.

These findings suggest that the calmodulin-and microfilament-dependent process may be involved in the proliferation of HL-60 cells, but not in the differentiation induced by 1,25-$(OH)_2D_3$ (2). Active vitamin D_3 analogues and calmodulin antagonists are reported to have anti-tumor activity in vivo. TRIF was found to enhance drug sensitivity of leukemic cells resistant to adriamycin treatment. Our results raise the possibility that differentiation-inducing drugs might be used in combination with anti-calmodulin drugs and other DNA sythesis-inhibitory drugs for the therapeutic use in vivo. Because calmodulin antagonists inhibit DNA synthesis as excess thymidine does (3).

References:

1. Matsui, T., Nakao, Y., Kobayashi, N., Kishihara, M., Ishizuka, S., Watanabe, S. and Fujita, T. (1984) Int. J. Cancer, 23:193-202.
2. Matsui, T., Nakao, Y., Kobayashi, N., Koizumi, T., Nakagawa, T., Kishihara, M. and Fujita, T. (1985) Cancer Res. 45:311-316.
3. Hidaka, H., Sasaki, Y., Tanaka, T., Endo, T., Ohno, S., Fujii, Y. and Nagata, T. (1981) Proc. Natl. Acad. U.S.A. 78: 4354-4357.

1,25-DIHYDROXYCHOLECALCIFEROL IN HORMONALLY-INDUCED DIFFERENTIATION OF MOUSE MAMMARY GLAND IN CULTURE

*G. Mezzetti, B. Barbiroli, T. Oka**
Istituto di Chimica Biologica, Università di Modena, Modena, Italy
*Laboratory of Biochemistry and Metabolism, NIADDK, National Institutes of Health, Bethesda, MD, 20205 USA

Introduction

Under appropriate hormone conditions, the mammary gland in culture can undergo structural and functional changes comparable to those which occur during several physiological states in the intact animal (1). When mammary explants from pregnant mice are cultured in the presence of lactogenic hormones (insulin, cortisol and prolactin) express their differentiation function by producing milk proteins such as casein (1). We report here that 1,25-dihydroxycholecalciferol (1,25$(OH)_2D_3$) augments milk protein synthesis induced by lactogenic hormones and that this effect is mediated by receptor mechanism.

Materials and Methods

Mouse mammary explants prepared from the abdominal glands of pregnant mice (Swiss Wos strain) were cultured for 4 days as previously described (2). Both insulin and prolactin were used at a concentration of 5 μg/ml of medium, and cortisol was used at 1 μg/ml. The amount of casein synthesized was detected by indirect immunoprecipitation (2). The 1,25$(OH)_2D_3$ receptor activity was examined by the sucrose density gradient technique after charging the cytosol with 0.8 nM 1,25$(OH)_2$[^{3}H]D_3 (160 Ci/mmol) in the presence or absence of 500 fold excess of radioinert steroid (3, 4).

Results and Discussion

Mammary explants were first cultured in the presence of insulin and cortisol for 3 days to deplete endogenous 1,25$(OH)_2D_3$. As shown in Table 1 these explants synthesized increasing amounts of casein in the presence of prolactin (ICP), whereas casein production occurred at very low level in the absence of this lactogenic hormone (IC). As it appears the addition of 10^{-9} M 1,25$(OH)_2D_3$ to these cultures selectively and dramatically augmented casein production in ICP system while it had no effect in IC system. This stimulatory effect was dose-dependent, and quite specific, since a variety of structurally related vitamin D analogs were completely uneffective (4).

Table 1. Effect of 1,25$(OH)_2D_3$ on casein synthesis in cultured mammary explants. 1,25$(OH)_2D_3$ (10^{-9}M) or vehicle were added to the culture for 24 h.

Incubation conditions	Casein production cpm x 10^{-3}/mg tissue
IC (3 days) + vehicle (1 day)	0.91 ± 0.02
ICP (3 days) + vehicle (1 day)	2.70 ± 0.21
IC (3 days) + 1,25$(OH)_2D_3$ (1 day)	0.92 ± 0.02
ICP (3 days) + 1,25$(OH)_2D_3$ (1 day)	4.10 ± 0.32

Vitamin D. A Chemical, Biochemical and Clinical Update

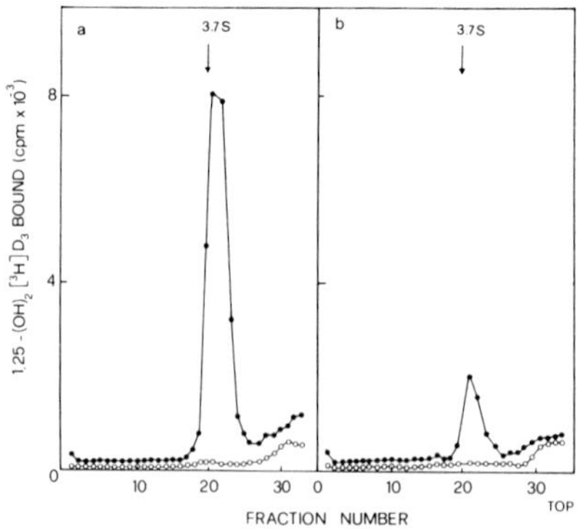

Figure 1. Sucrose density gradient analysis of $1,25(OH)_2D_3$ receptor in cultured mammary explants. Cytosol protein (280 μg) was incubated with 0.8 nM $1,25(OH)_2[^3H]D_3$ alone (●) or plus 400 nM radioinert $1,25(OH)_2D_3$ (o). Culture conditions were the same as for Table 1; (a) insulin, cortisol and prolactin; (b) insulin and cortisol.

Sucrose density gradient analysis, as well as studies on vitamin D_3 displacement and saturation of the binding sites have indicated that mammary tissue contains specific $1,25(OH)_2D_3$ receptors (4, 5). In fig. 1 is depicted the gradient centrifugation pattern of cytosol receptor from mammary explants cultured in the presence of insulin, cortisol and prolactin (a), or in the presence of insulin and cortisol (b). In this experiment the same amount of cytosol protein was added to each gradient so that changes in the peak area were likely to be indicative of change in receptor activity. As it is apparent $1,25(OH)_2D_3$ receptor activity was dramatically increased when all three lactogenic hormones were present in the culture medium. This fact is in good agreement with the responsiveness of the mammary gland to $1,25(OH)_2D_3$ that was maximal under the same culture condition.

It is known that prolactin regulates $1,25(OH)_2D_3$ synthesis in the kidney, and that the plasma concentration of the hormone is increased during lactation. Our results suggest that prolactin may also control mammary gland response to circulating $1,25(OH)_2D_3$ through a modulation of its receptor activity.

References

1. Topper, Y.J. and Freeman, C.S. (1980) Physiol. Rev. *60*, 1049-1106.
2. Ono, M. and Oka, T. (1980) Cell *19*, 473-480.
3. Mezzetti, G., Bagnara, G., Monti, M.G., Bonsi, L., Brunelli, M.A. and Barbiroli, B. (1984) Life Sciences *34*, 2185-2191.
4. Mezzetti, G., Barbiroli, B. and Oka T. (1985) J. Biol. Chem., submitted.
5. Colston, K., Hirst, M. and Feldman, D. (1980) Endocrinology *107*, 1916-1922.

MONONUCLEAR PHAGOCYTES RESORB BONE CHIPS IN RESPONSE TO LYMPHOKINES AND 1,25-DIHYDROXYVITAMIN D_3.

M.S. Cohen, R.L. Kaplan, C.N. D'Amico, R.C. Dodd, R.G. Snipes, D.E. Mesler, and T.K. Gray. Department of Medicine, UNC, Chapel Hill, NC 27514. USA

INTRODUCTION:

Bone resorption is a complex process which is mediated by osteoclasts and/or macrophages (1-3). Both cells have the ability to resorb bone in vitro, and respond to calcitropic hormones. Human monocytes and monocytic cell lines can be cultured so as to enhance their microbicidal and tumorcidal activity, and to resemble osteoclasts (4). The present studies were performed to identify incubation conditions which enhance bone resorption in vitro, and to study resorptive mechanism(s).

METHODS:

U937 cells, a human monoblastic line, were cultured as previously described (5). Human monocytes were separated from whole blood by dextran sedimentation and ficoll-hypaque separation. ^{45}Ca release from bone chips ranging in size from 25-45m was measured by the method of Teitelbaum et al (3). 1,25-dihydroxyvitamin D_3 (1,25-D_3) was provided by M. Uskokovic, Hoffmann-La Roche. Recombinant interferon gamma (IFN-γ) and lymphokines were purchased from Meloy Laboratories, Springfield, Va.

RESULTS AND COMMENTS:

Monocytes and U937 cells released 31% of the total ^{45}Ca during a 3 day incubation. This value was significantly greater than cell free control (p 0.01). Monocytes were activated by IFN-γ or 1,25-D_3, both of which lead to formation of polykaryons and increased competence for H_2O_2 secretion (4). As shown in Figure I, activation of cells with 1,25-D_3 did not enhance bone resorption, and pretreatment of monocytes with IFN-γ significantly inhibited their resorptive capacity.

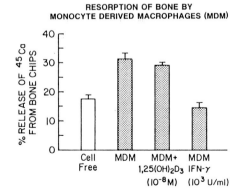

Fig. 1

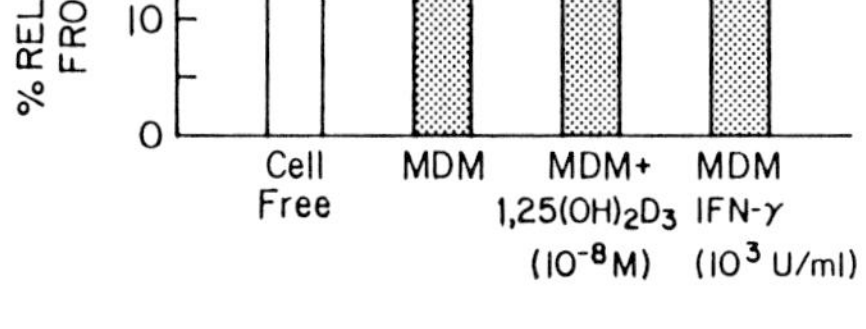

Vitamin D. A Chemical, Biochemical and Clinical Update

U937 cells could be activated with a combination of 1,25-D_3 and lymphokines. This combination increased competence of cells for formation of O_2 reduction products (Figure 2), as well as bone resorption (Table 1).

Fig. 2. Luminol-dependent luminescence in U937 cells stimulated with phorbol myristate acetate (100ng/ml)

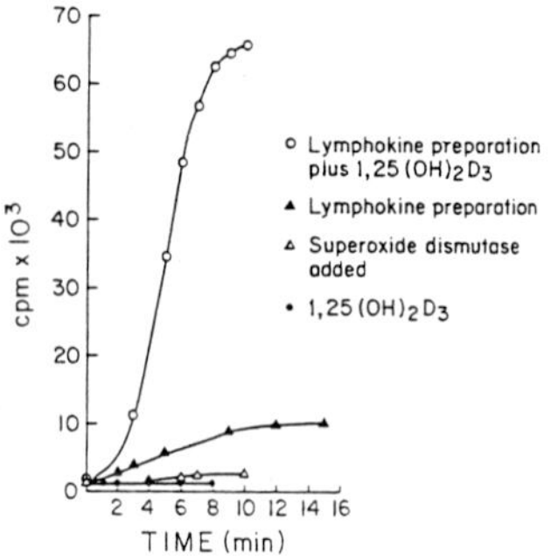

TABLE I
EFFECT OF U937 ACTIVATION ON % OF TOTAL ^{45}Ca RELEASED

Expts.	Media	Untreated Cells	Lymphokine	1,25-D_3 and Lymphokine
1	13.2±1	15.8±0.9*	17.5±1.3	23.7±2.2**
2	11.8±0.7	20.3±2.3*	25.2±2.5*	28.3±2.2**
3	15.2±0.9	21.0±1.5*	21.5±2.0*	39.2±1.4**

* $p<0.05$ from cell free control, ** $p<0.05$ from other conditions examined

Neutrophils did not resorb bone even when stimulated maximally with phorbol myristate acetate, or during ingestion of opsonized zymosan. Fibroblast cell lines grown to confluency also increased ^{45}Ca release relative to control. These findings show that phagocytosis of bone chips is neither necessary or sufficient for bone resorption *in vitro*. However, U937 cells secreted a soluble substance which released ^{45}Ca independent of changes in the medium pH, consistent with an earlier report in which human monocytes were employed (2). These results show that resorptive capacity of some monocytic phagocytes can be enhanced by activation with 1,25-D_3 and lymphokines. However, activation for bone resorption cannot be correlated with competence for formation of O_2 reduction products. Bone resorption *in vitro* results from the actions of stable, O_2-independent substances(s).

REFERENCES

1. Ibottson, K.J., Roodman, G.D., McManus, L.M. and Mundy, G.R. (1984) J. Cell. Biol. 99, 471-480.
2. Mundy, G.R., Altman, A.J., Gondek, M.D., and Bandelin, J.G. (1977) Science 196,1109-1111.
3. Teitelbaum, S.L., Stewart, C.C., and Kahn, A.J. (1979) Calif. Tiss. Intl. 27,255-261.
4. Weinberg, B.I., Hobbs, M.M., and Misukonis, M.A. (1984) Proc. Natl. Acad. Sci. 81, 4554-4557.
5. Dodd, R.C., Cohen, M.S., Newman, S.L., and Gray, T.K. (1983) Proc. Natl. Acad. Sci. (USA) 80, 7538-7541.

1,25-DIHYDROXYCHOLECALCIFEROL ENHANCES THE INTERFERON-γ-INDUCED EXPRESSION OF CLASS II MAJOR HISTOCOMPATIBILITY ANTIGENS IN MYELOMONOCYTIC CELLS (WEHI-3)

P. MOREL*, D. PROVVEDDINI+, D. WEGMANN°, J. CHILLER°, AND S. MANOLAGAS+
*Dept. Immunology, Scripps Clinic a Res. Fnd., +Endocrine Sect., U. of Calif., San Diego, V.A. Med. Ctr., and °Lilly Res. Labs, La Jolla, CA.

INTRODUCTION

The effects of $1,25(OH)_2D_3$ on immune phenomena mediated by activated lymphocytes have been recently appreciated (1,2). In addition, there is evidence that $1,25(OH)_2D_3$ exerts prodifferentiation effects on monocytes (3,4). Monocytes/macrophages are involved in the process of T-lymphocyte activation because they present antigen to these cells. In order to be able to present antigens to T cells (5), macrophages require Ia antigen on their surface and it is well known that interferon-gamma (IFN-γ) (a product of activated T cells) induces the expression of Ia antigens on macrophages (6). In the present studies we have used the murine monocytic line WEHI-3 which is known to be induced by IFN-γ to express Ia (7) and observed the modulation of this function by $1,25(OH)_2D_3$.

MATERIALS AND METHODS

The identification and characterization of $1,25(OH)_2D_3$ receptors in WEHI-3 cells was done by means of sucrose gradients, Scatchard analysis and DNA-cellulose chromatography. Ia expression was studied by indirect immunofluorescence and flow cytometry. The ability of the induced cells to present antigen was examined by an assay of the IL-2 production by a T cell hybrid (CAK1-22); this hybrid produces IL-2 only in the presence of a specific antigen (KLH) and the appropriate Ia molecule (Ia^d). The effect of IFN-γ, $1,25(OH)_2D_3$ and $24,25(OH)_2D_3$ on the proliferation of WEHI-3 cells was assessed by thymidine uptake measurements after 24 and 48 hours of culture.

RESULTS AND DISCUSSION

Sucrose gradient analysis demonstrated that WEHI-3 cells contain a $1,25(OH)_2D_3$ binding protein that sediments at 3.3S. Scatchard plots showed that this binding protein has a high affinity for $1,25(OH)_2D_3$ ($Kd=3.3 \times 10^{-10}M$). DNA-cellulose chromatography showed that the receptor ligand complexes bind to DNA-cellulose and can be eluted from the column with a KCl gradient. These characteristics are similar to those of classical $1,25(OH)_2D_3$ receptors. IFN-γ (25 U/ml) had no effect on the thymidine uptake of WEHI-3 cells whereas $1,25(OH)_2D_3$ ($10^{-8}M$) reduced it by 30%. Moreover, when IFN-γ and $1,25(OH)_2D_3$ were combined there was a 70% reduction in thymidine uptake. Cell cycle analysis indicated the cells were arrested in G1 of the cell cycle following treatment with both IFN-γ and $1,25(OH)_2D_3$. $24,25(OH)_2D_3$ ($10^{-8}M$) did not affect the proliferation of WEHI-3 cells either alone or in conjunction with IFN-γ. After 48 hours incubation with 50 U/ml IFN-γ, 50% of WEHI-3 cells were expressing IA^d antigens compared to less than 5% with 10 U/ml IFN-γ (Table 1a). $1,25(OH)_2D_3$ ($10^{-8}M$; $10^{-10}M$) had no effect on IA^d induction alone. However, when

Vitamin D. A Chemical, Biochemical and Clinical Update

$1,25(OH)_2D_3$ and IFN-γ were both present there was a marked enhancement of IA^d expression. $24,25(OH)_2D_3$ had no effect in these experiments.

Table 1a

	% Cells Positive for IA^d			
IFN-γ (U/ml)	Medium	1,25 (10^{-8}M)	1,25 (10^{-10}M)	24,25 (10^{-8}M)
0	1	1	1	1
10	4	60	11	4
50	51	93	79	40

Table 1b

	IL-2 Units/ml Produced by CAK1-22	
% Con A SN	Medium	$1,25(OH)_2D_3$ (10^{-8}M)
0	-	-
0.1	-	80
0.3	20	160
1	80	160
3	80	160

The IA^d detected by immunofluorescence was also able to function in antigen presentation (Table 1b) and the same enhancement of the IFN-γ effect was seen especially at limiting concentrations of IFN-γ. These data suggest that the $1,25(OH)_2D_3$ modulation of IFN-γ induction of Ia antigens might promote monocytes to function more efficiently as antigen presenting cells. However, in view of the immunosuppressive actions of the hormone in the T cell system, further studies will be essential in order to determine the overall impact of the hormone on the immune response. From our studies WEHI-3 cells seem to be good models and $1,25(OH)_2D_3$ an interesting tool for the study of Ia induction.

REFERENCES

1. Provveddini, D.M., Tsoukas, C.D., Deftos, L.J., and Manolagas, S.C. (1983) Science. 221:1181-1183.
2. Tsoukas, C.D., Provveddini, D.M., and Manolagas, S.C. (1984) Science. 224:1438-1440.
3. Abe, E., Miyaura, C., Sakagani, M., Takedu, H., Konno, K., Yamazaki, T., Yoshiki, S., and Suda, T. (1981) Proc. Natl. Acad. Sci. U.S.A. 78:4990-4995.
4. Amento, E.P., Bhalla, A.K., Kurnick, J.J., Kradin, R.L., Clemens, T.L., Holick, S.A., Holick, M.F., and Krane, S.M. (1984) J. Clin. Invest. 73:731-739.
5. Shevach, E., and Rosenthal, A. (1973) J. Exp. Med. 138:1213-1229.
6. Pace, J.L., Russell, S.W., Schreiber, R.D., Altman, A., and Katz, D.H. (1983) Proc. Natl. Acad. Sci. U.S.A. 80:3782-3786.
7. Walker, E.B., Lanier, L.L., and Warner, N.L. (1982) J. Exp. Med. 155:629-634.

INDUCTION OF SPERMIDINE N^1-ACETYLTRANSFERASE BY $1\alpha,25(OH)_2D_3$ AS AN EARLY COMMON EVENT IN THE TARGET TISSUES OF VITAMIN D

T. Shinki and T. Suda
Department of Biochemistry, School of Dentistry, Showa University, Tokyo 142, JAPAN

It is well known that synthesis of polyamines (putrescine, spermidine, and spermine) is closely related to the rate of cell growth and differentiation. We reported that the duodenal ornithine decarboxylase (ODC) activity and tissue content of putrescine increase markedly after a single i.v. injection of $1\alpha,25(OH)_2D_3$ into D-deficient chicks (1). The ODC activity began to increase 2 h after $1\alpha,25(OH)_2D_3$ injection and it attained a maximum in 6 h. The enhancement of the ODC activity occurred in parallel with that of the intestinal calcium absorption, suggesting that polyamine(s) is somehow involved in the intestinal calcium transport mechanism. We report here that the duodenal putrescine synthesis induced by $1\alpha,25(OH)_2D_3$ occurs by pathways from both ornithine and spermidine.

Duodenal tissues were rapidly excised from D-deficient chicks and washed thoroughly. The ODC and S-adenosylmethionine decarboxylase (SAMDC) activities were determined by measuring the release of $^{14}CO_2$ from [1-^{14}C]ornithine and S-adenosyl-[carboxyl-^{14}C]methionine, respectively (1, 2). Polyamine analysis was measured by the modification of the method of Tabor et al. Spermidine N^1-acetyltransferase (SAT) activity was measured by the method of Libby. Intestinal calcium transport activity was measured by the method of Omdahl et al.

Effect of α-difluoromethyl ornithine (α-DFMO), a specific irreversible inhibitor of ODC, on $1\alpha,25(OH)_2D_3$-induced duodenal activities of ODC, SAMDC, and calcium transport and duodenal contents of polyamines are presented in Fig. 1. The duodenal ODC activity was markedly increased by a single i.v. injection of $1\alpha,25(OH)_2D_3$. Administration of α-DFMO did not suppress the increase of the duodenal putrescine levels induces by the vitamin, though it inhibited ODC activity completely. Administration of $1\alpha,25(OH)_2D_3$ caused a slight decrease in the duodenal spermidine content. Concurrent treatment with $1\alpha,25(OH)_2D_3$ and α-DFMO further decreased spermidine content. The duodenal calcium transport activity increased in parallel with the increase of ODC activity but it was not affected by the treatment with α-DFMO. These results suggest that the duodenal putrescine is generated not only from ornithine but also from other sources.

Then, we examined the effect of $1\alpha,25(OH)_2D_3$ on SAT activity, a rate-limiting enzyme catalysing the conversion from spermidine to putrescine. The duodenal SAT activity began to

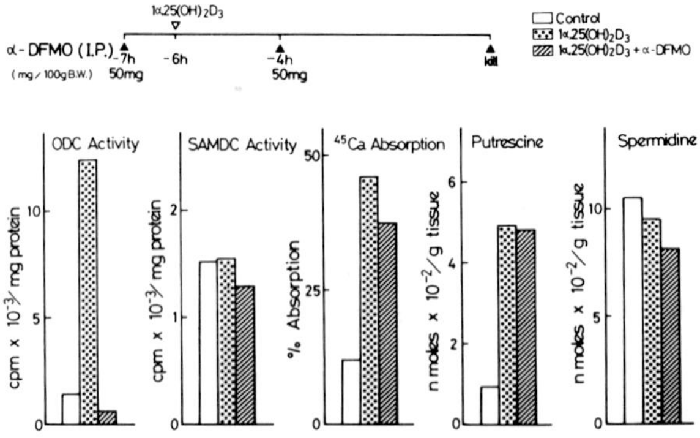

Fig. 1 Effect of α-DFMO on duodenal ODC, SAMDC, and calcium absorption activities and polyamine contents induced by 1α,25$(OH)_2D_3$. 1α,25$(OH)_2D_3$ was injected i.v. into D-deficient chicks. α-DFMO, 50 mg/100 b.w. i.p. 1 h before and 2 h after 1α,25$(OH)_2D_3$ (625 ng) injection. Animals were killed 6 h after 1α,25$(OH)_2D_3$ injection. Values represent means of two experiments.

increase 30 min after a single i.v. injection of 1α,25$(OH)_2D_3$ and it attained a maximum in 2 h. 1α,25$(OH)_2D_3$ induced ODC activity only in intestine (1), whereas it stimulated SAT activity in a number of tissues of the target organs of vitamin D including intestine, kidney, pancreas, and bursa of fabricius (3).

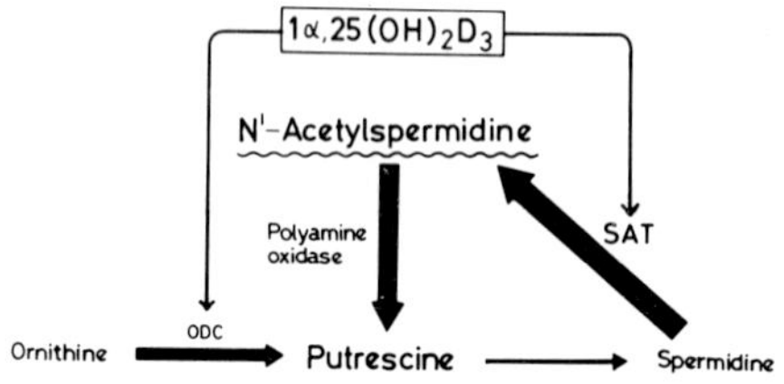

Fig. 2 Putrescine synthesis and sites where 1α,25$(OH)_2D_3$ stimulates it.

In summary, 1α,25$(OH)_2D_3$-induced synthesis of putrescine occures by pathways from both ornithine and spermidine (Fig. 2). Role of putrescine on the 1α,25$(OH)_2D_3$ action in intestine is under investigation in our laboratory.

REFERENCES

1. Shinki, T., Takahashi, N., Miyaura, C., Samejima, K., Nishii, Y. and Suda, T. (1981) Biochem. J. 195, 685-690.
2. Takahashi, N., Shinki, T., Kawate, N., Samejima, K., Nishii, Y. and Suda, T. (1982) Endocrinology 111, 1539-1545.
3. Shinki, T., Takahashi, N., Kadofuku, T., Sato, T. and Suda, T. (1985) J. Biol. Chem. 260, 2185-2190.

CHANGES IN LIPID METABOLISM IN CONNECTION WITH THE INDUCTION OF FUSION AND CYTOTOXICITY OF MOUSE ALVEOLAR MACROPHAGES BY 1α,25-DIHYDROXYVITAMIN D_3 [1α,25$(OH)_2D_3$]

C. Miyaura, E. Abe and T. Suda
Department of Biochemistry, School of Dentistry, Showa University, 1-5-8 Hatanodai, Shinagawa-ku, Tokyo 142, JAPAN

In 1981, we reported that 1α,25$(OH)_2D_3$ induces differentiation of mouse myeloid leukemia cells (M1) into monocyte-macrophages (1). Since then, we have extended this original observation to other types of hematopoietic cells. 1α,25-$(OH)_2D_3$ induces fusion of mouse alveolar macrophages forming multinucleated giant cells (2). In addition, the vitamin activates alveolar macrophages: it increases glucose consumption, the number of Fc receptors and cytotoxicity (3). However, the mechanism of the action of 1α,25$(OH)_2D_3$ in inducing fusion and activation of alveolar macrophages is not known. In this report, we show that lipid metabolism is involved in the 1α,25$(OH)_2D_3$-induced fusion and/or activation of alveolar macrophages.

MATERIALS AND METHODS: Alveolar macrophages were collected from ddy strain mice by the tracheobronchial lavage method and cultured for 1-3 days in modified MEM containing 5% human serum. Fusion rate and cytotoxicity of macrophages were determined as previously reported (2, 3). To analyze lipid metabolism, alveolar macrophages (5.6 x 10^5 cells) were cultured for 1-3 days with [^{14}C]-oleic acid (3 μCi/ml), [^{14}C]-acetic acid (40 μCi/ml) or [^{32}P]-phosphate (20 μCi/ml) in the growth medium with or without 5 ng/ml of 1α,25$(OH)_2D_3$. Lipids extracted with chloroform/methanol (2:1) were separated and analyzed by thin layer chromatography (TLC) and autoradiography. For the assay of diglyceride acyltransferase, macrophages (1.2 x 10^7 cells) cultured with or without 1α,25$(OH)_2D_3$ were homogenized in Tris-buffer. The homogenate was centrifuged at 20,000 xg for 20 min and the resulting cytosol fraction was used as a crude enzyme preparation. The reaction mixture contained 5 μM [1-^{14}C]-oleoyl-Co A, 0.2 mM 1,2-diolein and 50-80 μg of the crude enzyme preparation. After incubation for 30 min at 37°C, lipids were extracted and isolated by TLC. Radioactive spots of triglycerides on the TLC gel were scraped and counted.

RESULTS AND DISCUSSION: 1α,25$(OH)_2D_3$ directly induced fusion and cytotoxicity of alveolar macrophages, as previously reported (2, 3). Addition of 5 ng/ml of 1α,25$(OH)_2D_3$ caused about 60% of the cells to fuse and about 30% to exhibit cytotoxicity against B16 melanoma cells on day 3. Retinoic acid (300 ng/ml) and LPS (5 μg/ml) also induced cytotoxicity, but both compounds did not induce fusion at all. Retinoic acid, however, significantly enhanced the 1α,25$(OH)_2D_3$-induced

Vitamin D. A Chemical, Biochemical and Clinical Update

fusion of macrophages, whereas LPS inhibited it completely.

1α,25(OH)$_2$D$_3$ enhanced incorporation of [^{32}P]-phosphate into phospholipids of alveolar macrophages in a time-dependent manner. In the control macrophages, incorporation of ^{32}P into phosphatidylcholine (PC) was the highest (about 50% of the total phospholipids), followed successively by phosphatidylethanolamine (PE), phosphatidylserine (PS) and phoaphatidylinositol (PI). The order of the ^{32}P incorporation was not changed by incubation with 1α,25(OH)$_2$D$_3$.

1α,25(OH)$_2$D$_3$ markedly enhanced incorporation of [^{14}C]-oleic acid and [^{14}C]-acetic acid into triglycerides (TG) but not into diglycerides (DG). A significant increase in the [^{14}C]-oleic acid uptake into TG was recognized as early as 12 h, whereas induction of fusion and cytotoxicity was first observed 48 h after incubation with 1α,25(OH)$_2$D$_3$. Retinoic acid and LPS also stimulated TG synthesis. Simultaneous treatment with 1α,25(OH)$_2$D$_3$ and either retinoic acid or LPS exhibited cooperative effects in inducing TG synthesis. These results suggest that the 1α,25(OH)$_2$D$_3$-induced TG synthesis is associated with the induction of cytotoxicity rather than fusion. The activity of DG-acyltransferase was much higher in the macrophages cultured with 5 ng/ml of 1α,25(OH)$_2$D$_3$ than in the control macrophages. The maximal enhancement of DG-acyltransferase activity apparently preceded the induction of cytotoxicity, suggesting that the 1α,25(OH)$_2$D$_3$-induced TG synthesis is mediated by activating DG-acyltransferase (Fig. 1). These results clearly indicate that the enhancement of neutral lipid metabolism is involved in the induction of activation of mouse alveolar macrophages. The possibility whether the changes of phospholipid metabolism is involved in the induction of fusion and/or cytotoxicity is being explored in our laboratory.

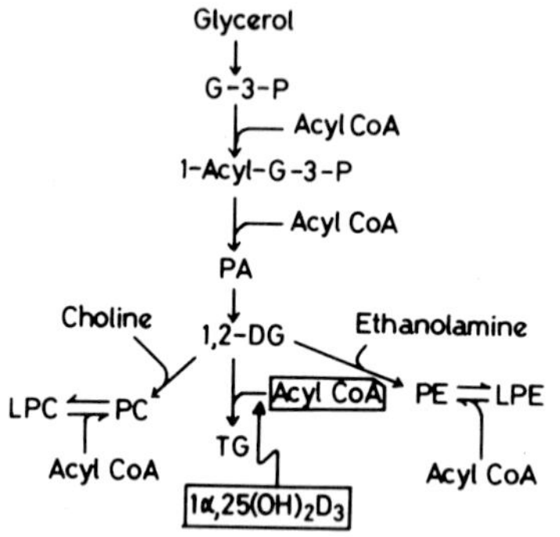

Fig. 1 The metabolic pathway of TG synthesis and a site where 1α,25(OH)$_2$D$_3$ stimulates TG synthesis.

REFERENCES

1. Abe, E., Miyaura, C., Sakagami, H., Takeda, M., Konno, K., Yamazaki, T., Yoshiki, S. and Suda, T. (1981) Proc. Natl. Acad. Sci. USA 78, 4990-4994.

2. Abe, E., Miyaura, C., Tanaka, H., Shiina, Y., Kuribayashi, T., Suda, S., Nishii, Y., DeLuca, H. F. and Suda, T. (1983) Proc. Natl. Acad. Sci. USA 80, 5583-5587.

3. Abe, E., Shiina, Y., Miyaura, C., Tanaka, H., Hayashi, T., Kanegasaki, S., Saito, M., Nishii, Y., DeLuca, H. F. and Suda, T. (1984) Proc. Natl. Acad. Sci. USA 81, 7112-7116.

1,25 DIHYDROXYVITAMIN D_3 INCREASES THE NUMBER OF HUMAN PROMYELOCYTIC LEUKAEMIA (HL-60) CELLS IN G_1/G_0 PHASE OF THE CELL CYCLE

C. PAUL DANIEL[1], A. PARREIRA[2] & D.M. McCARTHY[3], [1] Endocrine Unit and [2] MRC Leukaemia Unit (supported by the Gulbenkian Foundation, Portugal), Royal Postgraduate Medical School, [3] Department of Haematology, Westminster Hospital, London, England.

We have previously reported that 1,25 dihydroxyvitamin D_3 ($1,25(OH)_2D_3$) induces monocytic differentiation in normal and leukaemic haemopoietic cells including the human promyelocytic cell-line HL-60 (1,2). Differentiation in these cells is accompanied by a reduction in their rate of proliferation, but the degree of interdependence between these responses is not known. Early changes in growth-rate can be detected using a fluorescence-activated cell sorter (FACS) to analyse the proportion of cells in each phase of the cycle. We have therefore used FACS analysis to assess the relationship between the induction of differentiation in HL-60 cells by $1,25(OH)_2D_3$ and the reduction in their rate of growth.

Figure 1 shows the proportion of HL-60 cells showing markers of differentiation during treatment with 10 nM $1,25(OH)_2D_3$ for 4 days. Cells became capable of nitro blue tetrazolium (NBT) reduction after 24h. This was followed by a decrease in the proportion of S phase cells and an increase in those in G_1/G_0 after 48h (Fig. 2), while non-specific esterase activity was not detected until day 3. The absolute numbers of G_1/G_0 cells continued to increase until day 4 (Fig. 3). This accumulation of cells in G_1/G_0 phase was accompanied by a reduction in their ability to form clones in semi-solid methyl cellulose in the absence of $1,25(OH)_2D_3$

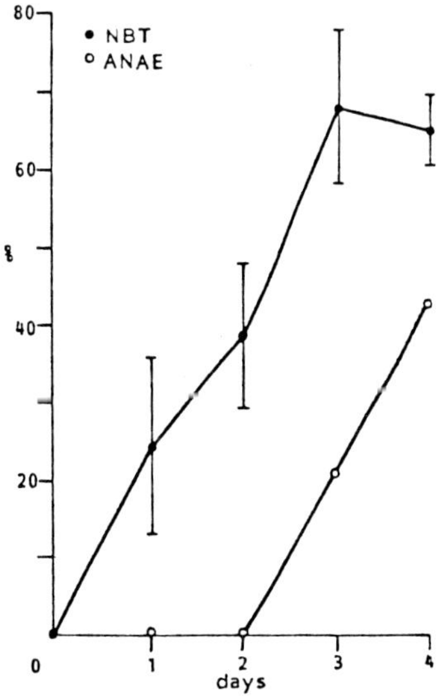

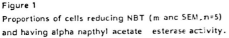

Figure 1
Proportions of cells reducing NBT (m anc SEM, n=5) and having alpha napthyl acetate esterase activity.

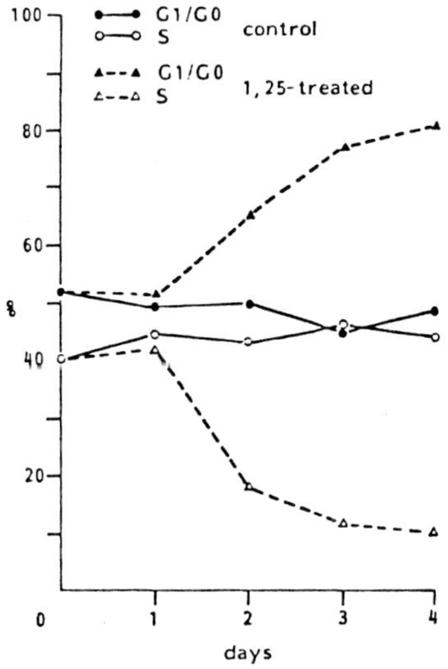

Figure 2
Proportions of cells in G1/G0 and S phase measured by FACS analysis.

Vitamin D. A Chemical, Biochemical and Clinical Update

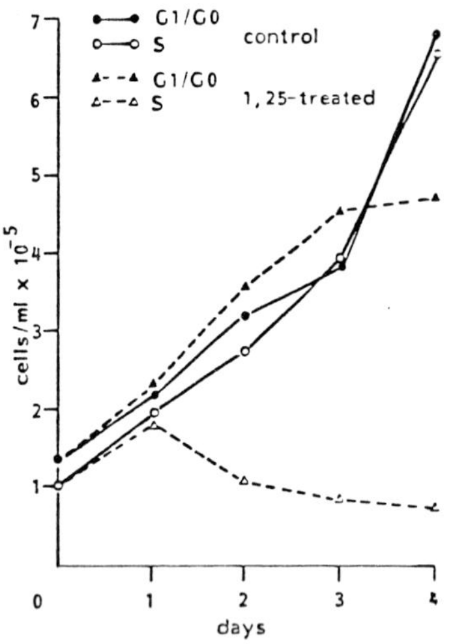

Figure 3
Numbers of cells in G1/G0 and S phase measured by FACS analysis.

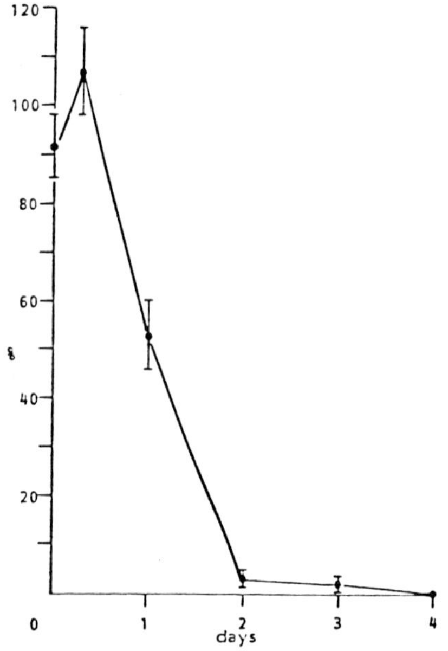

Figure 4
Proportion of cells forming clones in methyl cellulose after prior treatment with $1,25(OH)_2D_3$ in liquid culture. Results are expressed as a % of the number of clones derived from untreated cells. (m and SEM, n=6).

(Fig. 4). There was no reduction in the cloning efficiency of cells treated in liquid culture with $1,25(OH)_2D_3$ for up to 6h and then transferred to semi-solid medium without the hormone. After 24h, however, the proportion of cells capable of forming clones was reduced by half compared to control cells and by 48h it had fallen below 5%. Less than 1% of cloned cells reduced NBT compared to 40% of the cells treated with $1,25(OH)_2D_3$ for 48h, from which they were derived (Fig. 1). The clones, therefore, probably grew from the subpopulation of cells in liquid medium which were not visibly affected by $1,25(OH)_2D_3$ treatment.

These data are consistent with the hypothesis that HL-60 cells which begin differentiation become trapped in G_1/G_0 and hence are incapable of further division. Apart from the obvious parallelism between the appearance of markers of differentiation and the increase in the G_1/G_0 fraction, this conclusion is supported by the observation that cells which remained capable of clonal growth also retained the undifferentiated phenotype.

REFERENCES

1. McCarthy, D.M., San Miguel, J.F., Freake, H., Rodrigues, B., Andrews, C., Catovsky, D. and Goldman, J.M. (1984) Int. J. Cell Cloning 2, 227-242.

2. McCarthy, D.M., San Miguel, J.F., Freake, H.C., Green, P.H., Zola, H., Catovsky, D. and Goldman, J.M. (1983) Leuk. Res. 7, 51-55.

1,25$(OH)_2D_3$ ACTIVATES H_2O_2 SECRETION BY HUMAN MONOCYTE DERIVED MACROPHAGES.

M.S. Cohen, D.E. Mesler, R.G. Snipes, and T.K. Gray, Department of Medicine, UNC, Chapel Hill, NC 27514. USA.

INTRODUCTION:

Capacity for secretion of reactive oxygen intermediates by mononuclear phagocytes has been closely correlated with their tumorcidal and microbicidal activity (1). Monocytes, after 3 days in culture, express maximal secretion of H_2O_2 which decays unless cells are exposed to lymphokines such as interferon-γ (2). Recently, several investigators have demonstrated effects of 1,25$(OH)_2D_3$ on phagocytic cells (reviewed in Reference 3). The present study was undertaken to determine the effects of 1,25$(OH)_2D_3$ on the capacity of monocytic phagocytes to form and secrete H_2O_2.

METHODS:

Peripheral blood monocytes were isolated from normal adults by dextran sedimentation and ficoll-hypaque gradient separation. Non-adherent lymphocytes were removed by vigorous washing after two hours of incubation and the remaining cell population (greater than 90% mononuclear phagocytes) was incubated in culture medium containing 10% autologous serum, penicillin (100U/ml.) and streptomycin (100μg/ml per ml). Recombinant human interferon-γ (IFN-γ) (Biogen Laboratories, Cambridge, Mass. and Meloy Laboratories, Springfield, Mass.) or 1,25$(OH)_2D_3$ (provided by M. Uskokovic, Hoffman-LaRoche) was added to the medium. H_2O_2 secretion was determined in 96-well plates by the method of Pick and Keisari (4). Cell stimulation was produced with addition of phorbol myristate acetate (PMA, 100ng/ml).

RESULTS:

The effects of 1,25$(OH)_2D_3$ were compared with IFN-γ, a lymphokine believed to be critical for the activation of macrophage oxidative metabolism. Peak effects were noted at 10^{-8}M concentration of 1,25$(OH)_2D_3$ and 500-1000U/ml IFN-γ. The results obtained are summarized in Table 1.

Table 1. nmoles $H_2O_2/10^6$ MDM/60

H_2O_2 Secretion	-Day 3-		-Day 7-	
	Resting	Stimulated	Resting	Stimulated
Control	4.2 ± 3.2	21.7 ± 3.5	4.1 ± 1.4	12.1 ± 3.1
1,25-D_3	10.4 ± 5.8	57.0 ± 9.2*	6.3 ± 3.5	23.9 ± 6.4
IFN-γ	11.3 ± 3.2*	52.7 ± 3.1*	12.0 ± 5.0*	37.1 ± 8.0*

* $p<0.05$, Wilcoxon sign rank test

H_2O_2 secretion by resting monocyte derived macrophages incubated with either IFN-γ or 1,25$(OH)_2D_3$ was greater than control cells at both 3 and 7 days. Macrophages stimulated with PMA demonstrated enhanced secretion of H_2O_2. Cells incubated with 1,25$(OH)_2D_3$ at 3 days demonstrated a significant increase in H_2O_2 secretion relative to control cells, and were equivalent to cells exposed to IFN-γ. After 7 days in culture, macrophages demonstrated reduced ability (relative to younger cells) to secrete H_2O_2 in response to PMA.

Vitamin D. A Chemical, Biochemical and Clinical Update

Both IFN-γ and 1,25(OH)$_2$D$_3$ significantly offset decay of H_2O_2 secretion by these cells. Macrophages incubated with 24,25(OH)$_2$D$_3$ and 25(OH)D$_3$ demonstrated enhanced secretion of H_2O_2, but maximal effects were noted at higher concentrations than required for 1,25(OH)$_2$D$_3$. The combination of 1,25(OH)$_2$D$_3$ and IFN-γ did not further enhance secretion of H_2O_2 (Fig. 1).

FIG. 1

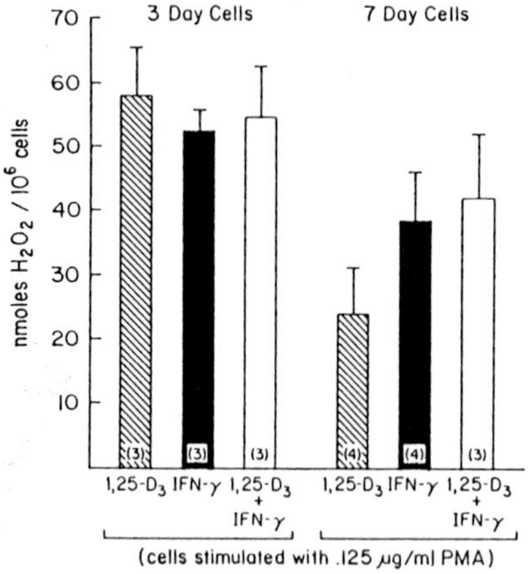

COMMENTS:

These results demonstrate another important effect of 1,25(OH)$_2$D$_3$. Monocyte activation and competence for secretion of oxygen reduction products is essential for normal host defenses. Although it seems clear that IFN-γ enhances activation of oxygen metabolism in these cells (2) our results show that 1,25(OH)$_2$D$_3$ is nearly equivalent to IFN-γ in this regard. Recently Honma et al have shown that 1,25(OH)$_2$D$_3$ enhances survival of mice innoculated with M1 tumor cells (5). 1,25(OH)$_2$D$_3$ also enhances the tumorcidal activity of murine alveolar macrophages (6). It seems likely that macrophage activation mediated by 1,25(OH)$_2$D$_3$ is involved in explaining these latter results, and suggests that 1,25(OH)$_2$D$_3$ plays a role in normal host immune function.

REFERENCES:

1. Nathan, C.F., Murray, H.W., and Cohn, Z.A. (1980) New England J. Med. 303:622-627.
2. Nathan, C.F., Murray, H.W., Wiebe, M.E. and Rubin, B.Y. (1983) J. Exp. Med. 158:670-689.
3. Gray, T.K., and Cohen, M.S. (1985) Vitamin D, Phagocyte Differentiation and Immune Function. Survey of Immunologic Research (in press)
4. Pick, E. and Keisari, Y. (1980) J. Immunol. Methods: 38:161-170.
5. Honma, Y., Hozumi, M., Abe, E., Konno, K., Fukushima, M., Hata, S., Nishii, Y., DeLuca, H.F., and Suda, T. (1983) Proc. Natl. Acad. Sci. (USA) 80:201-204.
6. Abe, E., Shiina, Y., Miyaura, C., Tanaka, H., Hayashi, T., Kanegasaki, S., Saito, M., Nishii, Y., DeLuca, H.F., and Suda, T. (1984) Proc. Natl. Acad. Sci. (USA) 81:7112-7116.

1,25-DIHYDROXYVITAMIN D_3-RELATED IONIC PERMEABILITIES IN THE CHICK SMALL INTESTINAL EPITHELIUM

H. S. CROSS, R. A. CORRADINO* and M. PETERLIK
Department of General and Experimental Pathology, University of Vienna Medical School, Vienna, Austria, and *Department of Physiology, New York State College of Veterinary Medicine, Cornell University, Ithaca, N.Y.

The continuous renewal of the small intestinal epithelium in the embryonic chick requires the proliferation of stem or crypt cells as well as their subsequent differentiation into mature enterocytes. Between embryonic day 15 and 20, different stages of epithelial maturation can be distinguished by the increasing number of differentiated absorptive, and also specialized, e.g. goblet, cells. Utilizing organ cultures of developing embryonic small intestine (1) we have shown that the action of vitamin D on Na^+-coupled membrane transport systems, like that of P_i or D-glucose, is tightly controlled by the degree of enterocyte differentiation (2). Also, 1,25-dihydroxyvitamin D_3 (1,25$(OH)_2D_3$) may itself be instrumental in advancing maturation, since the sterol increases the number of goblet cells during culture of embryonic jejunum (3). 1,25$(OH)_2D_3$ has also been shown to induce differentiation of some malignant hematopoetic cell lines (4) and to inhibit proliferation in others (5). Increased cellular Na^+ transport, either by stimulation of Na^+ influx or/and activation of the Na^+ pump, is an early response to mitogenic stimuli (6), whereas the anti-proliferative action of amiloride has been linked to inhibition of Na^+/H^+ antiport (7). Since 1,25$(OH)_2D_3$ is capable of modulating intestinal Na^+ transport, either by reduction of luminal Na^+/H^+ antiport and voltage-sensitive Na^+ flux (8) or by activation of the Na^+/K^+-ATPase (9), this study examined the influence of 1,25$(OH)_2D_3$ on pathways of cellular Na^+ transport during maturation of embryonic small intestinal epithelium.

Results:

1,25$(OH)_2D_3$ increased the activity of the Na^+ pump, as determined by ouabain-sensitive $^{86}Rb^+$ uptake, at all stages of embryonic development, though particularly during final embryonic differentiation (Fig. 1). The 1,25$(OH)_2D_3$ stimulation of Na^+ pumping, however, did not seem to be the consequence of increased Na^+ influx into enterocytes: although 1,25$(OH)_2D_3$ apparently stimulates Na^+ uptake at the mucosal surface, there was no consistent relation between Na^+ and Rb^+ uptake (Fig. 1). In addition, a large fraction of Na^+ uptake as measured probably proceeds via the paracellular route. This assumption is supported by the finding that 1,25-$(OH)_2D_3$ also increases luminal uptake of K^+ and Rb^+, utilized as ionic probes for paracellular permeability (10). When the stimulatory action of 1,25$(OH)_2D_3$ on Ca^{++} transport (1,2) was mimicked by the ionophore A23187, luminal uptake of Na^+ was significantly reduced (Fig. 2). This suggests that also in the intestine Na^+ entry is under negative feed-back control by intracellular Ca^{++} (cf. 11). When intracellular Ca^{++} was maximally raised by the combined effect of A23187 and 1,25$(OH)_2D_3$, Na^+ uptake was not further reduced but markedly stimulated (Fig. 2). These findings suggest, that 1,25$(OH)_2D_3$, through stimulation of Ca^{++} accumulation, interferes with Na^+ transfer across the brush border membrane, while the sterol simultaneously increases the junctional permeability of the epithelium for Na^+.

Conclusions:

By its influence on luminal Ca^{++} and Na^+ permeability as well as by its effect on basolateral Na^+/K^+ pumping, $1,25(OH)_2D_3$ provides multiple means for the joint regulation of proliferation and differentiation in intact intestinal epithelium. In addition, the possible influence of $1,25(OH)_2D_3$ on development of junctional ionic permeability may lead to the characteristic "leakiness" of small intestinal epithelium.

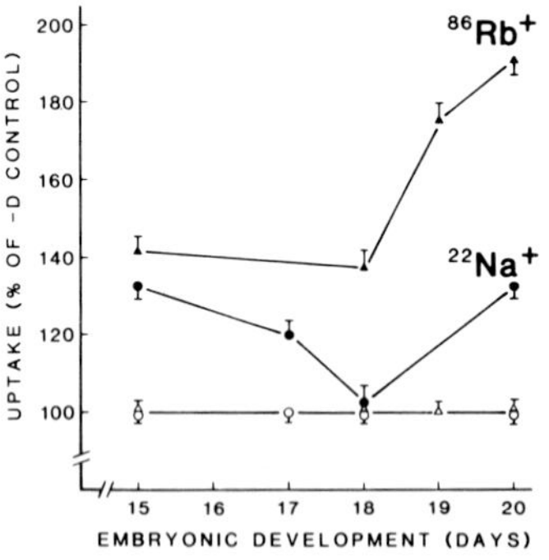

Fig. 1: Effect of $1,25(OH)_2D_3$ on Na/K-ATPase and Na uptake in embryonic jejunum. Culture time 48 h.△,O: $-1,25(OH)_2D_3$.▲,●: 110 nM $1,25(OH)_2D_3$. Incubation in KH buffer (0.1 mM RbCl, 30 min; 143 mM Na^+, 2 min)

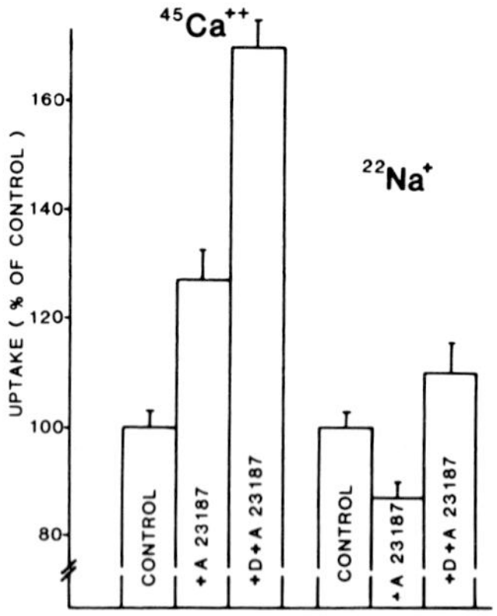

Fig. 2: Ca^{++} and Na^+ uptake in day 20 jejunum. Culture time 48 h. +D: 110 nM $1,25(OH)_2D_3$. +A23187: 50 nM. Ca uptake: ref. 1; Na uptake: cf. Fig. 1

This work was supported by the Austrian Science Foundation (Grant No. 4422) and the Anton Dreher-Gedächtnisschenkung (Grant No. 7/82).

References:

1. Corradino,R.A. (1973) J. Cell Biol. 58: 64-78
2. Cross,H.S., Peterlik, M. (1982) Horm. Metab. Res. 14: 649-652
3. Cross,H.S., Gazda,H., Stekel,H., Peterlik,M. (1984) J. Embryol. Exp. Morphol. 82: 248 (Suppl.)
4. Tanaka,H., Abe,E., Miyaura,C., Shiina,Y., Suda,T. (1983) Biochem. Biophys. Res. Comm. 117: 86-92
5. Miyaura,C., Abe,E., Honma,Y., Hozumi,Y., Nishii,Y., Suda,T. (1983) Arch. Biochem. Biophys. 227: 379-385
6. Rozengurt,E., Mendoza,S. (1980) Ann. N.Y. Acad. Sci. 339: 175-190
7. Smith,N.,Sparks,R.,Pool,T.,Cameron,I. (1978) Cancer Res. 38: 1952-2059
8. Fuchs,R., Graf,J., Peterlik,M., submitted for publication
9. Cross,H.S., Peterlik,M. (1983) FEBS Lett. 153: 141-145
10. Cross,H.S., Peterlik,M., in Phosphate and Mineral Metabolism, ed. S.G. Massry et al., p. 163-171, Plenum Press, New York 1984
11. Taylor,A.,Windhager,E.E. (1979) Am. J. Physiol. 236: F505-F512

TIME-RELATED VARIATIONS IN SERUM 1,25-$(OH)_2$ VITAMIN D (1,25-$(OH)_2D$) CONCENTRATIONS IN HUMANS.

M.E. Markowitz, J.F. Rosen, M.F. Holick, N. Hannifan and D.B. Endres
Dept. of Peds. and CRC, Einstein Coll. Med., Montefiore Medical Center, Bronx, NY 10467; Endocrine Unit, Mass. Gen. Hosp., Boston, MA 02114; and Nichols Institute, San Juan Capistrano, CA 92675.

Introduction: We have demonstrated previously that blood ionized calcium concentrations fluctuate with circadian rhythmicity in humans (1). A study of 1,25-$(OH)_2D_3$-treated hypoparathyroid children indicated that this hormone may modulate the calcium rhythm (2). We examined, therefore, the possibility that serum 1,25-$(OH)_2D$ concentrations also undergo rhythmical variations. In a preliminary report, we described wide diurnal swings in serum 1,25-$(OH)_2D$ concentrations that occurred (on average) every 3-4 hours in 3 healthy men (3). Subsequently investigations by others failed to confirm the wide fluctuations, the ultradian rhythm or both (4,5). The present study was undertaken to enlarge our data base and examine the etiology of our original observations (3).

Methods: Four healthy men, 25-40 years of age, were admitted to the Clinical Research Center the night prior to blood sampling. Blood was obtained via an indwelling venous catheter every 30 minutes for a period of 12 hours (1). Baseline biochemical determinations (Ca, P_i) were normal.

15 ml of blood were drawn at each time point and allowed to clot in glass tubes. After centrifugation, two separate 2.2 ml serum aliquots were pipetted into plastic tubes and frozen. The tubes from each subject (48 samples) were coded and sent to the Nichols Institute. Twelve sequential samples from one study (S.L.) were sent to the laboratory of Dr. Holick.

At Nichols Institute, a competitive chick cytosol binding radioassay was employed (6). All sera from a subject were run in a single assay. The interassay CV based on serum pools was 10-12%. In Dr. Holick's laboratory, samples underwent lipid extraction and sep-pak chromatography before final purification by HPLC (7). Determinations of 1,25-$(OH)_2D$ concentrations were then made using a modified bovine thymus assay (8).

Results were decoded in N.Y. The mean of the duplicates from each time point were plotted (Figure). The differences between the duplicates were used to calculate the error of the method (9):

$$\text{error} = \text{standard deviation of the mean of the differences}/\sqrt{2}$$

The 12-hour 1,25-$(OH)_2D$ mean, ranges, and assay errors were similar for all subjects. None of the four subjects had outlier values (defined as ±2 SD from the 12-hour mean, and/or, >75 pg/ml - the upper limit of normal for this assay based on random samples in healthy adults) that were confirmed on the duplicate sample.

Comparison of duplicate samples run in both assays (chick and thymus) yielded similar means ($n = 12$; $\bar{x}$ chick = 25 pg/ml vs $\bar{x}$ thymus = 28 pg/ml), ranges (chick: 19-29 vs thymus: 16-37 pg/ml) and error of the method based on differences between duplicate samples (chick: 3.2 pg/ml vs chick-thymus: 4.9 pg/ml).

An ultradian rhythm with low amplitude oscillation may be present in some of the subjects (L.C., T.M., K.S.). However, a longer time series would be required for formal statistical analyses.

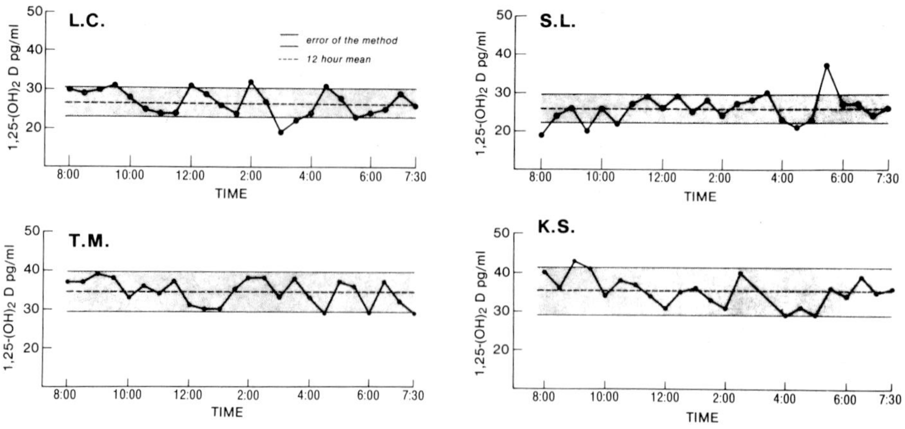

Discussion: We failed to duplicate the wide diurnal variations described earlier (4). Study conditions were similar: subject's age and sex, location, diet, activity and sleep wake cycle. Sample handling was identical. The determinations of serum 1,25-$(OH)_2D$ concentrations were performed in different laboratories but employed similar methods, the chick cytosol binding assay (7). Validation of the current results were obtained by analyses of duplicate samples in a different assay in a second laboratory (thymus assay).

One difference between study designs was the use of duplicate samples from each time point to calculate the value at that time rather than reliance on a single serum sample. In the few instances (average of 2/12-hr run) where one serum sample was >2 SD from the mean of the 12 hr run, the duplicate was always nonconfirmatory. Thus, random error of the assay could lead to spurious interpretation of the data. The fact that 1,25-$(OH)_2D$ peaks described in the first study occurred rhythmically argues against chance occurrence (3).

Another explanation is that the adult population is heterogenous; some subjects may have wide diurnal fluctuations in serum 1,25-$(OH)_2D$ values while others do not. A larger sample size and repeated study of the same individual are necessary to resolve whether and to what extent serum 1,25-$(OH)_2D$ values may fluctuate.

1. Markowitz, M.E., Rotkin, L., Rosen, J.F. (1981) Science 213, 672-674.
2. Markowitz, M.E., Rosen, J.F., Smith, C., DeLuca, H.E. (1982) J. Clin. Endocrinol. Metab. 55, 727-733.
3. Markowitz, M.E., Rosen, J.F., Laxminarayan, S., Smith, C., DeLuca, H.F. in Proceedings of the 5th Workshop on Vitamin D, 1982, pp. 707-709.
4. Halloran, B.P., Portale, A.A., Morris, R.C., Castro, M., Murphy, M., Goldsmith, R.G. in Endocrine Control of Bone and Calcium Metabolism, NY, Elsevier Science, 1984, pp. 369-372.
5. Manolagas, S.C., Deftos, L.J. (1985) N. Engl. J. Med. 312, 122-123.
6. Endres, D., Lu, J., et al. (1982) see ref. 3 above, pp. 812-819.
7. Adams, J.S., Clemens, T.L., et al. (1982) N. Engl. J. Med. 306,722-724.
8. Reindardt, T.A., Horst, R.L., Orf, J.W., Hollis, B.W. (1984) J. Clin. Endocrinol. Metab. 38, 91-99.
9. Winer, B.J. (1981) Statistical Principles in Experimental Design, McGraw Hill.

COMPARATIVE EFFECTS OF 1 ,25$(OH)_2D_3$, 24,24 DIFLUORO-1 , 25-$(OH)_2D_3$ AND 1 ,25-$(OH)_2$-24(R) FLUORO-D_3 ON HUMAN BONE CELLS IN CULTURE.

R. Vaishnav, J.A. Gallagher, D.F. Guilland-Cumming, J.A. Kanis and R.G.G. Russell.
Department of Human Metabolism and Clinical Biochemistry, University of Sheffield Medical School, Beech Hill Road, Sheffield S10 2RX.

Introduction

We have previously described methods for the culture of cells derived from human bone which express osteoblast-like characteristics and are responsive to 1,25$(OH)_2D_3$ (1). Low concentrations stimulate proliferation whereas high doses are inhibitory (2) coincident with stimulation of the bone-derived proteins, alkaline phosphatase and osteocalcin. Vitamin D metabolites with difluoro substitutions have been reported to be more potent inducers of calcium binding protein in the duodenal organ culture system than the natural metabolite (3). In this study on human bone cells, we have compared the effects of 1,25$(OH)_2D_3$ with those observed with two fluorinated analogues 1,25,$(OH)_2$-24R fluoro-D_3 or 24,24,-difluoro-1,25$(OH)_2D_3$.

Materials and Methods

Cells were cultured from explants of human bone by previously described methods (1). In brief, trabecular fragments from human bone were plated out into tissue culture dishes and cultured in Eagles minimum essential medium containing 10% fetal calf serum (FCS). These cells were subcultured after 4-5 weeks when a confluent monolayer was formed. All experiments were conducted at first passage in 6 well Falcon multiwells. Cell growth was assessed by measuring the incorporation of ^{3}H thymidine into DNA. Osteocalcin was measured by a specific radioimmunoassay using an antibody raised in rabbits against purified bovine osteocalcin. Alkaline phosphatase was determined by using the substrate 4-dinitrophenyl disodium orthophosphate in a glycine buffer. Protein synthesis was estimated by the method of Lowry.

Results

1,25-dihydroxy -24R fluoro D_3 and 24,24 difluoro - 1,25$(OH)_2D_3$ significantly inhibited proliferation of human bone cells in a dose-range of 10^{-10}-10^{-6}M when compared with controls. 1,25$(OH)_2D_3$, the naturally occurring biologically active metabolite of vitamin D_3, also inhibited proliferation of human bone derived cells over a similar dose range (fig 1). However, at 10^{-8}M and 10^{-6}M the inhibitory effect observed with the fluoro derivatives was significantly less than that observed with 1,25$(OH)_2D_3$. In contrast, the stimulation of the bone specific protein osteocalcin was markedly increased by the fluorinated metabolites and by 1,25$(OH)_2D_3$ (fig 1). 24,24 difluoro-1, 25,$(OH)_2D_3$ appeared to the most potent stimulator of osteocalcin synthesis over the dose range 10^{-10}-10^{-8}M. The maximal response with 1,25$(OH)_2D_3$ occurred at 10^{-8}M. Measurement of alkaline phosphatase activity showed significant stimulation with all three metabolites. The response was dose dependent (fig 1), and 1,25-dihydroxy-24R fluoro-D_3 was the most potent.

Discussion

This study indicates that fluorinated analogues have similar qualitative effects to those of 1,25$(OH)_2D_3$ on human bone cells in culture. The fluorinated analogues stimulated the synthesis of bone specific proteins.

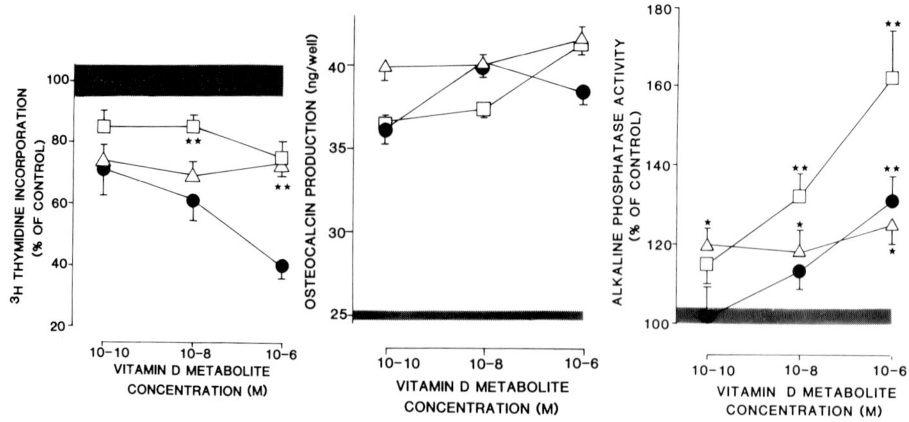

Figure 1: Effects of 1,25$(OH)_2D_3$ ●-●, 24,24 difluoro-1,25-$(OH)_2D_3$ △-△ and 1,25$(OH)_2$-24(R) fluoro-D_3 □-□ on ^3H thymidine incorporation, osteocalcin synthesis and alkaline phosphatase activity in cultured human bone cells. Values significantly different from control $P<0.05$ *, $P<0.01$**. In the case of thymidine incorporation, ** significantly ($P<0.01$) different from 1,25$(OH)_2D_3$.

At certain doses however, they showed a greater stimulatory effect then the natural hormone whilst affecting cell proliferation to a lesser degree. These findings are in accord with the high potency of 24,24, difluoro-1,25-$(OH)_2D_3$ already described in the chick (4) and the rat (5). The relative potencies of the analogues on target tissue, particularly on osteoblast-like cells, suggest that they might be of value in bone losing disorders such as osteoporosis.

Acknowledgements

We are grateful to Dr M. Uskokovic, Hoffmann-La Roche for supplies of the vitamin D analogues, and to the YCRC for supporing this work.

References

1. Beresford, J.N., Gallagher, J.A., Poser, J.N. and Russell, R.G.G. (1984) Metab.Bone.Dis.Rel.Res, 5, 229-234.
2. Skjodt, H., Gallagher, J.A., Beresford, J.N, Couch, M., Poser, J.W. and Russell, R.G.G. (1985) J.Endocr. (in press).
3. Corradino, R.A., Ikekawa, N. and DeLuca, H.F. (1981) Arch.Biochem. Biophys, 208, 273-277.
4. Corradino, R.A. (1984) In Vitamin D Basic and Clinical Aspects. Kumar, R, (ed). Martinus Nijhoff Publishing, Boston, 325-341.
5. Okamoto, S., Tanaka, Y., DeLuca, H.F., Kobayashi, Y. and Ikekawa, N. (1983). Am.J.Physiol, 224, E159-E163

EFFECTS OF 1,25-DIHYDROXYVITAMIN D_3 ON THE FUNCTION OF RAT ANTERIOR PITUITARY CELLS IN PRIMARY CULTURE.

S.D. Rose and M.F. Holick, Department of Applied Biological Sciences, M.I.T., Cambridge, MA, 02139, U.S.A.

Introduction:

The function of the putative receptor for 1,25-dihydroxyvitamin D_3 (1,25-$(OH)_2$-D_3) in pituitary cells has thus far only been investigated in rat pituitary tumor cell lines, and the reported results have been inconsistent. 1,25-$(OH)_2$-D_3 has been reported to both stimulate (1) and inhibit (2) prolactin (PRL) secretion by various strains of GH cells, under a variety of cell culture conditions. We have examined the effects of 1,25-$(OH)_2$-D_3 on the synthesis and secretion of PRL and thyrotropin (TSH) by non-transformed rat anterior pituitary cells in primary culture. These cells were found to have high affinity cytosolic specific binding proteins for 1,25-$(OH)_2$-D_3 (K_d=6.0x10^{-10} M; B_{max}=37fmol/mg protein) exhibiting a sedimentation coefficient of 3.5-3.7 S.

Methods:

Primary cultures of enzymatically dispersed rat anterior pituitary cells were prepared essentially as described by Vale, et al. (3). Cell cultures were seeded at a concentration of 3-5x10^5 cells/ml, in 1.5 ml culture medium (85% Ham's F10, 12.5% horse serum, 2.5% fetal bovine serum, supplemented with penicillin and streptomycin) in 35mm wells, and incubated for 4 days at 37°C, in an atmosphere containing 95% air and 5% CO_2. The conditioned medium was then removed, and the cells were washed with a serum-free test medium (Ham's F10). 1.5 ml of the test medium was then added to each culture, and the cells were returned to the incubator for a 1 hour pre-incubation period. Cultures were then treated with various concentrations of 1,25-$(OH)_2$-D_3 or its vehicle, for a variety of time periods. Cell and media samples were collected at each time point, and subsequently assayed for TSH and PRL content via radioimmunoassay, using kits provided by the NIADDK. Cellular protein content was determined by the method of Lowry (4).

Results:

No consistent significant effect was observed on either cellular or media PRL content (figure 1). Although cellular TSH content was also not appreciably altered, media TSH content was significantly elevated following 24 hours (157% control) and 48 hours (140% control) of incubation in the presence of 10^{-8} M 1,25-$(OH)_2$-D_3 (figure 2). This effect was found to be dose dependent, with an ED_{50} between 10^{-9} and 10^{-8} M at the 48 hour time point (figure 3).

Discussion:

These results indicate that 1,25-$(OH)_2$-D_3 is capable of stimulating TSH secretion by a direct action on rat thyrotropes, and for the first time confirm that the specific binding protein for 1,25-$(OH)_2$-D_3 present in non-transformed rat pituitary cells acts as a true receptor, in the classical pharmacological sense. They further suggest that 1,25-$(OH)_2$-D_3 may act in vivo as one of many factors involved in the complex regulation of TSH secretion. This speculation is consistent with several findings

Vitamin D. A Chemical, Biochemical and Clinical Update

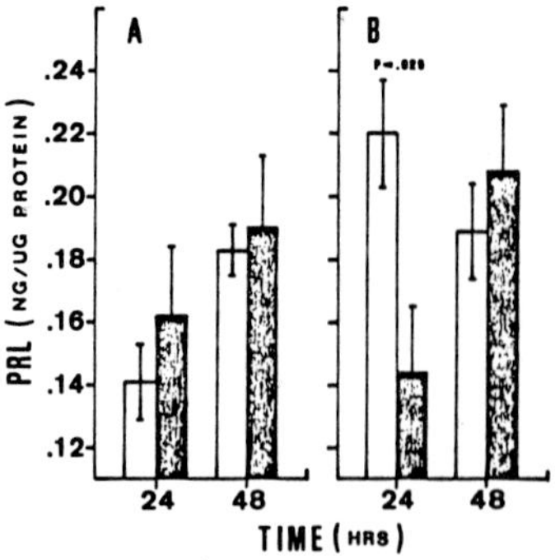

FIGURE 1: EFFECTS OF 10^{-8}M 1,25-$(OH)_2$-D_3 ON CONTENT OF PRL IN MEDIA AND CELL SAMPLES. A) MEDIA CONTENT (n=5/GROUP); B) CELLULAR CONTENT (n=3/GROUP). SOLID BARS ARE 1,25-$(OH)_2$-D_3, OPEN BARS ARE VEHICLE. ALL VALUES ARE MEAN ± SEM.

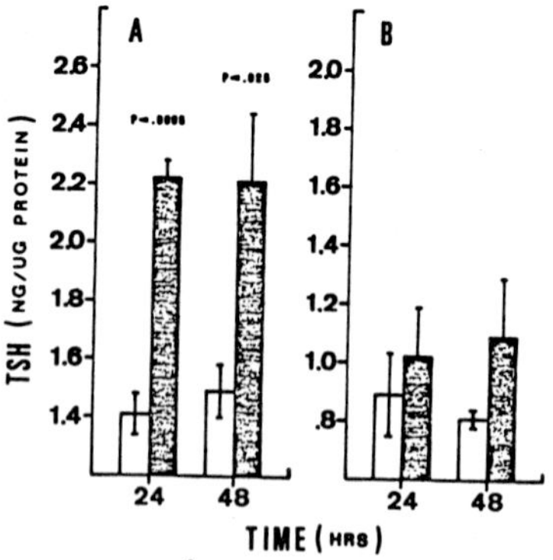

FIGURE 2: EFFECTS OF 10^{-8}M 1,25-$(OH)_2$-D_3 ON CONTENT OF TSH IN MEDIA AND CELL SAMPLES. A) MEDIA CONTENT (n=5/GROUP); B) CELLULAR CONTENT (n=3/GROUP). SOLID BARS ARE 1,25-$(OH)_2$-D_3, OPEN BARS ARE VEHICLE. ALL VALUES ARE MEAN ± SEM.

previously reported, including: exclusive localization of ^{3}H-1,25-$(OH)_2$-D_3 in nuclei of rat thyrotropes, as determined by combined autoradiography and immunohistochemistry (5); increased serum levels of TSH following acute injection of 1,25-$(OH)_2$-D_3 to rats in vivo (6); the requirement of thyroid hormones for normal bone growth, and to observe maximal effects of PTH and 1,25-$(OH)_2$-D_3 on bone calcium mobilization in vitro (7); and inhibition of renal 25-OH-D_3-1-hydroxylase activity in vitro by TSH, T_3, and T_4 (8). In addition, these results suggest that previously observed inconsistent effects of 1,25-$(OH)_2$-D_3 on PRL secretion may have resulted from the tumor cell models employed in these studies, and may not be of physiological relevance.

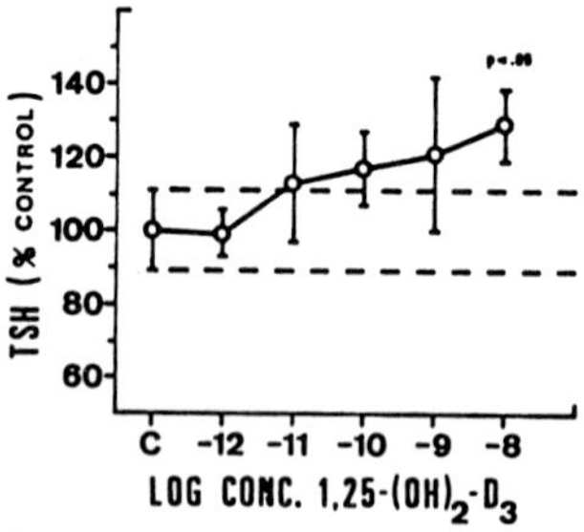

FIGURE 3: CONTENT OF TSH IN MEDIUM FOLLOWING 48 HOURS INCUBATION WITH VARIOUS DOSES OF 1,25-$(OH)_2$-D_3. ALL VALUES ARE MEAN ± SEM; n=4/GROUP.

References:

1. Wark, J.D., and Tashjian, Jr., A.H. (1982). Endocr. 111:1755-1757.
2. Murdoch, G., and Rosenfeld, M.G. (1981). J. Biol. Chem. 256:4050-5.
3. Vale, W., Grant, G., Amass, M., Blackwell, R., and Guillemin, R.(1972) Endocr. 91:562-572.
4. Lowry, O.H., Rosebrough, N.J., Farr, A.L., and Randall, R.J. (1951). J. Biol. Chem. 193:265-275.
5. Sar, M., Stumpf, W.E., and DeLuca, H.F. (1980). Cell Tissue Res. 209:161-166.
6. Sar, M., Miller, W.L., and Stumpf,W.E. (1981). The Physiologist 24:70
7. Williams, R.H. (ed.), Textbook of Endocrinology, 6th ed., (1981), pp. 211,935,962, W.B.Saunders Co., Philadelphia.
8. Kano, K., and Jones, G. (1984). Endocr. 114:330-336.

1,25-DIHYDROXYVITAMIN D_3 STIMULATES DIFFERENTIATION AND 24-HYDROXYLASE ACTIVITY IN CULTURED HUMAN KERATINOCYTES. E.L. Smith and M.F. Holick, Dept. of Applied Biological Sciences, MIT, Cambridge, MA 02139, USA.

INTRODUCTION

Numerous tissues have been shown to have receptors for 1,25-dihydroxyvitamin D_3 (1,25(OH)$_2$D). The presence of receptors in cultured human keratinocytes and dermal fibroblasts is suggestive that these cells are targets for 1,25(OH)$_2$D (1). In addition, we have demonstrated that this hormone inhibits the growth of cultured dermal fibroblasts (1), and others have demonstrated that 1,25(OH)$_2$D stimulates 25-OH-D-24-hydroxylase in these cells (2). 1,25(OH)$_2$D has been shown to affect the growth and/or differentiation of various normal and tumor cell types (1,3-4). With this knowledge, the effect of 1,25(OH)$_2$D on the differentiation of cultured human keratinocytes was investigated.

METHOD

Human keratinocytes were obtained from surgically-removed skin and plated according to the method of Rheinwald and Green (5). Keratinocytes were grown under serum-free conditions to prevent the interference of serum factors. Cells were incubated in the presence of 1,25(OH)$_2$D at 10^{-8} M or vehicle alone (<0.1 % absolute ethanol), and were redosed with each feeding (3x/wk). Methodology for the various indexes of morphological differentiation, proportion of different keratinocyte cell types (3), cornified cells (6), and cellular density (7), have been previously described by other investigators. Transglutaminase activity was measured by quantitating incorporation of ^{3}H-putrescine into casein (8). 25-OH-D-24-hydroxylase activity was quantitated after incubation of cells with ^{3}H-25-OH-D and measurement of incorporation into a metabolite that co-migrated on hplc with synthetic standard 24,25(OH)$_2$D (2).

RESULTS

A. MORPHOLOGICAL DIFFERENTIATION

There was a shift in the proportion of different cultured keratinocyte cell types after incubation with 1,25(OH)$_2$D (10^{-8} M) (Fig 1). After 2 wk there was a 1.6-fold decrease in the percentage of basal cells and an increase in the percentage of squamous (2-fold), cornified (6.3-fold), and floater (6.0-fold) cells. The effect on keratinocyte density was measured, and resulted in a shift to a more-differentiated state (i.e. lower cellular density).

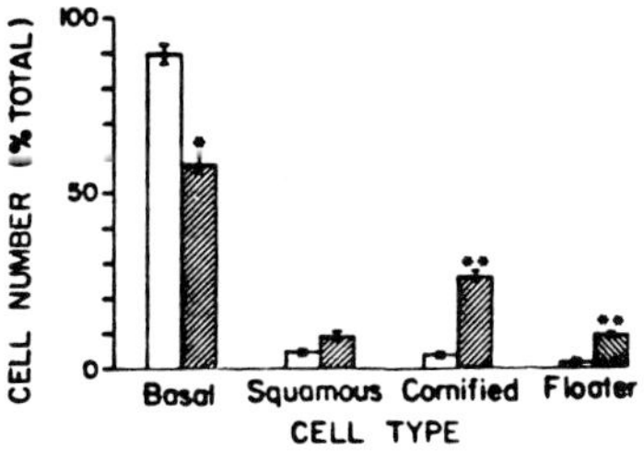

Fig 1. Proportion of Cultured Human Keratinocyte Cell Types Under Control (open bars) and 1,25-(OH)$_2$D-dosed (hatched bars) Conditions. Values represent mean of triplicate determinations ± SEM (*, $p<0.01$; **, $p<0.001$).

B. TRANSGLUTAMINASE ACTIVITY

After incubation with 1,25(OH)$_2$D at 10^{-8} M for 10 days, there was a highly significant increase in the transglutaminase activity of cultured human keratinocytes (Fig 2). Incorporation of ^{3}H-putrescine into casein after incubation with enzyme extract from 1,25(OH)$_2$D-dosed cells was greater than twice that of control values.

Vitamin D. A Chemical, Biochemical and Clinical Update

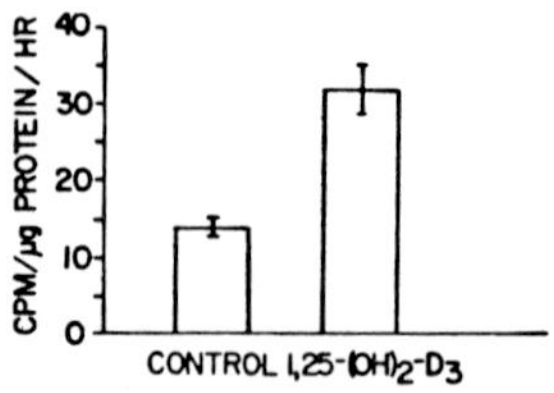

Fig 2. Transglutaminase Activity of Cultured Human Keratinocytes. Values represent mean of triplicate determinations ± SEM ($p<0.001$).

C. 25-OH-D-24-HYDROXYLASE ACTIVITY

Conversion of ^3H-25-OH-D into a tritiated metabolite that comigrated on hplc with synthetic $24,25(OH)_2D$ was much greater in samples from cells preincubated with $1,25(OH)_2D$, 11.0 ± 0.8% (mean ± SEM) (Fig 3B), than in control samples, 2.2 ± 0.2% (Fig 3A). In boiled control samples, cells preincubated with $1,25(OH)_2D$ and boiled prior to incubation with ^3H-25-OH-D, the precent conversion was less than 0.5 ± 0.05%. There was no radioactive incorporation into metabolites that comigrated with synthetic $25,26(OH)_2D$ or $1,25(OH)_2D$, suggesting that neither of these compounds is synthesized in amounts detectable by hplc.

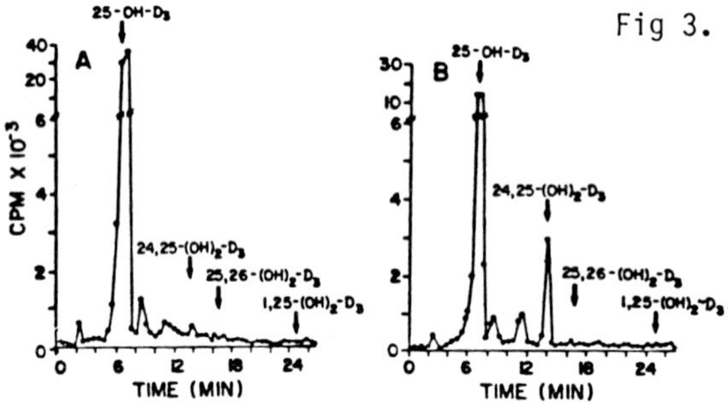

Fig 3. Hplc Profiles of Lipid Extracts of Cultured Human Keratinocytes After Incubation with ^3H-25-OH-D. Fig 3A: Cells preincubated with vehicle alone. Fig 3B: Cells preincubated with $1,25(OH)_2D$. Arrows indicate retention time of synthetic, unlabelled standard.

CONCLUSIONS

These data demonstrate that $1,25(OH)_2D$ is a potent stimulator of morphological and biochemical differentiation in cultured human keratinocytes. Although the physiological role of $1,25(OH)_2D$ in epidermal differentiation is not known, it may play an important role in the normal differentiation of skin during development or may be useful in understanding clinical disorders of differentiation.

REFERENCES

1. Clemens TL, Adams JS, Horiuchi N, Gilchrest BA, Cho H, Tsuchiya Y, Matsuo N, Suda T, and Holick MF (1983) J Clin Endocrinol Metab. 56, 824-830.
2. Feldman D, Chen T, Cone C, Hirst M, Shani S, Benderli A, and Hochberg Z (1982) J Clin Endocrinol Metab. 55, 1020-1022.
3. Hosomi J, Hosoi J, Abe E, Suda T, and Kuroki T (1983) Endocrinol. 3, 1950-1957.
4. Colston K, Colston MJ, Feldman D (1981) Endocrinol. 108, 1083-1086.
5. Rheinwald JG, and Green H (1975) Cell 6, 331-344.
6. Sun T-T, and Green H (1976) Cell 9, 511-521.
7. Simon M, and Green H (1984) Cell 26, 827-834.
8. Rice RH, and Green H (1979) Cell 18, 681-694.
9. This work was supported in part by NIH grants AM27334 and AG02918.

IDENTIFICATION OF A PHAGOCYTE DERIVED METABOLITE OF 25-HYDROXYVITAMIN D_3 AND MECHANISM OF FORMATION

T.K. Gray, M.S. Cohen, R.G. Snipes, D.E. Mesler, D. Millington and B.I. Weinberg, University of North Carolina at Chapel Hill and Duke University, North Carolina, U.S.A.

Phagocytes metabolized 25-hydroxyvitamin D_3 (25OH-D) to several more polar metabolites (1, 2), one of which have been identified by mass spectroscopy. The mechanism of their formation and their biological relevance is presently unknown.

METHODS:

U937 cells and human peripheral blood mononuclear cells were cultured as previously described (3). Human neutrophils (PMN) and monocytes were isolated from whole blood by ficoll-hypaque separation. Recombinant interferon gamma (IFN) was obtained from Biogen, Cambridge, M.A. Metabolites of 25OH-D were isolated by high performance liquid chromatography as previously described (3). 19-nor, 10-keto, vitamin D_3 was provided by M. Uskokovic, Ph.D., Hoffmann-LaRoche, Nutley, N.J. 4×10^7 cells were cultured in presence of 25OH-D (10^{-6}M) for 24 hours and the polar metabolites isolated. The metabolite previously designated as Peak III (1) was submitted for spectral analysis. In some experiments hydrogen peroxide (H_2O_2) formation by cells was measured by established techniques.

RESULTS AND COMMENTS:

In all of these experiments three metabolites of 25OH-D were seen. These metabolites were formed in equimolar amounts. Because peak III co-eluted on some chromatographic systems with 1,25-dihydroxyvitamin D_3, it was the first metabolite submitted for mass spectroscopy (MS/MS). The pattern observed with MS/MS was identical to that for 19 nor, 10 keto-25OH-D_3 as reported by Napoli and his associates.

Phagocytes use oxygen to make reduction products such as O_2- and H_2O_2 which are critical for the microbicidal and tumoricidal action of these cells. Several approaches were used to determine whether these products were involved in the formation of 19 nor, 10 keto-25OH-D. First, glucose was incubated with glucose oxidase in concentrations sufficient to generate H_2O_2 in amounts comparable to PMNs stimulated by phorbal myristate acetate (PMA, 0.1 ng-ml.) Under these conditions 25OH-D was not metabolized. Next, PMNs from two patients with chronic granulomatous disease of childhood known to make 7-20% of normal H_2O_2 were incubated with 25OH-D. No difference between these cells and normal PMNs in terms of 19 nor, 10 keto 25OH-D formation was observed. PMNs incubated in an anaerobic chamber for 1-3 hrs and stimulated by PMA produced 20% of the H_2O_2 formed by aerobic control cells. However, 19 nor, 10 keto 25OHD formation was identical under aerobic and anaerobic conditions. The addition of scavengers

Vitamin D. A Chemical, Biochemical and Clinical Update

for superoxide (SOD) and H_2O_2 (catalase) did not block synthesis of 19 nor, 10 keto 25(OH)D. Lastly, human monocytes exposed to IFN (10^3 u/ml) for 3 - 7 days in vitro increased H_2O_2 formation > 200 % of control, but did not significantly alter 19 nor, 10 keto 25(OH)D formation. In the latter experiments the synthesis of $1,25(OH)_2D_3$ was not observed.
The metabolite designated as Peak III is 19 nor, 10 keto, $25(OH)D_3$, a finding consistent with recent reports describing formation of this metabolite by HL-60 cells (4, 5). We have observed its formation by human PMNs and monocytes as well as U937 cells (1).
Formation of 19 nor, 10 keto $25(OH)D_3$ in vitro was not correlated with changes of O_2 reduction products. Given previous evidence that its formation is not enzymatic, it appears that synthesis involves either very small concentrations of O_2 reduction products or a unique oxidation reaction. Incubation of U937 cells in the presence of 19 nor, 10 keto 25(OH)D (10^8 M) lead to inhibition of cellular proliferation and enhanced differentiation (unpublished observations), similar to that observed with HL-60 cells (4). These findings suggest a biological action for 19 nor, 10 keto $25(OH)D_3$, which was previously thought to be inactive. It is possible that the differentiation induced by 25(OH)D (3) is caused by 19 nor, 10 keto 25(OH)D formed in vitro during the incubation of U937 cells with 25(OH)D.

REFERENCES:

1. Cohen, M.S. and Gray, T.K. (1984), PNAS 80: 1538
2. Adams, J.S. and Gacad, M.A. (1985), Abstracts of the Sixth Workshop on Vitamin D, p. 425, Merano, Italy
3. Dodd, R.S., et.al. (1983), PNAS 79
4. Teitelbaum, S.L., Bar-Shavit, Z., Perry, H.M., Welgus, H.G. Kahn, A.J., Reitsma, P., Gray, R., Horst, R. (1985), Abstracts of Sixth Workshop on Vitamin D, p. 64
5. Matsui, T., Nakao, Y., Fujita, T., Okabe, T., Ishizuka and Norman, A.W. (1985) Abstracts of Sixth Workshop on Vitamin D, p. 13.

METABOLISM OF 24(R)25-$(OH)_2D_3$ IN HUMAN PROMYELOCYTIC LEUKEMIA CELLS (HL-60)

ISOLATION AND IDENTIFICATION OF 19-NOR-10-KETO-24(R)25-$(OH)_2D_3$

S. Ishizuka[1], T. Matsui[2], Y. Nakao[2], T. Fujita[2], and A.W. Norman[3]

1) Teijin Institute for Bio-Medical Research, Tokyo, Japan, 2) Department of Medicine, University of Kobe, Kobe, Japan, and 3) Department of Biochemistry, University of California, Riverside, CA 92521, U.S.A.

Recently it is established that the hormonal form of vitamin D_3, 1α,25-$(OH)_2D_3$, can induce in vitro differentiation of the murine myeloid leukemic cell line (M1 cell) and human promyelocytic leukemia cell line (HL-60 cell) into monocyte-macrophages [1-4]. 24(R)25-$(OH)_2D_3$ also can mediate induction of the differentiation of HL-60 cells into monocyte-macrophages when present at 50 time the concentrations of 1α,25-$(OH)_2D_3$ [4]. It is yet unclear whether induction of differentiation of HL-60 cells is by 24(R)25-$(OH)_2D_3$ itself or by its metabolites. To solve this problem we investigated the metabolism of 24(R)25-$(OH)_2D_3$ in HL-60 cells. In this report, we demonstrate that HL-60 cells metabolize 24(R)25-$(OH)_2D_3$ to two unidentified metabolites during in vitro incubation. These two metabolites are identified as 5(Z)- and 5(E)-19-nor-10-keto-24(R)25-$(OH)_2D_3$.

<u>Incubation of 24(R)25-$(OH)_2D_3$ with HL-60 cells</u>
The HL-60 cells (1 x 10^7 cells) were washed with serum-free RPMI-1640 medium and incubated with 0.2 μCi of [^{3}H]24(R)25-$(OH)_2D_3$ (22 Ci/mmol) in 10 ml of serum-free RPMI-1640 medium for 1 min at 37°C in a humidified atmosphere of 5 % CO_2 in air. The reactions were terminated by adding two volumes of chloroform:methanol (1:1) to the cells and medium. To determine the structure of the metabolites of 24(R)25-$(OH)_2D_3$, 370 μg of 24(R)25-$(OH)_2D_3$ were incubated with HL-60 cells (2.8 x 10^9cells) in 3 liters of serum-free RPMI-1640 medium at 37°C for 60 min, and then the metabolites were extracted with two volumes of chloroform:methanol (1:1).

<u>Separation and purification of the metabolites by column chromatography</u>
The chloroform phase was evaporated and the residue was dried by ethanol azeotrope. The chloroform extracts were chromatographed on a 1.5 x 25 cm Sephadex LH-20 column eluted with 120 ml of chloroform:n-hexane (65:35). And then the column eluted with chloroform:n-hexane:methanol (75:23:2). The 24(R)25-$(OH)_2D_3$ metabolite fraction (32-120 ml) from the Sephadex LH-20 column was concentrated and then subjected to HPLC equipped with a 4.6 x 250 mm Zorbax Sil column, and eluted with 17 % isopropanol in n hexane. The eluate was continuously monitored by ultraviolet absorption at 310 nm, and the ultraviolet absorbing metabolite 1 and metabolite 2 eluted just before the elution position of 1α,24,25-$(OH)_3D_3$ and immediately after the elution position of 1α,24,25-$(OH)_3D_3$, respectively. The metabolite 1 and metabolite 2 were further purified by HPLC using a Zorbax Sil column eluted with 3 % methanol in dichloromethane. The metabolite 1 was eluted just before the elution position of 1α,25-$(OH)_2D_3$ and the metabolite 2 was eluted immediately after the elution position of 1α,25-$(OH)_2D_3$. According to these isolation and purification procedures, the total amounts of 1.92 μg of metabolite 1 and 8.07 μg of metabolite 2 were calculated, assuming an ε of 27,000 cm^{-1}.

Vitamin D. A Chemical, Biochemical and Clinical Update

Metabolism of [^{3}H]24(R)25-$(OH)_2D_3$ in HL-60 cells

HL-60 cells metabolized [^{3}H]24(R)25-$(OH)_2D_3$ to two new radioactive metabolites of 24(R)25-$(OH)_2D_3$, metabolite 1 and metabolite 2. We investigated the time-course experiment of [^{3}H]24(R)25-$(OH)_2D_3$ metabolism by HL-60 cells. Using 9.1×10^{-9} M of [^{3}H]24(R)25-$(OH)_2D_3$ as a substrate, the production of metabolite 1 and metabolite 2 reached the maximum level within 60 sec. and thereafter as time went by the metabolites were gradually decreasing till 60 min; this demonstrates that 24(R)25-$(OH)_2D_3$ metabolism by HL-60 cells was remarkably rapid.

Identification of the two metabolites of 24(R)25-$(OH)_2D_3$ by HL-60 cells

The structural confirmation of the two metabolites of 24(R)25-$(OH)_2D_3$ was carried out as follows: (i) anomalous chromatographic behavior of the isolated two metabolites resembled to that of 5(Z)- and 5(E)-19-nor-10-keto-25-OH-D_3 [5,6]; (ii) metabolite 1 and metabolite 2 isomerized each other; (iii) the ultraviolet absorption spectra of the two metabolites display both the unique chromophore with λmax=310 nm; (iv) the mass spectral fragmentation patterns of the two isolated metabolites give both m/e 418, 400, 375, 357, 341, 315, 273, 177 and 133; (v) the molecular weight of 418 and the loss of C_3H_7 fragments are mass spectral characteristics unique to 19-nor-10-ketovitamin D_3 derivatives [5,6]; (vi) the FT-IR spectra of the metabolite 1 and metabolite 2 indicate the very intense absorbance at 1680 cm^{-1} and 1678 cm^{-1}, respectively, which is indicative of carbonyl group conjugated double bonds. From these results, the structure of the two isolated metabolites of 24(R)25-$(OH)_2D_3$ was unequivocally determined to be 5(Z)-19-nor-10-keto-24(R)25-$(OH)_2D_3$ and 5(E)-19-nor-10-keto-24(R)25-$(OH)_2D_3$, respectively.

These unique metabolites, 5(Z)- and 5(E)-19-nor-10-keto-24(R)25-$(OH)_2D_3$, did not bind specifically to the chick intestinal 3.7 S receptor for 1α,25-$(OH)_2D_3$. It therefore appears that the 19-nor-10-keto-24(R)25-$(OH)_2D_3$ is in a pathway of vitamin D_3 metabolic deactivation. The biological and physiological functions of the two new metabolites still remain undefined. However, 19-nor-10-keto-24(R)25-$(OH)_2D_3$ metabolites may possibly show some biological activities other than calcium metabolism, because they are produced in cancer cells.

REFERENCES

1. Abe, E., Miyaura, C., Sakagami, H., Takeda, M., Konno, K., Yamazaki, T., Yoshiki, S., and Suda, T. (1981) Proc. Natl. Acad. Sci. 78, 4990-4994
2. Tanaka, H., Abe, E., Miyaura, C., Shiina, Y., and Suda, T. (1983) Biochem. Biophys. Res. Commun. 117, 86-92
3. Matsui, T., Nakao, Y., Kobayashi, N., Kishihara, M., Ishizuka, S., Watanabe, S., and Fujita, T. (1984) Int. J. Cancer 33, 193-202
4. Yoshida, M., Ishizuka, S., and Hoshi, A. (1984) J. Pharm. Dyn. 7, 962-968
5. Ishizuka, S., Norman, A.W. Matsui, T., Nakao, Y., Fujita, T., Okabe, T., Fujisawa, M., Watanabe, J., and Takaku, F. submitted to J. Biol. Chem.
6. Napoli, J.L., Sommerfeld, J.L., Pramanik, B.C., Gardner, R., Sherry, A.D., Partridge, J.J., Uskokovic, M.R., and Horst, R.L. (1983) Biochemistry 22, 3636-3640

EVIDENCE FOR A MONOCYTE-DEPENDENT MECHANISM IN THE CALCITRIOL INHIBITORY EFFECT ON LYMPHOCYTE PROLIFERATION

M. T. Zarrabeitia, J. A. Riancho, M. C. Farinas, V. Rodriguez-Valverde, J. Gonzalez-Macias
Dept. of Internal Medicine and Section of Rheumatology. National Hospital "M. Valdecilla". School of Medicine. Santander. Spain.

Specific calcitriol receptors have been identified in peripheral blood monocytes and in activated lymphocytes (1,2). A calcitriol inhibitory effect on lymphocyte proliferation, related to interleukin-2 (IL-2) production has been recently reported (2,3). This study was undertaken to asses the relation of monocytes and prostaglandins (PG) to this effect.

MATERIALS AND METHODS

Peripheral blood mononuclear cells (PBMC) were isolated from normal adult volunteers by Ficoll-Hypaque gradient. Cells were cultured in medium RPMI 1640 supplemented with antibiotics, L-glutamine and 10% fetal calf serum in microtiter plates at a concentration of $1x10^6$ cells/ml. Phytohemagglutinin was added at a final concentration of 1 µg/ml. Calcitriol was solubilized in ethanol and added to culture medium as a 0.025% solution in concentrations ranging from 10^{-10} to 10^{-8}M. Control PBMC were cultured in 0.025% ethanol. After cultured under 5% CO_2 at 37 C for 72 h, cell proliferation was evaluated by H^3-thymidine incorporation. The effect of calcitriol was studied under several culture conditions: 1) standard medium; 2) IL-2 addition; 3) monocyte depletion (by adherence to Petri dishes); 4) monocyte depletion plus IL-2 addition; 5) indomethacin addition (125 ng/ml); 6) indomethacin and IL-2 addition. Each study was performed with PBMC obtained from four donors and assayed in triplicate. Statistical analysis of the data was performed by paired t test.

RESULTS AND DISCUSSION

The results are summarized in the table below. They are expressed as percent of cell proliferation under standard culture conditions (mean±S.D.)

Calcitriol concentration

Culture	Without calcitriol	10^{-10}M	10^{-9}M	10^{-8}M
Standard medium	100	80.6±8.4	53.0±16.1	26.2±5.6
with IL-2	94.4±11.7	102.4±20.1	-	60.5±21.2
Monocytes depleted	92.1±9.2	96.3±19.6	80.5±11.8	64.9±7.8
Monocytes depleted+IL-2	96.3±7.4	91.2±15.8	-	73.5±8.7
with Indometacin	118.6±19,6	-	89.8±14.2	-
Indometacin + IL-2	113.2±22.3	-	96.6±7.3	-

Vitamin D. A Chemical, Biochemical and Clinical Update

The results obtained showed that calcitriol decreased lymphocyte proliferation in a dose dependent fashion ($p < 0.05$ at 10^{-10}M, $p < 0.01$ at 10^{-9} and 10^{-8} M vs. control). The addition of IL-2 significantly diminished the effect of calcitriol (102.4 $\pm$ 20.1 vs. 80.6 $\pm$8.4% at 10^{-10} M, $p < 0.05$; 60.5$\pm$21.2 vs. 26.2$\pm$5.6% at 10^{-8} M, $p < 0.05$). These findings corroborate that the diminution of IL-2 previously reported (2) has a role in the inhibitory effect of calcitriol on the cell proliferation.

Although monocyte depletion did not modify cell proliferation under standard conditions, it partly decreased the calcitriol inhibitory effect. This was statistically significant when 10^{-9} and 10^{-8}M calcitriol concentration cultures were evaluated ($P < 0.01$). This was not so for 10^{-10}M cultures.

Monocytes are known to produce several substances, including PG, which modulate the lymphocytic response to mitogens. In order to evaluate the possible intervention of PG we studied the inhibitory effect of calcitriol in the presence of indomethacin. Although indomethacin addition to standard medium does not significantly modify cell proliferation, we found that it decreased the inhibitory effect of calcitriol (89.8$\pm$14.2 vs. 53.0 $\pm$16.1%, $p < 0.01$).

These results suggest that IL-2, monocytes and PG play a role in the effect of calcitriol on lymphocyte proliferation. IL-2 addition, however, did not modify the calcitriol effect in monocyte-depleted cultures (91.2 $\pm$19.8 vs.96.3$\pm$ 19.6% at 10^{-10}M, N.S.; 73.5$\pm$ 8.7 vs.64.9$\pm$7.8% at 10^{-8}M,N.S) nor in indomethacin added cultures (96.6$\pm$7.3 vs. 89.8$\pm$14.2% at 10^{-9}M,N.S.).

These findings suggest that monocytes and PG exert their actions through IL-2 inhibition, since an additive effect would be expected if they acted independently. Therefore, we propose the following speculative sequence of events:

calcitriol → [monocytes] → ↑PG → [lymphocytes] → ↓IL-2 → ↓proliferation.

REFERENCES:

1.Bhalla, A. K., E. P. Amento, T. L. Clemens, M. F. Holick, and S. M. Krane. (1983). J. Clin. Endocrinol. Metab. 57:1308-1310.

2.Provvedini, D. M., C. D. Tsoukas, L. J. Deftos, and S. C. Manolagas. 1983. Science (Wash. DC) 221:1181-1183.

3.Lemire, J. M.;J.S. Adams; R. Sakai and S. C. Jordan (1984). J. Clin. Invest. 74:657-661.

Biological Actions for $24,25(OH)_2D_3$

1,25-DIHYDROXYVITAMIN D_3 INHIBTS LYMPHOCYTE PROLIFERATION AND ANTIGEN INDUCED LYMPHOCYTE ACTIVATION

A.K.BHALLA, E.P.AMENTO, B. SEROG and L.H. GLIMCHER
Department of Medicine, Harvard Medical School and the Arthritis Unit, Massachusetts General Hospital, Boston, MA 02114

A potential immunoregulatory role for 1,25-$(OH)_2D_3$ has been suggested by the finding of specific 1,25-$(OH)_2D_3$ receptors in activated but not resting T lymphocytes (1,2). The activation of normal T lymphocytes requires monocytes and the monocyte factor interleukin 1. Following activation, T lymphocytes produce interleukin 2 (IL2) which is necessary for their proliferation. Since 1,25-$(OH)_2D_3$ receptors are present in monocytes, any observed effects of 1,25-$(OH)_2D_3$ on lymphocyte proliferation may be indirect through an initial interaction with monocytes. To minimise complicating interactions inherent in heterogenous cell population, we examined the regulatory action of 1,25-$(OH)_2D_3$ on lymphocyte proliferation and activation using a murine model of cloned autoreactive and antigen-specific T cell hybridomas (3). These hybridomas secretive but do not utilise IL2 when 1) co-cultured with I-region matched stimulator (TA3) cells in the presence of the appropriate foreign antigen or 2) cultured with lectins or anti-Thy-1 monoclonal antibody (anti-Thy-1Ab) in the absence of TA3 cells.

Methods

An allogeneic mixed lymphocyte response (MLR) was generated by culturing irradiated BALB/C spleen cells with B10.A lymph node responder cells. After 5d in culture lymphocyte proliferation was determined by $[^3H]$ thymidine uptake. Antigen-primed lymph node cells (LNC) were co-cultured with antigen and with or without 1,25-$(OH)_2D_3$ and lymphocyte proliferation determined (4). T cell hybridomas were activated either with TA3 cells, lectins, or anti-Thy-1 Ab for 24 h in the presence or absence of vitamin D_3 metabolites or dexamethasone. Supernatants were collected and assayed for IL2 content using CTLL cells (4). T cell hybridoma were pretreated for 24 h with 100 nM 1,25-$(OH)_2D_3$, washed, and activated with varying numbers of TA3 cells. Similarly pretreated TA3 cells were used to activate untreated T cell hybridomas. Cytosols from T cell hybridomas and TA3 cells were examined for 1,25-$(OH)_2D_3$ receptors (1,4).

Results

In heterogenous cell populations 1,25-$(OH)_2D_3$ inhibited both an allogeneic MLR and the proliferation of antigen-primed LNC. This effect was apparent at physiological concentrations (0.01-0.1 nM) of 1,25-$(OH)_2D_3$. 25-$(OH)_2D_3$ was ineffective except at 100 nM. 1,25-$(OH)_2D_3$ inhibited IL2 production by several T cell hybridomas. In 1% FCS inhibition of IL2 production was seen at 0.1 nM 1,25-$(OH)_2D_3$ (Table I). No inhibition was seen with 25-$(OH)_2D_3$.

The inhibition of T cell hybridoma activation and IL2 production by 1,25-$(OH)_2D_3$ could be overcome by increasing the number of stimulator cells. 1,25-$(OH)_2D_3$ failed to inhibit T cell activation by lectins or anti-Thy-1 Ab. In contrast, dexamethasone inhibited the activation of T cell hybridoma by anti-Thy-1 Ab (Table II).

Vitamin D. A Chemical, Biochemical and Clinical Update

Table I

Activation of T Cell Hybridomas is Inhibited by 1,25-$(OH)_2D_3$

1,25-$(OH)_2D_3$ [nM]	[^{3}H] Thymidine Incorporation by CTLL cells (cpm) T cell Hybridoma	
	E8.A1	HEL C10
Control	59,713 ± 14,180	47,260 ± 2,129
0.1	24,517 ± 2,139	42,717 ± 2,070
1	23,324 ± 3,440	36,303 ± 5,016
10	19,184 ± 2,303	31,470 ± 4,271

Table II

Dexamethasone Inhibits T cell Activation by Anti-Thy-1 Ab

Dexamethasone [nM]	CTLL[^{3}H] Thymidine Incorporation (cpm)
0	254,255 ± 10,747
1	161,688 ± 14,635
10	141,059 ± 8,268
100	99,273 ± 8,299

To ascertain that 1,25-$(OH)_2D_3$ acted directly on T cell hybridomas pretreatment studies were done. The ability of T cell hybridomas pretreated with 1,25-$(OH)_2D_3$ to produce IL2 in the presence of untreated TA3 cells was diminished. Pretreated TA3 cells did not inhibit the activation of untreated T cell hybridomas. Furthermore, receptors for 1,25-$(OH)_2D_3$ were present only in T cell hybridomas but not in TA3 cells.

Discussion

Physiological concentrations of 1,25-$(OH)_2D_3$ inhibited lymphocyte proliferation as well as the activation of and IL2 production by T cell hybridomas. 1,25-$(OH)_2D_3$ acted directly on the T cell hybridomas and not on the stimulator TA3 cells as shown by pretreatment data. 1,25-$(OH)_2D_3$ unlike dexamethasone failed to inhibit IL2 production when the T cell hybridomas were activated by lectins or anti-Thy-1 Ab. Inhibition of T cell activation could be overcome by increasing the number of stimulator cells present. These results suggest that one mechanism by which 1,25-$(OH)_2D_3$ inhibits IL2 production might be through interference with early signals of T cell activation by antigen.

References

1. Bhalla A.K., Amento, E.P., Clemens, T.L., Holick, M.F. and Krane,S.M. (1983) J. Clin. Endocrinol. Metab. 57, 1308-1310.

2. Provvedini, D.M., Tsoukas, C.D., Manalagas, S.C. and Deftos, L.J. (1983). Science. 221, 1181 - 1183.

3. Glimcher, L.H. and Shevach, E.M. (1982) J. Exp. Med. 156, 640-645.

4. Bhalla, A.K., Amento, E.P., Serog, B. and Glimcher, LH. (1984) J. Immunol. 133 1748-1754.

Cultured Human Skin Fibroblasts from Patients with Psoriasis do not Repond to Physiological Doses of 1,25-$(OH)_2$-D_3

J.A. MacLaughlin, W.Gange, D. Taylor, M.F.Holick
Vitamin D Laboratory Massachusetts General Hospital, Boston, MA 02114

Introduction

Incubation of normal human fibroblasts with physiologic concentrations of 1,25-$(OH)_2$-D_3, increases cell generation time.[1] If the binding of 1,25-$(OH)_2$-D_3 to its receptor is defective, as reported in patients with a vitamin D-dependent rickets Type II, the 1,25-$(OH)_2$-D_3 does not increase cell generation time.[1] Inasmuchas 1,25-$(OH)_2$-D_3 has been shown to modulate epidermal cell differentiation in mouse[2] and human[3] keratinocytes, and increase the cell generation time in human fibroblasts, we wondered whether in a hyperproliferative disease, viz. psoriasis, the dermal fibroblasts would respond in a dose-dependent fash-fashion to 1,25-$(OH)_2$-D_3.

Patients and Methods

Dermal fibroblasts were obtained from 4mm punch biopsies taken from normal and psoriatic volunters. The culturing and harvesting of the fibroblasts was performed as previously described.[1] Normal and psoriatic fibroblasts were plated in triplicate into 35mm dishes in DMEM containing 5% fetal calf serum. After 12-15 hours, the media was removed and replaced with either 1,25-$(OH)_2$-D_3 (10^{-10} to 10^{-4}M) or EtOH (0.1%) alone. At several different times (0,1,2,3,5,7,9,days), the cells were trypsinized, centrifuged, resuspended and counted by hemacytometer. Methodology for sucrose density gradient centrifugation, DNA-cellulose chromatography and Scatchard analysis were performed as previously described.[1]

Results

As demonstrated in figure 1, normal fibroblasts incubated with a physiologic dose of 1,25-$(OH)_2$-D_3 (10^{-8}M) demonstrated a 30% increase in cell generation time in comparison to the normal EtOH controls. Incubation with 10^{-6}, 10^{-5} and 10^{-4}M 1,25-$(OH)_2$-D_3 increased the cell generation time by 59%, 72% and 92% respectively. There was no significant difference in cell generation time between the EtOH controls and fibroblasts incubated with 10^{-10}M 1,25-$(OH)_2D_3$. In comparison, the psoriatic fibroblasts incubated with 10^{-10} 10^{-8} and 10^{-6} did not show a significant difference from their EtOH controls. However, Incubation with 10^{-5} and 10^{-4}M increased the cell generation time approximately 40-50% and 95% respectively. To determine whether the response of psoriatic fibroblasts to 1,25-$(OH)_2$-D_3 was due to the absence of a receptor or to a defective receptor, we analyzed and compared the cytosols of normal and psoriatic fibroblasts with sucrose density centrifugation, Scatchard analysis and DNA cellulose chromatography. A 3.7S macromolecule (1,25-$(OH)_2$-D_3 receptor) was present in both normal and psoriatic fibroblasts. Scatchard analysis produced a Kd of 0.01nM and 0.014nM and an n_{max} of 22 and 20 fmoles of 1,25-$(OH)_2$-D_3 bound per mg of protein, for normal and psoriatic fibroblasts respectively. DNA cellulose chromatography provided evidence that both the 1,25-$(OH)_2$-D_3 receptors bind to chromatin comparable to that found in normal cells.

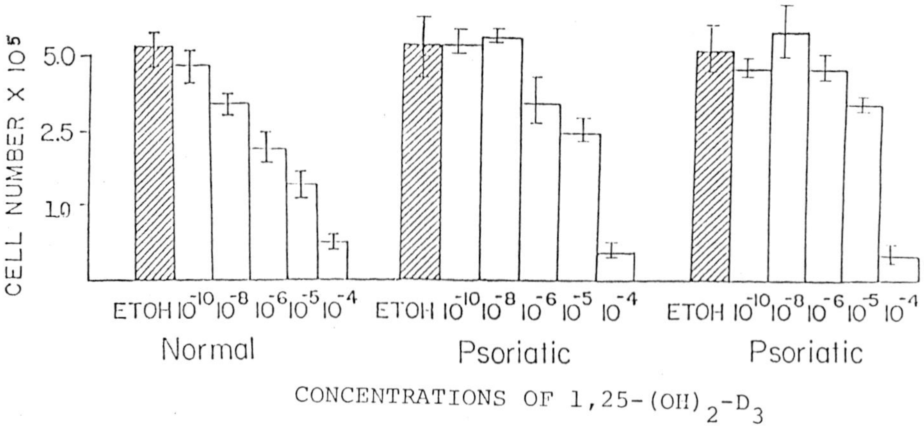

CONCLUSION

The present studies demonstrate the presence of a receptor for $1,25-(OH)_2-D_3$ in psoriatic fibroblasts with properties resembling those of normal fibroblasts. $1,25-(OH_2)-[^3H]D_3$ binding activity of the psoriatic fibroblasts was saturable and displayed similar affinity and specificity characteristics sedimented at 3.7S on linear 4-20% sucrose gradient, and eluted from DNA-cellulose at 0.22M KCl. Evidence that normal human skin fibroblasts are responsive to $1,25-(OH)_2-D_3$ in vitro was provided by our laboratory[1] and showed amarked increase on cell generation time. The same report demonstrated the absence of a specific saturable binding of $1,25-(OH)_2-D_3$ in keratinocytes and fibroblasts from a patient with DDR-II indicating that these cells lack an effective cytosolic receptor protein for the hormone or a receptor protein that is defective in binding $1,25-(OH)_2-D_3$. Correlated with this defect is perhaps the expression of an analogous genetic defect in other target tissues, such as intestine and bone which could explain the extreme resistance in these individuals to vitamin D. We now present another human skin fibroblast that by all parameters tested has a receptor which binds $1,25-(OH)_2-D_3$ and yet no biologic manifestation(increase in cell generation time) is observed with concentrations of $1,25-(OH)_2-D_3$ that markedly effect normal fibroblasts(10^{-8} and 10^{-6}).

REFERENCES

1. Clemens, T.L., J.A. Adams, N.Horiuchi, B.Gilchrest, H.Cho, Y. Tsuchiya, N.Matsuo, T. Suda and M.F.Holick(1983) J.Clin Endo and Met. 56, pp. 824-830.
2. Hosomi, J., J. Honsol, E. Abe, T. Suda, and T. Kuroki(1983) Endocrinology, 3, pp. 1950-1957.
3. Smith, E., M.F. Holick. Vitamin D 6th Workshop (1985).

This report was funded in part by NIH grants AM27334 & AG02918

HISTOLOGIC RESPONSE TO 24,25 $(OH)_2$ VITAMIN D IN RENAL OSTEO-DYSTROPHY.

D.J. SHERRARD, S.M. OTT, D.L. ANDRESS AND J.W. COBURN,
From the Veterans Administration Medical Center, Seattle, Washington, and West Los Angeles, California.

Introduction:
The 24,25 dihydroxy metabolite of vitamin D remains controversial. It is produced normally by kidney cells and bone cells(1). Tissue culture studies have shown that it enhances bone growth in the femur(2). Animal studies are conflicting with data from avian species(3), man(4) and rodents(5) supporting its role as necessary for some aspect of bone or body growth. On the other hand a large number of negative reports(7-9) imply that this substance has no physiologic activity.

In the midst of these arguments we set out to see if 24,25-$(OH)_2$ vitamin D (24,25 D) would be of beneficial in the refractory osteomalacia seen in patients with renal failure. At the time these studies were initiated it was not widely recognized that this lesion could be caused by aluminum. It soon became clear that aluminum, when present in high concentrations in the water, could cause this disorder (in this situation aluminum entered patients by a parenteral route via the dialysate water). Only later was it appreciated that aluminum also passed across the gastro-intestinal tract could therefore reach toxic levels as a result of oral administration as well(10).

Thus, these patients were not evaluated at the outset for aluminum toxicity. The presence of aluminum has been subsequently determined histochemically. In this report we describe the histologic and clinical response of 32 patients treated for one or more years with 24,25 D who had biopsies at the end of their treatment.

Methods

Patient selection:
There was no attempt to "select" patients for this study in a formal sense. Patients were largely referred to centers in 4 locations (Minnesota, Hawaii, California, Washington State). Although most of the patients came from the geographic area of the center, many did not. Patients were referred because of bone pain and/or fractures which usually had failed to respond to calcitriol and/or parathyroidectomy. Approximately twice as many patients entered the study as completed it.

Vitamin D. A Chemical, Biochemical and Clinical Update

Clinical status:
Patient's symptoms were classified according to the "global disability scale" described by Coburn(11). Changes noted in this report are based on that scale.

Parathyroid hormone (PTH) status:
Patients were referred from a wide geographic area. Although one PTH assay was used most commonly, at least 3 other assays were also used. For these assays the degree of elevation associated with hyperparathyroid bone disease in uremia is generally known. It is not clear, however, what lesser degrees of elevation or "normal" levels mean for these different assays. Therefore, in this report the values are reported as "elevated" if they are in the range for the assay usually associated with hyperparathyroidism. Values below that range are reported as "not elevated".

Bone histology:
Bones were assessed by quantitative histomorphometric techniques as previously described(10). Most patients took time spaced tetracycline labels for determination of dynamic bone parameters. Aluminum staining was also done and patients classified as having minimal (<0.5mm of surface aluminum/mm^2 tissue area), mild (0.5-1.0mm), moderate (1.0-2.0mm) or heavy (>2.0mm) aluminum staining.

Major changes in bone histology were seen in osteoid area and bone dynamic parameters in addition to aluminum. Osteoid area was noted as changed only if the change was greater than 5%. Bone mineralization rate was noted as changed if values changed from one group (low, normal or high bone mineralization) to another. Aluminum levels were noted as changed if patients moved from one group to another and changed more than 0.4mm of surface/mm^2 of tissue area.

Drug dosage:
These patients were treated with 10 to 20 micrograms of 24,25 D daily. Eighteen patients received 0.25 to 0.50 micrograms of 1,25 $(OH)_2$ vitamin D as well, while 14 were treated only with 24,25 D.

Results

Patient characteristics at onset of study:

Parathyroid status:
Five patients had values in the range associated with hyperparathyroid bone disease in renal patients (all >7 times the upper limit for normals). Eleven patients had values in the usual range for dialysis patients (all 1.0 to 3.5 times the upper limit for normal subjects). Sixteen had values in the normal range for patients without renal disease. As all these assays measured the carboxy-terminal end of the PTH molecule, these values are abnormally distributed to the low side for patients on dialysis.

Bone histology:
Osteoid area was normal (<10% of total bone area) in 5 subjects, moderately increased (10-15% of total bone area) in 8 subjects, markedly increased (15-30%) in 14 subjects and very markedly increased (>30%) in 5 subjects. Mineral apposition rate was low in 16 patients and increased in 2.

Aluminum staining:
Seven patients had minimal, 7 mild, 1 moderate, and 7 heavy aluminum staining.

Changes with treatment:

Symptoms:
Eighteen of the 32 patients improved their activity during treatment. Since limitation of activity due to pain was the major complaint, this represented a clear improvement.

Bone histology:
Sixteen of 32 patients showed improvement mineralization (decreased >5 percent of osteoid), or mineral apposition or both. Twelve patients had no significant change in osteoid area and four showed histologic deterioration. Curiously, one patient whose osteoid area increased healed several previously unhealing fractures and improved symptomatically as well. Another patient whose osteoid area did not change also healed one fracture that had previously remained unhealed for one year. She too improved symptomatically. Both of these patients had improved bone mineralization rates.

Aluminum staining:
Histochemical stain revealed that aluminum deposits decreased in 6 patients, did not change in 18 patients, and worsened in 7 patients. One patient had iron present in large amounts, preventing accurate quantitation of aluminum change. PTH values did not change during the year of treatment.

Clinical, biochemical, pathological relationships:
Of the 16 patients whose bone improved 9 had PTH values less than the upper limit for a normal population, 7 PTH values between 1.0 and 3.5 times the upper limit of normal and one patient had a very high value (8.5 times upper limit of normal).

In these 16 patients who improved histologically 4 increased, 4 decreased and 7 did not change aluminum deposits as determined by staining. The one patient with heavy iron deposits whose aluminum change could not be measured also showed histologic improvement.

Curiously, 11 of 12 patients who did not have "elevated" PTH levels responded symptomatically to 24,25 D alone. Ten of these had histologic improvement as well. The one patient whose bone histology failed to improve was one of the two mentioned above who demonstrated fracture healing despite the lack of histologic improvement.

Discussion:

Though a large number of patients are described the highly selected, heterogeneous nature of the group makes these observations anecdotal. None of the changes described are statistically significant. Whether they are clinically significant is another matter. At the time this study was started patients with "refractory osteomalacia(5)" or "fracturing osteodystrophy(12)" became progressively disabled and died. No therapy was helpful. It seems unlikely that half of such a group would have improved. Thus, we are of the opinion that 24,25 benefitted a proportion of these patients that would probably have done well otherwise.

Before 24,25 D could be studied in a controlled fashion, however, it became clear that this form of renal osteodystrophy was caused by aluminum(10). Chelation therapy (using deferoxamine) has proven highly effective(13) and clearly is the treatment of choice for aluminum related bone disease in these patients.

What then can be said for the role of 24,25? While this report does not substantiate benefit in any known conditions, it does appear that this agent had a beneficial effect on the bones of many of these patients. Reductions in excess osteoid, improved bone mineralization rate and decreased bone pain occurred in half the subjects.

At the doses used one would expect plasma levels several times normal(14). Whether such high levels would be required in other situations is not known. Nonetheless, no toxicity was noted in patients treated.

In addition to the effects noted in regards to the bones 2 other observations were made about this agent's activities. First, several patients with hypercalcemia became normocalcemic. In some patients 1,25 $(OH)_2$ vitamin D could be given at doses that had caused hypercalcemia prior to the use of 24,25 D.

The other effect noted related to a bizarre arthralgia seen in some long term renal dialysis patients. This arthralgia is characterized by severe stiffness in all joints and, may be severely debilitating. Five patients noted dramatic relief of this arthralgia with 24,25 D. On stopping the drug stiffness recurred. In 2 patients the drug was re-instituted and the stiffness again disappeared.

Thus, there may be several potential uses for this interesting agent. Further study is certainly indicated.

Acknowledgement:
Supported by Funds from the General Medical Research Service of the Veterans Administration.

References:

1. Howard, G.A., Turner, R.T., Sherrard, D.J., Baylink, D.J. (1981) J Biol Chem 256:7738-7740.
2. Howard, G.A., Carlson, C.A., Baylink, D.J. (1982) in Factors and Mechanisms Influencing Bone Growth, Dixon AD, Sarnat BG, eds Alan R. Liss, Inc. New York, pp. 259-274.
3. Henry, H.L., Norman, A.W. (1978) Science 210:835-837.
4. Bordier, P.A., Rasmussen, H., Marie, P., et al (1978) J Clin Endocrinol Metab 46:284-294.
5. Hodsman, A.B., Wong, E.G.C., Sherrard, D.J., et al (1983) Am J Med 74:407-414.
6. Goodman, W.G., Baylink, D.J., Sherrard, D.J. (1984) Calcif Tissue Int 36:206-213.
7. Ameenuddin, S., Sunde, M., DeLuca., et al (1982) Science 217:452-453.
8. Muirhead, N., Adami, S., Sandler, L.M., et al (1982) Quart J Med 51:427-444.
9. Evans, R.A., Hills, E., Wong,S.Y.P., et al (1982) in Vitamin D: Chemical, Biochemical and Clinical Endocrinology of Calcium Metabolism. Norman, A.W., et al, eds, Walter de Gruyter, New York, pp. 835-840.

10. Ott, S.M., Maloney, N.A., Coburn, J.W., et al (1982) N Engl J Med 307:709-714.
11. Coburn, J.W., Brickman, A.J., Sherrard D.J., et al (1977) Proc Europ Dial Transpl Assoc 14:442-450.
12. Parkinson, I.S., Ward, M.K., Feest, T.G., et al (1979) Lancet 1:406-409.
13. Ott, S.M., Andress, D.L., Nebeker, H.G., et al (1985) Kidney Int (in press).
14. Popovtzer, M., Personal communication.

BIOLOGICAL ACTIVITY AND CELLULAR BINDING OF $1,25(OH)_2D_3$ AND $24,25(OH)_2D_3$ IN CULTURED GROWTH PLATE RABBIT CHONDROCYTES IN A DIVIDING AND A STATIONNARY PHASE.

A. ULMANN, M. BRAMI, M.F. DUMONTIER, J. BOURGUIGNON, L. TSAGRIS and M.T. CORVOL,
INSERM U90 and U30, Hôpital Necker-Enfants Malades, 161, rue de Sèvres, 75730 Paris Cedex 15, FRANCE.

Introduction :

Since the first report by Coon (1) showing that articular chondrocytes can be grown in culture, several laboratories have been using the technique to study the morphological and metabolic behaviour of articular cartilage cells in vitro (2). It has been also shown that chondrocytes from growth plate (GP) cartilage of long bones behave differently in culture than AR chondrocytes (3). GP chondrocytes grow as small chains of cells forming multilayered colonies.

Vitamin D metabolites have previously been demonstrated to be metabolized in articular cells (4) and some of them have a biological effect on these cells in vitro (5,6). The aim of the present work was to study the morphological aspects of GP cells in culture and their responsiveness to vitamin D metabolites ($1,25(OH)_2D_3$ and $24,25(OH)_2D_3$) at different stages of the culture.

Materials ans methods

Chondrocyte culture

Growth plate chondrocytes from prepubertal Fauve de Bourgogne rabbits (300 g BW) were grown in culture, as described previously (3). GP chondrocytes in culture divide until day 18-20 of the culture forming multilayered colonies. In the present work, cells were studied at two successive stages : 1) on days 12 to 15, corresponding to the dividing phase, and 2) on days 17 to 21 when cells stop dividing and reach a stationnary phase.

Vitamin D. A Chemical, Biochemical and Clinical Update

Morphological study

During the culture, living cells were observed under phase contrast microscope. In some cases, cells were fixed with 1.6 % glutaraldehyde and colored with Toluidine Blue.

For the electron microscopic study, the cells were fixed, stained and embedded in situ in the culture flask, as described by Brinkley (7) and by Eguchi and Okada (8).

Morphometric study

Ultrathin cellular sections were observed at a x 13500 final magnification. Using a Digiplan (Kontron), cell diameter and surface, as well as the surface of the different cytoplasmic components were evaluated. A comparative study was performed between the dividing and stationnary culture stages.

Measurement of ^{35}S.sulfate incorporation into proteoglycans in response to vitamin D metabolites

Growth-plate chondrocytes at the two culture stages were used after 20 h incubation in serum-free medium.

$1,25(OH)_2D_3$ or $24,25(OH)_2D_3$ were added to cell culture medium at concentrations ranging from 1 pM to 1 nM which were previously shown to be effective on cultured chondrocytes (5). The culture medium used was sulfate-free Dulbecco's medium to which was added 1.5 uCi $^{35}SO_4$-sulfate per ml. The incubation lasted for 20 h at 37°C under 10 % CO_2 in air. Proteoglycans from the cellular layers and from the medium were then extracted separately with 3 M guanidinium hydrochloride and purified after dialysis against 8 M urea and chromatographied on DEAE cellulose column, as previously described (9). Sulfated proteoglycan subunits were eluted in 2 M NaCl. Aliquots were counted in Biofluor.

The sum of the ^{35}S.sulfate incorporation measured in the medium and in the cell layer was determined. Results, calculated as total dpm per ug DNA, are expressed as a percentage over the control value (in the absence of vitamin D metabolites).

An aliquot of the cell pellet was used to measure DNA as described by Burton (13).

DNA polymerase activities

At each of the two phases of the culture, some of the GP cells were deprived of FCS during 20 hours, and treated with $1,25(OH)_2D_3$ or $24,25(OH)_2 D_3$ (1 to 100 pM) in the presence of 1 % FCS during an additive 24 hour period. Cells were then scrapped off the culture flasks (4 identical flasks per group) and homogenized in 50 mM Tris HCl buffer pH 7.4 containing 10 mM KCl, 1 mM MgCl and 0.33 M Sucrose. The subcellular polymerase extracts were then prepared according to Bertazzoni et al (10). DNA polymerase activities were evaluated by incorporation of $[^3H]$-TMP into acid-insoluble material (freshly DNAse-activated calf thymus DNA). Results are expressed as dpm of $[^3H]$-TMP incorporated per mg protein and per hour.

Preparation of total cellular protein extracts

Cells were deprived of FCS during 20 hours and carefully rinsed, prior to be scrapped off the culture flasks in 0.4 M KCl buffer (50 mM Tris HCl, 0.1 mM EDTA, 5 mM Dithiothreitol, pH 7.4, 10 mM sodium molybdate pH 7.4) and containing 0.5 % Triton X-100. Cells were vortexed and sonicated at low speed during 3 x 10 sec. Total cytosolic and nuclear cellular proteins were recovered after centrifugation at 100 000 g during 60 min. Protein concentration in cellular extract ranged between 0.2 and 2.00 mg per ml (usually 0.9 mg/ml).

Assay of steroid receptors in cellular extracts

Aliquots of cellular extracts (0.5 ml) were incubated with either $[^3H]$ $1,25(OH)_2D_3$ spec. act. 140 Ci/mmole, or $[^3H]24,25(OH)_2 D_3$ spec. act. 168 Ci/mmole, (0.1 to 10 nM) with and without 500-fold molar excess of the corresponding unlabeled steroid for 3 h at room temperature. Bound and free labeled steroid were separated using dextran charcoal and evaluated by counting an aliquot in a Packard Tricarb with 45 % efficiency of tritium. Maximal binding capacity and K_D were calculated according to the method of Scatchard (11).

Protein concentration was determined by the method of Lowry et al. (12) using BSA as standard. DNA was measured according to Burton (13). In some experiments, bound and free steroid fractions were layered on the top of a 5-20 % surrose gradient made in the same 0.4 M KCl buffer. Samples were sedimented in SW 56 rotor at 300 000 g for 16 hours. Gradients were collected from the top in 8-drop fractions into counting vials.

Results and discussion

Morphological aspect of GP chondrocytes in primary culture

The morphological caracteristics of GP chondrocytes in culture are in favor of an intense metabolic activity with an important endoplasmic reticulum, numerous ribosomes and a well developped Golgi apparatus. All cells are embedded in an extracellular matrix composed of proteoglycan granules and sometimes a thin network of collagen fibers. Some changes appear during the cycle. During the 23 days of primary culture of GP chondrocytes one can observe a progressive increase in cellular diameter: 9 to 13 microns from day 3 to day 10, 22 ± 5 microns between days 10 and 18 and 36 ± 8 microns on day 23 of the culture. In addition to this increase in cellular size, there is a modification in the surface of each cytoplasmic component with the age of the culture. Since intracellular lipid droplets decrease with the age of the culture, there is a progressive increase in the surface of endoplasmic reticulum and Golgi apparatus as correlated with the total cell surface. Finally, between days 19 to 23, GP chondrocytes contain numerous lysosomal vacuoles (Table 1).

Table 1 : Cytoplasmic component surface area (in % of total cell surface)

Cultured Growth Plate Chondrocytes	n	Lipids	E.R.	Golgi	Mitochondria	Lysosomes
Division Phase (15 days)	100	2.3	7.7	11.4	2.2	0.6
Hypertrophic Phase (21 days)	125	0.05	7.7	10.4	1.6	1.8

These morphological changes are in agreement with the in vivo observations made by Brighton et al (14) who studied the intracellular composition of chondrocytes from the resting zone to the hypertrophic zone of growth plate cartilage in rats. Therefore, in our culture condition, GP chondrocytes seem to present a progressive morphological maturation resembling the in vivo growth plate chondrocytes maturation.

Metabolic activities and effect of vitamin D metabolites during culture cycle

In cultured GP chondrocytes, three succesive stages of metabolic activities were observed : 1) A resting phase when cells stick to the bottom of the flask. They do not synthetize DNA neither they synthetize sulfated proteoglycans. This stage corresponds to the first 8 days in culture, 2) A division phase with high DNA polymerase activities and low proteoglycan synthesis from day 8 to 15, 3) A stationnary phase with low DNA polymerase activities and high proteoglycan synthesis between days 18 and 23.

The biological effect of $1,25(OH)_2D_3$ and $24,25(OH)_2D_3$ was studied at the second and the third stages of GP cell maturation.

For each metabolite, results depended on the culture stage : $1,25(OH)_2D_3$ (400 pmole/10 ml flask) increases DNA polymerase activities in dividing GP cells but not in mature GP chondrocytes. In such mature cells, $1,25(OH)_2D_3$ (400 pmole/10 ml flask) inhibits DNA polymerase activities. $24,25(OH)_2D_3$ (1 pmole to 1 nmole/10 ml flask) has no effect on DNA synthesis at any stage of cell maturation. In contrast, both 1,25(OH) D and $24,25(OH)_2D_3$ (400 pmole/10 ml flask) enhance sulfate incorporation into proteoglycans synthetized by mature cells. This last result has also previously been observed in cultured articular chondrocytes (5).

These observations suggest that $1,25(OH)_2D_3$ and $24,25(OH)_2D_3$ have different effects on cartilage cells depending on their degree of maturation or differenciation.

Specific binding of vitamin D_3 metabolites to GP chondrocyte proteins at the two successive culture stages

Total 0.4 M KCl chondrocyte proteins were extracted at the dividing and stationnary culture phases, and incubated in the presence of tritiated metabolites.

Both dividing and mature GP chondrocytes contain a macromolecule which specifically binds $[^3H]$-1,25$(OH)_2D_3$. Scatchard analysis shows a single class of high affinity binding sites with a K_D of 0.12 nM and a number of sites which does not vary during culture cycle. $[^3H]$24,25$(OH)_2D_3$ binds to a macromolecule with a K_D of 0.29 nM in 12-15 days GP chondrocytes. In mature chondrocytes, K_D of the binding decreases to 0.14 nM, a value not significantly different to that for $[^3H]$1,25$(OH)_2D_3$ in GP chondrocytes at the same culture stage (0.11 nM). In the meantime, a significant decrease in maximal binding capacity for $[^3H]$24,25$(OH)_2D_3$ is observed. In preliminary experiments, we were not able to demonstrate by sucrose gradient technique a binding site for $[^3H]$24,25$(OH)_2D_3$ in dividing GP chondrocytes although unlabeled 24,25$(OH)_2D_3$ partially displaced $[^3H]$1,25 $(OH)_2D_3$ from its binding site in the same cells. In contrast,in mature cells, sucrose gradient experiments indicated well individualized binding peaks for both sterols.

In conclusion, prepubertal rabbit growth plate chondrocytes in culture present a progressive morphological and metabolic maturation during the 23 days of primary culture which resembles the in vivo chondrocytes maturation of growth plate cartilage. The cells possess binding sites for both 1,25$(OH)_2D_3$ and 24,25$(OH)_2D_3$. However, during the culture cycle, modifications in the characteristics of 24,24(Oh) D occur, while 1,25 $(OH)_2D_3$ binding appears unmodified. Such modifications could be related to the observed morphological and metabolic changes during cell maturation.

REFERENCES

1. Coon H.G. (1966) Proc. Nat. Acad. Sci. 55-66.
2. Green Jr W.T. (1971) Clin. Orthop. Relat. Res. 75: 248.
3. Corvol M.T., Dumontier M.F., Rappaport R. (1975) Biomedicine 23: 103.
4. Garabedian M., Bailly Du Bois M. Corvol M.T., Pezant E., Balsan S. (1978) Endocrinology 102: 1262.
5. Corvol M.T., Dumontier M.F., Garabedian M., Rappaport R. (1978) Endocrinology 102: 1269.
6. Harmand M.F., Thomasset M., Rouais F., Ducassou D. (1984) J. of Cellular Physiology 119: 359-365.
7. Brinkley B.R., Murphy P., Richardson L.C. (1979) J. Cell. Biol. 35: 279.
8. Eguchi G., Okada T.S. (1971) Develop Growth and Differentiation 12: 297.
9. Corvol M.T., Dumontier M.F., Rappaport R., Guyda H., Posner B. (1978) Acta Endocrinologica, 89: 263.
10. Bertazzoni U, Scovassi A, Brum G. (1977) Eur. J. Biochem 81: 237.
11. Scatchard G. (1949) An. NY Acad. Sci. 51: 660.
12. Lowry O.H., Rosebrough N.J., Farr A.L., Randall R.J. (1951) J. Biol. Chem. 265.
13. Burton K. (1956) Biochem J. 62: 315.
14. Brighton C.T., Sugioka Y., Hunt R.M. (1973) J. Bone Joint Surg. 55A: 771.
15. Corvol M.T., Ulmann A., Garabedian M. (1980) FEBS Lett. 116: 273.

$24,25(OH)_2D_3$ ATTENUATES THE CALCEMIC EFFECT OF $1,25(OH)_2D_3$ IN RATS WITH REDUCED RENAL MASS

D. Rubinger, T. Cojocaru and M.M. Popovtzer

Hadassah University Hospital, Jerusalem, Israel

$1,25(OH)_2D_3$, the active metabolite of vitamin D, exerts a calcemic action by stimulating intestinal transport and skeletal mobilization of calcium. In contrast, clinical and experimental evidence suggests that $24,25(OH)_2D_3$ may enhance bone mineralization with no change in the serum calcium level (1,2). Furthermore, $24,25(OH)_2D_3$ has been shown to attenuate the calcemic effect of $1,25(OH)_2D_3$ and to suppress the hypercalcemia induced by acute bilateral nephrectomy in rats (3). The present study was undertaken to evaluate the effect of administration of $24,25(OH)_2D_3$ and its interaction with $1,25(OH)_2D_3$ in rats with reduced renal mass, respective to plasma calcium and urinary calcium excretion.

Experimental Groups and Methods

The experiments were performed in white adult male rats of the Hebrew University strain. The rats underwent 5/6 nephrectomy in two stages and were studied 4 weeks after surgery. The animals were placed in metabolic cages, were fed standard pruina chow and drank tap water ad libitum. The experimental animals were divided in 4 groups: 1) rats receiving a daily s.c. injection of 54 ng $1,25(OH)_2D_3$ in 1-2 propanediol; 2) rats receiving a daily s.c. injection of 54 ng $24,25(OH)_2D_3$ in 1-2 propanediol; 3) rats receiving both $1,25(OH)_2D_3$ and $24,25(OH)_2D_3$ in a daily s.c. injection of 54 ng each; and 4) control animals receiving the vehicle only. Urine output was measured at 24 h intervals for 8 consecutive days. Blood was drawn at the beginning of the experiment and after 1, 4 and 8 days of vitamin D metabolite administration. The results are presented as mean$\pm$SE and the statistical evaluation was performed using the student's paired and unpaired t-test.

Results

The plasma calcium level and the urinary calcium excretion of the control and experimental animals after 24 h of administration of the various vitamin D metabolites are shown in Table 1. The serum calcium level in the $24,25(OH)_2D_3$-treated group was similar to the level of the control animals. A mild calcemic and calciuric effect was seen in both $1,25(OH)_2D_3$ and combined $1,25(OH)_2D_3$+$24,25(OH)_2D_3$-treated groups.

Table 1

Exp. Groups	Control	$1,25(OH)_2D_3$	$24,25(OH)_2D_3$	$1,25+24,25(OH)_2D_3$
P_{Ca} (μE/ml)	5.16±0.09	5.48±0.07*	5.08±0.12	5.57±0.17
$U_{Ca}V$ (μE/24h)	11.01±1.59	22.5±4.62**	13.93±3.18	28.63±9.22***

*p<0.02 vs. control; **p<0.05 vs. control; ***p<0.001 vs. control.

Vitamin D. A Chemical, Biochemical and Clinical Update

Table 2 shows the plasma calcium and the urinary calcium excretion in the 4 groups of animals after 5 days of treatment with vitamin D metabolites. Plasma calcium remained unchanged in the control and 24,25(OH)$_2$D$_3$ group. In contrast, significant hypercalcemia was seen in the 1,25(OH)$_2$D$_3$ and in the combined therapy group. Plasma calcium, however, was lower in the combined therapy animals as compared to the 1,25(OH)$_2$D$_3$ group.

Table 2

Exp. Groups	Control	1,25(OH)$_2$D$_3$	24,25(OH)$_2$D$_3$	1,25+24,25(OH)$_2$D$_3$
P_{Ca} (μEq/ml)	5.33±0.06	7.13±0.32*,a	5.22±0.05	6.27±0.15*
$U_{Ca}V$ (μE/24h)	39.55±10.28	426.62±49*	52.2±10.1	379.2±28.45*

*p<0.001 vs. control; a 1,25(OH)$_2$D$_3$ vs. 1,25+24,25(OH)$_2$D$_3$, p<0.05.

After 8 days of administration, hypercalcemia persisted in both 1,25(OH)$_2$D$_3$ and 1,25(OH)$_2$D$_3$+24,25(OH)$_2$D$_3$ groups. Again, plasma calcium was lower in animals receiving both metabolites than in those receiving 1,25(OH)$_2$D$_3$ alone. The hypercalcemia in 1,25(OH)$_2$D$_3$ and combined therapy groups was accompanied by a similar increase in urinary calcium excretion. No change in the urinary excretion of calcium was seen in the other groups of animals. During all experimental periods, the creatinine clearance was stable in all rats. Plasma phosphate and the fractional excretion of phosphate (C_P/C_{Cr}) were not affected by the vitamin D metabolites.

Discussion

In rats with reduced renal mass, administration of 24,25(OH)$_2$D$_3$ alone was not associated with changes in plasma calcium or urinary calcium excretion. In contrast, 1,25(OH)$_2$D$_3$ and combined 1,25+24,25(OH)$_2$D$_3$ administration resulted in significant hypercalcemia and hypercalciuria. After combined administration of 1,25(OH)$_2$D$_3$ and 24,25(OH)$_2$D$_3$ to rats with reduced renal mass, plasma calcium was significantly lower than after the administration of 1,25(OH)$_2$D$_3$ alone. The urinary excretion of calcium was similar in 1,25(OH)$_2$D$_3$ and combined therapy in animals. Thus, 24,25(OH)$_2$ attenuates the calcemic affect of 1,25(OH)$_2$ in rats with a reduced nephron population, without a concimitant increase in the urinary calcium excretion. It is suggested that the attenuation of the calcemic effects of 1,25(OH)$_2$D$_3$ may result, at least partly, from a direct action of 24,25(OH)$_2$D$_3$ on the bone.

References

1. DeLuca, H.F. and Schnoes, H.K. (1976) Ann Rev. Biochem. 58:631-666.
2. Kanis, J.A., Guilland-Cunning, D., Peterson, A.D. and Russell, R.G.G. (1982) In: Vitamin D: Chemical, Biochemical and Clinical Endocrinology of Calcium Metabolism. Ed. A.W. Norman et al. de Gruyter, Berlin, pp 157-167.
3. Pavlovitch, J.H., Cournet-Witman, G., Bourdeau, A., Balsan, S., Fischer, J.A. and Heynen, G. (1981) J. Clin. Invest. 68: 803-810.

A COMPARISON OF THE RESPONSES TO 24R,25$(OH)_2D_3$ AND 1,25$(OH)_2D_3$ BY DEVELOPING SKELETAL TISSUE

D. Sömjen, Y. Weisman*, E. Berger, N. Fine, A.M. Kaye** and I. Binderman
Hard Tissues Unit and *Vitamin Research Laboratory, Ichilov Hospital, Tel Aviv 64239, and **Department of Hormone Research, The Weizmann Institute of Science, Rehovot 76100, Israel.

INTRODUCTION

Vitamin D serves as a precursor or prohormone for more polar metabolites, two of which, 1,25-dihydroxy vitamin D_3 (1,25$(OH)_2D_3$) and 24R,25 dihydroxy vitamin D_3 (24R,25$(OH)_2D_3$) are the principal mediators of the spectrum of biological responses attributed to the parent compound. There is substantial evidence that the mechanism of action of 1,25$(OH)_2D_3$ and of 24R,25$(OH)_2D_3$ is similar to that of other steroid hormones. The first step in the mechanism of action of each of these seco-steroid metabolites is interaction with its specific intracellular receptors. The tight association of the steroid-receptor complex with specific chromatin loci in the nuclei of responsive cells leads to the modulation of mRNA synthesis for specific proteins which have been shown to be involved in the biological responses of vitamin D metabolites (1).

1,25$(OH)_2D_3$ has a major role in calcium homeostasis through its effects on calcium absorption in the intestine (2-8) and on bone mineral mobilization (10-11). However, many more organs were found to have receptors for 1,25$(OH)_2D_3$ (1,9), leading to the realization that the vitamin D endocrine system extends far beyond its original classic sites of action (1). Furthermore, recent studies indicate that vitamin D metabolites are associated with cell proliferation and differentiation (1). In recent years, attention was drawn to another renal metabolite of vitamin D, 24R,25$(OH)_2D_3$, which was shown to have important roles in development of endochondral bone (12-14) and hatching of chick embryos (15). Specific receptors for this compound were identified in parathyroid gland (16), chondrocytes (17), epiphyseal growth plate (18) and limb bud mesenchymal cells (19).

In this paper we review our recent data, which support the notion that the activities of 24R,25$(OH)_2D_3$ make this metabolite a unique hormone, completely distinguishable from 1,25$(OH)_2D_3$ in regulating development of embryonic bone and possibly other tissues (20).

Vitamin D. A Chemical, Biochemical and Clinical Update

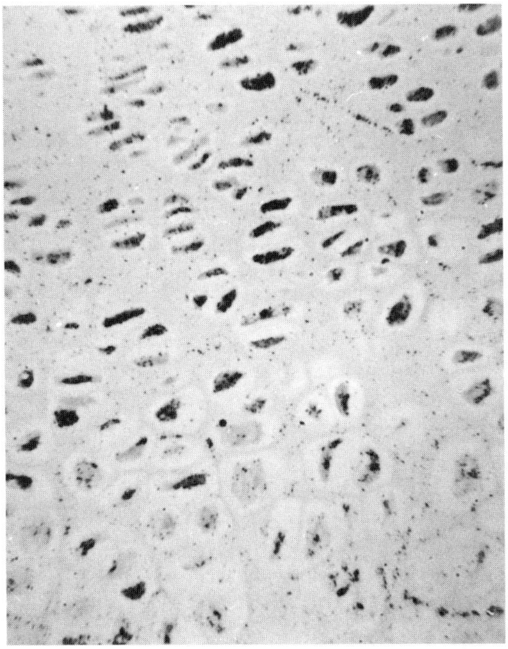

Fig. 1: Longitudinal section of proximal epiphyseal cartilage of a tibia from 4-day old vitamin D deficient rat pups incubated in MEM medium containing $[^3H]24R,25(OH)_2D_3$ (8.4 nM, 140 Ci/mmole) for 60 min. Note that radioactivity is concentrated in the nuclei and there is poor incorporation in the hypertrophic zone (bottom of figure). H & E x700.

EXPERIMENTAL SYSTEMS

Two experimental model systems were used in these studies.

a) Vitamin D depleted rats were used for *in vivo* studies. Female Wistar rats (4 weeks old) were raised in the dark on a vitamin D deficient diet containing 0.75% Ca and 0.5% P_i. They were mated with normal males to produce vitamin D depleted newborn rats (18).

b) Micro-mass cultures of embryonic chick limb bud mesenchymal cells were used for *in vitro* studies (19). These cultures are an advantageous system since they can undergo chondrogenesis within 4 days. Their differentiation and calcification may be regulated by manipulation of the growth medium (21,22). This *in vitro* system also has the advantage that no further hepatic or renal metabolism of the vitamin D metabolites can occur.

I. AUTORADIOGRAPHIC LOCALIZATION OF 24R,25$(OH)_2D_3$ RECEPTORS IN RAT TIBIAE

Localization of $[^3H]$ 24R,25$(OH)_2D_3$ by autoradiography in proximal epiphyses of the tibiae in 4 day old vitamin D depleted rats was performed as described elsewhere (23) by incubation of tibiae with $[^3H]$24R,25$(OH)_2D_3$ *in vitro*. Cytoplasmic and nuclear concentration of radioactivity was revealed in all cell layers of the epiphyseal cartilage, except for the hypertrophic cartilage zone, with the highest activity in the proliferating chondroblasts of the columnar zone (Fig. 1). Both cytoplasmic and nuclear labeling was diminished when the incubation was performed in the presence of a 100 fold molar excess of unlabeled 24R,25$(OH)_2D_3$ but not in the presence of unlabeled 25$(OH)_2D_3$ or 1,25$(OH)_2D_3$. Experiments performed with $[^3H]$ 1,25$(OH)_2D_3$ showed no specific labeling of epiphyseal cartilage (23).

These results extend previous biochemical data from our laboratory showing the existence of specific receptors for 24R,25$(OH)_2D_3$ in cartilage from rat (18) and chick (19). The localization of the receptors in the proliferating and differentiating zone of the columnar cartilage parallels the biochemical responses found to 24R,25$(OH)_2D_3$ in vitamin D depleted rats (Tables 2-4).

II. ENHANCEMENT OF PROTEIN SYNTHESIS BY 24R,25$(OH)_2D_3$ IN CHICK EMBRYO CELLS

For quantitation of protein synthesis in chick embryo limb bud cell cultures, cells were treated with 12 nM of either 25$(OH)_3$ or 1,25$(OH)_2D_3$ or 24R,25$(OH)_2D_3$ for 4 h and labeled for the last 2 h with $[^3H]$leucine (5 µCi/ml, 40-60 Ci/mmole). Protein content and radioactivity were assayed in

TABLE 1. Stimulation of $[^3H]$leucine incorporation into protein by vitamin D metabolites in chick embryo limb bud cell cultures (24). The ratios of experimental to control values are given in parenthesis.

Treatment (4 h)	$[^3H]$Leucine incorporation into protein (cpm/µg protein)	
Control	2250	
25$(OH)D_3$	3307	(1.47)
1,25$(OH)_2D_3$	2857	(1.27)
24R,25$(OH)_2D_3$	5400	(2.40)

each experiment (24). 12 nM 24R,25$(OH)_2D_3$ increases total cellular protein synthesis 2.4-fold, while the other metabolites had no significant effects (Table 1).

III. STIMULATION OF ORNITHINE DECARBOXYLASE (ODC) ACTIVITY IN RAT AND CHICK

Vitamin D depleted rats were injected i.p. with either 1,25$(OH)_2D_3$ (1.2 ng/g), 25$(OH)D_3$ (50 ng/g), 24R,25$(OH)_2D_3$ (6 ng/g) or 24S,25$(OH)_2D_3$ (6 ng/g). After 5 h, the animals were sacrificed and ODC was extracted from epiphyses or diaphyses and assayed (25). 24R,25$(OH)_2D_3$ caused a 6-fold increase in enzyme activity in epiphyses while 1,25$(OH)_2D_3$ caused a 3-fold increase in activity in diaphyses (Table 2). 24S,25$(OH)_2D_3$, the synthetic isomer, found to be inactive in other systems, did not affect ODC activity (Table 2).

Micro mass cultures of embryonic chick limb bud mesenchymal cells were incubated for 4 h with 12 nM of test metabolite (26). 24R,25$(OH)_2D_3$, but neither of the other metabolites tested, caused a 2-fold increase in ODC activity (Table 2). The increase in ODC activity in the rat epiphyses was both time and dose dependent (25).

TABLE 2. Stimulation of ODC activity by vitamin D metabolites in long bones of vitamin D depleted rats and in chick embryo limb bud cell cultures (25). Results are given as means ± SEM for $n \geq 5$. The ratios of experimental to control values are given in parenthesis. Significant differences (by t test) are indicated by *, $p < 0.005$; **, $p < 0.001$.

	ODC activity (pmol $^{14}CO_2$/h/mg protein)		
Treatment	Rat epiphyses	Rat diaphyses	Chicken limb bud cultures
Untreated	540±50	570±40	1060±150
25$(OH)D_3$	490±40 (0.90)	520±260 (0.91)	1360±290 (1.29)
1,25$(OH)_2D_3$	390±40 (0.72)	1810±410** (3.18)	830±140 (0.79)
24R,25$(OH)_2D_3$	3470±360** (6.43)	730±100 (1.27)	1890± 70* (1.79)
24S,25$(OH)_2D_3$	540 (1.00)	570 (1.00)	-

IV. STIMULATION OF DNA SYNTHESIS

Using the same protocol as for ODC induction (Section III above), vitamin D depleted rats were injected with each of 4 vitamin D metabolites. After 22 h, slices of epiphyses or diaphyses were incubated for 2 h with [^{3}H]thymidine (5 μCi/ml; 5 Ci/mmol). The rate of [^{3}H]thymidine incorporation into acid insoluble material and the content of DNA were measured (25). 24R,25(OH)$_2$D$_3$ increased DNA synthesis in epiphyses nearly 2-fold, while 1,25(OH)$_2$D$_3$ increased DNA synthesis in diaphyses 1.5-fold (Table 3).

In experiments using chick embryos, micro mass cultures of limb bud mesenchymal cells were incubated for 24 h, in the presence of vitamin D metabolites as described for ODC induction. Labeling with [^{3}H]thymidine and determination of the rate of DNA synthesis was performed as described previously (24). 24R,25(OH)$_2$D$_3$ but not the other metabolites tested caused a 2-fold increase in DNA synthesis in chondrocytes (Table 3). Increased concentration of phosphate in the medium, which by itself stimulated cell proliferation (22), did not alter the dose dependent effect (24) of vitamin D metabolites on DNA synthesis.

TABLE 3. Stimulation of DNA synthesis (25) by vitamin D metabolites in long bones of vitamin D depleted rats (26) and in chick embryo limb bud cell cultures. Results are given as means ±SEM for n≥3. The ratios of experimental to control values are given in parenthesis. Significant differences (by T test) are indicated by *, p<0.01; **, p<0.005.

	[^{3}H]thymidine incorporation into DNA (cpm/μg DNA)		
Treatment	Rat epiphyses	Rat diaphyses	Chicken limb bud cultures
Untreated	46±7	98±8	376±41
25(OH)$_2$D$_3$	-	-	259±59 (0.69)
1,25(OH)$_2$D$_3$	45±6 (0.97)	147±20* (1.50)	306±47 (0.81)
24R,25(OH)$_2$D$_3$	85±9** (1.85)	91±8 (0.90)	824±59* (2.19)
24S,25(OH)$_2$D$_3$	48 (1.01)	98 (1.00)	-

V. STIMULATION OF CREATINE KINASE (CK) ACTIVITY IN RAT AND CHICK

Vitamin D depleted rats were treated according to the protocol described for DNA synthesis. 24 h after injection, the soluble CK from epiphyses and diaphyses was assayed (26). 24R,25$(OH)_2D_3$ caused a 2.6-fold increase in CK activity in epiphyses, while 1,25$(OH)_2D_3$ caused a 1.5-fold increase in enzyme activity in diaphyses (Table 4).

In *in vitro* experiments, micro mass cultures of embryonic chick limb bud mesenchymal cells were incubated according to the method described for DNA synthesis. The enzyme was extracted, and assayed as described previously (27). CK was increased in this culture (2.4-fold) only by 24R,25$(OH)_2D_3$ (Table 4). The synthetic isomer 24S,25$(OH)_2D_3$ had no effect on enzyme activity (Table 4). When limb-bud mesenchymal cells were induced to differentiate into fibroblasts (22), they lost their response to 24R,25$(OH)_2D_3$ (27), as well as their specific 24R,25$(OH)_2D_3$ binding activity (19).

CK isozymes from both *in vivo* and *in vitro* experiments were separated by DEAE-cellulose chromatography (28). The iso-

TABLE 4. Stimulation of CKBB activity by vitamin D metabolites in long bones of vitamin D depleted rats (26) and in chick embryo limb bud cell cultures (27) The ratios of experimental to control values are given in parenthesis. Significant differences (by t test) are indicated by *, $p<0.01$; **, $p<0.005$.

	Creatine kinase activity (µmoles/min/mg protein)		
Treatment (24 h)	Rat epiphyses	Rat diaphyses	Chicken limb bud cultures
Control	4.4±0.2	4.5±0.1	0.10±0.05
25$(OH)_2D_3$	-	-	0.11±0.01 (0.10)
1,25$(OH)_2D_3$	4.9±0.1 (1.10)	7.0±0.6* (1.51)	0.14±0.03 (1.40)
24R,25$(OH)_2D_3$	11.4±1.2** (2.60)	4.8±0.3 (1.00)	0.24±0.04* (2.40)
24S,25$(OH)_2D_3$	-	-	0.15±0.01 (1.50)

form in both systems, or hormonal treatment, was the brain type isozyme of creatine kinase (CKBB) (26,27). The increase in CKBB activity in both systems was time and dose dependent (26,27) as well as dependent on protein synthesis.

GENERAL CONSIDERATIONS AND CONCLUSION

The localization of receptors for vitamin D metabolites shows cell type specificity (29,30). Receptors for $24R,25(OH)_2D_3$ are localized in developing chondroblasts while receptors for $1,25(OH)_2D_3$ are found in developing osteoblasts.

Biochemical and autoradiographic analysis of the specific binding of $24R,25(OH)_2D_3$ demonstrate specific receptors for this hormone in rat epiphyseal cartilage (18) and in chondrocytes from chick embryo limb bud cell cultures (19). The localization of binding sites in the proliferating and differentiating cells of the columnar zone, parallels the results of biochemical studies (9,24,25). In bone, specific receptors for $1,25(OH)_2D_3$ were demonstrated biochemically (29), and by autoradiography, but no receptor for $24R,25(OH)_2D_3$ was found (9). Therefore, we suggest that $24R,25(OH)_2D_3$ has a specific role in the development of the epiphyseal growth plate. Other laboratories have also found that $24R,25(OH)_2D_3$ has a role in bone development (13,14,31), and is capable of stimulating DNA and proteoglycan synthesis in cultured rat and rabbit chondrocytes (32).

We have presented evidence that $24R,25(OH)_2D_3$ can stimulate protein and DNA synthesis both <u>in vivo</u> and <u>in vitro</u> (24,25), and induce specific enzymes such as ODC (33,34) and CKBB (35) in chondrocytes, while $1,25(OH)_2D_3$ stimulates these parameters in bone cells in the diaphyses region. Both CK and ODC are involved in cell growth and proliferation (33-37). Unlike intestinal calcium binding protein, which is stimulated specifically by $1,25(OH)_2D_3$ (38), no specific $24R,25(OH)_2D_3$ dependent calcium binding protein has yet been found.

Induction of either ODC or CKBB are not unique responses to vitamin D metabolites since many hormones can stimulate these enzymes in their responsive tissues (39-41). The finding that CKBB is induced by vitamin D metabolites in cells having the appropriate receptors provides a convenient and sensitive marker for vitamin D action. CK is necessary for ATP regeneration (37), and the activity of the BB isozyme is correlated with ATP utilizing processes (37), such as ion transport and cell division, two processes in which vitamin D metabolites are apparently involved.

$24R,25(OH)_2D_3$ may be converted to $1,24,25(OH)_2D_3$ (42) in vitamin D depleted animals and theoretically this could be the active metabolite affecting epiphyseal cartilage.

However, there is no evidence that 24R,25(OH)$_2$D$_3$ is further metabolized to 1,24,25(OH)$_2$D$_3$ in limb bud mesenchyme cells. Even if 1,24,25(OH)$_2$D$_3$ produced in vivo is found to be active it still would show the absolute requirement for the presence of OH in the C-24 position in order for the metabolite to be active in epiphyseal cartilage.

We have recently found (20) that during postnatal development of rat kidney, specific receptors for 24R,25(OH)$_2$D$_3$ are predominant from 7-15 days after birth, while receptors to 1,25(OH)$_2$D$_3$ predominate in mature rat kidneys (from 3 weeks after birth). Moreover, the specific interaction between vitamin D metabolites and their appropriate receptors in kidney cells at different stages of development leads to the stimulation of CKBB activity (20).

The observation that chondroblasts respond to 24R,25(OH)$_2$D$_3$ while bone cells respond to 1,25(OH)$_2$D$_3$ suggests specific roles for each metabolite in developing bone, in which 24R,25(OH)$_2$D$_3$ is more active in the cartilage stage of early development.

We therefore conclude that 24R,25(OH)$_2$D$_3$ has an essential role in the development of vitamin D responsive tissues such as bone and kidney.

REFERENCES

1. Henry, H.L., and Norman, A.W. (1984) Ann. Rev. Nutr. 4, 493-520.
2. Tsai, H.C., and Norman, A.W. (1973) J. Biol. Chem. 248, 5697-5675.
3. Lawson, D.E.M., and Wilson, P.W. (1974) Biochem. J. 144, 573-583.
4. Zerwekh, J.E., Lindell, T.J., and Haussler, M.R. (1976) J. Biol. Chem. 251, 2388-2394.
5. Fraser, D.R. (1980) Physiol. Rev. 60, 551-613.
6. Wasserman, R.H., and Taylor, A.N. (1966) Science 152, 791-793.
7. Haussler, M., Nagode, L., and Rassmussen, H. (1970) Nature (London) 228, 1199-1305.
8. Wilson, P., and Lawson, D. (1978) Biochem. J. 173, 627-631.
9. DeLuca, H.F. (1980) Nutr. Rev. 38, 163-193.
10. Raisz, L.G., Trummel, C.L., Holick, M.F., and DeLuca, H.F. (1972) Science 176, 1146-1148.
11. Brommage, R., Neuman, W.F. (1979) Am. J. Physiol. 237, E113-E120.
12. Ornoy, A., Goodwin, D., Noff, D., and Edelstein, S. (1978) Nature (London) 276, 517-519.
13. Endo, H., Kiyoki, M., Kawashima, K., Naruchi, T., and Hashomoto, Y. (1980) Nature (London) 286, 262-265.

14. Malluche, H.H., Henry, H., Meyer-Saballek, W., Sherman, S., Massry, S.G., Norman, A.W. (1980) Am. J. Physiol. 238, E494-E496.
15. Henry, H.L., and Norman, A.W. (1978) Science 201, 835-837.
16. Merke, J., and Norman, A.W. (1981) Biochem. Biophys. Res. Commun. 100, 551-558.
17. Corval, M.M., Ulmann, A., and Garabedian, M. (1980) FEBS Lett. 116, 273-276.
18. Sömjen, D., Sömjen, G.J., Weisman, Y. and Binderman, I. (1982) Biochem. J. 204, 31-36.
19. Sömjen, D., Sömjen, G.J., Harell, A., Mechanic, G.L. and Binderman, I. (1982) Biochem. Biophys. Res. Commun. 106, 644-651.
20. Sömjen, D., Weisman, Y., Kaye, A.M., Earon, Y., and Binderman, I. (1985) Proceedings of the VI International Workshop on Calcified Tissue, Kiryat Anavim (in press).
21. Osdoby, P., and Caplan, A.I. (1976) Develop. Biol. 52, 283-299.
22. Binderman, I., Greene, R.M., and Pennypacker, J.P. (1979) Science 206, 222-225.
23. Fine, N., Binderman, I., Sömjen, D., Earon, Y., Edelstein, S., and Weisman, Y. (1985) Metab. Bone Dis. and Rel. Res. (in press).
24. Binderman, I., and Sömjen, D. (1984) Endocrinology 115, 430-432.
25. Sömjen, D., Binderman, I., and Weisman, Y. (1983) Biochem. J. 214, 293-298.
26. Sömjen, D., Weisman, Y., Binderman, I., and Kaye, A.M. (1984) Biochem. J. 219, 1037-1041.
27. Sömjen, D., Kaye, A.M., and Binderman, I. (1984) FEBS Lett. 167, 281-284.
28. Kaye, A.M., Reiss, N., Shaer, A., Sluyser, M., Iacobelli, S., Amroch, D., and Soffer, Y. (1981) J. Steroid Biochem. 15, 69-75.
29. Manolagas, S.C., Taylor, C.M., and Anderson, D.C. (1979) J. Endocrinol. 80, 35-40.
30. Narbaitz, R., Stumpf, W.E., Sar, M., Huang, S., and DeLuca, H.F. (1983) Calcif. Tissue Int. 35, 177-182.
31. Zusman, I., Hirsch, B.E., Edelstein, S., and Ornoy, A. (1981) Acta Anat. 111, 343-351.
32. Corval, M., Dumontier, M.F., Garabedian, M. and Rapport, R. (1978) Endocrinology 102, 1269-1274.
33. Russell, D., and Snyder, S.H. (1968) Proc. Natl. Acad. Sci. USA 60, 1420-1427.
34. Pegg, A.E., and Williams-Ashman, H.G. (1968) Biochem. J. 108, 533-539.
35. Reiss, N.A., and Kaye, A.M. (1981) J. Biol. Chem. 256, 1899-1904.
36. Höltta, E. and Jänne, J. (1972) FEBS Lett. 23, 117-121.
37. Kenyon, G.L., and Reed, G.H. (1983) Adv. Enzymol. 54, 367-426.

38. Haussler, M.R., and McCain, T.A. (1977) N. Engl. J. Med. 297, 974-983.
39. Morris, D.R., and Fillingame, R.H. (1974) Ann. Rev. Biochem. 43, 303-325.
40. Bachrach, U. (1984) Cell Biochem. Function 2, 6-10.
41. Kaye, A.M., Reiss, N.A., Weisman, Y., Binderman, I. and Sömjen, D. (1985) in Cellular Bioenergetics and Compartmentalization, (Brautbar, N., ed.) Plenum Press Corp., New York (in press).
42. Holick, M.F., Kleiner-Bossaller, A., Schones, H.K., Kasten, P.M., Boyle, I.T., and Deluca, H.F. (1973) J. Biol. Chem. 248, 6691-6696.

1a,25-DIHYDROXYVITAMIN D_3 AND 24R,25-DIHYDROXYVITAMIN D_3 ARE BOTH NECESSARY FOR BONE COMPOSITION OF INTRAMUSCULAR IMPLANTS OF DEMINERALIZED MATRIX IN RATS

S. Vukičević, B. Krempien, Č. Bagi, G. Vujičić and A. Stavljenić

Departments of Anatomy and Biochemistry, School of Medicine, University of Zagreb, Department of Analytical Chemistry, Faculty of Sciences, University of Zagreb, Yugoslavia and Institute of Pathology, University of Heidelberg, West Germany

Introduction:

The importance of 1,25-dihydroxyvitamin D_3 (1,25-DHCC) for bone remodelling and growth is well established. But two views exist in regard to the biological importance of 24R,25-dihydroxyvitamin D_3 (24R,25-DHCC). One view regards 24R,25-DHCC, in the presence of 1,25-DHCC, as essential for certain vitamin D dependent biological responces (1,2,3,4). The second view is based on experiments using synthesized 24R,24-difluoro-25 hydroxyvitamin D_3 (24R,24-F_2-25-OHD_3) (5,6). It was concluded that there is no evidence that 24-hydroxylation of vitamin D plays an important physiological role (7,8,9).

Material and Methods:

Marrow-free cylinders of 0.6 N HCl demineralized diaphyseal cortical bone matrix, prepared from 110 adult Fisher male donors rats were implanted in the anterior abdominal muscles of each of 130 recipient rats. Recipient rats were divided into four randomized groups of 30-40 male rats and received daily injections of either propan-1,2-diol as a vehicle, or vitamin D metabolites as follows: 30 ng 24R,25-DHCC, 10 ng 1a,25-DHCC, 10 ng 1a,25-DHCC and 30 ng 24R,25-DHCC in combination. At intervals ranging from 5 to 35 days after implantation the rats were sacrificed by exanguination under ether anesthesia and the implants were removed, freed of adhering tissue and then frozen in liquid nitrogen.

For alkaline phosphatase activity determination, 80-90 cylinders per group were lyophilized and homogenized as described previously (10). For bone mineral determinations the hydrolizates were analyzed for total calcium, phosphorus, magnesium, zinc and strontium by Inductively coupled plasma atomic emission spectrometry with a ARL-35000 C spectrometer (11). Bone carbonate measurements were provided by injecting liberated CO_2 directly into the ICP-AE spectrometer where the carbon was measured and time dependent CO_2 liberating diagram was obtained. The measurement provided data on the amount of bone CO_3 with the detection limit of 0.2 µg/mg tissue. For the statistical analysis the student's two-tailed t-test for nonpaired variates was used.

Results:

Alkaline phosphatase activity of implants was significantly increased ($p<0.001$) in animals treated with 1a,25-DHCC and 1a,25-DHCC+24R,25-DHCC between 18th and 23 day after implantation. In rats treated with 1a,25-DHCC the carbonate content steadily increased starting with the 14 day after implantation and reached 2.82 per cent d.w. on the 35 experimental day. The values for 1a,25-DHCC treated animals were significantly higher when compared to the controls. On the contrary, 24R,25-DHCC treated rats had significantly lower carbonate content (0.9%, $p<0.001$) of intramuscular implants. Time necessary for obtaining maximal CO_2 values was significantly delayed in 1a,25-DHCC treated animals ($p<0.01$). Calcium content increased gradually in all groups of animals being higher in 1a,25-DHCC treated rats only at day 10 ($p<0.01$). Phosphorus increased rapidly in parallel with the calcium values. In the 1a,25-DHCC treated rats the phosphorus content was lower throughout the experimental period ($p<0.01$).

Vitamin D. A Chemical, Biochemical and Clinical Update

Even in maximally advanced implants, when more than 85 per cent of the matrix was replaced, Ca/P molar ratio in 1a,25-DHCC treated animals exhibits values much higher than in other experimental groups. Magnesium content incresed also gradually, with high values in 1a,25-DHCC treated rats throughout the the experiment ($p<0.001$). The zinc values did not increase over time as did the other meqsured elements. They rose 4 fold between 14 and 20 day and then fell again to the previous values. When plotted against time the diagrams for both the values for zinc and the activity distribution of the measured enzymes have a similar appearance. The strontium content of implants in all animals gradually increased with time, showing an equal pattern of appearance in all treated groups of rats.

Conclusions:

We have shown that 1a,25-DHCC and 24R,25-DHCC are jointly needed for preserving normal bone composition during early mineralization. 1a,25-DHCC applied alone altered the composition of bone implants by stimulating incorporation of magnesium, increasing bone carbonate and calcium values, and decreasing the phosphorus content. Additionaly our results reveal that 1a,25-DHCC as well as 24R,25-DHCC have antagonistic effects on the bone carbonate content. Different time intervals in the appearance of peak values of liberated CO_2 could indicate a carbonate differently bound to the bone mineral in 1a,25-DHCC treated animals. Our results suggest that increased carbonate in 1a,25.DHCC treated rats probably occupy phosphate sites: as indicated by decreased phosphate content, increased carbonate content, and the Ca/P molar ratios. Magnesium content was extremely high in animals treated with 1a,25-DHCC. It therefore seems that 1a,25-DHCC alone could alter the nature of the early mineral deposited. On the other side, alternative effects of 24R,25-DHCC on the bone, opposite to 1,25-DHCC, clearly exist, and could be important factors in the protection of bone from different agents, as well as for the nature of early mineral deposited.

References:

1. Henry,H.L., Taylor,A.N.,Norman,A.W. (1977) J. Nutr. 107, 1918-1926.
2. Ornoy,A.,Goodwin,D.,Noff,D.,Edelstein,S. (1978) Nature 276, 517-519.
3. Norman,A.W.,Henry,H.L.,Malluche,H.H. (1980) Life Sci. 27, 229-237.
4. Malluche,H.H.,Henry,H.L.,Meyer-Sabellek,W.,Sherman,D.,Massry,S.G.,Norman,A.W. (1980) Am. J. Physiol. 238, E494-E498.
5. Kobayashi,Y.,Taguchi,T.,Terada,T.,Oshida,J.,Morisaki,M.,Ikekawa,N. (1979) Tetrahed. Lett. 22, 2023-2026.
6. Yamada,S., Ohmari,M., Takayama,H. (1979) Tetrahed. Lett. 21, 1859-1962.
7. Jarnagin,K.,Brommage,R.,DeLuca,H.F.,Yamada,S.,Takayama,H. (1983) Am. J. Physiol. 244, E290 E297.
8. Brommage,R.,Jarnagin,K.,DeLuca,H.F.,Yamada,S.,Takayama,H. (1983) Am. J. Physiol. 244, E298-E304.
9. Parfitt,A.M.,Mathews,C.H.E.,Brommage,R.,Jarnagin,K.,DeLuca,H.F. (1984) J. Clin. Invest. 73, 576-586.
10. Vukičević,S.,Stavljenić,A,Bagi, Č.,Vujičić,G.,Kračun,I.,Vinter,I. (1985). Clin. Orthop. 195, in press.
11. Barnes,R.M. (1984) Biol. Trace Element Res. 6, 93-103.

STUDY ON THE BIOLOGICAL ACTION OF 24R,25$(OH)_2D_3$
- HYPOCALCEMIC EFFECT IN RATS -

H. Orimo, Department of Geriatrics, Faculty of Medicine, University of Tokyo, Hongo, Tokyo, Japan.

Introduction:

Since the physiological role of 24R,25$(OH)_2D_3$ is still controversial, we have investigated the role of 24R,25$(OH)_2D_3$ in the regulation of serum Ca in rats with normal and abnormal Ca metabolism.

Materials and Methods:

Exp. 1. Male Wistar rats of 7 weeks old were divided into the following two groups (10 animals per each group):

i) control group in which only vehicle was orally administered.

ii) K-DR (24R,25$(OH)_2D_3$ of Kureha, Japan), 200μg/kg, treated group.

Blood samples were taken before and at 24 hours after treatment for the analysis of serum Ca.

Exp. 2. Male Wistar rats of 7 weeks old pretreated with 3mg/kg of V-D_3 for 7 days were divided into the following 2 groups. (6 - 8 animals per each group):

i) control group as in Exp. 1.

ii) K-DR, 200μg/kg, treated group

Blood samples were taken before, at 24 and 36 hours after treatment for the analysis of serum Ca.

Exp. 3. Thyroparathyroidectomized male Wistar rats (TPTx rats of 7 weeks old were divided into the following 4 groups (10 animals per each group):

i)	1α$(OH)D_3$ 150μg/kg treated group	(control group)
ii)	"	+K-DR 50μg/kg treated group
iii)	"	+K-DR 200μg/kg "
iv)	"	+K-DR 800μg/kg "

Blood samples were taken before, at 12, 24 and 36 hours after treatment for the analysis of serum Ca.

Results:

1. K-DR caused no changes in serum Ca in normal rats.

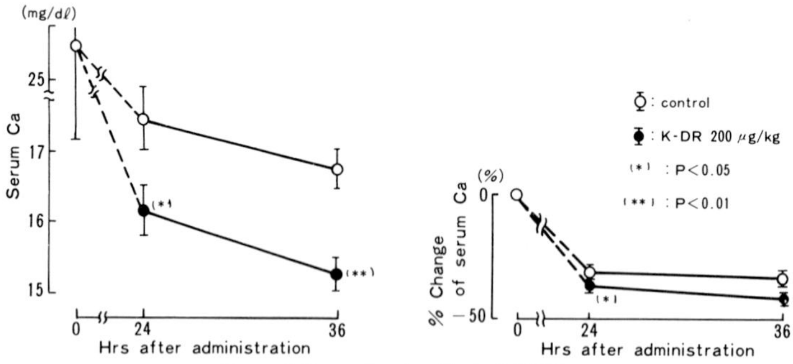

Figure 1 Hypocalcemic effect of K-DR in V-D_3 treated rats

Vitamin D. A Chemical, Biochemical and Clinical Update

2. Serum Ca levels at 24 and 36 hours in the control group treated with vitamin D_3 were 17.5±0.4mg/dl and 16.8±0.3 mg/dl respectively, while those of the group treated with K-DR were 16.2±0.3mg/dl ($P<0.05$) and 15.3±0.2mg/dl ($P<0.01$) respectively.
3. In the TPTx rats, serum Ca levels at 12 and 24 hours in the control group were 6.6±0.2mg/dl and 9.2±0.2mg/dl respectively, while those of the rats treated with K-DR were 6.1±0.2mg/dl ($P<0.05$) and 8.4±0.3mg/dl ($P<0.01$) respectively.

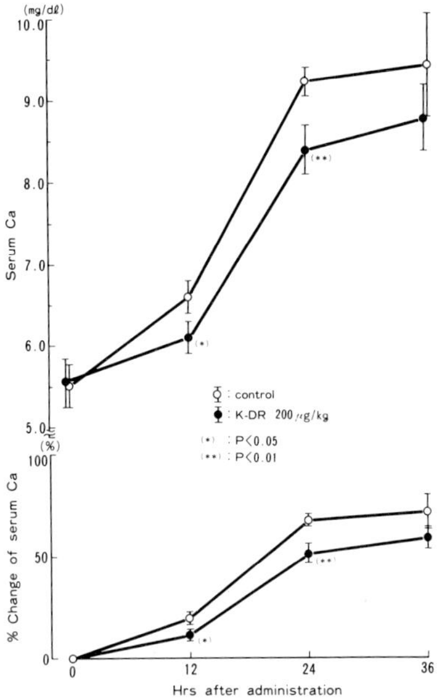

Figure 2 Effect of K-DR on serum Ca in TPTx rats treated with $1\alpha(OH)D_3$

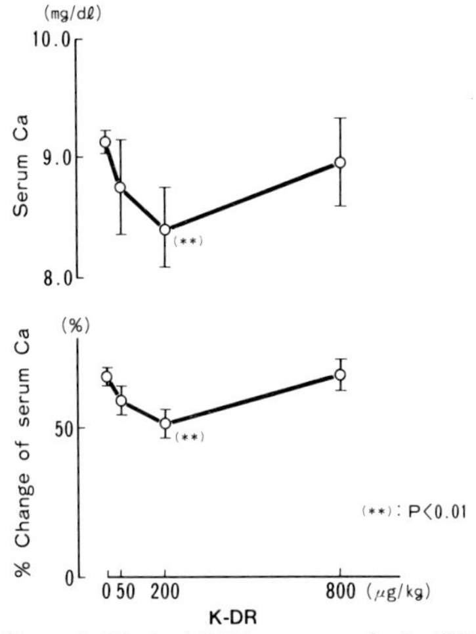

Figure 3 Effect of K-DR on serum Ca in TPTx rats treated with $1\alpha(OH)D_3$ (Dose response curve at 24 hr)

Conclusions:

$24R,25(OH)_2D_3$ has hypocalcemic effect in rats pretreated with V-D or $1\alpha(OH)D_3$. It appears that $24R,25(OH)_2D_3$ has antagonistic effect against the action of $1\alpha,25(OH)_2D_3$ on bone. Since the hypocalcemic effects of $24R,25(OH)_2D_3$ were also observed in TPTx rats, calcitonin may not be involve in the mechanism of hypocalcemic action of $24R,25(OH)_2D_3$ in rats.

SYNERGISTIC EFFECTS OF 1,25(OH)$_2$D$_3$ AND 24,25(OH)$_2$D$_3$ IN RACHITIC CHICKS

W.A. Rambeck, R. Goralczyk, C. Tröger and H. Zucker.
Institute for Physiology, Physiological Chemistry and Nutrition Physiology, Veterinary Faculty, University of Munich, Germany.

Introduction:

There exists considerable controversy as to whether 24,25(OH)$_2$D$_3$ plays a unique role distinct from that of 1,25(OH)$_2$D$_3$ and whether both metabolites or only 1,25(OH)$_2$D$_3$ are necessary to produce the complete spectrum of vitamin D dependent biological responses. While Norman and his group provided evidence supporting a biological role of 24,25(OH)$_2$D$_3$ (1), DeLuca and his collaborators find no evidence for the idea that 24,25(OH)$_2$D$_3$ has a significant in vivo role (2). In a recent study vitamin D deficient rats were given 24,24-F$_2$-25OHD$_3$ for two generations (3). Since growth, development, reproductive function and skeletal mineralization appeared normal in every respect it was assumed that only 1 - hydroxylation but not 24-hydroxylation of vitamin D is necessary.

On the other hand a recent report on the influence of vitamin D metabolites on fracture repair in chicks showed that the callus formation was most emphasized when a combination of 24,25(OH)$_2$D$_3$ and 1,25(OH)$_2$D$_3$ was administered (4). The therapeutic antirachtic activity in chicks was also highest, when both metabolites were given (5). In this study we compared the influence of 1,25(OH)$_2$D$_3$ alone or together with 24,25(OH)$_2$D$_3$ on CaBP synthesis and per cent bone ash in rachitic chicken and on the calcium excretion via the egg shell of Japanese quails.

Material and Methods

Newly hatched male broiler chicks were fed a vitamin D deficient diet for 10 days followed by a diet containing the vitamin D-metabolites for 6 days. CaBP has been determined by the ion exchange procedure according to Wasserman et al. (6) and is expressed as the percentage of radio activity in the supernatant from total radioactivity. The Japanese quail egg shell test was performed as described elsewhere (7).

Results and discussion.

From Table 1 the influence of 1,25(OH)$_2$D$_3$ in the diet on CaBP and percent bone ash can be seen. 24,25(OH)$_2$D$_3$, which has only a small effect when administered alone increases CaBP and bone ash dramatically when added together with 1,25(OH)$_2$D$_3$. This synergistic effect is also seen when the two metabolites are administered in combination to Japanese quails. Calcium excretion via egg shell is significantly higher when 24,25(OH)$_2$D$_3$ is administered additionally, as compared to 1,25(OH)$_2$D$_3$ alone (Results not shown in this paper).

Table 1. Duodenal CaBP and bone ash per cent in rachitic chicken after the administration of 1,25(OH)$_2$D$_3$ alone or together with 24,25(OH)$_2$D$_3$. Values are means $\pm$ SD (n = 10).

Addition per kg of diet	CaBP	Bone ash %
——— (neg. control)	1.98 $\pm$ 0.56	29.3
1.5 µg 1,25(OH)$_2$D$_3$	4.67 $\pm$ 1.15	33.7
15 µg 24,25(OH)$_2$D$_3$	2.33 $\pm$ 0.44	30.5
1.5 µg 1,25(OH)$_2$D$_3$+15 µg 24,25(OH)$_2$D$_3$	8.54 $\pm$ 1.56	39.3
20 µg Vitamin D$_3$	8.56 $\pm$ 1.01	39.4

The synergistic effect of 1,25(OH)$_2$D$_3$ and 24,25(OH)$_2$D$_3$ seems to be highest, when the two vitamin D metabolites are given at a molar ratio of 1 : 10 (8). A reinforcing effect of 24,25(OH)$_2$D$_3$ on 1,25(OH)$_2$D$_3$ bioactivity might allow to reduce the 1,25(OH)$_2$D$_3$ dosage in renal osteopathy therapy.

References

1. Norman, A.W., Roth, J. and Orci, L. (1982). Endocrine Rev. 3, 331-366.
2. DeLuca, H.F. and Schnoes, H.K. (1983). Ann. Rev. Biochem. 52, 411-439.
3. Jarnagin, K., Brommage, R., DeLuca, H.F., Yamada, S. and Takayama, H. (1983). Am. J. Physiol. 244, E290-E297.
4. Dekel, S., Salama, R. and Edelstein, S. (1983). Clin. Sci. 65, 429-436.
5. Babarykin, D.A., Baumann, V.K., Valinietse, M.J. and Rosental, R.L. (1982) in: Vitamin D, ed. Norman, A.W., de Gruyter, Berlin, New York, p. 1201-1203.
6. Wasserman, R.H., Corradino, R.A. and Taylor, A.N. (1968) J. Biol. Chem. 243, 3978-3986.
7. Rambeck, W.A., Weiser, H. and Zucker, H. (1984). Int. J. Vit. Nutr. Res. 54, 25 - 34.
8. Rambeck, W.A. and Zucker, H. (1985). Biochem. Biophys. Res. Comm. in press

COMPARATIVE STUDY OF 24,25(OH)$_2$D$_3$ AND 1,25(OH)$_2$D$_3$ ACTIONS ON TOTAL URINARY cAMP IN CONTROL, RACHITIC AND HYPOMAGNESEMIC RATS.

M.L.TRABA, C.de la PIEDRA, M.BABE and A.RAPADO.
Unidad Metabólica, Fundación Jiménez Díaz. Avda. Reyes Católicos, 2. Madrid-28040. SPAIN.

INTRODUCTION

We have studied the effects of 24,25(OH)$_2$D$_3$ and 1,25(OH)$_2$D$_3$ on total urinary cAMP, an index of PTH activity in different experimental conditions.

Although 24,25(OH)$_2$D$_3$ was considered as the initial event in inactivation of vitamin D, there is evidence of its biological actions, because receptors for this metabolite has been identified in parathyroid glands (1) chondrocytes (2) and endochondrial bone(3). Several reports have appeared suggesting that this metabolite has a specific function in calcification (4,5) intestinal absorption(6) and supression of PTH secretion(7). On the other hand, it is accepted that 1,25(OH)$_2$D$_3$ is the most active form of vitamin D. Intestinal calcium absorption(8), mobilization(9) and mineralization bone calcium processes(9), distal tubular calcium reabsorption(10), proximal tubular phosphorous reabsorption(11) among others physiological processes are mediated by 1,25(OH)$_2$D$_3$.

It has been calculated that in normal subjects 20-40 % of the urinary excretion of cAMP is produced by the effects of PTH on the nefrogenous production of cAMP. Thus, some physiological action that produces a variation in PTH levels, could be reflected by a variation in the urinary excretion of cAMP.

Previous works have indicated that 24,25(OH)$_2$D$_3$ suppresses iPTH(12,13, 14,15). Controversial findings have been reported on the actions of 1,25(OH)$_2$D$_3$ on PTH secretion. Increased(10,17,18) suppressed (19) or unchanged(17,20,21) PTH secretion has been found.

Rachitic and hypomagnesemic rats were selected in order to see more clear effects of 24,25(OH)$_2$D$_3$ and 1,25(OH)$_2$D$_3$ on total urinary cAMP, because rachitic rats are vitamin D depleted and we have found in previous determinations that the levels of 1,25(OH)$_2$D$_3$ in hypomagnesemic rats are decreased compared to control rats.

METHODS

Male Sprague-Dawley rats weighing about 90 g. were divided into 3 groups: A, B and C. Rats were housed in individual metabolic cages with free access to water and diet.

Group A received a control diet(mg/100 g of diet Ca:600, Mg:30, P:400 and standard vitaminic mixture). Group B received a Mg-deficient diet (mg/100 g of diet Ca:600, Mg:3, P:400 and standard vitaminic mixture). Group C received a rachitogenic diet(mg/100 g of diet Ca:600, Mg:30, P:100 and standard vitaminic mixture vitamin D free). Diets were supplied by Pan-Lab laboratories, Paris, France. After 8 days group A was subdivided into A_1, A_2, A_3 and group B into B_1, B_2, B_3 and B_4.

The degree of hypomagnesemia developed in groups B was assessed from blood samples obtained from the tail vein(serum Mg: 1.3 $\pm$ 0.1 mg/dl). These animals exhibited irritability, allopecia and peripheral vasodilatation.

Forty days after the beginning of the experiment group C was divided into 4 groups, C_1, C_2, C_3 and C_4. In order to assess the degree of rickets, bone-X-ray and calcium serum levels were determined(serum Ca: 7.4 $\pm$ 1.0 mg/dl).

Vitamin D. A Chemical, Biochemical and Clinical Update

TABLE I. MINERAL PARAMETERS IN SERUM OF: NORMAL(CONTROL),HYPOMAGNESEMIC AND RACHITIC RATS.

GROUP	Ca mg/dl	Mg mg/dl	$25(OH)D_3$ ng/ml	$1,25(OH)_2D_3$ pg/ml
CONTROL RATS	9.8 ± 0.4 (7)	2.1 ± 0.1 (6)	13.2 ± 4.9 (6)	68.7 ± 25.1 (4)
HYPOMAGNESEMIC RATS	10.3 ± 0.7 (12)	1.3 ± 0.2 (8)	9.8 ± 0.2 (6)	38.9 ± 10.3 (5)
RACHITIC RATS	7.4 ± 1.0 (5)	2.3 ± 0.2 (5)	1.4 ± 0.9 (4)	

TABLE II.TOTAL URINARY cAMP (nmol/100 ml GFR)

SUBGROUP	TREATMENT	A-CONTROL RATS	B-HYPOMAGNESEMIC RATS	C-RACHITIC RATS
1	vehicle	12.64 ± 1.19 (12)	8.04 ± 0.54 (10) B_1-A_1 $p< 0.001$	11.18 ± 2.30 (4) C_1-A_1 N.S.
2	$24,25(OH)_2D_3$	7.75 ± 1.40 (7) A_2-A_1 $p< 0.01$	6.02 ± 0.82 (6) B_2-B_1 $p< 0.01$	6.19 ± 0.85 (6) C_2-C_1 $p< 0.0025$
3	$1,25(OH)_2D_3$	11.10 ± 2.20 (6) A_3-A_1 N.S.	16.35 ± 3.60 (6) B_3-B_1 $p< 0.01$ B_3-A_1 N.S.	9.92 ± 0.26 (4) C_3-C_1 N.S.
4	$24,25(OH)_2D_3$ + $1,25(OH)_2D_3$	————	5.65 ± 1.60 (6) B_4-B_1 $p< 0.025$	4.23 ± 0.20 (6) C_4-C_1 $p< 0.001$

TABLE III.SERUM CALCIUM LEVELS (mg/dl)

SUBGROUP	TREATMENT	A-CONTROL RATS	B-HYPOMAGNESEMIC RATS	C-RACHITIC RATS
1	vehicle	9.8 ± 0.44 (7)	10.27 ± 0.67 (12) B_1-A_1 $p< 0.05$	7.40 ± 1.01 (4) C_1-A_1 $p< 0.001$
2	$24,25(OH)_2D_3$	9.38 ± 0.41 (9)	10.75 ± 1.02 (6) B_2-B_1 N.S. B_2-A_1 $p<0.05$	8.13 ± 0.62 C_2-C_1 N.S.
3	$1,25(OH)_2D_3$	9.86 ± 0.35 (6)	11.35 ± 1.37 (7) B_3-B_1 $p< 0.05$ B_3-A_1 $p< 0.01$	9.15 ± 0.52 (4) C_3-C_1 $p< 0.0125$
4	$24,25(OH)_2D_3$ + $1,25(OH)_2D_3$		10.85 ± 0.57 (6) B_4-B_1 $p< 0.05$ B_4-A_1 $p< 0.05$	9.95 ± 0.35 (6) C_4-C_1 $p< 0.0025$

STATISTICAL SIGNIFICANCE: Student's t-test. In brackets: number of rats.

From these subdivisions subgroups 2 received during 7 days a daily oral dose of 24,25$(OH)_2D_3$ (25 ng/200 µl ethanol).The subgroups 3 received 25 ng of 1,25$(OH)_2D_3$ and the subgroups 4 received a mixture of 25 ng of 24,25$(OH)_2D_3$ and 25 ng of 1,25$(OH)_2D_3$ in the same way.The subgroups 1 received during 7 days 200 µl of ethanol.The last day the animals were maintained in a fasting state and 24 hours urine was collected in ice-cooled containers.The next day,rats were killed under penthobarbital(Nembutal) anaesthesia,50 mg/Kg,and serum samples were obtained.

Urinary cAMP was determined by protein binding assay(22),25$(OH)D_3$ was determined by a protein binding assay(23),1,25$(OH)_2D_3$ by RIA(24) and calcium and magnesium by atomic absorption spectrophotometry..

RESULTS AND CONCLUSIONS

Table I shows the levels of calcium,magnesium,25$(OH)_2D_3$ and 1,25$(OH)_2D_3$ in serum from A_1,$B_1$and C_1 subgroups.These values show that experimental models are correctly obtained.

Table II shows the levels of total urinary cAMP in the three experimental groups.A decrease in total urinary cAMP was observed in control, hypomagnesemic and rachitics rats treated with 24,25$(OH)_2D_3$ when compared to their respective untreated groups.These results agree with above mentioned previous works(12-15).The administration of 1,25$(OH)_2D_3$ does not produce a significant change in the urinary cAMP of the control and rachitic rats,in agreement with other reports(17,20,21).A decrease in total urinary cAMP in hypomagnesemic rats(B_1) was found,but after 1,25$(OH)_2D_3$ treatment(B_3)these levels returned to those of control rats(A_1).These findings suggest that 1,25$(OH)_2D_3$ acts on cAMP secretion in hypomagnesemic rats,because these rats have decreased basal levels of 1,25$(OH)_2D_3$ (see table I).In a previous work we have found a decrease in the synthesis of ^{3}H-1,25$(OH)_2D_3$ in kidney,intestine and bone of hypomagnesemic rats 40 hours after the intravenous administration of ^{3}H-25$(OH)D_3$(16).

Table III shows serum calcium levels of the different groups after their respective treatments

The decrease produced by 24,25$(OH)_2D_3$ in urinary cAMP excretion appears to be mediated by a decrease of PTH,and independent of calcium serum levels.Urinary cAMP stimulation by 1,25$(OH)_2D_3$ in hypomagnesemic rats could be mediated by an effect on PTH secretion and/or action on target organs.The latter effect could be carried out directly by the 1,25$(OH)_2D_3$ or by calcium,because in the hypomagnesemic rats treated with 1,25$(OH)_2D_3$ a clear hypercalcemia was observed(see table III).

After the simultaneous administration of 24,25$(OH)_2D_3$ and 1,25$(OH)_2D_3$, the levels of total urinary cAMP decreased similarly as in the case of 24,25$(OH)_2D_3$ administration despite the fact that in the hypomagnesemic group 1,25$(OH)_2D_3$ administration increased urinary cAMP.

REFERENCES

1.Merke,J.,Norman,A.W.(1981)Biochem.Biophys.Res.Commun.100:551-558.
2.Corvol,M.T.,Dumontier,M.I.,Ulmann,A.,Garabedian,M.,Witmer,G.In Vitamin D:Basic Research and its clinical application,Ed.Norman et al.Walter de Gruyter,Berlin,New York,1979, p 419-424.
3.Sömjem,D.,Sömjen,G.J.,Weisman,Y.,Binderman,I.(1982)Biochem.J.204:31-36.
4.Rasmussen,H.,Bordir,P.(1978)Metabolic bone disease and Related disease 1:7-13.
5.Ornoy,A.,Goodwin,D.,Noff,D.,Edelstein,S.(1978)Nature 276:517-519.
6.Kanis,J.A.,Heynen,G.,Russell,R.G.G.,Smith,R.,Walton,r.j.,Warner,G.T.In Vitamin D,Bioche-

mical,Chemical and Clinical Aspects related to Calcium metabolism,Ed Norman et al,Waler de Gruyter,Berlin,1977,p 793-795.
7.Henry,H.L.,Taylor,A.N.,Norman,A.W.(1977),J.Nutr.107:1918-1926.
8.Norman,A.W.Vitamin D.The calcium homeostatic steroid hormone.Academic Press,New York, 1979,p.303-351.
9.See reference 8. p.374-402.
10.See reference 8. p.352-373.
11.Egel,J.,Pfanstial,J.,Puschett,J.B.(1985)Mineral Electrolyte Metab.11:62-68.
12.Canterbury,J.M.,Lerman,S.,Claflin,A.J.,Henry,H.,Norman,A.,Reiss,E.(1978) J.Clin.Invest. 61:1375-1383.
13.Care,A.D.,Bates,R.F.L.,Pickard,D.W.,Peacock,M.,Tomlinson,S.,Riordan,J.L.H.,Mawer,E.B., Taylor,C.M.,DeLuca,H.F.,Norman,A.W.(1977)Calcif.Tiss.Res.21:142-146.
14.Gueris,J.L.,Bordier,P.J.,Rassmussen,H.,Gravlet,A.M.,Marie,P.,Miravet,L.,Norman,A.W., (1977) 6th Parathyroid Conference,Vancouver,Canada,127(Abstr).
15.Canterbury,J.M.,Gavellas,G.,Bourgoignie,J.J.,Reiss,E.See ref 2 p.297-304.
16.Traba,M.L.,de la Piedra,C.,Marin,A.,Babé,M.,Rapado,A.Im Proceedings of I European Congress on Magnesium,Portugal,1983,Karger A.G., Basel(1984),in press.
17.Mallet,E.,Basuyan,J.P.,Tonan,M.C.,Vaudry,H.See reference 2.p.279-283.
18.Shen,F.H.,Barylink,D.J.,Werdegal,J.E.,Sherrard,D.J.,Norman,A.W.(1974)Clin.Res.22:479.
19.Chertow,B.S.,Baylink,D.J.,Werdegal,J.F.,Su,M.H.H.,Norman,A.W.(1975)J.Clin.Invest.56: 668-678.
20.Okano,K.,Nakai,R.,Tomori,T.,Nishii,Y.,Yashikawa,M.See reference 14,67(Abstr.).
21.Llach,F.,Coburn,J.W.,Brikman,A.S.,Kurokawa,K.,Norman,A.W.,Canterbury,J.M.,Keiss,E.(1977) J.Clin.Endocrinol. and Metab.44:1054-1060.
22.The cyclic AMP assay.CAT. No.TRK 432 The Radiochemical Center.Amersham,England.
23.Traba,M.L.,Quesada,M.,Marin,A.,de la Piedra,C.,Babé,M.,Navarro,F.(1984)Rev.Esp.Fisiol. 40:69-76..
24.1,25 Dihydroxyvitamin D_3 by RIA.CAT NO 6000 Immuno Nuclear Corporation.Stillwater. Minnesota.

ACTIVITY OF ORNITHINE DECARBOXYLASE (ODC) AND CREATINE KINASE (CK) IN SOFT AND HARD TISSUE OF VITAMIN D DEFICIENT (-D) CHICKS FOLLOWING PARENTERAL APPLICATION OF 1,25-DIHYDROXY-CHOLECALCIFEROL (1,25-DHCC) OR 24,25-DIHYDROXYCHOLECALCIFEROL (24,25-DHCC).

T. H. ITTEL, F. P. ROSS and A. W. NORMAN
Department of Biochemistry, University of California, Riverside, CA 92521, USA and Department of Internal Medicine II, University of Aachen, D 5100 Aachen, FRG

Introduction:

Recently evidence has been provided that the activity of ODC and of CK is stimulated by 1,25-DHCC and by 24,25-DHCC in -D animals. In the epiphysis of -D rats 24,25-DHCC caused an increase in ODC activity, while there was no effect on the ODC activity in the diaphysis and in the duodenum (1). Vice versa 1,25-DHCC enhanced the ODC activity in the duodenum and in the diaphysis, but had no influence on the epiphysis. Similarly 24,25-DHCC increased the activity of CK-BB in cultured chick cartilage cells and in the epiphysis of -D rats (2,3). 1,25-DHCC stimulated CK-BB activity in the diaphysis and in the kidney of rats, though it failed to alter the CK activity in the duodenum. However, other investigators could not confirm these results in -D chicks and the stimulation of ODC by 1,25-DHCC was confined to the duodenum (4,5). The present study has been undertaken, therefore, to investigate the effects of both vitamin D metabolites on the activity of ODC and CK in a wide spectrum of potential target organs in -D chicks.

Methods:

White Leghorn cockerels obtained on the day of hatch were raised for 4 weeks on a standard rachitogenic diet (6). The -D chicks received single i.m. injections of either 1,25-DHCC or 24,25-DHCC in a dose range from 1.6 - 6500 pmol 5 h prior to decapitation or the maximum dose was used and the time between administration and decapitation varied from 1 h to 72 h. Tissue homogenates of duodenal mucosa, pancreas, liver, kidney, lung, heart, brain, and diaphysis and epiphysis of the long bones were prepared according to (1). The activity of ODC was measured using a modification of a method described by Russell and Snyder (7). CK activity was measured spectrophotometrically at 340 nm using a modified coupled assay (8).

Results:

Following the administration of 1,25-DHCC the activity of ODC was enhanced in duodenum, pancreas, and bone. The increase in ODC activity became significant after 3 h in the duodenum and after 5 h in the pancreas. Peak values were measured after 5 h in both tissues and the ODC activity had declined back to baseline levels after 24 h and 48 h in pancreas and duodenum respectively. The enhancement of ODC was dose-dependent and doses as little as 19.5 pmol were effective in the duodenum.

Vitamin D. A Chemical, Biochemical and Clinical Update

Near maximum activities could be achieved with 195 pmol in both tissues, while 24,25-DHCC had no effect up to 6500 pmol. Furthermore 1,25-DHCC affected the hard tissues: the ODC activity, but not the CK activity was stimulated in the diaphysis and in the epiphysis and both sites responded equally well displaying a biphasic time course. Following an early increase after 1 h the ODC activity dropped back to the baseline and showed a second, higher peak after 24 h. 24,25-DHCC did not alter the activity of ODC or CK, neither in the epiphysis nor in the diaphysis. The activity of CK was stimulated in kidney, liver, and lung by injection of 1,25-DHCC. The enhancement showed dose-dependency, though maximum increases could only be demonstrated with 6500 pmol 1,25-DHCC in lung and kidney. In the liver 195 pmol were sufficient to produce a maximum response. The stimulation of CK activity was characterized by a time course which was markedly different from the time course of ODC activity. Following the administration of 1,25-DHCC significantly elevated CK activities were noted after 3 h in the lung and the liver, and after 5 h in the kidney. Thereafter the CK activities remained elevated over 72 h without a gradual decline towards the baseline. Moreover, CK activities in the lung reached a second peak after 48 h, which exceeded the previous activities. Again 24,25-DHCC failed to alter the activity of CK in any of the soft tissues. In heart and brain CK and ODC activities were not affected by either vitamin D metabolite.

Conclusions:
1. 1,25-DHCC but not 24,25-DHCC is an effective stimulator of ODC activity in pancreas and duodenum, and of CK activity in liver, kidney, and lung of -D chicks. 2. Epiphysis and diaphysis of long bones both respond to 1,25-DHCC with an increase in ODC activity and neither site of the bone responds to 24,25-DHCC. The CK activity in bone is not affected by either vitamin D metabolite. 3. There is no coincidence of stimulation of CK and ODC in the same tissue, and dose-dependency and time course of both enzymes differ considerably.

References:
1. Sömjen, D., Binderman, I. and Weisman, Y. (1983) Biochem. J. 214, 293-298
2. Sömjen, D., Kaye, A.M. and Binderman, I. (1984) FEBS Lett. 167, 281-284
3. Sömjen, D., Weisman, Y., Binderman, I. and Kaye, A.M. (1984) Biochem. J. 219, 1037-1041
4. Shinki, T., Takahashi, N., Miyaura, C., Samejima, K., Nishii, Y. and Suda, T. (1981) Biochem. J. 195, 685-690
5. Takahashi, N., Shinki, T., Kawate, N., Samejima, K., Nishii, Y. and Suda, T. (1982) Endocrinology 111, 1539-1545
6. Norman, A.W. and Wong, R.G. (1972) J. Nutr. 102, 1709-1718
7. Russell, D.H. and Snyder, S.H. (1969) Molec. Pharmacol. 5, 253-262
8. Reiss, N.A. and Kaye, A.M. (1981) J. Biol. Chem. 256, 5741-5749

EFFECT OF 24,25-DIHYDROXYVITAMIN D_3 ON PARATHYROID FUNCTION IN HUMANS

H.Asscheman,J.C.Netelenbos,P.Lips,W.J.F.van der Vijgh, M.J.M.Jongen,F.van Ginkel and W.H.L.Hackeng.
Department of Internal Medicine, Academisch Ziekenhuis der Vrije Universiteit, 1007 MB Amsterdam, The Netherlands.

Introduction:

Primary hyperparathyroidism (PHP) is a common endocrine disorder, for which effective drug treatment is not available (1). In animal (2) and some human experiments (3) a suppressive effect of 24,25-dihydroxyvitamin D_3 on parathyroid function is suggested. We investigated the long term effect of pharmacologic doses of 24,25$(OH)_2D_3$ orally on parathyroid function in patients with PHP.
Additionally the effect of one intravenous injection of 24,25$(OH)_2D_3$ was investigated in 4 volunteers with normal parathyroid function. The effect of 24,25$(OH)_2D_3$ on the other main vitamin D metabolites was also studied.

Methods:

Nineteen patients with PHP (total serum calcium >2.55 mmol/l, inappropriately elevated serum iPTH levels, decreased renal tubular phosphate threshold <0.81 mmol/l and creatinin clearance >40 ml/min) were followed for nine months. The first three months basal values were obtained. Thereafter they were randomized to treatment with placebo or 25 µg 24,25$(OH)_2D_3$ p.o., daily for three months. During the last three months the treatment was crossed over.
Monthly blood samples were drawn for iPTH(1-84) and midregion assay (4), ionized calcium and vitamin D metabilites (5).
Four volunteers received 25 µg 24,25$(OH)_2D_3$ intravenously and blood samples for iPTH, ionized calcium and vitamin D metabolites were collected at 0, 5, 10, 30, 60, 180 and 480 minutes and at day 1, 2, 3, 4, 7, 10 and 14.
Statistical analysis was performed with ANOVA.

Results:

Table 1

		basal	placebo	24,25$(OH)_2D_3$	p
iPTH(midregion)	pmol/l	10.9±3.5	12.6±4.6	12.1±4.5	ns
iPTH(1-84)	pmol/l	0.46±0.23	0.45±0.22	0.46±0.29	ns
ionized calcium	mmol/l	1.41±0.03	1.41±0.03	1.41±0.03	ns
24,25$(OH)_2$D	nmol/l	1.4±2.2	2.6±2.7	37.6±11.1	.01
1,25$(OH)_2$D	pmol/l	169±50	165±49	160±46	ns
25(OH)D	nmol/l	30±15	29±14	31±13	ns

Mean ± SD in three different periods in 19 PHP patients.

As shown in Table 1, serum concentrations of iPTH, ionized calcium, 25(OH)D and 1,25$(OH)_2$D did not change significantly.

Vitamin D. A Chemical, Biochemical and Clinical Update

The effect of the i.v.injection of 25 µg 24,25(OH)$_2$D$_3$ is shown in figure 1 and 2. Again the serum levels of iPTH, ionized calcium, 25(OH)D and 1,25(OH)$_2$D did not change significantly.

Figure 1

Mean ± SD
4 volunteers

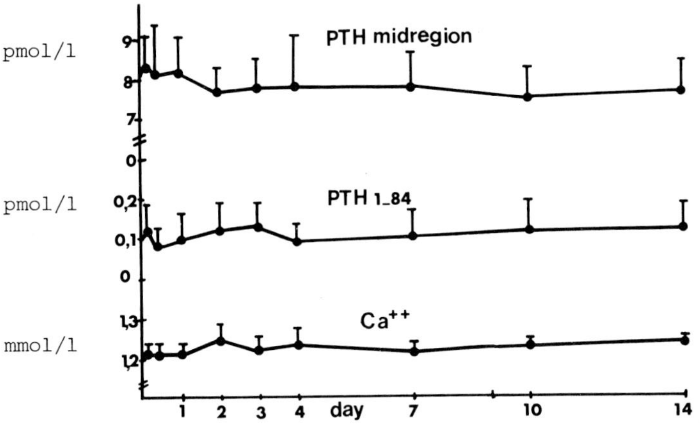

Figure 2

Individual values
4 volunteers

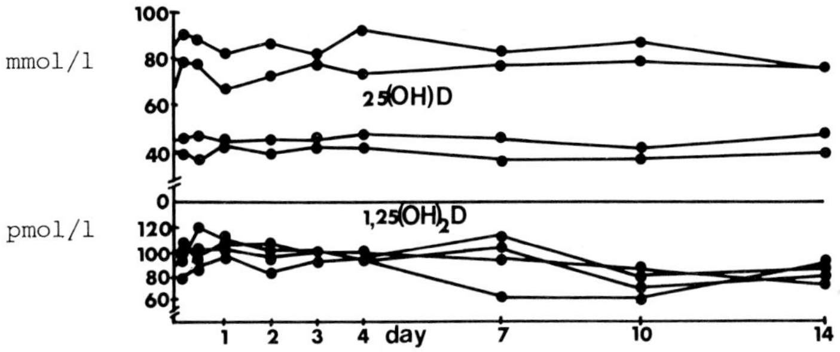

Conclusion:

In this long term double blind cross-over study with pharmacologic does of 24,25(OH)$_2$D$_3$ in patients with PHP and in the acute study in normal volunteers no effect on parathyroid function was observed. No effect of 24,25(OH)$_2$D$_3$ was observed on the serum levels of 25(OH)D and 1,25(OH)$_2$D in both studies. We conclude that 24,25(OH)$_2$D$_3$ does not affect parathyroid function in patients with PHP.

References:

1. Heath,H.,Hodgson,S.F.,Kennedy,M.A.(1980)N.Engl.J.Med.302: 189-193.
2. Canterbury,J.M.,Gavellas,G.,Bourgoignie,J.J.,Reiss,E. (1980)J.Clin.Invest.65: 571-576.
3. Miravet,L.,Guéris,J.,Rebel,J.,Norman,A.,Ryckewaert,A. (1981)Calcif.Tissue Int.33:191-194.
4. Lips,P.,Hackeng,W.H.L.,Jongen,M.J.M.,van Ginkel,F.C., Netelenbos,J.C.(1983)J.Clin.Endrocrinol.Metab.57:204-206.
5. Jongen,M.J.M.,van der Vijgh,W.J.F.,Willems,H.J.J., Netelenbos,J.C.,Lips,P.(1981)Clin.Chem.27:1757-1760.

DOES 24R,25(OH)$_2$D$_3$ HAVE A BENEFICIAL EFFECT IN OSTEOPOROSIS

H. Orimo[1], C. Tsutsumi[2], S. Moriuchi[3]
[1]Department of Geriatrics, Faculty of Medicine, University of Tokyo, Hongo, Tokyo, Japan, [2]Department of Nutrition, School of Health Sciences, Faculty of Medicine, University of Tokyo, Bunkyo-ku, Tokyo, Japan, [3]Department of Food and Nutrition, Faculty of Home Economics, Japan Women's University, Bunkyo-ku, Tokyo, Japan.

Introduction:

The biological role of 24R,25(OH)$_2$D$_3$ in bone metabolism is still controversial. We investigated the effects of 24R,25(OH)$_2$D$_3$ on experimental osteoporosis.

Materials and Methods:

Female SD rats of 7 weeks old, ovariectomized bilaterally 1 week before were divided into the following 7 groups (9 - 12 animals per each group)
K-DR (24R,25(OH)$_2$D$_3$ of Kureha, Japan) (1, 10, 100μg/kg.day), 1α,25(OH)$_2$D$_3$ (0.001, 0.01, 0.1μg/kg.day) or vehicle were given orally for 6 months.
Serum Ca, i-P, Alp, c-PTH, CT, osteocalcin, defatted dry bone weight, contents of ash, hydroxyproline and osteocalcin in the femurs were measured and contact of tibiae were taken after 6 months treatment.

Results:

1. Ash/def. D.W. of the femur was significantly greater in K-DR 1μg/kg and in 1α,25(OH)$_2$D$_3$ 0.01μg/kg treated groups.
2. Osteocalcin content of the femur was significantly greater in K-DR 1μg/kg and 10μg/kg treated groups than in control.
3. Decrease in travecular bone was significantly prevented by K-DR, 100μg/kg treated group.

Table 1 Changes in bone parameters in ovariectomized rats

	Ash/def. D.W.	Hypro/def. D.W.	Osteocalcin
K-DR 1 μg/kg	↑	→	↑
K-DR 10 μg/kg	→	→	↑
K-DR 100 μg/kg	→	→	→
1α, 25(OH)$_2$D$_3$ 0.001 μg/kg	→	→	→
1α, 25(OH)$_2$D$_3$ 0.01 μg/kg	↑	→	→
1α, 25(OH)$_2$D$_3$ 0.1 μg/kg	↑	→	→

→ : not significantly different from control
↑ : significantly increased from control

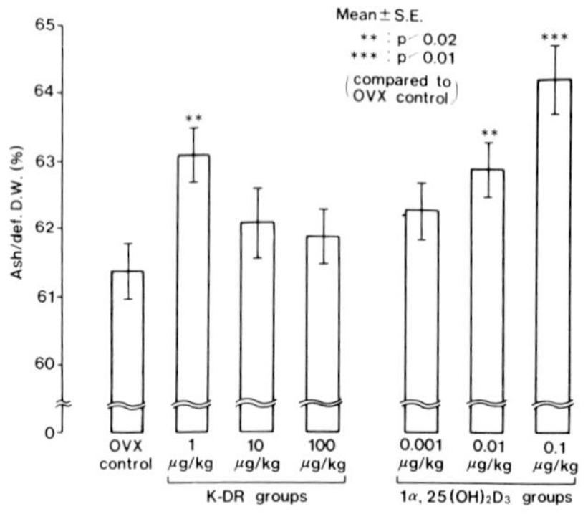

Figure 1 Ash content of the femur in ovariectomized rats

Vitamin D. A Chemical, Biochemical and Clinical Update

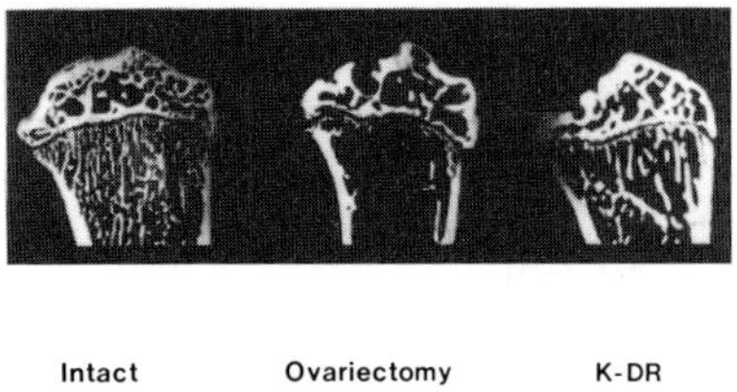

Figure 2 Contact microradiograms of longitudinal sections from the rat tibia

4. Significant positive correlation was observed between osteocalcin content and hydroxyproline/def. D.W. of the femur.

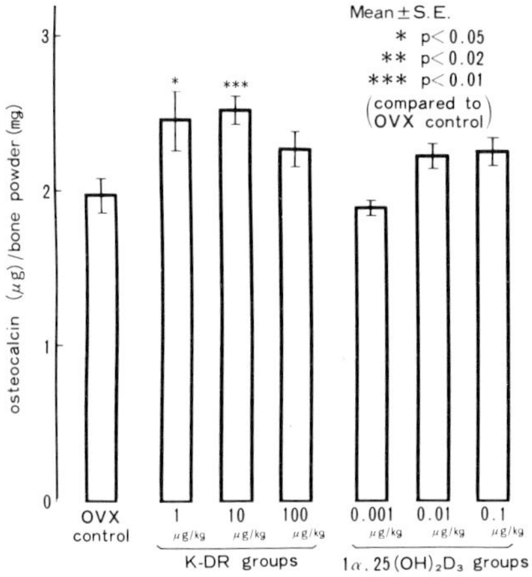

Figure 3 Osteocalcin content in the femur of ovariectomized rats

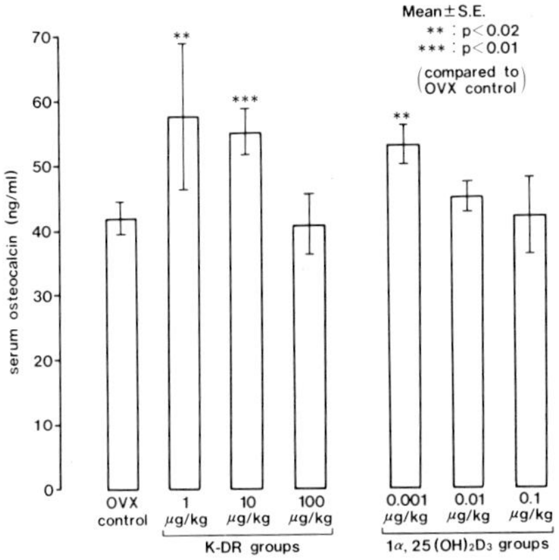

Figure 4 Serum osteocalcin levels in ovariectomized rats

5. Serum osteocalcin levels was significantly higher in K-DR 1μg/kg, 10μg/kg and 1α,25$(OH)_2D_3$ 0.001μg/kg treated groups than in control.
6. No significant changes in serum Ca, i-P, Alp, c-PTH and calcitonin levels were observed.
7. No significant correlation was found between serum osteocalcin level and bone or serum parameters.

Conclusions:

K-DR and 1α,25$(OH)_2D_3$ showed different dose dependency with respect to ash/def. D.W. and osteocalcin content in the bone. These results suggested that the mechanism of action of 24R,25$(OH)_2D_3$ was different from that of 1α,25$(OH)_2D_3$.

EFFECT OF 24,25(OH)2-VITAMIN D AND ALUMINUM ON BONE FORMATION

Susan M. Ott, Elmer Feist, Allen C. Alfrey, Guy A. Howard
University of Washington, Seattle, Washington; University of Colorado, Denver, Colorado; and American Lake Veteran's Administration Medical Center, Tacoma, Washington, U.S.A.

In a previous study (1), patients with renal osteodystrophy were treated with 24,25 (OH)2-Vitamin D (24,25-D). Half of the patients with osteomalacia had evidence of clinial and histologic improvement. Patients with osteitis fibrosis who were given 24,25-D either deteriorated or did not change (2). Recently aluminum had been identified as an element which will cause osteomalacia in animals (3,4) and which is closely associated with osteomalacia in dialysis patients (5). It is therefore a possibility that 24,25-D could play a role in reversing certain cases of aluminum toxicity. This was tested in a rat model.

Methods

Weanling male Holzman rats were used in all studies. In the first study, 6 groups of rats (N=6) were given daily intraperitoneal injections of the following: Groups 1-3: Water, aluminum (.2 mg/day), or 24,25-D (200 ng/day) for 53 days, then sacrificed. Group 4 was given water (1cc) for 75 days. Groups 5-6 were given aluminum (.2mg/day) for 53 days, then water or 24,25-D ,respectively, for 21 days, then sacrificed. Rats were given tetracycline injections 10 days apart, and tibial sections were examined for osteoid and tetracycline uptake. Aluminum was measured by flameless atomic absorption. Two rats died in groups 3 and 6.

In the second study, 6 groups (N=10) were given injections of: normal saline (1cc), 24,25-D (200 ng), 24,25-D + aluminum (1.6 mg/kg), 24,25-D + aluminum (10 mg/kg), aluminum (1.6 mg/kg), and aluminum (10 mg/kg). Only 4 rats each survived in the two groups given the high dose of aluminum; the remaining groups had 7-10 rats. Tibial sections as well as vetebral body sections were examined. Rate of bone formation was calculated by multiplying the length of the tetracycline labels by the distance between labels, per cross-sectional area of bone tissue. This was measured on a computerized digitizer.

Results

In both studies, there were no significant differences in the serum calcium, creatinine, or phosphate. There were also no differences in the total bone area, the periosteal tetracycline labelling, the osteoid width or osteoid length within the groups of each study. In the first study, the rats given 24,25-D either with or after the aluminum had lower bone aluminum than the rats given aluminum alone or aluminum followed by water. There were differences seen on endosteal surfaces of the rats in the first part of the first study. The group given 24,25-D +aluminum had more tetracycline label than either controls the group given aluminum only. However, in the second study these differences were not apparent. The trabecular surfaces also did not show any differences between rats given 24,25-D and saline or aluminum controls.

Vitamin D. A Chemical, Biochemical and Clinical Update

Study 1 Days 1-53	54-75	Endosteal label (% surface)	Periosteal apposition (u/day)	Bone area (mm^2)	Bone aluminum (mg/kg)
Water	--	16 ± 11	3.6 ± .5	4.4 ± .1	1.8 ± .64
Aluminum	--	16 ± 16	3.5 ± .7	4.6 ± .6	36.3 ± 4.6
Al + 24,25	--	57 ± 3#	4.3 ± .2	4.2 ± .4	14.0 ± 2.2*
Water	Water	11 ± 10	2.4 ± .4	4.9 ± .7	2.1 ± 1.3
Aluminum	Water	8 ± 8	2.5 ± .2	4.5 ± .5	53.2 ± 16
Aluminum	24,25	12 ± 9	2.3 ± .1	4.4 ± .2	13.5 ± .58*
Study 2					
Saline		15 ± 6	1.8 ± .3	4.8 ± .2	
24,25		22 ± 10	1.9 ± .3	4.8 ± .4	
25,25+Al(lo dose)		25 ± 14	2.0 ± .3	4.6 ± .5	
Aluminum		14 ± 9	1.8 ± .3	4.6 ± .6	

*=p<.01, #=p<.05, 24,25 vs. Aluminum alone Mean ± S.D.

Discussion

Although the aluminum accumulated in bone in rats given aluminum, there were no ill effects on bone formation. In rats given higher doses of aluminum for 9 weeks, we found decreased tetracycline uptake on endosteal and trabecular, but not periosteal, surfaces (6). The addition of 24,25-D resulted in a lower bone aluminum. The renal excretion of aluminum could have been enhanced, or the distribution within the body could have changed. Further studies are needed to determine the mechanism for the lowered bone aluminum.

There were few histological differences between controls and rats who received aluminum alone or with 24,25-D. In the first study the endosteal surfaces of 24,25-D treated rats had more tetracycline labels. This could result from increased formation or decreased resorption at that surface. The net effect was not large, since the total bone area was not different. This effect was not reproduced in the second study, with similar (but not identical) conditions. Furthermore, the trabecular surfaces did not show a difference in bone formation. Thus, although 24,25-D may enhance bone formation under certain pathological conditions, it did not cause increased bone formation in normal rats with mild aluminum levels.

1. Ott,S.M.,Recker,R.R.,Coburn,J.W.,Sherrard,D.J.(1983) Kidney Int.23:107.
2. Muirhead,N.,Adami,S.,Sandler,L.M.,Fraser,R.A.,Catto,G.R.D., Oriordan J.L.H.(1982) Quarterly J. Med. 51:427-444.
3. Goodman,W.G.,Gilligan,J.,Horst,R.(1983) J.Clin.Invest. 73:171-181.
4. Robertson,J.A.,Felsenfeld,A.J.,Haygood,C.C.,Wilson,P.,Clarke,C., Llach,F.(1983) Kidney Int. 23:327-335.
5. Ott,S.M.,Maloney,N.A.,Coburn,J.W.,Alfrey,A.C.,Sherrard,D.J.(1982) New Engl.J.Med. 307:709-713.
6. Ott,S.M.,Feist,E.,Howard,G.A.,Andress,D.L.,Alfrey,A.C.,Liu,C.C., Sherrard,D.J.(1984) Calcified Tiss.Int. 36:496.

$24,25(OH)_2D_3$ ENHANCES THE CALCEMIC EFFECT OF $1,25(OH)_2D_3$: EVIDENCE FOR HYPOCALCIURIC ACTION OF $24,25(OH)_2D_3$

H. Wald, T. Hayek and M.M. Popovtzer

Hadassah University Hospital, Jerusalem, Israel

The metabolite $1,25(OH)_2D_3$, the active form of vitamin D, is more potent than $25(OH)D_3$ both in enhancing the gut transport and in augmenting the skeletal mobilization of calcium (1,2). In contrast to $25(OH)D_3$ and $1,25(OH)_2D_3$, both of which exhibit a calcemic action, $24,25(OH)_2D_3$ does not alter the serum calcium concentration (3,4). Experimental evidence has been advanced implying that $24,25(OH)_2D_3$ may act to augment bone formation and bone mineralization (5-7). In a previous study by Pavlovitch et al (8) a single dose of $24,25(OH)_2D_3$ has been shown to suppress the hypercalcemia induced by acute bilateral nephrectomy and to attenuate the hypercalcemic effect of $1,25(OH)_2D_3$ in acutely nephrectomized rats. The present study was undertaken to examine the effect of $24,25(OH)_2D_3$ on the hypercalcemia induced by $1,25(OH)_2D_3$ in intact rats.

Materials and Methods

White male rats of the Hebrew University strain weighing 200-250 g were studied. Twenty-four rats of comparable age and weight were housed in metabolic cages and fed Purina pellet chow and tap water ad libitum for several days for acclimatization. On the first day of the study the rats were divided into four groups:

1) Control rats receiving the vehicle 1,2 propanediol s.c. only.
2) Rats receiving a daily s.c. injection of 54 ng $1,25(OH)_2D_3$.
3) Rats receiving $24,25(OH)_2D_3$ in the same dose and same manner.
4) Rats receiving $1,25(OH)_2D_3$ + $24,25(OH)_2D_3$ in the same dose and same manner.

Urine output and food intake was measured at 24 h intervals for 5 consecutive days and blood was drawn at the end of one and 5 days. In a separate group of 24 rats the same experiment was performed for 10 days and blood was drawn at the end of 10 days. Ca^{++}, Pi and creatinine excretion rates in 24 h urine collections and in plasma were measured. Serum albumin was also measured. Vitamin D metabolites were a gift of Hoffman-La Roche and Co., Basel, Switzerland. Results are presented as mean$\pm$SE and compared by the student's t-test.

Results

After 24 h S_{Ca}^{++} increased from 5.8$\pm$0.07 to 6.39$\pm$0.09 mEq/l ($p<0.005$) with $1,25(OH)_2D_3$, and to 6.33$\pm$0.11 ($p<0.005$) with $1,25(OH)_2D_3+24,25(OH)_2D_3$, while $24,25(OH)_2D_3$ alone did not change S_{Ca}^{++}, $U_{Ca}V$ after 24 h increased from 42$\pm$3.9 to 132$\pm$11 μEq/24 h ($p<0.001$) with $1,25(OH)_2D_3$; $24,25(OH)_2D_3$ did not change the $U_{Ca}V$, while with the combination $1,25(OH)_2D_3+24,25(OH)_2D_3$, $U_{Ca}V$ 94.6$\pm$12.3, was significantly lower than with $1,25(OH)_2D_3$ ($p<0.025$). It should be noted that the fall in urinary Ca^{++} excretion caused

Vitamin D. A Chemical, Biochemical and Clinical Update

by the addition of $24,25(OH)_2D_3$ to $1,25(OH)_2D_3$ compared to $1,25(OH)_2D_3$ alone, was not due to decreased serum Ca^{++} level, which as mentioned above was the same as with the administration of $1,25(OH)_2D_3$ alone. After 5 days of $1,25(OH)_2D$, S_{Ca}^{++} was 6.29 ± 0.08 whereas $1,25(OH)_2D_3$+$24,25(OH)_2D_3$ affected a greater increase in S_{Ca}^{++} up to 6.63 ± 0.09 ($p<0.01$). $24,25(OH)_2$ alone did not change S_{Ca}^{++}. $U_{Ca}V$ after 5 days of treatment with $1,25(OH)_2D_3$ rose to 673 ± 54 µEq/24 h; a similar increment was observed with the combination in spite of the greater increase observed in serum Ca^{++}. After 10 days of $1,25(OH)_2D_3$ S_{Ca}^{++} was 6.17 ± 0.15 mEq/l while with the combination S_{Ca}^{++} rose to 6.74 ± 0.2 ($p<0.025$). $24,25(OH)_2D_3$ alone did not change S_{Ca}^{++}.

No significant changes in creatinine clearance were observed after 24 h or 5 days of treatment with vitamin D metabolites. In all cases the clearances ranged between 0.9-1.1 ml/min which represent normal values for rats of about 200 g of weight. Fractional excretion of phosphate after 24 h was similar in all groups. After 5 days of treatment with $1,25(OH)_2D_3$ and with the combination of $1,25(OH)_2D_3$+$24,25(OH)_2D_3$ marked and similar phosphaturia was observed. $24,25(OH)_2D_3$ alone cause a mild but significant phosphaturic effect. There were no measurable changes in serum levels of phosphate after 24 hours or 5 days of treatment with vitamin D metabolites. Serum albumin concentrations and daily food intake did not differ between the 4 groups studied.

Conclusions

1) $24,25(OH)_2D_3$ alone does not alter S_{Ca}^{++} in normal rats.
2) Combined administration of $1,25(OH)_2D_3$+$24,25(OH)_2D_3$ enhances the hypercalcemic response to $1,25(OH)_2D_3$ without a parallel increase in $U_{Ca}V$.
3) It is suggested that the effect of $24,25(OH)_2D_3$ on serum Ca^{++} level may at least partly result from its hypocalciuric effect.

References

1. DeLuca, H.F. and Schnoes, H.K. (1976) Ann Rev. Biochem. 45: 631-666.
2. Favus, M.J. (1978) Med. Clin. North Am. 62: 1291-1317.
3. Llach, F., Brickman, A.S., Singer, F.R. and Coburn, J.W. (1979) Metab. Bone Dis. Rel. Res. 2: 11-15.
4. Miravet, L., Redel, J., Qucille, M.L. and Bordier, P. (1976) Calcif. Tissue Res. 21: 145-152.
5. Bordier, P., Rasmussen, H., Marie, P., Miravet, L., Quenis, J. and Ryckwaert, A. (1978) J. Clin. Endocrin. Metab. 46: 284-294.
6. Kanis, J.A., Cundy, T., Bartlett, M., Smith, R., Heyen, G., Warner, G.T. and Russell, R.G.G. (1978) Br. Med. J. 1: 1382-1386.
7. Russell, R.G.G., Kanis, J.A., Smith, R., Adams, N.D., Bartlett, M., Cundy, T., Cochran, M., Heynen, G. and Warner, G.T. (1978) Adv. Exp. Med. Biol. 103: 487-503.
8. Pavlovitch, J.H., Cournet-Witman, G., Bourdeau, A., Balsan, S., Fischer, J.A. and Heynen, G. (1981) J. Clin. Invest. 68: 803-810.

EFFECTS OF INTRAEPIPHYSEAL INJECTION OF VITAMIN D METABOLITES ON HEALING OF RICKETS IN CHICKS.

A. Ornoy[1], C. Lidor[2], I. Atkin[1,3] and S. Edelstein[2]. [1]Dept. of Anatomy and Embryology, Hebrew Univ.-Hadassah Med. School, Jerusalem, Israel, [2]Dept. of Biochemistry, Weizman Institute of Science, Rehovot, Israel and Morphology Unit [3]Ben Gurion University of the Negev, Beersheba, Israel.

The effect of vitamin D to promote normal bone and cartilage calcification has been generally attributed to increases in serum Ca and P concentrations associated with the effects of $1,25(OH)_2D_3$ on intestinal absorption and on bone mineral mobilization[1]. Recently, however, it has been suggested that $25(OH)D_3$ and $24,25(OH)D_3$ may also be directly involved in bone metabolism[2]. In an attempt to further define the nature of the active metabolite in bone, we designed the following experiments to ascertain which metabolite administered locally in vivo into the epiphyseal growth plate of the proximal tibia of rachitic chicks, could cure unilaterally the rachitic lesions thus, excluding any further renal metabolic transformations of the administered sterol.

One-day-old male chicks were made vitamin D deficient by feeding them a vitamin D-deficient diet for 4 weeks. The chicks were then divided into four groups and injected intraepiphyseally every 3 days with either vehicle alone (arachis oil) or vehicle containing 1µg of $1,25(OH)_2D_3$, 3µg of $24,25(OH)_2D_3$ and 5µg of $25(OH)D_3$. The sterols were injected into the right tibia while simultaneously the left tibia was injected with the vehicle only. Two additional groups of chicks served as non-treated controls; a group of -D chicks, and a group of vitamin D supplemented chicks. On the third day, following a course of 3 intraepiphyseal injections of the sterols the chicks were killed and plasma prepared for determining Ca levels and of the metabolites of cholecalciferol. The tibiae were removed from the chicks and non-decalcified longitudinal sections were prepared routinely and examined by light microscopy.

Rachitic chicks receiving either $1,25(OH)_2D_3$ or $24,25(OH)_2D_3$ maintained low plasma concentrations of calcium, similar to non-treated -D chicks. Furthermore none of the hydroxylated metabolites of cholecalciferol were detectable in the plasma of these chicks indicating that the locally injected sterol failed to leak into the blood stream. In contrast, chicks injected with $25(OH)D_3$ showed normal plasma concentration of Ca and detectable levels of the hydroxylated vitamin D metabolites although significantly lower than the levels measured in the +D group. Histological examination of all groups revealed that the upper tibial epiphyses was still cartilaginous consisting of reserve, proliferative and hypertrophic zones. In the control (+D) chicks the various zones were well defined, while the -D chicks revealed typical signs of rickets, manifested by elongated proliferative and hypertrophic zones, wide osteoid seams and reduced mineralization of the cartilage and bone and an increased number of osteoclasts. Treatment with $1,25(OH)_2D_3$ did not reduce the severity of the rickets and these animals resembled the -D group (Fig. 1). In contrast to this $24,25(OH)_2D_3$ caused almost complete recovery of the injected lesions. (Fig. 2). Injection of $25(OH)D_3$ was followed by recovery from rickets in both the injected right leg and to a lesser extent in the contralateral non-injected leg. Treatment with either sterol resulted in a significcant increase in the

Vitamin D. A Chemical, Biochemical and Clinical Update

number of osteoclasts as compared to +D chicks. Low doses of 0.1 μg or 0.3μg of $1,25(OH)_2D_3$ and of 0.3μg or 1μg of $24,25(OH)_2D_3$ failed to heal the rachitic lesions in the injected legs as well as in the vehicle injected tibiae. However at this low dose $24,25(OH)_2D_3$ induced a slight reduction in the osteoid width in the metaphysis.

Our findings suggest that $24,25(OH)_2D_3$ when injected locally into rachitic chicks has a direct effect on cartilage and bone in chicks while $1,25(OH)_2D_3$ has no such effect. This is consistent with other data[3,4] suggesting that $24,25(OH)_2D_3$ is a more potent metabolite for healing of rickets and probably plays a direct role in endochondral bone formation. Furthermore it appears possible to conclude from this study that $24,25(OH)_2D_3$ affects directly cartilage cells, enabling normal maturation of chondrocytes, later to be replaced by bone. In addition the healing effects observed in both legs following injection with $25(OH)D_3$ imply that this metabolite undergoes absorption into the circulation and is probably subsequently converted by the kidney into both active metabolites $1,25(OH)_2D_3$ and $24,25(OH)_2D_3$. This does not rule out the possibility that following local injection of $25(OH)D_3$, there may also be some in situ conversion of this metabolite into $24,25(OH)_2D_3$ as reported previously[5].

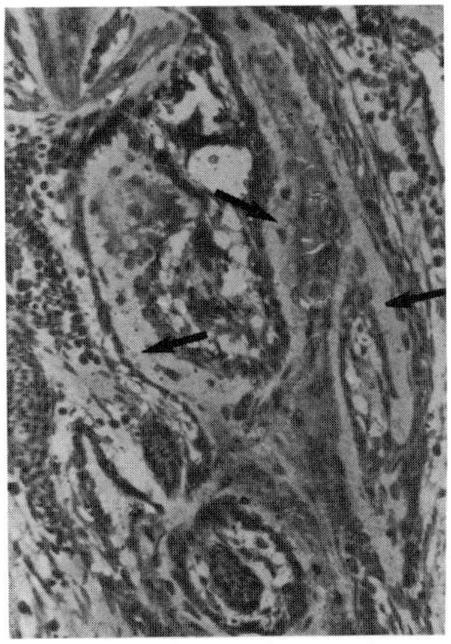

Fig. 1. Metaphyseal trabeculae from a tibia injected with 1μg of $1,25(OH)_2D_3$ to show wide osteoid seams (arrows) Tol. blue x420.

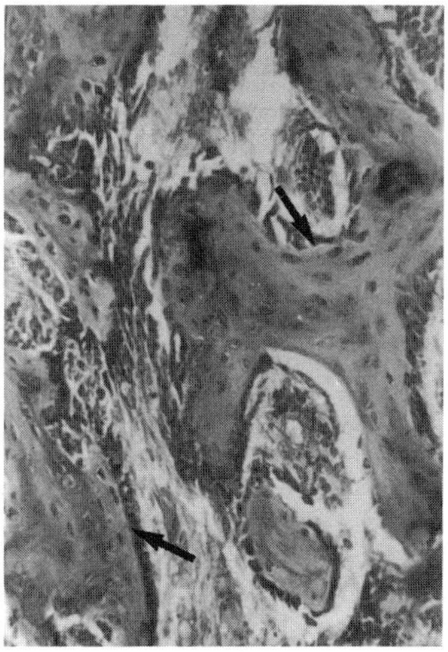

Fig. 2. Metaphyseal trabeculae from a tibia injected with 3μg of $24,25(OH)_2D_3$ to show thin osteoid seams (arrows) Tol. blue x420.

References

1. Bordier, P.A., Rasmussen, H., Marie, P., Miravet, Z. Gueris, J. and Rychwacat, A.J. (1978) J. Clin. Endocrinol. Metab. 48, 284-294.
2. Kanis, J.A., Cundy, T., Baetlett, M., Smith, R., Heynew, G., Warner, G.T. and Russell, R.G.G. (1978) Br. Med. Jr. 1, 1382-1386.
3. Ornoy, A., Goodwin, G., Noff, D. and Edelstein, S. (1978) Nature, 276, 517-519.
4. Goodman, W.G., Baylink, D.J. and Sherrard, D.J. (1984) Cal. Tissue Int. 36, 206-213.
5. Garabedian, M., Bailly Du Bois, M., Corvol, T., Pezant, E. and Balsan, S. (1978) Endocrinology, 102, 1262-1268.

THE DIRECT EFFECTS OF VITAMIN D METABOLITES ON BONE MODELLING IN FETAL MICE LONG BONES GROWN IN VITRO. A. Ornoy[1], Z. Schwartz[2], I. Atkin[1] and W.A. Soskolne[2], Dept. of Anatomy and Embryology[1] and of Periodontics[2], Faculties of Medicine and of Dentistry, Jerusalem, Israel.

Controversy still exists as to the possible role of $24,25(OH)_2D_3$ on bone. Several investigators have proposed a direct role of $24,25(OH)_2D_3$ in cartilage differentiation and maturation as well as bone formation[1] while others are of the opinion that the major active metabolite of vitamin D is $1,25(OH)_2D_3$[2], emphasizing the well defined role of this metabolite in stimulation of bone resorption.

We have recently developed an in vitro system for the study of bone modelling of fetal mice long bones. In this system, bone growth and remodelling is obtained for periods up to 6 days[3]. 16 day old radii and ulnae, prelabelled with ^{45}Ca one day before removal from the uterus were cultured for 48 hours in BGJ medium supplemented either with 10% fetal calf serum, or with 4mg/ml of human serum albumin (in this case serving as a chemically defined medium). In this system, bone growth and remodelling is obtained for periods up to 6 days[4]. We used this system to study the direct effects of $1,25(OH)_2D_3$ and $24,25(OH)_2D_3$ on growth, formation calcification and resorption of the fetal bones. Bone growth was determined by measuring the total bone length and the length of the diaphysis, determining the hydroxyproline content and studying nondecalcified sections of the bones by light microscopy. Calcification was studied by determining bone Ca and P content and resorption was estimated as the percent of total ^{45}Ca released into the medium.

$24,25(OH)_2D_3$ stimulated bone growth and mineralization at concentrations of 10^{-8} to 10^{-10}M and inhibited bone growth and mineralization at 10^{-6}M. ^{45}Ca release was significantly higher at 10^{-6}M when compared to control bones but was not different from controls at lower concentrations (Table 1). $1,25(OH)_2D_3$ inhibited growth and mineralization already at 10^{-8}M with the highest effect at 10^{-10}M and was dose dependent. ^{45}Ca release was significantly higher, at a dose dependent curve (Table 1). Hydroxyproline content was significantly increased in the bones exposed to $24,25(OH)_2D_3$ at concentrations of 10^{-9} and 10^{-10}M but was decreased by the addition of $1,25(OH)_2D_3$ or of 10^{-6}M $24,25(OH)_2D_3$ (Table 1).

Our morphological studies have shown that $24,25(OH)_2D_3$ stimulated new bone growth in vitro. There were more mesenchymal cells undergoing differentiation than in controls and the metaphysis and diaphysis was surrounded by a relatively thick periosteal bone collar. Bones grown in the presence of $1,25(OH)_2D_3$ revealed diaphyseal bone having few, short, and thin trabeculae with numerous osteoclasts (Fig. 1). Our results suggest that $24,25(OH)_2D_3$ at physiological doses has a direct stimulatory effect on bone formation in vitro but in pharmacological doses may enhance bone resorption. $1,25(OH)_2D_3$ is a potent bone resorber at concentrations higher than 10^{-11}M. This metabolite was not seen to directly enhance bone formation at the concentrations used by us. Our results on the direct action of $24,25(OH)_2D_3$ and of $1,25(OH)_2D_3$ are also in line with previous studies which showed a transplacental stimulatory effect of $24,25(OH)_2D_3$ on bone formation in rat fetuses as well as severe inhibition of fetal bone formation by high doses of $1,25(OH)_2D_3$[4].

Vitamin D. A Chemical, Biochemical and Clinical Update

TABLE 1

THE EFFECT OF DIFFERENT CONCENTRATIONS OF $24,25(OH)_2D_3$ AND OF $1,25(OH)_2D_3$ ON FETAL MICE LONG BONES IN VITRO: RESULTS OF A TYPICAL EXPERIMENT.

Treatment	Diaphyseal length±SE (mm)	Hydroxyproline/protein ± SE	Ca ± SE µg/bone	P ± SE µg/bone	% 45Ca releasae
		$24,25(OH)_2D_3$			
---	1.06±0.06	0.078±0.002	5.95±0.22	2.41±0.10	24.67±0.52
10^{-6} M	0.95±0.05	0.056±0.004*	4.11±0.32*	2.08±0.12*	34.27±2.26*
10^{-7} M	1.25±0.06	N.D	6.40±0.41	2.57±0.10	23.13±4.50
10^{-8} M	1.33±0.08*	0.092±0.010	6.75±0.27*	2.85±0.12*	28.13±4.50
10^{-9} M	1.37±0.06*	0.112±0.015*	7.00±0.21*	2.91±0.10*	29.04±1.01
10^{-10} M	1.34±0.07*	0.090±0.009	6.55±0.50	2.95±0.16*	27.21±2.38
		$1,25(OH)_2D_3$			
---	1.48±0.04	0.146±0.006	9.85±0.71	3.72±0.26	27.33±0.91
10^{-8} M	1.20±0.07*	0.082±0.004*	7.32±0.67*	2.65±0.20*	52.67±5.15*
10^{-9} M	1.24±0.08	0.098±0.007*	7.85±0.91*	3.05±0.37	42.79±2.50*
10^{-10} M	1.39±0.05	N.D	9.12±0.78	3.40±0.15	39.96±3.02*
10^{-11} M	1.40±0.06	0.148±0.009	10.10±0.66	3.71±0.31	29.80±1.29
10^{-12} M	1.49±0.06	0.136±0.012	11.15±1.62	3.73±0.30	27.32±0.49

Each value is the mean ± SE of 6 bones.

* Significantly different from control $P<0.05$

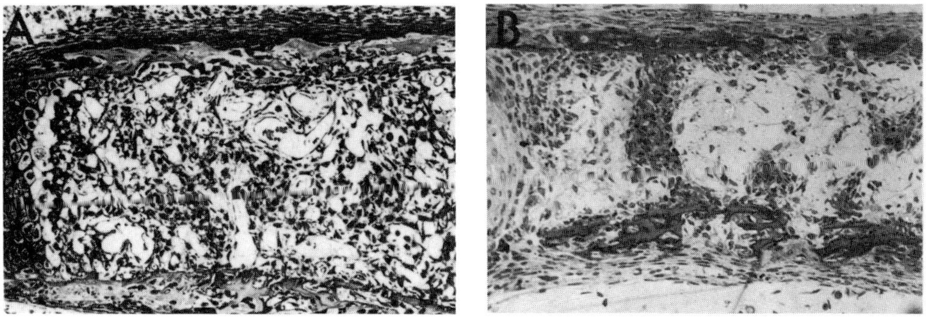

Fig. 1. 16 day old fetal mouse bone grown for 48 hrs. A) control, B) $1,25(OH)_2D_3$ at 10^{-8}M showing fewer diaphyseal trabeculae (Tol. blue x200)

References

1. Ornoy, A., Goodwin, G., Noff, D. and Edelstein, S. (1978) Nature, 276, 517-519.
2. Tanaka, Y., DeLuca, H.F., Kobayashi, Y., Taguchi, T., Ikekawa, N. and Monsaki, M. (1979) J. Biol. Chem. 254, 7163-7167.
3. Schwartz, A., Ornoy, A. and Soskolne, A.W. (1985) Acta Anat. in press.
4. Zusman, I., Hirsh, B.E., Edelstein, S., Ornoy, A. (1981) Acta Anatomica 111, 343-351.

Calcium Binding Proteins – Chemistry Physiology / Molecular Biology

NOMENCLATURE OF THE VITAMIN D-INDUCED CALCIUM-BINDING PROTEINS

R.H. Wasserman

The vitamin D-induced calcium-binding protein (CaBP) was first identified in chick intestine and subsequently isolated and extensively characterized (1). This protein has a molecular weight of about 28,000 daltons, binds 4 Ca^{2+} atoms per molecule with high affinity ($k_a \sim 2 \times 10^6 M^{-1}$), and is present in a number of tissues in the chick (e.g., kidney), pancreas, brain). A similar immunologically cross-reactive protein of about 28,000 daltons also occurs in mammalian tissues, prominently in the kidney and brain of some species.

Smaller CaBPs were also identified in the intestine of the rat and other mammalian species. These mammalian CaBPs have a molecular weight of about 9,000 daltons, bind two Ca^{2+} atoms per molecule with high affinity ($k_a \sim 2 \times 10^6 M^{-1}$) and is prominently present in the intestine, but also occurs in other mammalian tissues (e.g., kidney, bone tissue, teeth). The amino acid sequence of the 9kd intestinal proteins from the pig, cow and rat and the 28kd intestinal protein from the chick indicate their homology with the calcium-binding proteins of the troponin C super family, which include parvalbumin, calmodulin and troponin C. Each of these proteins contain the E-F hand configuration of the calcium-binding site in accordance with the "rules" of Kretsinger (2).

The function of the CaBPs in epithelial tissues is unknown at present although a quantitative relation exists between the degree of intestinal calcium absorption and intestinal CaBP concentrations. Suggestions have been put forth as to its mechanism of action (diffusional facilitator, activator of enzymes, intracellular calcium buffer) but an absolute definition of their function is still lacking. Also unknown is the function of the CaBPs in non-epithelial-type tissues, such as the brain and pancreas.

With this base of information, a group comprised of C.S. Fullmer, W.E. Stumpf, T. Freund, S. Christakos, M. Thomasset, A.W. Norman, A.K. Hall, O. Parkes, K. Baimbridge, V. Leathers, D. Pansu, E.M.W. Maunder, S. Ferrari and R.H. Wasserman met during the 6th Workshop on Vitamin D to discuss nomenclature of the CaBPs. The following designations were proposed and generally agreed upon by the group.

For the 28,000 dalton protein:

Calbindin-D_{28K}

For the 9,000 dalton protein:

Calbindin-D_{9K}

The "hyphen D" designates its dependency on vitamin D or a metabolite of vitamin D, and the subscript, the approximate molecular weight to differentiate the smaller from the larger protein.

CaBP remains as the appropriate abbreviation for both types of protein which could be made more specific with the relevant subscripts ($CaBP_{28K}$, $CaBP_{9K}$).

This nomenclature includes two of their important properties, i.e. high affinity calcium-binding and their dependency on vitamin D, and does not imply a function, the

Vitamin D. A Chemical, Biochemical and Clinical Update

latter still not precisely known. When a function has been defined, a more appropriate name could be proposed.

1. Background information can be found in R.H. Wasserman and C.S. Fullmer, "Vitamin D-Induced Calcium-Binding Protein", in Calcium and Cell Function (Ed. W.Y. Cheung), Academic Press, N.Y., Vol. II: 175-216, 1982. The sequence homology of Calbindin-D_{9K} and Calbindin-D_{28K} with other calcium-binding proteins is given by Fullmer and Wasserman (this volume). Other reports in this volume further define other properties and characteristics of the Calbindin-D's.

2. Kretsinger, R.H. Structure and function of calcium-modulated proteins. CRC Crit. Rev. Biochem. 8: 119-174, 1980.

VITAMIN D-INDUCED INTESTINAL CALCIUM-BINDING PROTEIN FROM THE CHICK: TENTATIVE AMINO ACID SEQUENCE

C.S. Fullmer and R.H. Wasserman
Department of Physiology, New York State College of Veterinary Medicine, Cornell University, Ithaca, New York 14853

Introduction:

The vitamin D-induced calcium-binding proteins (CaBP) represent the best defined molecular expression of the vitamin D endocrine system. Whereas considerable information is available regarding their physicochemical properties as well as their physiological relationships to vitamin D, their precise function in the process of calcium metabolism remains unknown.

Two types of vitamin D-induced CaBPs have been recognized which are species and tissue specific and within each type, additional primary structural variability exists.

Representative of the first type are the 9 kd mammalian intestinal CaBPs as well as those from bovine and porcine kidneys which bind 2 Ca atoms per molecule with high affinity. artial or complete primary structures are presently available for the bovine (1), porcine (2) and rat (3) proteins which, while not identical, (structurally or immunologically) exhibit considerable homology. These 9 kd proteins have been demonstrated to be members of the troponin C superfamily of high affinity calcium-binding proteins together with troponin C, calmodulin and the parvalbumins. Despite similarities in size and calcium-binding properties, the 9 kd vitamin D-induced CaBPs and the parvalbumins do not share significant overall structural similarities.

The second type of vitamin D-induced CaBPs, present in avian intestine, kidney, uterus (shell gland), rat and human kidney and in both avian and mammalian brain, are approximately 28 kd, bind 4 Ca atoms per molecule and have immunological properties in common. Primary structural determination has not been reported for this type and, therefore, their relationship to each other, to the 9 kd vitamin D-induced CaBPs and to calmodulin and troponin C remain unknown.

We report here the tentative amino acid sequence of the vitamin D-induced chick intestinal CaBP as representative of the 28 kd type.

Materials and Methods:

Chick intestinal CaBP was purified essentially as described previously (4). All preparations were subjected to reverse phase high performance liquid chromatography (HPLC) as the final purification step and to remove bound Ca^{2+} and buffer salts. Procedures for amino acid compositional analyses and automated sequence determination were as previously described (1).

All enzymatic digestions were conducted in 0.2 N N-ethylmorpholine acetate buffer (pH 8.0) at 37°C for the time periods indicated, with enzyme to protein ratio of about 1/100 (w/w). Peptide separations of the enzymatic digests were achieved by reverse phase HPLC, essentially as described (5), using a Waters Associates Z-Module fitted with an 8 mm C18 μBondapak (10 μ) Radial Pak cartridge. Separations were performed at room temperature at a flow rate of 2 ml/min and at operating pressures of 400 psi or less. Collected peptides were dried under a stream of nitrogen at 30°C for compositional, sequence and other analyses.

Vitamin D. A Chemical, Biochemical and Clinical Update

CHICK INTESTINAL CALCIUM-BINDING PROTEIN
TENTATIVE PRIMARY STRUCTURE

*(Thr,Ala)-Glu-(Thr-Glu-Gly-Val-Leu-His)-Glu-(Ser,Glu,Ala,Ala,Ile)-Phe-Phe-Glu-Ile-Trp-His-His-Tyr-Asp-Ser-

Asp-Gly-Asn-Gly-Tyr-Met-Asp-Gly-Lys-Glu-Leu-Gln-Asn-Phe-Ile-Gln-Glu-Leu-Gln-Gln-Ala-Arg-Ala-Gly-Leu-

Asp-Leu-Thr-Pro-Glu-Met-Lys-Ala-Phe-Val-Asp-Gln-Tyr-Gly-Lys(Asp,Thr,Gly,Ala,Leu,)-Lys-Ile-Gly-Ile-Val-

Glu-Leu-Ala-Gln-Val-Leu-Pro-Thr-Glu-Glu-Asn-Phe-Leu-Leu-Phe-Phe-Arg-Cys-Gln-Gln-Leu-Lys-Ser-Ser-Glu-

Asp-Phe-Met-Gln-Thr-Trp-Arg-Lys-Tyr-Asp-Ser-Asp-His-Ser-Gly-Phe-Ile-Asp-Ser-Glu-Glu-Leu-Lys-Ser-Phe-

Leu-Lys-(Asp,Glu,Ala,Leu,Leu,)-Lys-Gln-Ile-Glu-Asp-Ser-Lys-Leu-Thr-Glu-Tyr-Thr-Glu-Ile-Met-Leu-Arg-Met-

Phe-Asp-Ala-Asn-Asn-Asp-Gly-Lys-Leu-Glu-Leu-Thr-Glu-Leu-Ala-Arg-Leu-Leu-Pro-Val-Gln-Glu-Asn-Phe-Leu-

Ile-Lys-Phe-Gln-Gly-Val-Lys-Met-Cys-Ala-Lys-Glu-Phe-Asn-Lys-Ala-Phe-Glu-Met-Tyr-Asp-Gln-Asp-Gly-Asn-

Gly-Tyr-Ile-Asp-Glu-Asn-Glu-Leu-Asp-Ala-Leu-Leu-Lys-Asp-Leu-Cys-Glu-Lys-Glu-Leu-Asp-Ile-Asn-Asn-Leu-

Ala-Thr-Tyr-Lys-Lys-Ser-Ile-Met-Ala-Leu-Ser-Asp-Gly-Gly-Lys-Leu-Tyr-Arg-Ala-Glu-Leu-Ala-Leu-Ile-Leu-

Cys-Ala-Glu-Glu-Asn-OH

Cysteine residues were blocked in the reduced CaBP by alkylation with 4-vinyl pyridine to form the S-β-(4-pyridylethyl) cysteine (PEC) derivatives, as recently detailed (5).

Results and Discussion:

Direct automated sequencing of the chick CaBP was precluded by the presence of an N-terminal blocking group, a property shared by all members of the troponin C superfamily investigated to date. Enzymatic cleavage was initiated with TPCK-trypsin. Peptide separation by HPLC produced 21 tryptic peptides (Fig. 1), 19 of which were sequenced to completion or near completion (Table 1). Two additional peptides, designated as T-24 (34 residues) and T-27 (49 residues) could not be sequenced and were tentatively assigned to the N-terminus. Tryptic peptide T-27 was later shown to be an incomplete cleavage product containing the sequence, T24 →T-21. Similarly, peptide T-25 was found to be identical to T-22, but containing 5 additional residues at the C-terminus.

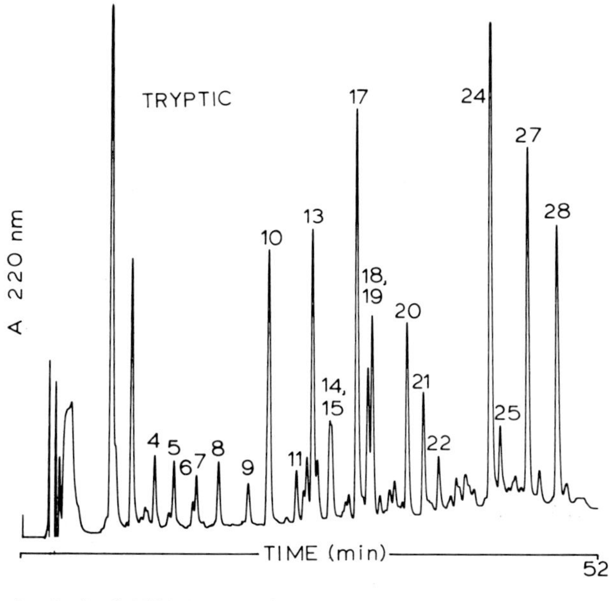

Figure 1. Analytical HPLC peptide map of 1 hour tryptic digest of native chick CaBP (100 μg). Unresolved peaks were isolated under special run conditions from the preparative map (not shown).

While this initial tryptic map provided peptides to account for the bulk of the protein sequence, only 227 of the expected ∿ 250 residues were found. In addition, only one cysteine residue was identified (peptide T-25, in low yield) from a predicted total of three, based on compositional analysis of performic acid oxidized CaBP. These results suggested either the existence of disulfide linkage in the native protein or some degree of oxidation of sulfhydryl groups during the mapping procedure with possible subsequent formation of mixed disulfides. Since all peptides contained at least one Lys or Arg residue, no C-terminal assignment could be made.

TABLE I

CHICK CABP - SEQUENCE OF TRYPTIC PEPTIDES

T-4	Q-I-E-D-S-K	(6)
T-5	E-F-N-K	(4)
T-6	L-Y-R	(3)
T-7	F-Q-G-V-K	(5)
T-8	D-L-L-Q-K	(5)
T-9	S-F-L-K	(4)
T-10	A-F-V-D-Q-Y-G-K	(8)
T-11	S-I-M-A-L-S-D-G-G-K	(10)
T-13	K-Y-D-S-D-H-S-G-F-I-D-S-E-E-L-K	(16)
T-14	A-G-L-D-L-T-P-E-M-K	(10)
T-15	E-L-D-I-N-N-L-A-T-Y-K-K	(12)
T-17	S-S-E-D-F-M-Q-T-W-R	(10)
T-18	L-T-E-Y-T-E-I-M-L-R	(10)
T-19	M-F-D-A-N-N-D-G-K-L-E-L-T-E-L-A-R	(17)
T-20	L-L-P-V-Q-E-N-F-L-I-K	(11)
T-21	E-L-Q-N-F-I-Q-E-L-Q-Q-A-R	(13)
T-22	A-F-E-M-Y-D-Q-D-G-N-G-Y-I-D-E-N-E-L-D-A-L-L-K	(-)
T-24	(D_4,T_2,S_2,E_5,G_4,A_3,V,M,I_2,L,Y_2,F_2,H_3,W,K)	(34)
T-25	A-F-E-M-Y-D-Q-D-G-N-G-Y-I-D-E-N-E-L-D-A-L-L-K-D(E,L,C)-K	(28)
T-27	(D_5,T_2,S_2,E_{11},G_4,A_4,V,M,I_3,L_3,Y_2,F_3,H_3,W,K,R)	(-)
T-28	I-G-I-V-E-L-A-Q-V-L-P-T-E-E-N-F-L-L-F-F-R	(21)
		(227)
PEC_T-1	M-C-A-K	(4)
PEC_T-2	C-Q-Q-L-K	(5)
PEC_T-3	D-L-C-E-K	(-)
PEC_T-3a	A-F-E-M-Y-D-Q-D-G-N-G-Y-I-D-E-N-E-L-D-A-L-L-K-D-L-C-E-K	(-)
PEC_T-4	A-E-L-A-L-I-L-C-A-E-E-N	(12)
		(248)

In any event, it was decided to break any existing disulfide bonds and block and protect all sulfhydryl groups. Numerous techniques exist for deactivating cysteine sulfhydryls, most of which introduce additional difficulties in subsequent procedures. We chose a method, originally described in conjunction with cysteine compositional determination, which employs alkylation of the completely reduced protein with 4-vinyl pyridine to form the S-β-4 pyridylethyl cysteine derivative (6). This was shown to be an excellent derivative for compositional and sequence analyses and to introduce a reporter group (254 nm) which provides for the facile and instantaneous identification of cysteine-containing peptides during HPLC mapping (5).

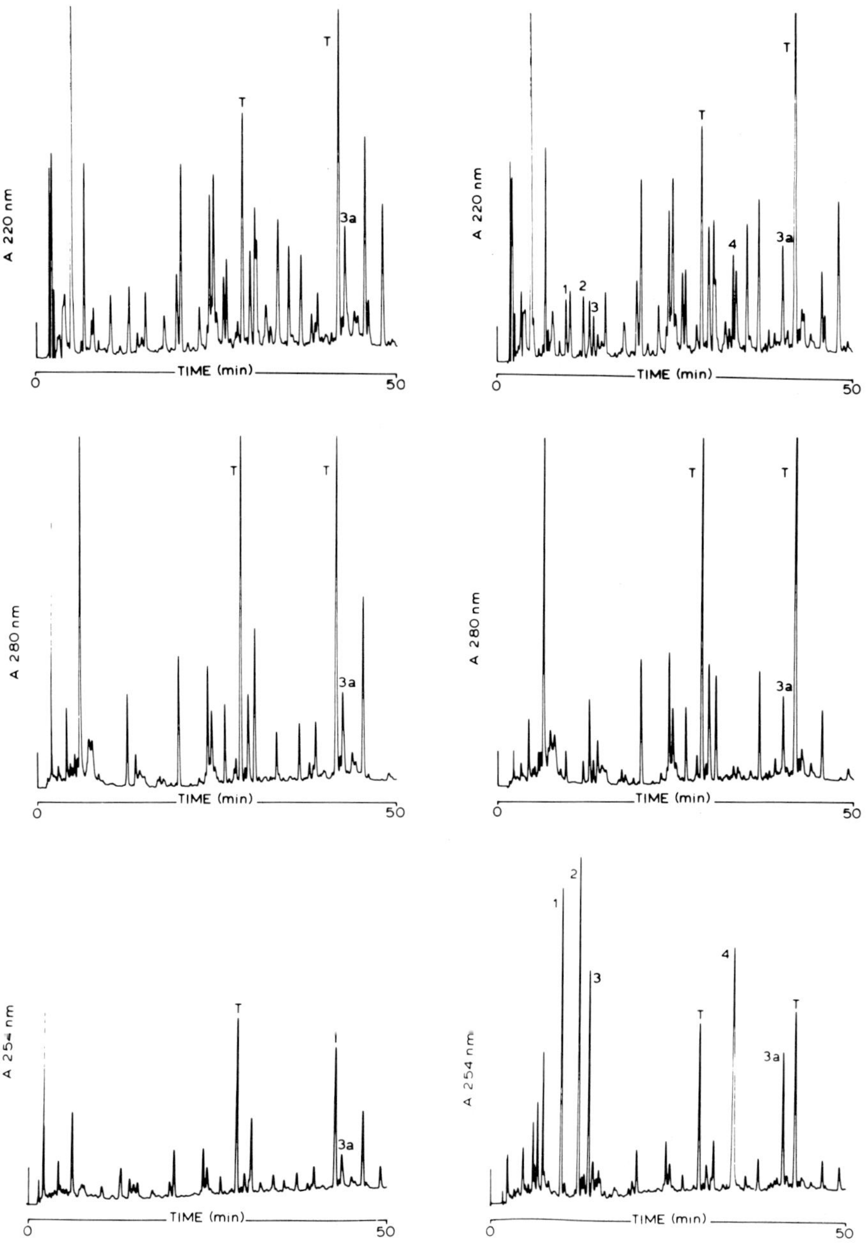

Figure 2. Analytical HPLC maps of 2 hour tryptic digests of chick CaBP (20 μg) with simultaneous effluent monitoring at 220, 280, and 254 nm. Left, native CaBP and right, PEC-CaBP. Tryptophan-containing peptides denoted by (T).

Following tryptic digestion of the S-pyridylethylated CaBP (PEC-CaBP), we could now identify and isolate, in high yield, 4 new tryptic peptides (Fig. 2), each of which was shown to contain 1 mole of PE-cysteine per mole of peptide. The sequences of these peptides (Table 1) were shown to be mutually exclusive, establishing the existence of 4 cysteine residues in the chick CaBP. In addition, one of these peptides (PEC_T-4), was shown to contain neither Lys or Arg and was tentatively assigned to the C-Terminus of the protein. From this point on, all cleavages were conducted on the PEC-CaBP only.

Partial tryptic digestion was employed as a means of obtaining larger fragments to aid in grouping and overlapping the original tryptic peptides. In this case, tryptic digestion was for 1 hour at pH 7.4 in the presence of 5 mM $CaCl_2$, followed by HPLC mapping (Fig. 3). This approach resulted in a number of tryptic peptides identical to those present in the map from the complete digest, some of which were recovered quantitatively. However, 4 large fragments (PTD 1-4) were isolated which subsequently aided in the overlapping. Fragment PTD 1 was shown to be identical to peptide T-27, whereas fragments PTD 2-4 were not previously

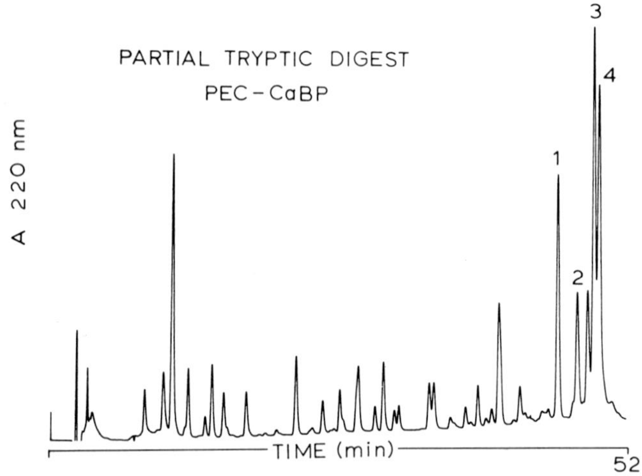

Figure 3. Analytical HPLC map of the partial tryptic digest (PTD) of PEC-CABP (100 µg).

encountered. Each of these fragments was subjected to complete tryptic digestion and HPLC mapping to ascertain the grouping of original tryptic peptides within each. Subsequent analyses of fragments PTD 1-4 were conducted in a similar fashion and provided less complicated maps than could be obtained from the intact CaBP. Due to space restrictions, fragment PTD 1 will serve as an example of the overlapping strategy. Fragment PTD 1 (blocked) was shown to be composed of T-24 (blocked) and T-21 (Fig. 4). Fragment PTD 3 also contained peptides T-24 and T-21 and, in addition, peptides T-10, T-14 and T-28. Fragment PTD 2 contained peptides T-17, T-4, T-9, T-13, T-18 and T-19 and fragment PTD 4 was identical except it also contained peptide T-20. These two pairs of overlapping fragments accounted

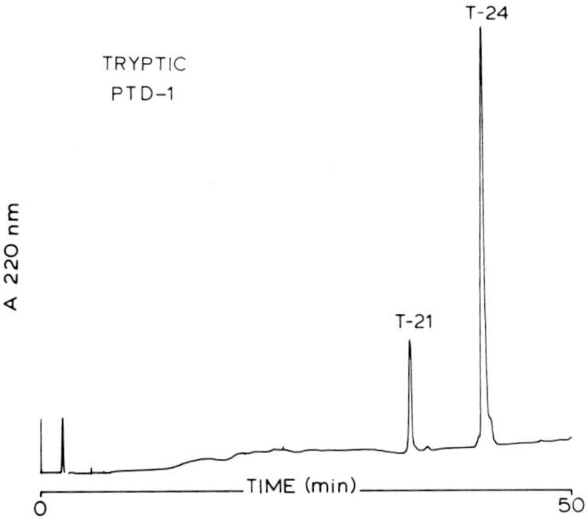

Figure 4. Analytical HPLC map of the complete tryptic digest (16 hours) of PTD 1 (20 µg).

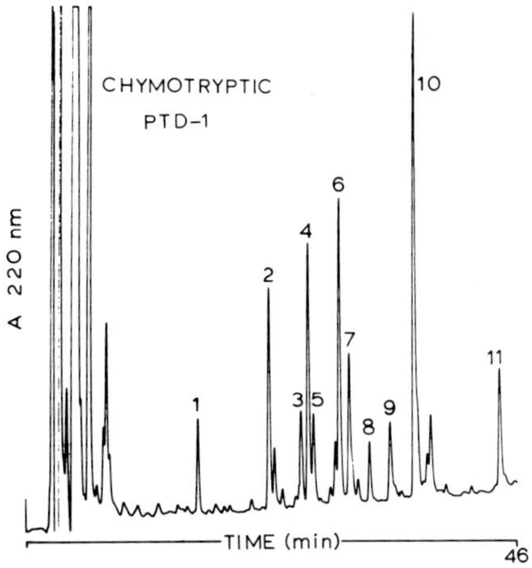

Figure 5. Analytial HPLC map of the chymotryptic digest (2 hours) of PTD 1 (40 µg).

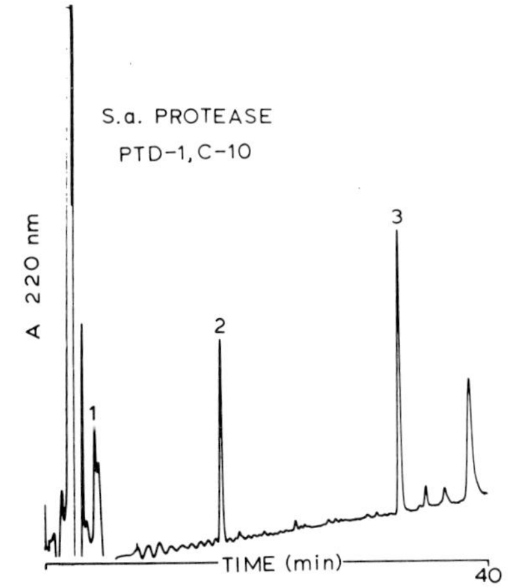

Figure 6. Analytical HPLC map of the S. aureus protease digest (16 hours) of PTD 1, C-10 (20 µg).

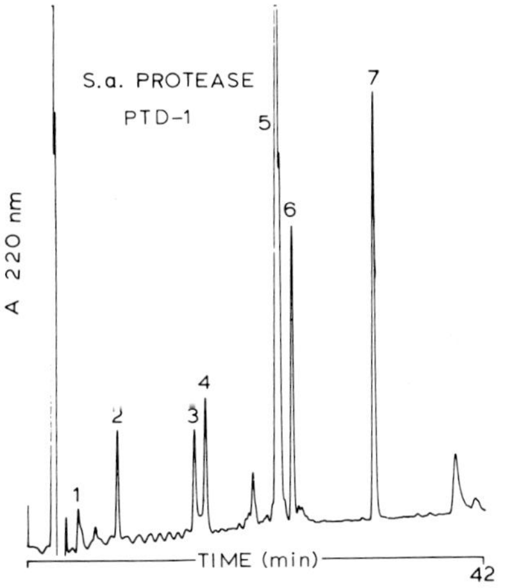

Figure 7. Analytical HPLC map of the S. aureus protease digest of PTD 1 (40 µg).

for about two-thirds of the protein sequence (160 residues) with the remainder cleaved completely to the constituent peptides. No Cys-containing peptides were present in fragments PTD 1-4.

Chymotryptic digestion of PTD 1 produced 11 peptides (Fig. 5). All were sequenced with the exception of PTD 1, C-8 (16 residues) and PTD 1, C-10 (17 residues) which were blocked and differed only by one Phe residue. S. aureus protease cleavage of PTD 1, C-10 yielded three peptides (Fig. 6), the sequences of which are yet to be determined, but are aligned at the N-terminus. S. aureus protease cleavage of PTD 1 (Fig. 7) completed the overlapping (Fig. 8). In this manner, overlaps were also established in PTD 2-4.

```
PTD-1              *(D,D,D, D,T,T,S,S,E,E, E,E,E,G,G, G,G,A,A,A,V,M,I,I,L,Y,Y,F,F,H,H,H,W)K-E-L-Q-N-F-I-Q-E-L-Q-Q-A-R
                   *(T,A-E)(T,E,G,V,L,H-E)(S,E,A,A,I)-F-F-E-I-W-H-H-Y-D-S-D-G-N-G-Y-M-D-G-K-E-L-Q-N-F-I-Q-E-L-Q-Q-A-R

CHYMOTRYPTIC  (1)                                                                                  I-Q-E-L-Q-Q-A-R
              (2)                                                    D-S-D-G-N-G-Y
              (3)                                                                  M-D-G-K-E-L-Q-N-F
              (4)                                        E-I-W
              (5)                                        E-I-W-H-H-Y
              (6)                                              H-H-Y-D-S-D-G-N-G-Y-M-D-G-K-E-L-Q-N-F
              (7)                                        E-I-W-H-H-Y-D-S-D-G-N-G-Y-M-D-G-K-E-L-Q-N-F
              (8) *(T,T,S, E,E,E,E,G,A,A, A,V,I,L,H, F)
              (9)                                      F-E-I-W
             (10) *(T,T,S, E,E,E,E,G,A,A, A,V,I,L,H,F, F)
             (11)                                      F-E-I-W-H-H-Y-D-S-D-G-N-G-Y-M-D-G-K-E-L-Q-N-F

S.A. PROTEASE (1) *(T,A-E)
              (2)                                                                                          L-Q-Q-A-R
              (3)
              (4)       (T,E,G,V,L,H-E)
              (5)                                          I-W-H-H-Y-D-S-D-G-N-G-Y-M-D-G-K-E
              (6)                                                                            L-Q-N-F-I-Q-E
              (7)                     (S,E,A,A,I)-F-F-E
```

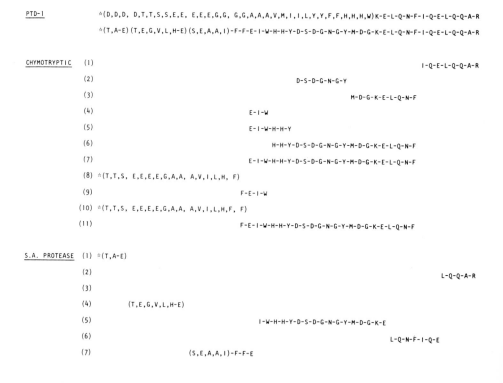

Figure 8. Established overlaps in fragment PTD 1 from chymotryptic and S. aureus protease digestions. Blocking group denoted by (*).

The remaining sequence overlaps are based on preliminary mapping of the chymotryptic (Fig. 9) and S. aureus protease (Fig. 10) digests from intact PEC-CaBP. The bulk of sequence missing from the partial tryptic digest was determined to be from the C-terminal one-third of the protein. In fact, only one of the original tryptic peptides (T_{PEC}-2) was positioned in the N-terminal two-thirds of the protein, overlapping PTD 3 and PTD 2. Also, two regions of sequence were identified subsequent to tryptic mapping which require sequence determination.

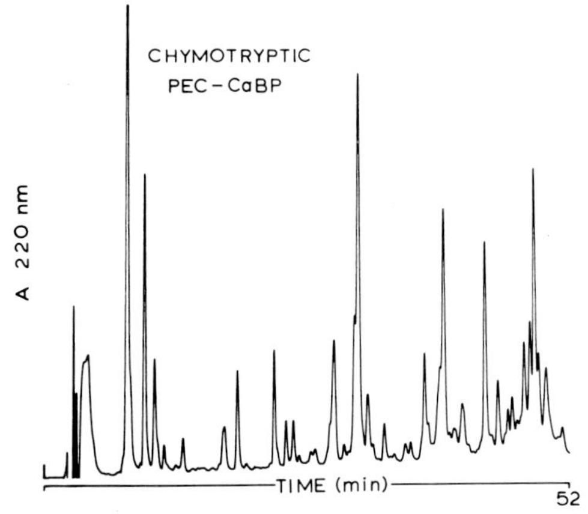

Figure 9. Analytical HPLC map of the chymotryptic digest (2 hours) of intact PEC-CaBP.

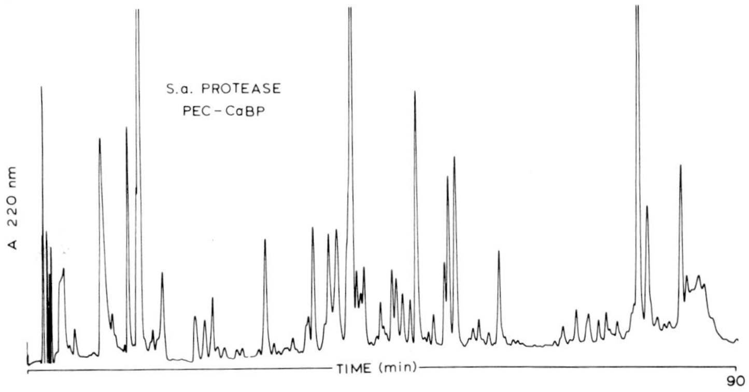

Figure 10. Analytical HPLC map of the S. aureus protease digest (16 hours) of the intact PEC-CaBP (100 µg).

While the amino acid sequence of chick CaBP presented here is tentative, pending confirmation of the C-terminal overlaps and determination of several short regions of sequence, several conclusions may be made regarding the overall primary structure. Four regions of homologous sequence exist in the chick CaBP (Fig. 11) which fit exactly the test sequence for "E-F Hand" type calcium-binding proteins (7) and are clearly homologous with the proposed calcium-binding regions in the vitamin D-induced mammalian CaBPs as well as calmodulin and Troponin C. However, aside from homology in these regions, there is insufficient overall similarity between the chick (28 kd) and mammalian (9 kd) CaBPs to point obviously to gene duplication.

	H	X*		Y*		Z*	GLY	-Y	H	-X*			-Z*	H
C CaBP - I	TYR	ASP	SER	ASP	GLY	ASN	GLY	TYR	MET	ASP	GLY	LYS	GLU	LEU
C CaBP - II	TYR	ASP	SER	ASP	HIS	SER	GLY	PHE	ILE	ASP	SER	GLU	GLU	LEU
C CaBP - III	PHE	ASP	ALA	ASN	ASN	ASP	GLY	LYS	LEU	GLU	LEU	THR	GLU	LEU
C CaBP - IV	TYR	ASP	GLN	ASP	GLY	ASN	GLY	TYR	ILE	ASP	GLU	ASN	GLU	LEU
MCBP - CD	GLY	ASP	SER	ASP	GLY	ASP	GLY	LYS	ILE	GLY	VAL	ASP	GLU	PHE
MCBP - EF	ILE	ASP	GLN	ASP	LYS	SER	GLY	PHE	ILE	GLU	GLU	ASP	GLU	LEU
STnC - I	PHE	ASP	ALA	ASP	GLY	GLY	GLY	ASP	ILE	SER	VAL	LYS	GLU	LEU
STnC - II	VAL	ASP	GLU	ASP	GLY	SER	GLY	THR	ILE	ASP	PHE	GLU	GLU	PHE
STnC - III	PHE	ASP	ARG	ASN	ALA	ASP	GLY	TYR	ILE	ASP	ALA	GLU	GLU	LEU
STnC - IV	GLY	ASP	LYS	ASP	ASN	ASP	GLY	ARG	ILE	ASP	PHE	ASP	GLU	PHE
CaM - I	PHE	ASP	LYS	ASP	GLY	ASN	GLY	THR	ILE	THR	THR	LYS	GLU	LEU
CaM - II	VAL	ASP	ALA	ASP	GLY	ASN	GLY	THR	ILE	ASP	PHE	PRO	GLU	PHE
CaM - III	PHE	ASP	LYS	ASP	GLY	ASN	GLY	TYR	ILE	SER	ALA	ALA	GLU	LEU
CaM - IV	ALA	ASN	ILE	ASP	GLY	ASP	GLY	GLU	VAL	ASN	TYR	GLU	GLU	PHE
B CaBP - II	LEU	ASP	LYS	ASN	GLY	ASP	GLY	GLU	VAL	SER	PHE	GLU	GLU	PHE
B CaBP - I	TYR	ALA	LYS	GLU	GLY	ASP	PRO	GLN	LEU	SER	LYS	GLU	GLU	LEU
	\ / ALA						\ / ASN							

Figure 11. Comparison of Ca-binding sites in chick CaBP with those of other calcium-binding proteins. H = hydrophobic; X,Y,Z = local coordinate system;; * = oxygen donor; C CaBP = chick CaBP; MCBP = carp muscle parvalbumin; STnC = skeletal troponin C; CaM = calmodulin; B CaBP = bovine CaBP. See reference 7 for details.

Acknowledgements:
This work supported by Grant AM-04652 from the National Institutes of Health.

References:

1. Fullmer, C.S. and Wasserman, R.H. (1981) J. Biol. Chem. 256, 5669-5674.
2. Hofmann, T., Kawakami, M., Hitchman, A.J.W., Harrison, J.E. and Dorington, K.H. (1979) Can. J. Biochem. 57, 737-748.
3. Desplan, C., Heidmann, O., Lillie, J.W., Auffray, C. and Thomasset, M. (1983) J. Biol. Chem. 258, 13502-13505.
4. Wasserman, R.H., Corradino, R.A. and Taylor, A.N. (1968) J. Biol. Chem. 243, 3978-3986.
5. Fullmer, C.S. (1984) Anal. Biochem. 142, 336-339.
6. Friedman, M., Krull, L.H. and Cavins, J.F. (1970) J. Biol. Chem. 245, 3868-3871.
7. Tufty, R.M. and Kretsinger, R.H. (1975) Science 187, 167-169.

CLONING OF cDNAs TO THE CHICK INTESTINAL 28K VITAMIN D-INDUCED CALCIUM BINDING PROTEIN (CaBP) mRNA AND THEIR USE TO STUDY THE REGULATION OF THE CaBP MESSAGE

G. Theofan, A. K. Hall, M. W. King and A. W. Norman, Dept. Biochem., University of California, Riverside, CA 92521, USA.

Introduction

The 28K calcium binding protein (CaBP) is the principal protein induced by $1,25(OH)_2D_3$ in the chick intestine, and it is also present in many other tissues. While the intestinal level of CaBP is proportional to intestinal Ca^{2+} transport, the exact biochemical function of CaBP remains unknown. CaBP is induced in the chick intestine by $1,25(OH)_2D_3$ via receptor-mediated induction of CaBP gene transcription. This is supported by the facts that $1,25(OH)_2D_3$ stimulation of CaBP production is inhibited by transcriptional inhibitors (actinomycin D and α-amanitin) and is correlated with increased polysomal CaBP-mRNA activity as well as increased nuclear, cytoplasmic, and total cellular CaBP-mRNA levels. In an effort to define the precise molecular responsibilities of $1,25(OH)_2D_3$ in mediating production of CaBP, we have synthesized and cloned cDNAs to CaBP-mRNA. These clones have been used as probes to study regulation of CaBP-mRNA under various conditions. In addition we have attempted to generate and sequence full length cDNAs to CaBP-mRNA in an attempt to determine the sequence of CaBP, which is still not completely known. Since CaBP has about 242 amino acids, the minimum message size to code for this protein would be about 726 nucleotides (not including 5' and 3' untranslated regions).

Cloning of cDNAs to CaBP-mRNA

Early attempts to generate cDNAs to CaBP-mRNA were hampered by the low abundance (0.1%) of this message in the chick intestine. By using polysome immunoprecipitation to enrich for CaBP-mRNA, and by screening the cDNA library with [^{32}P]-labeled cDNA probes prepared from this enriched mRNA preparation, it was possible to identify 26 clones as candidates for cDNAs to CaBP-mRNA. To determine whether any of these clones contained inserts complementary to CaBP-mRNA they were analyzed by hybridization selection and in vitro translation of the selected mRNAs. Using these procedures it was determined that 3 clones, designated pCI-CaBP-1, pCI-CaBP-2, and pCI-CaBP-26, did indeed contain sequences complementary to CaBP-mRNA (1).

Using these clones as probes in a "Northern" analysis of chick intestinal mRNA, it was determined that there were 3 species of CaBP-mRNA that were 2,000, 2,600 and 3,00 nucleotides long (see Fig. 2). Unfortunately the 3 clones were much smaller, only 200-400 base pairs each. It therefore became necessary to screen additional cDNA libraries in order to identify a clone(s) that would encompass the full length of the CaBP-mRNA. In order to optimize the synthesis of full length cDNA copies, the procedure of Gubler and Hoffman (2) was used. This procedure combines conventional first strand synthesis using reverse transcriptase with a novel second strand synthetic procedure using RNase H, DNA polymerase, and polynucleotide kinase. This eliminates the S_1-nuclease treatment which therefore optimizes the chance of obtaining full length cDNAs. The cDNAs

Vitamin D. A Chemical, Biochemical and Clinical Update

generated by these methods were then cloned in E. coli using pBR322 as the cloning vector. We used these methods to generate another cDNA library of approximately 13,000 clones (see Table 1 for cloning summary). After screening this library with the cDNA insert from pCI-CaBP-1 as a probe, we identified 3 additional clones which contained sequences complementary to CaBP-mRNA. One of these cDNAs was not excisable from the plasmid, the second was approximately 500 base pairs, and the third, designated pCI-CaBP-86, contained 1000 base pairs. This clone was further characterized by restriction mapping and was eventually sequenced in its entirety. The sequence of pCI-CaBP-86 overlapped with the 3 previous clones (pCI-CaBP-1, 2 and 26) which were also sequenced (see Fig. 1).

Table 1
Screening of Chick Intestinal cDNA Libraries

	Cloning		
	1st	2nd	3rd
Total Clones Screened	9,516	13,000	33,000
No. of clones with CaBP sequences	3	3	23
No. of "usable" cDNA probes	3	2	15

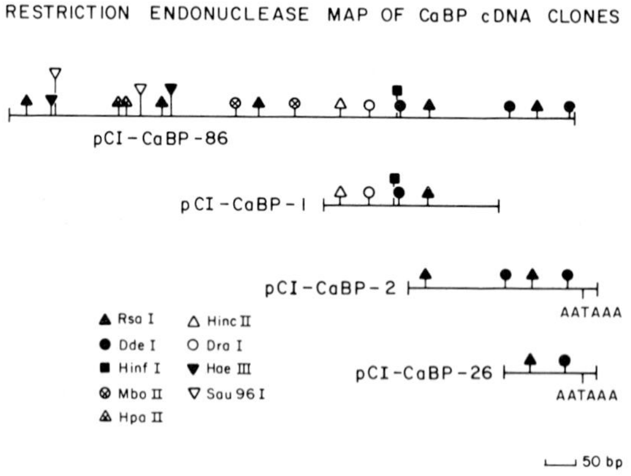

Fig. 1

Since our largest cDNA clone to this point still encompassed only half of the 2000 nucleotides of the CaBP-mRNA, we generated and screened a third, even larger cDNA library, again using the Gubler and Hoffman procedure (2). In an attempt to produce a greater number of positive clones, we used as the template poly A-mRNA prepared from intestinal RNA of chicks 5 hrs after a 6.5 nmole dose of $1,25(OH)_2D_3$. It had been determined in separate experiments that CaBP-mRNA levels are elevated significantly at this time (see Fig. 6). After screening this cDNA library with the cDNA insert from pCI-CaBP-86, 23 positive clones were identified (see Table 1). Three of these clones were larger than pCI-CaBP-86. The largest was designated pCI-CaBP-53, which encompassed 1700 base pairs, almost the full length of the CaBP message. Table 2 summarizes the CaBP-cDNA probes now available from screening all three cDNA libraries.

Table 2

Available cDNA Probes to the Chick Intestinal 28K-CaBP

Name	Length (bp)
pCI-CaBP-1	320
2	400
26	200
41	500
86	1000
53	1700
116	1600
207	1400
another 12 cDNAs	800-1000

We are now in the process of carrying out restriction mapping and sequencing of pCI-CaBP-53. Since this clone contains 1700 nucleotides of the 2000 nucleotide CaBP message, and since it would take approximately 720 nucleotides to code for CaBP, pCI-CaBP-53 should encompass at least more than half of the nucleotides which code for CaBP. It may be necessary to generate and screen additional CaBP-cDNA clones, perhaps by using primer extension techniques, to identify the 5' initiation site of the CaBP-mRNA. This would allow us to determine the entire sequence of CaBP, including the amino terminus which cannot be sequenced by conventional protein sequencing methods. In addition, we can generate 3' and 5'-cDNA probes which can be used to screen a chick genomic DNA library and allow us to begin studying the organization of the CaBP gene.

"Northern" Analysis of CaBP-mRNA Expression in Chick Intestine

In this series of experiments, total polyA-mRNA from chick intestine was separated by gel electrophoresis, then transferred to a nitrocellulose filter. This "Northern" blot was hybridized with one of the cDNA probes to CaBP-mRNA (labelled by nick translation), then subjected to autoradiography. Fig. 2 shows the results of a "Northern" hybridization analysis in which mRNA was isolated from intestine of vitamin D-deficient chicks at various times after receiving a dose of $1,25(OH)_2D_3$ (3.25 nmoles). The autoradiograph in Fig. 2A shows that there are 3 species of CaBP-mRNA which can hybridize to a specific cDNA probe. These 3 species were determined to be 2000, 2600, and 3100 nucleotides in length. Furthermore, all 3 species of the message are regulated similarly by 1,25$(OH)_2D_3$. None of the mRNAs are present in the absence of hormonal stimulation. All 3 start to accumulate by 60 min after the 1,25$(OH)_2D_3$ dose, and all 3 reach maximum accumulation at 24 hrs. The kinetics of these changes can be seen more easily in the densitometric tracing (Fig. 2B) of the "Northern" blot depicted in Fig. 2A. In addition, the maximal level attained by each of the 3 species is 1.3 to 1.4 fold above the level of each respective message in the chonic vitamin D-replete intestine.

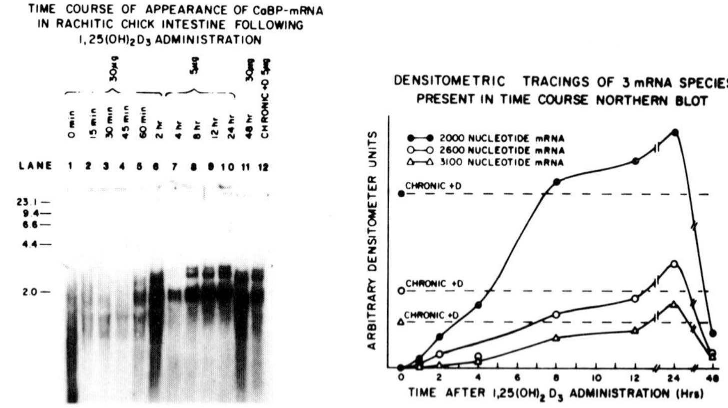

Fig. 2

There are several possible mechanisms to explain the existence of multiple forms of a particular message. One possibility is the existence of multiple CaBP genes, each of which produces a different size mRNA with similar nucleotide sequences. A "Southern" hybridization analysis of chick genomic DNA was carried out to determine the copy number of the CaBP gene (see Fig. 3). The results show that a [^{32}P]-labeled cDNA probe to CaBP-mRNA hybridized to only one PstI fragment, one EcoRI fragment, and two BamH1 fragments. This is strong evidence that the gene for CaBP is a unique gene in the chick genome, and therefore all 3 CaBP-mRNA species are transcribed from this single gene.

There are several other possible explanations for the existence of multiple forms of a message, a phenomenon which is not unique to CaBP-mRNA. The polymorphism seen in the message may result from differential processing at the 5' and/or 3' ends of the nuclear precursor mRNA, or, there could be multiple polyadenylation signal sequences at the 3' end of the gene. Multiple transcripts could also arise from the presence of more than one promoter sequence at the 5' end of the gene. Obviously, in order to determine the exact mode of production of the 3 CaBP-mRNA species, it will be necessary to know the complete nucleotide sequence of the CaBP gene. However, if there is any relationship of chick intestinal CaBP to calcium binding proteins in general, it is likely that the 3 species of CaBP-mRNA arise through multiple polyadenylation signals, as this is the situation for chick brain calmodulin mRNAs (3).

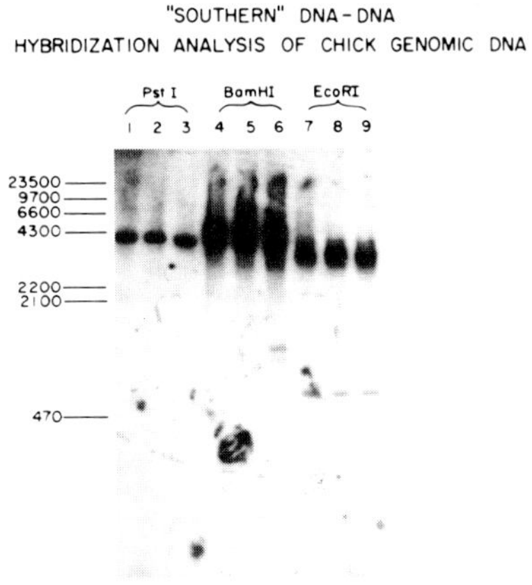

Fig. 3

Regulation of CaBP and CaBP-mRNA by 1,25$(OH)_2D_3$ in Chickens Fed Diets Varying in Calcium and Phosphorus Content

The availability of specific cDNA probes has allowed us to investigate the molecular responsibilities of 1,25$(OH)_2D_3$ at the level of the gene under a variety of physiological conditions. Preliminary experiments were directed towards mapping the temporal changes in intestinal CaBP-mRNA and CaBP as influenced by hormonal challenge with a pharmacological dose (6.5 nmoles) of 1,25$(OH)_2D_3$ *in vivo*. Groups of five birds were killed at intervals from 0 to 72 hrs following a single injection (6.5 nmoles, i.m.) of 1,25$(OH)_2D_3$. At these times, samples of intestinal mucosa were frozen in liquid nitrogen. Total cellular RNA was extracted by the guanidinium thiocyanate method (6) and blotted onto nitrocellulose filters which were hybridized with a cDNA probe prepared from pCI-CaBP-2 by nick translation. Hybridized filters were used to expose X-ray film and the autoradiographs were scanned densitometrically to quantitated the RNA in each dot. CaBP in the cytosolic fraction of intestinal homogenates was measured by an ELISA assay (7).

Initial experiments (Figs. 4A and 4B) revealed that rachitic intestinal mucosa did not contain statistically significant levels of CaBP-mRNA until 45 minutes after injection of 1,25$(OH)_2D_3$. To our knowledge, this is the earliest known effect of 1,25$(OH)_2D_3$ in relation to genome activation. CaBP-mRNA accumulation was maximal 12 hours after injection, then declined to reach near baseline levels by 72 hrs (Fig. 4A). CaBP accumulation was not maximal until 48 hrs following hormone stimulation and as such lagged well behind the peak of CaBP-mRNA accumulation (Fig. 4B). The reason(s) why CaBP accumulation has such an extended latency compared to CaBP-mRNA are puzzling, although it has been suggested that 1,25$(OH)_2D_3$ may regulate other genes (besides the CaBP gene), the products of which may in turn modulate translation of or processing of CaBP gene transcripts (8).

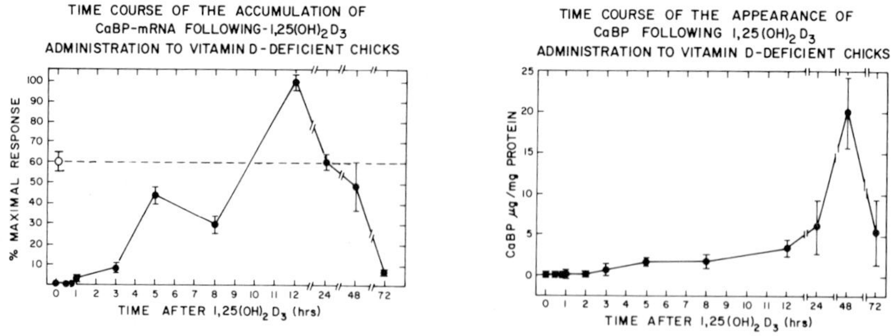

Fig. 4

Previous work (9,10), has indicated that serum Ca and P levels can be correlated with intestinal CaBP content in vitamin D-replete chick intestine. We therefore examined the effects of manipulating the dietary content of Ca and P on CaBP and CaBP-mRNA. Groups of chickens were raised on four separate D-replete diets containing low Ca (LCaNP), high Ca (HCaNP), low P (NCaLP) or normal Ca, normal P (NCaNP) diets for 14 days. Table 4 shows the levels of intestinal CaBP/serum calcium and phosphorus obtained in chicks subjected to these dietary manipulations. These values are in good accordance with those previously reported (9), in that the intestine adapts to changes in the serum calcium/phosphorus concentration by regulating CaBP levels. Fig. 5 shows a summary of the time course of the changes in CaBP-mRNA and CaBP levels after a dose of $1,25(OH)_2D_3$ in chicks maintained on the 4 diets.

Table 4

Levels of Intestinal CaBP, Serum Calcium and Phosphorus in Various Vitamin D-Replete Chickens

Dietary Manipulations	mg Calcium per 100 ml serum ±SD	mg Phosphorus per 100 ml serum ±SD	µg CaBP per mg protein ±SD
Normal Ca and P	8.1 ± 0.8	6.7 ± 1.3	10.0 ± 1.4
High Ca; normal P	13.5 ± 1.8	5.0 ± 1.1	6.7 ± 0.4
Low Ca; normal P	3.9 ± 0.5	9.5 ± 1.8	21.0 ± 0.2
Normal Ca; low P	11.6 ± 1.8	2.6 ± 0.5	28.6 ± 0.3

One of the most interesting features of the data that has emerged from these experiments was that none of the dietary manipulations altered the steady state level of CaBP-mRNA compared to the normal Ca, normal P diet (Fig. 5). Furthermore, while the nature of the initial (< 1 hr) response seems to vary according to diet, the magnitude of the stimulation above baseline is similar in all 4 dietary conditions, i.e. about a 1.4-1.5 fold increase in CaBP-mRNA at the maximum point, and in each case a drop back to baseline by 24 hrs. This is consistent with the data obtained by Northern analysis of the stimulation of the 3 forms of CaBP-mRNA in rachitic chick intestine after a dose of $1,25(OH)_2D_3$ (see Fig. 2B).

SUMMARY OF THE TIME COURSES OF $1,25(OH)_2D_3$ EFFECTS UPON INTESTINAL CaBP-mRNA AND 28K CaBP IN CHICKS FED VARIOUS D-REPLETE DIETS

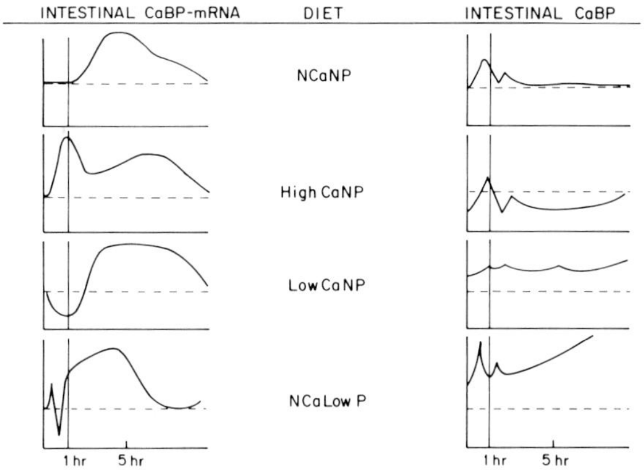

Fig. 5

Effects of α-Amanitin, Cycloheximide and $1,25(OH)_2D_3$ on Intestinal CaBP-mRNA in Chicks Subjected to Various Dietary Manipulations

As a logical extension of the previously described studies, we decided to examine the effects of a protein synthesis inhibitor (cycloheximide) and an RNA synthesis inhibitor (α-amanitin) on the ability of $1,25(OH)_2D_3$ to stimulate CaBP-mRNA and CaBP in chicks fed the four D-replete diets previously described. Preliminary experiments established optimal conditions (i.e. dose and times of treatment) for inhibiting RNA and protein synthesis as judged by the respective incorporation of $[^3H]$-uridine and $[^3H]$-leucine in the intestinal mucosa of chicks. α-Amanitin (20 µg/bird) and cycloheximide (600 µg/bird) were administered 2 hours prior to the injection of a standard dose (6.5 nmoles) of $1,25(OH)_2D_3$; mucosa was pooled and frozen 0, 15, 30, 60 and 120 minutes later. To our surprise dot blot analysis showed that cycloheximide but not α-amanitin inhibited CaBP-mRNA levels in all 4 dietary conditions. Fig. 6 shows a typical time course of CaBP-mRNA following $1,25(OH)_2D_3$ injection in chicks pretreated with cycloheximide and α-amanitin. There have been other reports (e.g., 5) that uninterrupted protein synthesis is a prerequisite for gene transcription which suggest that a protein(s) having a rapid turnover may be necessary for (i) processing of mRNA or (ii) direct/indirect stabilization of CaBP gene transcripts (e.g., by protection from nucleases).

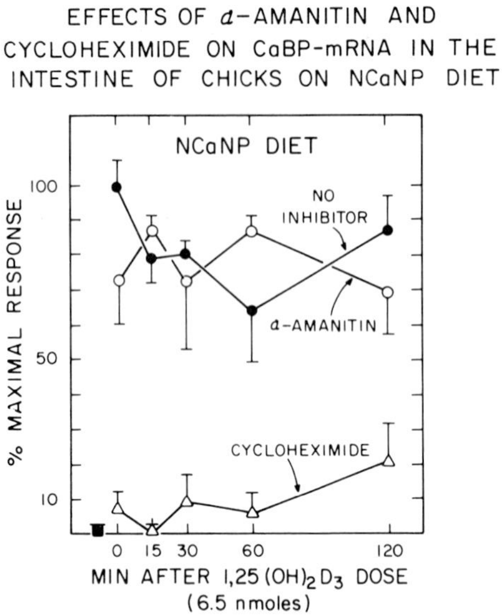

Fig. 6

The apparent absence of an in vivo effect of α-amanitin on intestinal CaBP-mRNA in these studies suggests that CaBP-mRNA must be stable for at least 4 hrs.

Fig. 7 shows the effects of the four dietary manipulations on intestinal CaBP when measured 100 minutes after $1,25(OH)_2D_3$ injection in cycloheximide and α-amanitin treated chicks. Consistent with data previously obtained in this laboratory (9,10) and with data already presented in this paper, low Ca and low P diets both stimulated CaBP levels while high Ca inhibited CaBP, compared to the level in normal Ca, normal P chick intestine. α-Amanitin had no effect on CaBP levels, while as expected, cycloheximide inhibited intestinal CaBP in all 4 dietary conditions.

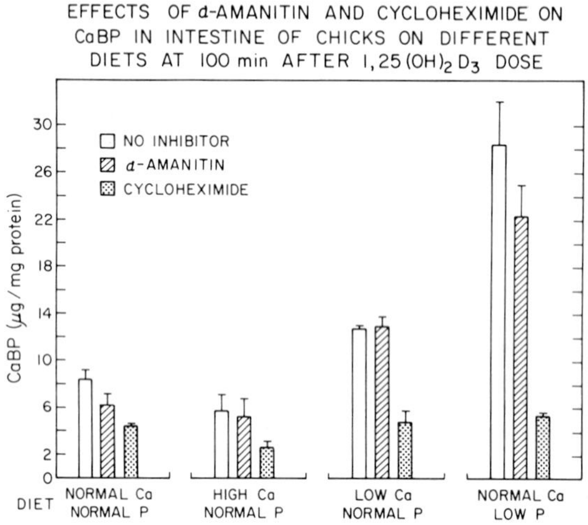

Fig. 7

Dose Response Studies of $1,25(OH)_2D_3$ Action on Intestinal CaBP and CaBP-mRNA in D-Replete and D-Deficient Chickens

In light of the previously described time course studies (Figs. 5A, 5B and Fig. 6) chickens were injected (i.m.) with a range of $1,25(OH)_2D_3$ doses (0 to 32.5 nmoles per bird) and killed 5 hrs later (D-replete) and 48 hours later (D-deficient); these were times at which CaBP-mRNA levels were maximally stimulated.

Stimulation of both CaBP (Fig. 8B) and CaBP-mRNA (Fig. 8A) by 1,25-$(OH)_2D_3$ was attenuated in D-replete intestine and was, for CaBP at least, independent of the injected dose of the hormone. More extensive studies indicated that very high pharmacological doses (13 to 65 nmoles/bird) exerted inhibitory effects on both CaBP and CaBP-mRNA accumulation (see Hall and Norman, this volume). CaBP formation was stimulated in a clearly defined dose-dependent fashion by $1,25(OH)_2D_3$ in D-deficient chick intestine (Fig. 8B) when measured 48 hours after injection; maximal stimulation was obtained with 5.85 to 13 nmoles per bird. CaBP-mRNA synthesis mimicked the changes seen with CaBP in these D-deficient animals (Fig. 8A).

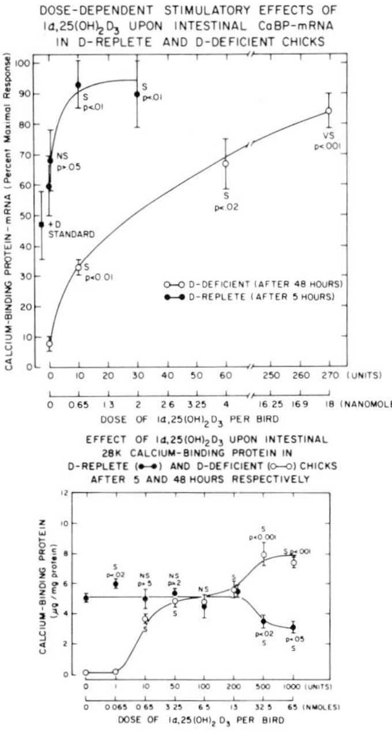

Fig. 8

It might be speculated that the "differential response" to $1,25(OH)_2D_3$ seen in +D and -D intestine may be due to (i) end organ metabolism of 1,25-$(OH)_2D_3$; (ii) altered functionality of the occupied $1,25(OH)_2D_3$ receptor (i.e. interaction with/translocation to the DNA acceptor sites). Any one or combination of these (and other undefined) mechanisms may mediate the differential responsiveness phenomenom that is associated with D_3 status.

Summary

We have cloned DNA complimentary to a vitamin D-dependent CaBP-mRNA and have used these cDNAs to show that (i) the chick CaBP gene is present as a single copy (by "Southern" analysis); (ii) that a polymorphism of the CaBP-mRNA exists (by "Northern" analysis)--there are 3 distinct messages of 2000, 2600 and 3100 nucleotides in many tissues of the chick; (iii) CaBP-mRNA is detectable in the -D chick intestine as early as 45 minutes after $1,25(OH)_2D_3$ administration in vivo; (iv) dietary manipulation of Ca and P modifies intestinal CaBP content but does not alter the ambient level of gene transcription in +D chicks; (v) CaBP-mRNA is stable in vivo for at least 4 hrs as shown by the inability of α-amanitin to block tissue accumulation of CaBP gene transcripts; (vi) vitamin D status modulates sensitivity of chick intestinal CaBP-mRNA and CaBP to $1,25(OH)_2D_3$.

Acknowledgements
This work was supported in part by USPHS grant AM-09012.

References

1. Hunziker, W., Siebert, P. D., King, M. W., Stucki, P., Dugaiczyk, A., and Norman, A. W. (1983) Proc. Natl. Acad. Sci. 80, 4228-4232.
2. Gubler, U., and Hoffman, B. J. (1983) Gene 25, 263-269.
3. Putkey, J. A., Ts'ui, K. F., Tanaka, T., Lagace, L., Stein, J. P., Lai, E. C., and Means, A. R. (1983) J. Biol. Chem. 258, 11864-11873.
4. Amara, S. G., Jonas, V., Rosenfeld, M. G., Ong, E. S., and Evans, R. M. (1982) Nature 298, 240-245.
5. Vannice, J. L., Taylor, J. M., and Ringold, G. M. (1984) Proc. Natl. Acad. Sci. 81, 4241-4245.
6. Chirgwin, J. M., Przybyla, A. E., MacDonald, R. J., and Rutter, W. J. (1979) Biochemistry 18, 5295-5299.
7. Miller, B. E., and Norman, A. W. (1983) Methods in Enzymology 102, 291-296.
8. Spencer, R., Charman, M., Wilson, P., and Lawson, D. E. M. (1976) Nature 263, 161-163.
9. Friedlander, E. J., Henry, H. L., and Norman, A. W. (1977) J. Biol. Chem. 252, 8677-8683.
10. Christakos, S., Friedlander, E. J., Frandsen, B. R., and Norman, A. W. (1979) Endocrinology 104, 1495-1503.

VITAMIN D-DEPENDENT CHICK INTESTINAL CaBP: CALCIUM DEPENDENT INTERACTIONS AS ASSESSED BY PHOTOAFFINITY LABELING.

V. L. Leathers and A. W. Norman,
Dept. Biochemistry, Univ. of California-Riverside, Riverside, CA 92521

Introduction: The mechanism by which vitamin D induces intestinal calcium absorption is believed to involve the participation of vitamin D-dependent calcium binding protein (CaBP). However, the function of this protein remains unknown. A photoaffinity probe for the 28K chick intestinal CaBP has been prepared (1). Preliminary data has suggested a heterologous calcium dependent interaction occuring between the chick intestinal 28K-CaBP and bovine intestinal alkaline phosphatase (BIAP) (1). The present study includes a further evaluation of the calcium-dependent crosslinking interactions of the CaBP-photoaffinity probe as well as putative homologous interactions between chick intestinal CaBP and chick intestinal brush border membrane proteins.

Methods: Iodine-125-labeled chick intestinal CaBP (2) was modified by covalent attachment of the heterobifunctional photoaffinity reagent methyl-4-azidobenzoimidate (MABI) as previously described (1). Bovine intestinal alkaline phosphatase was commercially obtained, and chick intestinal brush borders and brush border membranes were isolated by the method of Putkey, et al., (3). Unmodified CaBP was utilized for ELISA (4). Phosphatidylinositol-specific phospholipase C from *Staphylococcus aureus* was provided by Dr. Martin G. Lan and membranes were digested as described by Yusufi, et al. (5). Incubations of the photoaffinity probe were conducted in the presence (1mM $CaCl_2$) or absence (1mM EGTA) of calcium with the exception of the chick intestinal BBM which were incubated with ^{125}I-CaBP-MABI depleted of Ca^{2+} by prior incubations with EGTA and elution on a Sephadex G-25 column. Following incubation of 2 hrs for purified anti-CaBP IgG and 45 min with BIAP and membrane preparations, UV irradiation (2 min) resulted in crosslinking between ^{125}I-CaBP-MABI and neighboring proteins. Gradient 7-20% SDS-PAGE, autoradiography and densitometric scanning were utilized to visualize crosslinked products.

Results and Discussions: The specificity of crosslinking between the CaBP photoaffinity probe (28K) and BIAP (67K) was previously illustrated by the lack of interaction between *E. coli* A'Ptase as well as the calcium dependent nature of the conjugate species (1). Specificity is further demonstrated by the diminished crosslinking in the presence of excess unlabelled CaBP (Fig. 1). The calcium dependent manner in which anti-CaBP IgG recognize CaBP was illustrated by photoaffinity labeling and ELISA. As seen in Fig. 2, the standard curve for the ELISA is significantly altered by the addition of 1mM $CaCl_2$, suggesting a need for optimization of assay conditions due to calcium dependent conformational changes in CaBP. The calcium dependency of CaBP photoaffinity crosslinking was further illustrated by the homologous interactions present between chick intestinal BBM and ^{125}I-CaBP-MABI. As seen in Fig. 3 conjugates occur at 180K and 90K corresponding to proteins of 150K and 60K respectively (chick intestinal A'Ptase has a MW of approximately 140K).

The use of PI-PLC for specific release of A'Ptase was previously used by Yusufi, et al. in the rabbit kidney system (5). Less than 25% of the chick intestinal BBM A'Ptase activity was released by PI-PLC as compared to greater than 85% in rabbit and chick kidney BBM. However, the protein released into the supernatant was sufficient to result in crosslinking between ^{125}I-CaBP-MABI and proteins of 130K and 60K. Collectively these data demonstrate the calcium dependent nature by which CaBP interacts with neighboring proteins and suggests the presence of specific target proteins in the intestinal BBM which may be involved in the biological functioning of CaBP.

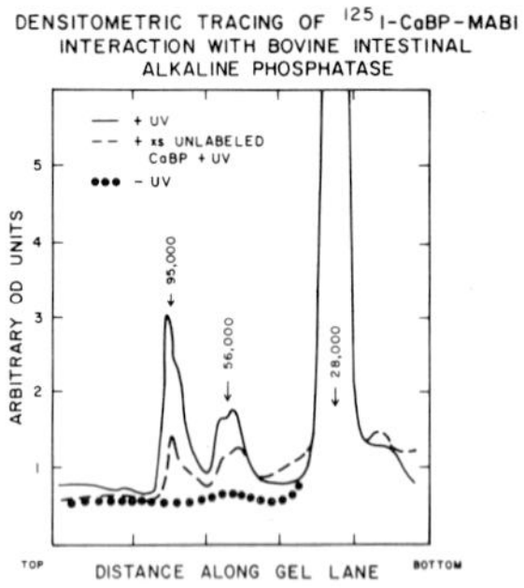

Fig. 1

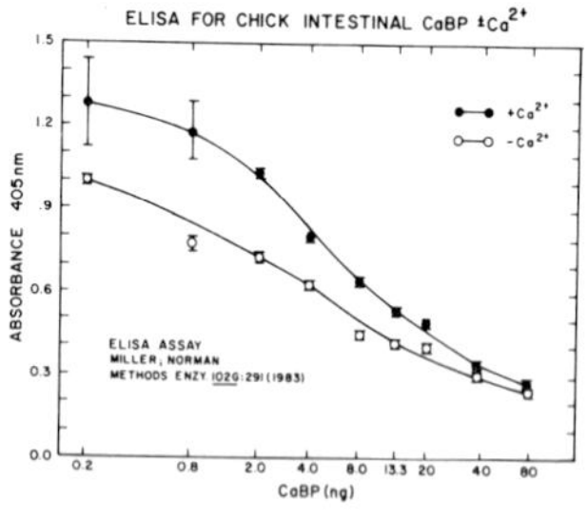

Fig. 2

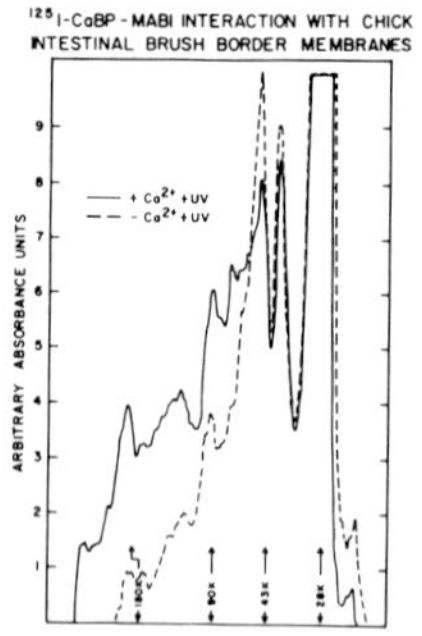

Fig. 3

References:

1. Norman, A. W. and Leathers, V. L. (1982) Biochem. Biophys. Res. Comm. 108, 220.
2. Friedlander, E. J., and Norman, A. W. (1980) Methods in Enzymology 67, 540.
3. Putkey, J. A., Spielvogel, A. M., Sauerheber, R. D., Dunlap, C. S., and Norman, A. W. (1982) Biochim. Biophys. Acta 688, 177.
4. Miller, B. E., and Norman, A. W. (1983) Methods in Enzymology 102, 291.
5. Yusufi, A. N. K., Low, M. G., Turner, S. T., and Dousa, T. P. (1983) J. Biol. Chem. 258, 5695.

CHARACTERIZATION OF RAT CHOLECALCIN (9000 MW CHOLECALCIFEROL-INDUCED CaBP) mRNA AND GENE USING A SPECIFIC cDNA.

C. PERRET, C. DESPLAN and M. THOMASSET
INSERM U.120, 44 Chemin de Ronde - 78110 Le Vésinet, France.

INTRODUCTION

The rat posesses two cholecalciferol-induced calcium-binding proteins, the cholecalcins (CaBP). The 9-kDa CaBP is mainly concentrated in the duodenum while 28-kDa CaBP is located in the kidney and cerebellum (1). Recently we reported that about 10% of the mRNA isolated from the duodenum of growing rats directs the synthesis of authentic rat 9-kDa cholecalcin in a cell-free system (2). Complementary DNA copies of rat intestinal cholecalcin (9-kDa CaBP) mRNA were inserted into the Pst I site of pBR322 and cloned in E. Coli (3). Recombinant plasmids coding for 9-kDa CaBP mRNA were selected by differential screening using ^{32}P-cDNA (synthesized from enriched or low 9-kDa CaBP mRNA preparations) as a probe.
We now report the use of this cloned cDNA to rat 9-kDa CaBP to characterize the corresponding messenger and gene.

MATERIALS AND METHODS

Animals. Male Sprague-Dawley rats 5 to 8 weeks old, fed a diet containing 0.5% calcium, 0.36% phosphorus, and 2000 IU of vitamin D_3/kg,were used.
Tissue preparation. The duodenal mucosa, kidneys and the cerebella were collected and immediately frozen in liquid nitrogen.
Extraction and purification of RNA. Total RNA was extracted from the tissues with phenol-chloroform at pH 9 and purified by LiCl precipitation as previously described (2). Ten percent of total RNA were stored at -80°C for cDNA hybridization. Poly(A^+) RNA was then purified by chromatography on oligo (dT)-cellulose T7 (2).
Preparation of cloned 9kDa CaBP cDNA. The cloned cDNA inserted at the PstI site of chimeric plasmid pBR322, pC109 (4) was obtained from bacterial cells by alkali extraction following chloramphenicol amplification. The plasmid was digested by PstI restriction enzyme.
Hybrid-selected translation. 8µg of cDNA was hybridized with 100 µg poly (A^+) RNA according to Parnes & al (5). The hybridized poly (A^+) RNA was translated in a rabbit reticulocyte lysate mixture.
Cell-free translation and specific immunoprecipitation. Details of the in vitro translation system in rabbit reticulocyte lysate containing ^{35}S methionine have been published (2). 9kDa cholecalcin was immunoprecipitated using specific rabbit anti-rat duodenal CaBP serum (1,2) and anti-rat goat IgG.
Preparation of the ^{32}P cDNA probe. The cDNA fragment was nick-translated (6). The specific activity of the cDNA probes was about 2 x 10^8cpm/µg.
Northern hybridization. Poly(A^+) RNA incubated with glyoxal was electrophoresed on 1.3% horizontal agarose gel and transfered to nitrocellulose filter as described by Southern (7).
Preparation of rat genomic DNA and Southern blotting. High-molecular-mass DNA prepared from liver as described by Blin and Stafford (8) was digested with an excess of restriction enzyme, run on 0.8% agarose gel, denatured with alkali and transfered to nitrocellulose filters as described by Southern (7).

RESULTS

Vitamin D. A Chemical, Biochemical and Clinical Update

Nucleotide sequence of 9-kDa cholecalcin cDNA. The nucleotide sequence analysis of the longest cDNA insert (375 bp) permits the assignement of 207 nucleotides in the coding region and 104 nucleotides of the entire 3' -non coding region of 9kDa cholecalcin mRNA (fig. 1) (4). The deduced amino acid sequence for rat intestinal cholecalcin (fig. 1) contains two "EF hand" domains, described by Kretsinger (9) and corresponding to the two calcium-binding sites (I and II) : residues 5 to 44 site I ; residues 45 to 75 site II. The analysis of nucleotide sequence homologies between the coding and non coding region of the 9kDa cholecalcin messenger shows a strong homology between site I structure and the region located just before and after the stop codon (residues 199 to 238) (4).
This suggests that rat 9kDa cholecalcin messenger contains the remains of an untranslated calcium-binding site III-like-structure (4) and raises the question of the specificity of the cDNA probe used.

*10

Pvu II

Poly G AAG AGC ATT TTT CAA AAA TAT GCA GCC AAA GAA GGC GAT CCA AAC CAG CTG TCC AAG GAG
Lys Ser Ile Phe Gln Lys Tyr Ala Ala Lys Glu Gly Asp Pro Asn Gln Leu Ser Lys Glu

Xba I

GAG CTG AAG CTG CTG ATT CAG TCA GAG TTC CCC AAC CTC CTG AAG GCT TCA AGT ACT CTA
Glu Leu Lys Leu Leu Ile Gln Ser Glu Phe Pro Asn Leu Leu Lys Ala Ser Ser Thr Leu

EcoR I

GAC AAT CTC TTT GAA GAG CTG GAT AAG AAC GAT GAT GGA GAA GTT AGC TAT GAA GAA TTC
Asp Asn Leu Phe Glu Glu Leu Asp Lys Asn Asp Asp Gly Glu Val Ser Tyr Glu Glu Phe

*210

GAA GTT TTC TTC AAA AAG TTA TCA CAA TGA AGC CAG AAG AAG GAG CTC CGA CAC CAC CTA
Glu Val Phe Phe Lys Lys Leu Ser Gln

Bgl II

CTG ATT GAA TCC TAT CCA ATC CCA AAG ATC TAG CTG TGA GAG CAA GAT ACT GTT AAT AAA

GCA AAT TCT GAG AC AAAAAAAAAAAAAAAAAAAAAAAAAAAA Poly C

Fig. 1 - Nucleotide and deduced amino acid sequences of rat intestinal cholecalcin (4)

Absence of homology with 28-kDa cholecalcin mRNA. Total RNA and Poly(A^+) RNA were extracted from duodenal mucosa, kidney and cerebellum of 5-8 week old Sprague Dawley rats. Poly(A^+) RNA hybridized to the cDNA probe were analyzed by cell-free protein synthesis. Poly(A^+) RNA was also analyzed by Northern hybridization using the ^{32}P cDNA probe.
Analysis of the cDNA-hybridized mRNA by cell-free protein synthesis. Poly (A^+)-rich RNA, extracted from duodenum, kidney and cerebellum, was hybridized to the rat 9-kDa cholecalcin cDNA (pC109) and analyzed by cell-free translation. Gel electrophoresis analysis of the total translated products obtained from cDNA-hybridized mRNA isolated from duodenum (fig.2) shows that only one major protein band comigrated with purified ^{125}I-labelled rat duodenal cholecalcin under denaturing conditions. However, a 2000-Da larger protein, representing about 10% of the major protein band (fig. 2 , lane 2), was also present. Both proteins were immunoprecipitated by anti-(rat duodenal cholecalcin) serum (not shown).

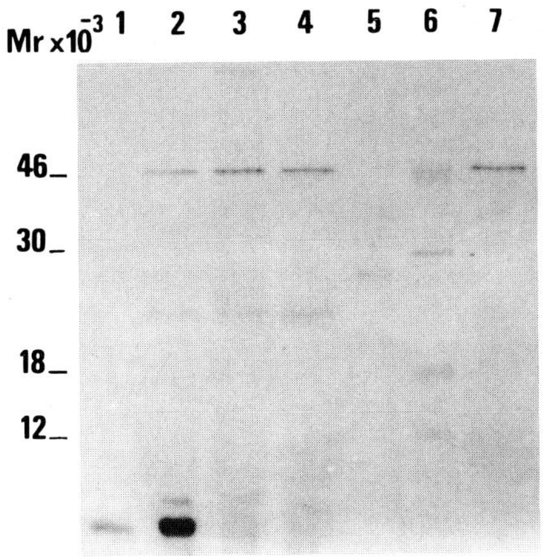

Fig. 2 - Analysis of total products of cell-free translation of cDNA hybridized mRNA prepared from rat duodenal renal and cerebellar mRNA by gel electrophoresis. cDNA-hybridized mRNA obtained from : 2, duodenum ; 3, kidney ; 4, cerebellum ; 1, ^{125}I-purified duodenal CaBP ; 5, ^{125}I-purified renal CaBP ; 7, translation without exogenous mRNA.

Nucleotide sequence analysis of the cDNA pC109 shows the presence of two stop codons, TGA and TAG at positions 207 and 271, respectively, of the 3' untranslated region (fig. 1). The UGA codon has been reported to be "leaky" allowing synthesis of a full-length protein (10).
In order to verify this hypothesis the UGA-suppressing serine tRNA was added to the *in vitro* translation assay. Fig. 3 indicates that the addition of UGA-suppressor tRNA enhanced the production of the larger-molecular-mass protein. Such a read-through, occuring *in vivo*, could explain the presence of two CaBPs initially isolated from rat intestinal mucosa (11).

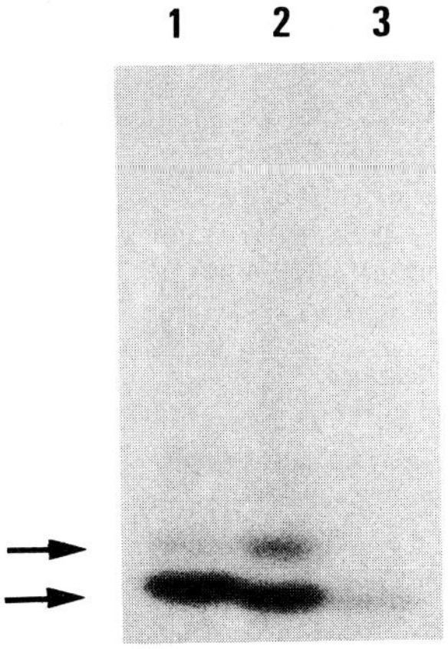

Fig. 3 - Analysis by SDS polyacrylamide gel electrophoresis of cell-free translation products of duodenal cholecalcin poly(A)-rich RNA in the presence of a UGA-suppressor tRNA. 1, immunotranslated products in the absence of UGA-suppressor tRNA. 2, as 1, in the presence of UGA-suppressor tRNA ; 3, 9-kDa ^{125}I-cholecalcin.

Poly(A)-rich RNA, extracted from kidney and cerebellum, were also analyzed by hybrid translation. No immunoprecipitable protein bands were detected when the translated products from cDNA-hybridized mRNA, isolated from kidney and cerebellum were treated with anti-(28-kDa cholecalcin) serum (not shown). These results demonstrate that the cDNA probe does not hybridize to the mRNA encoding 28-kDa cholecalcin.

Northern analysis mRNA hybridized to the cDNA. A single mRNA species was retained on the nitrocellulose filter under high stringency hybridization conditions (fig. 4a,lane 1). This size homogeneity was also observed under low stringency conditions (fig. 4b).

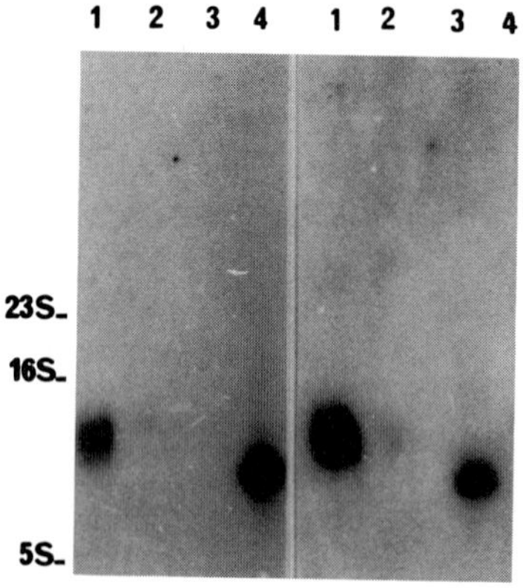

Fig. 4 - Analysis of Northern hybridization of mRNA isolated from duodenum, kidney and cerebellum. Stringent conditions : a) Strong b) low
cDNA-hybridized mRNA from lane 1, duodenum ; lane 2, kidney and lane 3, cerebellum. The size scale was determined by co-electrophoresis of ribosomal E. Coli RNA (23 S, 16 S and 5S) and denatured 9-kDa cholecalcin cDNA (lane 4).

There was a notable absence of a large mRNA species encoding 28-kDa cholecalcin, which is largely concentrated in the rat cerebellum and kidney (fig. 4a, 4b).

This absence of cross-hybridization, clearly indicates that there is very little homology between 9-kDa and 28-kDa cholecalcin mRNAs. This lack of homology is not inconsistent with the previously reported model for the evolution of the intracellular CaBPs (4). Thus 9-kDa cholecalcin could have arisen as a result of the transcription of a larger molecule containing four calcium-binding sites (28-kDa cholecalcin ?), with subsequent gene duplication of this sequence. But, to be consistent with the observed lack of cross-hybridization, this event must have occured early in their evolutionary development, since which time they have evolved independently. *A fortiori* mRNAs of other members of the intracellular CaBP family, such as calmodulin or troponin could not hybridize since their evolutionary divergence probably began even earlier than that of the 28-kDa and 9-kDa cholecalcin.

Southern blot analysis of rat liver genomic DNA. Plasmid pC109 was hybridized to Southern blots of rat liver genomic DNA digested with three restriction endonucleases to detect the homologous sequences after high-stringency washing (fig. 5). It was found that the cDNA probe hybridizates to a single 5000-base Hind III fragment and a single 4600-base XbaI fragment. Neither enzyme cuts within the pC109 sequence. Moreover, only two pieces of genomic DNA (3600 and 900 bases) were revealed after digestion by EcoRI, which shows a single restriction site in the pC109. Analogous results were obtained after washing at low stringency (not shown).

Fig. 5 - Southern blot of restricted rat genomic DNA. Rat genomic DNA was digested by EcoRI (lane 1) HindIII (lane 2), XbaI (lane 3).

Human liver genomic DNA had a very similar restriction pattern when digested with the same three enzymes (data not shown).

CONCLUSION

All these findings demonstrate that there is no cross-hybridization between 9-kDa CaBP mRNAs and indicate that there are distinct genes coding for each rat cholecalcin.
Only when the sequences of the downstream 3' region of the 9-kDa cholecalcin gene and that of the 28-kDa cholecalcin gene are both known can the relationship between the two be adequately described.

REFERENCES

1. Thomasset, M. ; Parkes, C.O. and Cuisinier-Gleizes, P. (1982) Am. J. Physiol. 243,E483-E488.
2. Thomasset, M. ; Desplan, C. and Parkes, C.O. (1983) : Eur. J. Biochem. 129, 519-524.
3. Desplan, C. ; Thomasset, M. and Moukhtar, M.S. (1983) : J. Biol. Chem. 258, 2762-2765.
4. Desplan, C. ; Heidmann, O. ; Lillie, J.W. ; Auffray, C. and Thomasset M. (1983) : J. Biol. Chem., 258, 13502-13505.
5. Parnes, J.R. ; Velan, B. ; Felsenfeld, A. ; Ramanathan, L. ; Ferrini, U. ; Appela, E. and Sidman, J.G. (1981) : Proc. Natl Acad. Sci. USA 78, 22-53
6. Rigby, P.W.J. ; Dieckmann, H. ; Rhodes, C. and Berg, P. (1977) : J. Mol. Biol., 113, 237-251.

7. Southern, E.M. (1975) : J. Mol. Biol., 98, 503-517.
8. Blin, N. and Stafford, D.W. (1976) : Nucleic Acids Res., 3, 2303-2311.
9. Kretsinger, R.H. (1976):Annu. Rev. Biochem., 45, 239-266.
10. Model, P. ; Webster, R.E. and Zinder, N.D. (1969) : J. Mol. Biol., 43, 117-190.
11. Drescher, D. and Deluca, H.F. (1971) : Biochemistry 10, 2308-2311.

Acknowledgments. We are grateful to N. Gouhier, for expert technical assistance and L. Castéra and INSERM S.C.6 for the preparation of the manuscript This work was supported by grants from CNRS (gene molecular biology 033.107) and UER Xavier Bichat 1985 Paris VII University.

IDENTITY BETWEEN RAT RENAL AND CEREBELLAR CHOLECALCINS (28,000 MW CHOLECALCIFEROL-INDUCED CaBP). COMPARISON WITH BOVINE BRAIN CALIGULIN.

S. INTRATOR[1], J. BAUDIER[2], J. ELION[1], M. THOMASSET[3] and A. BREHIER[3].

[1]Biochimie B Faculté Bichat, [2]ERA CNRS 551 Strasbourg and [3]INSERM U.120 78110 Le Vésinet, France.

INTRODUCTION

Mammals possess two biochemically and immunologically distinct types of cholecalcins (cholecalciferol induced calcium binding proteins) (1). 9-KDa cholecalcin is most abundant in the duodenum and larger 28-KDa cholecalcins are found mainly in the kidney and cerebellum. One of the basic characteristics of cholecalcins is their vitamin D dependence. While this has been well documented for the 9-KDa protein and the renal 28-KDa cholecalcin, no such dependence has been demonstrated for the cerebellar CaBP. As a result, the relationship between renal and cerebellar 28-KDa cholecalcins remains unclear, and we now report some elements suggesting the identity of the two proteins.

Caligulin, a new calcium binding protein from bovine brain (2) has been recently purified and characterized. We here describe some properties of caligulin and suggest that caligulin migh be related to 28-KDa cholecalcins.

MATERIELS AND METHODS

Purification of rat 28-KDa cholecalcins. Renal and cerebellar cholecalcins were purified using heat precipitation, gel filtration chromatography, chromatofocusing and gel-permeation HPLC.

Immunological methods. A specific antiserum directed to the pure rat renal cholecalcin was raised in rabbits. Immunocross reactivity was examined by Ouchterlony double immuno diffusion or radio immunoassay using iodinated renal cholecalcin.

Electrophoresis. Polyacrylamide gel electrophoresis under denaturing conditions and two dimensional isoelectric focusing/electrophoresis were performed.

Amino acid analysis. 5 nmoles of proteins were hydrolyzed and amino acid analysis were performed on a chromatospeck.

Peptide mapping. Tryptic and chymotryptic digestions were performed for 16h at 37°C and the resulting peptides were chromatographed on reversed phase HPLC.

N-terminal sequence. Manual Edman degradation was used and the resulting amino acids were separated and identified by thin layer chromatography after treatment according to Chang (3).

RESULTS AND DISCUSSION

28-KDa cholecalcins from kidney and cerebellum were eluted in identical positions during each of the chromatographic stages of purification. The final products obtained appeared as single band on SDS/PAGE, migrating with apparent molecular weights of 26-KDa.

By Outcherlony double immunodiffusion, homogenates of kidney and cerebellum tested against the antiserum to purified renal cholecalcin gave single precipitin bands which were perfectly fused, suggesting that a single immunologic species is present in both tissues. Such immuno cross-reactivity was also supported by the radioimmunoassay data.

Vitamin D. A Chemical, Biochemical and Clinical Update

Two dimensional isoelectric focusing/electrophoresis using a 3.5 to 10 pH gradient revealed identical behaviour of the two cholecalcins. The pI of 4.3 in the absence of calcium become less acidic (4.5) in the presence of 1mM calcium. The aminoacid composition of rat renal and cerebellar cholecalcins are shown in the table. The overall contents are remarkably similar, and are characterised by high Asp and Glu.
The peptide mays obtained after tryptic and chymotryptic digestion in the absence of calcium are identical. The presence of 1mM CaCl2 in the tryptic digests did not prevent hydrolysis as already reported for calmodulin. The N-terminal sequences of both cholecalcins were identical, N-Gly-Gly-Val-Ser providing further evidence for the close similarity of the two proteins. The major difference is their vitamin D-dependence in the post-weaning rats and this could be a function of the specific cells in which they are found.

Amino Acid composition

	CEREBELLAR CHOLECALCIN	RENAL CHOLECALCIN	CALIGULIN
ASP	27	32	33
THR	13	13	12
SER	16	15	13
GLU	37	39	38
PRO	3	4	8
GLY	24	23	17
ALA	16	20	15
VAL	5	5	7
MET	8	5	5
ILE	10	10	11
LEU	31	31	33
TYR	7	6	7
PHE	13	11	12
HIS	7	4	4
LYS	19	20	22
ARG	10	7	6
CYS	4	6	4
TRY	++	++	1

Caligulin exhibits several properties in common with 28-KDa cholecalcins including molecular weight, high thermal stability, and amino acid composition. They also share antigenic determinants. Therefore, there is no doubt that caligulin is related to the mammalian 2-kDa cholecalcins.

1. Thomasset, M. ; Parkes, C.O. and Cuisinier-Gleizes, P. (1982) Am. J. Physiol. 243, 483-488.
2. Waisman, D.M. ; Muranyi, J. and Ahmed, D.M. (1983) FEBS Letts. 164, 80-84.
3. Chang, J.Y. ; Brauer, D. and Wittman-Liebold, B. (1978) FEBS Lett. 93, 205-214.

REGULATION OF VITAMIN D-DEPENDENT 28K-CALCIUM BINDING PROTEIN (CaBP) AND MESSENGER RNA (mRNA) FORMATION IN THE CHICK INTESTINE BY 1,25-DIHYDROXY-VITAMIN D_3.

A. K. HALL and A. W. NORMAN
Dept. Biochemistry, Univ. of California, Riverside, CA 92521, USA

Introduction:

1,25-Dihydroxyvitamin D_3 [1,25$(OH)_2D_3$] is the principal active vitamin D_3 metabolite and acts in a manner that is characteristic of other more traditional steroid hormones. As a major target tissue for 1,25$(OH)_2D_3$, the intestinal epithelial cell responds to this seco-steroid with increased formation of (amongst other proteins) a 28K-calcium binding protein (CaBP) which is thought to play a pivotal role in the modulation of calcium transport. Stimulation of CaBP synthesis by 1,25$(OH)_2D_3$ is believed to involve an action of this hormone at the level of gene expression.

Work in this laboratory (1) has resulted in the construction of a recombinant library of cloned cDNA corresponding to a vitamin D_3-dependent CaBP-messenger RNA sequence. This cDNA library contains several useful clones which we have used as molecular probes to investigate the genomic action of 1,25$(OH)_2D_3$ in regulating chick intestinal CaBP-mRNA synthesis as a function of vitamin D_3 status.

Methods:

Animal Treatments

One day old White Leghorn cockerels were raised on a rachitogenic diet for 14 days prior to being maintained on either D-replete or D-deficient diets for a further 14 days. D-replete and D-deficient chicks then received a range of doses of 1,25$(OH)_2D_3$ (0 to 54 nmoles per bird), then were killed 5 and 48 hr later respectively. Blood was collected whilst intestinal mucosa was scraped, pooled and frozen in liquid nitrogen.

Isolation of RNA and Measurement of CaBP-mRNA:

Total cellular RNA was extracted from pooled mucosal scrapings by the guanidinium thiocyanate method. Nick-translated [^{32}P]-labelled cDNA (pCaBP-2, a 350 bp insert in pBR322) was hybridized to RNA immobilized on nitrocellulose paper filters which were then used to expose X-ray film at -70°C with intensifying screens. Exposed films were then quantitated using a scanning densitometer.

Measurement of Calcium-Binding Protein:

Samples of pooled intestinal mucosa were homogenized in 4 volumes of a buffer containing Tris-HCl, EDTA and dithiothreitol. CaBP was determined in the cytosolic fraction (100,000xg) by an enzyme-linked immunosorbent assay (ELISA).

Results:

The effects of 1,25$(OH)_2D_3$ upon serum calcium (measured by atomic absorption), intestinal CaBP (by ELISA) and CaBP-mRNA (measured by cDNA probes) in D-replete (5 h values) and D-deficient (48 h values) chicks are summarized in the following table.

Vitamin D. A Chemical, Biochemical and Clinical Update

	Dose of $1,25(OH)_2D_3$ (nmoles)	Serum Calcium (mg%) (mean ± 1 SD)	CaBP µg per mg protein (mean ± 1 SD)	CaBP-mRNA % Maximal OD Response (mean ± 1 SD)
	0	8.7 ± 0.37	4.54 ± 0.6	45.5 ± 15.9
D-replete	0.003	8.2 ± 0.20	4.7 ± 1.5	68.69 ± 10.4
(5 h)	0.65	8.8 ± 0.6	4.6 ± 1.20	92.57 ± 7.90
	19.50	8.7 ± 0.20	4.11 ± 0.60	90.16 ± 11.7
	0	4.27 ± 0.4	0.12 ± 0.03	8.1 ± 1.4
	0.065	4.0 ± 0.4	0.81 ± 0.05	ND
D-deficient	0.65	4.2 ± 0.5	2.73 ± 0.21	33.1 ± 0.99
(48h)	3.90	5.1 ± 0.7	3.69 ± 0.33	66.9 ± 16.8
	17.55	7.2 ± 0.9	10.27 ± 0.03	84.61 ± 6.7
	52.65	7.6 ± 0.6	10.31 ± 0.05	ND*

(*ND--not determined)

Summary and Conclusion:

The D-deficient intestine displays a tardy, but superior response to hormonal challenge by $1,25(OH)_2D_3$. D-replete intestinal mucosa appears refractory to the stimulatory influence of $1,25(OH)_2D_3$, in terms of CaBP and displays a blunted response in terms of CaBP-mRNA.

Repetition of these experiments with a more extensive dose-range (0 to 65 nmol units/bird) revealed that CaBP formation was unaffected by physiological doses of hormone, but was apparently depressed by pharmacological doses of $1,25(OH)_2D_3$ in D-replete birds. Stimulation of CaBP-mRNA by $1,25(OH)_2D_3$ in D-replete intestine is not accompanied by a parallel enhancement of CaBP formation--this may suggest that in addition to a blunting of $1,25(OH)_2D_3$ action upon transcription, some post-transcriptional process is tightly regulating CaBP formation in the +D intestine.

A differential response to $1,25(OH)_2D_3$ therefore exists in D-replete versus D-deficient chicken intestine in terms of both CaBP and CaBP-mRNA formation. These different states of "sensitivity" to $1,25(OH)_2D_3$ may reflect or be attributable to (i) an extended biological half-life of the steroid in D-deficient birds; (ii) altered "receptor-performance" as a function of D_3-status; (iii) a vitamin D_3-induced conformational rearrangement of the CaBP-gene which somehow influences the masking/exposure of "acceptor-sites" for the DNA-binding moiety of the occupied $1,25(OH)_2D_3$ receptor.

References:

1. Hunziker, W., Siebert, P.D., King, M.W., Stucki, P., Dugaiczyk, A. and Norman, A.W. (1983) Proc. Nat. Acad. Sci. (USA) 80, p. 4228-4232.

(This work supported in part by grant AM-09012-020 and a Fulbright Award to A.K.H.).

EXPRESSION OF CHOLECALCIN (9000 MW CHOLECALCIFEROL-INDUCED CaBP) GENE IN RAT DUODENUM AND PLACENTA DURING GESTATION.

F. de Maintenant, C. Perret, P. Brun and M. Thomasset

INSERM U.120 44, chemin de ronde - 78110 Le Vésinet, France.

INTRODUCTION

The marked rise in intestinal absorption of calcium and in the placental transfer of this ion in rats during the last days of gestation is associated with an increase in CaBP 9K in the maternal duodenum and placenta (1). To go further in the study of the active process of 9-kDa cholecalcin biosynthesis during pregnancy we now report a comparative analysis of the expression of the 9-kDa cholecalcin gene in the maternal duodenum and in maternal and fetal parts of the placenta at different stages of the gestation using a specific cDNA probe (2).

MATERIALS AND METHODS

Investigations were made on pregnant rats fed ad libitum with a diet containing 0.92% Ca, 0.90% P and 4000 iu of vitamin D_3/kg at days 15,17,19 and 21 of gestation. Size analysis of the mRNA sequences was performed by electrophoretic fractionation on agarose gels and Northern hybridization to the ^{32}P cDNA probe. 9-kDa cholecalcin mRNA levels were assayed in the tissues by Dot-blot hybridization.

RESULTS

Northern analysis of mRNA hybridized to the cDNA.

A homogeneous 500-600 nucleotide mRNA species was shown when poly(A^+) RNA isolated from duodenum and placenta was hybridized under stroug and low stringent conditions (not shown)

9-kDa cholecalcin mRNA levels : Dot-blot hybridization.

The highest concentration of CaBP 9-kDa mRNA occured on the last day of gestation in both tissues. At this time, CaBP 9-kDa mRNA was 20-30 times less concentrated in fetal and maternal parts of placenta than in the maternal duodenum. Cholecalcin 9-kDa mRNA levels increased 7 fold from day 15 to day 21 in the fetal placenta (fig.1).
This rise in CaBP mRNA levels paralleled the increase in translational activity of CaBP 9K mRNA in this tissue.

CONCLUSION

This evolution of CaBP 9k mRNA (level and activity) in maternal duodenum and fetal placenta during pregnancy correlates well with cholecalcin concentration its and provides evidence for an active process of CaBP 9k biosynthesis associated with concomittant changes in calcium transfer in these tissues.

Vitamin D. A Chemical, Biochemical and Clinical Update

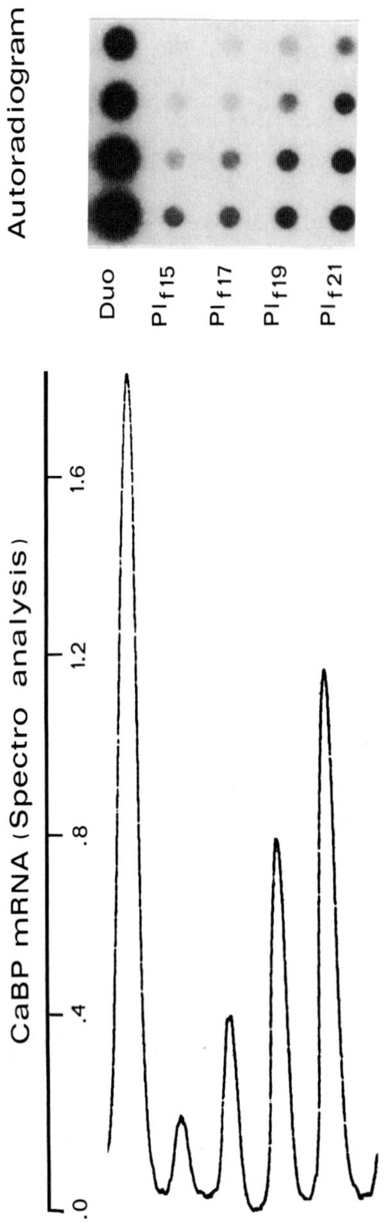

Fig. 1 9-kDa cholecalcin mRNA levels in the placenta.

Total RNA (10,5,2.5&1.25 ug, Lanes 1,2,3 & 4, respectively) was dotted on nitrocellulose filter and hybridized to the P cDNA probe (from 15,17,19&21 gestational days.

a. autoradiogram
b. spectrodensitometric curves of corresponding dots.

Aknowledgments: We are grateful to Pr. H. Mathieu and Dr. P. Cuisinier Gleizes for providing the required facilities. We thank N. Gouhier and M. Eb for their expert technical assistance.

THE ENDOCRINE CONTROL OF PLASMA CALCIUM BINDING PROTEIN LEVELS IN THE PIG

E.M.W. Maunder, A.V. Pillay, C. Chapman*, S. Tomlinson** and A.D. Care,
Department of Animal Physiology and Nutrition, Leeds University,
*Department of Nuclear Medicine, Leeds General Infirmary, Leeds,
and **Department of Medicine, University of Manchester, U.K.

Calcium binding protein (CaBP) which is produced in the intestine of pigs has also been found in the plasma (1). The role if any of CaBP in the plasma is not known. One suggested source of CaBP is simply a leak from the intestine (1). However, there is evidence to show that short term fluctuations of plasma CaBP occur during the day (2) and preliminary findings have indicated that plasma CaBP peaks may be stress related (3), which suggests that the levels of plasma CaBP may be controlled. The aim of this study was to determine which factors cause short term changes in plasma CaBP and to investigate the mechanism of the change.

Materials and Methods

Large White x Landrace and Yucatan minipigs of body weights (B.wt) varying from 25 to 60 kg were used for these experiments. Indwelling venous catheters were used to collect blood samples and administer drugs. Generally blood samples were collected at 15 minute intervals; three pre-treatment samples, then the experimental treatment was given and ten further blood samples taken.
The experimental treatments were as follows: insulin (0.25 U/kg B.wt) (n=11), insulin (0.25 U/kg B.wt) and glucose infusion (2 ml/min for 150 min of 50% glucose solution) (n=4), ACTH (20 µg/kg B.wt) (n=6) and cortisol sodium succinate (7.1 mg/kg B.wt) (n=6). Plasma was analysed for CaBP, by radioimmunoassay using a modification of the assay of Murray et al (4), for cortisol, by radioimmunoassay using a modification of the assay of Kane (5) and in some cases blood glucose was estimated, using glucose oxidase. Plasma levels of these parameters were compared with pre-treatment levels using Student's paired t-test.

Results and Discussion

The figures show the changes in plasma CaBP following each experimental treatment, for one typical experiment. Plasma CaBP and cortisol were significantly raised by insulin induced hypoglycaemia (155% and 500%, $P<0.001$ and $P<0.001$ respectively). But the continuous infusion of glucose following insulin injection, which prevented hypoglycaemia abolished the peaks in both CaBP and cortisol. This shows that the rise in plasma CaBP followed the hypoglycaemia rather than being a direct effect of insulin.

ACTH administration did lead to peaks in plasma CaBP and cortisol very similar to the one seen after insulin administration (170% and 480%, $P<0.05$ and $P<0.01$, respectively). It seemed possible therefore that cortisol was responsible for the effect on plasma CaBP, however the administration of pharmacological doses of cortisol did not alter plasma CaBP levels. Therefore if cortisol has any function it may affect plasma CaBP at physiological but not pharmacological doses, or it may exert a permissive effect. Alternatively ACTH has been shown to lead to other changes, e.g. a rise in plasma growth hormone (6) which might then lead to the peak in plasma CaBP. These hypotheses are being investigated.

Vitamin D. A Chemical, Biochemical and Clinical Update

We conclude that plasma CaBP can be significantly altered over a short period of time by certain endocrine changes i.e. insulin induced hypoglycaemia and ACTH.

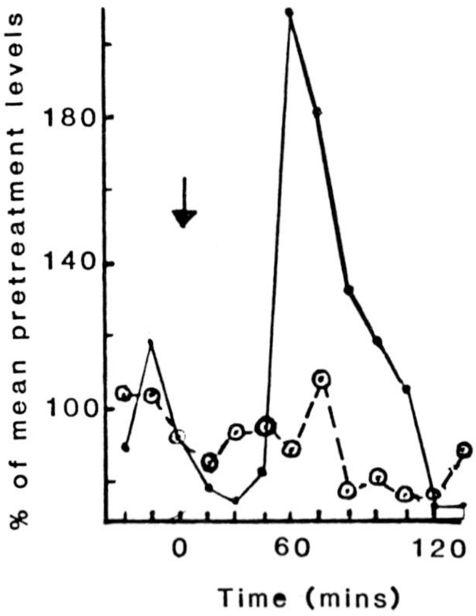

Figure 1. Plasma CaBP before and after intravenous administration of 0.25 U insulin/kg (↓) either alone (•——•) or followed by the continuous intravenous infusion of 50% glucose solution at 2 mls/min (⊙---⊙) in the pig.

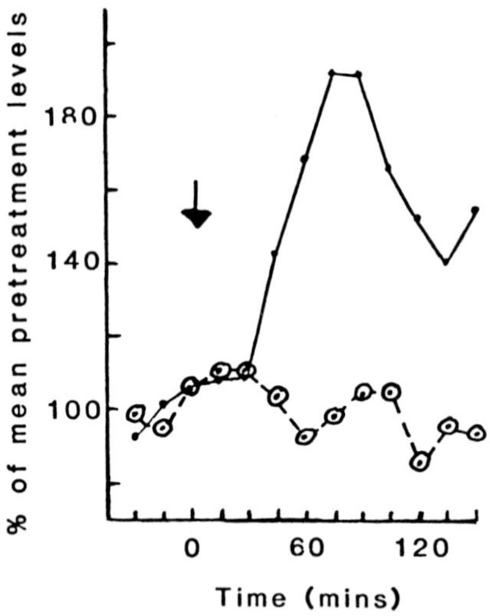

Figure 2. Plasma CaBP before and after intravenous administration of either 20 μg ACTH/kg (↓) (•——•) or 7.1 mg cortisol/kg (⊙---⊙) in the pig.

References

1. Arnold, B.M., Kuttner, M., Swaminathan, R., Care, A.D., Harrison, J.E. and Murray, T.M. (1975). Can.J.Phys.Pharm. 53, 1129-1134.
2. Ross, R., Maunder, E.M.W. and Care, A.D. (1982) in Vitamin D. Biochemical, Chemical and Clinical Aspects related to Calcium Metabolism (eds. A.W.Norman, K.Schaefer, D.V. Herrath and H.-G. Grigoleit), pp 265-266, DeGruyter, Berlin.
3. Murray, T.M., Brown, G., and Care, A.D. (1979). Proc. 61st Ann. Meeting Endocr. Soc.
4. Murray, T.M., Arnold, B.M., Tam, W.H., Hitchman,A.J.W. and Harrison, J.E. (1974). Metabolism 23, 829-837.
5. Kane, J.W. (1979). Ann. Clin. Biochem. 16, 209-212.
6. Lee, P.A., Keenan, B.S., Migeon, C.J. and Blizzard, R.M. (1973). J.Clin.Endocrinol.Metab. 37, 389-396.

28-kDa CHOLECALCIN (CaBP) LEVELS IN CEREBELLA OF MUTANT MICE

C. O. PARKES, J. MARIANI and M. THOMASSET
Physiology Dept., UBC, Vancouver, Canada, INSERM U120, Le Vésinet, France & Dept. de Biol. Moleculaire, Institut Pasteur, Paris, France.

Calcium is involved in the modulation of neuronal activity in many parts of the central nervous system (CNS) but the mechanism of its intra-neuronal regulation remains unclear. Several intracellular calcium-binding proteins are present in the CNS, including calmodulin, the S-100 proteins and the vitamin D-dependent calcium-binding protein, 28-kDa cholecalcin (CaBP). While the cerebellum contains by far the largest concentration of CaBP, the protein also occurs in the hippocampus, olfactory bulb, optic and auditory systems.

Cerebellar CaBP is restricted to the Purkinje (P) cells (1), implying that the protein is involved in the action of these cells. It is not known, however, whether CaBP is an intrinsic feature of all P cells or if its presence is an expression of their normal physiological activity. As CaBP synthesis in the post-weanling animal is apparently not vitamin D dependent (2), we have examined the CaBP level in the abnormal cerebella of mutant mice.

MATERIALS AND METHODS

Mutant Mice Seven mutant strains, raised at the Pasteur Institute, were studied: weaver (wv), staggerer (sg), Purkinje cell degeneration (pcd), reeler (rl), nervous (nr), hyperspiny Purkinje cell (hpc) and nodding (nd). Mutant animals were recognized clinically. Controls were homozygous +/+ mice of the same strain and age as the mutants.

CaBP measurements Mice were killed by decapitation and the cerebella dissected out, weighed, quick-frozen in liquid nitrogen and stored at -20 °C until assayed. CaBP was measured by radioimmunoassay (2).

DISCUSSION

The main result of our study is that the total cerebellar CaBP content of mutant mice appears to be a function of the size of the P cell population. P cells are present in the agranular cerebella of wv and rl mutants in apparently almost normal numbers, although they have reduced dendritic trees and the rl P cells are packed into a central mass below a greatly reduced cerebellar cortex. In spite of these abnormalities, the content of CaBP is within the normal range. However, the CaBP level is almost zero in mutants such as adult pcd or nr, in which P cells are lost (99% in pcd and 90% in nr).

The CaBP content is also dramatically reduced in the cerebella of sg mice, in which 60-90% of the P cells are lost. The remaining P cells exhibit marked abnormalities, including a lack of calcium spikes. The P cells of hpc and nd are malformed, having such juvenile characteristics as dendritic spines on the cell bodies and proximal dendrites, but the CaBP level is only slightly reduced (50-52%).

Vitamin D. A Chemical, Biochemical and Clinical Update

It is unlikely that the CaBP content of P cells is modulated by synaptic influence as sg, wv and rl have massive losses of granule cells, and thus a greatly depleted number of synapses between parallel fibres and P cells. Neither is multiple innervation a factor in inducing CaBP as all three of the above mutants also show multiple P cell climbing fibre innervation.

Thus, the CaBP content of P cells is characteristic of the cells themselves, no matter what their innervation, or developmental state.

RESULTS

Mutant	n	cerebellum wt (mg)	CaBP/protein ug/mg	CaBP/cerebellum ug
nervous (age = 105 d)				
test	5	39.4 +/- 1.75*	n.d.	n.d.
cont	5	50.6 +/- 3.47	10.26 +/- .39	19.0 +/- 3.1
pcd (age = 50 d)				
test	5	27.2 +/- 1.46	0.94+/- .26	1.12 +/- 0.37
cont	5	53.8 +/- 3.17	11.02+/- 1.73	11.9 +/- 1.47
staggerer (age = 22 d)				
test	9	7.5 +/- 0.32	0.09 +/- .01	0.015
cont	10	46.6 +/- 3.37	10.54 +/- 0.86	16.0 +/- 1.94
weaver (age = 25 d)				
test	5	14.6+/- 0.68	25.2 +/- 2.67	16.8 +/- 1.18
cont	5	49.0 +/- 1.64	9.9 +/- 0.69	14.0 +/- 2.16
reeler (age = 150 d)				
test	5	21.9 +/- 1.40	20.64 +/- 2.41	12.8 +/- 2.09
cont	5	57.3 +/- 0.61	11.06 +/- 1.03	17.8 +/- 2.05
hyperspiny Purkinje cell (age = 60 d)				
test	5	62.0 +/- 2.23	7.94 +/- 0.52	8.07 +/- 0.47
cont	5	85.5 +/- 1.86	10.63 +/- 0.50	15.39 +/- 0.52
nodding (age = 160 d)				
test	5	62.4 +/- 2.59	8.52 +/- 1.15	9.96 +/- 0.61
cont	5	84.6 +/- 1.54	13.34 +/- 0.86	19.97 +/- 0.91

* all values are means +/- SE; n.d.= not detectable

REFERENCES

1. Baimbridge, K.G. & Parkes, C.O. Cell Calcium, 2 (1981) 65-76.
2. Jande, S.S., Maler, L. & Lawson, D.E.M. Nature, 294 (1981) 765-767.
3. Legrand, C., Thomasset, M., Parkes, C.O., Clavel, M-C. and Rabié, A. Cell Tissue Res., 233 (1983) 389-402.
4. Thomasset, M., Parkes, C.O. & Cuisinier-Gleizes, P. Am. J. Physiol., 234 (1982) E483-E488.

LOCALIZATION OF CHOLECALCIN (9,000 MW CHOLECALCIFEROL-INDUCED CaBP) MESSENGER RNA IN RAT DUODENUM AND PLACENTA BY *IN SITU* HYBRIDIZATION.

M. WAREMBOURG, C. PERRET* and M. THOMASSET*,
INSERM U.156, Place de Verdun - 59045 Lille Cédex and *INSERM U.120 - 44, chemin de Ronde 78110 Le Vésinet, France.

INTRODUCTION

The cholecalcins (CaBPs), are high-affinity intracellular calcium-binding proteins. The duodenum of the rat contains a 9 000Mr cholecalcin (9-kDa CaBP) whose concentration in dependent upon $1,25(OH)_2D_3$, the hormonal form of vitamin D (1). We recently reported the molecular cloning of a cDNA fragment synthesized from rat duodenal mRNA coding for 9kDa cholecalcin (2) and the nucleotide sequence analysis of a resulting 375 base-pair cDNA clone, pC109 (3). We now report the use of this cloned cDNA to study the cytological distribution of 9-kDa cholecalcin mRNA in the rat duodenum and placenta by *in situ* hybridization.

MATERIALS AND METHODS

Animals - Pregnant Sprague Dawley rats (21 d), fed normal diet containing 4,000 IU of vitamin D_3/kg ad libitum, were used in all experiments.

Preparation of ^3H-cDNA probe - The cloned cDNA fragment (375 bp) was nick-translated using ^3H dCTP and ^3H dGTP. The specific activity of the cDNA probe was about 10^7 cpm/ug.

In situ hybridization - Tissue sections, fixed in ethanol:acetic acid, were hybridized to the ^3H-cDNA probe and processed for radioautography.

RESULTS

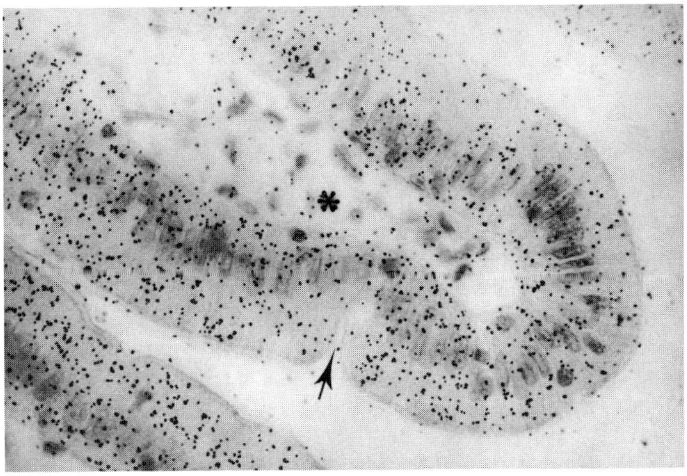

Fig. 1 : Radioautograph of rat duodenum
Villus tip. The silver grains are primarily over the absorptive epithelial cells with very few grains over the brush borders. The stroma of the villus (*) and goblet cells (arrow) show no selective labeling. Exposure time : 24 d. X530.

Vitamin D. A Chemical, Biochemical and Clinical Update

Duodenum (figure 1) - Cholecalcin mRNA, visualized by silver grains, was found only in the absorptive epithelial cells. The cholecalcin mRNA was observed mainly in the cytoplasm of the columnar cells and rately in the nuclei. Labeling was not seen over the brush border, goblet cells or their mucus secretion.

Placenta (figure 2) - The trophoblastic epithelium of the labyrinth zone was found to have intensive labeling. Silver grains were predominantly localized over the cytoplasm of the syncytial cells. The region between the labyrinth and the decidua basilis contained a small amount of radioactivity.

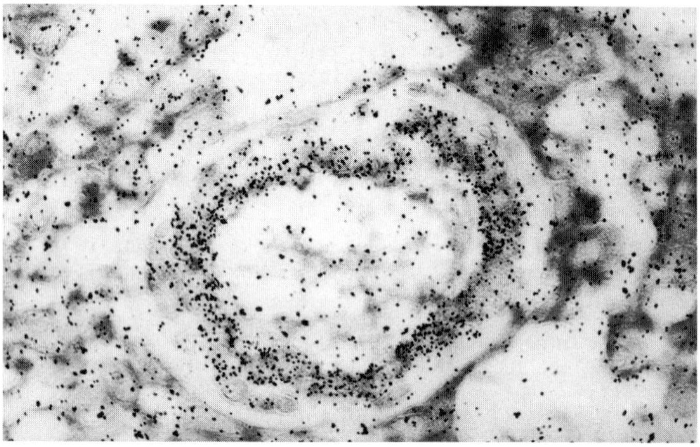

Fig. 2 : Radioautograph of rat placenta
Labyrinth zone. The trophoblastic epithelium is intensely labeled. Exposure time : 30 d. X530.

CONCLUSION

This demonstration of the 9 kDa CaBP gene activity in restricted areas, the columnar epithelial cells of the rat duodenum and the trophoblastic epithelium of the placental labyrinth zone, is in agreement with the immunocytochemical localization of cholecalcin itself and illustrates the usefulness of *in situ* hybridization for studies on the mechanism of steroid hormone action.

REFERENCES

1. Thomasset, M. ; Cuisinier-Gleizes, P. and Mathieu, H. (1979) FEBS Lett. 107, 91-94.
2. Thomasset, M. ; Parkes, C.O. and Cuisinier-Gleizes, P. (1982) Am. J. Physiol. 243,E483-E488.
3. Thomasset, M. ; Desplan, C. and Parkes, C.O. (1983) Eur. J. Biochem. 129, 519-524.

Supported in part by grant from CNRS (gene molecular biology 033.107)

EFFECT OF 1,25(OH)$_2$D$_3$, VERAPAMIL AND EDTA-INFUSION ON THE THYROLIBERIN-INDUCED THYROTROPIN RELEASE

K. TÖRNQUIST and C. LAMBERG-ALLARDT
Endocrine Research Laboratory, University of Helsinki
Minerva Foundation, Helsinki, Finland

Introduction:

The role of the pituitary on the vitamin D homeostasis is obvious. Both prolactin and growth hormone affect the hydroxylation of 25-hydroxycholecalciferol (25OHD$_3$) to 1,25-dihydroxycholecalciferol (1,25(OH)$_2$D$_3$) (1). Receptors for 1,25(OH)$_2$D$_3$ are found in the pituitary (2) and in cloned rat pituitary cells (GH$_3$-cells) secreting both prolactin and growth hormone (3). Sar et al. (4) showed that in rat pituitaries, thyrotrophes are target cells for 1,25 (OH)$_2$D$_3$. It has also been shown that 25OHD$_3$ elevates basal serum thyrotropin (TSH) levels (5). There is also investigations suggesting a role for the thyroid on the formation of 1,25(OH)$_2$D$_3$ (6). In the present study we investigated the effect of 1,25(OH)$_2$D$_3$, verapamil and EDTAinfusion on the thyroliberin (TRH) induced TSH release.

Materials and Methods:

Female Wistar rats (180-220 g) in groups of six received 20 % ethanol in saline (control), 1,25(OH)$_2$D$_3$ (0.05 µg/kg/day), verapamil (25 mg/kg/day) or 1,25(OH)$_2$D$_3$ + verapamil in two doses per day for three days. Ten hours after the last dose the rats were anaesthetized with pentobarbital and the jugular vein and the carotic artery were canulated. TRH (20 µg/animal) was injected i.v. and blood was drawn every ten minutes for forty minutes. In the EDTA-infusion experiments EDTA (30 mg/kg/100 min) was infused through a tail vein, starting 60 minutes before TRH was injected. TSH was assayed using a NIAMDD rat TSH kit. Calcium was determined using a flame atomic absorption spectrometer.

Results:

In the normal test, basal TSH values showed no significant differences between the experimental groups and the control group. In the groups receiving 1,25(OH)$_2$D$_3$ or 1,25(OH)$_2$D$_3$ + verapamil, peak TSH values increased significantly ($p<0,01$ respectively $p<0,001$; fig. 1a). EDTA-infusion changed the relationship between the peak TSH values after 1,25(OH)$_2$D$_3$ and 1,25(OH)$_2$D$_3$ + verapamil treatment, both groups still showing significant increases in the TSH secretion ($p<0,001$ respectively $p<0,01$; fig. 1b). Serum Ca was increased in the groups receiving 1,25(OH)$_2$D$_3$ ($p<0,01$, fig. 2a). The difference was diminished after EDTA-infusion (fig. 2b). Pituitary protein concentrations were also increased in the rats receiving 1,25(OH)-$_2$D$_3$. Basal TSH level in the verapamil-EDTA-infusion group showed a significant decrease compared to the control group ($p<0,01$).

Conclusions:

The results obtained in this investigation suggest that 1,25(OH)$_2$D$_3$ directly affects the secretion of TSH-from the rat pituitary during the TRH-test. Whether 1,25(OH)$_2$D$_3$ affects the synthesis or the secretion of TSH (or both) still remains unsolved. The elevated serum Ca exhibits a slight

Vitamin D. A Chemical, Biochemical and Clinical Update

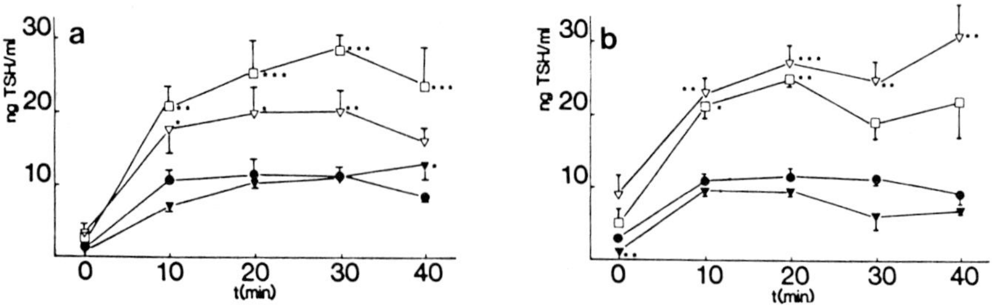

Fig. 1. Effect of 1,25(OH)$_2$D$_3$ (▽), verapamil (▼) and 1,25(OH)$_2$D$_3$ + verapamil on the TRH induced TSH secretion. Control (●). a) normal assay, b) with EDTA-infusion. ($\bar{x}$ ± SEM)

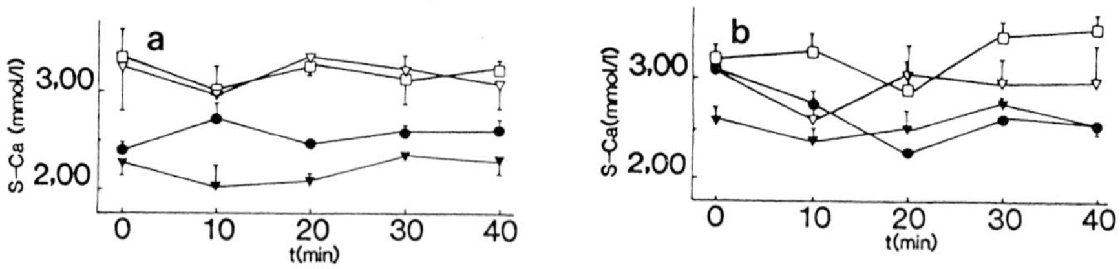

Fig. 2. Serum Ca-levels. Control (●), verapamil (▼), 1,25(OH)$_2$D$_3$ (▽) and 1,25(OH)$_2$D$_3$ + verapamil (□). a) normal assay, b) with EDTA-infusion ($\bar{x}$ ± SEM)

inhibitory effect, probably through release of dopamine from hypothalamic dopaminergic neurons (7). This effect is countracted by verapamil. Infusion of EDTA also has the same effect. An effect of verapamil on the TSH secretion could not be seen.

References:

1. Norman, A.W., Roth, J. and Orci, L. (1982) Endocrinol. Rev. 3:331-366.
2. Stumpf, W.E., Sar, M., Reid, F.A. and Tanaka, Y. (1979) Science 206:1188-1190.
3. Haussler, M.R., Manolagas, S.C. and Deftos, L.J. (1982) J. Steroid Biochem. 16:15-19.
4. Sar, M., Stumpf, W.E. and DeLuca, H.F. (1980) Cell. Tissue Res. 209:161-166.
5. Zofkova, J., Blahos, J. and Bednar, J. (1981) Endocrinologie 78:118-120.
6. Bouillon, R., Muls, E. and De Moor, P. (1980) J. Clin. Endocrinol. Metab. 51:793-797.
7. Röjdmark, S. and Andersson, D.E.H. (1982) J. Clin. Endocrinol. Metab. 54: 998-1001.

CONTROL OF CHOLECALCIN (9000 MW CHOLECALCIFEROL-INDUCED CaBP) GENE EXPRESSION BY $1,25(OH)_2D_3$ IN RAT INTESTINE.

C. PERRET, C. DESPLAN, J.M. DUPRE and M. THOMASSET.
INSERM U.120, 44 Chemin de Ronde - 78110 Le Vésinet, France.

INTRODUCTION

As a part of our study on the mechanism of the hormonal action of cholecalciferol we now report the distribution of the 9-kDa cholecalcin mRNA and its control by $1,25(OH)_2D_3$ along the digestive tract of the growing rat using a specific ^{32}P cDNA probe. We have also examined the rate at which concentrations of this mRNA increase in response to $1,25(OH)_2D_3$ injected into vitamin D-deficient rats (-D) fed a low (0.03%) calcium diet.

RESULTS

Distribution of 9-kDa cholecalcin mRNA along the digestive tract.
Total RNA (10,5, 2.5 and 1.25μg ; lanes 1,2,3 and 4 respectively in the insert fig.1 was assayed by dot blot hybridization

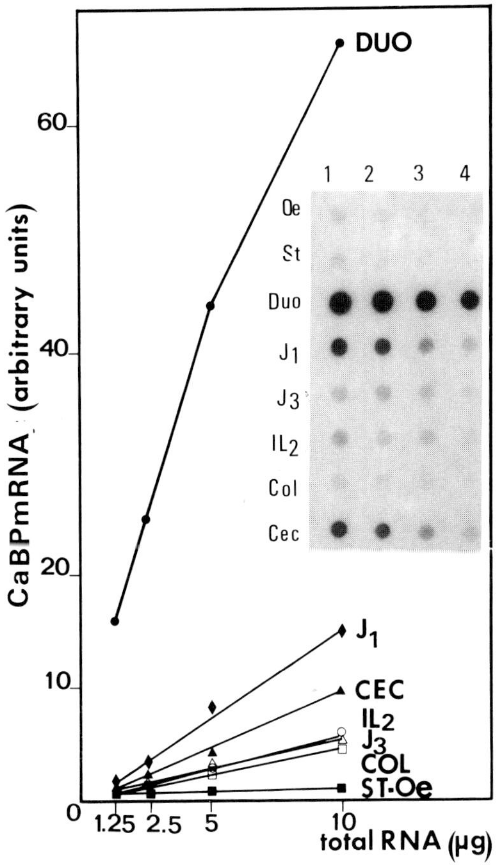

Fig.1 - 9-kDa cholecalcin mRNA levels along the digestive tract.

Vitamin D. A Chemical, Biochemical and Clinical Update

In rats fed a normal Ca (0.36%) and vitamin D-supplemented diet (2,000 iu/kg) the highest concentration of CaBP mRNA was found in the duodenum (fig. 1). The proximal jejunum and cecum contained 5 and 8 less than the duodenum respectively. The CaBP 9K mRNA was about 15 times less concentrated in the distal jejunum ; ileum and colon as compared to the duodenum. The observed differences in 9-kDa cholecalcin mRNA levels correlate well with both the in vivo variations in cholecalcin itself (not shown) and with the known intestinal sites of calcium absorption.

Northern analysis of 9-kDa cholecalcin mRNA along the digestive tract. Northern hybridization showed that the cDNA probe hybridized to a homogeneous 500-600 nucleotide mRNA species all along the intestine (not shown).

Vitamin D-dependence of cholecalcin mRNA in the rat intestine. CaBP mRNA contents decreased in (-D) animals throughout the intestine (fig. 2a, 2b). A single 1,25$(OH)_2D_3$ injection (200ng) to (-D) rats resulted in a return to the normal CaBP mRNA level in the duodenum (fig. 2a) and in an elevation of CaBP mRNA to supranormal levels in the distal intestine (not shown) and cecum (fig. 2b) 3 and 24 h after treatment.

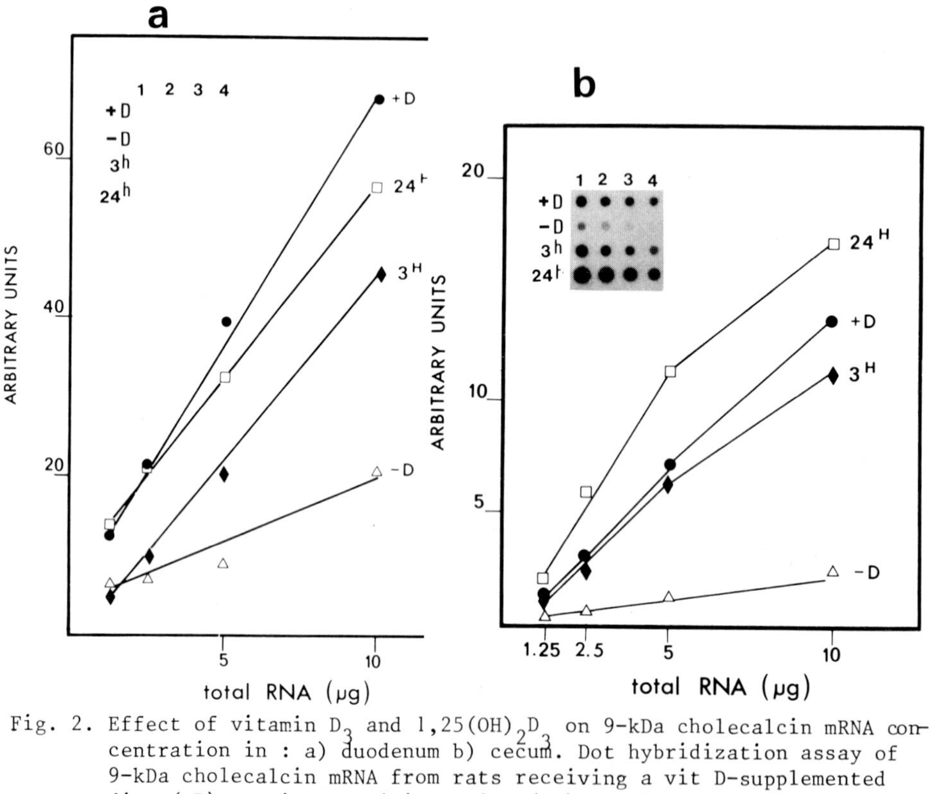

Fig. 2. Effect of vitamin D_3 and 1,25$(OH)_2D_3$ on 9-kDa cholecalcin mRNA concentration in : a) duodenum b) cecum. Dot hybridization assay of 9-kDa cholecalcin mRNA from rats receiving a vit D-supplemented diet (+D), a vit D-deficient diet (-D), a vit D-deficient diet and a single 1,25$(OH)_2D_3$ injection 3 hours (3 H) or 14 hours (14 H) before killing.

CALCIUM-BINDING PROTEIN DISTRIBUTION AND POSSIBLE FUNCTIONS IN RODENT AND PRIMATE BRAIN

K.G. Baimbridge and J.J. Miller
Department of Physiology, Faculty of Medicine, University of British Columbia, 2075 Wesbrook Mall, Vancouver, B.C., Canada V6T 1W5

Since the first observation of the presence of Vitamin D dependent calcium-binding protein (CaBP, M.W. = 28Kd) in the chick brain (14) a number of groups have reported the presence of a similar protein in the CNS of mammals, including primates, (2,3,4,7,8,11,12). In all species so far examined the protein retains it's 28Kd form in the brain, unlike the mammalian gut version of CaBP which is smaller and only binds two calcium ions per mole (10). When immunohistochemical techniques are used to locate CaBP in the CNS all neuronal elements, (cell bodies, dendrites and axons), of CaBP positive neurons are stained since the protein is highly soluble and occupies the entire cell volume. This particular property has made CaBP a useful tool for tracing neuroanatomical projections in the CNS. For example, analysis of the complex interconnections of the basal ganglia using CaBP immunohistochemistry reveals positively labelled cells in the Substantia nigra pars compacta corresponding to the A9 dopamine-containing neurons as well as a dense plexus of their terminal fibers throughout the striatum. Neurons exhibiting a heavy staining for CaBP in the striatum belong to the medium spiny cell population and their projection fibers terminating in the Substantia nigra pars reticulata are clearly visualized.

The distribution of CaBP in the rat brain has not revealed a clear correlation with any particular neuronal function or neurotransmitter. Examples of CaBP coexisting with almost all putative transmitters can be seen, e.g. the magnocellular cells of the Nucleus basalis of Meynert (Acetylcholine) and Supraoptic nucleus (oxytocin and vasopressin), cerebellar Purkinje cells (GABA); cells in the medial compacta zone of the Substantia nigra (Dopamine); dentate granule cells in the hippocampal formation (glutamate and an opiate peptide); and the medium spiny cells of the striatum (substance P).

Attempts to assign a function to CaBP in the CNS would be aided if it were possible to manipulate the concentration of this protein in cells which contain it. We have, recently demonstrated that if rats are stimulated to the point of inducing seizures, using the kindling paradigm (9), a highly specific loss of CaBP occurs from the dentate granule cells of the hippocampal formation (12).

Vitamin D. A Chemical, Biochemical and Clinical Update

Such an effect is progressive with the number of stimulations given and precedes the onset of full seizure activity (5). We have speculated that the function of CaBP may be to act as an intracellular buffering system in neurons and computer modelling studies of calcium channel activity in snail neurons (which contain a protein which cross-reacts with antibodies to human CaBP) have supported such a role (6). Specifically, the presence of a protein with the calcium-binding properties and intracellular concentration of CaBP can greatly enhance the open time of active calcium channels since the intracellular calcium ion concentration is buffered and prevented from inactivating it's own channels. Each high frequency stimulation used in the kindling experiments would most likely have resulted in a large uptake of calcium ions into the stimulated neurons (1) but the loss of CaBP from the dentate granule cells might result in the paradoxical effect (for tissue prone to seizure activity) of reducing the excitability of the cells by reducing their calcium currents. While clearly speculative, experimental support has been obtained which does in fact demonstrate a reduced activity of dentate granule cells in kindled rats (13).

References

1. Baimbridge, K.G. and Miller, J.J. (1981) Brain Research 221:299-305
2. Baimbridge, K.G. and Parkes, C.O. (1981) Cell Calcium 2:65-77
3. Baimbridge, K.G., Miller, J.J. and Parkes, C.O. (1982) Brain Research 239:519-525
4. Baimbridge, K.G. and Miller, J.J. (1982) Brain Research 245:223-229
5. Baimbridge, K.G. and Miller, J.J. (1984) Brain Research 324:85-90
6. Chad, J.E. and Eckert, R. (1984) Biophys. J. 45:993-999
7. Feldman, S.C. and Christakos, S. (1983) Endocrinology 112:290-302
8. Garcia-Segura, L.M., Baetens, D., Roth, J., Norman, A.W. and Orci, L. (1984) Brain Research 296:75-86
9. Goddard, G.V., McIntyre, D. and Leech, C. (1969) Exp. Neurol. 25:295-330
10. Hitchman, A.J.W. and Harrison, J.E. (1972) Can. J. Biochem. 50:758-765
11. Jande, S.S., Maler, L. and Lawson, D.E.M. (1981a) Nature 294:765-767
12. Jande, S.S., Tolnai, S. and Lawson, D.E.M. (1981b) Histochemistry 71:99-116
13. Miller, J.J. and Baimbridge, K.G. (1983) Brain Research ;278:322-326
14. Oliver, M.W. and Miller, J.J. (1985) In press.
15. Taylor, A.N. and Brindak, M.E. (1974) Arch. Biochem. Biophys. 161:100-108

ENZYME MODIFICATION BY RENAL CALCIUM BINDING PROTEINS

T. S. FREUND* and S. CHRISTAKOS
*Department of Biochemistry, FDU School of Dentistry, Hackensack, NJ 07601 and Department of Biochemistry, UMDNJ, Newark, NJ 07103, USA.

INTRODUCTION:

Although a specific function for them has remained elusive the vitamin D-dependent calcium binding proteins (CaBP) are widely distributed and generally accepted as possessing roles in transcellular calcium transport. Of the several functions which these proteins might play (1), as buffer or as enzyme modifier, we have concentrated our efforts in studying the latter role. Over the past several years, several preliminary reports have appeared which indicate that the CaBP isolated from the rat intestine (2) binds to and activates both the brush border alkaline phosphatase (AP) and the baso-lateral Ca-Mg ATPase (CMATP) while that from the chick (3,4, 5) binds to brush border membrane proteins. In order to develop a more universal hypothesis, as to the action of CaBP as a membrane enzyme effector we have examined the larger mammalian CaBP from the rat kidney in its possible role as a participant in the activity of the kidney membranous AP and CMATP.

MATERIALS AND METHODS:

CaBP was isolated from kidney as described (6). For the binding studies, some of the kidney CaBP had been radioactively labeled (7).

Membranes: A crude microsomal fraction of membranes obtained from kidney cortex containing both brush borders (AP) and baso-lateral (CMATP) membranes was used for this study. Following homogenization in a buffer containing 50 mM imidazole HCl (pH 7.4); 100 mM NaCl; 5 mM dithiothreitol; 0.5 mM EGTA and 0.1 mM phenylmethyl sulfonyl fluoride, the microsomal fraction was separated by differential centrifugation (15-30,000g). The pellet was resuspended in the same buffer, at a concentration of 1.5 mg protein per ml for use.

Enzyme Assays: Aliquots of assay mixture (50 uL each) were analyzed for AP activity (p-nitrophenol release at pH 8.5) and CMATP activity (inorganic phosphate release from Mg-ATP at pH 7.4).

CaBP Binding to membranes was measured by a Millipore filtration technique following incubation for 20 minutes with shaking at room temperature.

FIG. 1. CaBP Binding to Kidney.

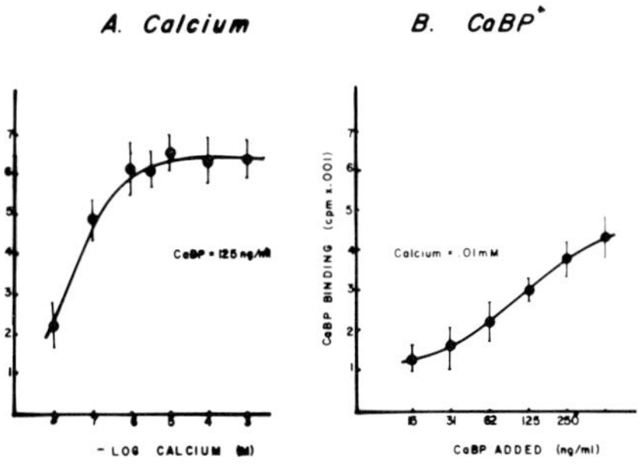

FIG. 2. CaMg ATPase Activity.

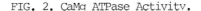

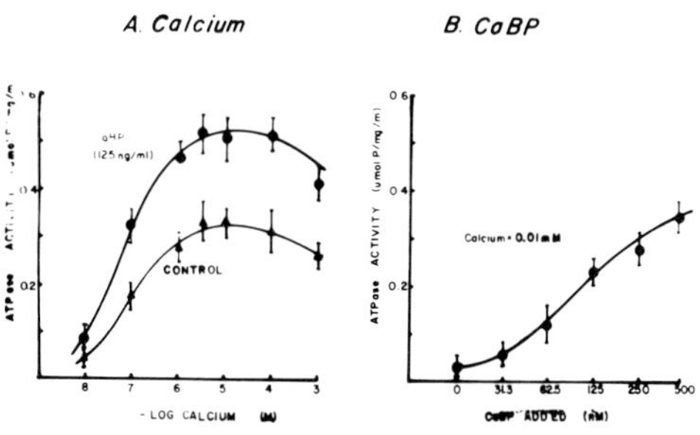

Vitamin D. A Chemical, Biochemical and Clinical Update

RESULTS:

The binding of the renal CaBP to the kidney microsomes is depicted in figure 1. While the binding in the presence of calcium was saturable in the micromolar range, saturation was only approached when CaBP was added at the maximum concentration tested (250 ng/50 ug membranes).

When compared to the activation of the CMATP (Figure 2) it is interesting to note the parallelism with binding. At a calcium concentration of 1 mM, the CMATP demonstratres the expected inhibition. However, the binding of CaBP does not follow, implying that the calcium inhibition may occur by an alternative mechanism.

Although not shown, the activation of the AP does occur in a similar fashion to that of the CMATP, but to a lesser degree (only 33% stimulation) with saturation at an increased calcium (100 uM). It should also be noted that, wheras 125 ng CaBP produces one-half maximal response for the CMATP a higher concentration (250 ng) is required for the AP.

Neither calmodulin (CaM) at a concentration of lug/ml nor serum albumin (a low affinity calcium binder) at 100 ug/ml demonstrated any significant competition with the binding of the CaBP. CaM did activate the CMATP, but to a lesser degree.

CONCLUSIONS:

Our data support the hypothesis that CaBPs are able to exert their physiological influence by binding to and activating membrane enzymes involved in calcium transport.

REFERENCES:

1. Wasserman, R.H, Shimura, F, Meyer, S.A. and Fullmer, C.S. (1983) in Calcium Binding Proteins 1983. de Bernard, et.al. eds, Elsevier, New York 183-188.

2. Freund, T. S. (1982) in Vitamin D, Chemical, Biochemical and Clinical Endocrinology of Calcium Metabolism. Norman, A. W. et.al. eds, De Gruyter, New York, pp. 249-251.

3. Moriuchi, S., Shidoji, Y., Mizuno, K., and Hosoya, N. (1980) in Calcium Endocrinology. Yoshitoshi, Y. and T. Fujita, eds, Chugai Igabu Co., Tokyo. pp. 221-233.

4. Norman, A. W., and Leathers V. L. (1982) Biochem. Biophys. Res. Comm. 108: 220-226.

5. Shimura, F. and Wasserman, R. H. (1984) Endocrinology 115: 1964-1972.

6. Pansini, A. R., and Christakos, S. (1984) J. Biol. Chem. 259: 9735-9741.

7. Sonnenberg, J., Pansini, A. R., and Christakos, S. (1984) Endocrinology 115: 640-648.

SQUID BRAIN CALCIUM BINDING PROTEIN: BIOCHEMICAL SIMILARITY TO 28,000 M_r VITAMIN D DEPENDENT CALCIUM BINDING PROTEIN

S. CHRISTAKOS, A. SORI, L. MALKOWITZ and S. C. FELDMAN[†]

Departments of Biochemistry and [†]Anatomy, UMDNJ-New Jersey Medical School, Newark, New Jersey USA

Squid brain CaBP was purified from postmicrosomal supernatants by gel filtration on Sephadex G-75 followed by preparative gel electrophoresis in the presence or absence of 1 mM EDTA and recovery of protein by reverse polarity elution (1, 2). The SDS polyacrylamide gel electrophoretic patterns at the various stages of purification are shown in Fig. 1A. A single band was observed after both SDS (Fig. 1A, B) and native gel electrophoresis (Fig. 1C) suggesting the homogeneity of the preparation.

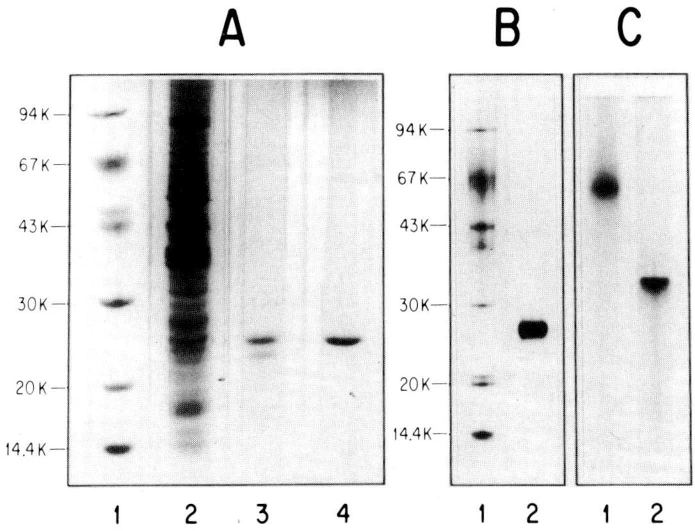

Fig. 1. Electrophoretic analysis at various stages of purification. A. SDS gel electrophoresis. 1, molecular wgt. standards; 2, crude cytosol; 3, after gel filtration on Sephadex G-75; 4, after preparative gel electrophoresis. B. Silver stain, SDS gel electrophoresis. 1, mol. wgt. standards; 2,5 µg purified squid CaBP. C. Analytical polyacrylamide gel electrophoresis. 1, the sample and gel buffer contained 1 mM Ca^{++}; 2, the sample and gel buffer contained 1 mM EDTA.

The molecular weight of squid CaBP determined from Ferguson plots was calculated to be 26,000 (Fig. 2A). Although the mobility of calmodulin during SDS-polyacrylamide gel electrophoresis is altered by the presence of

Vitamin D. A Chemical, Biochemical and Clinical Update

calcium, a similar mobility shift was not observed for either purified squid CaBP or vitamin D dependent rat renal CaBP (Fig. 2B, C).

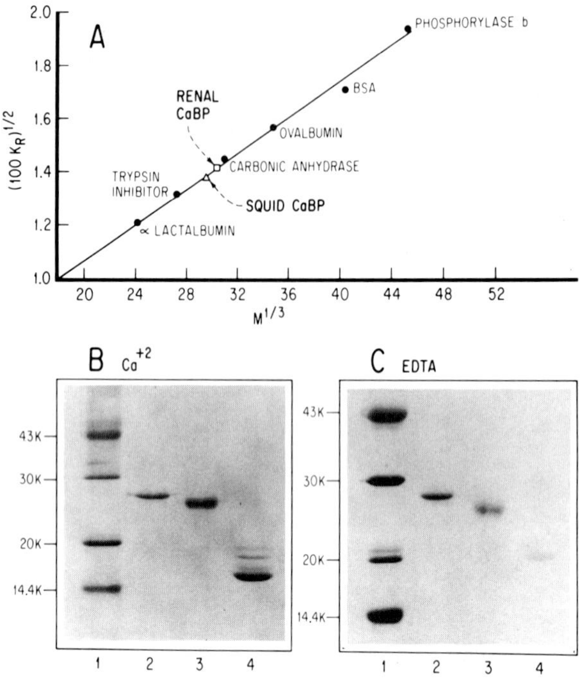

Fig. 2. Estimation of mol. wgt. of squid CaBP from Ferguson plots and SDS slab gel electrophoresis. A, Ferguson plot of the square root of retardation coefficient (K_R) and cube root of the molecular weights obtained by linear regression. B and C, SDS slab gel electrophoresis. 1, mol. wgt. standards; 2, renal CaBP; 3, squid CaBP; 4, calmodulin.

Also squid CaBP (up to 10 µg) does not cross in the calmodulin RIA and does not stimulate phosphodiesterase (data not shown). Amino acid analysis of squid CaBP revealed a high content of glutamic and aspartic acid and a low level of methionine and histidine, similar but not identical to the vertebrate 28,000 M_r CaBP. This study represents the first purification from an invertebrate of a calcium binding protein which is biochemically similar to vitamin D dependent CaBP.

1. Pansini, A. R. and Christakos, S. (1984) J. Biol. Chem. 259, 9735-9741.

2. Abramovitz, A. S., Randolph, V., Mehra, A. and Christakos, S. (1984) Preparative Biochemistry 14, 205-221.

CHOLECALCIN (28-kDa CaBP) : A KEY COMPONENT IN SENSORY PATHWAYS ?

A. Rabié, C.O. Parkes*, Ch. Legrand and M. Thomasset*

Laboratoire de Physiologie comparée, UA 653 CNRS, 34060 Montpellier, France ; * INSERM U 120, 44 Chemin de Ronde, 78110 Le Vésinet, France.

The intracellular calcium-binding protein cholecalcin or vitamin D-dependent calcium-binding protein (CaBP), was first described in chickens where it was found in tissues involved in the transepithelial transport of calcium, intestine, uterus and kidney (1,2). It was subsequently detected in certain avian and mammalian neurones, notably the cerebellar Purkinje cells (2,3) and hippocampal pyramidal cells (4), whose dendrites are known to produce calcium spikes. However, the precise role of cholecalcin in the neurones is still not known, neither is its relationship to vitamin D within the central nervous system clear. We now report on the presence of cholecalcin in specific cells of the three major sensory systems of the rat.

Immunocytochemical localization of cholecalcin in the brain and sensory organs of young rats was performed by the Sternberger peroxidase method using rabbit anti human 28-kDa cholecalcin serum as the primary antibody.

Olfactory system (Fig. 1) Cholecalcin was found in the periglomerular cells of the olfactory bulb, i.e. in the interneurones which modulate the function of the first synaptic contact of the olfactory pathway (4).

Auditory system (Fig. 2) Cochlear and vestibular hair cells also contain cholecalcin (5). Once again, the protein is present at the level of the first synaptic contact of the sensory tract. While cholecalcin is present throughout the cytoplasm of the hair cells, it appears most concentrated in the area of the cuticular plate (arrow). This cytoskeletal anchoring point of the stereocilia is said at the origin of the mechanochemical coupling in hearing and vestibular function. Its structure is also reminiscent of the intestinal brush border terminal web, where calmodulin and cholecalcin are concentrated.

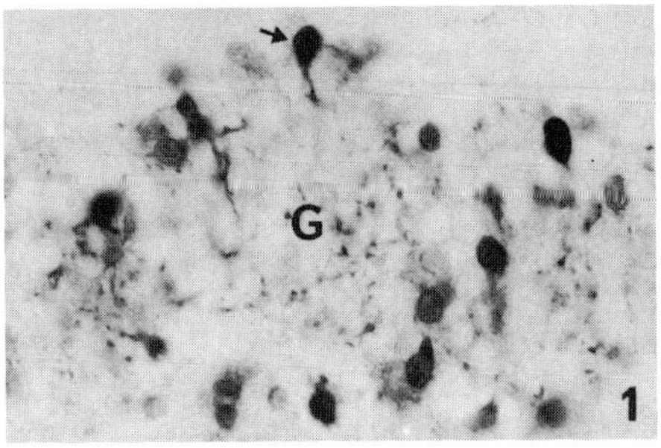

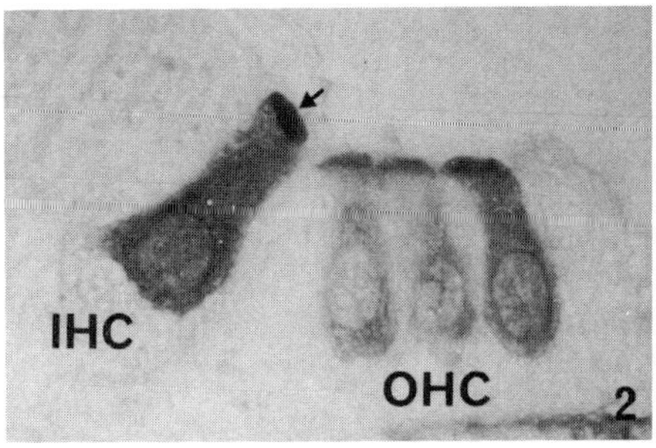

Fig. 1 : Olfactory bulb of 14-day-old rat (x 200). Periglomerular cells show intense staining for cholecalcin both in cell bodies (arrow) and in dendrites penetrating the glomerulus (G).

Fig. 2 : Cochlea of 3-day-old rat (x 910), showing hair cells containing cholecalcin. Note that staining is more intense in inner hair cell (IHC) than in the outer hair cells (OHC). The cuticular plate (arrow) is more intensely stained than the rest of the cytoplasm.

Vitamin D. A Chemical, Biochemical and Clinical Update

Visual system (Fig. 3) The horizontal cells of the retina contain cholecalcin. The protein is present throughout the cytoplasm and can be seen in the cell processes running in the outer plexiform layer. Thus, once again, cholecalcin is present in the interneurones modulating the first step in the sensory pathway.

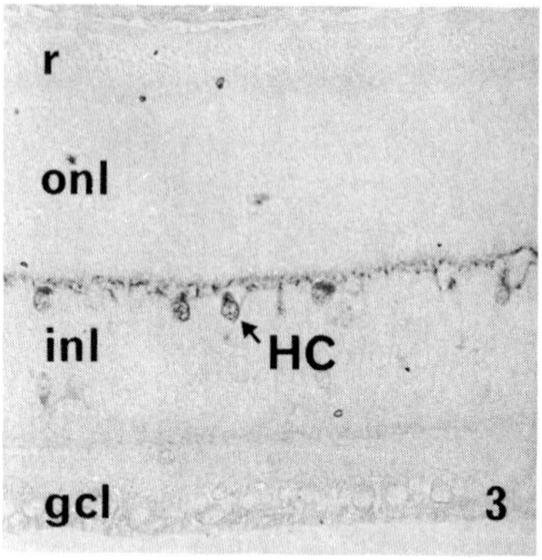

Fig. 3 : Retina of 19-day-old rat (x 205). The layer of horizontal cells (HC) contains cholecalcin. The protein is mainly in the cytoplasm, including the cell processes. Receptor cells (r), outer nuclear layer (onl), inner nuclear layer (inl) and ganglion cell layer (gcl) are not labelled.

High concentrations of cholecalcin are, therefore, present in specific cells at the very first steps of all three sensory pathways. Although the functions of the three types of cells appear to be quite different, all may have a modulatory involvement of calcium, as in, for example, the retinal horizontal cells which produce no impulses but develop sustained graded potentials depending on the intensity of retinal stimulation. Modulation of calcium-regulated mechanisms involving actin, myosin and other calcium-dependent proteins may also be the major role of cholecalcin in the hair cells. Whether, in this modulating action, cholecalcin acts merely as an intracellular calcium buffer, or has a more active role, remains to be demonstrated. The widespread, but specific, distribution of this protain, which in other organs is vitamin D-dependent, would also suggest that vitamin D has an, as yet unspecified, action upon the central nervous system.

(This work was supported by INSERM, PRC 135 016 and CRL 82.40024).

References

1- *Taylor, A.N. and Wasserman, R.H. (1967) Arch. Biochem. Biophys. 119, 536-540.*

2- *Jande, S.S., Tolnai, S. and Lawson, D.E.M. (1981) Histochemistry 71, 99-116.*

3- *Legrand, Ch., Thomasset, M., Parkes, C.O., Clavel, M.C. and Rabié, A. (1983) Cell Tissue Res. 233, 389-402.*

4- *Baimbridge, K.G. and Miller, J.J. (1982) Brain Res. 245, 223-229.*

5- *Rabié, A., Thomasset, M. and Legrand, Ch. (1983) Cell Tissue Res. 232, 691-696.*

6- *Rabié, A., Thomasset, M., Parkes, C.O. and Clavel, M.C. (1985) Cell Tissue Res., in press.*

PRESENCE OF VITAMIN D-DEPENDENT CALCIUM-BINDING PROTEIN (CaBP 9-kDa CHOLECALCIN) IN CALCIFYING CARTILAGE.

N. Balmain, M. Thomasset, P. Cuisinier-Gleizes, H. Mathieu
INSERM U.120, 44, chemin de Ronde - 78110 Le Vésinet, France.

INTRODUCTION

There are two intracellular vitamin D-dependent calcium-binding proteins, cholecalcins, in the rat. The smaller, 9-kDa protein (CaBP) is found mainly in the small intestine (1,2) and its location has been described immunohistochemically in the soft tissues of a number of species (3,4,5) and in teeth (6). This study describes the distribution of 9-kDa CaBP in the epiphyseal cartilage of the rat.

MATERIAL AND METHODS

The proximal tibial ends of 21 day-old Sprague Dawley derived female rats were fixed in Carnoy's fluid or formaldehyde (pH 7.4), frozen in CO_2 and either cryosectioned or embedded in methylmethacrylate and sectioned undecalcified. Immunohistochemical localization was performed using immunofluorescence (FITC) or protein-A-coupled peroxidase. Resin was removed with acetone, prior to immunohistochemistry. Specific antiserum raised in rabbits against rat duodenal 9-kDa CaBP, was diluted 10-80 fold before use. Controls consisted of non immune rabbit antiserum ; specific primary antiserum linked to an excess of the corresponding antigen ; specific antiserum followed by non-labeled protein A and protein A-peroxidase ; estimation of the autofluorescence.

RESULTS AND DISCUSSION

Immunoreactive material was detected throughout the zone of epiphyseal cartilage located beneath the proliferative zone (fig.1). 9-kDa CaBP was found

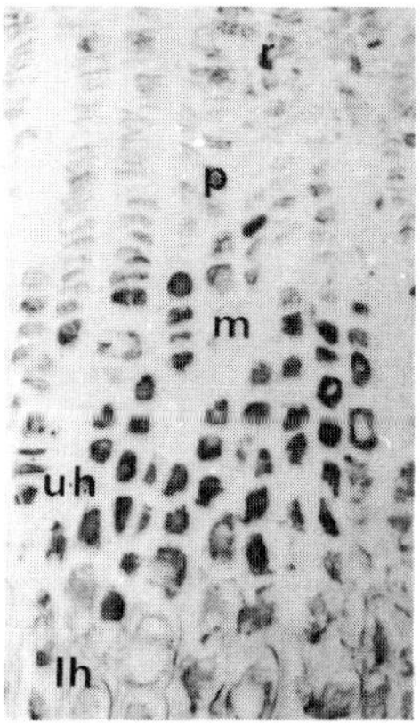

Fig.1.Epiphyseal cartilage. Protein A-peroxidase; resting zone (r), proliferative zone (p), maturing zone (m), upper hypertrophic zone (u.h.), lower hypertrophic zone(l.h)x170

Fig.2.Immuno control. Antiserum linked to CaBP in excess.

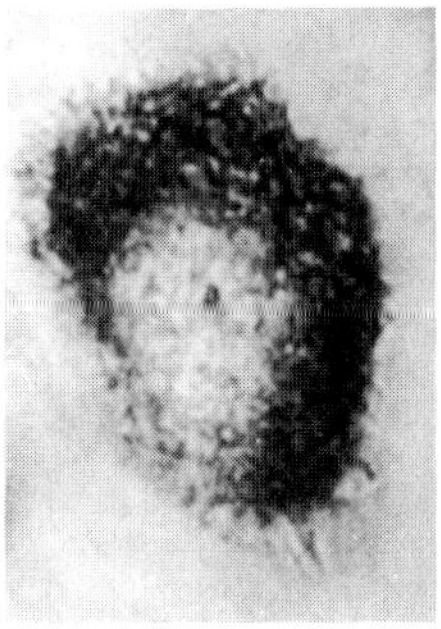

Fig.3.Chondrocyte of the maturing zone (m) ; protein A-peroxidase. Positive cytoplasm. Nucleus unstained X 1,700.

Vitamin D. A Chemical, Biochemical and Clinical Update

exclusively in the cytoplasm of chondrocytes of the maturing zone (fig.3) ; here the chondrocytes are in the process of maturation and are actively synthesizing the cartilage matrix which will, later, be calcified. 9-kDa CaBP can be seen in the region of the rough endoplasmic reticulum (RER). In the upper hypertrophic zone, CaBP was found in both the cytoplasm and the cytoplasmic processes of chondrocytes. As the chondrocytes become more hypertrophied, in the lower hypertrophic zone, the intracellular concentration of CaBP progressively decreases and appears in an extracellular region on the lateral edges of the calcifying longitudinal septa (fig. 4). It is in these areas that matrix vesicles are known to occur.

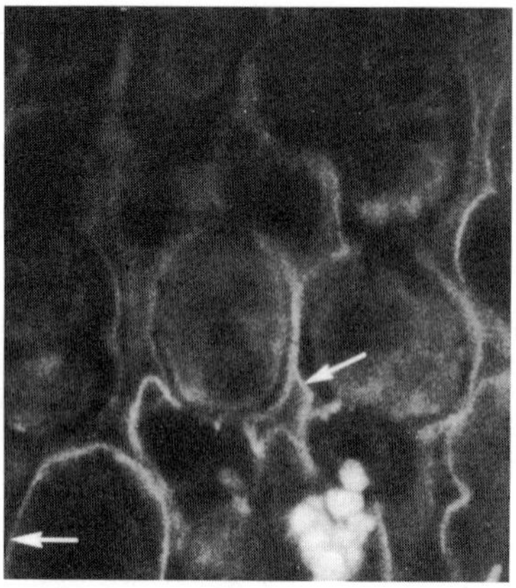

Fig.4.Calcifying hypertrophic cartilage. Immunofluorescence (FITC).
Positive staining for CaBP on the lateral edges of the longitudinal calcifying septa (arrows) X850

Fig.5.Control : specific antiserum linked to CaBP in excess.

CONCLUSION

The cytoplasmic localization of 9-kDa CaBP in the mature chondrocytes of the epiphyseal plate together with its detection in those extracellular regions were matrix vesicle mineralization is initiated, suggest that the protein may be involved in matrix vesicle associated process of cartilage calcification.

REFERENCES

1. Wasserman, R.H. , Taylor, A.N. (1966) Science 152:791-793
2. Delorme, A.C. , Marche, P. and Garel, J.M. (1979) J. Develop. Physiol. 1:181-194.
3. Taylor, A.N. (1981) J. Histochem. Cytochem. 29:65-73.
4. Delorme, A.C. , Cassier, P. , Geny, B. and Mathieu, H. (1983) Placenta 4:263-270.
5. Schreiner, D.S. , Jande, S.S. , Parkes, C.O. , Lawson, D.E.M. and Thomasset, M. (1983) Acta Anat. 117:1-14.
6. Taylor, A.N. (1983) In : Calcium-binding proteins, B. de Bernard and al. ed. Elsevier Science Publishers B.V., 207-213.

DEVELOPMENT AND CHARACTERIZATION OF MONOCLONAL ANTIBODIES TO THE VITAMIN D-DEPENDENT CHICK INTESTINAL CALCIUM BINDING PROTEIN.

B. E. MILLER and A. W. NORMAN
Dept. Biochem., Univ. Calif., Riverside, CA 92521, USA.

Introduction: The first reported vitamin D_3-inducible protein was the 28,000-Dalton calcium binding protein isolated from the chick intestine (1). Since then, vitamin D_3-dependent CaBPs have been isolated from a variety of chick tissues, as well as from species other than the chick (2). While the chick intestinal CaBP has been extensively characterized, little is currently known regarding its function. Nor has the structural similarities between the vitamin D_3-dependent CaBPs isolated from various chick tissues, as well as from different species, been examined. To facilitate such studies we have prepared monoclonal antibodies (MAb) against the 28,000 dalton chick intestinal calcium binding protein.

Methods: Spleen cells from a non-immunized BALB/c mouse were *in vitro* immunized with 4.5 µg purified chick intestinal CaBP (3). These spleen cells were then fused (4) with mouse plasmacytoma cell line MPC11 45.6TG1.7 using 35% polyethylene glycol 4000, 5% DMSO. The fused cells were grown over a macrophage feeder layer, and were maintained as described by Fazekas De St. Groth and Scheidegger (5). Hybridoma colonies were assayed for antibody production by a solid phase radioimmunoassay, a modification of our ELISA technique for the chick intestinal CaBP (6). In this solid phase radioimmunoassay, antibodies to the chick intestinal CaBP are detected by the addition of a goat antimouse immunoglobulin antibody to which [^{125}I] has been coupled. Those colonies screening positive for the production of antibodies against chick intestinal CaBP were subsequently cloned twice by limiting dilution to obtain MAb. These MAb were then classified with respect to immunoglobulin subclass, and epitope and antigen specificities. The immunoglobulin class determination was achieved using a commercially available identification kit. Epitope specificity was determined by biosynthetically labeling the MAb with [^{75}Se]-methionine. These labeled MAb were then competed with nonradioactively labeled MAb for binding to chick intestinal CaBP. The antigen specificity of these MAb was examined using our solid phase radioimmunoassay technique. The antigens screened included purified vitamin D-dependent CaBPs from the chick, bovine, baboon, and rat intestines, bovine brain calmodulin, bovine and human serum albumin, ovalbumin, and *E. coli* alkaline phosphatase.

Results and Discussion: Fifty-three hybridomas were obtained which produced MAb specific for the vitamin D-dependent chick intestinal CaBP. Eight of these MAb were randomly selected for characterization. Classification of these MAb with respect to immunoglobulin subtype revealed that all eight are immunoglobulin M. Seven of these MAb were observed to inhibit binding to chick intestinal CaBP by each of the other MAb, suggesting that these antibodies are recognizing the same epitope. However, in view of the differing antigen specificities displayed by these antibodies, this is not likely. Alternatively the binding of one MAb may sterically inhibit the binding of the second MAb, suggesting adjacent epitopes are being recognized. The antigen specificity studies

Vitamin D. A Chemical, Biochemical and Clinical Update

revealed that three MAb (2049, 2052, and 2056) were highly specific for the chick intestinal CaBP; while four of the MAb (2013, 2019, 2023, and 2037) recognized, to varying extents, the vitamin D-dependent intestinal CaBP from the cow, rat and baboon, and calmodulin. This suggests that these MAb are recognizing complex epitopes, portions of which are present on the four other CaBPs examined. One of these five MAb (2037) highly cross-reacted with the vitamin D-dependent CaBP from rat intestine (87% of its reactivity with chick CaBP) and to a lesser extent (64% of its reactivity with chick CaBP) to baboon CaBP. Apparently the epitope being recognized by this MAb is highly conserved in the vitamin D-dependent intestinal CaBPs from chick, rat, and baboon. Finally four of the MAb (2013, 2019, 2037, 2046) cross-reacted with alkaline phosphatase. However, the physiological and biochemical significance of this interaction is unclear.

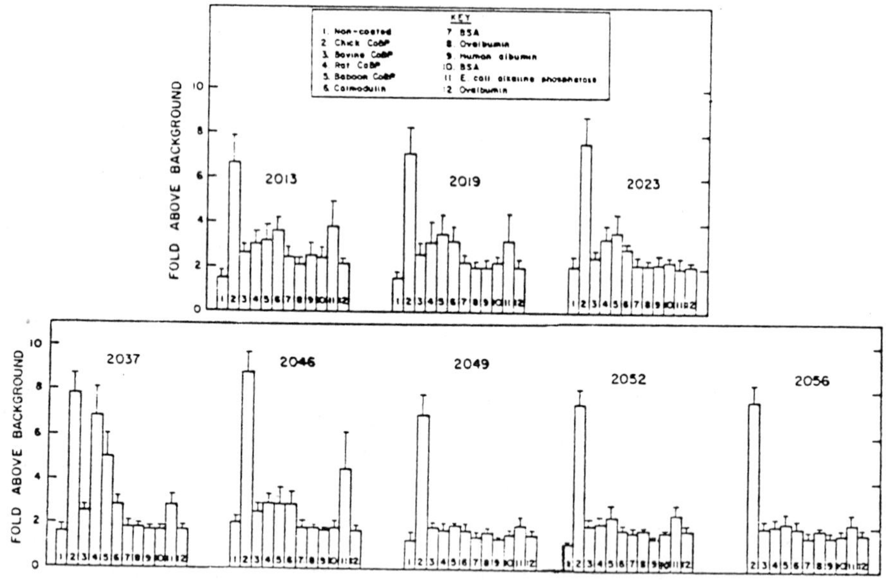

Fig. 1. Antigen Specificity of MAb to Chick Intestinal CaBP.

References:

1. Taylor, A. N., and Wasserman, R. H. (1965) Nature (London) 205, 248-250.
2. Henry, H. L., and Norman, A. W. (1984) Ann. Rev. Nutr. 4, 493-520.
3. Luben, R. A. and Mohler, M. A. (1980) Mol. Immol. 17, 635-639.
4. Luben, R. A., Mohler, M. A., and Nedwin, G. E. (1979) J. Clin. Invest. 64, 337-341.
5. Frazekas De St. Groth, S., and Scheidegger, D. (1980) J. Immunol. Meth. 35, 1-21.
6. Miller, B. E., and Norman, A. W. (1983) Methods in Enzymology: Hormone Action, Academic Press, NY. 102, 291-296.

PROTEIN SYNTHESIS INHIBITORS BUT NOT TRANSCRIPTION INHIBITORS BLOCK $1,25(OH)_2D_3$-INDUCED CaBP and $CaBP_{28K}$-mRNA EXPRESSION IN CHICK INTESTINE.

G. Theofan and A. W. Norman, Dept. Biochem., University of California, Riverside, CA 92521, USA.

Introduction: Calcium binding protein (CaBP) is induced in the chick intestine by the action of $1,25(OH)_2D_3$ via receptor-mediated induction of transcription of the CaBP gene. We have previously demonstrated that administration of 6.5 nmoles of $1,25(OH)_2D_3$ to vitamin D-replete chicks results in an increase in intestinal CaBP-mRNA levels 5 hrs later. The present study was undertaken to determine the short-term effects of $1,25(OH)_2D_3$ administration in vitamin D-replete chicks maintained on diets containing varying amounts of Ca and P, with or without pretreatment with α-amanitin or cycloheximide.

Methods: Two week old white leghorn cockerels were placed on one of 4 vitamin D-replete diets for 2 additional weeks: normal Ca and normal P, high Ca and normal P, low calcium and normal P or normal Ca and low P. Chicks were divided into 3 groups; the control group received no inhibitor, one group was dosed i.m. with 20 µg of α-amanitin, and the third group was dosed i.m. with 600 µg of cycloheximide. These doses of the inhibitors were shown in preliminary experiments to inhibit by 85%-95% $[^3H]$uridine incorporation into RNA or $[^3H]$leucine incorporation into protein, respectively. Two hrs after inhibitor treatment, all chicks were dosed i.m. with 6.5 nmoles of $1,25(OH)_2D_3$. Duodenal mucosa was collected from 5 chicks/time point at 0, 15, 30, 60 and 120 min. Total RNA was isolated and analyzed by dot blot hydridization, and CaBP levels were quantitated by ELISA assay.

Results and Discussion: Altering the dietary Ca and P levels had no effect on the steady state level of CaBP-mRNA in chick intestine [compared to CaBP-mRNA levels in chicks maintained on normal Ca and P diets (□)] (Fig. 1), while CaBP levels were affected by the dietary changes in a manner similar to that described previously by this laboratory (1). That is, low Ca and low P diets resulted in elevated levels of CaBP, while high Ca decreased intestinal CaBP levels (compared to the normal Ca, normal P group) (Fig. 2). These results indicate that regulation of CaBP by Ca and P occurs at a post-transcriptional level, i.e., without affecting rate of transcription of the CaBP gene. Varying Ca and/or P levels may regulate CaBP itself in a number of ways; for example, there may be an effect on the stability or half-life of CaBP, or possibly an effect on the efficiency of translation of CaBP-mRNA. There is evidence for the involvement of $1,25(OH)_2D_3$ in the initiation of polypeptide synthesis in chick intestine (2). Altered Ca and P levels may affect this interaction directly or by modulating levels of $1,25(OH)_2D_3$. Fig. 1 shows that α-amanitin had no effect on chick intestinal CaBP-mRNA levels irrespective of dietary Ca and P levels. CaBP levels were partially inhibited by α-amanitin in chicks maintained on the normal Ca and P diet, but were unaffected in the other 3 dietary conditions (Fig. 2). This indicates that CaBP-mRNA is stable for at least 4 hrs. Cycloheximide significantly inhibited CaBP (Fig. 2) as well as CaBP-mRNA (Fig. 1) in all 4 dietary groups. This indicates that $1,25(OH)_2D_3$-induced expression of CaBP-mRNA is dependent on ongoing protein synthesis of a rapidly turned-over protein. This protein may function as an RNA processing

Vitamin D. A Chemical, Biochemical and Clinical Update

factor that allows production of stable transcripts. This may occur by several possible mechanisms: (a) the protein may stabilize CaBP-mRNA transcripts by binding directly to them; (b) it may be a processing protein that is required for maturation of the primary transcripts; (c) the protein may inhibit a nuclease which specifically breaks down CaBP-mRNA. The existence of such a protein would also allow for tissue-specific processing of transcripts from the same gene. There is evidence from other steroid-regulated systems for the existence of such a processing protein, based on the necessity of continual protein synthesis for production/accumulation of specific transcripts (3,4,5).

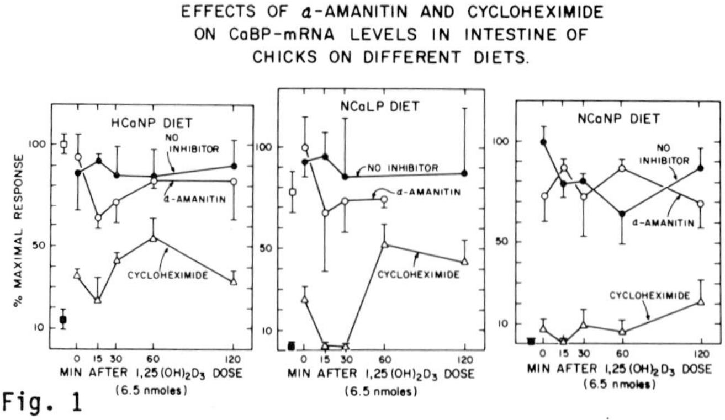

Fig. 1

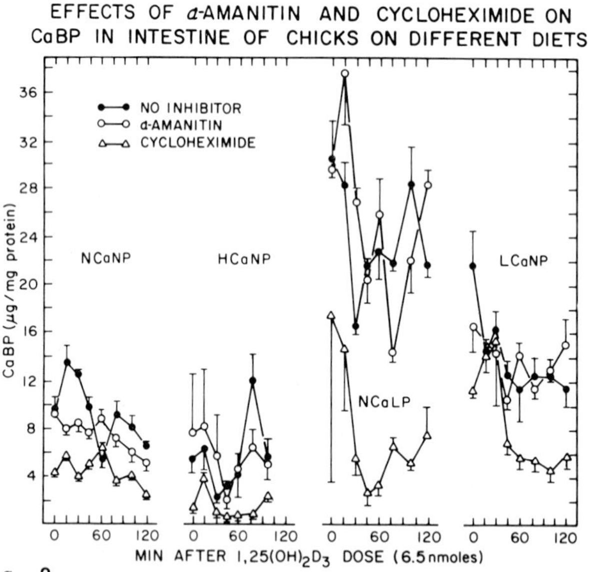

Fig. 2

References:

1. Friedlander, E.J., Henry, H.L., and Norman, A.W. (1977) J. Biol. Chem. 252, 8677-8683.
2. Mezzetti, G., Moruzzi, M., and Barbiroli, B. (1984) Biochem. J. 219, 99-106.
3. Vannice, J.L., Taylor, J.M., and Ringold, G.M. (1984) Proc. Natl. Acad. Sci. 81, 4241-4245.
4. Baumann, H., Firestone, G.L., Burgess, T.L., Gross, K.W., Yamamoto, K.R., and Held, W.A. (1983) J. Biol. Chem. 258, 563-570.
5. McKnight, G.S. (1978) Cell 14, 403-413.

PRESENCE OF A CALCIUM BINDING PROTEIN (N-CaBP) IN NECTURUS KIDNEY.

M.RIZK, M.BOUTHIER, A.EDELMAN, F.MOUNIER, T.ANAGNOSTOPOULOS and S.BALSAN.
INSERM U.30-CNRS UA.583 et INSERM U.192, Hôpital des Enfants-Malades, 75015 PARIS, FRANCE.

INTRODUCTION

Calcium binding proteins (CaBP) with a molecular weight of 28,000 have been localized in the mammalian (1), avian (2), and reptile kidney (3). The expression of such proteins, in amphibia a transitional stage from fish to reptile has not been reported. The present study was initiated in order to assess whether CaBP is present in Necturus kidney (Necturus maculosus) a common model for ion transport studies.

MATERIAL AND METHODS

Animals : Five adult Necturi were utilized. Their kidneys were perfused 10 min with a physiologic Ringer's solution to wash out the blood, then the kidneys were removed and weighted. Homogenization was performed in cold water using a motor-driven potter homogener. The homogenate was centrifuged at 100,000 g for 60 min, and the pellet reextracted again. Clear supernatants were combined and lyophilized.

Detection and purification: Cytosolic proteins were dissolved in 2.5 ml of a 20 mM ammonium acetate buffer solution, pH=8.0 and fractionated on Sephacryl S200 column (2.5x85cm), previously equilibrated with protein markers to estimate the molecular weight of the eluted proteins. Fractions were collected,analyzed for their calcium binding activity using Chelex resin assay, and separated by sodium dodecyl (SDS)-polyacrylamide slab gel electrophoresis (10%-polyacrylamide slab gel electrophoresis).

Fractions presenting high calcium binding activity were lyophilized. Further purification of the CaBP fractions were obtained using DEAE-SEPHADEX A-25 ion exchange chromatography in a buffer containing 0.02M imidazole,0.02M NaCl, 0.001 M EDTA, pH=7.4,and a linear 0.02-0.7M NaCl gradient. Final purification and desalting was carried out by filtration of obtained pooled protein peaks, on Sephacryl S200 column equilibrated with 20 mM ammonium acetate buffer pH=8.0. Fractions were collected and analyzed as above. The N-CaBP peak was lyophilized.

Vitamin D. A Chemical, Biochemical and Clinical Update

Antiserum obtention : Antiserum to purified N-CaBP was raised in rabbit. The presence of anti N-CaBP, its specificity, and cross reactivity were tested using Ouchterlony's double immunodiffusion technique and ELISA assay. For immunohistochemical localization, 5 µm sections of kidneys were tested for indirect immunoperoxidase technique.

RESULTS

When the 100,000 g supernatant of Necturus kidney homogenate was chromatographed on Sephacryl S200 and the calcium activity of the different fractions analyzed, 2 peaks were observed. Peak I appeared at the void volume, and peak II appeared in the molecular weight 14,000 region. After ion exchange chromatography the N-CaBP from peak II was eluted in the higher anionic form at 0.3M NaCl. After final filtration and desalting on Sephacryl S200 column, the electrophoretic pattern of the pooled fraction with a calcium binding protein activity, showed a single protein band with a molecular weight estimated to 14,000±2,000 Da. The specificity of the rabbit antiserum was shown by a single precipitation line in Ouchterlony's double immunodiffusion technique, when the kidney extract and purified N-CaBP were reacted with this antiserum. Rat intestinal, renal and skin CaBP did not cross react with the antiserum to N-CaBP. Immunohistology on Necturus kidney sections with this N-CaBP antiserum gave strong irregular cytoplasmic staining in distal and collecting tubular cells.

CONCLUSIONS

1) A novel kidney CaBP has been purified from Necturus kidney. 2) The molecular weight of this N-CaBP is close to 14.0 ± 0.2 Kd. 3) N-CaBP is immunologically different from rat intestine, kidney and skin CaBP proteins. 4) This N-CaBP seems to be localized mainly in distal tubular cells.

REFERENCES :

1. Rhoten, W.B., and Chirstakos, C. (1981) Endocrinology. 109, 981-983.

2. Christakos, S., Brunette, M.G., and Norman A.W. (1981) Endocrinology. 109, 322-324.

3. Rhoten, W.B., Lubit, B., and Christakos, S. (1984) Gen. Comp. Endocrinol. 55, 96-103.

THE CRYPT-VILLUS DISTRIBUTION OF CALCIUM BINDING PROTEIN IN BIOPSIES OF HUMAN JEJUNUM MEASURED BY AN ENZYME-LINKED IMMUNO-ADSORBENT ASSAY.

Michael Staun, Medical Department P, Division of Gastroenterology, Rigshospitalet and Biochemical Department C, The Panum Institute, University of Copenhagen, Denmark.

Introduction

The transepithelial calcium transport in the proximal part of the small intestine is an important process in the calcium homeostasis. A cytosolic calcium binding protein (CaBP) regulated by 1,25 dihydroxycholecalciferol and expressed in the epithelial cells is considered to play a significant role in the calcium absorption. CaBP was first discovered in the small intestine of the chick and has later been studied in mammalian species. We have purified a 10 kDa CaBP from human small intestine. Very little is known about human intestinal CaBP as no method to measure this protein specifically has been available. An enzyme-linked immunoadsorbent assay (ELISA)was therefore established. The method is applicable to measure CaBP in small intestinal biopsies and thus allows studies concerning distribution, physiological and clinical significance of human intestinal CaBP.

The differentiation of mitotically active intestinal epithelial crypt cells to active absorptive cells takes place as the cells migrate up the villus. Information about the distribution of CaBP along the villus-crypt axis may thus lead to a better understanding of the role of CaBP in the intestinal calcium absorption.

Methods

A piece of proximal jejunum was obtained from a necro-kidney donor 25 minutes after the patient died. Biopsies of 6 mm in diameter were punched out (at 4°C) and frozen to a chryostat chuck by using solid CO_2. The edge of the biopsies were trimmed with a scalpel and then cutted with a cryostat at -20°C in 8 µm thick slices (about 90 slices per biopsy). To verify that biopsies were cut perpendicular to the villus crypt axis and to estimate the distribution of villi, crypts and connective tissue every tenth slice was stained and immediately inspected in a stereo microscope. Intermediate slices were pooled with corresponding slices from other biopsies. The tissue was then homogenized at 4°C in 40 µl of 0.9% NaCl containing 0.1 mM PMSF, 2.8 µg/ml of aprotinin and 1% Triton X-100. After an incubation period of 15 min the homogenate was centrifuged at 40°C for 45 min at 50000 g and the supernatant was analysed by using a competitive ELISA. Polystyrene microtestplates were coated with purified CaBP (80 ng). Standard amounts of CaBP (5-50 ng) or test samples then compete for binding a limiting amount of a rabbit anti-CaBP antibody. The amount of antibody attached to the solid-phase antigen is quantitated using a peroxidase-labeled second antibody. The assay measures

Vitamin D. A Chemical, Biochemical and Clinical Update

CaBP in the range 5-50 ng (in 150 µl) and has an interassay variation coefficient of 9.6%. For comparison alkaline phosphatase activity was determined with p-nitrophenylphosphate as substrate and aminopeptidase N was measured using alanine p-nitroalanilide as substrate. Protein was determined using a Bio Rad kit with bovine serum albumin as standard.

Results and discussion

The results obtained by analysis of the sectioned biopsies are shown in Table I. The microscopic inspection of every tenth slice proved that biopsies were cut horizontally. The amount of CaBP/mg of protein were highest at the villus tip and decreased steeply in the upper villus region. In fractions corresponding to the lower villus region and crypts the decrease in CaBP/mg of protein paralleled the percentage distribution of villi indicating that very low amounts of CaBP were present in the crypt cells. The amount of CaBP correlated well with the amount of alkaline phosphatase and aminopeptidase with the exception that specific activity of both enzymes had maximum in fractions corresponding to the upper villus region. The present study demonstrates that human small intestinal CaBP has a distribution very similar to two brush border enzymes present in the highest amount in the most differentiated cells. These are also likely to be the most active in calcium absorption and thus the present study supports a role of CaBP in this process.

Table I. Crypt-villus distribution of marker enzyme activities and CaBP in tangentially sectioned biopsies of human jejunum. The relative percentage distribution between villi, crypts and connective tissue in the microscopic sections is also indicated.

Fraction no.		Villi	Crypts	Connec. tissue	CaBP µg/mg protein	Alkaline phosphatase activity U/mg protein	Aminopeptidase Activity U/mg protein
		% of total area					
Villus	1	00	0	0	7.3	302	125
	2	100	0	0	4.3	503	158
	3	100	0	0	3.5	289	82
	4	95	5	0	3.4	245	101
	5	90	10	0	2.5	237	85
	6	47	45	5	2.2	211	40
↓	7	33	51	20	2.0	107	22
Crypt	8	12	42	50	1.3	84	8
	9	2	21	80	0.4	85	0

25-OH-D_3 INHIBITS CALMODULIN-ACTIVATED PHOSPHODIESTERASE

H. Van Baelen, H. Van Belle, F. Wuytack and R. Bouillon
Laboratorium voor Experimentele Geneeskunde en Endocrinologie, Gasthuisberg, B-3000 Leuven and Laboratory of Biochemistry, Janssen Pharmaceutica, B-2304 Beerse, Belgium.

Recently, a high affinity binding between calmodulin (CAL) and 25-OH-D_3 has been described by Reddy and Johnson (1). In their study these authors followed the fluorescence increase produced by vitamin D analogs in dansylchloride labeled CAL. Whether this new CAL interaction influences its biological activity was not investigated. Therefore, we examined seven vitamin D analogs and four classical steroids at two different concentrations for their ability to inhibit CAL-activated phosphodiesterase (PDE). The source of CAL and PDE as well as the experimental assay conditions have been described in detail by Van Belle (2). As shown in the table only 24,25-$(OH)_2$-D_3, 25,26-$(OH)_2$-D_3 and 25-OH-D_3 emerge as potent inhibitors at a concentration of 5 μM. At a concentration of 0.5 μM the inhibition produced by 25-OH-D_3 is only slightly decreased whereas a pronounced decrease is observed for 24,25-$(OH)_2$-D_3 and to a lesser extent for 25,26-$(OH)_2$-D_3. None of the vitamin D analogs (at 0.5 μM) and steroids (at 5 μM) inhibited the PDE activity in the absence of CAL.

PERCENTAGE INHIBITION OF CALMODULIN-ACTIVATED PHOSPHODIESTERASE

Inhibitor concentration	5 μM	0.5 μM
vitamin D_2	0	3.9
vitamin D_3	5.4	1.0
25-OH-D_3	60.4	55.2
1,25-$(OH)_2$-D_3	35.6	2.6
24,25-$(OH)_2$-D_3	78.6	4.6
25,26-$(OH)_2$-D_3	77.2	21.0
1,24,25-$(OH)_3$-D_3	5.7	2.6
estradiol	7.7	N.D.
testosterone	2.3	N.D.
progesterone	4.1	N.D.
cortisol	1.8	N.D.

N.D. = not determined

The dose response curve for 25-OH-D_3 (Fig. 1,△) shows that this compound is unable to completely inhibit CAL-activated PDE. A maximal inhibition of about 80% was obtained routinely. The concentration for 50% inhibition was 0.26 μM. There was no influence of 25-OH-D_3 on the basal activity of PDE at every concentration investigated. A similar dose response curve was obtained when 25-OH-D_3 was preincubated for 15 minutes in the reaction vessel before addition of CAL and PDE. For compound R24571 which is the most potent inhibitor known up till now complete inhibition could be achieved and the concentration for 50% inhibition was 10 nM (Fig. 1,O). The presence of 0.8 μM human vitamin

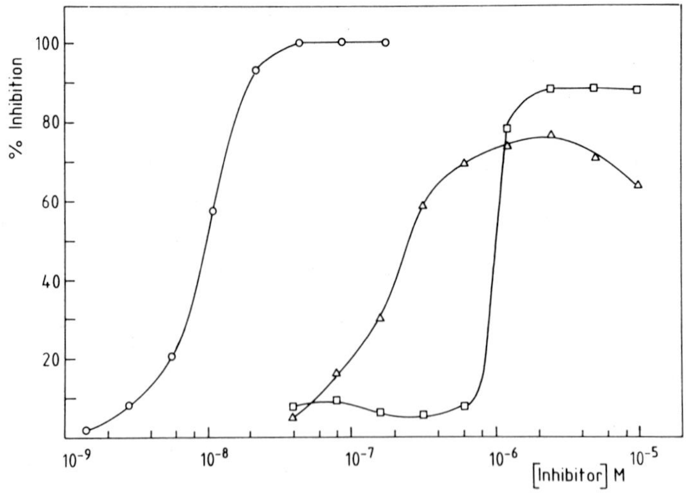

Fig. 1. Dose response curves for compound R24571 (○), for 25-OH-D_3 (△) and for 25-OH-D_3 in the presence of 0.8 μM DBP (□) on phosphodiesterase activated with 6 nM calmodulin.

D-binding protein (DBP) in the assay system results in a completely different dose response curve (Fig. 1,□). At 25-OH-D_3 concentrations below the DBP concentration the inhibitory effect of 25-OH-D_3 is almost completely abolished. At concentrations exceeding the DBP concentration the inhibition increases sharply to reach a maximal value of about 90%. Similar dose response curves were obtained after preincubating 25-OH-D_3 for 15 minutes with DBP or with CAL before addition of the other substances of the assay. The addition of DBP had no influence neither on the basal activity of PDE nor on the dose response curves for CAL and R24571. Sucrose gradient ultracentrifugation experiments of mixtures of CAL and DBP preincubated with tritium labeled 25-OH-D_3 reveal that the affinity of 25-OH-D_3 for CAL is at least 100 times lower than for DBP. We conclude that CAL is a specific intracellular binding protein with low affinity for 25-OH-D_3 and that this new CAL interaction influences its biological activity. Whether 25-OH-D_3 could reach intracellular levels high enough to modulate CAL activity in vivo remains hypothetical.

(1) Reddy, G.S. and Johnson, J.D., VIII Int. Conf. on Calcium Regulating Hormones, abstract P-4, Workshop Tokyo, Japan, Oct. 1983.
(2) Van Belle, H. (1981) Cell Calcium 2, 483-494.

VISUALIZATION OF VITAMIN D-DEPENDENT CALCIUM-BINDING PROTEIN (CaBP 28-kDa CHOLECALCIN) IN RAT EPIPHYSEAL CARTILAGE.

N. Balmain, A. Brehier, P. Cuisinier-Gleizes and H. Mathieu
INSERM U.120, 44 Chemin de Ronde - 78110 Le Vésinet, France.

INTRODUCTION

The calcium binding protein (CaBP), cholecalcin, which is considered to be a molecular expression of the action of $1,25(OH)_2D_3$, was first found in chick duodenal mucosa by Wasserman and Taylor (1) and has now been detected in numerous other organs and tissues (2). 28-kDa CaBP has been demonstrated immunohistochemically in the soft tissues of a number of species and recent reports have shown its presence in ameloblasts (3,4) and calcified cartilage (4). We now report the localization of 28-kDa in rat epiphyseal cartilage using a specific rabbit antiserum to rat renal CaBP (5).

MATERIAL AND METHODS

Tibial epiphyseal cartilages from 21 day-old female Sprague Dawley rats were dissected on ice, fixed in Carnoy's solution at 4°C, washed with PBS-0.5% BSA and frozen in CO_2. Cryosections were incubated with diluted antiserum (1:10 - 1:80) followed with peroxidase-conjugated protein A. Controls included non immune rabbit serum,protein A-peroxidase complex alone, specific antiserum followed by non-labeled protein A and protein A-peroxidase.

RESULTS

Brown staining specific for 28-kDa CaBP was found in the nuclei of the chondrocytes. These was no specific staining in the cytoplasm (fig. 1 and 3).

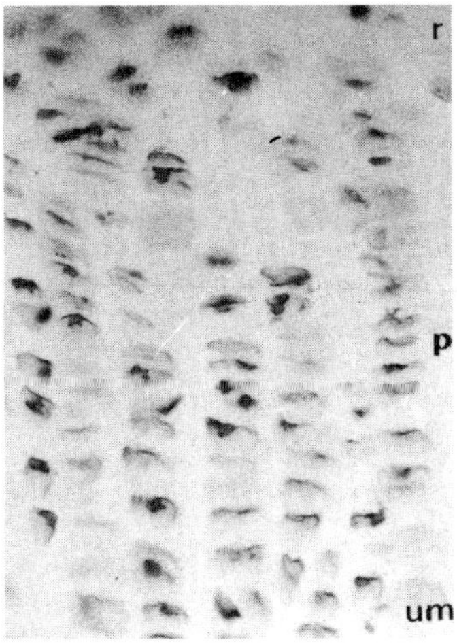

Fig.1.Immunocytochemical localization of 28-kDa CaBP in epiphyseal cartilage

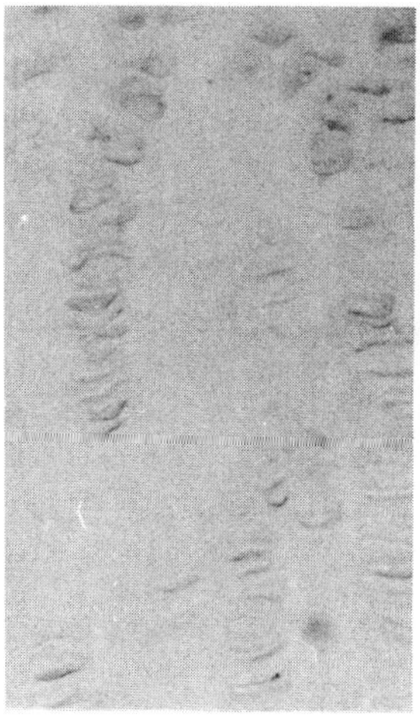

Fig.2.Immunocontrol : non immune rabbit serum.

Resting zone (r), proliferative zone (p) upper maturing zone (um). X420

Vitamin D. A Chemical, Biochemical and Clinical Update

Immunoreactive material was not uniformly distributed throughout the epiphyseal cartilage, but was restricted to the chondrocytes of the resting zone, the proliferative zone and the upper maturing zone (fig. 1 and 3). No staining for 28-kDa CaBP was detected in the chondrocytes of the hypertrophic zone (fig. 4). All the controls were negative.

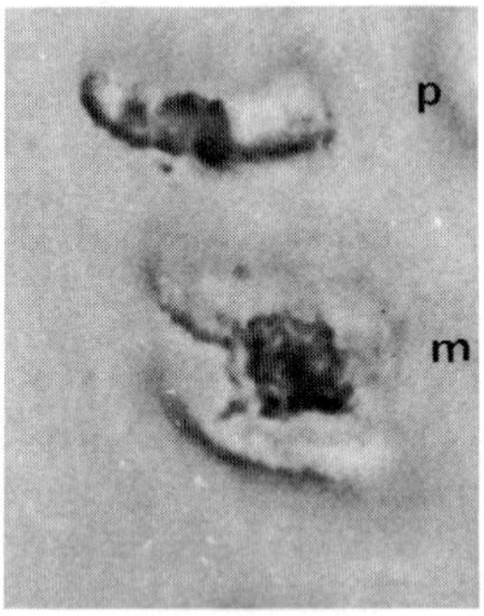

Fig. 3. Proliferative (p) and maturing (m) chondrocytes : X 1,700
Positive nuclei.

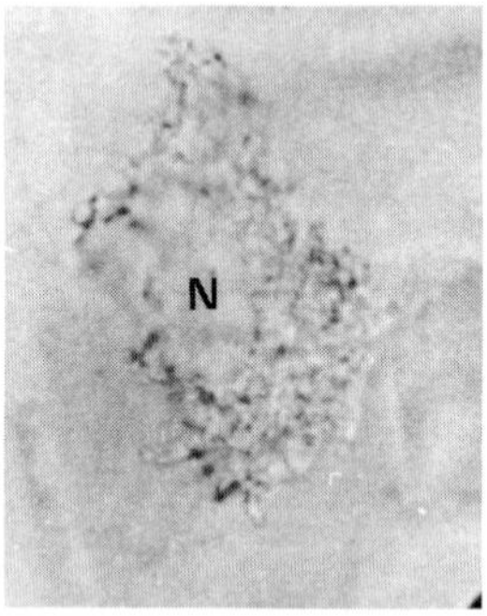

Fig.4. Hypertrophic chondrocyte : X 1,700
Unstained nucleus (N).

CONCLUSIONS

The data show the exclusive intranuclear localization of 28-kDa CaBP in chondrocytes implicated in proliferative activity. These findings raise the possibility that 28-kDa CaBP may be involved in mitotic activity in which intranuclear calcium is known to be implied, acting in the regulation of the proliferation process via intranuclear calcium. Furthermore, the localization of 28-kDa CaBP, which is different from that of 9-kDa CaBP (see preceeding manuscript) suggests a specific role for each protein in the epiphyseal cartilage.

REFERENCES

1. Wasserman, R.H. , Taylor, A.N. (1966) Science 152:791-793
2. Thomasset, M. , Parkes, C.O. and Cuisinier-Gleizes, P. (1982) Am. J. Physiol. 243:E483-E488.
3. Taylor, A.N. (1984) J. Histochem. Cytochem. 32:159-164
4. Celio, M.R. , Norman, A.W. and Heizmann, C.W. (1984) Calcif. Tissue Int. 36:129-130
5. Brehier, A. , Elion, J. and Thomasset, M. (1983) Calcium Binding Proteins in Health and disease. De Bernard et al. Elsevier Science, 389-390.

Intestinal
Ca and P Transport

RAPID CHANGES IN ENTEROCYTE MEMBRANE PHOSPHOLIPID CONTENT AND ION TRANSPORT INDUCED BY 1,25 DIHYDROXYVITAMIN D3 (CALCITRIOL)

T. Drüeke, B. Lacour, P.A. Lucas, G. Karsenty, F. Mauriat, INSERM U90, Hôpital Necker, Paris, France

Several recent reports suggest that calcitriol exerts an early direct effect on epithelial cell membranes in addition to its well established genomic effect. In the intestine, calcitriol has been shown to increase Ca (1-3) and inorganic phosphate (Pi) (4-6) transport as well as to stimulate CAMP levels (7) and alkaline phosphatase activity (8) within 30 min of its addition to the incubation medium. Such rapid effects may occur independently of de novo protein synthesis.

The purpose of the present study was to investigate whether the in vitro incubation of isolated enterocytes with calcitriol could alter the kinetics of Ca uptake and the phospholipid composition of the intestinal epithelium.

Non fasted normal male Wistar rats weighing 100-180 g were used. They were fed the standard lab. diet. Enterocytes were obtained as previously described (5). The working buffer was of the following composition (mM) : NaCl, 120 ; Tris, 20 ; $MgCl_2$, 1.0 ; $CaCl_2$, 1.0 ; glucose, 10 ; K_2HPO_4, 3.0. It contained 1 g/l BSA ; pH was 7.4 ± 0.1. Ca uptake was performed as previously described for Pi (5) except that 10 µCi 45-$CaCl_2$ were added and the influx velocity of Ca (iVCa) was determined between 1 and 30 min by linear regression. In these experiments isolated cells were obtained by collagenase digestion rather than mechanical vibration. Calcitriol (100 pM) or its vehicle solution (ethanol 0.2 %) was added to the incubation milieu 20 min prior to uptake or phospholipid studies. The membrane phospholipids, phosphatidyl choline (PC) and phosphatidyl ethanolamine (PE) were determined either in whole cell or brush border membrane (BBM) lipid extracts using thin layer chromatography and subsequent phosphorus measurement.

The addition of calcitriol (100 pM) to the incubation medium during 20 min led to a significant increase in iVCa of rat enterocytes when compared to control experiments : 1.27 ± 0.24 SEM versus 0.86 ± 0.17 (control) nmol/min.mg protein, n=9, $p < 0.02$, Student's paired t test. When repeating the study we found a similar increase though absolute iVCa's were lower : 0.31 ± 0.07 versus 0.28 ± 0.06 nmol/min.mg prot., n=7, $p < 0.02$. The difference between the two series or experiments could be due to the different batches of collagenase used. When replacing NaCl of the incubation medium by isomolar amounts of choline Cl, calcitriol (100 pM) still exerted its rapid enhancing effect on enterocyte iVCa : 83.3 ± 10.6 versus 76.5 ± 10.9 pmol/min.mg prot., n=6, $p < 0.05$. It must be noted that absolute Ca transport rates were markedly lower when Na was replaced by choline.

Whole enterocyte membrane phospholipids were also significantly modified after calcitriol (100 pM) addition. Thus, the PC/PE ratio increased from 0.98 ± 0.18 (control) to 1.16 ± 0.15 (calcitriol) (n=8, $p < 0.05$). Similarly, the phospholipid ratio of BBM increased markedly from 1.38 ± 0.12 to 2.67 ± 0.55 (n=4).

Vitamin D. A Chemical, Biochemical and Clinical Update

The early in vitro effects of calcitriol on enterocyte Ca transport observed in these experiments as well as the hormone's effect on enterocyte Pi transport previously reported by our group (5,6) favour an action at the membrane level, independent of de novo protein synthesis. The concomitant changes in brush border membrane phospholipid composition induced by calcitriol suggest that these events are somehow interrelated. Whether such changes reflect a liponomic type of action secondary to an increase in membrane "fluidity" as suggested by Rasmussen et al (9) remains highly controversial (10). Clarification of this issue requires further investigation.

REFERENCES

1. Nemere,I., Yoshimoto,Y. and Norman, A.W. (1984) Endocrinology 115 : 1476-1483

2. Nemere, I. and Szego, C.M. (1981) Endocrinology 108 : 1450-1462

3. MacLaughlin, J.A., Weiser, M.M. and Freedman, R.A. (1980) Gastroenterology 78 : 325-332

4. Birge, S.J. and Miller, R. (1977) J. Clin. Invest. 60 : 980-988

5. Karsenty, G., Lacour, B., Ulmann, A., Pierandreï, E. and Drüeke, T. (1985) Am. J. Physiol. 248 : G40-G45

6. Karsenty, G., Lacour, B., Ulmann, A., Pierandreï, E. and Drüeke, T. (1985) Pflügers Arch. 403 : 151-155

7. Corradino, R.A. (1978) J. Steroid Biochem. 9 : 1183-1187

8. Bachelet, M., Ulmann, A. and Lacour, B. (1979) Biochem. Biophys. Res. Comm. 89 : 694-700

9. Rasmussen, H., Matsumoto, T., Fontaine, O. and Goodman, D.B.P. (1982) Fed. Proc. 41 : 72-77

10. Bikle, D.D., Whitney, J. and Munson, S. (1984) Endocrinology 114 : 260-267

MECHANISMS BY WHICH 1,25-DIHYDROXYVITAMIN D REGULATES CALMODULIN BINDING TO THE DUODENAL BRUSH BORDER MEMBRANE.

D.D. Bikle and S.J. Munson,
Department of Medicine, Veterans Administration Medical Center and University of California, San Francisco, Ca., USA

We (1) have recently demonstrated that $1,25(OH)_2D$ administration to vitamin D-deficient chicks results in an increase in the calmodulin (CaM) content of the duodenal brush border membrane (BBM) that parallels in time the stimulation by $1,25(OH)_2D$ of calcium transport in vivo and calcium uptake by purified BBM vesicles (BBMV) in vitro. We have observed that the increased CaM content in BBM can be attributed to the increased ability of certain BBM proteins to bind CaM in a fashion independent of calcium (2). The most prominent of these proteins has a molecular weight of 102 KD. We then evaluated whether $1,25(OH)_2D$ stimulated CaM binding to the 102 KD protein by stimulating synthesis of this protein or by altering its affinity for CaM through a process such as phosphorylation. To this end, we administered 625 pmol $1,25(OH)_2D$ to vitamin D-deficient chicks; 0, 4, 9, 12, 18, and 24 h later, the duodena were incubated in situ with ^{35}S-methionine or $^{32}PO_4$ for 15 min, following which the duodenal mucosae were obtained and BBMV prepared. The BBMV were subjected to SDS-PAGE and analyzed for newly synthesized or phosphorylated proteins by autoradiography. The autoradiograms were scanned by densitometry, and the results were expressed in densitometric units for ^{35}S or $^{32}PO_4$ incorporation into the 102 KD protein as shown below.

Table 1. The effect of $1,25(OH)_2D$ on ^{35}S-methionine or $^{32}PO_4$ incorporation into the 102 KD protein of BBMV.

	Hours after $1,25(OH)_2D_3$					
	0	4	9	12	18	24
^{35}S*	10.7	10.0	16.9	12.5	13.7	12.6
$^{32}PO_4$*	4.0	3.8	5.3	5.3	4.3	3.4

* The results are expressed in arbitrary densitometric units resulting from scans of autoradiograms of SDS-PAGE gels containing samples of BBMV from chick duodena incubated in situ with ^{35}S-methionine or $^{32}PO_4$. Only the results of a band with 102 KD molecular weight are shown.

These results suggest that $1,25(OH)_2D$ may have a modest stimulatory effect on 102 KD CaM-binding protein production which could account for the modest increase in phosphorylation. To test this possibility further, we blocked protein synthesis by administering cycloheximide (or vehicle), 20 µg intraperitoneally every four hours, beginning 1 h before the oral administration of 625 pmol 1,25(OH)$_2$D (or vehicle). Twelve hours after the administration of 1,25(OH)$_2$D, the chicks were killed, the duodena were either incubated with ^{35}S-methionine in situ to measure protein synthesis into BBMV, or were obtained immediately for BBMV preparation to analyze for calcium uptake, alkaline phosphatase, and CaM binding to the 102 KD protein. The results are shown below.

Table 2. The effects of cycloheximide on 1,25(OH)$_2$D-stimulated calcium uptake, alkaline phosphatase activity, protein synthesis, and CaM binding to the 102 KD protein in BBMV.

	Control	1,25(OH)$_2$D	Cyclo	1,25(OH)$_2$D cyclo
Alk Pase*	9.6 ± .3	27.4 ± 2.2	4.0 ± .3	5.6 ± .4
CaU †	7.1 ± .4	10.1 ± .6	7.7 ± .4	10.2 ± .2
^{35}S-Met ‡	7.1	7.8	2.2	<1
^{125}I-CaM §	28.7	78.6	32.5	76.9

* Alkaline phosphatase activity in nmol/min/µg protein.

† Calcium uptake by BBMV in nmol Ca/30 min/mg protein.

‡ ^{35}S-methionine incorporation into the 102 KD protein measured in arbitrary densitometric units from a scan of an autoradiogram of the SDS-PAGE gel containing these BBMV samples.

§ ^{125}I-CaM binding to the 102 KD protein measured in arbitrary densitometric units from a scan of an autoradiogram of the SDS-PAGE gel containing these BBMV samples that was incubated in ^{125}I-CaM according to the technique of Glenney and Weber (3).

These data indicate that although cycloheximide inhibits alkaline phosphatase activity and synthesis of the 102 KD protein, it does not inhibit calcium uptake or CaM binding to the 102 KD protein or block the stimulation by 1,25(OH)$_2$D of these activities.

Our data suggest that $1,25(OH)_2D$ stimulated the ability of BBMV to bind CaM by a mechanism independent of new protein synthesis, and that this mechanism may underlie the ability of $1,25(OH)_2D$ to stimulate calcium movement across the BBM.

References

1. Bikle, D.D., Munson, S., Chafouleas, J. (1984) FEBS Letters 174:30-33.

2. Bikle, D.D., Munson, S., Chafouleas, J. (1984) In: Epithelial Calcium and Phosphate Transport: Molecular and Cellular Aspects (Bronner, F., and Peterlik, M., eds) pp. 193-198, Alan R. Liss, New York.

3. Glenney, J.R., Jr. and Weber, K. (1980) J. Biol. Chem. 255:10551-10554.

INTESTINAL CALCIUM TRANSPORT IN THE SPONTANEOUSLY HYPERTENSIVE RAT: ROLE OF VITAMIN D.

H.P. SCHEDL, D.L. MILLER, R.L. HORST, H.D. WILSON, K. NATARAJAN, T. CONWAY
Veterans Administration Medical Center, Iowa City, IA 52242; National Animal Disease Laboratory, Ames, IA 50010.

Introduction

Plasma membrane functions related to Ca are abnormal in hypertensive diseases. For example, Ca binding to membranes of erythrocytes and adipocytes is decreased and the intracellular Ca pool is increased in adipocytes of the spontaneously hypertensive (SH) rat as compared with the normotensive Wistar-Kyoto (WKy) control. Since aberrations of Ca transport may be etiologic for hypertension, and the SH rat is the most widely studied model of essential hypertension, we measured Ca transport by proximal and distal small intestine in the WKy and SH rat (1). We found Ca transport in SH to be decreased in comparison with the WKy rat and 1,25-dihydroxycholecalciferol [1,25-$(OH)_2D_3$] concentration to be the same in both SH and WKy fed a diet adequate in Ca (1% by wt) and vitamin D (3.3 IU/gm). Since the decreased Ca transport is probably genetically determined and co-segregated with the genes for hypertension in the SH rat, it is possible that this Ca transport defect, if expressed in smooth muscle and nerve, could be etiologic for hypertension. To determine the mechanism of the depression in intestinal Ca transport, we examined the response of Ca transport and the vitamin-D-endocrine axis to Ca-depletion.

Methods

We used male weanling (3 wk old) SH and WKy rats from the colony of the University of Iowa Cardiovascular Center, Iowa City, Iowa. For *in vitro* studies at 5 wk of age, animals were fed either a normal (NCD, 1.2%) or low (LCD, 0.03%) Ca semisynthetic diet, adequate in vitamin D (10 IU/g) for 2 wk. For *in vivo* studies at 12 wk of age, animals were fed Purina Chow (1% Ca) for 7 wk post weaning and then fed NCD or LCD for 2 wk. Animals were randomly allocated for Ca transport studies or blood drawing.

Ca transport was measured *in vitro* in 5 wk old animals using the everted duodenal sac, i.e. the 8 cm of gut just distal to the pylorus. Ca conc. was 0.4 mM with tracer ^{45}Ca and the incubation period was 1 h (1). *In vivo* Ca transport by 12 wk old rats was measured by luminal perfusion of the most proximal 20 cm of intestine just distal to the pylorus and the most distal 20 cm segment just proximal to the cecum (1). The gut was perfused for 1 hr with Ca conc ranging from 0.6 to 13.6 mM containing tracer ^{45}Ca in isotonic saline solution. Blood drawn from the aorta of subgroups of each group of animals was analyzed for 1,25-$(OH)_2D$ (2). Blood pressure was measured by tailcuff manometry.

Results

Fig. 1 shows serosal-to-mucosal (S/M) concentration ratios of ^{45}Ca developed by 5 week old WKy and SH rats taking NCD or LCD. The S/M ratio was lower for SH than WKy rats for both diets. The S/M ratio increased in response to calcium depletion for SH but not WKy.

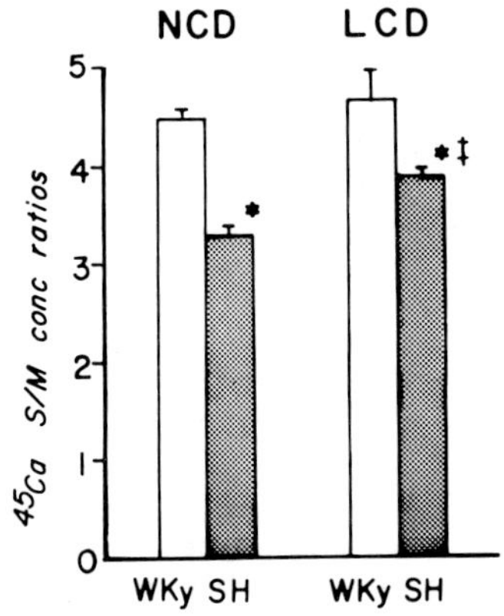

Fig. 1. Effect of Ca depletion on serosal/mucosal (S/M) conc ratio developed by everted duodenal sacs. NCD is normal Ca diet. LCD is low Ca diet. *S/M is lower in SH than WKy, $p < 0.05$. S/M is the same with NCD and LCD in WKy. S/M is greater with LCD than NCD in SH, $p < 0.05$.

In vivo Ca influx (flux of Ca out of the lumen into the animal) is shown in Fig. 2-5. The rate vs conc curves are the best fit to a rectangular hyperbola calculated from K_t and V_{max} values (Table 1) derived from the data points by the method of Lineweaver and Burk (3). Proximal segment data for WKy (Fig. 2) do not show a significant increase with Ca depletion (LCD), whereas the increase with SH (Fig 3) is significant, based on V_{max} values (Table 1). In the distal segment, both WKy (Fig. 4) and SH (Fig. 5) show a significant increase in Ca transport with Ca depletion, based on the increase in V_{max} with LCD.

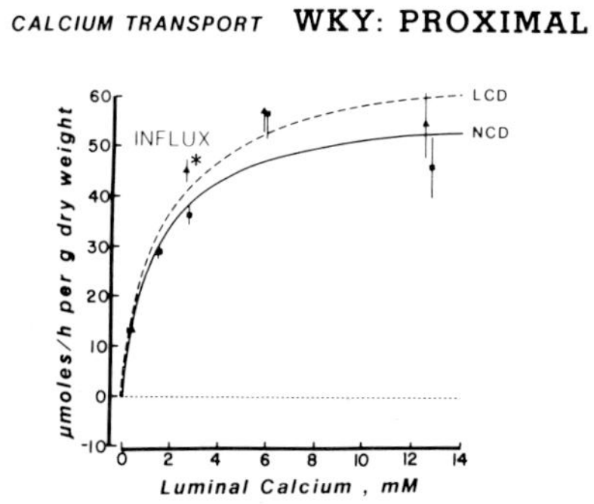

Fig. 2. WKy: Proximal segment. Ca influx in relation to luminal Ca conc. Influx is defined as unidirectional movement of Ca out of the lumen. The small increase in influx with Ca depletion (LCD) does not result in a significant increase in V_{max}. *For Figs. 2-5, designates LCD $>$ NCD, $p < 0.05$.

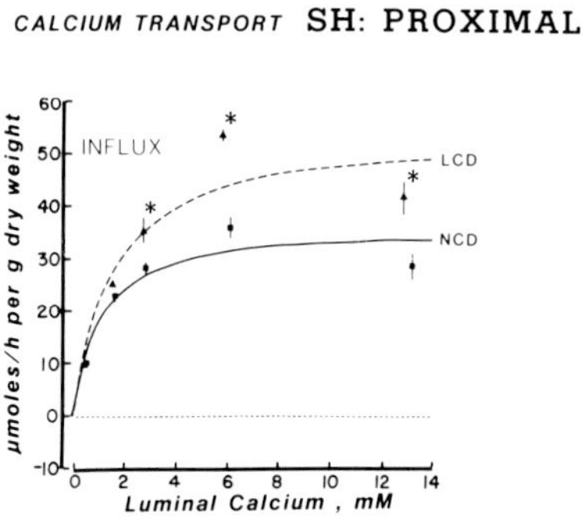

Fig. 3. SH: Proximal segment. Effect of Ca depletion on Ca influx V_{max} for LCD is greater than for NCD, $p < 0.05$. Table 1.

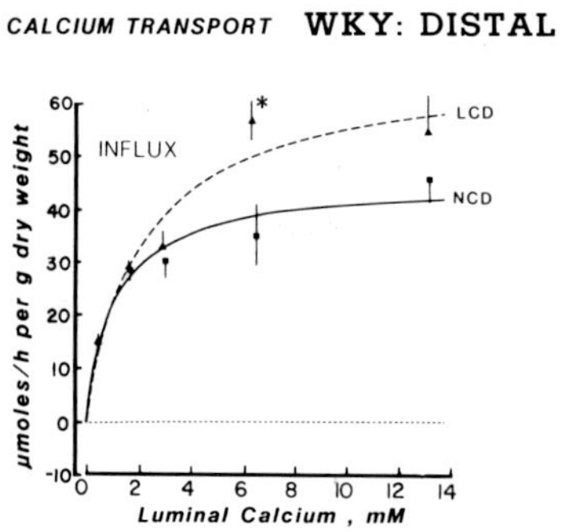

Fig. 4. WKy: Distal segment. Effect of Ca depletion on Ca influx. V_{max} for LCD is greater than for NCD, $p < 0.05$.

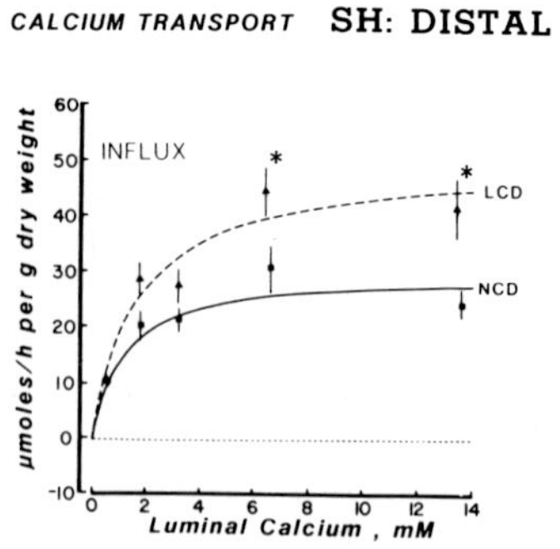

Fig. 5. SH: Distal segment. Effect of Ca depletion on Ca influx. V_{max} for LCD is greater than for NCD, $p < 0.05$.

Kinetic constants for calcium influx are summarized in Table 1. The mean values of V_{max} are lower in SH than WKy for both segments and for both diets. For NCD, V_{max} is significantly lower in both segments of the SH rat. V_{max} increased significantly in response to calcium depletion (LCD) in both segments of the SH rat but only in the distal segment of the WKy rat. All K_t values were similar.

Table 1. Kinetic Constants (Mean ± SE)

	Proximal		Distal	
	WKy	SH	WKy	SH
V_{max}, μmol/h per g:				
NCD	58 ± 7	36 ± 4*	46 ± 4	30 ± 4*
LCD	67 ± 6	55 ± 8†	67 ± 8†	50 ± 5†
K_t, mM:				
NCD	1.4 ± 0.6	0.9 ± 0.4	1.2 ± 0.4	1.0 ± 0.5
LCD	1.6 ± 0.4	1.6 ± 0.8	2.3 ± 0.8	1.7 ± 0.6

* Within a given diet group, SH < WKy; $p < 0.05$
† Within a given rat group, LCD > NCD; $p < 0.05$.

Table 2 shows serum conc of 1,25-$(OH)_2D_3$ in SH and WKy rats taking NCD and LCD at 5 and 12 wk of age. Conc of 1,25-$(OH)_2D_3$ were similar in WKy and SH taking NCD and increased similarly with LCD in both.

Table 2. Serum Concentrations of 1,25-$(OH)_2D_3$ (Mean ± SE)

Age, wk	WKy NCD	WKy LCD	SH NCD	SH LCD
5	95 ± 4	256 ± 22*	87 ± 5	336 ± 22*†
12	218 ± 7	513 ± 47*	166 ± 6†	484 ± 17*

* Within a given rat group, LCD differs from NCD; $p < 0.02$.
† Within a given diet group, SH differs from WKy; $p < 0.05$.

Blood pressure was significantly elevated in SH as compared with WKy under all study conditions and at all time periods.

In summary, in 5 wk old rats, the physiologic stimulus of Ca depletion increased in vitro transport only in SH. Ca transport was lower in the SH than the WKy rat under both basal and stimulated conditions. In 12 week old animals in vivo, V_{max} for Ca transport was lower in the SH than the WKy rat taking NCD. V_{max} increased with LCD in both the proximal and distal segment of the SH rat, but only in the distal segment in the WKy rat. Serum 1,25-$(OH)_2D_3$ increased in response to calcium depletion at both 5 and 12 weeks in both the WKy and SH rat. The SH rat is hypertensive and increases Ca transport in response to increased vitamin D activity. The SH rat remains hypertensive and blood pressure does not change with increased Ca transport. The WKy rat is normotensive, has limited response to increased vitamin D activity, and remains normotensive. Therefore, effects of 1,25-$(OH)_2D_3$ on Ca transport are unrelated to hypertension.

We conclude that 1) intestinal calcium transport is decreased in the SH as compared to the WKy rat; 2) the vitamin-D-endocrine axis is intact in both the SH and WKy rat; 3) the decreased calcium transport in the SH rat is not related to vitamin D and is consistent with a primary transport defect in the enterocyte; 4) although basal calcium transport rate is higher in WKy than SH, responsiveness to the physiologic stimulus of Ca depletion is lower; 5) the lower calcium transport in the enterocyte of SH as compared with the WKy rat could be related to abnormalities of calcium transport in smooth muscle in hypertension.

1. Schedl, H.P., Miller, D.L., Pape, J.M., Horst, R.L. and Wilson, H.D., (1984). J. Clin. Invest., 73, 980-986.
2. Horst, R.L., Littledike, E.T., Riley, J.L. and Napoli, J.L., (1981). Anal. Biochem. 116, 189-203.
3. Lineweaver, H. and Burk D., (1934). J. Am. Chem. Soc. 56, 658-666.

HYPOPHOSPHATAEMIA AND VITAMIN D METABOLISM IN SHEEP

E.M.W. Maunder, A.V. Pillay and A.D. Care
Department of Animal Physiology and Nutrition
University of Leeds, LEEDS LS2 9JT, U.K.

In ruminant animals phosphorus depletion leads to an increased efficiency of intestinal phosphorus absorption (1) but not calcium absorption (2) in contrast to nonruminants where both phosphorus and calcium absorption are increased (3,4). The role of 1,25 dihydroxyvitamin D (1,25$(OH)_2$D) in calcium absorption has been well established in non-ruminant animals (5,6). Plasma 1,25$(OH)_2$ concentrations have been shown to increase following dietary phosphorus depletion in non-ruminants (7). However, preliminary results from this laboratory suggest that this does not occur in ruminants (8). If this is confirmed, this might explain the different responses to hypophosphataemia in terms of calcium absorption in ruminants and non-ruminants. We have therefore investigated the effect of hypophosphataemia on plasma 1,25 dihydroxyvitamin D (1,25$(OH)_2$D) concentrations, metabolic clearance rate (MCR) and production rate (PR) in sheep.

Materials and Methods

Hypophosphataemia was induced in sheep by feeding a low phosphorus (LP) diet (0.07% P compared to 0.3% P in the normal phosphorus (NP) diet; both diets based on sugar beet pulp). The animals were allowed three weeks to stabilize on each diet. At this stage the plasma samples were analysed for calcium, phosphorus, 25 hydroxyvitamin D (25(OH)D) and 1,25$(OH)_2$D. Plasma 1,25$(OH)_2$D was measured by a modification of the radioimmunoassay of Clemens *et al* (9). The MCR of 1,25$(OH)_2$D was measured using the method of Fox, Ross & Care (7). The PR of plasma 1,25$(OH)_2$D was calculated from the MCR and plasma concentration. The sheep were initially given the NP diet, followed by the LP diet, and then returned to the NP diet.

Results and Discussion

The results are shown in the table below. They do not show any large changes in plasma 1,25$(OH)_2$D levels or metabolism in sheep during hypophosphataemia. This is in contrast to results obtained with pigs (7) and may explain the different responses in calcium absorption to hypophosphataemia, i.e. why ruminants do not show increased calcium absorption. These results indicate that adaptation of the efficiency of intestinal absorption of phosphate during dietary phosphorus depletion probably occurs in sheep largely independently of increased circulating levels of 1,25$(OH)_2$D.

Vitamin D. A Chemical, Biochemical and Clinical Update

Effect of normal phosphorus and low phosphorus diets for 3 weeks on plasma calcium, phosphate, 25(OH)D and $1,25(OH)_2D$ and the MCR and PR of plasma $1,25(OH)_2D$ (mean $\pm$ SE)

	NP Diet	LP Diet	Return to NP diet
Plasma PO_4 mM (n=4)	1.73 ± 0.19	0.54 ± 0.04**	2.13 ± 0.42*
Plasma Ca mM (n=4)	2.56 ± 0.07	2.76 ± 0.09	2.35 ± 0.11*
Plasma 25(OH)D ng/ml(n=4)	17 ± 4.7	15 ± 3.3	16 ± 0.6
Plasma $1,25(OH)_2D$ pg/ml(n=4)	57 ± 13.8	51 ± 1.1	59 ± 19.7
MCR of plasma $1,25(OH)_2D$ ml/min/$kg^{0.75}$	0.67 ± 0.06 (n=5)	0.59 ± 0.04 (n=5)	0.67 ± 0.05 (n=4)
PR of plasma $1,25(OH)_2D$ pg/min/$kg^{0.75}$	47 ± 9.9 (n=5)	39 ± 8.5 (n=5)	39 ± 10.0 (n=4)

Statistical analysis by Student's paired t-test (LP vs NP; Return to NP vs LP)
* $P<0.05$ ** $P<0.01$

References

1. Braithwaite, G.D. (1984). J. Agric. Sci. Camb. 102, 295-306.
2. Young, V. R., Richards, W.P.C., Lofgreen, G.P. & Luick, J.T. (1966). Br.J.Nutr. 20, 783-794.
3. Fox, J. and Care, A.D. (1978). J.Endocr. 77, 225-231.
4. Fox, J., Pickard, D.W., Care, A.D. and Murray, T.M. (1978). J.Endocr. 78, 379-387.
5. Fox, J., and Care, A.D. (1979). J.Endocr. 82, 417-424.
6. Ribovich, M.L. and DeLuca, H.F. (1975). Arch.Biochem.Biophys. 170, 529-535.
7. Fox, J., Ross, R. and Care, A.D. (1985). Metab. Bone. Res. In press.
8. Manas-Almendros, M., Ross, R. and Care, A.D. (1982). Quart. J. Exp.Phys.67, 269-280.
9. Clemens, T. L., Hendy, G. N., Papapoulos, S.E., Fraher, L.J., Care, A.D. and O'Riordan, J.L.H. (1979). Clin. Endocrinol. 11, 225-234.

BIOLOGICAL ACTIVITY AND CHARACTERISTICS OF 1α,25-$(OH)_2D_3$-26,23-LACTONE

S. Ishizuka, M. Kiyoki, H. Orimo* and A.W. Norman**

Teijin Institute for Bio-Medical Research, Tokyo, Japan, *Faculty of Medicine, University of Tokyo, Tokyo, Japan, and **Department of Biochemistry, University of California, Riverside, CA 92521, U.S.A.

1α,25-$(OH)_2D_3$-26,23-Lactone was isolated and identified as a main metabolite of 1α,25-$(OH)_2D_3$ in the serum of rats and dogs given large doses of 1α,25-$(OH)_2D_3$ [1-3]. This 1α,25-$(OH)_2D_3$-26,23-lactone can be produced from 1α,25-$(OH)_2D_3$ by the chick kidney or the rat intestine under in vitro conditions. The naturally-occurring 1α,25-$(OH)_2D_3$-26,23-lactone slightly stimulated intestinal calcium transport and decreased serum calcium levels in vitamin D-deficient rats fed a low calcium diet [4]. Associated with the reduction in serum calcium was a significant increase in urinary calcium excretion for 24 hr after the administration of the natural 1α,25-$(OH)_2D_3$-26,23-lactone [4]. Furthermore, prior administration of the natural 1α,25-$(OH)_2D_3$-26,23-lactone partially blocked the actions of a subsequently administered dose of 1α,25-$(OH)_2D_3$ in a increasing serum calcium levels, but did not affect the action of 1α,25-$(OH)_2D_3$ in stimulating intestinal calcium transport [4]. Recently, we have succeeded in chemically symthesizing four diastereoisomers of 1α,25-$(OH)_2D_3$-26,23-lactone [5]. We report the biological activity and characteristics of four diastereoisomers of 1α,25-$(OH)_2D_3$-26,23-lactone.

The stereochemical configuration of natural 1α,25-$(OH)_2D_3$-26,23-lactone

The four synthetic diastereoisomers of 1α,25-$(OH)_2D_3$-26,23-lactone could be separated into 3 peaks by high pressure liquid chromatography on a Zorbax Sil column using 12 % isopropanol in n-hexane. The naturally-occurring 1α,25-$(OH)_2D_3$-26,23-lactone isolated from dog serum and in vitro incubation of chick kidney homogenates comigrated with 23(S)25(R)-1α,25-$(OH)_2D_3$-26,23-lactone. The four diastereoisomers of 1α,25-$(OH)_2D_3$-26,23-lactone were tested against natural 1α,25-$(OH)_2D_3$-26,23-lactone to determine their relative competition in the 1α,25-$(OH)_2D_3$-specific receptor binding assay for 1α,25-$(OH)_2D_3$-26,23-lactone. Natural 1α,25-$(OH)_2D_3$-26,23-lactone was almost the same binding affinity that of 23(S)25(R)-1α,25-$(OH)_2D_3$-26,23-lactone. These data unequivocally demonstrate that the stereochemistry of the natural 1α,25-$(OH)_2D_3$-26,23-lactone has the 23(S) and 25(R) configurations [2,5].

Metabolic pathways from 1α,25-$(OH)_2D_3$ to 1α,25-$(OH)_2D_3$-26,23-lactone

To solve the metabolic pathway from 1α,25-$(OH)_2D_3$ to 1α,25-$(OH)_2D_3$-26,23-lactone, we investigated the production of 1α,25-$(OH)_2D_3$-26,23-lactone by incubating 6 μg of various vitamin D_3 metabolites with 1α,25-$(OH)_2D_3$-supplemented chick kidney homogenates. The results are as follows : 80 ng was from 1α,25-$(OH)_2D_3$, 280 ng from 1α,23(S)25-$(OH)_3D_3$, 150 ng from 1α,25(R)26-$(OH)_3D_3$, 1200 ng from 1α,23(S)25(R)26-$(OH)_4D_3$ and 3756 ng from 23(S)25(R)-1α,25-$(OH)_2D_3$-26,23-lactol. Above shows that 1α,23(S)25(R)26-$(OH)_4D_3$ is the key intermediate, in the metabolic pathway from 1α,25-$(OH)_2D_3$ to 1α,25-$(OH)_2D_3$-26,23-lactone. There are two metabolic pathways from 1α,25-$(OH)_2D_3$ to 1α,23(S)25(R)26-$(OH)_4D_3$. One is from 1α,25-$(OH)_2D_3$ to 1α,23(S)25(R)26-$(OH)_4D_3$ by way of 1α,23(S)25-$(OH)_3D_3$ and the other is by

Vitamin D. A Chemical, Biochemical and Clinical Update

way of 1α,25(R)26-$(OH)_3D_3$. 1α,23(S)25(R)26-$(OH)_4D_3$ is further metabolized to 1α,25-$(OH)_2D_3$-26,23-lactone via 23(S)25(R)-1α,25-$(OH)_2D_3$-26,23-lactol. The metabolic pathway by way of 1α,23(S)25-$(OH)_3D_3$ of the two is thought to be the main one.

Hypocalcemic action of 1α,25-$(OH)_2D_3$-26,23-lactone in rats

We previously reported that the natural 1α,25-$(OH)_2D_3$-26,23-lactone decreased the serum calcium concentrations in vitamin D-deficient rats [4]. Using 4 synthetic diastereoisomers of 1α,25-$(OH)_2D_3$-26,23-lactone, we investigated the reduction of the serum calcium levels in normal rats and in hypercalcemic rats which are given large doses of vitamin D_3. In normal rats, 23(S)25(S)- and 23(R)25(R)-1α,25-$(OH)_2D_3$-26,23-lactone slightly elevated the serum calcium concentrations. However, 23(S)25(R)- and 23(R)25(S)-1α,25-$(OH)_2D_3$-26,23-lactone significantly decreased the serum calcium levels 4 to 24 hr after the administration. The potency of 23(S)25(R)-1α,25-$(OH)_2D_3$-26,23-lactone in reducing the serum calcium concentrations was stronger than that of 23(R)25(S)-1α,25-$(OH)_2D_3$-26,23-lactone. Eel calcitonin also remarkably decreased in serum calcium levels 2 to 8 hr after the administration. These results indicate that eel calcitonin has rapid and short action, on the contrary 1α,25-$(OH)_2D_3$-26,23-lactone has gradual and long action. The same is true in the case of hypercalcemic rats.

Effect of 23(S)25(R)-1α,25-$(OH)_2D_3$-26,23-lactone on bone metabolism

We investigated the effects of 23(S)25(R)-1α,25-$(OH)_2D_3$-26,23-lactone on bone formation and bone resorption. The former is evaluated by the increase in alkaline phosphatase activity and stimulation of collargen synthesis using osteoblastic clone MC3T3-El cell culture and the latter by evaluation system of bone resorption using mouse calvaria in organ culture. 1α,25-$(OH)_2D_3$-26,23-Lactone stimulated alkaline phosphatase activity in MC3T3-El cells. The maximum of stimulated enzyme activity per mg protein was 1.8 times higher than that of control cultures at 200 pg/ml. 1α,25-$(OH)_2D_3$-26,23-Lactone also increased collagen synthesis about 1.5 times stronger than that of control level at 200 pg/ml. On the other hand, 1α,25-$(OH)_2D_3$-26,23-lactone decreased slightly but significantly ^{45}Ca mobilization, and blocked the resorptive action of 1α,25-$(OH)_2D_3$ and parathyroid hormone, in mouse calvaria [6]. These results strongly indicate that 1α,25-$(OH)_2D_3$-26,23-lactone has a direct stimulative effect on bone formation and an inhibitory effect on bone resorption.

REFERENCES

1. Ohnuma, N., Bannai, K., Yamaguchi, H., Hashimoto, Y., and Norman, A.W. (1980) Arch. Biochem. Biophys. 204, 387-391
2. Ishizuka, S., Yamaguchi, H., Yamada, S., Nakayama, K., and Takayama, H. (1981) FEBS Lett. 134, 207-211
3. Ishizuka, S., Ishimoto, S., and Norman, A.W. (1984) Biochemistry 23, 1473-1478
4. Ishizuka, S., Ishimoto, S., and Norman, A.W. (1984) J. Steroid Biochem. 20, 611-616
5. Ishizuka, S., Oshida, J., Tsuruta, H., and Norman (submitted)
6. Kiyoki, M., Kurihara, N., Ishizuka, S., Ishii, S., Kumegawa, M., and Norman, A.W. (1985) Biochem. Biophys. Res. Commun. (in press)

RAPID STIMULATORY EFFECT OF 1α-HYDROXYVITAMIN D_3 ON INTESTINAL TRANSPORT OF PHOSPHORUS IN CHICKS

V.K.BAUMAN, M.Y.VALINIETSE, Y.Y.GALVANOVSKY
Institute of Biology, Academy of Sciences of Latvian SSR, Salaspils, 229021, USSR

It has been recently reported (1,2) that 1,25-$(OH)_2D_3$ causes an early stimulatory effects - during the first 30 min - on the transport of inorganic phosphorus (P_i) in the small intestine of chicks and rats. These results are indicative of a direct action that hormone exerts on the plasmalemma of enterocytes and/or the activity of intracellular enzyme systems responsible for P_i transport. The purpose of the present study was to investigate rapid effect of a synthetic analog of 1,25-$(OH)_2D_3$ - 1α-hydroxyvitamin D_3 (1α-OHD_3).

Investigations were carried out on chicks raised on a vitamin D-deficient diet. At the age of 3.5-4 weeks, when severe rachitis was evident, chicks were used for experimentation. The transport of P_i was studied in vitro by means of everted gut sacs as described by Wilson and Wiseman (3) with some modifications. The sacs were incubated in Ringer solution (pH 7.0) for 30 min at 37°C and continuous gassing with oxygen. The net flux of P_i was determined from total change of P_i in the serosal solution. Action of 1α-OHD_3 on ^{32}P uptake by jejunum was studied by everted mucosal preparations (4) under conditions practically identical to those described for everted sacs. The single difference in this case was the presence of ^{32}P in the incubation solution (10 μCi/l). Incubation period was 5 min. The radioactivity of samples was determined on a liquid scintillation counter and P_i influx rate into enterocytes was calculated. Part of the chicks received 15 nmoles vitamin D_3 or 1α-OHD_3 dissolved in 0.1 ml of propylene glycol by intramuscular injection 30 min before use. The other group was repleated 72 hr prior to use with 32.5 nmoles of vitamin D_3. The control group received vehicle only.

The results obtained are summarized in the table.

Sterol and its administration	Flux of P_i, $nmol.min^{-1} . g^{-1}$ tissue	
	Net transport	Influx
None	9.5±1.5	84.0±5.2
Vitamin D_3, 72 hr before use	64.6±6.1	122.5±10.0
Vitamin D_3, intramuscularly 30 min before use	9.6±1.4	96.11±8.3
1α-OHD_3, intramuscularly 30 min before use	53.6±4.5	119.40±4.5

It is seen that intramuscular injection of 1α-OHD_3 to rachitic chicks significantly (5.6 times) increased the translocation rate of P_i across the intestinal wall, though the administration of vitamin D_3 under the same conditions did not cause any effect. Also the hydroxylated form of vitamin D_3 significantly stimulated (1.42 times, $p<0.002$) the influx rate of P_i into the intestine. Both characteristics of the transport process practically reached the level observed for chicks repleted with vitamin D_3 72 hr prior to experimentation.

Thus, the administration of 1α-OHD_3 to rachitic chicks as well as the administration of the hormone 1,25-$(OH)_2D_3$ affected a rapid increase of P_i absorption in the small intestine. The action of 1α-OHD_3 seems to be aimed at the apical membrane of enterocytes since the sterol affects entry of P_i into the intestinal cells.

1. Bauman, V.K., Valinietse, M.Y., Galvanovsky, Y.Y., Babarykin, D.A. (1983) Izvestiya Ac.Sc Latvian SSR, No.12, 94-97.
2. Bachelet, M., Lacour, B., Ulmann, A. (1982) Mineral Electrolyte Metab. 8, 261-266.
3. Wilson, T.H., Wiseman, G. (1954) J.Physiol., London, 123, 166-125.
4. Karasow, W.H., Diamond, J.M. (1983) J.Comp.Physiol. 152, 105-116.

ACTION OF VITAMIN D ON LEAD METABOLISM IN CHICKS

R.J.ANDRUSHAITE, V.K.BAUMAN
Institute of Biology, Academy of Sciences of Latvian SSR,
Salaspils, 229021, USSR

It is known that vitamin D enhances the assimilation of Pb in animals (1-4). The present study was designed to investigate the dose-dependence of vitamin D_3 action and its synthetic analog - 1α-hydroxyvitamin D_3 (1α-OHD_3) on Pb metabolism in chicks kept on a rachitogenic diet. Chicks, starting from the age of 8 days and up to 28 days, were fed a diet containing Pb acetate (500 mg/kg) and were dosed daily with vitamin D_3 or 1α-OHD_3. Various doses of sterols (162, 320, and 650 nmoles), dissolved in propylene glycol, were administered by intramuscular injection. At the end of the experimental period 7 chicks from each group were decapitated and blood samples collected and assayed for Pb and δ-aminolaevulinic acid (ALA). ALA in erythrocytes was determined colorimetrically using Erlich reagent. Pb content in tissues was determined by atomic absorption spectrophotometry after their ashing and dissolving in 6 N HCl. The results of these investigations are summarized in the table.

Sterol	Dose, nmoles	Bone-ash, %	ALA in erythrocytes, μg/ml	Pb content of blood, μg/ml	Pb content of dry bone, μg/g
Vit.D_3	162	34.9±1.6	4.5±0.4	5.4±0.7	184.6±12.4
- " -	325	37.1±0.9	5.8±0.6	6.5±0.4	253.7±16.4
- " -	650	40.8±2.4	7.4±1.1	7.6±0.7	308.2±22.4
1α-OHD_3	162	39.7±0.5	9.5±1.2	7.0±0.3	255.2±14.3
- " -	325	42.6±0.5	11.9±2.4	7.4±0.5	298.5±26.9
- " -	650	43.5±0.8	15.7±4.1	9.8±0.5	510.5±43.1
None	-	23.5±1.0	1.8±0.4	4.0±0.2	121.7±10.1

The represented data show that Pb accumulation in tissues is dependent on sterol dosage. However, the activity of 1α-OHD_3 is considerably higher than that of vitamin D_3. The toxic effect of 1α-OHD_3 as assayed according to ALA levels in erythrocytes is twice higher than that caused by the same dose of

Vitamin D. A Chemical, Biochemical and Clinical Update

vitamin D_3. The increased absorption of Pb in the small intestine was the cause of the vitamin D-induced enhance in toxicosis. Already 72 hr after the administration of 500 IU vitamin D_3 to rachitic chicks the absorption of Pb-210 in the duodenum increased twice in agreement with results of other authors (2, 4). Evidently, vitamin D stimulates Pb absorption through the specific vitamin D-dependent calcium-binding protein which binds with high affinity Ca as well as Pb (according to preliminary data $K_a = 0.61 \cdot 10^5 M^{-1}$). However, it can't be excluded that vitamin D acts indirectly on Pb assimilation preventing the formation of low-soluble Pb salts in the intestinal lumen due to increased Ca and P absorption (1).

In other experiment (experimental set-up similar to the previous one) chicks up to the age of 28 days were kept on a rachitogenic diet supplemented with Pb. A day before the administration of a single dose vitamin D_3 (32.5 nmoles) Pb was excluded from the diet, and chicks were decapitated 1, 3 and 7 days later. It was found that vitamin D affected a rapid and intensive release of Pb accumulated in soft tissues. Particulary high decrease was observed in kidneys where the Pb content, 7 days after the dosing with vitamin D, was almost twice lower than that in controls. However, vitamin D together with stimulation of bone mineralization increased Pb accumulation in that tissue (by 34%).

Thus, vitamin D exerts a twofold effect on Pb metabolism: sterol stimulates lead absorption in intestine and increases its excretion in kidneys.

1. Andrushaite, R.J., Bauman, V.K. (1984) Voprosi pitaniya, No.6, 46-49.
2. Barton, J.C., Conrad, M.E., Harrison, L., Nuby, S. (1980) Amer.J.Physiol. 238, 124-130.
3. Mykkänen, H.M., Wasserman, R.H. (1982) J.Nutr. 112, 520-527.
4. Smith, C.M., DeLuca, H.F., Tanaka, Y., Mahaffey, K.R. (1978) J.Nutr. 108, 843-847.

VITAMIN D-DEPENDENT, ATP-DRIVEN CA^{2+}-TRANSPORT IN CHICK DUODENAL BASAL-LATERAL MEMBRANE VESICLES.

J.S. CHANDLER, S.A. MEYER AND R.H. WASSERMAN, New York State College of Veterinary Medicine, Cornell University, Ithaca, NY 14853 (USA)

Current evidence suggests that calcium transfer across the duodenal basal-lateral plasma membrane involves, in part, an active calcium pump. In rat duodenum, a high affinity Ca^{2+}-ATPase activity has been implicated as the enzymatic expression of this membrane calcium transport system (1). We have previously reported that purified basal-lateral membrane vesicles (BLMV) isolated from chick duodenum transport calcium in an ATP-dependent fashion and that calcium uptake by these vesicles is responsive to cholecalciferol (D_3) and 1,25-dihydroxycholecalciferol (1,25$(OH)_2D_3$) treatment (2). Calcium uptake by these BLMV preparations is characterized by a K_m of about 0.33 μM. Vitamin D_3 or 1,25$(OH)_2D_3$ repletion of rachitic birds increases the rate of calcium uptake (2-2.5 fold). Vesicle orientation in these BLMV preparations was determined by monitoring the latent expression of Na/K-ATPase activity and a ouabain-insensitive Mg^{2+}-ATPase activity in saponin-permeabilized vesicles. These results indicated that BLMV were enriched 7-10 fold in Na/K-ATPase activity (relative to initial homogenates) and 60-70% of the vesicles were sealed. Approximately 50% of the sealed vesicles are considered to be "inside-out" (Io) and it is this fraction that exhibits ATP-dependent calcium uptake. Importantly, vitamin D_3 treatment does not significantly alter BLMV orientation.

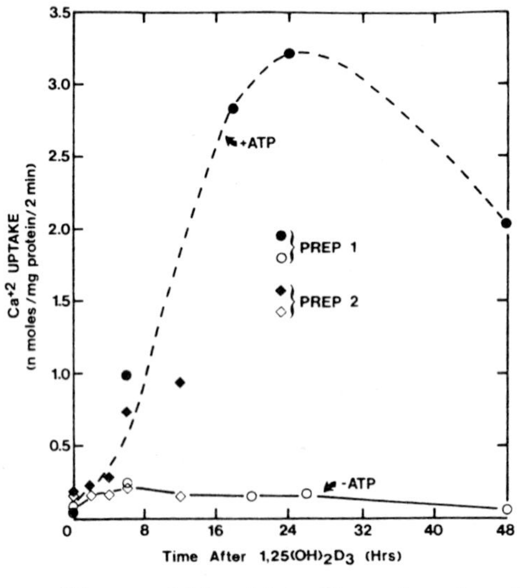

Figure 1: Temporal induction of BLMV calcium-uptake by 1,25-$(OH)_2D_3$ (0.5 μg), intracardial) in 6-week rachitic chicks. Each group contained 6 chicks and the data are the means of triplicate determinations in the presence (closed symbols) or absence (open symbols) of 5 mM ATP. BLMV were prepared essentially as described in (3) except that EDTA was omitted. ^{45}Ca-uptake was performed as in (4).

When rachitic chicks (4 weeks of age) are supplemented with cholecalciferol (12.5 μg, intramuscular) or 1,25$(OH)_2D_3$ (0.5 μg,intracardial) the maximum rates of calcium uptake by Io BLMV from rachitic, 1,25$(OH)_2D_3$-treated and vitamin D_3-treated chicks are 1.25 nmoles/mg/min, 2.82 nmoles/mg/min, and 3.02 nmoles/mg/min, respectively. A brief summary of our findings relating to BLMV calcium uptake are as follows: a) Ca^{2+}-uptake specifically requires ATP, other

Vitamin D. A Chemical, Biochemical and Clinical Update

nucleotides (AMP, ADP, GTP, CTP, ITP, UTP) do not support uptake; b) $1,25(OH)_2D_3$-induced Ca^{2+}-uptake can be detected within 2-4 hours following a pulse dose (0.5 μg, intracardial) of $1,25(OH)_2D_3$ and a maximal effect is observed between 18 and 30 hours (Fig. 1); c) $1,25(OH)_2D_3$-induced BLMV Ca^{2+}-uptake is dose-dependent (Fig. 2); and d) actinomycin D and cycloheximide appear to block a portion of the $1,25(OH)_2D_3$-mediated response. BLMV calcium uptake is sensitive to inhibition by vanadate and is virtually abolished in the presence of 10 μM vanadate. Inclusion of sodium (100 mM) in the calcium uptake assay medium inhibits (∿50%) BLMV Ca^{2+}-uptake, indicative of the presence of a Na^+/Ca^{2+} exchange mechanism (4) in the chick duodenal basal-lateral membrane.

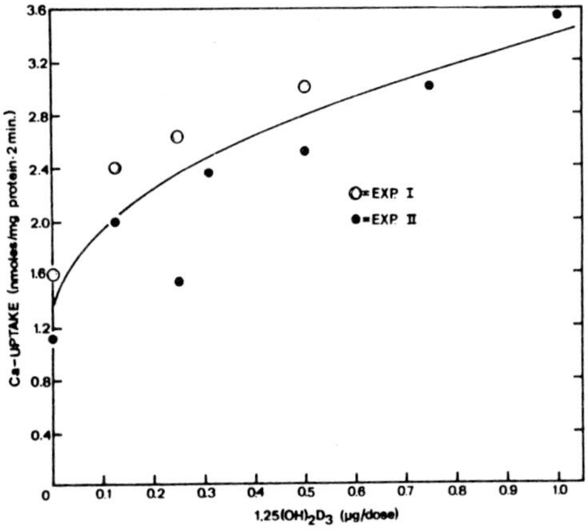

Figure 2: Dose-dependent induction of ATP-dependent calcium uptake in BLMV by $1,25(OH)_2D_3$. Four-week-old chicks (6/group) were treated with the indicated amounts of $1,25(OH)_2D_3$ (intracardially) and sacrificed 18 hours later. BLMV preparation and Ca^{2+}-uptake were as in Figure 1.

Analysis of ATP-hydrolysis by BLMV from rachitic or $1,25(OH)_2D_3$-treated chicks revealed that Na/K-ATPase and Mg^{2+} -ATPase activities are unaffected by hormone treatment. However, a high-affinity Ca^{2+}-activated ATP-ase activity (Ca^{2+}-ATPase), assayed at low levels (0.5-2.0 μM) of "free" calcium, increases following hormone treatment (2.92 ± 0.74 vs 3.49 ± 0.435 μmoles Pi/mg/hour). This Ca^{2+}-ATPase activity reflects only a small fraction (∿1-3%) of the total ATP hydrolysis observed in these BLMV preparations. We are currently attempting to isolate this Ca^{2+}-ATPase to further study its regulation by vitamin D. (Supported by NIH Grant AM-04652).

References

1. Ghijsen, W.E.J.M., DeJong, M.D. and Van Os, C.H. (1982) Biochim. Biophys. Acta, 689, 327-336.
2. Chandler, J.S., Meyer, S.A. and Wasserman, R.H. (1984) Fed. Proc. 43, 985.
3. Mircheff, A.K. and Wright, E.M. (1976) J. Membrane Biol. 28, 309-333.
4. Gmaj, P., Murer, H. and Kinne, R. (1979) Biochem. J. 178, 549-557.

VITAMIN D, CA TRANSPORT AND ALTERATION OF FATTY ACID COMPOSITION IN THE RAT.

T. S. FREUND and A. M. MARINO
Department of Biochemistry and OHRC, Fairleigh Dickinson University, School of Dentistry, Hackensack, NJ 07601, USA.

INTRODUCTION:

Recent studies have indicated that the widely distributed vitamin D-dependent calcium binding proteins (CaBP) may function by interacting with components of membranous calcium transport systems (1,2), interacting with lysolecithin (3) and that vitamin D-administration alters membrane lipid composition (4,5,6) in the chick.

In an effort to examine the extent that lipid alterations exist and might play a role in transcellular calcium movement in the rat, we analyzed the fatty acid composition of rat tissues with particular emphasis on the state of saturation and geometric isomerism.

MATERIALS AND METHODS:

Animals Wealing Spraque- Dawley derived rats were maintained on normocalcemic (0.5%) diets containing either no (-D) or 2000i.u. vitamin D2/kg diet (+D) or on Purina rat chow.

Preparation of extract. Freshly obtained rat tissues were either used immediately or frozen in liquid nitrogen for storage. Tissues were homogenized (20%) and extracted in chloroform: methanol (3:1). Following filtration and drying a portion of the lipid extract was separated, taken up in methanol: diethylether and refluxed with 5N NaOH under nitrogen.

The free fatty acids in the aqueons layer were converted to methyl ester (FAME) by refluxing in methanolic boron trichloride and extracted into hexane.

Fatty acid methyl ester analysis was accomplished on a Perkin-Elmer G.C. equipped with a Sigma-1 analyzer (flame ionization detector). A liquid phase of 10% Silar 10C with a stationary phase 100/120 gas chrom A utilizing a temperature program (145·C to 190·C at 2·C/minute) allowed for the successful separation of the FAMEs. The technique allowed for a recovery of 87% of an added external standard (Tricosamoic acid).

Lipid geometry was examined following infrared analysis (Perkin-Elmer IR 283B) of KBr pellets or evaporated chloroform methanol extracts on NaCl plates. Isomers containing "trans" unsaturation demonstrated an absorption at 970 cm-1 while the "cis" form absorbs at 770 cm^{-1}. Samples were compared by calculating the area under the curves at the respective wavenumbers.

RESULTS:

Analysis of the FAMEs from all three tissues indicated that Palmitic acid (C16:0), Palmitolcic acid (C16:1) Stearic acid (C18:0), Oleic acid (C18:1), Linolaic acid (C18:2) and Arachidonic acid (C20:4) were present as the major components (The data for the intestine are illustrated in Figure 1). Vitamin D-deficiency lead to several alterations, none of which were statistically significant. For the intestine, the saturated (C-16 and C-18) and unsaturated (C16:1) increased in weight percentage while the polyunsaturated arachidonic acid (C20:4; a known precursor for prostaglandins) decreased in weight percentage. The liver demonstrated a

Vitamin D. A Chemical, Biochemical and Clinical Update

similar effect, which was not carried on to the kidney.

The increased C20:4 fatty acids in the vitamin D replete animal can be correlated to the increased "cis" geometry of the double bonds (Fig. 2) seen in only the intestine and liver.

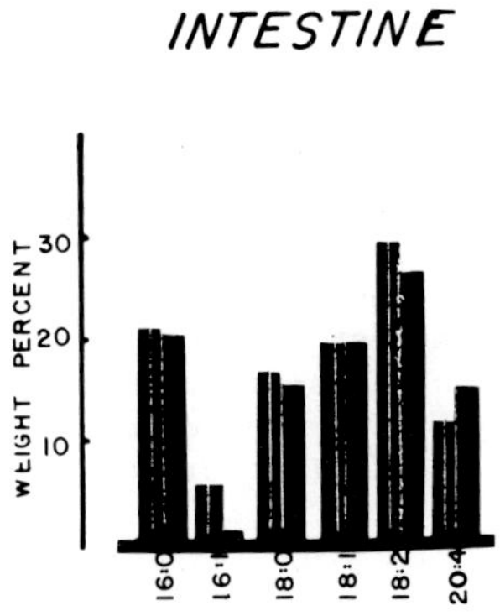

FIG. 1. Fatty Acid Composition

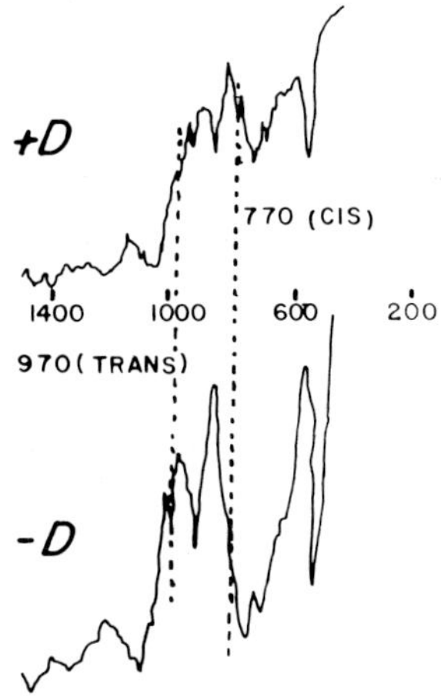

FIG. 2. Lipid Geometry

CONCLUSIONS:

In going from the vitamin D-deficient rat to the D-replete state in both the intestine and liver, the fatty acid composition, characterized by a decrease in saturation with a rise predominently in arachidonic acid with increased "cis" geometry, reflects an increase in membrane fluidity. Our data suggest, which requires further work to examine, that vitamin D may, in addition to proteins synthesis, alter lipid composition related to prostaglandin action which could have it effect reflected in an early rise in calcium transport.

REFERENCES:

1. Freund, T. S. (1982) in Vitamin D, Chemical, Biochemical and Clinical Endocrinology of Calcium Metabolism. Norman, A.W. et.al. eds. De Gruyter, New York, pp. 249-251.

2. Freund, T. S. and Christakos, S. (1985) This volume.

3. Wasserman, R. H. (1970) Biochem. Biophys Acta. 20: 176-179.

4. O'Doherty, P.J.A. (1979) Lipids 14:75.

5. Matsumoto, T., Fontaine, O., Rasmussen, H. (1981) J. Biol. Chem. 256: 3354.

6. Armbrecht, H. J., Wise, R. W. and Wasserman, R. H. (1984) Fed. Proc 1176 abs.

THE NORMAL RAT DUODENAL VILLUS/CRYPT GRADIENT OF Ca TRANSPORT BY BASOLATERAL MEMBRANES IS ABSENT IN VITAMIN D-DEFICIENCY.

J.R.F. WALTERS and M.M. WEISER
Division of Gastroenterology, SUNY Department of Medicine, Buffalo General Hospital, 100 High Street, Buffalo, NY 14203, USA.

Introduction:

Calcium transport in the small intestine is the result of several subcellular processes - at the microvillus membrane, in the cytosol and at the basolateral membrane (BLM). The vitamin D-dependence of many of these steps is well established and recently it has been shown that the rate of ATP-dependent Ca-transport by BLM vesicles is reduced in vitamin D-deficient rats [1,2]. Most data, such as the villus/crypt distributions of alkaline phosphatase and Ca-binding protein, suggest that vitamin D-dependent Ca absorption occurs primarily in the villus-tip cells; consequently we have investigated the villus/crypt distribution of duodenal BLM Ca-transport in normal and vitamin D-deficient or repleted rats.

Methods:

Five to eight week-old male Holtzman rats were fed either a vitamin D-deficient or a control, vitamin D-sufficient diet. Repleted animals were given $1,25(OH)_2D_3$ 125ng IV 6h before death. Five fractions of cells were isolated sequentially from 15cm of duodenum using a modification of the method of Weiser [3]. These fractions were similar in size (about 20% protein each) and showed selective enrichment for alkaline phosphatase activity (villus-tips) and in vivo ^3H-thymidine incorporation (crypts). Microscopy confirmed sequential removal of cells. BLM were prepared from cell-fractions pooled from 10-12 animals using sorbitol density-gradient centrifugation as described previously [4]. Similar purifications of BLM Na/K-ATPase activities were found for all cell-fractions. Ca-transport was measured by incubating membranes with ^{45}Ca, 0.5mM EGTA, 3mM ATP, 5mM Mg, 135mM KCl in a 10mM imidazole-acetate buffer at pH 7.5 and $25^{o}C$ (0.5uM free Ca). Ca-uptake was determined by millipore filtration after 1 and 2 min and Ca-binding in the presence of A23187 was subtracted. Vanadate was shown to abolish ATP-dependent Ca-transport.

Results:

In normal, control animals, there was a large villus/crypt gradient of BLM Ca-transport rates which were two-fold higher in BLM vesicles prepared from villus-tip compared to crypt cells ($p<0.001$) [Figure]. In vitamin D-deficient rats, the BLM Ca-transport villus/crypt gradient was greatly diminished; villus-fraction rates were reduced to that of crypts of normal and vitamin D-deficient animals. The upper and mid-villus fractions were significantly lower than controls. In the animals repleted for 6h with $1,25(OH)_2D_3$, a significant increase occurred in the BLM Ca-transport rate of the mid-villus fraction. No change was seen in the villus-tip fractions.

Vitamin D. A Chemical, Biochemical and Clinical Update

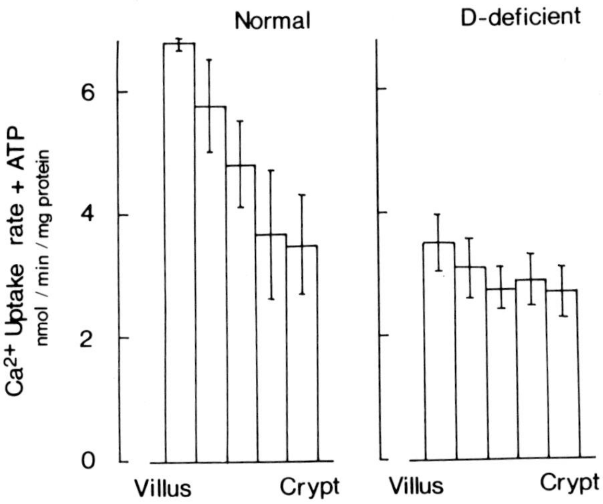

Figure. ATP-dependent Ca-transport rates in basolateral membranes prepared from 5 equal cell-fractions obtained from duodenal villus/crypt gradients of normal or vitamin D-deficient rats. Free Ca = 0.5uM. Mean ± SEM, n = 5-6 expts.

Conclusions:

1. A significant villus/crypt gradient of Ca-transport by BLM vesicles is present in normal rat duodenum. These findings differ from those of van Corven and van Os [5].
2. The gradient is not found in vitamin D-deficient animals indicating that vitamin D is necessary for the increased BLM transport as the cell differentiates.
3. 6h after $1,25(OH)_2D_3$ repletion, a significant increase in BLM Ca-transport occurs in the mid-villus, but not in the villus-tip fraction which presumably is too differentiated to respond further.
4. The distribution of duodenal basolateral membrane Ca-transport suggests that vitamin D-dependent Ca-absorption occurs predominantly in the upper villus.

References:

1. Ghijsen, W.E.J.M., and van Os, C.H. (1982) Biochim. Biophys. Acta 689, 170-172
2. Walters, J.R.F., Horvath, P.J., and Weiser, M.M. (1984) in Epithelial Calcium and Phosphate Transport (Bronner, F., and Peterlik, M., eds) pp. 187-192, Alan R. Liss, New York
3. Weiser, M.M. (1973) J. Biol. Chem. 248, 2536-2541
4. Freedman, R.A., Weiser, M.M., and Isselbacher, K.J. (1977) Proc. Natl. Acad. Sci. USA 74, 3612-3616
5. van Corven, E.J.J.M., and van Os, C.H. (1984) in Epithelial Calcium and Phosphate Transport (Bronner, F., and Peterlik, M., eds) pp. 295-299, Alan R. Liss, New York

THE ROLE OF DECREASED RENAL 25-HYDROXYVITAMIN D-1-HYDROXYLASE ACTIVITY IN GASTROINTESTINAL MALABSORPTION OF CALCIUM IN THE AGING RAT: A REAPPRAISAL.

B. Lobaugh, R. Cooper, M.K. Drezner, L.S. Birnbaum, S.A. Schuette and D.V. Havlir.

Departments of Surgery, Physiology and Medicine, Duke University Medical Center, Durham, North Carolina, USA and the National Institute of Environmental Health Science, Research Triangle Park, North Carolina, USA.

Introduction:

Previous studies in rats indicate that diminished gastrointestinal absorption of calcium associated with aging results from decreased 25-hydroxyvitamin D-1-hydroxylase (1-OHase) activity (1,2). These conclusions are based on measurement of [^{3}H]-25-hydroxyvitamin D conversion to [^{3}H]-1,25-dihydroxyvitamin D in cortical slices from vitamin D and calcium deficient young and adult animals. In the present study we evaluated the adequacy of the assay previously employed and determined if the enzyme abnormality exists in aged rats kept under basal conditions.

Methods

We studied male Fisher F-344 and Long-Evans hooded rats of three ages (Young: 1-3 mo.; Middle: 11-14 mo.; Aged: 18-30 mo.). Gastrointestinal calcium absorption was measured by an *in situ* recirculating perfusion technique (3) and we employed our sensitive assay of mammalian 1-OHase activity (4) to assess enzyme function. This method utilizes the chick intestinal cytosol binding protein assay to quantify the 1,25-dihydroxyvitamin D produced *in vitro* by crude renal homogenate to which sufficient 25-hydroxyvitamin D substrate has been added to both saturate the inhibitory protein present in mammalian kidney and allow for measurement of enzyme V_{max}.

Results and Discussion

In preliminary studies we observed that use of [^{3}H]-25-hydroxyvitamin D as substrate and separation of reaction products by traditional techniques (LH-20 chromatography [chloroform:hexane 65:35] and/or straight phase HPLC [2-propanol:redistilled hexane 10:90]) results in comigration of a tritiated metabolite with [^{3}H]-1,25-dihydroxyvitamin D. Indeed, up to 75% of the apparent 1,25-dihydroxyvitamin D is a contaminant which elutes separately upon reverse phase HPLC (methanol:water 75:25). Moreover, the relative insensitivity of the renal slice method mandates prestimulation of 1-OHase to measurable levels by inducing vitamin D/calcium depletion. Such treatment confounds the role(s) of age and other dietary and metabolic factors in modifying enzyme activity. The use of our assay confers the sensitivity needed to measure 1-OHase in animals maintained on a basal diet and is

Vitamin D. A Chemical, Biochemical and Clinical Update

unaffected by the coeluting metabolite.

A significant reduction in the gastrointestinal absorption of calcium was observed in the Middle and Aged groups of both F-344 and Long-Evans hooded male rats (Young: 22.2 ± 2.5; Middle:8.9 ± 1.8; Aged: 7.6 ± 0.8 μmol/g intestine/hr). This finding is in agreement with previously published reports (1,2,5). However, despite this malabsorption in older animals, we found that under basal conditions 1-OHase activity is similar in all age groups of both strains (Young: 1.3 ± 0.1; Middle: 1.1 ± 0.1; Aged: 1.3 ± 0.2 fmol 1,25-dihyrdroxyvitamin D produced/mg kidney/min).

These data indicate that separation of $[^3H]$-1,25-dihydroxyvitamin D from tritiated contaminants should be demonstrated when methods which employ scintillation counting or determination of area under an HPLC peak to quantify 1-OHase reaction products are chosen. Further, while it remains possible that 1-OHase reserve may differ with age, our observations offer clear evidence that the calcium malabsorption of age cannot be explained on the basis of reduced enzyme activity.

References:

1. Armbrecht, H.J., Zenser, T.V., and Davis, B.B. (1980) J. Clin. Invest. 66, 1118-1123.
2. Armbrecht, H.J., Wongsurawat, N., Zenser T.V., and Davis, B.B. (1982) Endocrinology 111, 1339-1344.
3. Eastin, W.C., Wilson, H.D., and Schedl, H.P. (1980) Proc. Soc. Exp. Biol. Med. 163, 553-557.
4. Lobaugh, B. and Drezner, M.K. (1983) Anal. Biochem. 129, 416-424.
5. Horst, R.L., DeLuca, H.F., and Jurgenson, N.A. (1978) Metab. Bone Dis. and Rel. Res. 1, 29-33.

1,25-DIHYDROXYVITAMIN D INCREASES THE INTRACELLULAR FREE CALCIUM CONCENTRATION OF DUODENAL EPITHELIAL CELLS

D.D. Bikle, D.M. Shoback, and S.J. Munson,
Department of Medicine, Veterans Administration Medical Center and University of California, San Francisco, Ca., USA

In previous studies using radioisotope techniques and electron microscopy, we concluded that the administration of 1,25-dihydroxyvitamin D ($1,25(OH)_2D$) to vitamin D-deficient chicks results in a transient (4-8 h) increase in the total amount of intracellular Ca in the duodenal mucosa; this level returns to baseline by 18 h despite a continued increase in Ca transport across the duodenum. These findings suggested that the stimulation by $1,25(OH)_2D$ of Ca entry into the cell across the brush border membrane (BBM) preceded the stimulation of Ca removal at the basolateral membrane (BLM). Since the intracellular free Ca concentration is at least one determinant of the activity of the Ca pump at the BLM, we measured this concentration (using the fluorescent probe QUIN-2) in duodenal epithelial cells eluted from the distal portion of the villus of vitamin D-replete chicks and vitamin D-deficient chicks given $1,25(OH)_2D$ 0, 4, or 18 h before removal of the duodenum and elution of the cells. In these experiments, the cells were eluted by everting each duodenum over a glass rod and incubating for 10 min at $37^{\circ}C$ in 96 mM NaCl, 1.5 mM KCl, 8 mM KH_2PO_4, 5.6 mM Na_2HPO_4, 27 mM Na citrate, 0.1 mM PMSF, pH 7.3 (these cells were discarded), then for 10 more min in 154 mM NaCl, 10 mM NaH_2PO_4, 1.5 mM EDTA, 0.5 mM dithiothreitol, 0.1 mM PMSF, pH 7.3 (these cells were collected). This fraction of cells originating from the distal 1/3 of the villus and excluding (>95%) trypan blue, was then incubated with 70-100 μM Quin-2AM in 1 mM NaH_2PO_4, 125 mM NaCl, 1 mM $CaCl_2$, 1 mM $MgSO_4$, 1 mM K_2HPO_4, 25 mM HEPES, 5.5 mM glucose, 0.1 mM PMSF, 1 mg/ml BSA, pH 7.47, and the fluorescent signal in 10×10^6 cells/ml was determined. We observed that the intracellular free Ca concentration was higher (125 ± 20 nM) in cells 18 h after $1,25(OH)_2D$ administration than in cells from vitamin D-deficient controls (71 ± 11 nM) or in cells 4 h after $1,25(OH)_2D$ administration (62 ± 5 nM). The intracellular free Ca concentration in duodenal epithelial cells from chicks raised for 6 weeks on a vitamin D-replete diet (130 ± 5 nM) was comparable to that of cells from vitamin D-deficient chicks given $1,25(OH)_2D$ 18 h prior to measurement of the intracellular free Ca concentration. We conclude that the intracellular free Ca concentration is higher in duodenal epithelial cells from vitamin D-replete chicks, and that this facilitates transcellular Ca transport by stimulating the Ca pump at the BLM.

Vitamin D. A Chemical, Biochemical and Clinical Update

EFFECT OF 1,25$(OH)_2D_3$ ON THE SUBCELLULAR REDISTRIBUTION OF LYSOSOMAL HYDROLASES AND POTENTIAL RELATION TO CALCIUM TRANSPORT.

I. NEMERE and A. W. NORMAN.
Dept. of Biochemistry, Univ. of California, Riverside, CA 92521, USA.

Introduction: Earlier work (1-4) with both normal (+D) and vitamin D-deficient (-D) animals, has suggested a role for lysosomes in 1,25-$(OH)_2D_3$-mediated effects on intestinal cells. More recently, vascular perfusion of +D chick duodena has demonstrated a rapid effect of 1,25-$(OH)_2D_3$ on calcium transport that is inhibited by the anti-microtuble agent colchicine (5). These cytoskeletal elements are associated with lysosomes, and most likely act to facilitate transport of the membrane-delimited organelles (6,7). In the current report, analysis of acid hydroxylase distribution in subcellular fractionS prepared from -D chicks treated with vehicle or 650 pmols of 1,25$(OH)_2D_3$ *in vitro*, suggested additional perfusion studies to test the effects of various inhibitors of membrane-related events.

Materials and Methods: Previously published procedures were used for isolation of intestinal membranes (8), determination of acid phosphotase (AcP) and cathepsin (CB) activities (3), perfusion studies in +D duodena (5), *in vitro* incubation conditions of viable intestinal cells isolated from +D duodena and preparation of particle-free supernatant (3,4).

Results and Discussion: Analysis of whole mucosal homogenates prepared from duodena of -D chicks treated with vehicle or 650 pmols of 1,25-$(OH)_2D_3$ *in vivo* prior to sacrifice, revealed a substantial increase in CB specific activity: 176% and 217% of control levels at 2h and 10h, respectively, after injection of the secosteroid. In contrast, AcP in the same homogenates was only 72 and 87% of controls, 2 h and 10 h after 1,25$(OH)_2D_3$, respectively. The subcellular distribution of these hydrolases in isolated membrane fractions is shown in Fig. 1. Both CB and AcP are elevated in Golgi membranes 2 h after 1,25$(OH)_2D_3$ *in vivo*, but only CB undergoes an apparent redistribution to basal-lateral membranes with time, and to a smaller extent, brush borders. These results prompted studies of the relationship of protease activity to ^{45}Ca transport in vascularly perfused duodenal loops. Figure 2 illustrates that 1 mM leupeptin (an inhibitor of CB)substantially reduced the rapid effect of 1,25-$(OH)_2D_3$ on ^{45}Ca transport. The small increase in ^{45}Ca transport in the presence of leupeptin was found to be due to a stabilizing effect of the inhibitor in duodena vascularly perfused with control medium. Similar studies conducted

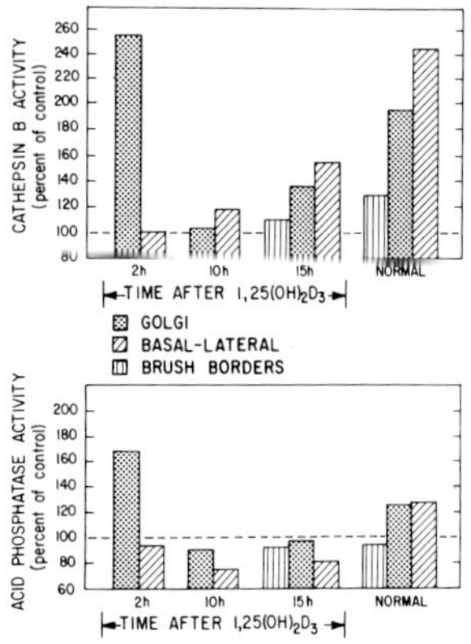

Fig. 1: Distribution of two lysosomal hydrolases in isolated intestinal membranes.

Vitamin D. A Chemical, Biochemical and Clinical Update

with 1 mM lumenal pepstatin (a cathepsin D antagonist), failed to abolish 1,25(OH)$_2$D$_3$-enhanced ^{45}Ca transport (data not shown).

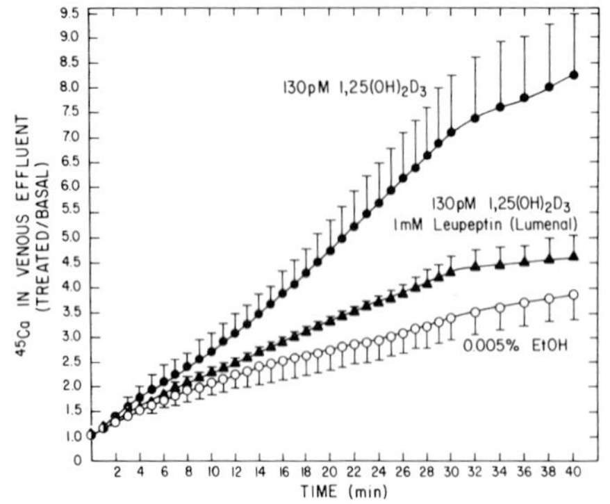

Fig. 2: Transport of ^{45}Ca in chick duodena perfused with 130 pm 1,25(OH)$_2$D$_3$ (P) = 0.05 to 0.04, relative to controls at 20-40 min) and inhibition by leupeptin (P > 0.1 to 0.2, relative to controls at 20-40 min).

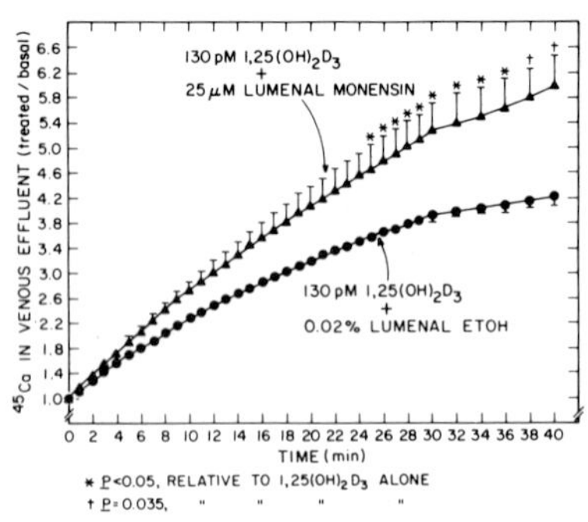

Fig. 3: Transport of ^{45}Ca in duodena vascularly perfused with 1,25(OH)$_2$D$_3$ and enhancement by 25 µM monensin (P > 0.5 to 0.035, relative to 1,25(OH)$_2$D$_3$ alone at 25-40 min).

In an attempt to assess the contribution of vesicular flow through the Golgi, vehicle or 25 µM monensin was added to the lumenal medium. Subsequent vascular perfusion with 1,25(OH)$_2$D$_3$ resulted in a monensin-enhanced ^{45}Ca transport (Fig. 3). In control perfusions, monensin had no effect (data not shown). These seemingly paradoxical results were later found to correlate well with enhanced release of AcP from isolated intestinal cells treated with monensin and 1,25(OH)$_2$D$_3$ *in vitro*, and lack of effect of monensin in the absence of the seco-steroid (Table 1).

Table I. Monensin-enhanced release of acid phosphatase activity from isolated intestinal cells treated with 130 pM 1,25(OH)$_2$D$_3$ *in vitro*

		ACID PHOSPHATASE (nmols/min/mg cell protein)			
EXPERIMENT	TREATMENT min:	0	10	20	30
1	1,25(OH)$_2$D$_3$[a]	1.38	1.57	1.22	1.12
	1,25(OH)$_2$D$_3$ +M[b]	1.33	1.56	1.52	2.20
2	1,25(OH)$_2$D$_3$[a]	1.80	1.75	1.67	1.85
	1,25(OH)$_2$D$_3$ +M[b]	1.65	1.99	1.85	2.16
3	1,25(OH)$_2$D$_3$[a]	1.58	2.45	2.59	3.03
	1,25(OH)$_2$D$_3$ +M[b]	1.94	3.28	3.12	3.27
(Av % OF CONTROL		103	119	119	127)
4	Control[a]	1.62	1.38	1.75	2.20
	Control +M[b]	1.62	1.60	1.82	1.96
5	Control[a]	1.22	1.24	1.33	1.94
	Control +M[b]	1.23	1.40	1.39	1.73
(Av % OF CONTROL		101	114	104	89)

[a] Received an equivalent volume of vehicle
[b] 25 µM monensin (M)

References:

1. Jande, S. S. and Brewer, L. M. (1974) Z. Anat. Entwickl.-Gesch. 144, 249-265.
2. Davis, W. L. , Jones, R. G. and Hagler, H. K. (1979) Tiss. Cell. 11, 127-138.
3. Nemere, I. and Szego, C. M. (1981) Endocrinology 108, 1450-1462.
4. Nemere, I. and Szego, C. M. (1981) Endocrinology 109, 2180-2187.
5. Nemere, I., Yoshimoto, Y. and Norman, A. W. (1984) Endocrinology 115, 1476-1483.
6. Szego, C. M. (1974) Rec. Prog. Hormone Res. 30, 171-233.
7. Collot, M., Louvard, D. and Singer, S. J. (1984) Proc. Natl. Acad. Sci., U.S.A. 81, 788-792.
8. Putkey, J. A., Spielvogel, A. M. Sauerheber, R. D., Dunlap, C. S. and Norman, A. W. (1982) Biochim. Biophys. Acta. 688, 177-190.

EFFECTS OF VITAMIN D INTAKE UPON MINERAL UTILIZATION, INTESTINAL CaBP AND PHOSPHATASES IN PIGS FED A PHYTIC PHOSPHORUS DIET.

A. POINTILLART, N. FONTAINE and M. THOMASSET,
Nutrition CNRZ-INRA, Jouy-en-Josas and INSERM U.120 Le Vésinet. France.

Introduction

The diets of pigs usually contains at least two thirds of phosphorus in the form of phytates. Phytic phosphorus utilization is not well understood. High phytate-P diets are known to decrease calcium absorption and to provoke mineral metabolism disorders such as hypocalcemia, hypercalciuria, hypophosphatemia and decreased bone mineralization. Two intestinal enzymes, alkaline phosphatase (AP) and phytase, which are vitamin D-sensitive, could be involved in phytic P-absorption. The effects of dietary vit.D upon the two intestinal phosphatases, CaBP, Ca and P metabolism and hormonal control in pigs fed high phytate diets are reported here.

Material and methods

Fourteen D-depleted growing pigs (plasma $25OHD_3$ levels: 1.7 ± 0.1 ng/ml) were divided into 2 groups fed the same cereal-meal basal diet : 0.6% P, of which 80% is phytic, and 0.6% Ca. One group (+D) was supplemented for one month with vit.D_3 (1000 IU/kg diet) while the other was not (-D). Plasma concentrations of Ca, inorganic P, PTH, vit.D metabolites and plasma AP activity were determined 2 weeks prior to the experiment, 4 days and 2 weeks later and at slaughter. Twenty cm segments of proximal, mid and distal duodenum, mid-jejunum, distal ileum, proximal cecum and colon were collected at slaughter to evaluate CaBP contents and both phosphatase activities. A 10-day balance was carried out on both groups to measure Ca and P absorption, urinary and fecal excretions and retention. Fibula and tibia were removed to determine bone mineral contents, weight, length and density (X-rays). Most of the above determinations have been previously described (1).

Results

Table 1. Calcium (and phosphorus) balances (g/day)

	Intake	Absorbed	Urinary	Retained
-D	5.7(5.1)	0.8(1.3)	0.4(0.07)	0.5(1.2)
+D	6.7(5.9)	3.7*(2.4*)	0.6(0.05)	3.1*(2.4*)

* $P < 0.01$, t test +D vs -D

In +D pigs, Ca-absorption and P-absorption were 4 and 2 times higher, respectively, than those of -D pigs (table 1). Tibia density, length and weight, spongy bone (tibial metaphysis) calcium, whole fibula Ca were greater in +D pigs. The vit.D supplementation progressively increased plasma Ca and Pi levels, but much more rapidly and drastically plasma levels of 25OHD and $1,25(OH)_2D$, which reached maximal values 2 weeks after introducing +D diet. In -D pigs plasma Ca, 25OHD, $1,25(OH)_2D$ decreased whereas plasma alk. phosphatase activity and PTH level increased.

Unexpectedly, there was no effect of D-supplementation upon the two mucosal enzymes, alk. phosphatase and phytase, whatever the segment

Vitamin D. A Chemical, Biochemical and Clinical Update

tested (table 2). Vit.D supplementation increased the CaBP content of all intestinal segments ; the effect was greater in jejunum (X12) ileum (X4) cecum (X7) and colon (X4) than in proximal or distal duodenum (X2, +D vs -D) (table 2).

Table 2. Intestinal CaBP and phosphatase activities

	Duodenum[1]	jejunum	ileum	cecum	colon
CaBP, µg/mg mucosal protein					
-D	14.4 (18.8)	1	0.5	0.9	1
+D	33.6*(37.1*)	12.5*	2.1*	6.8*	4.1*
A.P. (and phytase) mIU/mg mucosal protein					
-D	70(0.7)	240(0.9)	100(0.4)	10(0.7)	10(0.6)
+D	90(0.8)	250(1.2)	130(0.6)	10(0.6)	12(1.0)

1 proximal (and distal) : CaBP, mid : phosphatases. * $P < 0.01$ -D vs +D

Discussion

Vitamin D supplementation improves phytate P absorption in pigs, as it does in chicks (2) and rats (3). However, as in rats fed phytic P diets (4), the increased phytate P-absorption is not related to intestinal phosphatase activities. Thus, in pigs in contrast to rats (3) or birds (2), both intestinal alkaline phosphatase and phytase seem to be independent of vitamin D status. Nevertheless, this is in agreement with previous results in D-deficient (5) or D-replete pigs (1). Vit.D-improved Ca-absorption might be related to the increase in intestinal CaBP content as was also shown in pigs fed low Ca-diets (6). This increased D-dependent CaBP agrees with the increased plasma $1,25(OH)_2D$ levels as classically reported (7). In addition, the very low 25OHD values found in -D pigs (0.2-0.4 ng/ml) coexisting with fairly high values of $1,25(OH)_2D_3$ (65-84 pg/ml) suggest an increased renal 1α hydroxylase activity, as already demonstrated in vit.D-deficient pigs (8). This is also supported by the very high levels of plasma $1,25(OH)_2D_3$ observed in +D pigs (initial values X 1.6-3.3). In -D pigs, decreased bone scores might result from both bone decreased formation and increased resorption as shown by greatly reduced Ca and P retentions and increased PTH secretion.

References

1. Pointillart, A., Fontaine, N., and Thomasset, M. (1984) Nut. Rep. Intl. 29, 473-483.
2. Davies, M., Ritcey, G., and Motzok, I. (1970) Poultry Sci., 49, 1280-1286.
3. Roberts, A. and Yudkins, J. (1961) Brit. J. Nutr. 15, 457-471.
4. Moore, R. and Veum, T. (1983) Nut. Rep. Intl. 27, 1267-1275.
5. Pointillart, A., Jay, M.E., and Fontaine, N. (1985) Jour. Rech. Porcine en France, 17, 463-472.
6. Thomasset, M., Pointillart, A., Cuisinier-Gleizes, P., and Guéguen, L. (1979) Ann. Biol. anim. Bioch. Biophys. 19, 769-773.
7. Wasserman, R., Taylor, A., and Fullmer, C. (1974) Biochem. Soc. Spec. 3, 55-74.
8. Littledike, E.T., and Engström, G. (1984) Calcif. Tissue Int. 36, 518.

PHOSPHATE–BINDING PROTEIN FROM KIDNEY AND INTESTINE BRUSH–BORDER MEMBRANE

H.Debiec, R. Lorenc

Child's Health Center, 04-736 Warsaw, Al,Dzieci Polskich 20, Poland

Introduction. The existence of Na^{+}gradient-dependent phosphate / Pi / transport in the kidney and intestinal brushborder membrane/B B M/ is a well established phenomenon /1,2/. However, the transport system per se still remains largely uncharacterized. In rabbit kidney BBM a low molecular weight proteolipid that binds Pi has been demonstrated /3/Previously we have isolated from rat kidney BBM proteolipid fraction that specifically binds Pi. Our data indicated that a sulfhydryl and a lysyl residue are required both for the Na^{+} - dependent Pi uptake into brush-border membrane vesicles and for the binding of Pi by the proteolipid fraction. This evidence suggests that proteolipid may be involved in the Pi transport mechanism in the kidney BBM.It is also possible that a similar proteolipid exists in intestinal BBM and is responsible for Pi transport.Therefore. we tried to isolate purify and characterize the proteolipid from rabbit kidney and intestinal BBM.

Methods . BBM were prepared from renal cortex and intestinal mucosa by the magnesium precipitation method and differential centrifugation. Proteolipids from these membranes were extracted with chloroform: methanol 2 : 1 and precipitated by diethyl ether. The obtained precipitate is later refered as crude proteolipid. The dependence of Pi-binding by the crude proteolipid on Pi concentration was tested and kinetic parameters were calculated. The influence of lysyl and sulfhydryl resudues on the Pi-binding activity of the crude proteolipid were tested by using an aminoreactive reagent 2,4,6 trinitrobenzene sulfonate / TNBS / and a sulfhydryl reagent 5,5 dithiobis-2-nitrobenzoic acid / DTNB /. The crude proteolipid was preincubated for 30 min with 0.5 mM TNBS or DTNB before measuring the Pi binding activity. In order to determine whether a lysyl or sulfhydryl residue is present at the binding site, the time course of chemical modification of the proteolipid by TNBS and DTNB in the presence of Pi was measured spectrophotometrically. The partially delipidated on Sephadex LH-20 proteolipid was dissolved in Hepes-NaOH buffer pH 7.8 with or without Pi. Then TNBS or DTNB were added and the increase in absorbance at 346 nm or 412 nm, respectively were monitored continously. In the next step of experiment the crude proteolipid from the kidney and intestine were purified by chromatography on a Extrelute /Kisielghur/ column.The column was eluted with the following sequence of solvents. chloroform,.methanol 20 . 1 , chloroform : methanol 10 : 1, chloroform : methanol 1:1 , methanol. Pi-binding activity was determined by the partition test in an aqueous organic system/ 3/. Protein content was estimated by the Lowry method modified by Lees and Paxman /4/.Protein composition of the active proteolipid fraction eluted from the column was analyzed by polyacrylamide gel electrophoresis.Gels contained. 6M urea, 9.6%aerylamide 0.3:bisacrylamide and 0.1%SDS and were stained with silver nitrate.The presence of lipids in these active fractions was checked by thin-layer chromatography/TLC/on Silicagel ,using chloroform: methanol: water 80:25:4 as eluent. Lipids were visualized with phosphomolybdic acid spray.

Results and Discussion The crude proteolipid isolated from the kidney and from the intestine brush-border membrane show a high affinity for phosphate. The 0.5 for Pi binding by the crude proteolipid from kidney and intestine was estimated as 12,5 uM and 17.8 uM respectively. DTNB inhibited Pi binding by the kidney and intestine proteolipids up to 45%, whereas TNBS within the range 80-90%. The time course of chemical modification of the sulfhydryl residues of the proteolipid by DTNB in the presence of Pi was not significantly different from that in its absence.However, a marked protection of lysyl residues by Pi against the TNBS modification was observed.It indicates that lysyl residues are essential for the binding of Pi by the proteolipid both from the kidney and intestine.

Separation of the crude proteolipid on two active components was achieved by Extrelute chromatography. The elution profiles of the kidney and intestine proteolipid were similar. The first active fraction of proteolipid was eluted with chloroform: methanol 10: 1 , the second one with chloroform. methanol 1:1. Urea SDS polyacrylamide gel electrophoresis of the protedipid from the active fraction shows a single with molecular weight of about 15.500 for intestine and about 3000 for kideny. The second active fraction on the contrary shows a double band near molecular weight of 67000 irrespective of origin.

Vitamin D. A Chemical, Biochemical and Clinical Update

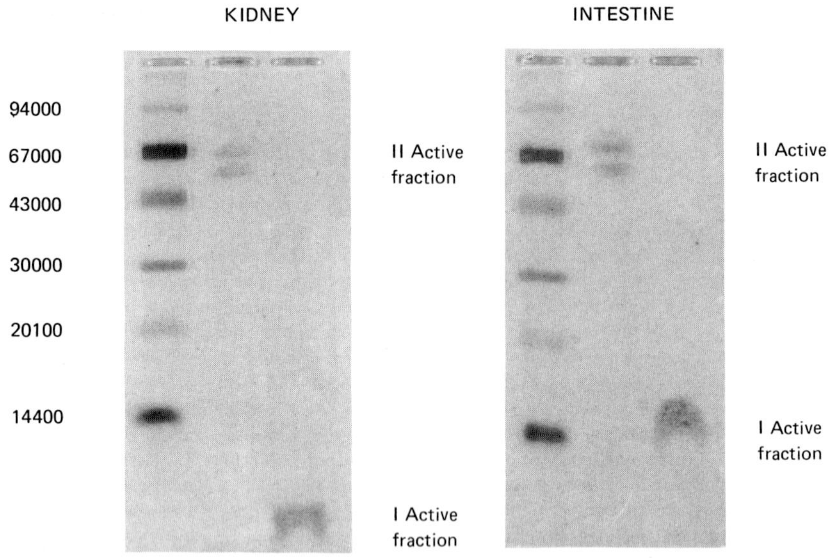

Fig. 1. Polyacrylamide gel electrophoresis of proteolipid fractions.

Analysis on TLC indicated that the main lipids associated with the low molecular weight proteolipids are cardiolipin and phosphatidylethanolamine while with the high molecular weight proteolipid phophatidylinositol. The different mobilities in electrophoresis of low molecular weight proteolipids from the kidney and intestine indicate on organ specificity for these Pi transporters. However, it should be mentioned that the amount of associate lipids can alter the electrophoretic mobility. since the difference could be a function of the contaminating lipids.

On the basis of the presented data we conclude that both kidney and intestine BBM contain the low molecular weight and high molecular weight proteolipids that can be involved in Pi transport.

Literature.

1.Danisi, G.,Murer,H., Straub,R.W./1984/Am. J.Physiol. 246:G 180-186.
2. Chang, L.Sactor, B. 1981J.Biol.Chem. 256: 1556-1564.
3. Kessler, R.J.Vaughn, D.A.Fanestil, D.D./1982/J.Biol.Chem. 257: . 14311-14317.
4.Lees, M.B.,Paxman, S. 1972 Anal.Biochem 47' 184-192.

Acknowledgment The work parltly supported by Wroclaw Politechnics under R.I.9.

POSSIBLE ROLE OF CALMODULIN IN $1,25(OH)_2D_3$-MEDIATED CALCIUM TRANSPORT IN PERFUSED DUODENA FROM NORMAL CHICKS: STUDIES ON THE EFFECT OF TRIFLUOPERAZINE.

Y. Yoshimoto, I. Nemere and A. W. Norman
Dept. Biochem., Univiversity of California, Riverside, CA 92521, USA

Introduction:

Using an *ex vivo* duodenal perfusion system in vitamin D-replete chicks we have previously reported (1) that low doses of $1,25(OH)_2D_3$ when added to the vascular perfusate but not intestinal lumen can significantly stimulate (within 14 mins) an increase in the transfer of ^{45}Ca from the intestinal lumen to the vein. This "rapid effect" of $1,25(OH)_2D_3$ is not inhibited by actinomycin D but is inhibited by leupeptin and colchicine. Here we report the effects of trifluoperazine (TFP), a putative calmodulin antagonist, on basal and $1,25(OH)_2D_3$ mediated intestinal calcium transport in two systems; (i) in an *ex vivo* intestinal perfusion system in -D and +D chicks; and (ii) *in vivo* in both chicks.

Materials and Methods:

White leghorn cockerels were obtained on the day of hatch and maintained on a vitamin D-supplemented diet for 5-8 weeks to prepare normal vitamin D_3-replete chicks. When vitamin D-deficient chicks were employed, they were initially raised for 2 weeks on the vitamin D-suplemented diet and then placed on a rachitogenic diet for an additional 4-6 weeks. *Ex vivo* intestinal perfusion (1) and intestinal calcium absorption (ICA) (2) were done, respectively, as described previously.

Results:

Addition of 0.5 mM TFP to the perfusate had no effect on basal ^{45}Ca transport but decreased significantly ($P<0.001$) the 450 pM $1,25(OH)_2D_3$-mediated stimulation of intestinal lumen perfusate ^{45}Ca transport; further TFP (0.5-1 mM) in the lumen was without effect in an *ex vivo* perfusion system in +D chicks (Fig. 1). When TFP was administered (10 mg/100 g B.W. i.m.) before *ex vivo* perfusion, there were significant decreases in the absolute Ca transport 1 hr to 7 days after treatment in +D birds (Fig. 2) and in -D birds (data not shown). But basal and $1,25(OH)_2D_3$-mediated ^{45}Ca transport were significantly increased 1 hr after TFP treatment and their TFP given 1.5 hr to 7 days before perfusion resulted in inhibition of the $1,25(OH)_2D_3$-mediated ^{45}Ca transport in +D birds (Fig. 3). In -D chicks, TFP given 2-48 hours before perfusion significantly decreased ^{45}Ca transport ratios. In other experiments where ^{45}Ca absorption is measured *in vivo* in chicks, we have noted that prior treatment with TFP (10 mg/100 g B.W. i.m.) significantly enhances the ICA in both vitamin D-replete and D-deficient birds within 1-3 hours and inhibits it in both groups 24 hours before experiments (Fig. 4).

Conclusions and Discussion:

The experiments reported here confirm that TFP, a calmodulin antagonist, has an apparent biphasic effect on intestinal calcium transport. That is in the early periods after TFP treatment it increases intestinal calcium transport and later inhibits this process (3,4). Only vascular

Vitamin D. A Chemical, Biochemical and Clinical Update

perfusion with TFP, and not TFP in the lumen, abolished the rapid lumen-to-vascular effluent effect of 1,25$(OH)_2D_3$ on ^{45}Ca transport, which suggests that TFP acts mainly at the serosal side of the intestine where the Ca^{++}, Mg^{+}-ATPase is thought to be located (5). However, TFP inhibits both calmodulin-sensitive and calmodulin-insensitive ATPase activities in rat red blood cells (6) and also interacts with many cellular proteins (7). So results from calmodulin-inhibitor study must be interpreted judiciously.

Fig. 1.

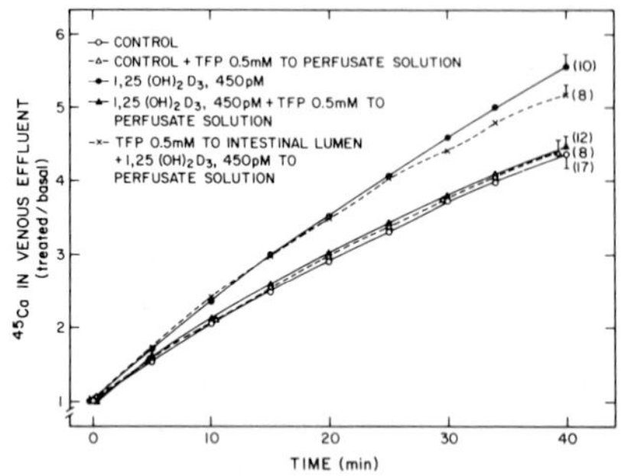

Fig. 2.

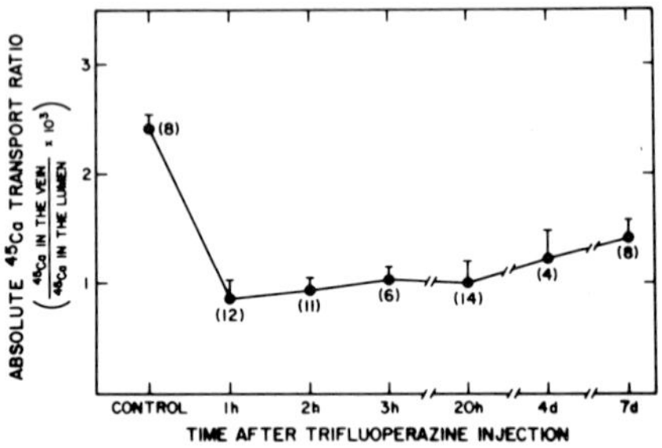

Fig. 3.

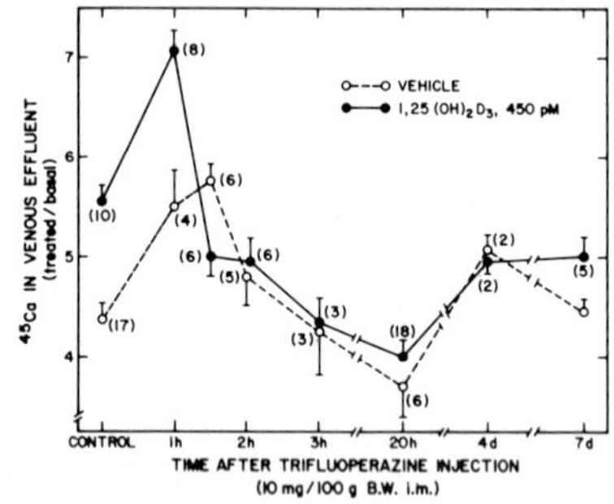

Fig. 4.

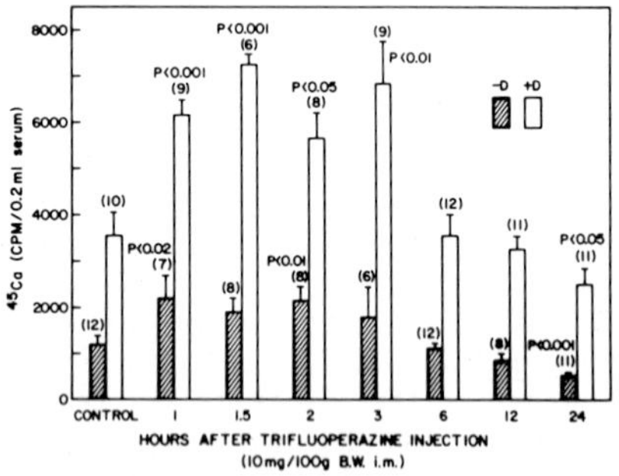

References:

1. Nemere, I., Yoshimoto, Y. and Norman, A.W. (1984) Endocrinology 115, 1476-1483.
2. Hibberd, K. A. and Norman, A. W. (1969) Biochem. Pharmacol. 18, 2347-2355.
3. Favus, M. J., Angeid-Backman, E., Breyer, M. D. and Coe, F. L. (1983) Am. J. Physiol., 244, G111-115.
4. Roche, C., Pansu, D. and Bronner, F. (1984) "Epithelial Calcium and Phosphate Transport: Molecular and Cellular Aspects" in Bronner, F. and Peterlik, M. (eds), 261-265.
5. Ghijsen, W. E. J. M., De Jong, M. D., and Ven Os, C. H. (1982) Biochim. Biophys. Acta. 689, 327-336.
6. Luthra, M. G. (1982) Biochim. Biophys. Acta. 692, 271-277.
7. Moore, P. and Dedman, J. (1982) J. Biol. Chem. 257, 9663-9669.

DUODENAL AND JEJUNAL TRANSPORT OF CALCIUM AND PHOSPHORUS: REGULATORY MECHANISMS

H. JUNGBLUTH and U. BINSWANGER
Section of Nephrology, Department of Internal Medicine, University of Zurich, Switzerland

Introduction:

1,25 $(OH)_2D_3$ does not affect intestinal calcium (Ca) and inorganic phosphorus (Pi) absorption in all segments of the intestine to the same extent (1). Thus, the duodenum is the most responsive segment in terms of increased Ca absorption, whereas Pi absorption is mainly stimulated in the jejunum (1). In contrast to absorption, much less is known about Ca and Pi secretion. We therefore investigated the effects of endogenously stimulated 1,25 $(OH)_2D_3$ synthesis as induced by dietary Pi depletion of the animals (2) as well as exogenous application of the hormone.

Methods:

Male albino Sprague-Dawley rats were obtained as weanlings (50 g) and were prepared by feeding a 0,3 % phosphorus diet for 2 weeks, followed by either the same diet [C] , a low phosphorus diet (0,03 % Pi [-P]), a low phosphorus diet plus EHDP treatment (40 mg/kg/d x 4 s.c. [-P -D]) or the same treatment but supplementation with 1,25 $(OH)_2D_3$ (500 pmol x 2 i.v. [-P -D +D]). Experimental diets were given for 3 weeks. By means of a modified Ussing technique (3) under short-circuit conditions unidirectional intestinal transport was investigated in vitro using ^{45}Ca and ^{32}Pi as tracers. Krebs-Ringer-Bicarbonat solution was used as buffer containing 1,25 mM Ca, 2,4 mM Pi and 11 mM D-Glucose. Fluxes of Ca and Pi were calculated using the method reported by Schultz and Zalusky (4). Net fluxes resulted from the difference of simultanously estimated mucosal-to-serosal (Jms) and serosal-to-mucosal fluxes (Jsm). Positive fluxes indicate net absorption and negative data indicate net secretion. For each piece of gut, tissue conductance (Gt) was monitored. Total plasma Ca was analyzed by atomic absorption spectrophotometry.

Results:

The results of duodenal and jejunal Ca and Pi transport as well as corresponding tissue conductance and plasma Ca concentration in vivo are demonstrated in the table. MS fluxes of Ca and Pi were correlated in the duodenum (r = 0,85) and changed according to the 1,25 $(OH)_2D_3$ status of the animals. SM transport of Ca and Pi was correlated as well (r = 0,92 and r = 0,89 for duodenum and jejunum, respectively). There was a close relationship between Jsm for Ca (Fig. 1) and Pi and tissue conductance in the duodenum (r = 0,75 and r = 0,77), and in the jejunum (r = 0,52 and r = 0,63). Furthermore tissue conductances of duodenum (Fig. 1) and jejunum were correlated to plasma Ca concentration in vivo (r = 0,82 and r = 0,50).

Conclusions:

Duodenal and jejunal MS transport of Ca and Pi changed in parallel dependent on the 1,25 $(OH)_2D_3$ status of the animal. In contrast, SM transport for Ca and Pi was independent from 1,25 $(OH)_2D_3$ but related to tissue conductance. The latter was dependent upon plasma Ca concentration in vivo. The mechanism by which Ca might alter tissue conductance is unclear.

Data suggest that changes in plasma Ca concentration in vivo might induce alterations of epithelial properties and by this way modulate diffusional ion fluxes.

References:

1. Walling, M.W. (1977) Am. J. Physiol. 233: E 488 - E 494.
2. Hughes, M.R., Brumbaugh, P.F., Haussler,M.R., Wergedal,J., Baylink,D.J. (1975) Science 190: 578 - 579.
3. Walling, M.W., Rothman, S.S. (1969) Am. J. Physiol. 217: 1144-1148.
4. Schultz, S.G., Zalusky, R. (1964) J. Gen. Physiol. 47: 567 - 584.

Intestinal Ca and Pi transport, tissue conductance (Gt), and plasma calcium concentration in vivo in experimental groups (M±SEM)

DUODENUM										
Expl Group	n	Calcium Flux ($nmol\cdot cm^{-2}\cdot h^{-1}$) Jms	Jsm	Jnet	Phosphorus Flux ($nmol\cdot cm^{-2}\cdot h^{-1}$) Jms	Jsm	Jnet	Gt ms ($mS\cdot cm^{-2}$)	Gt sm	plasma calcium (mmol/l)
C	9	86,9± 7,1	11,6±0,7	75,3± 6,9	13,8±2,7	20,7±0,9^{m}	-6,9±3,5	16,6±1,1	16,9±0,8	2,46±0,04
-P	9	168,6±15,4	17,8±1,1	150,9±14,9	43,7±5,5	36,1±3,9^{n}	7,6±4,8	23,5±1,2	23,4±1,4	2,83±0,07
-P -D	9	74,2±5,9	29,1±3,5	45,1± 5,8	12,7±1,0	45,6±7,5^{o}	-32,9±7,4	25,6±1,2	25,4±1,1	3,34±0,10
-P -D +D	8	218,6±5,8	30,1±1,4	188,5±6,3	60,6±6,3	56,7±4,7^{p}	3,9±9,3	33,1±1,3	33,0±1,5	3,95±0,07

JEJUNUM										
Expl Group	n	Calcium Flux ($nmol\cdot cm^{-2}\cdot h^{-1}$) Jms	Jsm	Jnet	Phosphorus Flux ($nmol\cdot cm^{-2}\cdot h^{-1}$) Jms	Jsm	Jnet	Gt ms ($mS\cdot cm^{-2}$)	Gt sm	plasma calcium (mmol/l)
C	10	19,1±1,0	25,9±2,3	-6,8±1,9	51,4±4,7	42,9±4,4	8,6±4,7	26,8±1,4	25,8±2,3	2,45±0,04
-P	10	38,0±3,8	24,5±2,3	13,5±4,5	67,9±6,4	34,7±4,1	33,2±6,1	25,4±1,1	26,5±2,7	2,78±0,06
-P -D	8	14,4±1,6	33,3±4,6	-18,9±3,3	45,5±13,8	42,8±7,5	2,5±6,8	28,7±2,5	28,7±2,6	3,51±0,09
-P -D +D	8	37,7±5,4	35,7±3,1	2,0±4,3	66,7±9.1	58,0±4,3^{o}	8,7±10,6	36,6±1,7	35,5±1,4	3,92±0,14

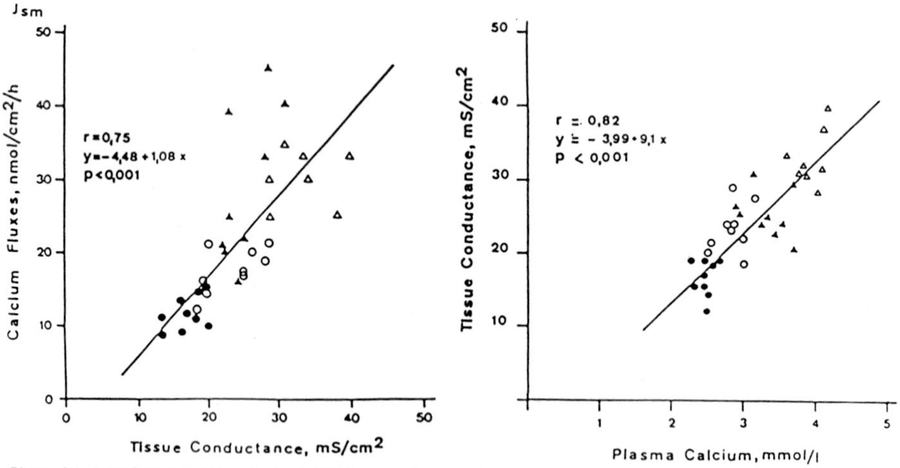

Figure 1: Correlation between duodenal SM fluxes of Ca and tissue conductance (left side) and between tissue conductance and plasma Ca levels in vivo (right side).
C: ●, -P: ○, -P -D: ▲, -P -D +D: △

RELATIVE IMPORTANCE OF BRUSH-BORDER AND BASOLATERAL CALCIUM TRANSPORT IN RAT DUODENUM

C.ROCHE, C.BELLATON, D.PANSU, and F.BRONNER.
EPHE and INSERM U 45 Lyon France and University of Connecticut Health Center Farmington Conn. USA

Purpose: the effect on duodenal Ca transport of trifluoperazine (TFP) a calmodulin inhibitor and theophylline,an inhibitor of alkaline phosphatase was explored at several levels of tissue and cell organization in order to determine the relative importance of brush-border-and basolateral membranes during the active Ca absorption.

Methods: two-month old rats were used.Everted duodenal sacs were instilled and incubated with a fructose buffer containing 0.25 or 1mM $CaCl_2$ with 45Ca.Ca transported at the serosal side and 45Ca of the tissue (Ca in transit) were measured after 90 min.Brush-border membrane vesicles (BBMV) and basolateral membrane vesicles (BLMV) were preincubated as described in (1) and (2).For Ca uptake vesicles were preincubated for 30 min with or without the drug, then incubated for 1 to 15 min with 1mMCa for BBMV or 0.1mM Ca for BLMV. BBMV uptake was corrected from the binding observed at 4°C,BBMV uptake was corrected from the uptake observed in the absence of ATP. Ouabain insensitive Ca Mg ATPase and ouabain sensitive Na K ATPase were measured according to (3)in the presence of 4mM EDTA. Low affinity Ca ATPase was measured according to (4) in the presence of 0.1 mM $CaCl_2$ and 2mM ouabain.

Results : are presented in Tables 1 and 2 and expressed as percentage of the control values.TFP induced a dose-dependent decrease of Ca transported without change of Ca in transit, suggesting an inhibition of extrusion. In BBM alkaline

		TRIFLUOPERAZINE CONCENTRATION							
	Ca Added	0	1μM	10μM	25μM	50μM	100μM	200μM	400μM
EVERTED SACS									
Ca transported	1mM	100 %	–	–	–	83 %	40 %	10 %	-14%
Ca in transit	1mM	100 %	–	–	–	99 %	81 %	56 %	46%
BRUSH-BORDER MEMBRANES									
Ca uptake by BBMV	1mM	100 %	125 %	106 %	–	116 %	78 %	—	—
Alk.Phosphatases	no	100 %	100 %	100 %	100 %	94 %	88 %	—	—
BASOLATERAL MEMBRANES									
Ca uptake by BLMV	0.1 mM	100 %	100 %	50%	—	0%	—	—	—
Ouabain insensitive CaMg ATPases	no	100 %	100 %	79 %	49%	33%	13%	—	—
Ouabain sensitive Na^+K^+ ATPases	no	100 %	100 %	100 %	87 %	10%	0%	—	—

Table 1 : Inhibiting effects of Trifluperazine .Results are expressed as per cent of the values obtained in the absence of TFP . Each experiment counted 4 to 8 assays for each concentration. Results for vesicular uptake are those observed after 15 min of incubation.

Vitamin D. A Chemical, Biochemical and Clinical Update

phosphatase and Ca uptake were unchanged .In BLMV Ca uptake was reduced by 50% in the presence of 10 µM and totally suppressed by 50 µM TFP.Inhibition of Ca Mg ATPase was dose-dependent from 10 to 100 µM.The inhibition was located at the serosal side and could be related with the inhibition of Ca Mg ATP ase.Theophylline inhibited in a dose-dependent manner alkaline phosphatase in both BBM and BLM and inhibited the low affinity Ca ATPaseas previously described by Ghijsen et al. (4).Ca uptake by the whole tissue and by vesicles were not significantl y decreased.The inhibition of transport in everted sacs of adult rats remains to be explained , Ca transport was not inhibited inyoung rats nor when duodenal sacs were incubated in the presence of cAMP or db cAMP.

	THEOPHYLLINE CONCENTRATION								
	Ca Added	0mM	0.3mM	0.6mM	1.25mM	2.5mM	5mM	10mM	20mM
EVERTED SACS									
Ca transported adult rats	0.25mM	100 %	–	–	–	92 %	52%	56%	26%
Ca transported young rats	0.25mM	100 %	–	–	98 %	91 %	96 %	98 %	–
BRUSH-BORDER MEMBRANES									
Ca uptake by BBMV	0.25mM	100 %	–	–	70 %	78 %	78 %	–	–
Alk.Phosphatases	1 µM	100 %	–	–	97 %	98 %	101 %	87 %	–
	1 mM	100 %	11	9	7	4	0	0	–
BASOLATERAL MEMBRANES									
Ca uptake by BLMV	0.1 mM	100 %	–	83 %	80 %	85 %	82 %	–	–
Alk.Phosphatases	no	100 %	–	–	66 %	44%	24%	10%	–
Low affinity Ca ATPases	0.1 mM	100 %	71 %	71 %	60 %	51%	46%	33%	–
Ouabain insensitive									–
CaMg ATPases	no	100 %	–	–	79 %	71 %	71 %	67 %	–
Ouabain sensitive									
Na^+K^+ ATPases	no	100 %	–	–	84 %	89 %	78 %	83 %	–

Table 2 : Inhibiting effects of Theophylline. Same legend as in Table 1.

Conclusion: The complete inhibition of alkaline phosphatase does not inhibit cellular Ca entry.

The active transcellular Ca transport involves events largely located at the basolateral membrane;

Support by NATO,the Kroc Foundation and the University of Connecticut Research Foundation.

References

(1) Miller,A;III, Bronner,F.,(1981) Biochem.j. 196,991-401.
(2) Miller,A.III, Bronner,F.,in Epithelial Calcium and Phosphat te Transport :Molecular and Cellular Aspects, Eds Bronner F. and Peterlik M. (1984) p 281-288.
(3) Quigley,J.P. ,Gotterer G.A.,(1967) Biochim.Biophys.Acta 173, 456-468.
(4)Ghijsen, W.E.J.M.,DeJong M.D.,Van Os C.H. (1980) Biochim. Biophys. Acta 599, G111-G115.

$1,25(OH)_2D_3$-MEDIATED INTESTINAL CALCIUM ABSORPTIVE MECHANISM: DIRECT INHIBITION BY LEAD IN DUODENAL ORGAN CULTURE

R.A. CORRADINO
Department/Section of Physiology, New York State College of Veterinary Medicine, Cornell University, Ithaca, New York 14853, USA

Previous work has indicated that vitamin D may stimulate intestinal lead absorption in intact, vitamin D-deficient animals (1-3), and that dietary lead interferes with intestinal calcium absorption (4,5). In those studies, it could not be determined, on the one hand, whether vitamin D-repletion directly stimulated an intestinal transport mechanism resulting in increased lead absorption, nor, on the other hand, whether lead ingestion directly inhibited the intestinal calcium transport mechanism. The present studies, using the embryonic chick, duodenal organ culture model system, were undertaken first, to assess the possibility that vitamin D (as $1,25(OH)_2D_3$) does directly stimulate lead absorption, and, second, to determine if lead directly inhibits the vitamin D-mediated, calcium absorptive mechanism.

METHODS

The techniques for duodenal organ culture (6,7), for assay of the vitamin D-induced calcium-binding protein (CaBP), and for measurement of calcium (as ^{45}Ca) absorption were performed exactly as previously described (6). Lead (as ^{203}Pb) absorption was assessed by the same procedures used for calcium absorption.

RESULTS AND DISCUSSION

Incubation of duodena in the presence of $1,25(OH)_2D_3$ (50 nM) resulted in a 2-2.5 fold increase in ^{45}Ca absorption, as expected, but, no effect of $1,25(OH)_2D_3$ on ^{203}Pb absorption was observed (see table). ^{203}Pb absorption was linear over a 1-30 minute absorption period: the two regression lines, $\pm$ 1,25, passed through the origin, their slopes were statistically indistinguishable, and their correlation coefficients were greater than 0.99. These results are in contrast to *in vivo* studies and afford no support for a direct action of vitamin D on intestinal lead absorption. An indirect role of vitamin D on lead absorption *in vivo* seems more reasonable, possibly in terms of the correction of one or more of the manifold morphologic, compositional, or biochemical abnormalities of the vitamin D-deficient intestine, rather than a direct action on a specific mechanism capable of transporting lead.

The addition of stable lead to a phosphate-free culture medium (lead phosphate is highly insoluble) resulted in the inhibition of the synthesis of the $1,25(OH)_2D_3$-induced CaBP and the $1,25(OH)_2D_3$ stimulated absorption of ^{45}Ca. The range of lead concentration producing these inhibitory effects without generalized cytotoxicity was 1-10 µM: at 10 µM both measures were inhibited about 60%. These observations are in accord with *in vivo* results, but clearly demonstrate an inhibitory action of lead *directly* on the intestinal calcium absorptive mechanism. The *in vivo* studies did not permit such a determination.

At 10 µM stable lead concentration in the culture medium, inhibition of both $1,25(OH)_2D_3$-stimulated CaBP and ^{45}Ca absorption occurred as early as 12 hr after the start of culture. Although CaBP synthesis continued through the 48 hr culture period, the final concentration was only about 40% of that seen in the absence of lead.

Lead inhibition of CaBP synthesis was partially prevented by pre-incubation, or co-incubation, in the presence of 2.5-5 mM calcium in the culture medium (see table).

Vitamin D. A Chemical, Biochemical and Clinical Update

EFFECTS OF $1,25(OH)_2D_3$, LEAD, AND/OR CALCIUM IN THE CULTURE MEDIUM ON CABP BIOSYNTHESIS AND ^{45}CA OR ^{203}PB ABSORPTION

1st 24 hr Ca^{2+} (mM)	1st 24 hr Pb^{2+} (μM)	2nd 24 hr Ca^{2+} (mM)	2nd 24 hr Pb^{2+} (μM)	CaBP (μg/100 mg duodenum)	Absorption (% change from minus $1,25(OH)_2D_3$ control) ^{45}Ca	^{203}Pb
0.5	0	0.5	0	73 ± 9[a]	+144[a]	-
2.5	0	2.5	0	73 ± 6[a]	+104[a]	-
0.5	10	0.5	0	28 ± 5[b]	+ 51[b]	-
2.5	10	2.5	0	31 ± 5[b]	+ 45[b]	-
0.5	0	0.5	10	32 ± 4[b]	+ 59[b]	-
2.5	0	2.5	10	52 ± 3[c]	+ 66[b]	-
0.5	0	0.5	0	74 ± 6[a]	-	-1[a]
5	0	5	0	70 ± 8[a]	-	+8[a]
0.5	10	0.5	10	30 ± 4[b]	-	-1[a]
5	10	5	10	50 ± 12[c]	-	-10[a]

Values: mean ± S.E.; 6-8 duodena/treatment. Values in each column followed by the same superscript were not significantly different.

The absorption of lead (as ^{203}Pb) was unaffected by the presence of $1,25(OH)_2D_3$, lead (10 μM) or calcium (0.5-5 mM) in the culture medium. These results, and other aspects of the present studies are summarized in the table.

Together, these studies provide no support for a direct action of vitamin D on intestinal lead absorption, nor for a direct influence of calcium or lead status of the intestine on lead absorption. In vivo results to the contrary are most likely explicable on the basis of indirect actions of vitamin D on overall intestinal cellular function, and/or an alteration of vitamin D metabolism with consequent indirect actions on the intestine.

The present results do provide strong support for a direct inhibitory action of lead on the vitamin D-mediated, intestinal calcium absorptive mechanism. The consequences of lead ingestion might, therefore, include an initial intestinal insult -inhibition of calcium absorption with consequences relating to calcium deprivation - in addition to what appears to be the unimpaired absorption of lead, with all its well known toxic effects.

REFERENCES

1. Smith, C.M., DeLuca, H.F., Tanaka, Y. and Mahaffy, K.R. (1978) J. Nutr. 108, 843-847.
2. Mykkanen, H.M. and Wasserman, R.H. (1982) J. Nutr. 112, 520-527.
3. Mykkanen, H.M. and Wasserman, R.H. (1981) J. Nutr. 111, 1757-1765.
4. Smith, C.M., DeLuca, H.F., Tanaka, Y. and Mahaffey, K.R. (1981) J. Nutr. 111, 1321-1329.
5. Edelstein, S., Fullmer, C.S. and Wasserman, R.H. (1984) J. Nutr. 114, 692-700.
6. Corradino, R.A. (1973) J. Cell Biol. 58, 64-78.
7. Corradino, R.A. (1984) in Vitamin D: Basic and Clinical Aspects, (Kumar, R., ed.) pp. 325-341, Martinus Nijhoff, Boston.

Renal Actions of D Metabolites

VITAMIN D AND STEROIDS : RAPID EFFECT ON MEMBRANE POTENTIAL OF HYPERTROPHIC CHONDROCYTES AND PROXIMAL TUBULAR CELLS.

A. EDELMAN, M. GARABEDIAN, T. ANAGNOSTOPOULOS and S. BALSAN.
INSERM U.192-CNRS UA.583, Hôpital des Enfants-Malades, 75015 Paris, FRANCE.

Evidence has been recently gathered supporting non-genomic action of 1,25-dihydroxyvitamin D (1,25-$(OH)_2D_3$). This vitamin D metabolite has been shown : (i) to act even in the absence of cell nucleus, e.g., on isolated brush border membrane vesicles in vitro (1,2) ;(ii) to act rapidly on intestinal cells,by modifying within 60 minutes the membraneous phospholipid content (3,4) or even by changing, within less than 30 minutes, the alkaline phosphatase activity and calcium transport (5,6) ; (iii) to alter within 1 min cell membrane potential (V_m) of intact cells studied in vitro (7,8).

Electrophysiological techniques are particularly suitable for the study of rapid changes of the membrane properties in intact cells without altering the cellular metabolism. We applied these techniques to different types of cell, i.e. rabbit hypertrophic chondrocytes, Necturus renal proximal cells and frog myocytes, to assess :

1/ whether different tissues are sensitive to vitamin D derivatives,

2/ whether different vitamin D derivatives affect to the same extent cell membrane potential in a given tissue,

3/ which are the mechanisms involved in this rapid action.

METHODS :

Most investigations were performed on the proximal tubule of Necturus kidney,in vivo, a model largely used for the study of ion transport (Fig.1). The proximal tubule was impaled with a

Vitamin D. A Chemical, Biochemical and Clinical Update

double barreled micropipette and perfused through one barrel with a Ringer's solution containing the metabolite solvent ; the second barrel was filled with the same solution plus the studied metabolite. The solutions could be easily exchanged in the tubular lumen by means of a gravimetric system. A single pipette was used to suck up the perfusate. Membrane potential was continuously monitored during luminal perfusion with control and metabolite-supplemented solutions, by means of a single microelectrode. In this way, each studied cell served as its own control with regard to cell membrane potential

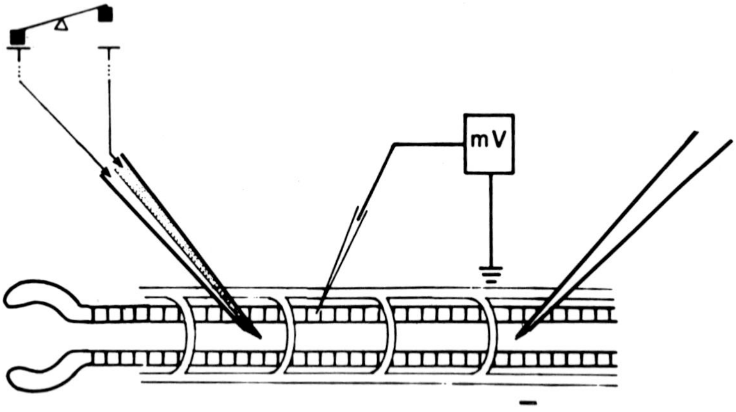

Figure 1: Schematic representation of the proximal tubule from Necturus kidney with the double barreled micropipette (on the left), the microelectrode (center of the figure), and the single pipette (on the right).

Figure 2 shows a typical recording of cell membrane potential and its variation during addition of 1,25-$(OH)_2D_3$ (A) or vitamin D_3 (B) in luminal perfusion fluid ; the experiment was performed in the Necturus kidney. Black bars indicate the period of exposure to 1,25-$(OH)_2D_3$ or vitamin D_3 ; in ordinate : V_m, in abcissa : the time. Both molecules were applied at 10^{-10}M.

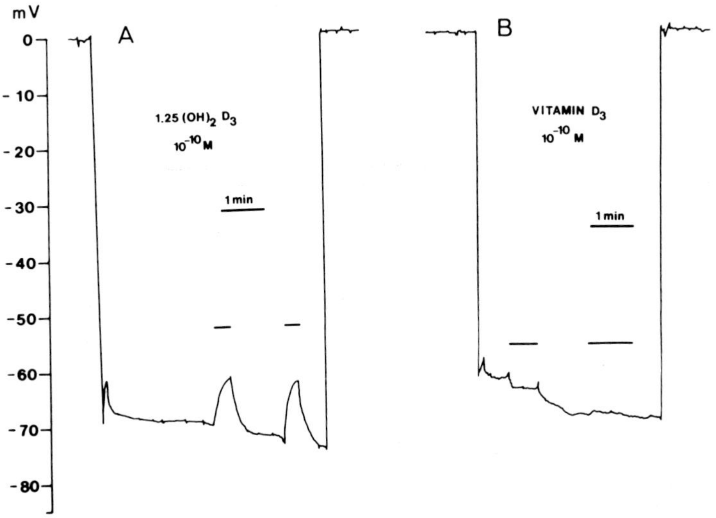

Figure 2

It is seen that 1,25-$(OH)_2D_3$ elicited a rapid and reversible membrane potential depolarization (cell potential became less negative as compared to reference). By contrast vitamin D_3 did not change of V_m.

1.CELL SPECIFICITY :

To test whether the observed membrane potential changes are specific of presumptive target cells for vitamin D we investigated the response of three tissues (Table 1). The rapid effects of vitamin D_3 and of three of its metabolites were searched for in rabbit cartilage, proximal tubule of Necturus kidney and frog muscle. 1,25-$(OH)_2D_3$ (10^{-10}M) and 24,25-$(OH)_2D_3$ (10^{-10}M) induced rapid changes of membrane potential in cartilage and proximal tubule but not in muscle. Therefore the effect seems to be specific of certain cells. Moreover the cell responses depend on the form of vitamin D studied : vitamin D_3 itself had no effect on membrane potential and 25-$(OH)D_3$ was only active in proximal tubular cells.

TABLE 1 : EFFECTS ON MEMBRANE POTENTIAL

METABOLITES / CELL TYPES	1,25-$(OH)_2D_3$ (10^{-10}M)	24,25-$(OH)_2D_3$ (10^{-10}M)	25-$(OH)D_3$ (10^{-10}M)	VITAMIN D_3 (10^{-10}M)
CARTILAGE (RABBIT)	+	+	0	0
PROXIMAL TUBULE (NECTURUS)	+	+	+	0
MUSCLE (FROG)	0	0	0	0

In other experiments (not shown) we demonstrated that the effect of vitamin D metabolites also depended on the absolute value of cell membrane potential. Therefore only those cells displaying a resting membrane potential of approximately -70 mV and which responded by a depolarization to the addition of vitamin D metabolites will be considered hereafter.

2.STEROID SPECIFICITY :

At $10^{-10}M$ $1,25-(OH)_2D_3$ but also $25-(OH)D_3$, $24,25-(OH)_2D_3$ and $5,6$-Trans-$25-(OH)D_3$, were able to modify the membrane potential(V_m) of tubular proximal kidney cells. By contrast 1α $-(OH)D_3$ and vitamin D_3 were ineffective (Fig.3).

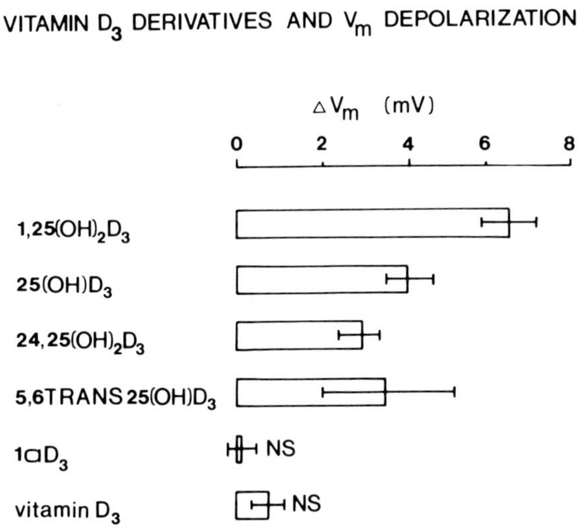

Figure 3

The effects of 5 steroids has also been tested (not shown): testosterone ($10^{-8}M$), œstradiol ($10^{-8}M$),and 19-diol cholesterol ($10^{-10}M$), but neither aldosterone ($10^{-8}M$) nor cholesterol ($10^{-10}M$) affected V_m.

Clearly, all the molecules, endowed with an OH-group on carbon seventeen or on the lateral chain attached to this carbon,modified the kidney cell membrane potential, and $1,25-(OH)_2D_3$ was the most potent among tested molecules.

3.POSSIBLE MECHANISM OF THE RAPID ACTION OF 1,25-$(OH)_2D_3$:

Cell membrane potential is a function of transmembrane ion distribution, partial ionic conductances and active transport. Assuming, in our experimental conditions, that the addition of metabolites in the luminal perfusate does not change luminal ion activities or basolateral active transport, and since change of intracellular ion activities are unlikely, V_m changes reflect most probably changes in ionic conductance(s). In kidney proximal tubules, the partial membrane conductances of sodium and chloride are negligible. Thus the observed V_m changes should reflect modifications of the potassium conductance. Nevertheless we verified that Na and Cl ions are not involved in the metabolite-induced V_m change by replacing Na by TMA (an impermeant cation) or Cl by methylsulfonate (an impermeant anion) in the perfusing solutions. 1,25-$(OH)_2D_3$ addition during such lumen perfusions altered V_m to the same degree as in NaCl containing solutions. Investigation of the 1,25-$(OH)_2D_3$ rapid action in the presence of barium (2 mM),a known blocker of the potassium conductance, or in the presence of quinine (0.5 mM), a putative inhibitor of Ca-dependent K conductance, suggests that 1,25-$(OH)_2D_3$ depolarizes the membrane by blocking the potassium conductance via a calcium dependent mechanism.

CONCLUSIONS :

Secosteroids and steroids which possess an OH-group on C_{17} or on the lateral chain attached to C_{17} are able to rapidly affect (in less than 1 minute) the membrane potential of hypertrophic chondrocytes and proximal tubular cells. 1,25-$(OH)_2D_3$ was the most potent among tested molecules. The low metabolite concentration required to obtain this effect in intact cells, as well as the observation of steroid specificity and cell specicity suggest that these changes may reflect a physiological rapid action of 1,25-$(OH)_2D_3$.

REFERENCES

1. Elgavish, A., Rifkind J. and Sactor, B. (1983) J. Memb. Biol. 72, 85-91.
2. Kurnik, B.R.C. and Hruska, K. (1984) Amer. Soc. Nephr. (Abst) 21A.
3. Matsumoto, T., Fontaine, O. and Rasmussen, H. (1981) J. Biol. Chem. 256 ; 3354-3360.
4. Wasserman, R.H., Brindak, M.E., Meyer, S.A. and Fullmer, C.S. (1982) Proc. Natl. Acad. Sci. USA 79, 7939-7943.
5. Bachelet, M., Ulmann, A., and Lacour, B. (1979) Biochem. Biophys. Res. Comm. 89 ; 694-700.
6. Nemere, I. and Norman, A.W. (1983) Fed. Proceed. (Abst) 42, 1179.
7. Druëke, T., Lacour, B., Lucas, P.A., Karsenty, G., and Mauriat, F. (1985) Sixth Workshop on Vitamin D, Merano, (Abst) Italy, 138.
8. Edelman, A., Thil, C.L., Garabédian, M., Anagnostopoulos, T., and Balsan, S. (1983) Biochem. Biophys. Acta 732, 300-303.
9. Edelman, A., Thil, C.L., Garabédian, M., Plachot, J.J., Guillozo, H., Fritsch, J., Thomas, S.R., and Balsan, S. (1985) Mineral and Electrolyte Metab. (in press).

BONE RESORPTION AND Ca^{+} MOVEMENTS IN BONE CELLS : EFFECTS OF A VITAMIN D_3 METABOLITE, A Ca INHIBITOR AND A CALCIUM AGONIST

By S.Y. LY, C. REBUT-BONNETON
U 18 INSERM, 6 rue Guy Patin 75010 Paris-France

Introduction

The relationship between bone resorption and Ca movements in bone cells was investigated using an inductor of bone resorption, 1,25 dihydroxycholecalciferol ($1{,}25(OH)_2D_3$), a calcium channel inhibitor, diltiazem and a Ca agonist, ionophore 23187. Bone resorption was measured in organ culture of mice calvaria and Ca movements were detected in a suspension of bone cells

Materials and Methods

Organ culture : the general method has previously been described in detail (1). The skeletons of newborn mice were prelabelled with ^{45}Ca (1 µCi) by subcutaneous injection 4 days before experiment. Separated calvaria were explanted on stainless grid at the interface of the 5 ml BGJb medium and the gas (CO_2 = 5 p. cent in air). Quantification of the change in bone resorption after treatment was done by counting the ^{45}Ca in the media from both treated and untreated paired explants by liquid scintillation. Bone radioactivity was measured after calcium solubilisation in formic acid 0,5 %. For the in vivo/in vitro experiment, 6-day-old mice prelabelled with ^{45}Ca were prepared as described above. They were injected with control solution or the test substance. At death, pairs of half explants were prepared from each mouse and one bone of each pair was cultivated at 4° C. Thus, the amount of cell mediated resorption was calculated from the difference in isotope release between 37° cultivated half minus 4° cultivated half.

Isolation of bone cells : bone cells were isolated from long bones of three day-old rat pups ; bones were minced in small pieces, then scrapped ; the larger pieces or calcified matrix were eliminated by simple filtration through a 35 µm/nylon net to remove large pieces. The cells were suspended overnight in minimum essential medium (HMEM, Flow laboratories) containing 10 % heat-inactivated calf serum and antibiotics.

Efflux studies : cells were incubated over night with medium labelled with ^{45}Ca (0,1 µCi/2 x 10^6 cells) ; products were added to the culture 2 hours before the efflux experiment. At short time intervals the cells suspension was removed from control and experimental tubes, the ^{45}Ca cells was extracted by 0,5 % formic-acid solution and cell associated supernatant radioactivity were determined using Picofluor 15 scintillation fluid (Packard). The results were used to calculate the initial radioactivity associated to the cells at time 0 (Co) as well as the one remaining in the cells at each time point (Ct). The cellular exchangeable calcium pool was calculated from the specific radioactivity of the medium used to label the cells

Results

In vitro effects of diltiazem in organ culture :

Diltiazem alone did not inhibit the ^{45}Ca release from untreated bone. In concentration above 5 µmol/l diltiazem was found to inhibit the release of ^{45}Ca stimulated by $1.25(OH)_2D_3$. This inhibition was not lineat in concentrations (Talbe 1). No significant differences were observed between 20, 50 and 100 µmol/l.

Table 1 : In vitro effects of diltiazem on bone resorption induced by $1.25(OH)_2D_3$ (1.2 nmol/l during 48 hours in culture. (resorption is expressed as percentage of bone isotope).

$$R = \frac{^{45}Ca \text{ release by } 1.25(OH)_2D_3 \text{ alone}}{^{45}Ca \text{ release by } 1.25(OH)_2D_3 + \text{diltiazem}}$$

Diltiazem concentration		R	
2 µmol/l	=	1.04 ± 0.10	(6)
5 µmol/l	=	1.25 ± 0.19**	(6)
20 µmol/l	=	1.39 ± 0.29***	(7)
50 µmol/l	=	1.27 ± 0.15*°	(7)
100 µmol/l	=	1.23 ± 0.24**	(7)

Results are mean ± SD (Number of experimentation in parenthesis)
Significantly different from the percent release by $1.25(OH)_2D_3$ alone :
**$p < 0.01$ (Student's t test), *° $p < 0.005$, *** $p < 0.001$

In vivo/in vitro effects of diltiazem : cell mediated bone resorption, as measured by the in vivo/in vitro technique, was not affected by diltiazem injection mice 18 hours before sacrifice (from 20 to 100 nmol/g, body weight). Cell mediated bone resorption was higher in the $1.25(OH)_2D_3$ treated group (Table 2) (0.480 pmol/g body weight) than in the control one. Injection of 100 nmol/g body weight of diltiazem simultaneously with $1.25(OH)_2D_3$, 18 hours before sacrifice, decreased significantly the increase in bone resorption due to $1.25(OH)_2D_3$. Calcium and phosphorus plasma concentrations remained as elevated in the $1.25(OH)_2D_3$ + diltiazem-treated group as in the $1.25(OH)_2D_3$ alone group. Injection of diltiazem 100 nmol/g body weight, 2 hours before sacrifice, when $1.25(OH)_2D_3$ had been injected 16 hours before was ineffective in reducing bone resorption (bone cells mediated resorption 14.77 ± 3.26 and 14.64 ± 3.31 %).

Table 2 : In vivo/in vitro effects of diltiazem on $1.25(OH)_2D_3$ increased bone resorption (treatment 18 hours before sacrifice).

	Resorption due to cellular activity %	
Control	7.74 ± 1.6	(11)
$1.25(OH)_2D_3$ 0.480 pmol/g body weight	14.0 ± 3.4	(7)
$1.25(OH)_2D_3$ + diltiazem 100 nmol/g body weight	10.1 ± 1.9*	(10)

Results are mean ± SD. Number of experimentation in parenthesis. *$p < 0.05$ between $1.25(OH)_2D_3$ + diltiazem and $1.25(OH)_2D_3$ alone.

Efflux experiments : The data, plotted on a logarithmic scale against time, revealed two different efflux rates. The analysis of ^{45}Ca efflux was done according to the equation derived from Borle (2). $^{45}Ca^{2+}$ efflux from bone cells can be adequatly described by the sommation of two exponential terms $E = Ae^{-k_A t} + Be^{-k_B t}$: k_A and k_B are the slopes of the curves and A, B the intercepts. The system of cells can be represented by compartments in a series. Our system was a closed one since the Ca which was released from the cells into medium could be rensed for a further influx.

	Rate constants of ^{45}Ca efflux(mn^{-1} (k_B))
Control	0,0033 ± 0,0016
$1,25(OH)_2D_3$ 10 ng/10^6 cells	0,0048 ± 0,000811*
diltiazem 40 nmol/10^6 cells	0,0039 ± 0,00024
$1,25(OH)_2D_3$ + diltiazem	0,0053 ± 0,00134*
Control	0,00244 ± 0,00055
ionophore	0,003813 (n = 3)*
ionophore + diltiazem	0,00393 (n = 3)*

*$p < 0.010$ compared with control, the results are mean $\pm$ SD

Discussion

$1,25(OH)_2D_3$ was shown to increase the rate of exchange of $^{45}Ca^{2+}$ between the slow and fast compartment in bone cells as it was demonstrated earlier (3). Some discrepancies exist between the results obtained in bone resorption and those in calcium movements : $1,25(OH)_2D_3$ effects on bone resorption which are antagonized by diltiazem are not modified on $^{45}Ca^{2+}$ kinetic in bone cells. It seems therefore difficult to hypothesize a simple relationship between bone resorption and Ca^{2+} movements in bone cells.

References

1 - Reynolds J.J., Holick M.F., Deluca H.F. (1973) Calcif. Tiss. Res. 12 : 295-301.
2 - Borle A., (1969) J. Gen. Physiol. 53 : 57-69.
3 - Edlam Y., Szydel N., Harell A. (1980) Mol. Cell. Endocrinol. 19 : 263-273.

SECONDARY HYPERPARATHYROIDISM, BUT NOT AMINOACIDURIA, IN VITAMIN D DEFICIENCY IS DEPENDENT ON DIETARY CALCIUM AND PHOSPHATE INTAKE.

S. Dabbagh, R.W. Chesney and E. Slatopolsky.
Department of Pediatrics, The University of Wisconsin, Madison, WI. USA and Department of Medicine, Washington University School of Medicine,
St. Louis, MO. USA

Introduction:

Secondary hyperparathyroidism is known to accompany vitamin D deficiency and this elevation of hormone secretion is known to be responsible for phosphaturia and resultant hypophosphatemia (1). Generalized aminoaciduria is also found and has been attributed to the influence of PTH on the proximal nephron (2). However, the possibility that vitamin D deficiency, per se, has a direct, PTH-independent effect has not been included. The purpose of this study is to examine the metabolic changes related to vitamin D deficiency in the rat and to determine how changes in the dietary intake of Ca and PO_4 influence both urinary PO_4 and amino acid excretory patterns.

Methods:

Sprague Dawley rats were placed in a room with tungsten lights and fed a series of vitamin D deficient diets for 4-6 weeks: (1) very low Ca (VLC) (0.02%); Low Ca (LC)(0.47%); high Ca (HC)(2.5%) and very low PO_4 (VLP) (0.1%). Control rats received 1.1% Ca and 0.74% PO_4 with 2.5µg vitamin D. A separate group of VLC rats received 500 pmoles of $1,25(OH)_2D$ for 2 days before sacrifice (VLC + 1,25). On the day before sacrifice rats were placed in metabolic cages for 14 to 17 hours with free access to water. Blood and urine were collected. Ca and PO_4 were measured by conventional methods. After deproteinization, amino acids were determined by amino acid analyzer in plasma, renal cortex and urine. Immunoreactive PTH was measured by Dr. Slatopolsky using a specific rat anti-PTH antibody.

Results:

All vitamin D deficient diets resulted in secondary hyperparathyroidism except the VLP diet where PTH was not different from normal. Plasma Ca was reduced (4.8 ± 0.1 to 8.8 ± 0.1 mg/dL) compared to control and VLP. Plasma PO_4 was significantly elevated in VLC, VLC + 1,25 and LC, and reduced in HC and VLP, where tubular reabsorption of PO_4 exceeded 99%. Urinary Ca/Cr was 0.72 ± 0.11 in VLP rats vs. under 0.05 in all other groups; VLC + 1,25 rats had significant reduction of Ca/Cr at 0.01 ± 0.01. Urinary cAMP excretion was elevated in all diets except VLP.

Vitamin D. A Chemical, Biochemical and Clinical Update

All vitamin D-deficient rats developed a generalized aminoaciduria irrespective of diet, but the levels of the following amino acids were unchanged in plasma and renal cortex; taurine, aspartic acid, threonine, serine, glutamine methionine, proline, glutamic acid, citrulline, glycine and alanine. No correlation between urinary taurine or proline and plasma Ca or PO_4 was found. Similarly, no correlation between aminoaciduria and iPTH and urinary cAMP was evident.

The acute (2 day) administration of $1,25(OH)_2D$ to rats receiving the VLC diet corrected phosphaturia, led to lower urinary Ca excretion and a rise in serum Ca, but did not alter the generalized aminoaciduria.

Discussion:
In this study of vitamin D deficiency, wide variation in the levels of calcium and phosphate were utilized. The intake of Ca and PO_4 had direct effects on the serum levels of Ca, PO_4 and iPTH as would be anticipated. In addition, dietary Ca and PO_4 intake also influenced urinary Ca, PO_4 and cAMP excretion. For example, the VLP diet was associated with a low iPTH level, a normal serum calcium, hypercalcuria, hypophosphatemia and no urinary PO_4 excretion as has been shown previously (3). However, despite these changes and the lack of a rise in iPTH, the generalized aminoaciduria is not different than that found after ingesting the VLC or LC diet.

Thus, the mechanism underlying the defect in the renal handling of amino acids in vitamin D-deficiency remains unclear, since it appears in all diets despite Ca or PO_4 content. Suggested mechanisms including hypercalcitoninemia (4) and alteration in the membrane phospholipid content (5) should be explored since vitamin D deficiency induces a generalized aminoaciduria which appears to be independent of creatinine clearance, plasma and tissue amino acid levels, iPTH, plasma Ca and PO_4 and urinary cAMP.

References:

(1) Arnaud, C., Glorieux, F. and Scriver, C.R. (1972) Pediatrics 49: 837-840.
(2) Fraser, D., Kooh, S.W. and Scriver, C.R. (1967) Pediatr. Res. 1:425-435.
(3) Brautbar, N., Walling, M.W. and Coburn, J.W. (1979) J. Clin. Invest. 63:335-341.
(4) McInnes, R.R. and Scriver, C.R. (1980) Pediatr. Res. 14:218-223.
(5) Fontaine, O., Matsumoto, T., Goodman, D.B.P. and Rasmussen, H. (1981) Proc. Natl. Acad. Sci. USA 78:1751-1754.

THE ANTIPHOSPHATURIC ACTION OF 25(OH)VITAMIN D3 IN RATS: EVIDENCE AGAINST INVOLVEMENT OF CYTOSOLIC MICROTUBULES

M.M. Friedlaender, H. Wald and M.M. Popovtzer

Hadassah University Hospital, Jerusalem, Israel

Previous studies from this laboratory have demonstrated that 25(OH)vitamin D_3, 1,25$(OH)_2$ vitamin D_3 and 24,25$(OH)_2$ vitamin D_3 acutely suppress the phosphaturic action of parathyroid hormone (PTH) and that this is associated with decreased urinary cAMP excretion (1,2). In vitro PTH-induced activation of renal adenylate cyclase is also suppressed by vitamin D. The mechanism of this effect is unknown. The rapidity of onset and its inhibition by cycloheximide suggest that post-transcriptional protein synthesis is involved (3). Since cytosolic microtubules are thought to be involved in several renal intracellular processes including the action of PTH and of vasopressin (4), we have examined whether colchicine, an alkaloid which disrupts cytosolic microtubules, might interfere with the action of vitamin D. Since colchicine has also been shown to abolish the rapid "membranophilic" action of vitamin D in the intestine (5), these experiments might examine whether such a mechanism may also be involved in the renal antiphosphaturic action of vitamin D.

Methods

Acute clearance studies were performed on male Sabra rats, 48 hours post-parathyroidectomy (PTX) and after pretreatment with i.p. colchicine in 0.45% sodium chloride, 0.25 mg 16 hours prior to the experiment and 0.25 mg prior to anaesthesia. Control rats received i.p. 0.45% sodium chloride. In vitro studies on renal cortical membrane fractions prepared from similar PTX, colchicine pretreated rats were performed.

Results

Colchicine pretreatment was associated with an increase in fractional excretion of phosphorus (FE_{Phos}) in PTX rats from 0.029 ± 0.005 to 0.102 ± 0.011 ($p<0.001$). Parathyroid hormone (PTH) infusion at 3 U/hour caused a rise of FE_{Phos} to the same maximum in both colchicine-pretreated and control rats.

In PTX PTH-infused rats pretreated with colchicine, addition of 25(OH)vitamin D_3 40 U/hour caused a decrease in FE_{Phos} compared to similar control rats not receiving vitamin D (0.344 ± 0.022 vs. 0.235 ± 0.026, $p<0.005$). Urinary cyclic AMP decreased similarly from 93.2 ± 11.0 to 69.0 ± 9.5 pmol/min ($p<0.025$). In vitro examinations of adenylate cyclase activity showed that colchicine pretreatment per se reduced the activity of basal adenylate cyclase with PTH 1 U/ml, and with PTH 1 U/ml $\pm$ 25(OH) vitamin D 1 µg/ml in the incubation medium. However, vitamin D had a similar significant inhibitory effect on PTH-induced adenylate cyclase activation both after colchicine pretreatment (activity reduced from 7.60 ± 0.45 to 4.47 ± 0.33 pmol cAMP/mg protein/min, $p<0.001$, Δ - 40.8 ± 4.1%) and without colchicine pretreatment (from 10.63 ± 0.69 to 5.93 ± 0.29 pmol cAMP/mg protein/min, $p<0.001$, Δ - 43.3 ± 3.2%). Thus whilst colchicine may partially blunt the adenylate cyclase mediated effect of PTH, it neither affects the antiphosphaturic action of vitamin D in vivo, nor the inhibitory affect of vitamin D on PTH-induced adenylate cyclase activation in vitro.

Conclusion

The antiphosphaturic action of 25(OH)vitamin D_3 does not appear to be mediated via cytosolic microtubules or by a rapid "membranophilic" action.

References

1. Friedlaender, M.M., Kornberg, Z., Wald, H. and Popovtzer, M.M. (1983) Am. J. Physiol. 244: F674-F678.
2. Popovtzer, M.M., Robinette, J.B., DeLuca, H.F., and Holick, M.F. (1974) J. Clin. Invest. 53: 913-921.
3. Brezis, M., Wald, H., Shilo, R. and Popovtzer, M.M. (1983) Pflugers Arch. 398: 247-252.
4. Dousa, T.P., Duarte, C.G. and Knox, F.G. (1976) Am. J. Physiol. 231: 61-65.
5. Norman, A.W., Nemere, I., Williams, G. and King, M. (1984) In: Endocrine Control of Bone and Calcium Metabolism. Elsevier Science Publ. pp. 316-319.

AN APPROACH TO THE PURIFICATION OF CYTOCHROME P_{450} FROM CHICK KIDNEY MITOCHONDRIA.

JOHAN-CHANH M. TRAN and HELEN L. HENRY, Department of Biochemistry, University of California, Riverside, CA 92521, U.S.A.

Introduction:

The major circulating metabolite of vitamin D_3, 25-OH D_3, is converted to the active $1,25(OH)_2D_3$ and to $24,25(OH)_2D_3$ in kidney mitochondria by 1α-hydroxylase and 24-hydroxylase, respectively. It is known that 1α-hydroxylase is a mixed function oxidase, but it is not clear what the mechanism of 24-hydroxylase is. However, both hydroxylase activities appear to be cytochrome P_{450}-dependent. In vitamin D-deficient chicks, the level of 1α-hydroxylase is high while in D-sufficient chicks, the level of 1α-hydroxylase activity is diminished and 24-hydroxylase activity is elevated (1,2). Our goal is to study the mechanism of regulation of the hydroxylase activities. During the course of these studies, we found that under certain conditions of mitochondrial extraction, a metabolite other than $1,25(OH)_2D_3$ is produced.

Methods:

Kidney mitochondria in 30 mM sodium phosphate buffer, pH 7.4, were subjected to 6 mM CHAPSO (3-[cholamidopropyl dimethylammonio]-2-hydroxy-1-propane-sulfonate) extraction for 30 min at 4°C. The resulting supernatant was dialyzed against Tris-acetate (Tris-OAc) buffer pH 7.4 and was used for reconstitution assay. The assay included 50 µl of the dialyzed CHAPSO extract, 1 µM adrenodoxin (Adx), 0.18 µM adrenodoxin reductase (AR), 0.1 mM NADPH, 2 mM glucose-6-phosphate (G6P), 0.2 u/ml G6P-dehydrogenase and 4 x 10^{-7} M ^3H 25-OH D_3 in 0.5 ml 25 mM HEPES or 30 mM Tris-OAc buffer pH 7.4. Dithiothreitol (DTT), when present, was 0.1 mM. After incubation, the assays were subjected to lipid extraction. High pressure liquid chromatography (HPLC) was used to separate and quantitate the radioactive metabolites.

Results:

HPLC in 7% isopropanol/hexane (IPA/hex) of the products of incubating CHAPSO extract with ^3H 25-OH D_3 showed the presence of an unknown radioactive peak migrating in fractions 9 and 10, which we called peak Alpha (Fig. 1a). Compound Alpha was collected and rechromatographed on 2% isopropanol/dichloromethane (IPA/DCM). From this column, Alpha eluted in fractions 10 and 11 (Fig. 1b). Alpha was again collected from the 2% IPA/DCM column and rechromatographed on a 15% water/methanol column where it eluted in fractions 18 and 19 (Fig. 1c). These chromatographic profiles resembled those of cis-19-nor-10-oxo-25-OH D_3, a novel vitamin D metabolite observed by Simpson et al. (3) in a primary culture kidney cell from -D rats and by Lester et al. (4) in cultured dog kidney cells. Alpha production was optimal in Tris-OAc assay buffer containing no DTT (Fig. 2), and was not dependent on added Adx, AR or NADPH (Fig. 3). When the CHAPSO extract was incubated with ^3H 1,25-$(OH)_2D_3$, there was no production of Alpha (Fig. 4). This indicated that Alpha was not a metabolic product of $1,25(OH)_2D_3$. Mitochondrial extracts from vitamin D-deficient chicks produced less Alpha (14.8 ± 3.1 %) than did extracts from D-replete chicks (25.7 ± 2.2 %).

Vitamin D. A Chemical, Biochemical and Clinical Update

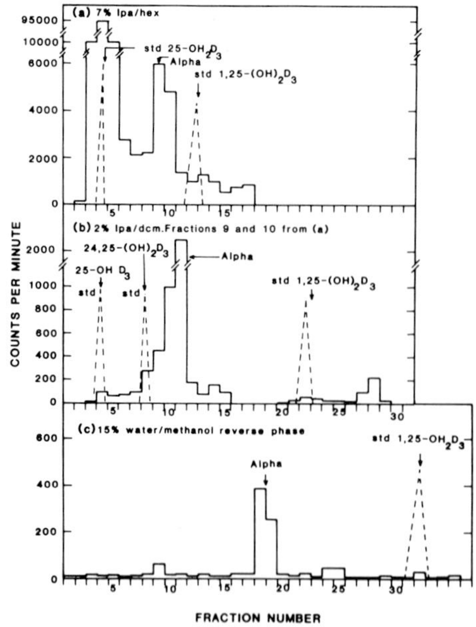

Figure 1. Chromatographic profile of the metabolites produced in the incubation of CHAPSO extract with ^3H 25-OH D_3 in Tris-OAc buffer.[^3H 25-OH D_3] was 4 x 10^{-7} M, 150 cpm/pmol. The dashed peaks indicate the elution positions of standard vitamin D metabolites. Fraction number: (a) and (b) 1.5 ml/0.5 min/fraction; (c) 1 ml/min/fraction.

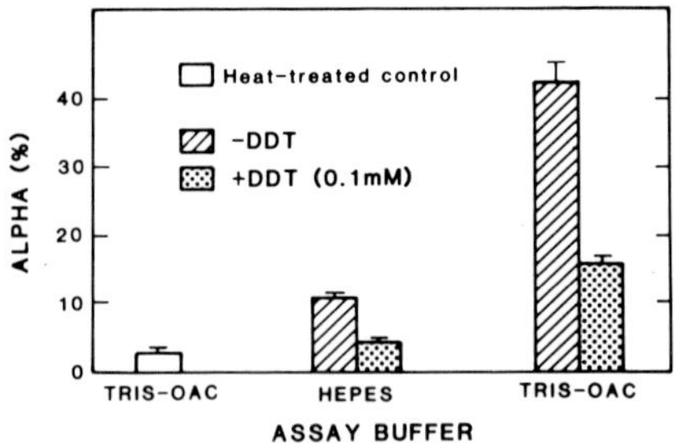

Figure 2. Alpha production as a function of assay buffer and the presence of dithiothreitol (DTT). The percentage represents the ratio of cpm as of Alpha to the total cpm recovered from HPLC, multiplied by 100. Values are the means ± SD, n = 3.

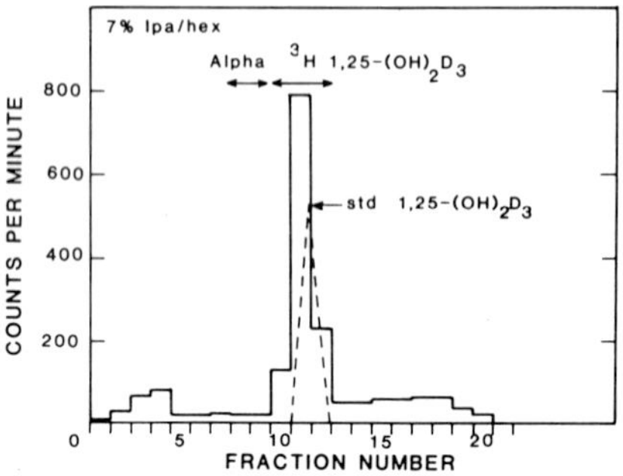

Figure 4. Chromatographic profile in 7% IPA/hex of the products of incubating the CHAPSO extract with ^3H 1,25$(OH)_2D_3$ as substrate. [^3H 1,25$(OH)_2D_3$] was 0.3 x 10^{-7} M, 420 cpm/pmol. The incubation was carried out in Tris-OAc buffer containing no DTT. Fraction number: 1.5 ml/0.5 min/fraction.

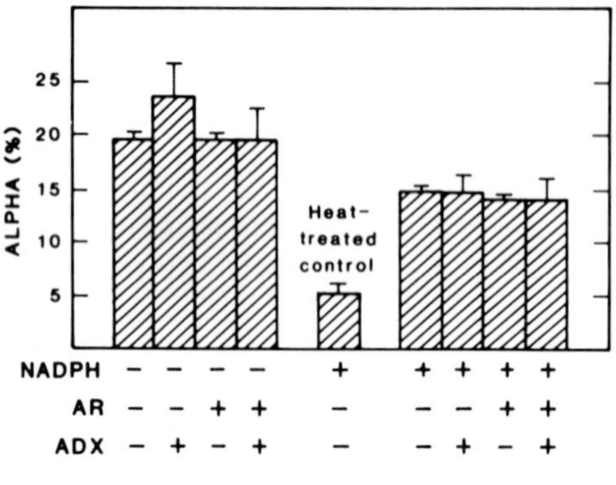

Figure 3. Dependency of Alpha production on adrenodoxin (Adx), adrenodoxin reductase (AR) and NADPH. The incubation was carried out in Tris-OAc buffer containing no DTT. Values are the means ± SD, n = 3.

1. Fraser, D. R. and Kodicek, E. (1970) Nature (London) 228:764-766.
2. Tanaka, Y., Lorenc, R. S. and DeLuca, H. F. (1975) Arch. Biochem. Biophys. 171:521-526.
3. Simpson, R. V., Wichmann, J. K., Paaren, H. E., Schnoes, H. F. and DeLuca, H. F. (1984) Arch. Biochem. Biophys. 230:21-29.
4. Lester, G. E., Horst, R. L. and Napoli, J. L. (1984) Biochem. Biophys. Res. Commun. 120:919-925.

Supported by USPHS Grant AM-21398.

EFFECT OF A SHORT-TERM TREATMENT WITH 1,25(OH)2D3 ON GLA PROTEIN IN HUMANS

R. Nuti, M. Galli, V. Turchetti, G. Righi and A. Caniggia
Institute of Clinical Medicine, University of Siena, 53100 Siena, Italy

The bone GLA protein (BGP) is a non-collagenous vitamin K dependent protein containing residues of gamma-carboxyglutamic acid; it is synthesized de novo in bone cells and found circulating in human blood. BGP may provide a more specific chemical index of bone turnover. Most of the evidence indicates that BGP is produced by the osteoblasts and reflects bone formation (1). It was demonstrated that both intracellular and serum BGP levels are increased by the active metabolite of vitamin D, 1,25(OH)2D3. The only study in man has been carried out by Gundberg et al. who have shown 1,25(OH)2D3 therapy to cause an increase in serum BGP in patients with rickets (2).

In order to answer the question if 1,25(OH)2D3 could directly influence in man the activity of osteoblasts, the effect of a short-term treatment with high dose of 1,25(OH)2D3 on serum levels of BGP was investigated.

Materials and methods

This study was carried out in eight healthy women, in two patients with Paget's disease of bone (one male and one female); their age ranged 21-65 yrs.
Synthetic 1,25(OH)2D3 was administrated orally at the dose of 2 µg/day for a period of ten days. Before and at the end of the study were evaluated the following parameters: serum GLA protein (radioimmunoassay procedure according to Price and Nishimoto, Immuno Nucl. Co.); plasma and 24h. urinary calcium (atomic absorption spectrophotometry, Perkin Elmer 2280); serum alkaline phosphatase, plasma and 24h. urinary phosphate, 24h. urinary hydroxyproline (standard methods). Paired Student's t tests were used in statistical analyses to examine the significance of differences.

Results and discussion

1,25(OH)2D3 treatment promoted in all normal subjects a statistically significant ($p < 0.01$) increase of serum levels of BGP, from basal value of 4.6 ng/ml ± 1.2 (mean ± SD) to 6.5 ng/ml ± 1.7 (Fig. 1). In two pagetic patients, the basal values of BGP were elevated (13 ng/ml and 22.1 ng/ml); after 1,25(OH)2D3 administration a noticeable increase of serum osteocalcin was also appreciated (15.4 ng/ml and 26.5 ng/ml). Fasting plasma calcium prior to the initiation of the therapy was in normal subjects 9.2 mg% ± 0.5; after 1,25(OH)2D3 a sustained increase (9.8 mg% ± 0.4) however not statistically significant, was noticed (Fig. 1). As it concerns 24h. urinary calcium, the mean basal value was in normal subjects 115 mg/24h. ± 63; a remarkable and significant increase (301 mg/24h. ± 104.6) was observed after the short-term treatment with 1,25(OH)2D3. Similar changes was appreciated in pagetic patients. The

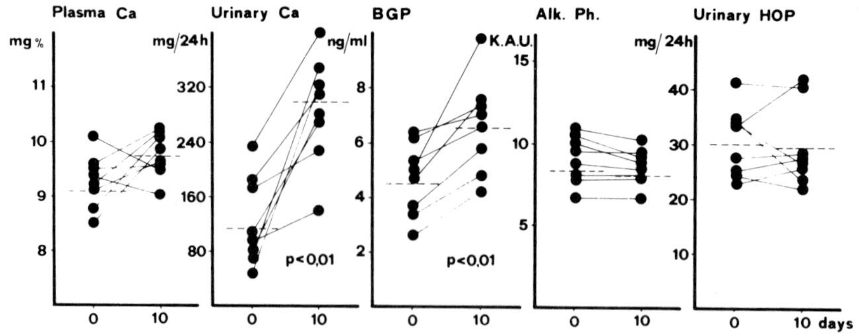

Figure 1. Changes in plasma calcium level, urinary calcium excretion (statistically significant), serum osteocalcin (statistically significant), serum alkaline phosphatase and urinary hydroxyproline (from the left) in normal subjects after 1,25(OH)2D3 administration.

serum alkaline phosphatase levels and the 24h.urinary excretion of hydroxyproline showed no change in normal subjects after 1,25(OH)2D3 administration (Fig. 1).

The efficacy of 1,25(OH)2D3 in restoring a normal intestinal calcium absorption had been demonstrated even in short-term studies (3,4). The results of the present paper concerning fasting plasma calcium and urinary calcium excretion must be considered as a consequence of the improved intestinal calcium transport. The finding that 24h. urinary hydroxyproline excretion was not influenced by the treatment rules out the possibility that osteoclast activity is stimulated by 1,25(OH)2D3. Animal studies indicate that increases in circulating osteocalcin are associated with new bone formation; it is also known that the protein is synthesized by the osteoblast. Otherwise BGP is a more sensitive index of osteoblast activity than alkaline phosphatase.

Our results carried out in healthy subjects demonstrate that 1,25(OH)2D3 is capable to promote an increase in BGP synthesis; this effect has been confirmed even in patients with Paget's disease, caractherized by a pathological target cell. The finding can be therefore interpreted as a consequence of osteoblast stimulation by the active vitamin D metabolite.

References:

1. Price, P.A. (1983) in Bone and mineral research (Peck, W.A., ed.), pp. 157-190, Excerpta Medica, Amsterdam.
2. Gunberg, C.M., Cole, D.E.C., Lian, J.B., Reade, T.M., Gallop, P.M. (1983) J. Clin. Endocrinol Metab. 56,1063-1067.
3. Caniggia, A., Vattimo, A. (1979) Clin. Endocrinol. 11, 99-103
4. Caniggia, A., Nuti, R., Loré, F., Vattimo, A. (1984) J. Endocrinol. Invest. 7,373-378.

INFLUENCE OF VITAMIN D STATUS ON THE ACTIVITY OF CARBONIC ANHYDRASE IN THE CHICK KIDNEY

J.DREWE, P.DIETSCH
Institut für Molekularbiologie und Biochemie,
Freie Universität Berlin, D-1000 Berlin 33, and
E.KECK
Medizinische Klinik C der Universität, D-4000 Düsseldorf, GFR

Introduction

Vitamin D deficiency in the chick leads to decreased cyclic AMP-dependent protein kinase activity in the kidney. This effect has not been found in other tissues. It is caused by increased concentrations of an endogenous inhibitor protein of the cyclic AMP-dependent protein kinase (1).
As had been shown by us (2), carbonic anhydrase (CA) is an interconvertible enzyme, which can be activated by the action of parathyroid hormone (PTH). In this way, some of the physiological actions of PTH on bone and kidney can be explained by the increased secretion of H^+-ions following the activation of CA.
We therefore investigated the activity of CA in kidney and epiphysis of vitamin D deficient chicks and studied the action of 1,25-$(OH)_2D_3$, 25-OH D_3 and 24,25-$(OH)_2D_3$ on the CA activity in the kidney.

Methods

Plasma calcium levels were determined by atomic absorption spectrophotometry. Protein bound calcium was separated by ultrafiltration with an Amicon MPS 1 system. PTH was assayed by RIA using an antibody which reacts with intact hormone or the C-terminal part. For the determination of 25-OH D and 24,25-$(OH)_2D$ a binding protein from rat serum was used; for 1,25-$(OH)_2D$ the binding protein was prepared from the cytosol of the intestinal mucosa of chicks. The metabolites were fractionated on a column of Sepharose LH 20 or by HPLC. The animals were sacrificed by decapitation under nembutal anaesthesia. Tissues were frozen immediately after preparation in liquid nitrogen. CA was prepared from 100 000 g supernatants of tissue homogenates by affinity chromatography on p-aminomethyl-benzene-sulfonamide linked Sepharose 4 B. From the homogenate DNA was determined by fluorescence photometry with 4',6-diamidino-2-phenylindol.
For the experiments with vitamin D deficient animals, chicks were raised for 6 weeks under red light on a diet devoid of vitamin D. Control animals were raised under normal conditions. A second group of chicks was raised under vitamin D deficiency as above and divided into four parts. For the following period of 7 days, they received a daily oral dose of: a) 0.5 ml of deionized, sterile water, b) 500 pg of 1,25-$(OH)_2D_3$ in 0.5 ml, c) 200 ng of 25-OH D_3 in 0.5 ml, d) 30 ng of 24,25-$(OH)_2D_3$ in 0.5 ml deionized, sterile water.

Vitamin D. A Chemical, Biochemical and Clinical Update

Results

After 6 weeks of treatment, vitamin D deficient chicks showed a marked hypocalcemia. In bone, the total CA activity had decreased to 40 % but was found unchanged when related to DNA content. The specific activity of the enzyme was nearly doubled. In this way, the diminished total activity caused by the lower cell number has been compensated by activation. After isolation of the enzyme by affinity chromatography and polyacrylamide gel isoelectric focussing, the distribution of isoenzymes and activated versus inactivated forms showed the picture as we find it after treatment of chicks with PTH. This means that under vitamin D deficiency, a secondary hyperparathyroidism has been developed.
None of the described changes could be found in the kidney. The specific activity of CA was even increased slightly (but not significantly).
After substitution of vitamin D deficient chicks with 1,25-$(OH)_2D_3$, 25-OH D_3 or 24,25-$(OH)_2D_3$, the following changes in the plasma levels of calcium, PTH and vitamin D metabolites had been found:

Table 1: Plasma concentrations of vitamin D deficient versus vitamin D treated chicks

treatment	calcium [mM]	iPTH [mU/ml]*	1.25- [pg/ml]	25- [ng/ml]	24,25- [ng/ml]
none	1.53 ± 0.07	3.24 ± 0.27	55	9	2
1.25-$(OH)_2D_3$	1.38 ± 0.10	2.11 ± 0.29	220	35	2
25-OH D_3	2.09 ± 0.09	3.44 ± 0.34	160	18	7
24,25-$(OH)_2D_3$	1.34 ± 0.05	2.70 ± 0.20	180	12	4

Values are mean $\pm$ SEM; SEM is not given for vitamin D metabolites because of lower number of experiments. *MRC standard

The specific activity of CA in the kidneys of the vitamin D treated chicks was more than doubled after 1,25-$(OH)_2D_3$ and 25-OH D_3. Even in the case of 24,25-$(OH)_2D_3$, there was an increase of 60 %. This may be due to relatively high levels of 1,25-$(OH)_2D_3$ which developed in these animals (Tab.1). Our experiments are a further proof for the activation of CA by a second messenger mechanism and confirm the results of Henry et al. about the inhibition of a cyclic AMP-dependent protein kinase in the kidney of vitamin D deficient chicks. Epiphyses show normal PTH response. 25-OH D_3 and 1,25-$(OH)_2D_3$ restore the protein kinase activity; 24,25-$(OH)_2D_3$ is partly active, perhaps by conversion to active vitamin D metabolites.

References

(1) H.L.Henry et al. (1983), Comp.Biochem.Physiol.74B, 715
(2) P.Dietsch and P.R.Siegmund (1984), Ann.N.Y.Acad.Sci.429, 243

THE INFLUENCE OF VITAMIN D DEFICIENCY ON RENAL AMINO ACID EXCRETION IS MANIFEST AT THE BRUSH BORDER SURFACE.

S. Dabbagh, R.W. Chesney and N. Gusowski, Department of Pediatrics, The University of Wisconsin, Madison, WI USA

Introduction:

Generalized aminoaciduria is common in vitamin D-deficiency rickets which has been ascribed to a "modulating" influence of PTH on the renal proximal tubule (1,2). However, the site and mechanisms responsible for this aminoaciduria are poorly understood. Other potential mechanisms include the influence of calcitonin on renal amino acid reabsorption, deficiency of intracellular Ca^{++} or/and changes in renal phospholipid content caused by vitamin D deficiency, similar to that found in intestinal brush border (3,4). The effect of vitamin D deficiency on brush border membrane accumulation of amino acids has not been explored. Since this surface is the site for the active accumulation of amino acids, it is pertinent to explore the vesicle accumulation of amino acids under the condition of vitamin D deficiency. We examined the uptake of proline, an α-amino acid, and taurine, a β-amino acid, by isolated BBMV.

Methods:

Weanling rats were placed on one of the following vitamin D deficient diets for 4-6 weeks: a) VLC 0.02% Ca, 0.3% P; b) VLC + $1,25(OH)_2D_3$ VLC + 500 pmoles 1,25 x 2d; c) LC 0.47% Ca, 0.3% P; d) HC 2.5% Ca, 0.3% P; e) VLP 1.2% Ca, 0.1% P. The control diet contained 1.1% Ca, 0.7% P and 2.5 μg vitamin D. Blood and urine were collected for Ca, P, iPTH, c-AMP and amino acid determination, according to previously described methods (5). BBMV were prepared according to Booth and Kenny (6) Purity and enrichment were verified enzymatically.

Results:

Vitamin D deficiency induced a generalized aminoaciduria which was independent of plasma Ca, PO_4, iPTH and urinary excretion of c-AMP, without changing the creatinine clearance of the animals. The uptake of ^{3}H-taurine and ^{3}H-proline by renal BBMV was sodium-dependent in the normal and vitamin D-deficient groups. The uptakes of the amino acids were reduced at the peak of the Na-dependent "overshoot" on each of the vitamin D deficient diets when compared to control. The decrease in the peak "overshoot" ranged between 22% and 40% for taurine, and 1% and 39% for proline. The difference was statistically significant. This defect corrected with acute supplementation of $1,25(OH)_2D_3$ when proline was studied (Table 1).

Uptake	Control	VLC	VLC+1,25	LC	HC	VLP
Proline (30 sec)	181±44	110±31	182±67	133±29	133±30	134±33
Taurine (360 sec)	50±6	37±6	28±8	39±7	38±7	39±4

Vitamin D. A Chemical, Biochemical and Clinical Update

There was no effect on Km of uptake (Table 2).

Diet	Km (Taurine) µM (@ 60 sec)	Km (Proline) µM (@ 15 sec)
Normal	39.75 ± 2.75 (7)	76.82 ± 7.27 (9)
VLC	39.78 ± 8.43 (7)	62.90 ± 4.44 (4)
VLC + 1,25$(OH)_2D_3$	36.36 ± 4.41 (10)	91.28 ± 12.35 (7)
LC	36.06 ± 3.51 (8)	76.70 ± 23.28 (8)
HC	37.34 ± 1.43 (8)	121.42 ± 23.28 (6)
VLP	40.95 ± 1.88 (8)	93.88 ± 8.87 (8)

There was a decrease in the initial rate of uptake (Vmax) for ^{3}H-taurine at 60 sec which corrected with supplementation, which was statistically significant. No such change was seen for ^{3}H-proline. No correlation was found between peak overshoot of uptake and plasma Ca, PO_4, iPTH and urinary c-AMP for taurine and proline. However, there was a correlation between taurinuria and the peak overshoot of ^{3}H-taurine uptake at 360 sec. ($r= -0.458$, $p<0.01$).

Conclusion:

The defect in renal aminoacid transport secondary to vitamin D deficiency is manifest at the renal cortical brush border membrane. These findings suggest that the aminoaciduria of vitamin D deficiency is an apical surface event for both α- and β-amino acids. Although the parameters of kinetics (Km_D Vmax) are not affected, there is a consistent and significant decrease in the peak overshoot of uptake of taurine and proline by the BBMV. The mechanism of this defect is not clear, but it seems to correlate with the aminoaciduria and to be independent of plasma Ca, PO_4, iPTH and urinary c-AMP. The pathogenic mechanism could involve decreased intracellular Ca^{++} affecting transport, or changes in the phospholipid composition of the brush border membrane secondary to vitamin D deficiency (1-4) and these possibilities are currently under investigation.

References:

(1) Arnaud, C., Glorieux, F. and Scriver, C.R. (1972) Pediatrics 49:837-840.
(2) Fraser, D., Kooh, S.W. and Scriver, C.R. (1967) Pediatr. Res. 1:425-435.
(3) Brautbar, N., Walling, M.W. and Coburn, J.W. (1979) J. Clin. Invest. 63:335-341.
(4) McInnes, R.R. and Scriver, C.R. (1980) Pediatr. Res 14:218-223.
(5) Dabbagh, S., Chesney, R.W. and Slatopolsky E. (1985) Proceedings Sixth Workshop On Vitamin D, in press.
(6) Booth, A.G. and Kenny, A.J. (1974) Biochem. J. 142:575-581.

THE INFLUENCE OF CYCLIC ADENOSINE - 3', 5'-MONOPHOSPHATE (cAMP) ON AMINO ACID ACCUMULATION BY RAT RENAL BRUSH BORDER MEMBRANE VESICLES (BBMV).

S. Dabbagh, R.W. Chesney and N. Gusowski.
Department of Pediatrics, The University of Wisconsin, Madison, WI. USA

Introduction:

The aminoaciduria and phosphaturia of vitamin D deficiency has been ascribed to the action of PTH on the renal tubule (1,2). Since PTH binds to the peritubular membrane, changes in the reabsorption of PO_4 at the apical surface of the proximal tubule are influenced by the generation of cAMP (3). Reduction in phosphate uptake is related to cAMP-dependent protein phosphorylation in canine brush border membrane vesicles (BBMV)(4). Previous studies in our laboratory indicate that the aminoaciduria of vitamin D deficiency is not related to plasma iPTH values or to urinary cAMP excretory patterns (5). In this study we have examined the influence of dibutyryl-cAMP on taurine uptake by rat renal BBMV.

Methods:

BBMV were prepared from adult Sprague-Dawley rats by a previously described method (6). The uptake of ^3H-taurine was measured at 15, 60, 360 and 2700 sec. by a Milipore filtration method in the presence of dbcAMP at values of 10^{-1} to 10^{-7} M. Since ATP is needed for the phosphorylation of membrane proteins in the presence of cAMP, we introduced 10μM dbcAMP, 25μM ATP and 10mM potassium fluoride by hypo-osmotic lysis according to the method of Hammerman et al (4). All studies examined Na^+-dependent taurine uptake.

Results:

Direct exposure of BBMV to external dbcAMP did not influence the initial (15 sec. and 60 sec.) uptake of taurine at 10^{-3} to 10^{-7} M dbcAMP. Only extraordinarily high levels (10^{-1} to 10^{-2} M) inhibited uptake. At the peak of the overshoot (360 sec.) dbcAMP at 10^{-4} to 10^{-7} M did not alter uptake. Again, non-physiologic, hyperosmolar levels of dbcAMP blocked uptake. No effect of varying temperature (4° to 40°) or preincubation time was evident.

Hypotonic lysis, allowing the entry of dbcAMP followed by isotonic resealing did not alter the uptake of taurine. Incubation in the presence of 10μM dbcAMP, 25μM ATP and 10mM KF led to an uptake of taurine of 30 ± 5.4 pmoles/mg protein/60 sec. vs 29.07 ± 7.2 pmoles/mg protein/60 sec. in lysed-resealed control membranes, N.S. All possible combinations of dbcAMP, ATP, KF and lysis did not alter taurine uptake (Figure 1).

Discussion:

Although PTH has been implicated in the pathogenesis of the

Vitamin D. A Chemical, Biochemical and Clinical Update

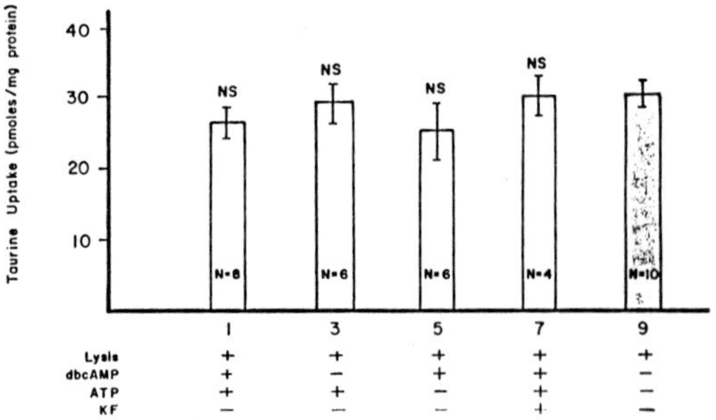

Figure 1: Effect of internal dbcAMP, ATP and KF, using hypotonic lysis on the initial rate of uptake of taurine by BBMV. (All results represent the mean ± SEM).

aminoaciduria of vitamin D deficiency via a modulating action of the adenylate cyclase-cAMP-dependent protein phosphorylation scheme (3,4) the data presented in this paper are inconsistent with the notion. Our previous studies have indicated that aminoaciduria occurs in vitamin D-deficiency all a variety of circulating levels of iPTH, being high in rats on a very low calcium diet and normal in rats on a low phosphate diet (5). In this study, we have examined an end-product of PTH action-cAMP-in order to directly examine vesicle uptake of amino acids. Under usual conditions with rats on a conventional diet, permitting them to be vitamin D sufficient, no evidence for cAMP-induced inhibition of taurine uptake was found. This lack of effect was evident both for internal and external cAMP and in the presence of adequate ATP to promote phosphorylation. Previous studies employing cortex slices had shown the same lack of effect of dbcAMP on taurine uptake (7). Hence, it appears unlikely that cAMP influences taurine transport at either the apical of anti-luminal surface and these data are consistent with the notion that the aminoaciduria of vitamin D-deficiency relates to modulation of tubule function by PTH.

References:

(1) Arnaud, C., Glorieux, F. and Scriver, C.R. (1972) Pediatrics 49:837-840.

(2) Fraser, D., Kooh, S.W. and Scriver, C.R. (1967) Pediatr. Res. 1:425-435.

(3) Sacktor, B., Cheng, L. and Noronha-Blob, L. (1984) Coupled Transport In Nephron 10-22.

(4) Hammerman, M.R. and Hruska, K.A. (1982) J. Biol. Chem. 257:992-999.

(5) Dabbagh, S., Chesney, R.W. and Slatopolsky E. (1985) Proceedings Sixth Workshop On Vitamin D, in press.

(6) Chesney, R.W., Gusowski, N. and Friedman, A.L. (1983) Kidney Int. 24:588-594.

(7) Chesney, R.W. and Jax, D.K. (1979) Pediat. Res. 13:861-867.

STIMULATION OF CREATINE KINASE BB, 25-OHD$_3$-24-HYDROXYLASE AND DNA SYNTHESIS BY 1,25(OH)$_2$D$_3$ IN A HUMAN KIDNEY CELL LINE.

Y. WEISMAN, N. JACCARD, E. BERGER, I. BINDERMAN, A.M. KAYE and D. SOMJEN
The Bone Disease and the Hard Tissues Unit, Ichilov Hospital, Tel Aviv and the Department of Hormone Research, The Weizmann Institute of Science, Rehovot, Israel.

Introduction

The kidney contains receptors for 1,25(OH)$_2$D$_3$ (1,2) and responds to 1,25(OH)$_2$D$_3$ by increased synthesis of vitamin D dependent calcium binding proteins (3,4). However, there are few data about the biological functions of vitamin D in the kidney. Creatine kinase (CK) participates in regulating the intracellular concentration of ATP. The brain type isozyme of creatine kinase (CK-BB) is an early marker for the action of various hormones (5,6). We have demonstrated recently that in the rat kidney, 1,25(OH)$_2$D$_3$ stimulates CK-BB activity (7). In this study, we show the effects of vitamin D metabolites on CK activity, on DNA synthesis and on 25-OHD$_3$-24-hydroxylase activity in a human kidney cell line.

Materials and Methods:

Human kidney cells (Tel-Aviv University human kidney cell line) growing in M-199 medium were incubated with various concentrations of vitamin D metabolites, for various times up to 24 h, in the presence or absence of cycloheximide (10 μg/ml). Enzyme extracts were prepared and assayed in a Gilford 250 automatic recording spectrometer at 340 nM using a coupled assay (7). Unit enzyme activity was defined as the amount yielding 1 μmole of ATP/min at 30°C. Creatine kinase isozymes were separated by a stepwise DEAE cellulose column chromatography (7).^{3}H-thymidine incorporation into DNA (7) and 25-OH-D$_3$-24-hydroxylase activity were determined as previously described (7).

Results and Discussion

1,25(OH)$_2$D$_3$ (1 nM), but not 24R,25(OH)$_2$D$_3$ or 25-OH-D$_3$ (1-10 nM) caused within 24 h a two fold stimulation of CK activity (Fig.), a parallel 1.7 fold increase in ^{3}H-thymidine incorporation into DNA and a 5 fold increase in 25-OHD$_3$-24-hydroxylase activity. The response of CK activity to 1,25(OH)$_2$D$_3$ was dose and time dependent showing maximal stimulation with 1 to 10 nM 1,25(OH)$_2$D$_3$ and significant increase at 4h and 24h, the longest time interval tested. Analysis by DEAE cellulose column chromatography showed that the predominant isozyme of CK was CK BB in both the unstimulated (80%) and stimulated (67%) cultures. 1,25(OH)$_2$D$_3$ failed to stimulate CK activity when cycloheximide was added to the medium (Fig.), consistent with the hypothesis that the stimulation of CK depends at least in part on activation of mRNA transcription. 1,25(OH)$_2$D$_3$-stimulated CK activity could be involved in the two major ATP-consuming functions of vitamin D: one, in transcellular Ca^{2+} transport, and the other, in events leading to cell division and differentiation. We propose that CK activity can serve as a useful marker for the study of the function and mode of action of vitamin D metabolites in the kidney.

Vitamin D. A Chemical, Biochemical and Clinical Update

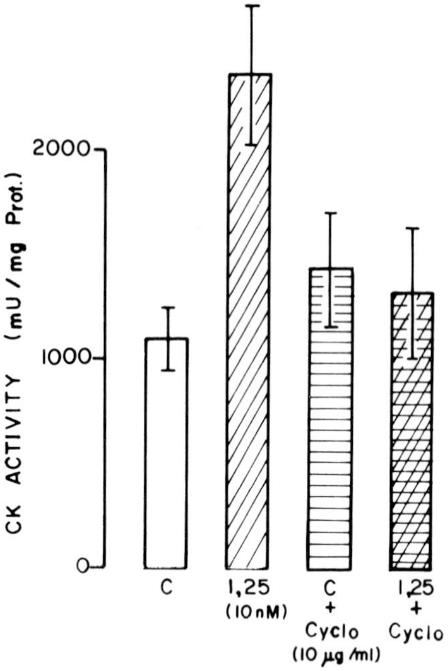

Figure: The effects of $1,25(OH)_2D_3$ and cycloheximide on creatine kinase activity in a human kidney cell line. c-control, 1,25-$1,25(OH)_2D_3$, cyclo-cycloheximide.

References

1. Chandler,J.S., Pike,J.W., Haussler,M.R. (1979) Biochem.Biophys.Res. Commun. 90:1057-1063.
2. Colston,K., Feldman,D. (1980) J.Biol.Chem. 255:7510-7513.
3. Rhoten,W.B., Christakos,S. (1981) Endocrinology 109:981-983.
4. Roth,J., Brown,D., Norman,A.W., Orchi,L. (1982) Am.J.Physiol. 243: F243-252.
5. Reiss,N.A., Kaye,A.M. (1981) J.Biol.Chem. 256:5741-5749.
6. Kaye,A.M., Reiss,N.A., Weisman,Y., Binderman,I., Somjen,D. 1984 in Cellular Bioenergetics and Compartmentation, Brautbar, N., Ed. Plenum Publ. Corp., New York (in press).
7. Somjen,D., Weisman,Y., Binderman,I., Kaye,A.M. (1984) Biochem.J. 219: 1037-1041.
8. Feldman,D., Chen, T., Cone,C., Hirst,M., Shani,A., Benderli,A., Hochberg,Z. (1982) J.Clin.Endocrinol.Metab. 55:1020-1022.

Skeletal Actions of D Metabolites

INHIBITION OF ALKALINE PHOSPHATASE BY LEVAMISOLE PREVENTS THE $1,25(OH)_2$VITAMIN D_3-INDUCED STIMULATION OF BONE MINERALIZATION IN THE MOUSE.

M.T. GARBA and P.J. MARIE
Unité 18 INSERM, Hôpital Lariboisière, 6 rue Guy Patin, 75010 Paris, France.

Introduction :

There is considerable evidence that the skeletal isoenzyme of alkaline phosphatase (AP) plays a critical role in the process of bone formation (1). However the precise role of AP in bone mineralization and the physiological function of the enzyme in vivo remains unknown. AP activity appears to be regulated by 1,25 dihydroxyvitamin D_3 ($1,25(OH)_2D_3$) but the effect of the hormone on AP appears to depend on the state of maturation of the osteoblastic cells(2).It remains unknown whether $1,25(OH)_2D_3$ influences AP activity in vivo. This study was undertaken 1) to determine the relation between AP and bone formation in vivo and 2) to test the hypothesis that the effects of $1,25(OH)_2D_3$ on bone mineralization are mediated by changes in AP activity.

Animals and Methods :

Two groups of 28 days old mice were injected daily for 7 days with L-tetramisole, a reversible specific inhibitor of AP activity (3). The compound was given at the doses of 40 or 80 mg/kg. Another group of 12 mice were infused with $1,25(OH)_2D_3$ using Alzet^R osmotic minipumps. The metabolite was given for 7 days at the dose of 0.05 µg/kg/day that has been shown previously to stimulate bone mineralization without rising serum calcium (4). Two other groups of mice were treated with levamisole at the doses indicated above combined with a concurrent infusion of $1,25(OH)_2D_3$ (0.05 µg/kg/day) while a control group received the solvent alone. At sacrifice , the mineral concentrations were measured in serum and bone ash, and serum alkaline phosphatase and $1,25(OH)_2D_3$ levels were determined. Skeletal changes were evaluated by histomorphometric analysis of caudal vertebrae after in vivo double ^{3}H-proline and double tetracycline labelings.Dynamic parameters of bone formation and mineralization were determined using conventional histomorphometric methods. Osteoclasts actively engaged in bone resorption were identified after histochemical detection of acid phosphatase activity.

Results :

The administration of levamisole produced no deleterious effects. The body weight gain was similar in treated animals (+ 18.7 - 33.3 %) compared to controls (+ 20 %) except in mice treated with 80 mg/kg of levamisole and $1,25(OH)_2D_3$ (+ 6 %). However, the skeletal growth evaluated by the tibia length was identical in all groups. Serum $1,25(OH)_2D$ levels rose by 20-93 % in mice infused with the vitamin D metabolite. Accordingly, the number of active osteoclasts increased in mice treated with $1,25(OH)_2D_3$. Serum calcium rose slightly by about 10 % only in the two groups of animals treated with levamisole combined to $1,25(OH)_2D_3$. Treatment with $1,25(OH)_2D_3$ alone resulted in a slight inhibition of AP activity compared to controls (Table1). The same dose of $1,25(OH)_2D_3$ infused for 28 days in mice was found previously to increase serum AP activity but this was associated with increased osteoblastic population (4).
The lower dose of levamisole produced a fall in serum AP while the larger dose markedly inhibited AP activity. The administration of $1,25(OH)_2D_3$ combined to levamisole amplified the inhibition of AP activity induced by either $1,25(OH)_2D_3$ or levamisole alone but this effect was not augmented at the higher dosage level. Treatment with levamisole alone or combined with $1,25(OH)_2D_3$ was associated with decreased serum phosphate (Table 1) By contrast a significant 10.9 - 37.4 % increase in bone phosphorus content was observed in all groups of mice treated with levamisole. The infusion of $1,25(OH)_2D_3$ increased the mineral apposition rate (MiAR) evaluated by the double tetracycline labeling method. No change in the matrix apposition rate (MaAR) determined by the double ^{3}H-proline labeling method was noted (Table 2). Treatment with levamisole decreased the bone MaAR at the lower dose given and decreased both the MaAR and MiAR at the higher dosage. Despite concurrent administration of levamisole at the low dosage level, the MiAR was still stimulated by $1,25(OH)_2D_3$ while at the higher dosage level, levamisole prevented the $1,25(OH)_2D_3$-induced stimulation of MiAR (Table 2). Because of the accelera-

Vitamin D. A Chemical, Biochemical and Clinical Update

ted mineralization rate and/or the reduced matrix apposition rate, the osteoid thickness was decreased in all treated groups.

Treatment	Change in serum alkaline phosphatase (% controls)	Change in serum phosphate (% controls)
$1,25(OH)_2D_3$	- 17.1[a]	- 1.5
Levamisole 40 mg/kg	- 18.4[a]	- 14.5[a]
80 mg/kg	- 61.3[a]	- 22.8[a]
$1,25(OH)_2D_3$ + Levamisole		
40 mg/kg	- 37.9[a]	- 18.1[a]
80 mg/kg	- 45.8[a]	- 13.9[a]

Table 1 : Changes in biochemical parameters (a: significant at the 1-5 % level)

Treatment	Change in bone MiAR(% controls)	Change in bone MaAR(% controls)	Change in osteoid thickness (% controls)
$1,25(OH)_2D_3$	+ 8.5[a]	+ 1.9	- 14.1[a]
Levamisole 40 mg/kg	+ 3.0	- 13.5[a]	- 23.2[a]
80 mg/kg	- 9.0[a]	- 27.9[a]	- 33.3[a]
$1,25(OH)_2D_3$ + Levamisole			
40 mg/kg	+ 9.0[a]	- 8.2	- 25.9[a]
80 mg/kg	- 18.5[a]	- 26.0[a]	- 30.6[a]

Table 2 : Changes in parameters of bone formation (a:significant at the 1-5 % level)

Discussion :

The skeletal isoenzyme form of AP can be identified on the basis of its sensitivity to the inhibitor levamisole (3). In our in vivo study, no toxic effect related to levamisole could be recorded at the doses given. Moreover, no change in the osteoblastic population could be found in any treated group. The administration of levamisole resulted in a 18-61 % inhibition of AP activity in serum which is mainly of skeletal origin in mice (5). A moderate (18-38 %) inhibition of AP activity resulted in inhibition of the bone matrix apposition rate. This effect was related to the fall in serum phosphate observed in all the levamisole-treated groups (Table 1). At this level of AP inhibition, the bone mineralization rate remained normal and the mineralizing effect of $1,25(OH)_2D_3$ was not inhibited. By contrast, a more severe inhibition of AP activity (46-61 %) resulted in alteration of both the matrix and mineral apposition rates. Moreover the stimulatory effect of $1,25(OH)_2D_3$ on bone mineralization was inhibited. This study shows that 1) inhibition of AP activity in vivo is associated with reduction of both bone matrix synthesis and mineralization rates. However, the AP activity must be decreased by about 50 % in order to observe changes in bone mineralization ; 2) inhibition of AP by about 50 % prevents the stimulatory effect of $1,25(OH)_2D_3$ on bone mineralization. This suggests that the in vivo mineralizing effect of $1,25(OH)_2D_3$ is in part mediated by AP activity.

References :

1 - White, M.P., in Clinical Disorders of Bone and Mineral Metabolism, Ed. Frame, P., Potts, J.T., Excerpta Medica, 1983, p 120-124.

2 - Rodan, G.A., Rodan, S.B., in bone and Mineral Research, Ed Peck, W.A., Elsevier Science Pub., 1983, p 244-285.

3 - Van Bell, H.(1972), Biochem. Biophys. Acta 289 : 158-168.

4 - Marie,P.J., Travers, R., (1983), Calcif. Tissue Int. 35, 418-425.

5 - Menahan, L.A., Sobocinski, K.A., Peter Austin, B. (1984). Comp. Biochem. Physiol.2;279-283

LONG-TERM CALCIUM INFUSIONS CAN CURE OSTEOMALACIA AND PROMOTE NORMAL MINERALIZATION IN HEREDITARY RESISTANCE TO 1,25-DIHYDROXY VITAMIN D.

S. BALSAN, M. GARABEDIAN, M. LARCHET, A.M. GORSKI, G. COURNOT, C. TAU, A. BOURDEAU, and C. RICOUR.
Laboratoire des Tissus Calcifiés (CNRS UA.583 - INSERM U.30) and Department of Pediatric Gastroenterology, Hôpital des Enfants-Malades, 149, rue de Sèvres, 75015 Paris, France.

We have reported (1) in a child with hereditary resistance to 1,25-dihydroxyvitamin D ($1,25(OH)_2D$) and alopecia who had been responsive to therapy with high-dosage vitamin D derivatives, the occurrence of a relapse at age 6 years. From 6 years to 9 years of age all therapeutic trials were unsuccessful despite serum $1,25(OH)_2D$ concentrations maintained at very high levels i.e. 11,012 $\pm$ 4,487 pg/ml (mean $\pm$ SD, n=14) during treatment with 5 mg/d of 25-hydroxyvitamin D_3. Three months after cessation of this treatment, a 6-month trial with a high-calcium (2,250 mg/d) high-lactose (62 to 82 g/d) diet was also ineffective. Then, the child was given a normal calcium diet and a program of nocturnal calcium infusions was initiated. This treatment providing from 08pm to 08am, via an intracaval catheter, 1g elemental calcium (calcium gluconate in 500 ml 5 % dextrose solution) during 4 months, then 0.75g calcium, was continued for $\sim$8 months (5 months nightly, subsequently thrice-weekly).

The initial data were the following : serum calcium 9.6 mg/dl; serum phosphorus 2.4 mg/dl; alkaline phosphatase 15,700 nkat/dl (normal: 1,500-5,000); serum iPTH-(53-84) 90 pg/ml (normal: 15-60 pg/ml). Serum 25(OH)D concentration was 21 ng/ml, serum $24,25(OH)_2D$ 0.9 ng/ml, and serum $1,25(OH)_2D$ 187 pg/ml (normal: 25(OH)D = 6-30 ng/ml; $24,25(OH)_2D$ = 1-3 ng/ml; $1,25(OH)_2D$ = 20-80 pg/ml). Skeletal radiograms and iliac crest bone biopsy showed overt lesions of rickets and osteomalacia. Primary cultures of her bone-derived cells demonstrated, in the

Vitamin D. A Chemical, Biochemical and Clinical Update

presence of $1,25(OH)_2D_3$ (10^{-9} and 10^{-6} M) a lack of activation of 25-hydroxyvitamin D - 24-hydroxylase.
Results of nocturnal calcium infusions: This treatment suppressed in two weeks the child's bone pains and muscular weekness. Serum calcium remained normal; serum phosphorus increased and remained normal beyond the 2nd month; serum alkaline phosphatase and iPTH were normalized on the 4th month. Skeletal radiograms showed initiation of healing after 3 weeks and disappearance of ricketic lesions after 5 months. A bone biopsy obtained after 4 months of therapy showed normalization of osteoid volume and width, and a normal pattern of mineralization (tetracycline uptake).

In conclusion, these results demonstrate that : (i) even in the absence of a normal $1,25(OH)_2D$ effector-receptor system in bone cells, normal mineralization can be achieved in humans if adequate serum calcium and phosphorus concentrations are maintained ; (ii) intermittent calcium infusions can be an efficient alternative for the management of patients with hereditary resistance to $1,25(OH)_2D$ unresponsive to large doses of vitamin D derivatives.

REFERENCE

1. Balsan, S., Garabédian, M., Liberman, U.A., Eil, C., Bourdeau, A., Guillozo, H., Grimberg, R., LeDeunff, M.J., Lieberherr, M., Guimbaud, P., Broyer, M. and Marx, S.J. (1983) J. Clin. Endocrinol. 57, 803-811.

HYPEROSTEOIDOSIS DUE TO LOW DOSES OF 1,25-DIHYDROXYCHOLECALCIFEROL [$1,25(OH)_2D_3$] IN MILD SUBACUTE UREMIA. Rogely Waite Boyce, Steven E. Weisbrode, and Charles C. Capen, Department of Veterinary Pathobiology, The Ohio State University, Columbus, Ohio (U.S.A.) 43210.

Osteodystrophy is a frequent and debilitating consequence of the profound alterations in mineral homeostasis associated with chronic renal failure. The specific mechanisms underlying renal osteodystrophy are complex and include intestinal malabsorption of calcium, phosphorus retention, and acidosis. Alterations in vitamin D metabolism which occur in uremia may be central in the development of renal osteodystrophy.

The objectives of this study were to determine the effects of low doses of exogenous $1,25(OH)_2D_3$ on the early development of uremic bone disease in young female Sprague-Dawley rats with experimentally-induced renal failure.

Materials and Methods

Female Sprague-Dawley rats (50-60 gm) were subjected either to a one-stage 5/6 nephrectomy (NX) or sham operation (SO). Post-operatively, all rats were fed *ad libitum* normal laboratory chow. Rats were divided into the following treatment groups: SO rats, placebo (n=6), NX rats, placebo (n=11), NX rats, 6.75 ng $1,25(OH)_2D_3$ (n=13), and SO rats, 6.75 ng $1,25(OH)_2D_3$ (n=13). Rats were treated daily with placebo (50 ul 95% ethanol, vehicle control) or $1,25(OH)_2D_3$ I.P. for 28 days commencing day 1 post-operatively. Three days prior to termination, all rats received (I.P.) 15 mg/kg oxytetracycline. Terminal serum was assayed for calcium, phosphorus and creatinine.

Tibial epiphyses and metaphyses were evaluated qualitatively for fibrosis of the marrow, amount and distribution of mineralized bone and osteoid, and relative changes in size and number of osteoblasts and osteoclasts. On six rats randomly chosen from each group, the total area of the epiphysis, area of mineralized osseous tissue of the epiphysis and area of osteoid of the epiphysis were determined. Growth plate width was determined on perpendicular sections of the proximal tibial epiphyseal plate. Longitudinal growth per day in mm was determined by measuring the distance of the fluorescent band from the top of the proximal tibial growth plate, subtracting the width of the plate, and dividing by the number of days from labeling to sampling. Quantitative data were analyzed by a two-way analysis of variance followed by a Duncan's multiple range test.

Results

$1,25(OH)_2D_3$ and placebo-treated NX rats had a significantly lower serum calcium compared with $1,25(OH)_2D_3$-treated SO rats. However, serum calcium in $1,25(OH)_2D_3$-treated SO rats was not significantly different from placebo-treated SO rats (Table 1).

No significant changes in serum phosphorus due to renal failure or $1,25\text{-}(OH)_2D_3$ treatment were seen.

Serum creatinine was significantly increased in both placebo- and 1-25-treated NX rats compared with placebo- and $1,25(OH)_2D_3$-treated SO rats. $1,25(OH)_2D_3$ treatment did not significantly increase serum creatinine in NX rats.

$1,25(OH)_2D_3$-treated NX rats weighed less than placebo and $1,25(OH)_2D_3$-treated SO rats but not less than placebo-treated NX rats.

Undecalcified sections of tibias from placebo-treated NX rats and $1,25(OH)_2D_3$-treated SO rats revealed no significant alterations in the amount, distribution and

Vitamin D. A Chemical, Biochemical and Clinical Update

organization of mineralized bone or osteoid compared with placebo-treated SO rats. There was no evidence of medullary fibrosis or apparent differences in numbers and size of osteoblasts and osteoclasts. Tibias from $1,25(OH)_2D_3$-treated NX rats had epiphyseal and metaphyseal hyperosteoidosis characterized by a mild to marked increase in numbers and width of osteoid seams. Seams in $1,25(OH)_2D_3$-treated NX rats were predominantly lined by hypertrophied osteoblasts compared with other groups. The distribution of the lesion in the epiphysis ranged from focal and confined to trabeculae adjacent to the growth plate to diffuse involvement of the majority of trabecular surfaces. In the metaphysis, widened seams varied in location between rats, involving either proximal mid and/or distal metaphysis.

$1,25(OH)_2D_3$ decreased longitudinal growth in both SO and NX rats but was significant only in NX rats (Table II).

TABLE I

EFFECT OF UREMIA AND 1,25 $(OH)_2D_3$ TREATMENT ON SERUM CALCIUM, PHOSPHORUS, AND CREATININE AND BODY WEIGHT. (Mean ± Standard Deviation; Means sharing the same letter are not significantly different from each other, $p < 0.05$.)

	SO placebo	SO 1,25 $(OH)_2D_3$	NX placebo	NX 1,25 $(OH)_2D_3$
	n = 6	n = 13	n = 11	n = 13
Calcium (mg/dl)	10.88 ± 1.00^{AB}	11.42 ± 1.03^{B}	10.20 ± 0.87^{A}	10.60 ± 0.72^{A}
Phosphorus (mg/dl)	10.28 ± 1.14^{A}	9.13 ± 1.24^{A}	9.58 ± 1.30^{A}	9.15 ± 1.28^{A}
Creatinine (mg/dl)	0.48 ± 0.16^{A}	0.38 ± 0.13^{A}	0.85 ± 0.10^{B}	0.73 ± 0.18^{B}
Body Weight (g)	181 ± 19^{A}	176 ± 9^{A}	155 ± 6^{AB}	124 ± 40^{B}

TABLE II.

EFFECT OF UREMIA AND 1,25 $(OH)_2D_3$ TREATMENT ON BONE PARAMETERS.

(Mean ± standard deviation; Means sharing the same letter are not significantly different from each other, $p < 0.05$.)

	SO placebo	SO 1,25 $(OH)_2D_3$	NX placebo	NX 1,25$(OH)_2D_3$
Longitudinal Growth mm/day	0.31 ± 0.05^{AB}	0.26 ± 0.05^{A}	0.32 ± 0.05^{A}	0.24 ± 0.09^{B}
Growth Plate Width mm	0.32 ± 0.03^{A}	0.29 ± 0.03^{A}	0.32 ± 0.03^{A}	0.24 ± 0.07^{B}
Total area of epiphysis mm^2	7.29^{A} ± 0.81	6.48^{A} ± 1.27	6.70^{A} ± 0.47	6.89^{A} ± 1.15
Mineralized osseous tissue area of epiphysis mm^2 (%)	$2.62\ (36.1)^{A}$ $\pm 0.40\ (5.5)$	$2.28\ (34.8)^{A}$ $\pm 0.60\ (3.1)$	$2.04\ (30.2)^{A}$ $\pm 0.43\ (5.1)$	$2.59\ (37.3)^{A}$ $\pm 0.96\ (11.8)$
Osteoid area of epiphysis mm^2 (%)	$0.02\ (0.31)^{A}$ $\pm 0.01\ (0.18)$	$0.04\ (0.65)^{A}$ $\pm 0.02\ (0.17)$	$0.03\ (0.38)^{A}$ $\pm 0.01\ (0.25)$	$0.44\ (6.55)^{B}$ $\pm 0.47\ (7.42)$

Growth plate width was significantly decreased in $1,25(OH)_2D_3$-treated NX rats.

The total area of the epiphysis (total area of osseous tissue and marrow space), and the absolute and relative area of mineralized osseous tissue (bone) of the epiphysis were not affected by renal failure or $1,25(OH)_2D_3$ treatment. The absolute and relative areas of osteoid in the epiphysis were significantly increased in $1,25(OH)_2D_3$-treated NX rats compared with all other groups.

Conclusions

1. One-stage 5/6 nephrectomy (NX) in 50-60 GM rats resulted in a mild but significant elevation in serum creatinine, no change in serum calcium or phosphorus, and no histologic bone lesions when compared with SO rats at 4 weeks post-NX.

2. Administration of low doses (6.75 mg) of $1,25(OH)_2D_3$ to 5/6 NX rats with mild renal failure produced tibial epiphyseal and metaphyseal hyperosteoidosis. This dose did not affect bone morphology in non-uremic rats. Hyperosteoidosis was present in various locations of the metaphysis and widespread in the epiphysis. The total area of the epiphysis and amount of bone were not affected by NX or $1,25(OH)_2D_3$ treatment. Therefore, the hyperosteoidosis in $1,25(OH)_2D_3$-treated NX rats reflects an increase in total osseous tissue.

3. Bone may be uniquely sensitive in mild uremia to the effects of low doses of exogeneous $1,25(OH)_2D_3$.

1,25(OH)$_2$D$_3$ AND ITS ANALOGUES INDUCE ALKALINE PHOSPHATASE ACTIVITY IN OSTEOBLASTIC CLONE MC3T3-E1, CELLS DRIVED FROM NEWBORN MOUSE CALVARIA.

M. Kumegawa, N. Kurihara[1)], K. Ikeda[1)], Y. Hakeda, M. Kiyoki[2)] and S. Ishizuka[2)]

Department of Oral Anatomy and Periodontology[1)], Josai Dental University, Sakado, Saitama 350-02, Japan. Institute for Bio-Medical Research[2)], Teijin Limited, Hino, Tokyo 191, Japan

1,25(OH)$_2$D$_3$ and its analogues at physiological concentrations have been reported to directly stimulate bone resorption. However, the cellular basis for the direct effect of vitamin D metabolites on bone remains unclear, perhaps due to the extreme heterogeneity of the tissue. Kodama et al. (1,2) have recently isolated osteoblastic clone MC3T3-E1 cells from newborn mouse calvaria, which cells have retained osteoblastic cellular functions. They also respond to PGE$_2$ (3) and PTH (4). Therefore, these cells must be useful for the study of the effect of vitamin D metabolites on osteoblastic cells in vitro.

Clone MC3T3-E1 cells, plated at an initial density of 5×10^4 cells in 35-mm dish containing α-MEM with 10% calf bovine serum, were cultured until nearly confulent. In order to examine the time-dependent effect of 1,25(OH)$_2$D$_3$ on alkaline, phosphatase (ALP) activity in the cells, they were further cultured in medium supplemented with 2% serum with or without 40 pg/ml of the hormone. ALP activity was significantly increased as early as 48 h and the greatest difference between the hormone-added and-free cultures were observed at 4 days (Fig. 1). Therefore, further experiments were carried out at 4 days after the hormone added. The hormone significantly increased ALP activity in a dose-dependent fashion up to a concentration of 50 pg/ml, at which dose the activity was approximately two-fold higher than that of controls (Fig. 2).

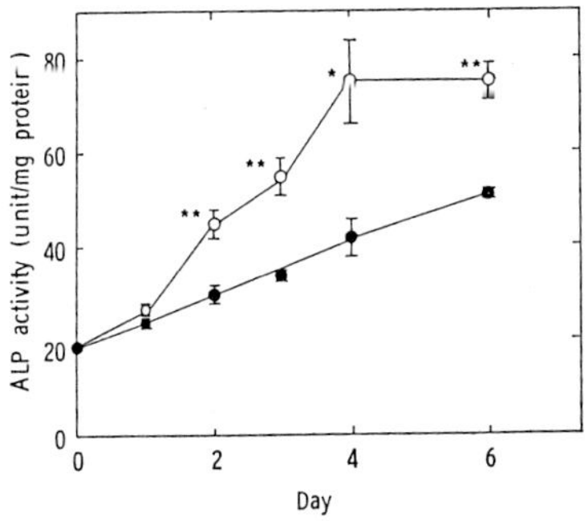

Fig. 1. Time course of the effect of 1α,25(OH)$_2$D$_3$ on ALP activity in clone MC3T3-E1 cells. Each plot shows the average of four independent cultures; the bars represent S.E.M. ●, control; ○, 1α,25(OH)$_2$D$_3$ (40 pg/ml); $^*p<0.05$, $^{**}p<0.01$ compared with control (Student's t test).

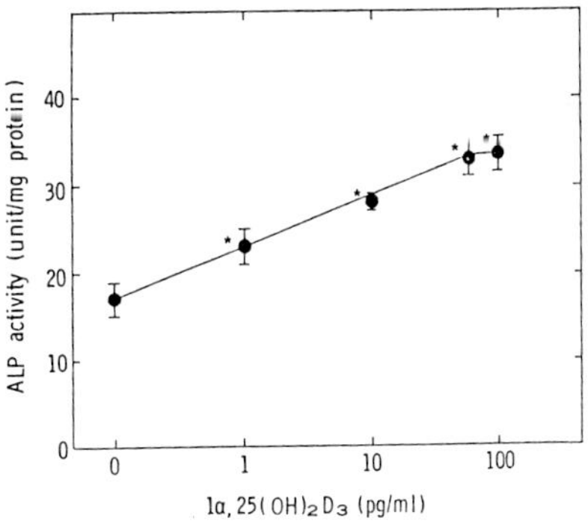

Fig. 2. Relationship between 1α,25(OH)$_2$D$_3$ concentration and ALP activity in clone MC3T3-E1 cells. The cells were transferred to medium containing various concentrations of 1α,25(OH)$_2$D$_3$ at day 5.

Vitamin D. A Chemical, Biochemical and Clinical Update

1,24R(OH)$_2$D$_3$, 1(OH)D$_3$ and 24R, 25(OH)D$_3$ also showed a does-dependent stimulation of ALP activity (Table 1). However their effective concentration was 100 or 1,000-fold greater than that of 1,25(OH)$_2$D$_3$. ALP activity in 1,25(OH)$_2$D$_3$-treated or control cells was the same as that of the enzyme from newborn mouse calvaria by heat-stability and amino acid inhibition tests. That is "bone-live-kidny" type.

TABLE I. Effects of vitamin D_3 analogues on ALP activity in clone MC3T3-E1 cells. After the cells had been cultured for 5 days in medium supplemented with 10% calf bovine serum, they were cultured for another 4 days in medium supplemented with 2% calf bovine serum containing various concentrations of hormones. Values are means ± S.E.M. from 5 cultures. Values in parentheses show percent activity of non-treated controls. ALP activity in cultures with 40 pg/ml of 1α,25(OH)$_2$ D$_3$ in the same experiment with 24R,25(OH)$_2$ D$_3$ was 62.4 ± 4.6.

Concentration	Alkaline phosphatase activity (units/mg protein)		
	1α,24(OH)$_2$ D$_3$	24R,25(OH)$_2$ D$_3$	1α(OH) D$_3$
Control (none)	23.4±1.6 (100)	29.9±1.7 (100)	25.9±3.3 (100)
1 ng/ml	41.0±2.5 (175)[b]	33.8±1.5 (113)	N.T.
10	51.8±7.4 (221)[b]	45.3±2.8 (151)[b]	34.0±4.3 (131)
100	51.0±1.3 (217)[b]	61.9±2.9 (207)[b]	41.6±4.4 (160)[a]

N.T., not tested. [a] $p<0.05$, [b] $p<0.01$ compared to control (Student's t test).

1,25(OH)$_2$D$_3$ receptors in clone MC3T3-E1 cells had the same binding affinity (Kd=1.47×10^{-11}M) and sedimentation coefficient (3.67S) as those in other mouse osteoblast cells and other organs. Moreover, 1,25(OH)$_2$D$_3$ receptor complex bound to nuclear chromatin temperature-dependently.

These results indicate that vitamin D$_3$ metabolites stimulate the differentiation of osteoblastic cells mediated by 1,25(OH)$_2$D$_3$ receptors in vitro. We thank you Dr. H. Kodama for the gift of clone MC3T3-E1 cells.

References

1. Kodama, H., Amagai, Y., Sudo, H., Kasai, S. and Yamamoto, S. (1981) Jpn. J. Oral Biol. 23, 899-901.
2. Sudo, H., Kodama, H., Amagai, Y., Yamamoto, S. and Kasai, S. (1983) J. Cell Biol. 96, 191-198.
3. Hakeda, Y., Nakatani, Y., Hiramatsu, M., Kurihara, N. Tsunoi, M., Ikeda, E. and Kumegawa, M. (1985) J. Biochem. 97, 97-104.
4. Nakatani, Y., Tsunoi, M., Hakeda, Y., Kurihara, N., Fujita, K. and Kumegawa, M. (1984) Biochem. Biophys. Res. Comm. 123, 761-771.

THE METABOLISM OF VITAMIN D DURING FRACTURE HEALING IN CHICKS.

C. Lidor, S. Dekel* and S. Edelstein

Biochemistry Department, The Weizmann Institute of Science 76100 Rehovot and The Department of Orthopedic Surgury*, Ichilov Hospital, Tel-Aviv, Israel.

The association of cholecalciferol (vitamin D_3) with bone formation is well known (1). The two-step hydroxylation of the vitamin yeilds $1,25(OH)_2D_3$ and $24,25(OH)_2D_3$ which are the most importent dihydroxylated metabolits under normal physiological conditions (2).

The mechanisms by which the active metabolites of cholecalciferol influences bone metabolism are not clearly defined (3,4).

Fracture healing is an active process of bone formation (5), which ends by actual reconstitution of the injured bone to its original form.

The objective of the present study was therefore to obtain furthur information about the involvment of these steroid hormones in bone formation.

Materials & Methods: One day old male chicks were fed on vitamin D - deficient diet but were supplemented with (1,2-^{3}H) cholecalciferol (specific radioactivity 0.2 mCi/mol). 1.8µg of the radioactive vitamin were injected 5 days. This procedure ensured steady state condition of measurable cholecalciferol metabolites.

At the end of 3-weeks period experimental fractures were performed in the mid-shaft of the right tibia. A small skin incision under sterile condition was made over the tibia, and a hole was drilled with the aid of a small dental burr. The skin was closed, and then the tibia was fractured by a light pressure with the fingers.

The chicks were killed at 1,3,5,7,9,11,14 and 21 days after the fracture had been performed.

Three experiments were carried out. In the first experiment the calluses formed in the fracture sites, the parallel regions in the unfractured tibiae of the contralateral legs, the proximal epiphyis of both legs, the kidneys, the duodenum and the serum were removed and extracted for lipids (6). The lipid extracts were analyzed for colecalciferol metabolites with the aid of HPLC.

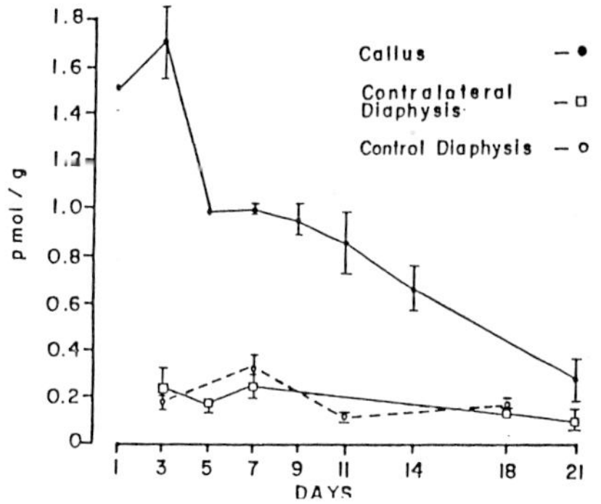

Fig. 1: The levels of $24,25(OH)_2D_3$ in callus in contralateral diaphysis and in diaphysis obtained from normal birds. (Each point represents mean±SEM of 6 chicks).

days after the fracture	$24,25(OH)_2D_3$ production pmol/g in 15 min	
	CONTROL	FRACTURED
3	3.9 ± 0.7 *	12.3 ± 2.9 [a]
7	3.0 ± 1.4	4.0 ± 0.5

* values are MEAN ± SEM of four chicks. a $p < 0.05$

Table 1: The renal production of $24,25(OH)_2D_3$ during fracture repair.

Vitamin D. A Chemical, Biochemical and Clinical Update

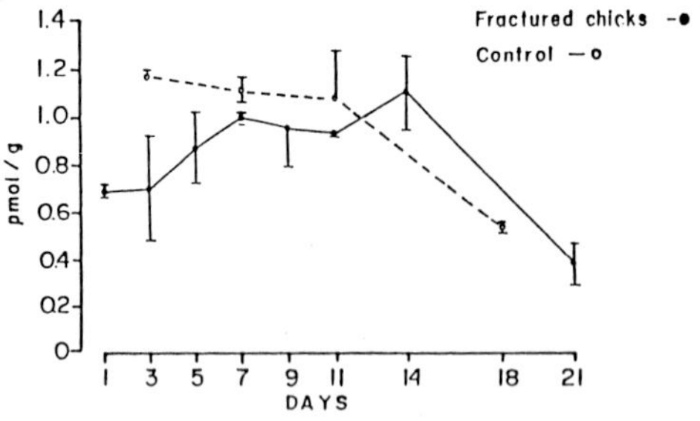

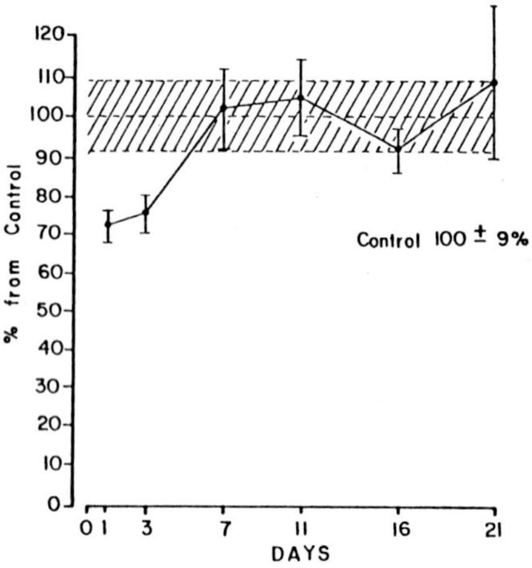

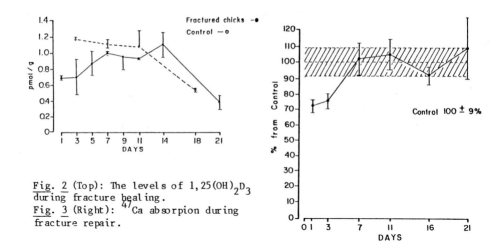

Fig. 2 (Top): The levels of 1,25$(OH)_2D_3$ during fracture healing.
Fig. 3 (Right): ^{47}Ca absorpion during fracture repair.

In the second experiment the duodenal absorption of ^{47}Ca was measured utilizing the ligated loop technique (7).

In the third - the renal production of the dihydroxylated metabolites were analyzed (8).

Results & Conclusions: The levels of the dihydroxylated metabolites were increased in the calluses with levels of 24,25$(OH)_2D_3$ (Fig. 1) coincided with the formation of cartilaginous tissue, (as shown by histological examination) and with the renal production of this steroid (Table 1).

In the duodenum of the fractured chicks, the levels of 1,25$(OH)_2D_3$ dropped significantlly during the first week following fracture (Fig. 2), coincided with reduction in the intestinal absorption of calcium (Fig. 3).

In the serum during those three weeks of healing process the levels of 1,25$(OH)_2D_3$ were far below normal (data not shown).

These findings indicate that during the process of fracture-repair, changes in the metabolism and expression of vitamin D are taking place in order to meet the new requirments of the body under stress condition of skeletal fracture.

References:

1. Raiz, L.G., Kream, B.E. (1983) N. Engl. J. Med. 309: 29-35; 83-89.
2. Kanis, J.A. (1982) J. Bone and Joint Surg. 64-B: 542-560.
3. Ornoy, A., Goodwin, D., Noff, D., Edelstein, S. (1978) Nature 276: 517-519.
4. Dekel, S., Ornoy, A., Sekeles, E., Noff, D., Edelstein S. (1979) Calcif. Tissue Int. 28: 245-251.
5. Sevitt, S. (1981) Bone Repair and Fracture Healing in Man. Churchill Livingstone.
6. Bligh, E.G., Dyer, W.J. (1959) Can. J. Biochem. Physiol. 37(8) 911-917.
7. Morrissey, R.L., Wasserman, R.H. (1971) Am. J. Physiol. 220: 1509-1515.
8. Fraser, D.R., Kodicek, D. (1973) Nature, New Biol. 241: 163-166.

OSTEOINDUCTIVE AND MITOGENIC ACTIVITIES ARE REDUCED IN DEMINERALIZED ALLOGENEIC BONE MATRIX FROM VITAMIN D DEFICIENT RATS

R.T. Turner*#, J. Farley+, J.J. Vandersteenhoven#, and N.H. Bell#

V.A. Hospital, Loma Linda, CA 92357*, Loma Linda University, Loma Linda, CA 92350+, and V.A. Medical Center, Charleston, SC 29402#.

The term osteoinduction is used to denote induced ectopic endochondral bone formation following implantation of demineralized allogeneic bone matrix (DABM) (1). The magnitude of osteoinduction was reduced when the DABM was prepared from the long bones of rats fed a diet containing vitamin D (+D) and implanted into vitamin D deficient (-D) rats (2). In order to determine whether the osteoinductive capacity of bone per se is altered by vitamin D status we raised rats from weanlings on a -D diet. After 4-5 months DABM was prepared from the long bones of the -D rats and implanted into rats fed a diet containing vitamin D. Figure 1a shows the histology of DABM implants from +D rats harvested 3 weeks postimplantation. Note the large resorption cavities (RC) in the implant matrix (IM) filled with marrow (M). There are extensive areas of new bone (NB) bounded by cement lines (CL). The surfaces of the implant matrix are lined by osteoblasts (OB) and osteoclasts (OC). In contrast, when DABM implants prepared from -D rats were examined (Figure 1b) there were no prominent resorption cavities and no new bone formation. No osteoblasts or osteoclasts were observed.

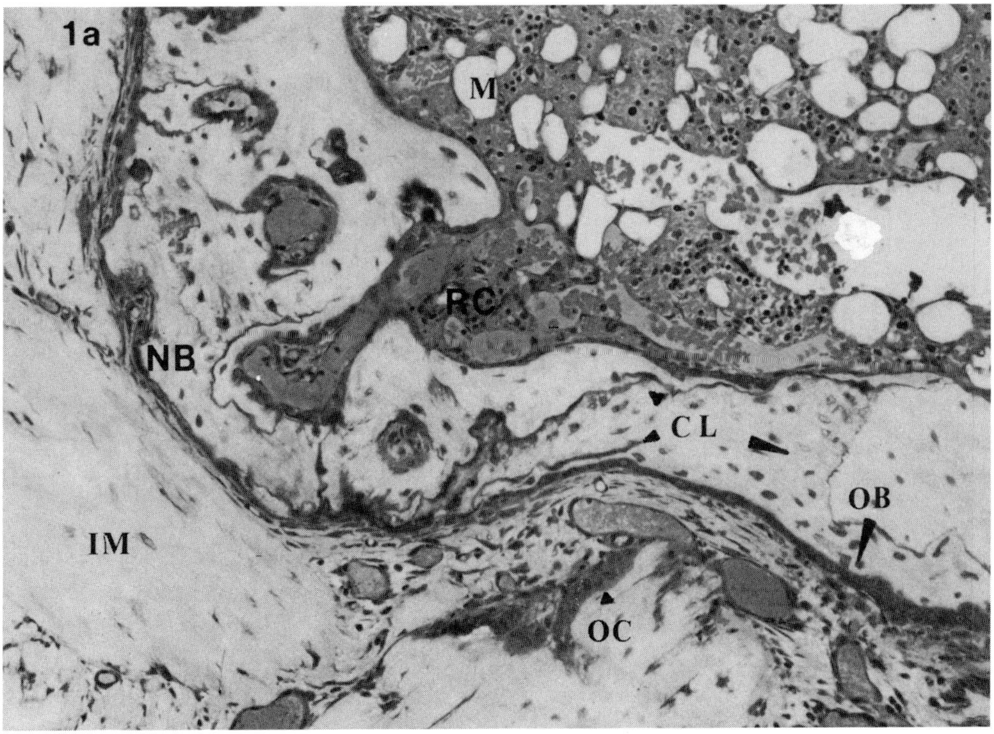

Vitamin D. A Chemical, Biochemical and Clinical Update

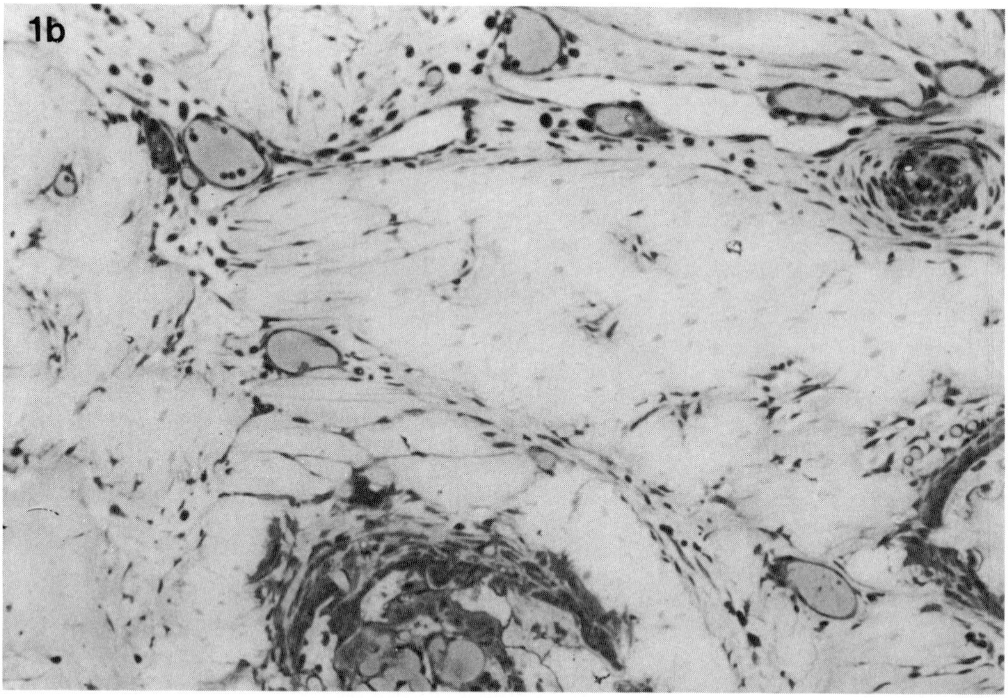

Mitogenic activity was determined in extracts of DABM-implants by stimulus of ^{3}H-thymidine incorporation into TCA-precipitable material in monolayer culture of chick calvarial cells (3). The mitogenic activity of DABM prepared from -D rats was only 32% of that from +D animals.

The results of the present studies that bone matrix from -D animals is abnormal in that it a) is ineffective in promoting osteoinduction and b) contains reduced mitogenic activity. Further studies are necessary to determine the precise relationship of mitogenic factors and osteoinduction.

References

1. Urist, M.R., DeLange, R.J., and Finerman, G.A.M. (1983). Science 220: 680:686.
2. Vandersteenhoven, J.J., Delustro, F.A., Bell, N.H., and Turner, R.T. (In press) Clin. Orthoed. Rel. Res.
3. Drivdahl, R.H., Puzas, J.E., Howard, G.A., and Baylink, D.J. (1981). Soc. Exp. Biol. Med. 166:113-122.

EFFECT OF $1,25(OH)_2D_3$ ON PHOSPHOLIPID METABOLISM IN OSTEOGENIC SARCOMA CELLS (UMR 106). RELATIONSHIP TO ITS ROLE ON BONE MINERALIZATION.

Toshio Matsumoto, Yumiko Kawanobe, Keiko Morita and Etsuro Ogata
Fourth Department of Internal Medicine, University of Tokyo School of Medicine, Tokyo 112, Japan.

Introduction

Acidic phospholipids, especially phosphatidylserine (PS), have been shown to be associated with bone mineralization process. PS can bind calcium (Ca) and phosphate (Pi) avidly to form Ca-PS-Pi complexes, and matrix vesicles are rich in Ca-PS-Pi complexes (1). In addition, these complexes can nucleate apatite formation from metastable Ca and Pi solutions (2). Previously, it was demonstrated that $1,25(OH)_2D_3$ alters phospholipid metabolism in the intestinal epithelial cells (3) and the renal tubular cells (4). Those results suggested that the resultant changes in phospholipid composition of the brush border membranes are the mechanism by which $1,25(OH)_2D_3$ alters trans-epithelial ion transport. The present study was undertaken to test the possibility that $1,25(OH)_2D_3$ has a direct effect on osteoblasts to stimulate bone mineralization by altering phospholipid metablism of osteoblasts, using a clonal rat osteogenic sarcoma cell line, UMR 106, with osteoblast-like nature (5).

Materials and Methods

UMR 106 cells were a gift from Dr. T.J. Martin, University of Melbourne, Australia. Cells were cultured in Eagle's minimum essential medium supplemented with 5% heat--inactivated fetal bovine serum. After treatment of the cells with $1,25(OH)_2D_3$ for 48h, the cells were double labeled with [^{3}H]ethanolamine and [^{14}C]serine, or [^{3}H]inositol and [^{14}C]choline for 1h. At the end of incubation, lipids were extracted and separated by two-step TLC. For the analyses of phospholipid contents, UMR 106 cells were culturd in a medium containing 50uM serine with or without $1,25(OH)_2D_3$.

Results and Discussion

As shown in Table I, when UMR 106 cells were treated with 10^{-8}M $1,25(OH)_2D_3$ for 48h, there was a marked increase in [^{14}C]serine incorporation into PS. At the same time, the incorporation of [^{3}H]ethanolamine, [^{3}H]inositol and [^{14}C]choline into PE, PI and PC respectively decreased by the treatment. Among them, the reduction in [^{3}H]ethanol-amine incorporation into PE was the largest. The effect of $1,25(OH)_2D_3$ on phospholipid contents is shown in Table II. Treatment with $1,25(OH)_2D_3$ significantly increased PS content and slightly reduced PE, PI and PC contents.

Vitamin D. A Chemical, Biochemical and Clinical Update

Table I. Effect of $1,25(OH)_2D_3$ on the incorporation of substrates into respective phospholipids in UMR 106 cells.

	[^{14}C]Serine into PS	[^{3}H]Ethanolamine into PE	[^{3}H]Inositol into PI	[^{14}C]Choline into PC
		dpm/10^{6} cells		
Control	431 ± 19	7622 ± 433	427 ± 30	6448 ± 299
$1,25(OH)_2D_3$	797 ± 12	2904 ± 169	349 ± 17	5452 ± 213

Thus, the changes in the incorporation of various substrates into phospholipids appear to be due to changes in the synthesis of these phospholipids. Because PS is synthesized mostly by a base exchange reaction of serine with the other phospholipid head groups, and because the most favorite substrate for the base exchange reaction of serine is shown to be PE (6), the present results suggest that $1,25(OH)_2D_3$ enhances PS synthesis by a stimulation of base exchange reaction in UMR 106 cells. In the light of these observations as well as the previous demonstration that PS stimulates bone mineralization through the formation of Ca-PS-Pi complexes, it is reasonable to speculate that $1,25(OH)_2D_3$ has a direct effect on osteoblasts to stimulate bone mineralization by enhancing the synthesis of PS in these cells.

Table II. Effect of $1,25(OH)_2D_3$ on phospholipid contents in UMR 106 cells.

	PS	PE	PI	PC
		μg phospholipid phosphorus / mg protein		
Control	0.95 ± 0.17	4.61 ± 0.18	1.01 ± 0.06	4.71 ± 0.30
$1,25(OH)_2D_3$	1.27 ± 0.07	4.32 ± 0.26	0.77 ± 0.16	4.52 ± 0.08

Supported in part by a Grant-in-Aid for Encouragement of Young Scientists and a Grant-in-Aid for Scientific Research from the Ministry of Education, Science and Culture of Japan, and a grant from Yamanouchi Foundation.

References

1. Wuthier, R.E. (1982) Clin. Orthop. Rel. Res. 169,219--242
2. Boskey, A.L. and Posner, A.S. (1977) Calcif. Tissue Res. 23,251-258
3. Matsumoto, T., Fontaine, O. and Rasmussen, H. (1981) J. Biol. Chem. 256,3354-3360
4. Tsutsumi, M., Alvarez, U.M., Kurnik, B., Avioli, L.V. and Hruska, K.A. (1984) Abstract of the 6th Annual Meeting of the ASBMR, A78
5. Partridge, N.C., Alcorn, D., Michelangeli, V.P. Ryan, G. and Martin, T.J. (1983) Cancer Res. 43,4308-4314
6. Holub, B.J. and Kuksis, A. (1978) Adv. Lipid Res. 16,1-125

EFFECT OF 1,25(OH)2D3 ON MINERALIZATION OF DENTIN

S.Matsumoto, M.Yamaguchi, M.Arai and T.Tsudyuki
Department of Pharmacology, School of Dentistry, Aichi-Gakuin University, Nagoya 464 JAPAN

We have previously reported the enhancement of dentin mineralization by parathyroid hormone (PTH) in the parathyroidectomized (PTXed) animals without affecting serum calcium level ([Ca]s), that is a potent regulatory factor of the process (S.Matsumoto et.al., 4th Workshop on Vitamin D 1979, 411-414). In this study, effects of the active Vitamin D3 (1,25(OH)2D3) on Ca s and mineralization of dentin were examined in two hypocalcemic rats, PTXed and Vitamin deficient (VDdef) ones.

MATERIALS AND METHODS

Male Wistar strain rats were used. In the first experiment, 8 weeks old animals were PTXed and fed a synthetic diet (0.3% Ca, 0.42% P and V.D free, 12 g/day, at 17:00). In the second one, 3 weeks old weanling rats were fed the same diet for 8 weeks. Hypocalcemia that was lower than 6 mg% was taken as the indication of successful operation in PTX or of Vitamin D deficiency.
1,25(OH)2D3 of four doses (0(vehicle), 2.5, 8, 25ng/day/head) were infused for 10 (in the first experiment) or 9 (in the second one) days by using 'osmotic mini-pumps'.
Blood samples were taken from tail vein of the rats and [Ca]s was determined by atomic absorption, spectrophotometry.
Small dose (3 mg/kg) of Lead-acetate (Pb) was injected (i.v.) to mark time in the dentin. Pb3 (the third injection of Pb, and so on) was injected at the beginning of the infusion. Pb4 and Pb5 were injected on the third and on the eight day of the infusion, respectively.
The rats were killed at the end of infusion, and histological sections of the dentins were prepared.

RESULTS AND DISCUSSION

1) Effects of 1,25(OH)2D3 in PTXed animals
As shown in Fig. 1, infused 1,25(OH)2D3 elevated [Ca]s, which has been decreased by PTX, in a dose dependent manner. At the highest dose applied (25 ng/day), [Ca]s reached at a hypercalcemic level (ca. 12 mg%) and the most obvious diurnal change of [Ca]s was observed.
The dentin was remineralized by the infusion of 1,25(OH)2D3. The Pb4 deposited at the beginning of the remineralized zone in the 8 ng group, and it was found within the zone in the 25 ng group. Periodical pattern which corresponded to the diurnal change of [Ca]s was observed in the remineralized zone of the sections. These results show the obvious dependency of the remineralization on the dose of 1,25(OH)2D3.

Vitamin D. A Chemical, Biochemical and Clinical Update

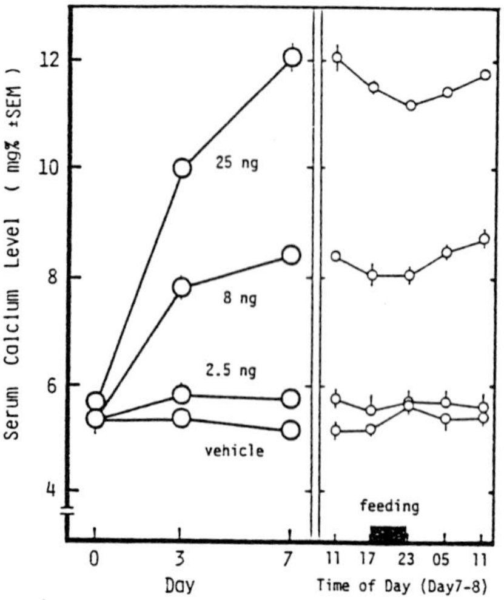

Fig.1 Effect of 1,25(OH)2D3 on Serum Calcium in Parathyroidectomized Rats

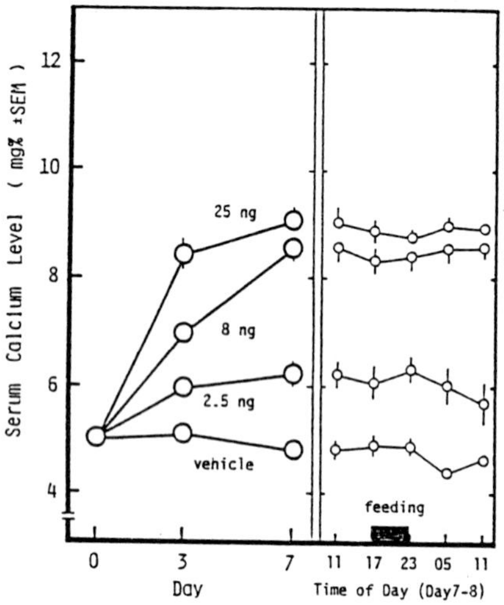

Fig.2 Effect of 1,25(OH)2D3 on Serum Calcium in Vitamin D-Deficient Rats

It is notable that weak but marked remineralization was induced even by the smallest dose of 1,25(OH)2D3 (2.5 ng/day) without significant increase of [Ca]s (Fig. 1). This observation would suggest a possible role of 1,25(OH)2D3 on direct regulation in the dentin (re)mineralization.
Judging from the difference in width of dentin of the four groups, the matrix formation of the dentin in PTXed animals seemed to be enhanced by the infusion of 1,25(OH)2D3.

2) Effects of 1,25(OH)2D3 in VDdef animals
Severe hypocalcemia (ca. 5 mg%) and suppressed dentin mineralization were also established by feeding young rats with a synthetic V.D free diet for 8 weeks (Fig.2). Elevation of [Ca]s by the infused 1,25(OH)2D3 was again dose dependent. The smallest dose of 1,25(OH)2DS (2.5 ng/day) significantly elevated [Ca]s in VDdef rats. However, effect of the highest dose of 1,25(OH)2D3 (25 ng/day) on [Ca]s was lesser in VDdef rats than that in PTXed ones.
1,25(OH)2D3 also induced the remineralization of dentin in the VDdef animals. The position where the Pb4 or Pb5 deposited clearly show the dependency of the effect on the dose of 1,25(OH)2D3. In the VDdef rats, however, the initiation of remineralization was later than that of PTXed ones which were given the same dose of 1,25(OH)2D3. These discrepancies might be explained by an unknown role of PTH in the metabolism of 1,25(OH)2D3.
Except the case of 2.5 ng group in the PTXed animals, it rather seemed that the initiation of remineralization was mainly controled by the [Ca]s.
The matrix formation of the dentin was not affected appreciably by the infusion of 1,25(OH)2D3 in VDdef animals. This might suggest a contribution of PTH released in response to the severe hypocalcemia on the matrix formation of dentin.

$1,25(OH)_2D_3$ INCREASES ALP ACTIVITY AND TYPE I COLLAGEN PRODUCTION IN OSTEOBLASTIC CLONE MC3T3-E1 CELLS IN SERUM-FREE MEDIA.

N. Kurihara, M. Kumegawa[1)], K. Ikeda, Y. Hakeda[1)], M. Kiyoki[2)] and S. Ishizuka[2)]

Department of Periodontology and Oral Anatomy[1)], Josai Dental University, Sakado, Saitama 350-02. Institute for Biomedical research[2)], Teijin Limited, Hino, Tokyo 191, Japan

We have previously demonstrated that $1,25(OH)_2D_3$ at physiological concentrations stimulated an increase in alkaline phosphatase (ALP) activity in osteoblastic clone MC3T3-E1 cells (1) in the presence of serum (2). However, in supplemented media a detailed analysis of the mechanism underlying vitamin D action on osteoblast differentiation is difficult because undefind factors in the medium may interfere. Therefore, cultivation of osteoblastic cells in serum-free medium should clarify how vitamin D effects the cell.

First, to know time-dependent response to the cells to $1,25(OH)_2D_3$, 3×10^4 cells were cultured in 35-mm dishes containing α-MEM with 10% fetal bovine serum or 1,2,3,5 and 10 days, and the cells were then transferred to media containing 0.1% BSA plus 5 pg/ml of $1,25(OH)_2D_3$. This hormone increased ALP activity in an early culture. Therefore, in further experiments the hormone was added to the cells which had been cultured for 2 days. $1,25(OH)_2D_3$ had a slight but significant effect on protein content, but not on DNA content(Table 1).

Table 1. Effect of $1,25(OH)_2D_3$ on DNA and protein contents and ALP activity in clone MC3T3-E1 cells

		DNA	protein	ALP activity	
		(μg/dish)	(mg/dish)	(units/μg DNA)	(units/mg protein)
Control		6.974±0.346	0.337±0.035	1.587±0.063	32.84±2.08
$1,25(OH)_2D_3$ (pg/ml)	0.2	6.662±0.350	0.329±0.048	1.798±0.099	36.41±1.98
	1.0	6.404±0.306	0.349±0.019	2.448±0.107*	44.95±6.43*
	5.0	6.256±0.414	0.383±0.022	4.455±0.245**	72.77±0.97**
	10.0	6.124±0.154	0.401±0.042	3.748±0.336**	57.23±3.52**

Values are means±SE for 5 dishes. *, $P<0.05$, **, $P<0.01$ compared to control

This hormone increased does-dependently ALP activity in the cells up to a concentration of 5 pg/ml which is one-tenth of those observed in the cells cultured in medium containing serum (2). The maximal effect was observed at 5 pg/ml of $1,25(OH)_2D_3$, being 2.2-fold above that of control cultures. $1,25(OH)_2D_3$ stimulated an increase in type I collagen production via an elevation of collagen synthesis but not an inhibition of collagen degradation (Table 2). Moreover, this hormone affected non-collagen protein synthesis to a less

Vitamin D. A Chemical, Biochemical and Clinical Update

extent than collagen synthesis, indicating that the hormone has a rather specific effect on collagen synthesis.

Table 2.

Effect of $1,25(OH)_2D_3$ on collagen and non-collagen protein syntheses in clone MC3T3-E1 cells

		Collagen synthesis (cpm 10^{-4}/dish)	Non-collagen protein synthesis (cpm 10^{-4}/dish)	Percent of collagen synthesis to protein synthesis
Control		5.10 ± 0.43	6.98 ± 0.36	11.9
$1,25(OH)_2D_3$ (pg/ml)	0.2	5.30 ± 0.27	6.73 ± 0.32	12.7
	1.0	8.90 ± 0.50**	8.52 ± 0.79*	16.2
	5.0	9.46 ± 0.55**	9.07 ± 0.85*	19.3
	10.0	7.14 ± 0.10*	7.48 ± 0.55	15.0

*, $P<0.05$; **, $P<0.01$ compared to control

Table 3.

Effect of $1,25(OH)_2D_3$ on collagen accumulation and content of free hydroxyproline in clone MC3T3-E1 cells.

	Accumulated Collagen ($dpm \times 10^{-3}$/dish)	Free Hydroxyproline ($dpm \times 10^{-3}$/dish)	Free Hydroxyproline / Accumulated Collagen
Control	14.9 ± 1.4	1.41 ± 0.10	95
$1,25(OH)_2D_3$	33.0 ± 1.5*	1.38 ± 0.06	42
$1,25(OH)_2D_3$/control	2.21	0.98	

*$P<0.01$

Finally, we examined the correlation between the binding ability of $1,25(OH)_2D_3$ receptor and DNA synthesis. The maximal binding ability of $1,25(OH)_2D_3$ receptors was observed at 3 day of cultures, its level being 2-fold above that in later cultures. The binding ability of $1,25(OH)_2D_3$ receptor was correlated with DNA synthesis and the response of the cells to the hormone.

Thus, to our knowledge, this is the first report that $1,25(OH)_2D_3$ alone stimulates increases in ALP activity and collagen production in osteoblasts *in vitro*. These results indicate a direct anabolic effect of $1,25(OH)_2D_3$ on the differentiation of osteoblast *in vitro*. We thank you Dr. H. Kodama for the gift of clone MC3T3-E1 cells.

References

1. Sudo, H., Kodama, H., Amagai, Y., Yamamoto, S. and Kasai, S. (1983) J. Cell Biol. 96, 191-198.
2. Haneji, T., Kurihara, N., Ikeda, K. and Kumegawa, M. (1983) J. Biochem. 94, 1127-1132.

HOW DO OESTROGENS MODULATE BONE RESORPTION?

R.M. FRANCIS, M. PEACOCK, G.A. TAYLOR, A.J. KAHN* and S.L. TEITELBAUM*
MRC Mineral Metabolism Unit, The General Infirmary, Leeds,UK.
*Washington University Medical Center, St Louis,Missouri, USA.

Introduction:

Oestrogens reduce bone resorption in vivo independent of the calcium regulating hormones (1). They also suppress bone resorption in organ culture but only at high concentrations (2) which suggests toxicity. Since oestrogen receptors have not been identified in bone cells, indirect mechanisms of action must be considered. Such an action may be on lymphocytes as they release bone resorbing lymphokines and have receptors for oestrogen, PTH and $1,25(OH)_2D$ (3). We have investigated the effects of oestrogen on the resorption of devitalized bone by macrophages (MØ), on monocytic differentiation of the promyelocytic leukaemia HL-60 cell line induced by $1,25(OH)_2D_3$ and on the release of bone resorbing factors from human mononuclear cells exposed to PTH or phytohaemagglutinin (PHA).

Methods:

MØ-mediated resorption: Rat peritoneal MØ's (5×10^5 cells/well) were incubated with radiolabelled devitalized bone particles (4) and the effect of 17-β oestradiol (E_2;10^{-9} to 10^{-4}M) on ^{45}Ca release determined.

Monocytic differentiation: HL-60 cells were treated with $1,25(OH)_2D_3$ 10^{-8}M ± E_2 10^{-6}M and the effect on proliferation and adherence to plastic observed (4). HL-60 cells were also screened for oestrogen receptors.

Mononuclear cell induced resorption: Human mononuclear cells from blood were cultured (2×10^6 cells/ml) with and without E_2 10^{-6}M for 1 day. The cells were then exposed to PTH (100 ng/ml) for 4 hours or PHA (5 μg/ml) for 6 days. After pH correction, conditioned media was then tested for its ability to stimulate ^{45}Ca release from radiolabelled mouse calvaria and MØ-mediated resorption. In the calvarial assay 4-5 day old mouse pups were injected with 3 μCi ^{45}Ca and killed a day later. 3 mm punch biopsies from each hemicalvarium were cultured with modified BGJ media + 10% horse serum diluted 1 to 1 with control or conditioned media and ^{45}Ca release measured at 96 hours.

Results:

E_2 (10^{-9} to 10^{-6}M) had no effect on mØ-mediated resorption; apparent inhibition occurred at 10^{-4}M but was associated with a corresponding reduction in cell number. The mØ oestrogen receptor status is unknown.

E_2 also had no effect on $1,25(OH)_2D$ stimulated monocytic differentiation of HL-60 cells, and oestrogen receptors were not found on these cells.

The effect of E_2 on the release of bone resorbing factors from mononuclear cells treated with PTH is shown (Fig.). Control media + PTH, stimulated calvarial resorption but

Vitamin D. A Chemical, Biochemical and Clinical Update

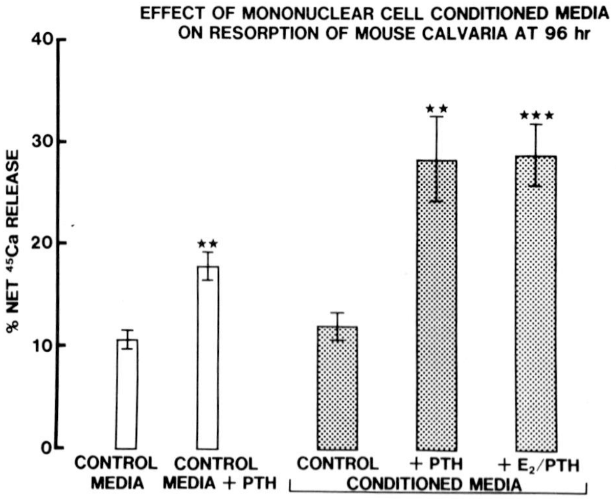

Fig.

conditioned media from cells exposed to the same concentrations of PTH showed a significantly ($p<0.05$) greater stimulation, which pretreatment with E_2 did not prevent. Media + PTH did not stimulate Mø-mediated resorption, but conditioned media from cells treated with PTH showed enhancement of resorption which was not reversed by pretreatment with E_2. PHA also stimulated the release of bone resorbing factors from mononuclear cells and this was also unaffected by E_2.

Summary:

1. The "inhibition" of bone resorption with E_2 in vitro is due to toxicity.
2. E_2 does not inhibit $1,25(OH)_2D_3$ stimulated monocytic differentiation of HL-60 cells suggesting that oestrogens do not inhibit osteoclast recruitment.
3. Circulating mononuclear cells release bone resorbing factors when exposed to PTH or PHA.
4. Pretreatment of these cells with E_2 does not alter the response to PTH or PHA.

References:

1. Peacock,M.,Selby,P.L.,Francis,R.M.,Taylor,G.A.(1985) This volume.
2. Peacock,M.,Taylor,G.A.,Norman,A.W., in Vitamin D:Biochemical and Clinical Aspects Related to Calcium Metabolism.Ed. Norman e.a., Walter de Gruyter,Berlin.1977,p411-413
3. Haussler,M.R.,Donaldson,C.A.,Allegretto,E.A.,Marion,S.L., Mangelsdorf,D.J.,Kelly,M.A.,Pike,J.W.,in Osteoporosis. Ed. Christiansen e.a. Dept.Clin.Chem.Glostrup Hospital,Denmark 1984,p725-736
4. Bar-Shavit,Z.,Teitelbaum,S.L.,Reitsma,P.,Hall,A.,Pegg,L.E., Trial,J.,Kahn,A.J.(1983) Proc.Natl.Acad.Sci.USA.80,5907-5911

CONTRASTING EFFECTS OF 1,25(OH)$_2$ VITAMIN D$_3$ AND AMINOHYDROXYPROPYLIDENE BISPHOSPHONATE (APD) ON BONE TURNOVER IN THE MOUSE.

P.J. MARIE, M. HOTT and M.T. GARBA
Unité 18 INSERM, Hôpital Lariboisière, 6 rue Guy Patin, 75010 Paris-France.

Introduction :

Whereas 1,25(OH)$_2$D$_3$ is known to be a potent stimulator of bone resorption, it remains unknown whether this metabolite exerts a direct or indirect effect on bone formation. It has been shown that stimulation of osteoclastic bone resorption following the continuous infusion of 1,25(OH)$_2$D$_3$ in mice results in increased bone mineralization without change in serum calcium level (1). In this study, we have investigated whether stimulation of bone mineralization results from a direct effect of 1,25(OH)$_2$D$_3$ or is secondary to stimulation of bone resorption. To test this hypothesis, bone resorption was inhibited by the bisphosphonate APD, administered prior to the concurrent infusion of 1,25(OH)$_2$D$_3$.

Animals and Methods :

32 days old mice from the C57BL/6J strain were divided into 8 groups of 8-15 animals. One group of mice was injected daily with APD for 10 days at the dose of 16 µmol/kg/day, a dosage level that has been shown to inhibit bone resorption (2). Three other groups were given the same treatment with the first injection of APD occurring 3 days prior to the continuous administration of 1,25(OH)$_2$D$_3$ at 3 different doses for 7 days. The metabolite was infused from Alzet^R osmotic minipumps at the doses of 0.06, 0.13 or 0.20 µg/kg/day that has been previously shown to stimulate bone resorption in mice (1). Another group of mice was infused with 1,25(OH)$_2$D$_3$ alone at the same doses and control animals were given the solvent alone. Biochemical and skeletal changes were assessed by determination of minerals in serum and bone ash and by histomorphometric analysis of undecalcified sections of caudal vertebrae after double ^{3}H-proline and double tetracycline labelings. The identification of osteoclasts was made after histochemical staining of acid phosphatase activity.

Results :

As expected, serum 1,25(OH)$_2$D$_3$ concentration increased in all groups of mice treated with the hormone. 1,25(OH)$_2$D$_3$ infusion at the highest dosage levels was associated with reduced body and skeletal growth of the treated mice. These deleterious effects were abolished in mice treated by 1,25(OH)$_2$D$_3$ and the concurrent administration of APD. Similarly, 1,25(OH)$_2$D$_3$ infusion for 7 days produced hypercalcemia and this effect was abolished in mice treated with 1,25(OH)$_2$D$_3$ combined with APD (Table 1). Compared to controls, APD alone at the dose given inhibited bone resorption as shown by the decreased number of acid phosphatase-stained osteoclasts (Table 1). APD alone also decreased all parameters of bone formation such as the amount of osteoid, the osteoblastic surface, serum alkaline phosphatase and the endosteal mineral apposition rate and matrix apposition rate (Table 2).

		Serum calcium (% of controls)	No of active osteoclasts/mm² (% of controls)
APD		+ 2.5	- 20.2[a]
1,25(OH)$_2$D$_3$	0.06[b]	+ 26.9[a]	+ 17.9[a]
	0.13	+ 27.3[a]	+ 29.7[a]
	0.20	+ 35.2[a]	+ 40.3[a]
APD + 1,25(OH)$_2$D$_3$	0.06	- 3.4	- 30.6[a]
	0.13	+ 6.0	- 25.9[a]
	0.20	+ 6.7	- 29.3[a]

Table 1 : Change in serum calcium and osteoclastic bone resorption (a : significant at the 5% level or better, b : µg/kg/day)

Vitamin D. A Chemical, Biochemical and Clinical Update

When given alone, 1,25$(OH)_2D_3$ increased the number of active osteoclasts (table 1). The endosteal mineral apposition rate increased with 1,25$(OH)_2D_3$ dosage while the matrix apposition rate was decreased at the two highest doses, causing a dose related decrease in the osteoid volume, surface and thickness (table 2).

		Osteoid thickness (% of controls)	Matrix apposition rate (% of controls)	Mineral apposition rate (% of controls)
APD		- 28.7[a]	- 40.8[a]	- 16.0[a]
1,25$(OH)_2D_3$	0.06[b]	- 19.7[a]	- 2.9	+ 25.1[a]
	0.13	- 26.4[a]	- 22.5[a]	+ 31.8[a]
	0.20	- 28.7[a]	- 34.3[a]	+ 27.0[a]
APD + 1,25$(OH)_2D_3$				
	0.06	- 36.8[a]	- 42.6[a]	0
	0.13	- 44.0[a]	- 43.8[a]	+ 5.8
	0.20	- 49.9[a]	- 64.5[a]	+ 1.6

Table 2 : Change in parameters of bone formation (a : significant at the 1 % level, b : µg/kg/day).

In mice treated with APD prior to 1,25$(OH)_2D_3$, the osteoclastic bone resorption was as much inhibited as in animals treated with APD alone (table 1). Accordingly, the mineralizing effect of 1,25$(OH)_2D_3$ was abolished and the mineral apposition rate was not augmented compared to controls (table 2). By contrast the matrix apposition rate and the amount of osteoid were further decreased compared to the groups treated with either APD or 1,25$(OH)_2D_3$ alone. The calcified bone volume was increased by 22 % after treatment with APD and this effect was abolished after the concurrent infusion of 1,25$(OH)_2D_3$.

Discussion :

This study shows that 1,25$(OH)_2D_3$-induced stimulation of bone turnover can be inhibited in vivo by the concurrent administration of APD. Pretreatment with APD prevented the deleterious effects produced by the high doses of 1,25$(OH)_2D_3$ on body growth. In addition, the bisphosphonate blocked the hypercalcemic as well as the bone resorbing effects of 1,25$(OH)_2D_3$. We also found that the bone mineralization rate was not augmented after treatment with APD and 1,25 $(OH)_2D_3$ despite increasing circulating 1,25$(OH)_2D_3$ level. These results demonstrate that the stimulatory effect of 1,25$(OH)_2D_3$ on bone minerelization is blocked when bone resorption is inhibited, which supports the hypothesis that 1,25$(OH)_2D_3$ promotes bone mineralization in the mouse mainly in response to stimulation of bone resorption.

References :

1 - Marie,P.J., Travers, R. (1983) Calcif. Tissue Int. 35,: 418-425.

2 - Reitsma, P.H., Bijvoet, O.L.M., Verlinden-ooms, H., Van der Wee-pals, L.J.A., (1980). Calcif. tissue Int. 32 : 145-147.

IS THERE A DIRECT RELATIONSHIP BETWEEN VITAMIN D AND BONE RESORPTION?

LEROY KLEIN AND KAM M. WONG

Department of Orthopaedics, Case Western Reserve University,
School of Medicine, Cleveland, Ohio 44106 U.S.A.

INTRODUCTION:

Interactions between vitamin D and bone have been observed by binding of D metabolites to nuclear receptors of cultured bone cells (1), increased release of ^{45}Ca from prelabelled fetal bones in organ culture (2), and by net increase of calcium and ^{45}Ca in blood from prelabelled rats and chicks that were treated with vitamin D (3). These observations have led to the conclusion (4) that vitamin D metabolites increase bone resorption. In the present report we demonstrate that under normal conditions where diurnal variation of plasma ^{45}Ca (5), ^{3}H-tetracycline, and 1,25-dihydroxycholecalciferol (1,25-DHCC) occurs in dogs there is a reciprocal relationship between the plasma levels of 1,25-DHCC and that of ^{45}Ca and ^{3}H-tetracycline suggesting that bone resorption was at a minimum when 1,25-DHCC was at a maximum. The effect of vitamin D or its metabolites were also studied in dogs or chicks under different experimental conditions.

METHODS AND RESULTS:

Young growing chicks or pups were prelabelled extensively with multiple injections of ^{45}Ca and ^{3}H-tetracycline over 2 to 6 weeks, respectively (5,6). Four weeks after the end of labelling when the dogs (n = 5) had approached an isotopic steady state for ^{45}Ca, they showed a diurnal variation in blood ^{45}Ca (35-40%) and ^{3}H-tetracycline (20-25%) that reached a minimum at 5 PM when blood 1,25-DHCC was at its highest level (200-300% of normal); blood calcium remained constant. Prelabelled dogs that were thyroparathyroidectomized (TPTX) showed no diurnal variation for blood ^{45}Ca or ^{3}H-tetracycline.

Oral administration of 1,25-DHCC (0.5 to 3 μg) to dogs prelabelled with ^{45}Ca (7) showed elevation of blood calcium in 5 normal dogs from 11.5 to 15 mg/dl and in 5 TPTX dogs from 7.3 to 12 mg/dl without significant increases in blood ^{45}Ca (dpm/ml). Dogs prelabelled with ^{45}Ca were placed on a rachitogenic diet for 2 months, whereby both 25-DHCC and 1,25-DHCC were markedly reduced. These dogs were treated by returning them to a normal diet which resulted in an exaggerated diurnal variation of blood ^{45}Ca and hypercalcemia as well as a prompt and very large decrease in blood ^{45}Ca (dpm/ml) which varied inversely with the marked increases in blood calcium.

When conditions of hypervitaminosis D are induced with large doses of vitamin D in young chicks prelabelled with ^{45}Ca, ^{3}H-tetracycline, and ^{3}H-proline (6), vitamin D induces a high blood calcium (16 mg/dl) and large losses of ^{45}Ca from bone (40%) within the first week of D treatment without increasing the loss of ^{3}H-tetracycline or ^{3}H-collagen from bone. A gradual decrease in the ratio of blood ^{45}Ca specific activity to that of bone indicates a gradual inhibition of bone resorption. Bone mineralization was markedly inhibited as seen by the total absence of bone oxytetracycline fluorescence or by the complete inhibition of ^{3}H-tetracycline in nonradioactive chicks treated with vitamin D.

DISCUSSION AND CONCLUSION:

The data derived from diurnal variation, 1,25-DHCC administration to normal or TPTX dogs, and the treatment of rachitic dogs with a normal diet suggest that 1,25-DHCC or its metabolites have little effect on increasing bone resorption under conditions that can mobilize calcium from the intestine. In hypervitaminosis D where large amounts of ^{45}Ca can be rapidly mobilized from bone and excreted, bone resorption is somewhat reduced instead of being increased. Under these conditions net bone resorption or mobilization of bone calcium into blood could be increased by a marked inhibition of bone mineralization rather than an increase in the absolute rate of bone resorption. These interpretations are consistent with vitamin D receptors being found in osteoblasts but not in osteoclasts (8), and 1,25-DHCC did not increase bone resorption when disaggregated rabbit osteoclasts were tested in vitro (9).

REFERENCES:

1. Walters, M.R., Rosen, D.M., Norman, A.W., Luben, R.A. (1982) J. Biol. Chem. 257: 7481-7484.
2. Raisz, L.G., Trummel, C.L., Holick, M.F., DeLuca, H.F. (1972) Science 175: 768-769.
3. Holick, J.F., Garabedian, M., DeLuca, H.F. (1972) Science 176: 1146-1147.
4. Norman, A.W. (1979) Vitamin D: The Calcium Homeostatic Steroid Hormone, Academic, New York, pp. 388-390.
5. Wong, K.M., Klein, L. (1984) Am. J. Physiol. 246: R688-R692.
6. Klein, L. (1980) Proc. Natl. Acad. Sci. 77: 1818-1822.
7. Klein, L., Wong, K.M. (1985) Can. J. Physiol. Pharmacol., in press.
8. Narbaitz, R., Stumpf, W.E., Sar, M., Huang, S., DeLuca, H.F. (1983) Calcif. Tiss. Intern. 35: 177-182.
9. Chambers, T.J., McSheehy, P.M.J., Thomson, B.M., Fuller, K. (1985) Endocrinology 116: 234-239.

A NORMAL DIETARY CALCIUM INTAKE OR HYDROCHLOROTHIAZIDE INHIBITS BONE RESORPTION WHEN SERUM 1,25-$(OH)_2$-D LEVELS ARE ELEVATED.

J. LEMANN, JR., R.W. GRAY, W.J. MAIERHOFER AND H.S. CHEUNG
Departments of Medicine and Biochemistry, MEDICAL COLLEGE OF WISCONSIN, Milwaukee, WI 53226 USA

We previously observed that experimental elevations of serum 1,25-$(OH)_2$-D concentrations caused negative Ca balances and increased urinary hydroxyproline excretion in healthy men fed diets providing only 4-5 mmol Ca/day (1,2). The present studies were undertaken to assess the effects of increasing dietary Ca intake or the administration of hydrochlorothiazide (HTZ) in the presence and absence of experimentally elevated serum 1,25-$(OH)_2$-D concentrations. We have evaluated the components of Ca balance, daily urinary hydroxyproline excretion and fasting urinary Ca/creatinine as indices of net bone resportion as well as serum 1,25-$(OH)_2$-D and PTH concentrations.

We studied healthy men fed diets containing either 4 mmol Ca/day (n = 14), 9 mmol Ca/day (n = 3) or 22 mmol Ca/day (n = 3). Subjects were studied while they either ate these diets alone or while they were also given calcitriol, 0.5 or 0.75 µg 6-hourly. Six subjects who ate the 4 mmol/day Ca diet were studied before and during the administration of HTZ, 25 mg 12-hourly; three of these subjects were also given calcitriol 0.5 µg 6-hourly during both the control and HTZ phases of their studies. Control observations were obtained beginning at least ten days after the adaptation to the standard diets. Experimental observations during the administration of either calcitriol or HTZ were obtained during periods beginning ten days after the initiation of calcitriol administration or after six days of ongoing HTZ administration. The analytic methods for the measurements of mineral and acid balances, Ca regulating hormones and hydroxyproline have been published (3,4).

When dietary Ca intake was only 4 mmol/day, net intestinal Ca absorption averaged -0.6 ± 1.2 SD mmol/day, urinary Ca excretion averaged 2.6 ± 1.3 mmol/day and Ca balance averaged -3.2 ± 1.5 mmol/day. When serum 1,25-$(OH)_2$-D levels were experimentally increased among subjects fed this low Ca diet, net intestinal Ca absorption increased to 2.4 ± 0.5 mmol/day; $p < 0.001$. However, urinary Ca excretion rose to a greater extent reaching 8.0 ± 2.0 mmol/day; $p < 0.001$. Thus, Ca balances became more negative averaging -5.7 ± 1.4 mmol/day, $p < 0.025$. Urinary hydroxyproline excretion also rose. By contrast, when dietary Ca intake was 9 or 22 mmol/day, experimentally increased serum 1,25-$(OH)_2$-D levels did not cause more negative Ca balances or an increase in urinary hydroxyproline excretion (3).

When HTZ was given to the six subjects fed only 4 mmol Ca/day (regardless of calcitriol administration), net intestinal Ca absorption did not change from control rates averaging 0.5 ± 2.2 mmol/day. Urinary Ca excretion fell as expected during HTZ by -1.4 ± 0.8 mmol/day; $p < 0.01$, so that Ca balances became less negative by -1.6 ± 1.0 mmol/day; $p < 0.025$. Daily urinary hydroxyproline excretion and fasting urinary Ca/creatinine also fell (5).

Serum PTH was suppressed in proportion to dietary Ca intake at any given plasma 1,25-$(OH)_2$-D concentration. Thus, the availability of

Vitamin D. A Chemical, Biochemical and Clinical Update

dietary Ca appears to protect the skeleton when serum 1,25-$(OH)_2$-D levels are high by suppressing PTH secretion. HTZ had no effect on serum PTH or 1,25-$(OH)_2$-D concentrations. It also did not effect urinary cAMP excretion. However, HTZ raised serum bicarbonate concentrations and blood pH by 2.7 ± 0.5 mEq/L; $p < 0.001$ and by 0.05 ± 0.02 units; $p < 0.005$, respectively. Thus relative alkalosis in response to HTZ may contribute to the mechanism by which HTZ inhibits net bone resorption.

Acknowledgements: Supported by USPHS AM 15089, AM 22014 and RR 00058.

REFERENCES

1. Adams, N.D., Gray, R.W., Lemann, J. Jr. and Cheung, H.S. (1982) Kidney Int. 21:90-97.
2. Maierhofer, W.J., Gray, R.W., Cheung, H.S. and Lemann, J. Jr. (1983) Kidney Int. 24:555-560.
3. Maierhofer, W.J., Lemann, J. Jr., Gray, R.W. and Cheung, H.S. (1984) Kidney Int. 26:752-759.
4. Lennon, E.J., Lemann, J. Jr. and Litzow, J.R. (1966) J. Clin. Invest. 45:1601-1607.
5. Lemann, J. Jr., Gray, R.W., Maierhofer, W.J. and Cheung. H.S. (1985) Kidney Int. 27:121.

VITAMIN A AND 1,25$(OH)_2D_3$ ARE BOTH ABLE TO INHIBIT BONE COLLAGEN SYNTHESIS AS WELL AS TO STIMULATE BONE RESORPTION.

I.R. DICKSON and J. WALLS,
Department of Medicine, University of Cambridge Clinical School, Addenbrooke's Hospital, Cambridge CB2 2QQ, England.

1,25$(OH)_2D_3$ and vitamin A (retinol) both can stimulate bone resorption in vitro (1,2). Both can stimulate secretion of collagenase and reduce the production of collagenase inhibitor by bone in culture (3). There is also evidence that 1,25$(OH)_2D_3$ can influence bone-forming as well as bone-resorbing cells since it can inhibit collagen synthesis by mammalian (4,5) and chick (6) bone in vitro. We have therefore investigated whether the ability to influence bone matrix synthesis is also possessed by retinol.

Two systems were used to study retinol action: cultures of 16-day-embryonic chick calvaria, which contain few osteoclasts and thus provide a convenient means to study bone-forming cells, and secondly, cultures of 4-day-old murine calvaria, which contain both bone-forming and bone resorbing cells. Bones were cultured, on grids of stainless-steel mesh, in petri dishes at 37°C and a gas phase of CO_2/air (1:19) with a modified BGJ_b medium containing ascorbic acid (150μg/ml) and bovine serum albumin (5mg/ml). Bones were labelled by the addition of 5μCi[^{3}H]-proline and 50 μg ascorbic acid per ml of medium 4h before the end of the culture period and afterwards were extracted with cold 5% TCA:10mM proline, acetone and ether before being air-dried, weighed and homogenised in 0.5M acetic acid. Synthesis of collagen and non-collagenous protein was estimated by measuring the degree of incorporation of [^{3}H]-proline into collagenase-digestible and collagenase non-digestible fractions of the homogenate by the procedure of Peterkofsky and Diegelmann (7). The experimental procedures used have been described in detail elsewhere (8).

Incubation of chick calvaria with retinol for 48h decreased collagen synthesis, as measured by incorporation of [^{3}H]-proline into collagenase-digestible protein. The effect increased with the concentration of retinol and synthesis of non-collagenous protein was relatively unaffected. Collagen synthesis, expressed as a percentage of total protein synthesis was 38% in control cultures and this proportion decreased progressively with increasing concentration of retinol above 2μg/ml to a value of 15% at 20 μg/ml. At lower concentrations of retinol (0.001-1μg/ml) the synthesis of collagen and non-collagenous protein was not significantly different from controls. The selective effect of retinol on collagen synthesis was similar to that observed with 1,25$(OH)_2D_3$.

Vitamin D. A Chemical, Biochemical and Clinical Update

Collagen synthesis was significantly lower than controls after 24h incubation with retinol and decreased progressively with the length of time in culture; non-collagenous protein synthesis was not significantly affected up to 4 days in culture. 1,25$(OH)_2D_3$ also significantly reduced collagen synthesis within 24h but longer periods of incubation did not produce a much greater response. The inhibitory effect on collagen synthesis produced by incubating chick bones with either retinol or 1,25$(OH)_2D_3$ could be reversed by a further period of incubation in control medium.

Retinol also selectively inhibited collagen synthesis by cultures of neonatal murine calvaria. The minimum concentration of retinol necessary to produce a statistically significant response was approximately one tenth of that required for chick calvaria. The murine and chick culture systems showed a similar difference in sensitivity with respect to the action of 1,25$(OH)_2D_3$ on collagen synthesis. The concentration of retinol necessary to produce an inhibitory effect on collagen synthesis by murine calvaria was similar to that required to stimulate resorption, the latter being estimated by release into the medium of ^{45}Ca by calvaria of mice that had been pre-labelled with that isotope in vivo.

These observations provide evidence that retinol can influence the metabolism of bone-forming cells and suggest that there are some similarities between retinol and 1,25$(OH)_2D_3$ in the way these compounds influence bone-forming as well as bone-resorbing cells. Further investigation of this relationship should help to establish the mechanisms by which these compounds act on bone.

References

1. Raisz, L.G. (1965) J. Clin. Invest. 44, 103-116.
2. Reynolds, J.J., Holick, M.F. and DeLuca, H.F. (1973) Calcif. Tissue Res. 12, 295-301.
3. Sellers, A., Meikle, M.C. and Reynolds, J.J. (1980) Calcif. Tissue Int. 31, 35-43.
4. Raisz, L.G., Maina, D.M., Gworek, S.C., Dietrich, J.W. and Canalis, E.M. (1978) Endocrinology 102, 731-735.
5. Bringhurst, F.R. and Potts, J.T. Jr. (1982) Calcif. Tissue Int. 34, 103-110.
6. Dickson, I.R. and Maher, P.M. (1985) J. Endocrinology (in press).
7. Peterkofsky, B. and Diegelmann, R. (1971) Biochemistry 10, 988-994.
8. Dickson, I.R. and Walls, J. (1985) Biochem. J. (in press).

REGULATORY EFFECT OF VITAMIN D_3 METABOLITES, CALCITONIN AND PARATHYROID HORMONE ON THE BGP SYNTHESIS AND/OR SECRETION IN CHICK EMBRYONIC CALVARIA IN VITRO.

C. TSUTSUMI, N. HOSOYA, H. ORIMO, K. HOSHIBA*, S. MORIUCHI*
Faculty of Medicine, University of Tokyo, Bunkyo-ku, Tokyo 113, Japan, *Japan Women's University, Bunkyo-ku, Tokyo 112, Japan.

Introduction

Since the discovery of the stimulatory effect of 1,25-dihydroxyvitamin D_3(1,25-$(OH)_2$-D_3) on the BGP(bone γ-carboxyglutamic acid containing protein) synthesis and/or secretion in rat osteosarcoma cell in culture(1), the regulation of BGP in bone has attracted special attention. To study this issue, the effect of calcium regulating hormones(1,25-$(OH)_2$-D_3, 24,25-dihydroxyvitamin D_3(24,25-$(OH)_2$-D_3), parathyroid hormone(PTH), calcitonin(CT)) on the synthesis and/or secretion of BGP in the chick embryonic calvariae were investigated in vitro.

Materials and Methods

Chick embryonic calvariae from 13 days' incubation were cultured in the Eagle's MEM supplemented with 10% fetal calf serum. As test substances, 1,25-$(OH)_2$-D_3(Teijin Pharmaceutical Company), 24,25-$(OH)_2$-D_3(Kureha Chemical Company), PTH(3300 U/mg) and CT(6 U/µg)(Toyo Jozo Chemical Company) were used. 1,25-$(OH)_2$-D_3 and 24,25-$(OH)_2$-D_3 were dissolved in 95% ethanol, PTH was in 0.1% bovine serum albumin and CT was in 0.1 mM citrate buffer(pH 6.0), respectively. The final concentration of vehicles was less than 0.25%. In the control group, only vehicle was added. Each substance or vehicle was added into culture media through a Millipore filter. Calvariae were cultured for 24, 48, 72 or 120 hours respectively in a humidified incubator (Hotpack Corp., USA) continuously supplied with 5% CO_2 in air at 37°C. After culture, calvariae and media were collected for the determinations of BGP contents. BGP was measured by a radioimmunoassay(2). Data were either expressed as µg BGP/mg bone dry powder for BGP contents in calvariae and those in media as ng BGP/mg wet weigtht of cultured calvaria or the ratio of BGP contents in calvariae or media of treated group over control.

Results and Discussion

In good agreement with the results from cell culture system of osteosarcoma cell line(ROS 17/2), the addition of 10^{-8}M 1,25-$(OH)_2$-D_3 into culture media of chick embryonic calvariae significantly stimulated the secretion of BGP in culture media. 1,25-$(OH)_2$-D_3 induced increase of BGP in

Vitamin D. A Chemical, Biochemical and Clinical Update

culture media was observed from 24 to 72 hours of culture and then became plateau at 120 hoursof culture. 1,25-$(OH)_2$-D_3 induced increase in BGP level in culture media after 72 hours was 4-5 times when compared with the controls. On the other hand, until 72 hours of culture, BGP content in calvaria was not affected by 1,25-$(OH)_2$-D_3 and significantly increased at 120 hours. It appears that the synthesized BGP in the calvaria by 1,25-$(OH)_2$-D_3 was immediately released into the medium up to 72 hours after culture, while BGP was accumulated in the calvaria and not released into the medium at 120 hours after culture. Our previous study(3) showed that increase in BGP following the injection of 1,25-$(OH)_2$-D_3 into developing 13-day chick embryos was preceded by the increase in serum BGP. A similar response for 1,25-$(OH)_2$-D_3 injection into normal rat was reported by Price *et al*(4). These facts may be explained by the change of the physiological property of the bone.
Subsequently, the effects of other calcium regulating hormones on the synthesis and/or secretion of BGP in chick embryonic calvariae were compared with those of 1,25-$(OH)_2$-D_3 *in vitro*. After a 72 hour culture, 1,25-$(OH)_2$-D_3 increased BGP contents in culture media at concentration of 10^{-10}M-10^{-7}M and the effect was maximum at 10^{-8}M. BGP contents in calvariae were not changed significantly by 1,25-$(OH)_2$-D_3. On the other hand, 24,25-$(OH)_2$-D_3 increased BGP contents in media and in calvariae only at 10^{-6}M. PTH caused biphasic change of BGP both in calvariae and media. PTH increased BGP contents in calvariae and media at low concentration(1 U/ml), while it decreased BGP contents at high concentrations(5 U-10 U/ml). CT had no effect on BGP contents in calvariae and media from 0.5 U/ml to 10 U/ml. These findings suggest that 1,25-$(OH)_2$-D_3 is the most potent regulator of BGP synthesis and/or secretion among calcium regulating hormones.

References

(1) Price, P.A. and Baukol, S.A. (1980) J.Biol.Chem. 255, 11660-11663.

(2) Tsutsumi, C., Hosoya, N. and Moriuchi, S. (1983) J.Nutr. Sci.Vitaminol. 29, 643-654.

(3) Tsutsumi, C., Hosoya, N. and Moriuchi, S. (1985) J.Nutr. Sci.Vitaminol. 31, 27-34.

(4) Price, P.A. and Baukol, S.A. (1981) Biochem.Biophys.Res. Commun. 99, 928-935.

INTERLEUKIN 1 AND CYCLOSPORIN A MODULATE ACTIONS OF 1,25-DIHYDROXYVITAMIN D_3 ON BONE IN VITRO

H.Skjodt,* J.N. Beresford,*, D.D. Wood+ and R.G.G. Russell*.
*Department of Human Metabolism and Clinical Biochemistry, University of Sheffield Medical School, Beech Hill Road, Sheffield S10 2RX, UK,
+Ayerst Research Lab., Princeton, NJ 08540, USA.

Introduction

There is increasing evidence that 1,25-$(OH)_2D_3$ influences skeletal homeostasis by regulating local cells involved in bone resorption as well as cells directing bone formation and mineralisation. Cells of the immune system may be directly involved in the local regulation of bone remodelling. Thus, several monokines and lymphokines have been reported to affect the activity of both the osteoclast or its putative precursors of the monocyte-macrophage lineage (1,2) and cells of the osteoblast stromal lineage (3,4). Although 1,25$(OH)_2D_3$ is clearly stimulating osteoclast-mediated bone resorption in vitro, specific 1,25$(OH)_2D_3$ receptors have not been demonstrated in osteoclasts. However, recent evidence has confirmed that 1,25$(OH)_2D_3$ not only promotes the differentiation of putative osteoclast precursor cells (5), but also regulates the production of several monocyte/macrophage- and T lymphocyte-derived cytokines which may all participate in the regulation of bone remodelling (6,7).

We have shown that the monokine, interleukin 1 (Il-1) antagonises 1,25$(OH)_2D_3$ induced osteocalcin production by human bone cells in vitro (4). In fact, the production of Il-1 can be enhanced by 1,25$(OH)_2D_3$ (6) and it is possible that Il-1 may be involved in the local modulation of 1,25$(OH)_2D_3$ action on bone. Thus, the above finding could represent a putative negative feedback modulation. In this study we addressed the question whether cyclosporin A (CSA) might modify actions of 1,25$(OH)_2D_3$ on bone in vitro. This immunomodulator exerts a highly selective blockage of the production of several T cell derived factors, incuding osteoclast activating factor (OAF, 8). Moreover, we have shown that actions of Il-1 on bone are antagonised by CSA (9). Thus, CSA could be a useful probe to test putative Il-1 dependent 1,25$(OH)_2D_3$ actions on bone.

Materials and Methods

Human bone cell monolayers were formed by cell outgrowth from explants of human trabecular bone. This cell population expresses certain putative phenotypic features of osteoblasts, as described earlier (4). All experiments were performed at first subculture. Osteocalcin was measured by a specific radioimmunoassay using an antibody raised in rabbits against purified bovine osteocalcin as reported previously (4).

Bone resorption assay. Newborn mouse calvaria were labelled with ^{45}Ca as described earlier (1). After a 48 hour test incubation ^{45}Ca release was measured and results were expressed as a treated/control ratio.

Partially purfified human Il-1 (MW 15000, neutral peak) was prepared from normal and transformed monocytes as described earlier (1). CSA was a generous gift from Sandoz Ltd, Switzerland.

Results and Conclusion

CSA antagonised 1,25$(OH)_2D_3$-dependent production of osteocalcin by human osteoblast-like cells in a dose dependent manner. During a 48 hour incubation period the net release of osteocalcin induced by 5×10^{-9} M 1,25$(OH)_2D_3$ was reduced by 10^{-8}M CSA to 71 $\pm$ 3% of control values

Vitamin D. A Chemical, Biochemical and Clinical Update

(n=5, P<0.01) and by 10^{-6}M CSA to 59 ± 1% of control values (n=5, P<0.01).

The results presented in Table 1 show that CSA can antagonise $1,25(OH)_2D_3$ stimulated bone resorption in a dose dependent manner. This effect was apparently independent of prostaglandin synthesis, as it was unaffected by the addition of indomethacin (data not shown). CSA did not in itself affect the basal ^{45}Ca release (Table 1).

Table 1
^{45}Ca release/48 h from prelabelled mouse calvaria in response to $1,25(OH)_2D_3$ and CSA.

Compound		Addition		n	Treated/control ratio
$1,25(OH)_2D_3$ 10^{-8}M		Medium alone		6	2.3 ± 0.21
		CSA	10^{-8}M	5	1.7 ± 0.09[a]
			10^{-7}M	5	1.5 ± 0.10[a]
			10^{-6}M	5	1.3 ± 0.06[b]
CSA	10^{-8}M	Medium alone		5	1.1 ± 0.05
	10^{-7}M			6	1.0 ± 0.09
	10^{-6}M			6	1.2 ± 0.12

[a] p<0.01; [b] p<0.001 (analysis of variance)

We conclude that effects of $1,25(OH)_2D_3$ on bone resorbing as well as bone forming cells may be modulated by CSA sensitive local factors, including Il-1. In fact, the bone resorbing activity of Il-1 is potently antagonised by CSA (9). In view of the possible enhancement of Il-1 release by $1,25(OH)_2D_3$ (6), Il-1 could be acting as a $1,25(OH)_2D_3$ agonist in terms of bone resorption although we have found no apparent synergism between the factors in preliminary studies. On the other hand, we reported previously that Il-1 could antagonise $1,25(OH)_2D_3$ dependent osteocalcin production, an effect which is partially reversed by CSA (9). Taken together with the present findings, it is possible that immune cell derived cytokines may have a role in $1,25(OH)_2D_3$ action on bone.

References

1. Gowen, M., Wood, D.D., Ihrie, E.J., McGuire, M.K.B. and Russell, R.G.G. (1983) Nature 306, 378-380.
2. Horowitz, M., Vignery, A., Gershorn, R.K., Baron, R. (1984) Proc.Nat. Adad.Sci USA, 81, 2181-2185.
3. Rifas, L., Shen, V., Mitchell, K., Peck, W.A. (1984) Proc.Nat.Acad.Sci USA, 81, 4558-4562.
4. Beresford, J.N., Gallagher, J.A., Gowen, M., Couch M., Poser, J.W., Wood, D.D., Russell, R.G.G. (1984) BBA 801, 58-65.
5. Abe, E., Miyaura, C., Tanaka, H., Shuna, Y., Kuribayashi, T., Suda, S., Nashi, Y., DeLuca, H.F., Suda, T. (1983) Proc.Natl.Acad.Sci USA, 80, 5583-5587.
6. Amento, E.P., Bhalla, A.K., Kurnick, J.T., Kradin, R.L., Clemens, T.L., Holick, S.A., Holick, M.F., Krane, S.M. (1984) J.Clin.Invest, 73, 731-739.
7. Hodler, B., Evequoz, V., Trechsel, U., Fleisch, H. (1984) Calc.Tiss.Int, 36, suppl 2, S40.
8. Horowitz, M., Baron, R., Mart, J., Andreoli, M., Vignery, A. (1984) Calc.Tiss.Int, 36,4,462.
9. Skjodt, H., Crawford, S., Elford, P.R., Ihrie, E., Wood, D.D., Russell, R.G.G. (1985) Brit.J.Rheum (in press).

THE ROLE OF VITAMIN D METABOLITES IN NON-UNION OF FRACTURE

S.A. HAINING, R.M. ATKINS, D.F. GUILLAND-CUMMING, W.J.W. SHARRARD, R.G.G. RUSSELL and J.A. KANIS,
Department of Human Metabolism and Clinical Biochemistry, University of Sheffield Medical School, Beech Hill Road, Sheffield S10 2RX

Introduction

There is increasing evidence that vitamin D metabolites have an important role in the healing of fractures. Vitamin D deficiency delays fracture repair in birds and mammals (1,2), but the role of specific metabolites is less clear. Both $1,25(OH)_2D_3$ and alfacalcidiol have been reported to promote fracture healing in D-deficient rats or chicks (3,4), suggesting that metabolites such as $25\text{-}OHD_3$ or $24,25(OH)_2D_3$ are not essential for this process. In contrast, the combination of $24,25(OH)_2D_3$ and $1,25(OH)_2D_3$ has been found to promote fracture repair more completely or more rapidly than either agent or alfacalcidiol alone (4). Moreover $24,25(OH)_2D_3$ is localised in high concentrations in the calluses of experimental chicks (5) and low values for $24,25(OH)_2D$ have been described following femoral neck fracture in the elderly (2). It has also been reported (4) that the serum $24,25(OH)_2D$ values are low in patients with non-union of fracture, and that its administration may promote healing (6). For these reasons we investigated serum concentrations of vitamin D metabolites and biochemical indices of skeletal metabolism in patients with established non-union of fracture.

Methods

We studied 15 patients with established non-union of fracture (14 males and 1 female, age range 19-82), and 15 control subjects matched for age and sex. Dihydroxylated metabolites were extracted from 3 ml of serum using hexane: n-butanol: isopropanol (93:4:3 v/v) and then partially purified on Sep-Pak C_{18} cartridges followed by separation on HPLC. $1,25(OH)_2D_3$ was assayed by radioimmunoassay using antiserum 02282 and $24,25(OH)_2D$ and 25-OHD with a competitive binding protein assay, using a 1:70,000 dilution of normal human serum. 25-OHD was measured on an ethanolic extract of 200 ul of serum followed by chromatography on silicic acid.

Results

Biochemical indices of bone turnover were normal in patients with non-union of fracture. The mean value of urinary hydroxyproline/creatinine, a marker of bone resorption, was 22 $\pm$ 2 umol/mmol (normal range 15-35 umol/mmol) and serum alkaline phosphatase activity, a marker of bone formation was 77 $\pm$ 5 U/l (normal range 35-105 U/l). There were no significant differences in the serum concentrations of the vitamin D metabolites between patients with non-union of fracture and controls (Fig. 1). To account for the seasonal variation in vitamin D metabolism, $24,25(OH)_2D$ concentrations were also expressed as a percentage of 25-OHD. Patients with non-union of fracture were found to have slightly but not significantly higher values (10.4 $\pm$ 1.3%), than controls; (7.3 $\pm$ 1.2%; $p>0.05$).

Vitamin D. A Chemical, Biochemical and Clinical Update

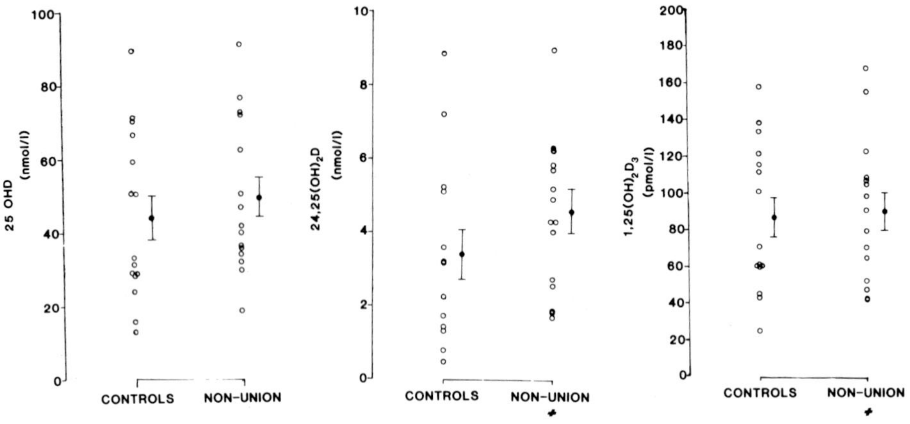

Figure 1: Vitamin D metabolite concentrations in serum from patients with established non-union of fracture and from controls.

Discussion

The serum concentrations of the vitamin D metabolites did not differ in patients with non-union from their age and sex matched controls. We, therefore, found no evidence to support the previous finding of low $24,25(OH)_2D$ concentrations in patients with non-union. Indeed, when $24,25(OH)_2D$ values were expressed as a percentage of 25OHD, this value was slightly higher in patients than controls. It is possible that the low values found by others were in patients with less established non-union, and in whom the metabolic effects of the fracture were still present. In our patients, the markers of bone turnover examined, urinary hydroxyproline excretion and serum alkaline phosphatase activity, showed no deviation from normal. We, therefore, find no evidence for defective production of $24,25(OH)_2D$, or other vitamin D metabolites in the maintenance of non-union of fracture.

Acknowledgments

We are grateful to the SERC and Teva Pharmaceutical Industries for their support, and to Hoffman La Roche for supplies of vitamin D metabolites and to Professor JLH O'Riordan for the antiserum 02282.

References:

1. Brumbaugh, P.F, Speer, D.P., Pitt, M.J. (1982) Am.J.Pathol. 106, 171-179
2. Weisman, Y., Salama, R., Harell, A., Edelstein, S. (1978) Brit.Med.J, (ii), 1196-1197.
3. Lindholm, T.S., Sevastikoglou, J.A. (1978) Acta Othop.Scand. 49, 485-491.
4. Dekel, S., Salama, R., Edelstein, S. (1983) Clin.Sci, 65, 429-436.
5. Dekel, S., Ornoy, A., Sekeles, E., Noff, D., Edelstein, S. (1979) Calcif. Tissue. Int. 28, 245-251.
6. Goodman, W.G, Baylink, D.J., Sherrard, D.J. (1984) Calcif.Tissue.Int. 36, 206-213.

HEPATIC OSTEODYSTROPHY: THE IMPORTANCE OF VITAMIN D DEFICIENCY or ALL THAT GLITTERS IS NOT GOLDNER

Irwin H. Rosenberg, M.D.
University of Chicago, Chicago, IL 60637, USA

In an effort to focus our evening discussion on the importance of vitamin D in the etiology, treatment, and prevention of osteodystrophy which commonly complicates cholestatic liver disease, we might ask the question posed in a recent editorial: "When is vitamin D responsive bone disease not osteomalacia?" (1). The editorial called attention to the trend of recent reports of series of patients with cholestatic liver disease in which bone biopsies failed to meet the diagnostic criteria of osteomalacia, though osteopenia was often advanced. A recent series that failed to show either osteomalacia or osteoporosis concluded rather that there was increased fractional resorbing surface as the major lesion (2), and the latest series, which also fails to diagnose osteomalacia, observes defective osteoblast function (3). There is little doubt that the histomorphometric criteria for the diagnosis of osteomalacia have grown tighter over the roughly 30 years that bone biopsies have been used to study this problem, but serious questions can be raised as to the extent to which these tightening diagnostic criteria add to our understanding of the etiology and pathogenesis of hepatic osteodystrophy. In particular, since vitamin D is the focus of this workshop, we might ask whether osteomalacia as currently defined in bone biopsy criteria is a satisfactory indicator of the participation of vitamin D in the complex etiology of the osteodystrophy that complicates cholestatic liver disease. Perhaps we have gone a bit too far in depending on biopsy criteria alone while we give too little weight to the clinical criteria which has historically been the basis for the diagnosis of osteomalacia. Further, although the use of tetracycline labeling has added a dynamic element to the evaluation of bone biopsies, I propose that an even more compelling advance beyond static diagnostic criteria would be the dynamic response of clinical indices of bone disease and parameters of bone biopsy evaluation to treatment with vitamin D or vitamin D metabolites.

Permit me to introduce our discussion by presenting a brief review of the various series of patients with cholestatic liver disease who have had both clinical and bone biopsy evaluations over the past thirty years. This review will demonstrate the trends in technique and evaluation of bone biopsies and the growing tendency to use exclusively histological criteria to classify the bone lesion. This review will include a smaller number of series in which repeat bone biopsies were performed after vitamin D therapy to permit a closer look at those measures which respond to vitamin D even though static values were not considered indicative of osteomalacia. Finally I will show some of the small experience, now growing, with the use of bone mineral density studies by photon absorptiometry which will almost certainly have to take the place of the assessments of trebecular bone volume on trephine biopsy as a way of looking at trends in bone mass in these patients.

Vitamin D. A Chemical, Biochemical and Clinical Update

Table 1

PREVALENCE OF "OSTEOMALACIA"
BY BIOPSY IN CHOLESTATIC LIVER DISEASE

SERIES	# PATIENTS	# "OSTEOMALACIA"	COMMENT
1956 Postgraduate London (4)	20	7	Wide osteoid seams, osteoporosis observed in 3
1978 Royal Free London (7)	25 /16	18	Histomorphometry
1980 St. Thomas London (8)	32 /17	4	Histomorphometry & toluidine blue
1980 Univ. of Chicago Chicago (9)	7 /5	5	No tetracycline labelling
1981 St. James Leeds (10)	15 /0	7	Toluidine blue, tetracycline
1982 Johns Hopkins Baltimore (11)	15 /1	0	Normal bone formation rate
1982 Tufts, MGH Boston (12)	10 /2	0	Selected for osteopenia
1983 Royal Infirmary Manchester (13)	5	3	Tetracycline
1984 Univ. of Texas Dallas (2)	11 /5	0	↑ bone resorptive surface
1985 Mayo Clinic Rochester (3)	15 /0	0	↓ bone formation rate with normal osteoblast/ osteoid surface

Table 1 lists representative series of bone disease in cholestatic patients dating back to the earliest studies in which bone biopsy was used for the characterization of the metabolic bone disease. The seminal 1956 study by Atkinson, Nordin, and Sherlock (4) used a combination of bone pathology and clinical criteria to arrive at an estimate of the prevalence of osteomalacia in their population of patients with primary biliary cirrhosis and related cholestatic syndromes. The figures presented in Table 1 describe osteomalacia based on bone biopsy criteria alone, in this case wide osteoid seams. Quantitative histomorphometric criteria were not used. It is of interest that only three patients in this series were diagnosed to have osteoporosis. Although there were intervening studies from the Royal Free Hospital in London which used similar bone biopsy criteria to arrive at the diagnosis of osteomalacia in 2 of 12 and 2 of 11 patients (5,6), the next major series from the Royal Free Hospital (7) added quantitative histomorphometry to the bone biopsy evaluation and found 18 of 25 patients met the static diagnostic criteria of osteomalacia. It is of interest that 16 of the 25 patients were under some form of vitamin D treatment. In the face of growing recognition that histological diagnosis of osteomalacia required some assessment of the activity of the calcification front, Compston and her coworkers at St. Thomas reported a series of 32 patients of whom four met the newer criteria for osteomalacia (8). Using similar techniques and criteria the group at Leeds reported a prevalence of osteomalacia of 7 of 15 patients (10). Our series at the University of Chicago used static histomorphometric criteria to identify 5 of 7 patients with osteomalacia (9). Tetracycline labeling was used in only two of those patients. However, this series added an additional dynamic dimension to the evaluation of bone biopsies by studying the response of histomorphometric indices over time to therapy which restored the serum 25-hydroxyvitamin D levels to normal or high normal. In the two studies which were reported in 1982 from Boston and Baltimore (11,12), osteoporosis was the only lesion recognized on bone biopsy by the diagnostic criteria employed. Two most recent series from the University of Texas in Dallas (2) and from the Mayo Clinic (3) similarly reported no patients who met the diagnostic criteria of osteomalacia. The Dallas study emphasized increased bone resorptive surface as the predominant lesion on these biopsies while the Mayo Clinic study emphasized decreased bone formation rate but failed to observe an increased osteoblast-osteoid surface. These studies must be viewed in the context of shifting techniques, variable patient selection, and evolving criteria for diagnosis. It is hard to conclude that osteomalacia or vitamin D deficiency is disappearing from this population. Are the current diagnostic criteria underemphasizing the participation of vitamin D deficiency in the pathogenesis of osteodystrophy in cholestatic patients?

Table 2

RESPONSE TO VITAMIN D THERAPY BY BONE BIOPSY

	Response to Vitamin D Therapy			
	Osteoid	TBV	Sr	$\overline{M}$
1980 Univ. of Chicago (9)	$\downarrow$ 5/6 = 1/6	$\downarrow$ 4/6 $\uparrow$ 2/6		
1982 Johns Hopkins (11)	Vos .0027-.0018	$\downarrow$ 13/15 $\uparrow$ 2/15		

1982	Tufts, MGH (12)	↓ 6/8 ↑ 2/8	↓ 3/8 ↑ 3/8 = 2/8		
1984	Univ. of Texas (2)	↓ 5/7 ↑ 1/7 = 1/7	↓ 3/7 ↑ 3/7 = 1/7	↓ 7/7	↓ 5/6 = 1/6

Vos = Osteoid Volume %
TBV = Trabecular bone volume
Sr = Fractional resorption surface
$\overline{M}$ = Trabecular appositional rate

One possible approach to the question of the importance of vitamin D deficiency in the pathogenesis of the bone lesion (and incidentally one which involves the clinician as well as the pathologist in the evaluation) is an examination of the response to vitamin D therapy. A response to vitamin D therapy might be seen either as correction of a lesion induced by vitamin D deficiency or as a pharmacologic effect of vitamin D therapy. There are four series in which the response to vitamin D can be judged by histomorphometric criteria. These data are reviewed in Table 2.

<u>Figure 1</u>

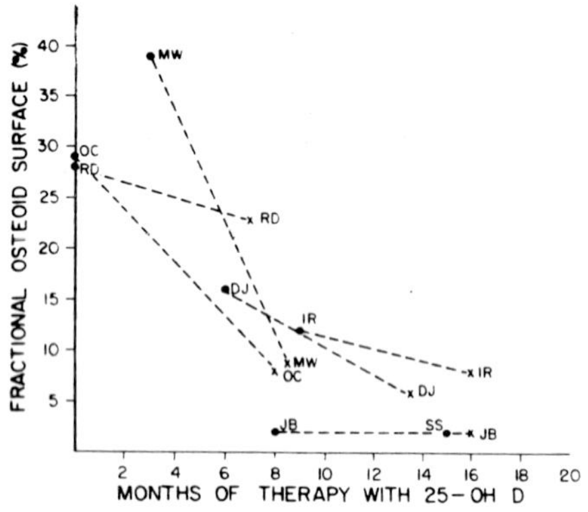

Correlation of duration of oral 25-hydroxyvitamin D therapy with improvement in osteomalacia, represented by change in fractional osteoid surface. The same change occurred in relative osteoid volume. Two of 7 patients (*OC, RD*) had not received 25-hydroxyvitamin D before the first biopsy (*closed circle*). Follow-up biopsy (×) was obtained in 6 patients.
Reed et al (9).

In the University of Chicago study, five of six showed a lessening of the increased fractional osteoid surface in the presence of vitamin D therapy while one patient with normal osteoid at the beginning of the study remained the same. Although there was no statistical change in the mean trabecular bone volume as a measure of osteopenia, it is of interest that two of the six patients showed a slight trend upward in trabecular bone volume while four showed decreases. It should be emphasized here that the sampling problems in respect to bone volume measurements are a major deterent to the use of this technique as a means of assessing the skeletal response to therapeutic intervention. The Johns Hopkins and Tufts/MGH studies are of interest in that they fail to recognize osteomalacia by their diagnostic criteria. Although individual data are not presented in the Hopkins study the mean osteoid volume decreased by 33% from .0027 to .0018 with vitamin D therapy while trabecular bone volume was. in general, decreasing inexorably. In the Boston study, six of eight patients showed a decreasing amount of osteoid with vitamin D therapy while changes in trabecular bone volume were almost random. Of special interest is the study from Dallas which concluded that there was no osteomalacia but rather an increased bone resorptive surface. Five of the seven patients studied with repeat biopsy showed a decrease in osteoid with vitamin D therapy. Seven of seven showed a sharp decrease in what was reviewed as the excessive bone resorptive surface, and five os six showed vitamin D responsive decreases in the bone appositional rate. We must be cautious not to conclude that a biopsy which does not meet criteria for osteomalacia at one point in time provides evidence that vitamin D deficiency has little or no part in the pathogenesis of the bone lesion and, by implication, in the management of these patients.

Finally, I would like to call attention to an additional clinical question. It has been clear since some of the early studies by Dr. Sherlock and her colleagues that bone disease in primary biliary cirrhosis will progress in spite of aggressive vitamin D therapy. How should we assess the impact of vitamin D prophylaxis or therapy in the face of osteomalacia, which may be subclinical, or osteoporosis which may be unresponsive, knowing that the assessment of changes in trabecular bone volume are confounded seriously be sampling difficulties. The current hope lies in non-invasive studies of bone mineral density by photon absorptiometry.

Table 3

BONE MINERAL DENSITY VALUES IN CHOLESTATIC LIVER DISEASE: RESPONSE TO VITAMIN D

		Response to Vitamin D	25OHD	Comment
1976	Univ. of Chicago (14)	6/7 ↓	3/7 ↑	single photon
1982	Tufts, MGH (12)	8/8 ↓		single photon
1984	Univ. of Texas (2)	7/7 ↓		single photon

Three studies in the literature have used single photon absorptiometry. Our study at the University of Chicago from 1976 (14) reported a difference in the response to oral 25-hydroxy D therapy versus the response to oral vitamin D therapy as measured by single photon absorptiometry of the metacarpal bone. Three of seven of the patients treated with 25-hydroxy D showed an improvement by this measure of bone density. The two subsequent studies from Boston and Dallas have shown progressive loss of bone mineral density in spite of vitamin D therapy by single photon absorptiometry of the radius. The only study which uses both single and dual photon absorptiometry, currently in press, from the Mayo Clinic may set the standard by which we will have to assess the bone mineral response to therapy. Issue of controls will be paramount and very difficult. We will certainly need to match trends in bone mineral content versus age and sex-matched controls. Will we be able to compare rates of bone mineral loss in the presence of vitamin D prophylaxis or therapy versus those periods or patients in whom vitamin D therapy is withheld?

Returning to the question, "When is vitamin D responsive bone disease not osteomalacia," Drs. S. D. Rao and M. Parfitt proposed a tentative answer: "When it is due to secondary hyperparathyroidism prior to the emergence of a significant mineralization defect." The role of secondary hyperparathyroidism in the hepatic osteodystrophy lesion remains uncertain. Most studies have not found significant elevations of iPTH in three patients with the notable exception of the Leeds study (3). Once again this may be a matter of patient selection. Early PBC, as in the Mayo study (3), is likely to be associated with minor degrees of vitamin D deficiency (4 of 15 patients has low 25-OH-vitamin D levels) and vitamin D deficiency may not be sufficiently severe or prolonged to result in a permanent PTH response.

Many questions remain to be resolved in relation to the role of vitamin D in Hepatic Osteodystrophy.

1. Will early intervention with vitamin D or 25-OH-vitamin D therapy retard the progressive loss of bone mass which is so commonly seen? What is the relative value of bone morphology vs. bone density states in this evaluation?

2. Should "prophylaxis" be used only in these patients who show early evidence of vitamin D depletion? If so, what are the best indices to use for initiation and monitoring of mophylaxis serum 25-OH_2-vitamin D, serum; PTH, urinary cAMP, serum 24,25-OH_2-vitamin D.

Perhaps some of these questions will have partial answers by the time of the 7th Vitamin D Workshop. Almost certainly some multi center and multidisciplinary studies will be required.

BIBLIOGRAPHY

1. Rosenberg, I.H. (1984) Hepatology 4, 157-158.

2. Cuthbert, J.A., Pak, C.Y.C., Zerwekh, J.E., Glass, K.D., and Combes, B. (1984) Hepatology 4, 1-8.

3. Hodgson, S.F., Dickson, E.R., Wahner, H.W., Johnson, K.A., Mann, K.G., and Riggs, B.L. (1985) Ann. Intern. Med. (In Press)

4. Atkinson, M., Nordin, B.E.C., and Sherlock, S. (1956) Quart. J. Med. 25(New Series), 299-312.

5. Kehayoglou, A.K., Agnew, J.E., Holdsworth, C.D., Whelton, M.J., and Sherlock, S. (1968) Lancet 1, 715-718.

6. Ajdukiewicz, A.B., Agnew, J.E., Byers, P.D., Wills, M.R., and Sherlock, S. (1974) Gut 15, 788-793.

7. Long, R.G., Meinhard, E., Skinner, R.K., Varghesa, Z., Wills, M.R., and Sherlock, S. (1978) Gut 19, 85-90.

8. Compston, J.E., Crowe, J.P., Wells, I.P., Horton, L.W.L., Hirst, D., Merritt, A.L., Woodhead, J.S., and Williams, R. (1980) Dig. Dis. and Sciences 25, 28-32.

9. Reed, J.S., Meredith, S.C., Nemchausky, B.A., Rosenberg, I.H., and Boyer, J.L. (1980) Gastroenterology 78, 512-517.

10. Dibble, J.B., Sheridan, P., Hampshire, R., Hardy, G.J., and Losowsky, M.S. (1982) Quart. J. Med. 51(new series), 89-103.

11. Herlong, H.F., Recker, R.R., and Maddrey, W.C. (1982) Gastroenterology 83, 103-108.

12. Matloff, D.S., Kaplan, M.M., Neer, R.M., Goldberg, M.J., Bitman, W., and Wolfe, H.J. (1982) Gastroenterology 83, 97-102.

13. Davies, M., Mawer, E.B., Klass, H.J., Lumb, G.A., Berry, J.L., and Warnes, T.W. (1983) Dig. Dis. and Sciences 28, 145-153.

14. Wagonfeld, J.B., Bolt, M., Boyer, J.L., Nemchausky, B.A., Vander Horst, J., and Rosenberg, I.H. (1976) Lancet 2, 391-394.

Vitamin D Hydroxylases (Hepatic + Renal): Biochemistry and Regulation

FURTHER STUDIES ON THE REGULATION OF 25-OH-D_3 METABOLISM IN KIDNEY CELL CULTURE

HELEN L. HENRY and EDEN M. LUNTAO,
Department of Biochemistry, University of California, Riverside, California, USA.

INTRODUCTION

The study of the regulation of the metabolism of 25-OH-D_3 has spanned the past dozen years and has been approached by a wide variety of experimental systems in a number of laboratories. Initially, attention was focused on delineating the factors which appeared to alter the production of 1,25$(OH)_2D_3$ and/or 24,25$(OH)_2D_3$ in vivo as well as characterizing the enzymatic properties of the 25-OH-D_3-1-hydroxylase, and to a lesser extent, the 24-hydroxylase, in isolated mitochondria. Several years ago it became apparent that an intermediate level of organization, intact kidney cells in culture, would bring advantages to the study of the regulation of 25-OH-D_3 metabolism which were not available in the whole animal or subcellular fractions. These include intact cellular structure, required for example, for the response to parathyroid hormone, and relatively close control over the immediate environment of the cell.

Utilizing such cell culture systems, it was demonstrated by several investigators (1-4) that the effect of vitamin D status, one of the most powerful determinators of 25-OH-D_3 metabolism in vivo, is brought about by a direct effect of 1,25$(OH)_2D_3$ on kidney cells in culture. The effect of the steroid is to decrease 1-hydroxylase activity and induce 24-hydroxylase activity, most likely through nuclear mediated events. Cultured kidney cells were also important in demonstrating that other factors which appear to regulate 25-OH-D_3 metabolism in vivo, e.g. estrogens, apparently do not do so through direct effects on the renal cell (5,6).

The study of kidney cells in culture has been useful to assess whether a variety of other possible modulators of 25-OH-D_3 metabolism act directly at the level of the intact kidney cell and the purpose of this paper is to review our more recent findings in this area.

METHODS

Kidney cells were isolated as described previously (1) by digestion of tissue from 2-3 week old vitamin D-deficient chicks with collagenase, hyaluronidase and trypsin. Cells were cultured in Minimal Essential Medium containing 5% fetal calf serum. All cultures were changed to serum-free medium 20-24 hours prior to the addition of ^3H-25-OH-D_3. The radioactive substrate was allowed to incubate with the cells for either 30 minutes or, when the effect of PTH was being assessed, 4 hours. Following extraction of the lipids, substrate and products were separated by HPLC and the eluted fractions were counted to determine the amount of radioactivity present as ^3H-1,25$(OH)_2D_3$ or ^3H-24,25$(OH)_2D_3$. In some experiments, the ^3H-1,25$(OH)_2D_3$ was sequentially rechromatographed in isocratic 8% IPA/hexane; 3% dichloromethane in IPA, and 15% water in methanol. Throughout this rechromatography, more than 90% of the radioactivity co-migrated with authentic $1,25(OH)_2D_3$.

EFFECTS OF PTH AND FORSKOLIN ON $25\text{-}OH\text{-}D_3$ METABOLISM

It had previously been shown (7) that the diterpene forskolin not only stimulates cyclic AMP formation in cultured chick kidney cells but, at concentrations below those required for this effect, also markedly enhances the response of the cells to PTH. For example, 0.05 µM forskolin brings about a 20-fold increase in the amount of cyclic AMP produced in response to 50 ng/ml PTH. The time course for elevation of cyclic AMP by forskolin alone is very similar to that of PTH (7).

Figure 1 documents that when chick kidney cell cultures are incubated for 4 hours in the presence of $^3H\text{-}25\text{-}OH\text{-}D_3$, $bPTH_{1\text{-}34}$ (10 ng/ml) increases the accumulation of $^3H\text{-}1,25(OH)_2D_3$ and depresses that of $^3H\text{-}24,25(OH)_2D_3$, which is substantial in control cultures due to the endogenous production of $1,25(OH)_2D_3$ during the 4-h incubation period. A low concentration of forskolin (0.05 µM) which alone has no effect on $^3H\text{-}25\text{-}OH\text{-}D_3$ metabolism (data not shown) markedly enhances this effect of PTH. As shown in Figure 2, higher concentrations of forskolin alone bring about similar changes in $^3H\text{-}25\text{-}OH\text{-}D_3$ metabolism.

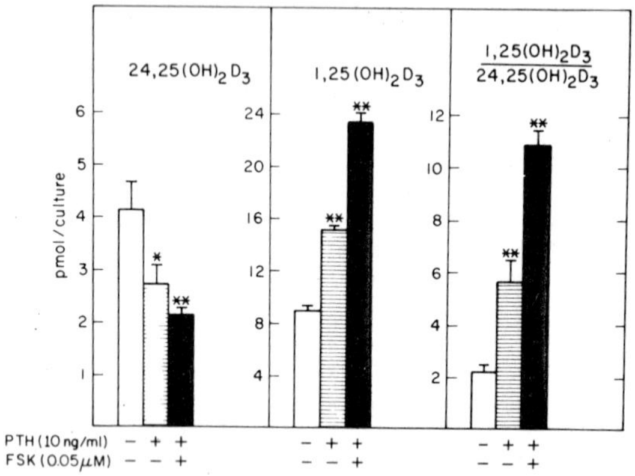

Figure 1. Effect of PTH with and without forskolin on $^3H\text{-}25\text{-}OH\text{-}D_3$ metabolism by chick kidney cell cultures. Cultures were incubated with 10 ng/ml PTH with and without 0.05 µM forskolin for 4 hours in the presence of $^3H\text{-}25\text{-}OH\text{-}D_3$. Values shown are the mean ± SD of four cultures. Asterisks indicate significant differences from control values: *, $p < 0.01$; **, $p < 0.001$; crosses (+) indicate significant differences from cultures treated with PTH only; +, $p < 0.05$; ++, $p < 0.001$.

To determine whether the effect of PTH and forskolin on $^3H\text{-}1,25(OH)_2D_3$ accumulation was due to increased production or decreased 24-hydroxylation, cultures were incubated with radioactive substrate for only 30 minutes following a 4-hour incubation with non-radioactive substrate, PTH and forskolin. The results are shown in Table 1. As expected and observed in several other experiments, there was no effect of PTH and forskolin on $^3H\text{-}25\text{-}OH\text{-}D_3$ metabolism when cells were not preincubated with either $25\text{-}OH\text{-}D_3$ or $1,25(OH)_2D_3$. Increased $^3H\text{-}1,25(OH)_2D_3$ and decreased $^3H\text{-}24,25(OH)_2D_3$ production in response to PTH was observed during the 30-minute incubation period when cultures were preincubated for 4 hours with nonradioactive $25\text{-}OH\text{-}D_3$. In other experiments in which cultures were incubated with $^3H\text{-}25\text{-}OH\text{-}D_3$ for 4 hours, there was not an appreciable difference between control and PTH-treated cultures in the concentration of $^3H\text{-}25\text{-}OH\text{-}D_3$ present at the end of the 4-hour incubation

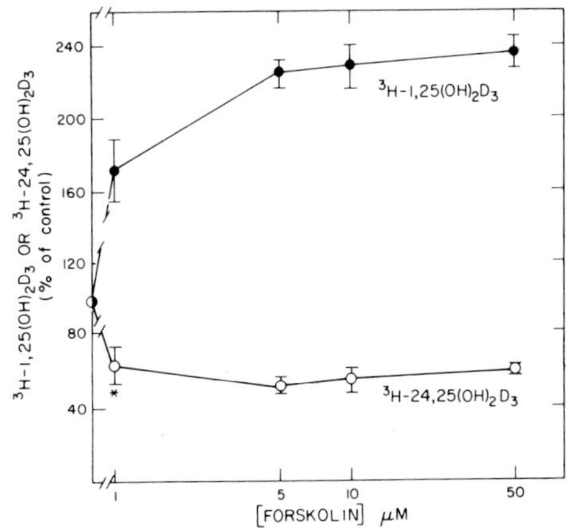

Figure 2. Effect of forskolin on ^{3}H-25-OH-D$_3$ metabolism. Chick kidney cell cultures were incubated with the indicated concentration of forskolin for four hours in the presence of ^{3}H-25-OH-D$_3$. Values are the mean ± SD of four cultures. Significantly different from control, $p < 0.05$; all other values for both metabolites were significantly different from control, $p < 0.001$.

Table 1. Effects of preincubation conditions on the subsequent response of 25-OH-D$_3$ metabolism to PTH and forskolin.

Steroid during Preincubation	PTH+FSK	^{3}H-1,25(OH)$_2$D$_3$	^{3}H-24,25(OH)$_2$D$_3$	1,25(OH)$_2$D$_3$ / 24,25(OH)$_2$D$_3$
		(pmol/culture)	(pmol/culture)	
None	-	21.2 ± 3.2	---	---
	+	20.9 ± 2.0	---	---
25-OH-D$_3$-4 hrs	-	8.3 ± 0.7	3.5 ± 0.4	2.4 ± 0.4
	+	11.5 ± 0.5*	2.2 ± 0.1*	4.9 ± 0.8*
1,25(OH)$_2$D$_3$-20 hrs	-	7.2 ± 0.6	3.9 ± 0.6	1.9 ± 0.3
	+	9.4 ± 1.9	3.6 ± 0.6	2.7 ± 0.6
25-OH-D$_3$-4 hrs	-	4.1 ± 0.1	6.0 ± 0.4	0.69 ± 0.06
+ 1,2(OH)$_2$D$_3$-20 hrs	+	4.4 ± 0.2	5.5 ± 1.0	0.86 ± 0.15

* Significantly different from appropriate control, $p < 0.002$.

Chick kidney cell cultures were incubated in serum-free medium for 20 h prior to the beginning of the experiment. 1,25(OH)$_2$D$_3$ (5 x 10^{-8} M) was present for the entire period and 25-OH-D$_3$ (5 x 10^{-8} M) was present for the final 4 h, as indicated, prior to the addition of ^{3}H-25-OH-D$_3$ for a 30-minute incubation. PTH (10 ng/ml) and forskolin (0.05 μM) were present for 4 h prior to the addition of ^{3}H-25-OH-D$_3$. Values are mean ± SD of four cultures.

period, so that the results in Table 1 cannot be attributed to a different total substrate concentration at the beginning of the 30-minute incubation period. Thus, PTH and forskolin stimulate ^3H-1,25$(OH)_2D_3$ accumulation over a 30 minute time period suggesting an effect on the production of this steroid.

As also shown in Table 1, when cultures were preincubated with 1,25$(OH)_2$-D_3 for 20 hours prior to the 30 minute incubation with PTH, there was only a slight and not statistically significant effect of PTH on the production of either ^3H-1,25$(OH)_2D_3$ or ^3H-24,25$(OH)_2D_3$. There are two possible explanations for this observation. One is that the effect of PTH, in order to be optimal, requires the presence of the substrate, 25-OH-D_3. This was tested by preincubating cultures with 1,25$(OH)_2D_3$ for 20 hours and including 25-OH-D_3 for the final 4 hours prior to the 30-minute incubation with ^3H-25-OH-D_3. As can be seen in Table 1, under these conditions there was no effect of PTH on either hydroxylase activity indicating that it is not the lack of substrate which prohibits maximal expression of the effect of PTH on 25-OH-D_3 metabolism when cells are preincubated with 1,25$(OH)_2D_3$. An alternative explanation is that when intracellular levels of 1,25$(OH)_2D_3$ are high, bringing about maximal suppression of 1-hydroxylase and induction of 24-hydroxylase activities, these effects cannot be overcome by the opposing action of PTH.

This possibility is supported by the observation that effects of PTH and forskolin on ^3H-25-OH-D_3 metabolism in chick kidney cells are dependent on the initial substrate concentration in the medium. This is illustrated by the data in Table 2. At the higher substrate concentration, the stimulatory effect of PTH on the accumulation of ^3H-1,25$(OH)_2D_3$ is

Table 2. Effect of ^3H-25-OH-D_3 concentration on the response of chick kidney cells to PTH and forskolin.

Group	Initial ^3H-25-OH-D_3: 5×10^{-8} M ^3H-25-OH-D_3	Initial ^3H-25-OH-D_3: 20×10^{-8} M ^3H-25-OH-D_3
	pmol ^3H-1,25$(OH)_2D_3$	
Control	2.7 ± 0.2	23.2 ± 1.7
PTH (10 ng/ml)	3.5 ± 0.5	20.0 ± 3.3
PTH/control	1.3 ± 0.2	0.8 ± 0.2*
FSK (10 µM)	6.1 ± 0.6	36.4 ± 3.6
FSK/Control	2.3 ± 0.2	1.6 ± 0.2*

Cultures which had been in serum-free medium for 20 hours were incubated with the indicated concentration of ^3H-25-OH-D_3 alone (control) or with the indicated concentration of $bPTH_{1-34}$ or forskolin.

* Significantly different from 5×10^{-8} M, $p < 0.02$.

completely abolished and that of forskolin is markedly reduced. This could be due to the increased absolute amount of endogenously produced $1,25(OH)_2D_3$ at the higher substrate concentration which is exerting its repressive effect on 1-hydroxylase activity. If this is indeed the explanation for the observed phenomenon, then this serves as another example of how the amount of $1,25(OH)_2D_3$ produced at any given moment is the result of a delicate balance between the prevailing levels of $1,25(OH)_2D_3$ and parathyroid hormone.

The above studies provide strong evidence that PTH alters $25\text{-}OH\text{-}D_3$ metabolism by increasing the rate of production of $1,25(OH)_2D_3$ and decreasing that of $24,25(OH)_2D_3$, an effect that supports the idea that, as originally proposed some years ago (8), the relative amount of these two dihydroxylated metabolites produced by the kidney is determined primarily by the effective ratio between $1,25(OH)_2D_3$ and PTH to which kidney cells are exposed. Furthermore, the fact that forskolin enhances and mimicks the effect of PTH (above and ref. 9) lends strong support to the concept that this effect of PTH is mediated through the elevation of intracellular cyclic AMP. This is also supported by the observation that the majority of the proteins phosphorylated in response to PTH in intact chick kidney cells appear to be substrates for cyclic AMP dependent protein kinases (10).

GLUCOCORTICOIDS

As part of our continuing effort to assess the potential of various hormones and other factors to directly modulate the metabolism of 25-OH-D_3 by cultured chick kidney cells, a number of experiments with glucocorticoids have been carried out. Dexamethasone decreases the production of $1,25(OH)_2D_3$ in cells which have not been treated with this steroid to depress the 1-hydroxylase and induce the 24-hydroxylase. A typical experiment is shown in Figure 3. Clearly, the longer time with dexamethasone brought about greater inhibition and 10^{-8} M dexamethasone was

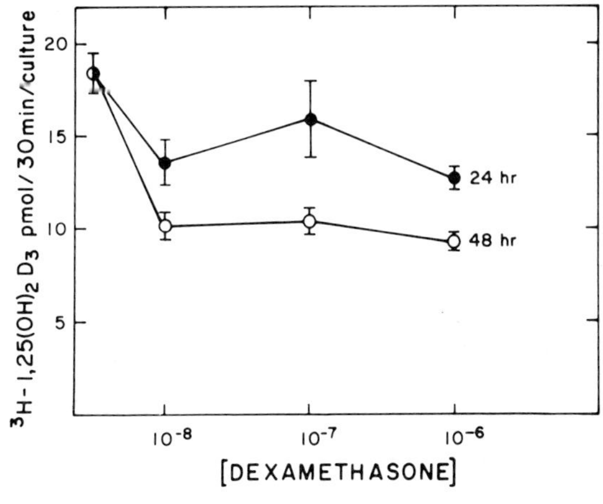

Figure 3. Effect of dexamethasone on ^3H-$1,25(OH)_2D_3$ production by chick kidney cell cultures. Dexamethasone was added to cultures either 24 hours prior to assay when cells were changed to serum-free medium or at this time as well as 24 hours previously, when cells underwent their initial medium change. Values are mean ± SD (n = 4).

about as effective as the higher concentration. There was no effect of dexamethasone on cell number under these conditions, as assessed by DNA content. Interestingly, $1,25(OH)_2D_3$ production was never reduced to less than approximately 50% of control levels. The glucocorticoid has no effect on 24-hydroxylase activity under these conditions, but brought about a 50% increase in the accumulation of ^3H-$24,25(OH)_2D_3$ when cultures were incubated with substrate for 4 hours (Figure 4). Since there was no effect of dexamethasone on $24,25(OH)_2D_3$ production when substrate was incubated with the cells for 30 minutes, it is possible that the increase seen during the 4-hour incubation period is actually due to a dexamethasone-induced decrease in 1-hydroxylation of $24,25(OH)_2D_3$, as well as 25-OH-D_3, rather than stimulation of 24-hydroxylation. As shown in Figure 4, dexamethasone did not substantially alter the effect of PTH on 25-OH-D_3 metabolism.

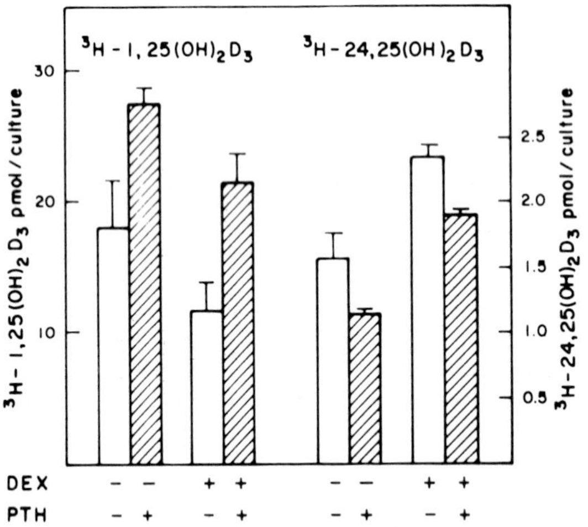

Figure 4. Effect of PTH and forskolin on ^3H25-OH-D_3 metabolism in the presence and absence of dexamethasone. Chick kidney cell cultures were incubated with 10^{-7} M dexamethasone in serum-free medium for 20 hours at which time $bPTH_{1-34}$ (10 μg/ml), forskolin (0.05 μM) were added. Four hours later, cells and medium were collected for lipid extraction and quantitation of tritiated metabolites. Values are the mean ± SD of four cultures.

In another series of experiments, the substrate concentration was varied for a 30-minute incubation with ^3H-25-OH-D_3 following treatment of the cultures with dexamethasone for 24 hours and the apparent K_m and maximal velocity were determined. These are tabulated in Table 3 and it is clear that, particularly at the higher dexamethasone concentration, both kinetic parameters are altered. Interestingly, the apparent K_m of the 1-hydroxylase for its substrate is decreased (which should result in an increase in initial velocity) but the V_{max} is decreased sufficiently to overcome this apparent increased affinity, the net result being inhibition of $1,25(OH)_2D_3$ production by dexamethasone. This apparent decrease in K_m may account for the fact that at the routine substrate concentra-

Table 3. Effect of dexamethasone on K_m and V_{max} of $1,25(OH)_2D_3$ production by chick kidney cell cultures.

Exp.	Dex	K_m ($x\ 10^{-7}$ M)	V_{max} (pmol/30 min/culture)
1	0	1.2	42
	10^{-7}	0.8	26
2	0	1.7	44
	10^{-6}	0.5	19

Kidney cell cultures were incubated with the indicated concentration of dexamethasone for 24 hours prior to assay with varying concentrations of ^3H-25-OH-D_3. K_m and V_{max} values were obtained from Eadie-Hofstee plots of the kinetic data.

tion, 5 x 10^{-8} M, maximum inhibition of $1,25(OH)_2D_3$ production obtained is approximately 50%. Perhaps at a saturating substrate concentration, a greater degree of inhibition would be obtained. Experiments are underway to test this hypothesis.

CALCIUM

One of the earliest appreciated correlations obtained from studies of the regulation of 25-OH-D_3 metabolism in vivo is the negative one between serum calcium levels and the circulating levels of and rate of production of $1,25(OH)_2D_3$. Whether this is a direct effect of calcium on the renal cell or whether the effect is mediated indirectly through PTH could not be determined from in vivo studies and we have therefore carried out a number of experiments to test the effect of the extracellular calcium concentration on 25-OH-D_3 metabolism in cultured chick kidney cells.

The results of two such experiments are shown in Figures 5 and 6. In Figure 5, cells were exposed to low (0.5 mM) or high (2.5 mM) calcium for 24 hours and the concentration dependency of the effect of $1,25(OH)_2D_3$ on ^3H-25-OH-D_3 metabolism was assessed. Calcium did not alter the quantitative pattern of metabolites formed in control cultures nor did it change the responsiveness of the cells to various concentrations of $1,25(OH)_2D_3$. In addition, the time course of the response to $1,25(OH)_2$-D_3 was not affected by medium calcium concentrations (data not shown). Similarly the extracellular calcium concentration of the medium did not affect the response of the cells to PTH, as can be appreciated from Figure 6. It has been reported that renal slices from rats (11) and cells from mice which were vitamin D replete (12) respond to elevated calcium concentrations with decreased $1,25(OH)_2D_3$ production. On the other hand, chick kidney cells cultured to confluence in low or high calcium showed no difference in 25-OH-D_3 metabolism (2) as was the case in the present report. This may represent a species difference or may indicate that the kidney requires exposure to vitamin D in vivo in order for cells to respond to altered calcium concentrations in vitro. This hypothesis is currently being tested.

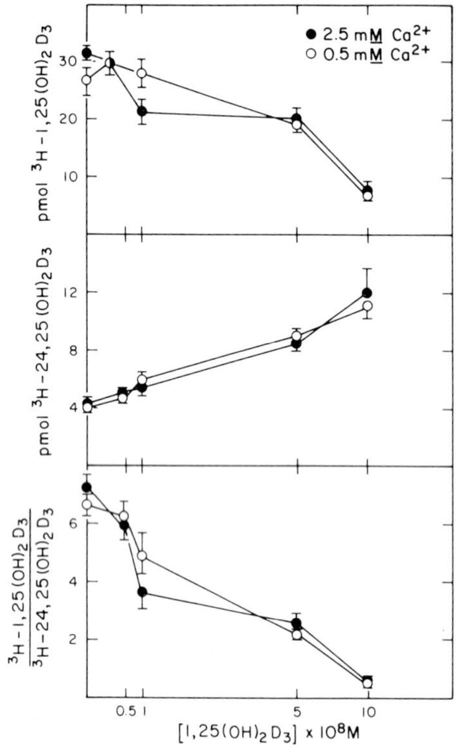

Figure 5. Lack of effect of medium calcium concentration on response of chick kidney cells to $1,25(OH)_2D_3$. Cells were exposed to serum-free medium containing 2.5 mM (●) or 0.5 mM (o) Ca^{2+} and the indicated concentration of $1,25(OH)_2D_3$ for 20 hours prior to a 30 minute incubation with ^3H-$1,25(OH)_2$-D_3. Values are the mean ± SD of four cultures.

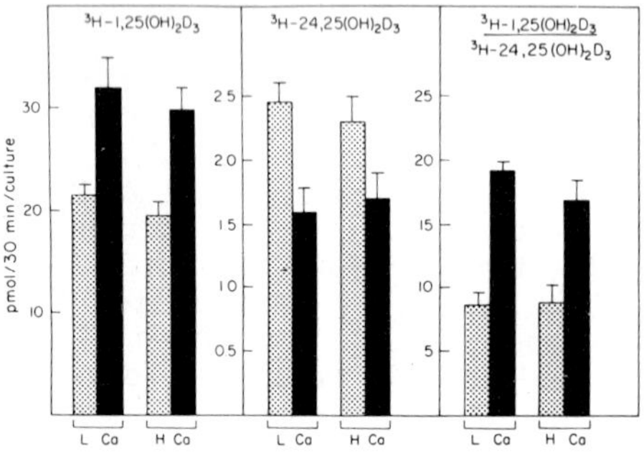

Figure 6. Effect of PTH on ^3H-25-OH-D_3 metabolism in media with low and high calcium concentrations. Chick kidney cell cultures were in serum-free medium containing 2.5 mM (H Ca) or 0.5 mM (L Ca) for 20 h prior to the addition of $bPTH_{1-34}$ (10 ng/ml), forskolin (0.05 μM) and ^3H-25-OH-D_3. Values shown are the mean ± SD of five cultures. Asterisks indicate significant differences from control values: *, $p < 0.05$; **, $p < 0.01$; ***, $p < 0.001$

ANTIMYCOTIC AGENTS

As an example of the utility of kidney cell culture to test the possible influence of compounds not previously implicated in the alteration of vitamin D metabolism, we carried out a series of experiments to extend the observation (13) that the antimycotic agent ketoconazole blocks steroidogenesis in adrenal cells and $24,25(OH)_2D_3$ production by LLC-PK_1 cells. As can be seen in Figure 7, ketoconazole inhibited the production of both $1,25(OH)_2D_3$ and $24,25(OH)_2D_3$ in cultured chick kidney cells. The K_i was approximately 1.9 µM (1 µg/ml). A related antimycotic, miconazole was also tested and found to be inhibitory as well, with somewhat less potency than ketoconazole. These data lend strong support to the idea that both the 1-hydroxylase and 24-hydroxylase are cytochrome P-450-dependent enzymes. These results underscore the utility of the chick kidney cell culture system for this type of investigation and suggest that compounds which are implicated in steroidogenesis in other tissues should be monitored for possible effects on vitamin D metabolism as well.

Figure 8 summarizes, in a qualitative manner, the current status of putative regulatory factors of 25-OH-D_3 metabolism based on a recent review of the literature (14) in which detailed citations can be found. By far the most consistently reported effects, which appear to be independent of experimental approach and to be exerted directly on the renal cell, are the opposing ones of $1,25(OH)_2D_3$ and PTH.

In summary, the primary kidney cell culture system has continued to yield important information relevant to the regulation of 25-OH-D_3 metabolism. It is clear that in order to understand on a molecular basis, the details underlying changes in the production of $1,25(OH)_2D_3$ and $24,25(OH)_2D_3$, the components of these enzyme systems must be isolated and studied. However, the cellular level of organization has and will continue to provide direction in terms of the questions to be asked at the molecular level.

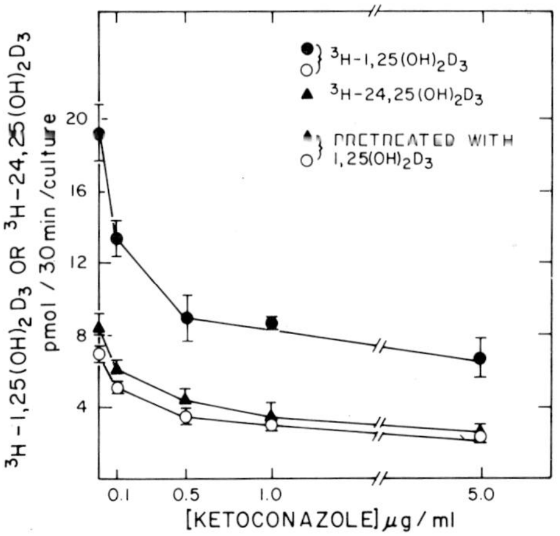

Figure 7. Effect of ketoconazole on ^3H-25-OH-D_3 metabolism in chick kidney cell cultures. Cultures were incubated with the indicated concentration of ketoconazole for 1 hour prior to the addition of ^3H-25-OH-D_3 for a 30 minute incubation. One set of cultures (○ , ▲) was pretreated with $1,25(OH)_2D_3$ for 20 hours to decrease 1-hydroxylase and increase 24-hydroxylase activity. Values are the mean + SD of four cultures.

	In vivo		In vivo→In vitro		In vitro	
	$1,25(OH)_2D_3$	$24,25(OH)_2D_3$	$1,25(OH)_2D_3$	$24,25(OH)_2D_3$	$1,25(OH)_2D_3$	$24,25(OH)_2D_3$
$1,25(OH)_2D_3$	↓	↑	↓	↑	↓	↑
PTH	↑	↓	↑	↓	↑	↓
CT	↑→		↑		↑↓→	(↑)
INCREASED Ca	↓	↑	↓	↑	(↓)→	(↑)→
DECREASED P	↑	↓	↑ →	→	→	→
ESTROGENS			↑	↓	→	→
PROLACTIN	(↑)→		↑		↑	→
GLUCOCORTICOIDS	↓ →		↓		↓	→

Figure 8. Observations in the literature have been classified according to the type of experimental protocol employed. On the left are experiments in which intact animals were used for both treatment and assessment of $25\text{-OH-}D_3$ metabolism. In the center of the figure are summarized experiments in which intact animals were treated and $25\text{-OH-}D_3$ metabolism was measured in vitro using intact cells, kidney homogenates, or isolated mitochondria. On the right are observations from systems in which both treatment and measurement of $25\text{-OH-}D_3$ metabolism were carried out in intact freshly prepared or cultured kidney cells. Detailed citations to the literature can be found in reference 14.

References

1. Henry, H. (1979) J. Biol. Chem. 254, 2722-2729.
2. Trechsel, U., Bonjour, P. J. and Fleisch, H. (1979) J. Clin. Invest. 64, 206.
3. Howard, G. A., Turner, R. T., Bottemiller, B. L. and Rader, J. I. (1979) Biochim. Biophys. Acta 587, 495-506.
4. Fukase, M., Birge, S. J., Rifas, L., Avioli, L. V. and Chase, L. R. (1982) Endocrinology 110, 1073-1075.
5. Henry, H. L. (1981) Am. J. Physiol. 240, E119-E124.
6. Spanos, E., D. I. Barret, D. I., Chong, K. T. and MacIntyre, I. (1978) Biochem. J. 724, 231-236.
7. Henry, H. L., Cunningham, N. S. and Noland, Jr., T. A. ((1983) Endocrinology 113, 1942.
8. Henry, H., Midgett, R. M. and Norman, A. W. (1974) J. Biol. Chem. 249, 7584.
9. Henry, H. L. (1985) Endocrinology 116, 503-510.
10. Noland, T. A., Jr., Henry, H. L. (1983) J. Biol. Chem. 256, 538.
11. Armbrecht, H. J., Wongsurawat, N., Zenser, T. V. and Davis, B. B (1983) Arch. Biochem. Biophys. 220, 52.
12. Fukase, M., Avioli, L. M., Birge, S. J. and Chase, L. R. (1984) Endocrinology 114, 1203.
13. Loose, D. S., Kan, P. B., Hirst, M. A., Marcus, R. A. and Feldman, D. (1983) J. Clin. Invest. 71, 1495-1499.
14. Henry, H. L. and Norman, A. W. (1984) Ann. Rev. Nutr. 4, 493-520.

Supported by USPHS grants AM-21398 and AM 23790.

RENAL 25OHD$_3$-1-HYDROXYLASE AND 24-HYDROXYLASES IN PATIENTS WITH RENAL DISEASE.

Y. SEINO, K. SATOMURA, Y. TANAKA* and H.F. DeLUCA**,
Department of Pediatrics, Osaka University School of Medicine, Osaka, Japan.
*Department of Biochemistry, University of Wisconsin-Madison, (Present address, VA Medical Center, Albany, N.Y. 12208).
**Department of Biochemistry, University of Wisconsin-Madison.

Introduction:

Vitamin D undergoes sequential 25-hydroxylation in the liver and 1-hydroxylation in the kidney to become an active form that regulates calcium and phosphorus metabolism (1). Although it is well accepted that 1,25-dihydroxyvitamin D (1,25(OH)$_2$D) is synthesized in vivo by the mammalian kidney, measurement of 25-hydroxyvitamin D$_3$-1-hydroxylase (1-hydroxylase) by kidney homogenates or mitochondria has not been possible in vitro. Past studies have demonstrated that a 25-hydroxyvitamin D (25OHD) binding protein reduces the availability of substrate to the enzyme and variably inhibits the measurable activity (2). Tanaka and DeLuca (3) have developed a technique for the measurement of mammalian renal 1-hydroxylase activity that uses substantial amounts of nonradioactive 25OHD$_3$ substrate to saturate the inhibitory protein. More recently, we have developed a microassay modification of that method for clinical use with small biopsy specimens (4).

In patients with renal disease, vitamin D and mineral metabolism may be impaired by reduction of the nephron mass and the effects of the administration of some drugs. Although the serum level of 1,25(OH)$_2$D has been studied in patients with renal disease, the 1-hydroxylase activity has not been measured. In this study, we have measured the 1-hydroxylase and 24-hydroxylase activities in patients with asymptomatic proteinuria and/or hematuria, in patients treated with prednisolone, and in patients with mild or severe renal insufficiency.

Materials and Methods:

We measured the enzyme activities in twelve patients with asymptomatic proteinuria and/or hematuria (Group A), four patients on prednisolone therapy (Group B) (two had lupus nephropathy and the others had idiopathic nephrotic syndrome), three patients with mild renal insufficiency (Group C), and three patients with severe renal insufficiency (Group D) on chronic hemodialysis or continuous ambulatory peritoneal dialysis. The patients of Group A had not received any agents which affect calcium or phosphorus metabolism. The patients in Group B were being treated with 15 to 20 mg of prednisolone

Table 1 Patients

Group A (n=12)	.....	Asymptomatic Proteinuria and/or Hematuria (Normal Renal Function)
Group B (n=4)	.....	Prednisolone Therapy (15-20 mg daily) (Normal Renal Function)
Group C (n=3)	.....	Mild Renal Insufficiency (GFR; 50-70 ml/min/1.73 m^2)
Group D (n=3)	.....	Severe Renal Insufficiency* (on HD or CAPD) *, treated with 1α-hydroxyvitamin D_3

daily for 45 to 105 days at the time of renal biopsy. The patients in Group D were treated with 1-hydroxyvitamin D_3 before renal transplantation for prophylaxis of renal osteodystrophy. Except in Group D, an ultrasound guided needle biopsy of the lower pole of the kidney was performed and the specimen was prepared for histological analysis. In the three patients with severe renal insufficiency, the kidney specimen was obtained during kidney transplantation. The parents of all children studied had given their informed consent for renal biopsy.

Blood samples were obtained in the fasting state for serum analysis and determination of renal function. Serum calcium, inorganic phosphorus, and creatinine levels were determined by automated methods. Urinary calcium, phosphorus, and creatinine were determined with an autoanalyzer using twenty-four-hour pooled urine.

Measurement of 1-hydroxylase activity was accomplished as follows (4): the remaining kidney specimen from the diagnostic procedure was used for enzyme assay.

A 2.5% homogenate of the kidney tissue was prepared in a Tris-acetate buffer (15 mM Tris-acetate, pH 7.4, 0.19 M sucrose, 2 mM EGTA, 2 mM DTT). Then 200 µl of the homogenate and 100 µl of a sodium succinate solution (0.75 mM sodium succinate in Tris-acetate buffer) were pipetted into each of two test tubes. The test tubes were placed in a water bath and shaken at 37°C. The reaction was initiated by the addition of 5 µg of $25OHD_3$ per mg of tissue to one of the test tubes and 95% ethanol to the other test tube. The reaction was terminated by the addition of 1.5 ml of methylene chloride and then labeled $1,25(OH)_2D_3$ (10000 dpm) was added to the assay tubes to monitor the recovery of $1,25(OH)_2D_3$. The methylene chloride phase was applied to high performance liquid chromatography (HPLC; Waters Associates, Milford, MA) in a solvent system of hexane-2-propanol (9:1, vol/vol), and the fraction containing $1,25(OH)_2D$ was collected. The fraction containing $24,25(OH)_2D_3$ was collected separately for further purification by HPLC. Duplicate samples were assayed for $1,25(OH)_2D$ or $24,25(OH)_2D$ by CPBA as described previously (5,6). The $1,25(OH)_2D$ or $24,25(OH)_2D$ detected in the tube incubated without substrate was subtracted from the value detected in the sample incubated with substrate.

Results and Discussion:

Laboratory findings

The stature and body weights of the patients in Group A were within the normal ranges. The serum calcium and inorganic phosphorus values were within the normal range, suggesting no evidence of impaired mineral metabolism.

In Group B normal levels of GFR suggest that there was no impairment of renal function. Although the mean serum $1,25(OH)_2D$ did not differ from that in Group A, the mean serum 25OHD was significantly lower than that in Group A.

Group C showed a mean value of GFR which was significantly lower than that in Group A. The mean serum 25OHD and $1,25(OH)_2D$ did not differ from their levels in Group A.

Table 2 Laboratory Findings (7)

	Group A (Proteinuria and/or hematuria)	Group B (Prednisolone)	Group C (mild RF)	Group D* (severe RF)
GFR	105.6±14.5	110.8±20.3	65.1±6.1**	
Blood				
Calcium (mg/dl)	9.2±0.4	9.1±0.8	9.0±0.7	9.2±0.6
Phosphorus (mg/dl)	4.7±0.5	4.3±1.0	4.6±1.0	8.5±1.2**
25OHD (ng/ml)	18.9±6.1	11.1±2.3**	15.9±3.6	25.8±9.8
$1,25(OH)_2D$ (pg/ml)	66.3±22.4	53.6±15.1	88.5±22.5	53.7±17.0
$24,25(OH)_2D$ (ng/ml)	2.22±0.52	2.13±0.73	1.14±0.34**	ND

Results are means±SD**, significantly different ($p<0.05$) from the value in Group A
GFR, glomerular filtration rate ($ml/min/1.73\ m^2$); ND, not detectable;
*, treated with 1α-hydroxyvitamin D_3

However, the mean serum 24,25$(OH)_2D$ was significantly lower than that in Group A.

In Group D (severe renal insufficiency treated with 1-hydroxyvitamin D_3) the mean serum 1,25$(OH)_2D$ was normal, but 24,25$(OH)_2D$ was not detectable.

In Group B, the mean value of TmP/GFR did not differ from that in Group A, while the ratio of urinary calcium/creatinine was significantly higher than that in Group A. On the other hand TmP/GFR in Group C was significantly lower than that in Group A.

Histological findings

In Group A, the histological study by light microscopy showed the tubules where 1-hydroxylase should be localized to be normal in these cases. The numbers of glomeruli and distribution of proximal tubules in the specimen in the low power field were similar to each other, indicating that the specimens from the 12 individuals were representative portions of cortical tissue where 1-hydroxylase is localized. In Group C (mild renal insufficiency), there was focal atrophy of the tubules. The histological study of Group D showed end stage kidney.

1-Hydroxylases (7)

The renal 1-hydroxylase activity in Group A was 83.2±37.7 pg/mg tissue/20 min. Since these patients did not show any impaired mineral metabolism or pathological changes in the renal tubules where 1-hydroxylase should be localized, we presume that this result for renal 1-hydroxylase activity indicates the normal value in children. The mean 1-hydroxylase activity in Group B (treated with prednisolone) did not differ from that in Group A, whereas the urinary excretion of calcium was increased. Therefore, these data suggest that glucocorticoid-induced changes in urinary calcium excretion may not be the result of a direct effect of prednisolone on renal 1-hydroxylase. The mean 1-hydroxylase activity in patients with mild renal insufficiency was not reduced. Probably an increased intracellular concentration of phosphorus in the proximal tubules in mild renal insufficiency (8) suppresses the activity of 1-hydroxylase, and the reduced nephron mass also reduces the enzyme activity. On the contrary, an increased serum level of parathyroid hormone in mild renal insufficiency may stimulate 1-hydroxylase activity. Therefore, it appears that the 1-hydroxylase activity remains at a normal level as a result of two oppossing factors. In severe renal insufficiency, however, the 1-hydroxylase activity seems to be reduced by the combination of an increased level of intracellular phosphorus and a markedly reduced nephron mass.

Table 3 Enzyme activities

	1-hydroxylase (7) (pg/mg tissue/20 min)	24-hydroxylase (ng/mg tissue/20 min)
Asymptomatic proteinuria and/or hematuria (Controls)	83.2 ± 37.7	0.51 ± 0.22
Patients treated with prednisolone	81.1 ± 27.1	0.43 ± 0.19
Mild renal insufficiency	75.4 ± 22.4	0.4 ± 0.07
Severe renal insufficiency	6.4 ± 3.0	ND

24-Hydroxylases

The renal 24-hydroxylase activity in Group A was 0.51±0.22 ng/mg tissue/20 min, representing the reference value for 24-hydroxylase in children. The mean 24-hydroxylase activity in Group B did not differ from that in Group A, suggesting no direct effect of prednisolone on renal 24-hydroxylase activity. The mean 24-hydroxylase activity in patients with mild renal insufficiency was reduced, but not significantly. However, no activity was detectable in the cases of severe renal insufficiency.

Summary:

First, prednisolone did not affect the renal 1 or 24-hydroxylase activity.

Second, in mild renal insufficiency the 1-hydroxylase activity remained normal, but the 24-hydroxylase activity was slightly low.

Third, in severe renal insufficiency, the 1 and 24-hydroxylase activities were markedly low.

References:

1. DeLuca, H.F. and Schnoes, H.K. (1976) Ann. Rev. Biochem. 45, 631-666.
2. Ghazarian, J.G., Kream, B., Botham, K.M., Nichells, M.W. and DeLuca, H.F. (1978) Arch. Biochem. Biophys. 189, 212-220.
3. Tanaka, Y. and DeLuca, H.F. (1981) Proc. Natl. Acad. Sci. 78(1), 196-199.
4. Tanaka, Y., DeLuca, H.F., Satomura, K., Yamaoka, K. and Seino, Y. (1983) J. Lab. Clin. Med. 102, 1010-1016.

5. Yamaoka, K., Seino, Y., Ishida, M., Ishii, T., Shimotsuji, T., Tanaka, Y., Kurose, H., Matsuda, M., Satomura, K. and Yabuuchi, H. (1981) J. Clin. Metab. 53, 1096-1100.
6. Shimotsuji, T., Hiejima, T., Seino, Y., Yamaoka, K., Ishii, T., Ishida, M., Matsuda, S., Ikehara, C. and Yabuuchi, H. (1980) Clin. Chim. Acta 106, 145-154.
7. Satomura, K. (in preparation).
8. Portale, A.A., Booth, B.E., Halloran, B.P. and Moris, R.C.Jr. (1984) J. Clin. Invest. 73, 1580-1589.

FAILURE OF SIMULATED ACIDOSIS TO INFLUENCE 25-HYDROXYVITAMIN D_3 (25OHD_3) METABOLISM BY KIDNEY CELL MONOLAYERS

J. Cunningham, G. Griffin and L.V. Avioli
Jewish Hospital and Washington University School of Medicine, St. Louis MO 63110, USA

Introduction

In many studies purporting to show an influence of pH on 25OHD3 metabolism in acidotic animals, secondary effects of acidosis on minerals and hormones make impossible the assignment of a role for pH per se to any observed changes in the metabolism of 25OHD3 (1-4). These drawbacks apply to all human studies, to animal studies performed in vivo and to those which have used in vitro methods to study fresh material from acidotic animals. In an attempt to overcome these problems, we have used cultured mouse kidney cells grown in serum-free medium, with assessment of 25OHD3 metabolism in the presence of acidosis or alkalosis simulated in vitro.

Methods

Kidney epithelial cells were obtained from collagenase/hyaluronidase digested pieces of renal cortex from C57BL6J mice (4-6 weeks old) and were grown to confluence in a serum-free medium (5). The medium was a 1:1 mixture of Ham's F12 and DMEM containing: Ca 1mM; Pi 1mM; glutamine 2mM; insulin 5 μg/ml; transferrin 5 μg/ml; prostaglandin E_1 50 ng/ml, at pH 7.4. Medium was changed every 2-3 days and confluence was reached at 8-11 days. 25OHD3-1-hydroxylase was assayed by measuring conversion of ^{3}H25OHD3 to ^{3}H1,25(OH)2D3. Approximately 60,000 dpm of ^{3}H25OHD3 was added to 25 cm^2 of confluent monolayer and incubated for 6 hours, at which point the reaction was stopped and lipid extracted. Vitamin D metabolites were separated by HPLC, using a Waters Rad-Pak Sil column eluted with methylene chloride:methanol (98:2). The ^{3}H1,25(OH)2D3 peak was then rechromatographed on a μ-Porasil column eluted with hexane:isopropanol (90:10) to verify cochromatography with authentic 1,25(OH)2D3 on this system also. The pH of the medium bathing the cells was perturbed EITHER immediately prior to the six hour assay, OR 24 hours prior to assay by adjusting bicarbonate concentration, using chloride as the balancing anion at constant Pco_2. Experiments were done at pH 6.8, 7.1, 7.4 and 7.7.

Results

Exposure of the cells to abnormally low or high pH (range 6.8 to 7.7) for periods of up to 30 hrs had no consistent effect on cell numbers or DNA content per dish. Conversion rate of 25OHD3 to 1,25(OH)2D3 was generally between 7% and 11%. There was no convincing evidence of production of 24,25$(OH)_2D_3$, 25,26$(OH)_2D_3$ or 1,24,25$(OH)_2D_3$.

pH	% conversion/100 μg DNA		% conversion/10^6 cells	
	6 hr simulation	30 hr simulation	6 hr simulation	30 hr simulation
6.8	9.5±0.6 (n=7)	11.3±0.7 (n=7)	2.5±0.2 (n=7)	2.7±0.2 (n=7)
7.1	11.7±1.1 (n=7)	11.5±1.0 (n=7)	3.3±0.4 (n=7)	2.9±0.2 (n=7)
7.4	11.4±0.4 (n=7)	10.5±0.7 (n=7)	3.0±0.1 (n=7)	2.5±0.4 (n=7)
7.7	11.7±0.4 (n=6)	11.4±1.2 (n=7)	3.0±0.2 (n=7)	2.5±0.4 (n=7)

Data are mean ± SEM of the indicated number of samples for each pH (either 6 hrs or 30 hrs duration). Each sample was derived from pooled lipid from 3 culture dishes.

Vitamin D. A Chemical, Biochemical and Clinical Update

When pH was altered at the beginning of the 6 hr assay, there was no discernable effect on $1,25(OH)_2D_3$ production, even at the pH extremes of 6.8 and 7.7. Likewise, no change resulted from pH alterations introduced 24 hours prior to the 6 hour assay (Kruskall-Wallis and Mann Whitney U tests).

Discussion

These results have shown that short term changes in extracellular pH in vitro have no detectable influence on the metabolism of $25OHD_3$ by mouse kidney cells cultured in serum-free medium. 1-hydroxylase remains active in the cells and is capable of responding to changes in the main controlling factors such as PTH, calcium and phosphate (5). Therefore disturbances of membrane receptors or transport function during the isolation or culture procedures are unlikely to be the explanation for the lack of response to altered pH.

In the first set of experiments, pH was perturbed only for the duration of the 1-hydroxylase assay. It was reasoned that if an effect of pH were to be the result of altered ionic regulation of 1-hydroxylase activity (6), changes in 1-hydroxylase activity should occur rapidly and therefore be readily detectable over the course of a 6 hr assay. When no pH effect could be shown under these circumstances, the possibility arose that pH might alter $1,25(OH)_2D_3$ production in a manner that required a change in enzyme synthesis or degradation, imposing a delay on the response. However, experiments in which pH was altered for 24 hrs prior to the beginning of the 1-hydroxylase assay also failed to show an effect of pH on enzyme activity.

The data indicate that previous reports of altered $25OHD_3$ metabolism following acid loading in vivo probably reflect indirect compensatory responses of the vitamin D endocrine system during acidosis. There is no evidence to support the contention that acidosis interferes directly with $25OHD_3$ metabolism, thereby leading to osteomalacia.

References

1. Lee, S.W., Russell, J. and Avioli, L.V. (1977). Science 195, 994-996
2. Sauveur, B., Garabedian, M., Fellot, C., Mongin, P. and Balsan, S. (1977). Calcif. Tissue Res. 23, 121-124.
3. Kawashima, H., Kraut, J.A. and Kurokawa, K. (1982). J. Clin. Invest. 70, 135-140.
4. Cunningham, J., Bikle, D.D. and Avioli, L.V. (1984). Kidney Int. 25, 47-52.
5. Fukase, M., Birge, S.J., Rifas, L., Avioli, L.V. and Chase, L.R. (1982). Endocrinology 110, 1073-1075.
6. Bikle, D.D. and Rasmussen, H. (1975). J. Clin. Invest. 55, 292-298.

INDUCTION OF RENAL 25-HYDROXYVITAMIN D_3-24-HYDROXYLASE (24-OHase) IN MOUSE KIDNEY: EFFECT OF THE X-LINKED Hyp MUTATION

H.S. Tenenhouse
MRC Genetics Group, McGill University-Montreal Children's Hospital Research Institute, Montreal, Quebec, Canada H3H 1P3

Introduction

The X-linked Hyp mouse, a murine homologue of X-linked hypophosphatemia in man, is characterized by hypophosphatemia, rickets, and decreased phosphate (Pi) transport across the renal brush border membrane (1). Recent studies have indicated that renal metabolism of 25-hydroxyvitamin D_3 (25-OH-D) is also disturbed in the Hyp mouse (2-5). Vitamin D replete Hyp mice have significantly elevated 24-OHase activity (2,3) and vitamin D and calcium deprived Hyp mice have significantly reduced 25-OH-D-1-hydroxylase (1-OHase) activity relative to normal littermates (4). Furthermore, the reduction in 1,25-dihydroxyvitamin D_3 (1,25$(OH)_2$D) synthesis in the mutant strain is associated with a decrease in Vmax for renal mitochondrial 1-OHase (6). The purpose of the present study was to establish whether vitamin D and calcium deprived Hyp mice can respond normally to regulators known to inhibit renal 1-OHase and induce renal 24-OHase activities.

Methods

Normal (+/Y) and mutant (Hyp/Y) male weanlings were fed a vitamin D deficient, low calcium diet for 40 days. Three days prior to sacrifice, groups of +/Y and Hyp/Y mice received (i) calcium gluconate (Ca) in drinking water (30 g/l) (ii) daily IP injections of 1,25$(OH)_2$D (1ng/g) or (iii) both Ca and 1,25$(OH)_2$D. Sera were analyzed for Pi and calcium and isolated renal mitochondria assayed for 1-OHase and 24-OHase activities as described previously (4,6).

Results and Discussion

The results are summarized in Table 1. Serum Pi is significantly lower than normal in all groups of Hyp mice and is only increased in mutants treated with 1,25$(OH)_2$D and Ca + 1,25$(OH)_2$D. Serum calcium is higher than normal in untreated Hyp mice, is increased in all groups of treated normal mice but only in Ca + 1,25$(OH)_2$D-treated mutants. Renal 1-OHase activity is significantly lower than normal in Hyp mice and is markedly reduced in all groups of treated +/Y and Hyp/Y mice. Finally, renal 24-OHase activity is significantly increased in 1,25$(OH)_2$D-treated +/Y mice and in Hyp/Y mice treated with 1,25$(OH)_2$D and Ca + 1,25$(OH)_2$D. Furthermore, in spite of similar serum calcium levels in both genotypes, renal 24-OHase activity is significantly higher in all three groups of treated Hyp/Y mice as compared to treated +/Y littermates.

Kinetic studies revealed that Vmax for induced 24-OHase is 8-fold greater than normal in Hyp mice whereas the apparent Km is not different in the two groups of Ca + 1,25$(OH)_2$D-treated mice.

The present results demonstrate that relative to normal littermates, vitamin D and calcium deprived Hyp mice have an exaggerated 24-OHase response to

Vitamin D. A Chemical, Biochemical and Clinical Update

Table 1. Effect of Treatment and Genotype on Serum Phosphate, Serum Calcium and Renal Mitochondrial 1-OHase and 24-OHase Activities in Vitamin D and Calcium Deprived Mice

		No Treatment	Ca	$1,25(OH)_2D$	Ca + $1,25(OH)_2D$
Serum Pi (mg/dl)					
	+/Y	7.00 ±0.31	6.67 ±0.99	7.92 ±0.43	7.91 ±0.45
	Hyp/Y	4.34 ±0.48[1]	4.78 ±0.40[1]	6.25 ±0.30[1,2]	5.80 ±0.45[1,2]
Serum Ca (mg/dl)					
	+/Y	6.18 ±0.21	8.85 ±0.480[2]	8.52 ±0.240[2]	9.54 ±0.17[2]
	Hyp/Y	8.15 ±0.21[1]	8.46 ±0.160	8.76 ±0.070	9.80 ±0.21[2]
1-OHase[3]					
	+/Y	0.454±0.026	0.212±0.020[2]	0.034±0.010[2]	0.047±0.013[2]
	Hyp/Y	0.067±0.016[1]	0.023±0.004[1,2]	0.028±0.006[2]	0.010±0.002[1,2]
24-OHase[3]					
	+/Y	0.002±0.001	0.003±0.003	0.274±0.126[2]	0.153±0.063
	Hyp/Y	0.002±0.002	0.060±0.006[1]	0.776±0.022[1,2]	1.154±0.061[1,2]

Each number is the M±SEM of values from 5 to 11 mice

1 Effect of genotype, $p < 0.001$ by Student's t test

2 Effect of treatment, $p < 0.01$ by ANOVA and Duncan's multiple range test

3 Expressed as pmoles/min/mg prot.

regulators known to inhibit renal 1-OHase and induce renal 24-OHase activities. The inhibitory control of 1-OHase activity, however, appears to be intact in Hyp mice. These findings indicate that the abnormality in the regulation of renal 25-OH-D metabolism in Hyp mice involves the induction of $24,25(OH)_2D_3$ synthesis as well as the previously reported deficit in $1,25(OH)_2D$ production in response to calcium and vitamin D deficiency (4,6). Further study will be required to elucidate the mechanism for abnormal regulation of renal 25-OH-D metabolism in the Hyp mouse and to determine whether this defect is a primary consequence of the mutant gene.

References

1. Tenenhouse H.S., Scriver C.R., McInnes R.R., and Glorieux F.H. (1978) Kidney Int. 14: 236.
2. Tenenhouse H.S. (1982) Vitamin D: Chemical, biochemical and clinical endocrinology of calcium metabolism. Walter de Gruyter, Berlin, p. 471.
3. Cunningham J., Gomes H., Seino Y. and Chase L.R. (1983) Endocrinol. 112: 633.
4. Tenenhouse H.S. (1983) Endocrinol. 113: 816.
5. Lobaugh B. and Drezner M.K. (1983) J. Clin. Invest. 71: 400.
6. Tenenhouse H.S. (1984) Endocrinol. 115: 634.

MODIFICATION OF 1 - HYDROXYLASE BY PROTEIN KINASE-CATALYZED PHOSPHORYLATION

A mechanism for the down-regulation of renal 1,25-dihydroxyvitamin D output

J.G. Ghazarian and D.M. Yanda

Department of Biochemistry, Medical College of Wisconsin, Milwaukee, Wisconsin 53226 USA

In our efforts to study the metabolic regulation of the 1-hydroxylase complex we have found that a partially purified chick kidney mitochondrial Type II protein kinase (specific activity of 1430 pmol of γ-phosphorus of ATP transferred per mg of protein per minute using calf thymus histone type II-A as acceptor substrate) can catalyze the phosphorylation of the cytochrome P-450 in the absence of the ferredoxin component of the monooxygenase (1, 2). Phosphorylation of vitamin D-deficient chich cytochrome in the absence of the ferredoxin component has no effect on the rate of $1,25(OH)_2D$ formation in vitro in a reconstituted assay system containing the phosphorylated cytochrome, chick kidney mitochondrial ferredoxin and chick kidney mitochondrial flavoprotein. The phosphorylation of the cytochrome in the absence of ferredoxin does not alter the spectral properties of the cytochrome from which the calculated concentrations of the cytochrome are found to remain unchanged. However, the inclusion of ferredoxin with the cytochrome during the phosphorylation reaction prior to activity assay of the cytochrome in the reconstituted system completely abolished $1,25(OH)_2D$ formation. Although cAMP-dependent protein kinase activity can be demonstrated in the purified kinase, the above findings appear to be cAMP-independent. It should be noted that the activities of the cAMP-dependent as well as the cAMP-independent kidney mitochondrial protein kinases are unaffected by the vitamin D status of the chicks.

To test the effects of protein kinase-mediated phosphorylation on the ability of the 1-hydroxylase to form $1,25(OH)_2D$ in a reconstituted assay system in vitro, 0.6 nmol of cytochrome P-450 (isolated from kidney mitochondria of vitamin D deficient chicks) serving as the phosphate acceptor substrate instead of histone was preincubated in the phosphorylating system described above containing 0.3 mg of the purified kinase. After 10 minutes at 30°C the reaction was interrupted in ice. To the reaction mixture were added 10 nmol chick renal mitochondrial ferredoxin, 210 µg of renal mitochondrial flavoprotein (NADPH-ferredoxin reductase with a specific activity of 12.7 nmol cytochrome c reduced per mg of protein per minute), 102,000 cpm ^3H-25 OH D (23.6 ng) (specific radioactivity of 1.5 Ci/mmol), 250 nmol NADPH, 7.5 µmol glucose 6-phosphate and 1 unit of yeast glucose 6-phosphate dehydrogenase. The mixture was incubated for an additional 60 minutes at 30°C then extracted for high pressure liquid chromatography. In other studies, the preincubation mixture during the phosphorylation reaction contained both the cytochrome and the renal ferredoxin prior to interruption on ice and the subsequent completion of the assay as above but without the further addition of ferredoxin. The results shown in Table I clearly indicate that the phosphorylation of the cytochrome in the absence of ferredoxin has no effect on the catalytic activity of the cytochrome in vitro while the presence of the ferredoxin component (also as in the control assays with protein kinase) entirely abolishes all in vitro activity of the cytochrome.

Vitamin D. A Chemical, Biochemical and Clinical Update

TABLE I

$1,25(OH)_2D$ formation *in vitro* by reconstituted 1-hydroxylase system containing cytochrome P-450 preincubated with protein kinase in the presence or absence of ferredoxin.

Preincubation conditions	pmol $1,25(OH)_2D$/nmol cytochrome P-450
Control (complete system without PK)	3.86
P-450 + PK - cAMP - Ferredoxin	3.95
P-450 + PK + cAMP - Ferredoxin	3.91
P-450 + PK - cAMP + Ferredoxin	0
P-450 + PK + cAMP + Ferredoxin	0
Control + PK - cAMP	0
Control + PK + cAMP	0

Can the above phosphorylation effects represent a viable biological mechanism for the control of the 1-hydroxylase activity and thus of renal $1,25(OH)_2D$ output? The answer lies in the proportion of the total mitochondrial cytochrome P-450 that is specifically active in the 1-hydroxylation reaction. If this proportion is very small, then a physicochemical modification of a very small proportion of the mitochondrial P-450 cytochromes should have a large impact (positive or negative) on the catalytic reaction in which the modified cytochromes participate. Under these circumstances one would not expect to detect changes in the gross spectral properties exhibited by the bulk of the cytochromes. While this explanation is tenable, it will require the assignment of function(s) to the bulk of the P-450 cytochromes present in the avian kidney mitochondria.

REFERENCES:

1. Pedersen, J.I., Ghazarian, J.G., Orme-Johnson, N.R., and DeLuca, H.F. (1976) J.Biol.Chem. 251, 3933-3941
2. Kulkoski, J.A., and Ghazarian, J.G. (1979) Biochem.J. 177, 673-678.

RELATIONSHIP BETWEEN CIRCULATING 25-OHD AND 1,25-$(OH)_2D$ IN END-STAGE RENAL FAILURE. EVIDENCE FOR AN EXTRA-RENAL PRODUCTION OF 1,25-$(OH)_2D$ IN MAN.

T. Storm, O.H. Sørensen, Bi. Lund, Bj. Lund, J.D. Thode, M. Brahm, M. Friedberg and S. Nistrup.
Department of Medicine, Sundby Hospital, Copenhagen, Denmark.

Introduction:

The kidney has been considered to be the only organ capable of converting 25-OHD to 1,25-$(OH)_2D$. Undetectable levels of circulating 1,25-$(OH)_2D$ have been found in anephric patients (1) with restoration towards normal after successful renal transplantation (2). Recent studies have, however, indicated, that an extra-renal production of 1,25-$(OH)_2D$ may occur in man (3,4, 5). The vitamin D metabolites were studied in hemodialysed patients exposed to sunshine or given a single injection of PTH.

Patients and Methods:

During the Danish winter time a 3 weeks´ vacation was arranged on the sunny Canary Islands for 9 patients with end-stage renal failure, hemodialysed 2-3 times per week. The vitamin D metabolites were measured before and after the vacation. The effect of a PTH injection (200 USP i.v.) on circulating 1,25-$(OH)_2D$ was studied in 6 hemodialysed patients: 2 with remaining kidneys, 1 with left nephrectomy and an aplastic right kidney and 3 anephric patients.
Vitamin D metabolites were measured by competitive binding assays. The 1,25-$(OH)_2D$ was chromatrographed on a Sephadex LH-20 column followed by HPLC. The lower detection limit was 3 pg/ml.

Results:

Sunshine exposure:

Mean serum 25-OHD was normal and increased after sun exposure (fig.1). Mean serum 1,25-$(OH)_2D$ remained low but a marked increase was observed in 2 patients with low starting values of 25-OHD which was normalized after sun exposure. An opposite pattern was observed in one patient who developed acute liver insufficiency: a pronounced decrease in serum 25-OHD accompanied by a fall in serum 1,25-$(OH)_2D$. The low serum 24,25-$(OH)_2D$ concentrations did not change (fig. 1).

PTH induced stimulation:

An increase in serum 1,25-$(OH)_2D$ following injection of PTH was seen in all 6 patients studied (fig. 2).

Conclusion:

The results indicate that changes in the delivery of substrate (25-OHD) to the renal 1-alpha-hydroxylase system might affect the production of 1,25-$(OH)_2D$ in the residual kidney tissue in patients with chronic renal failure. The increase in serum 1,25-$(OH)_2D$ observed in the 2 patients with remaining kidney tissue who were given PTH i.v. could be explained by a stimulation of the renal 1-alpha-hydroxylase. The small increases seen in the anephric patients receiving PTH may be due to a PTH-stimulated extra-renal production of 1,25-$(OH)_2D$. Since bilateral

Vitamin D. A Chemical, Biochemical and Clinical Update

nephrectomy is a rare procedure the number of patients studied has been small. We therefore found it of interest to add the present results indicating an extra-renal production of 1,25-$(OH)_2D$.

Fig. 1

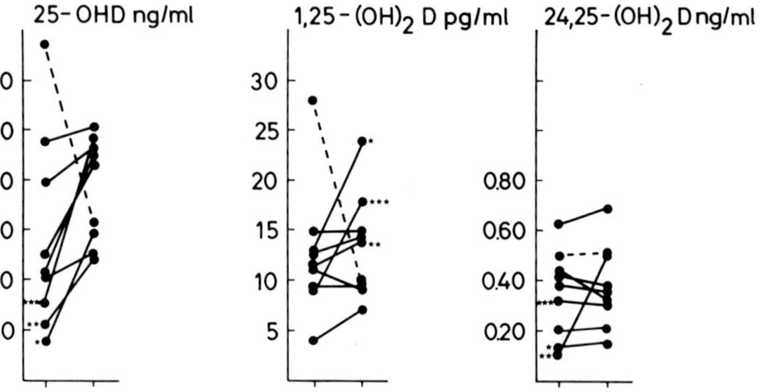

Serum levels before and after sun exposure
----- Acute liver insufficiency

Fig. 2

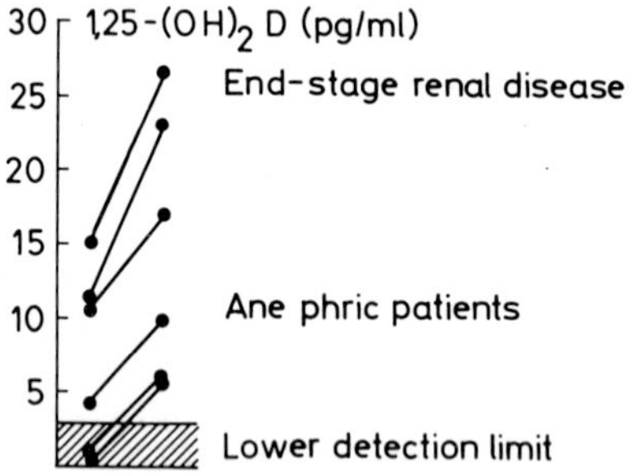

Serum 1,25-$(OH)_2$ D before and after 200 USP u of PTH i.v.

References:
1. Gray RW, Weber HP, Dominguez JH, Lemann J. (1974) J Clin Endocrinol Metab 39, 1045-1056.
2. Lund B, Clausen E, Friedberg M, Moskowics M, Nielsen SP, Sørensen OH. (1980) Nephron 25, 30-33.
3. Fraher LJ, Adami S, Papapoulos SE, McGonigle RJ, Sudan HL, Parsons V, O´Riordan JLH. (1983) Calcif Tiss Int suppl. 35, A47.
4. Barbour GL, Coburn JW, Slatopolsky E, Norman AW, Horst RL. (1981) New Engl J Med 305, 440-443.
5. O´Riordan JLH, Fraher LJ. VIII International Conference on Calcium Regulating Hormones 1983;abstr. F-17.

INVOLVEMENT OF IONISED CALCIUM AND CALMODULIN IN THE REGULATION OF 25OHD3 PRODUCTION BY SHEEP LIVER *IN VITRO*.

M.S. Chaudhary, A.D. Care and S. Tomlinson*, Department of Animal Physiology and Nutrition, University of Leeds, Leeds LS2 9JT, U.K. and *Department of Medicine, University of Manchester, M13 9WL, U.K.

INTRODUCTION

The present study was designed to evaluate the influence of [Ca^{2+}] on the 25-hydroxylation of vitamin D_3 in ovine liver *in vitro* and to investigate the possible involvement of calmodulin in the regulation of this enzyme.

METHODS

A 10% homogenate of fresh ovine liver was prepared in sucrose (0.3 M). Two ml homogenate was added to a phosphate buffer pH 7.4, containing Mg^{2+} ions and a NADPH generating system. The reaction was initiated by adding 0.4 pmoles ^3H-D_3 to the incubation medium along with the drug, the effect of which was to be investigated. After incubation for one hour at 37°C, the reaction was stopped by flash freezing and the incubate extracted by the method of Bligh and Dyer (1). The substrate and product were separated by silica Sep-pak chromatography.

RESULTS

The data from each experiment are reported as the means of five to six observations. Modulation of hepatic 25-hydroxylase was achieved by either the addition of Ca^{2+} (calcium gluconate) or partially depleting the incubation medium of Ca^{2+} by the addition of EGTA (Fig 1). The addition of 0.1 mM Ca^{2+} enhanced the 25OHD$_3$ production (2.3 ± 0.09 vs control 2.0 ± 0.07 pmoles/gram fresh liver/h). Further increase in [Ca^{2+}] resulted in reduced 25OHD$_3$ synthesis, a significant decrease being observed at 0.69 mM and a 50% inhibition at 1.38 mM Ca^{2+} (0.9 ± 0.06 vs control 2.0 ± 0.07 pmoles/gram fresh liver/h). The addition of EGTA also reduced the production of 25OHD$_3$, with a 50% decrease at about 40 µM EGTA (0.54 ± 0.08 vs control 1.4 ± 0.05 pmol/gram fresh liver/h 25OHD$_3$ $P<0.002$)

To examine the possible involvement of calmodulin in the synthesis of 25OHD$_3$ in ovine liver, the effects of several calmodulin antagonists were studied; the results are shown in Fig 2. The addition of 1 µM TFP significantly ($P<0.001$) inhibited 25OHD$_3$ production (0.45 ± 0.04 vs control 1.92 ± 0.06 pmoles/g/h), with a 50% inhibition at 0.5 µM TFP. W7, Calmidazolium and Compound 48/80 all inhibited 25OHD$_3$ production, with a 50% inhibition at 200 µM, 10 µM and 40 µg/ml of these drugs, respectively. The slow Ca^{2+} channel blockers verapamil and nifedipine also had inhibitory effects with a 50% reduction at concentrations of 25 µM and 160 µM, respectively.

DISCUSSION

These studies demonstrate that [Ca^{2+}] modulates the hepatic 25-hydroxylation of vitamin D_3 in vitamin D replete ovine liver *in vitro*, and is in agreement with a similar study using rachitic rat liver *in vitro* (2). The inhibiting effect of calmodulin antagonists on the

Vitamin D. A Chemical, Biochemical and Clinical Update

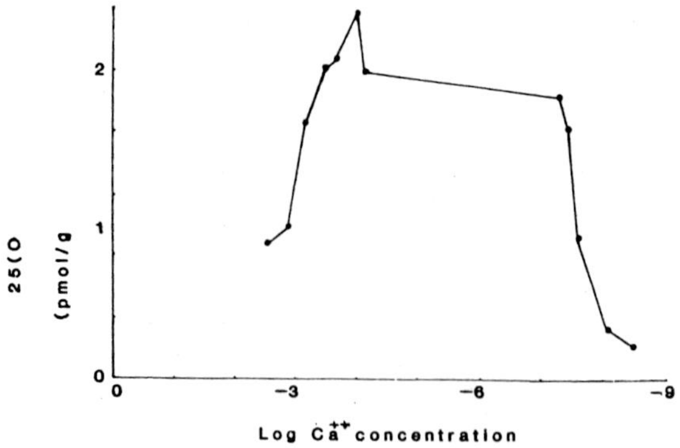

Fig 1. Effect of ionised $[Ca^{2+}]$ on the 25-hydroxylation of vitamin D_3 in ovine liver in vitro.

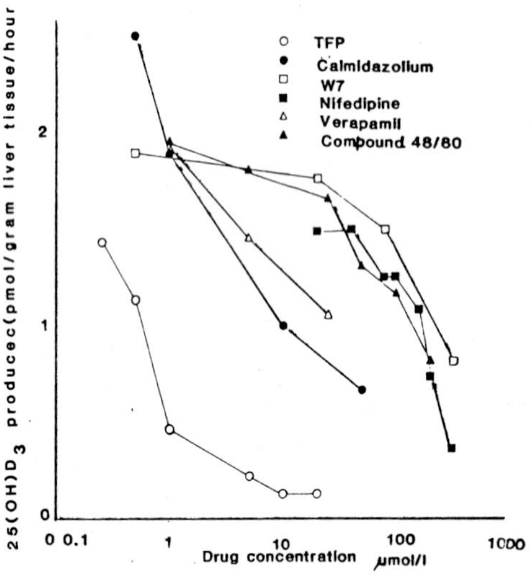

Fig 2. Effect of calmodulin antagonists and Ca^{2+} channel blockers on the 25-hydroxylation of vitamin D_3 in ovine liver in vitro.

hepatic 25-hydroxylation of vitamin D_3 in vitro demonstrates the possibility of involvement of this protein in the mechanism by which intracellular $[Ca^{2+}]$ mediates its effect on $25OHD_3$ production in liver. The more specific inhibitors of calmodulin action, W7, Compound 48/80 and Calmidazolium all showed effects on hepatic 25-hydroxylation similar to that shown by TFP. The inhibitory effects of verapamil and nifedipine on 25-hydroxylation are also in agreement with the report of Minocherhomjee and Roufogalis (3) that these calcium antagonists can also act as calmodulin antagonists. It is concluded that vitamin D 25-hydroxylase in sheep liver is calcium sensitive. The mechanism of this regulation may involve calmodulin.

REFERENCES

1. Bligh, E.G. and Dyer, W.J. (1959) Can.J. Biochem. 37, 911-917.
2. Baran, D. and Milne, M. (1983) Clinical Research 31, 693-A.
3. Minocherhomjee, M.A. and Roufogalis, B.D. (1984) Cell Calcium 5, 37-63

EFFECTS OF CHRONIC RENAL FAILURE, RENAL TRANSPLANTATION AND UNILATERAL NEPHRECTOMY ON 1,25 DIHYDROXYCHOLECALCIFEROL

P.A.Lucas, R.C.Brown, L.Bloodworth, C.R.Jones and J.S.Woodhead

Departments of Renal Medicine and Medical Biochemistry, University of Wales College of Medicine, Cardiff, U.K.

Introduction:

The discovery, over a decade ago, that the hormonally active form of vitamin D, 1,25-dihydroxycholecalciferol (1,25(OH)2D3), must be synthesised in the kidney enabled substantial advances to be made in our understanding of the disturbances in calcium metabolism associated with reduced renal function. It is generally agreed that by the time renal replacement therapy is needed, most patients are unable to sustain normal circulating levels of 1,25(OH)2D3. The situation obtaining in milder renal insufficiency is less clear and the level of renal function at which 1,25(OH)2D3 begins to fall remains controversial (1,2). This question has obvious implications in terms of replacement therapy. To gain insight into this problem as well as further to investigate determinants of 1,25(OH)2D3 other than glomerular filtration rate (GFR), we measured vitamin D3 metabolites in subjects with mild to moderate renal insufficiency with chronic renal failure (CRF) and after renal transplantation (RTX). In the latter group we investigated the relationship between 1,25(OH)2D3 levels and intestinal calcium absorption. We also studied the acute changes which followed unilateral nephrectomy (UN) in live related donors by frequent sampling in the week post UN.

Subjects and methods:

GFR was measured by single injection of 51-CrEDTA in 31 CRF subjects and by creatinine clearance in 6 post-UN and 34 RTX subjects. The latter had undergone RTX at least 3 months previously. No subject had proteinuria of greater than 1 g daily. No CRF or post-UN subject had received vitamin D or its metabolites and no RTX subject received such medication after RTX. Metabolites of vitamin D3 were measured in plasma from these subjects and in 10 RTX subjects in samples obtained both in winter and summer. Determination was by radioimmunoassay using the method of Clemens et al (3) with modifications. After the addition of tracer amounts of tritiated metabolites (Amersham International, UK) for determination of recovery, 2 ml of serum was extracted with 3 ml of acetonitrile. The fraction containing vitamin D3 metabolites was separated from the extract by chromatography on Sep-Pak C18 cartridges (Waters Instuments Ltd). The metabolites were then fractionated by high performance liquid chromatography (Partisil 5μ developed in hexane: 2-propanol: methanol, 90:5:5 v/v). Antiserum (02282) was kindly provided by Professor A.D.Care, University of Leeds, U.K. Normal 1,25(OH)2D3: 22-54 pg/ml, 25(OH)D3: 6-36 ng/ml. These metabolites were uncorrelated in 23 normal subjects.

Oral 47-Ca was given with 20 mg elemental calcium to 17 fasting RTX subjects, 15 of whom were taking corticosteroids (5-20 mg/day) with azathioprine or cyclosporine. Two subjects were taking cyclosporine alone. The fraction of administered radioactivity measured in plasma obtained 60 min later was taken as a measure of intestinal calcium absorption (4) (Normal: 0.6-2.3%). Serum iPTH was measured by immunoradiometric assay (5) which recognises the intact molecule, cross-reacting weakly with the commercially available fragment 1-34, but not with commercially available fragments 28-48, 44-68 or 53-84. The PTH standard was a partially purified preparation from human adenoma tissue which had been calibrated against NIBSC 75/549. Normal range for serum iPTH: <1 ng/ml.

Vitamin D. A Chemical, Biochemical and Clinical Update

Statistics:

2 tailed statistical tests were used throughout. The Mann-Whitney U test was used for all between-group comparisons. Results expressed as mean ± SEM.

Results:

CRF: A positive correlation was found between 1,25(OH)2D3 and GFR for GFRs 15-90 ml/min ($r=0.60$, $p<0.001$) and for GFRs 15-45 ml/min ($r=0.61$, $p<0.05$). Serum 1,25(OH)2D3 was 30.9±3.0 pg/ml in 11 subjects with early CRF (GFRs 50-90 ml/min; mean 69.5±3.0), 21.1±2.6 pg/ml in 18 subjects with more severe CRF (GFRs 20-50 ml/min; mean 36.1±2.3) compared with 38.0±1.6 pg/ml in 23 normal subjects ($p<0.05$).

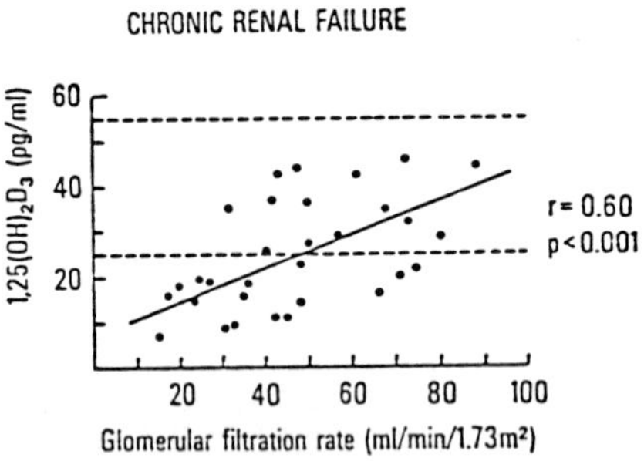

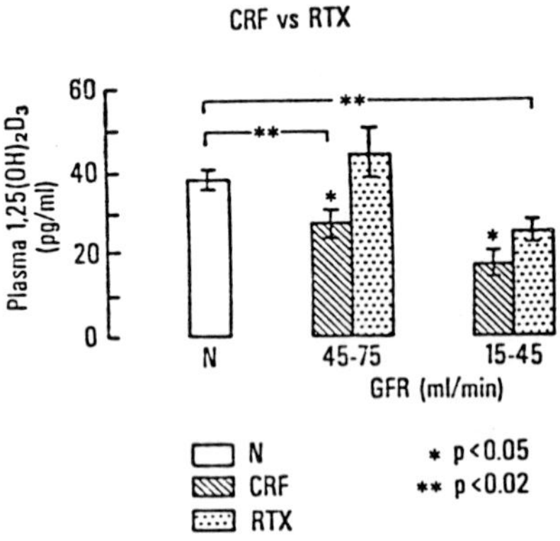

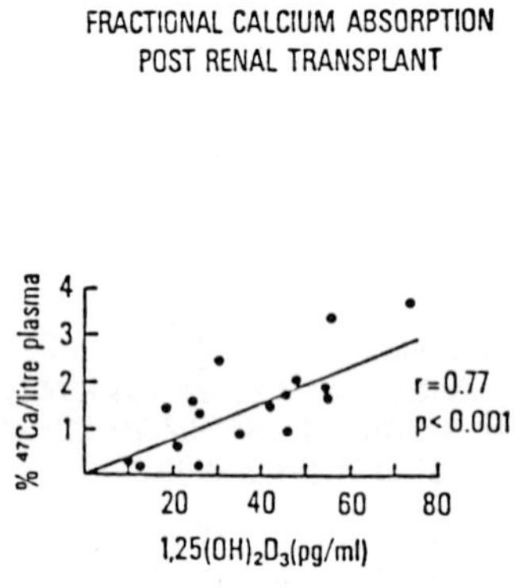

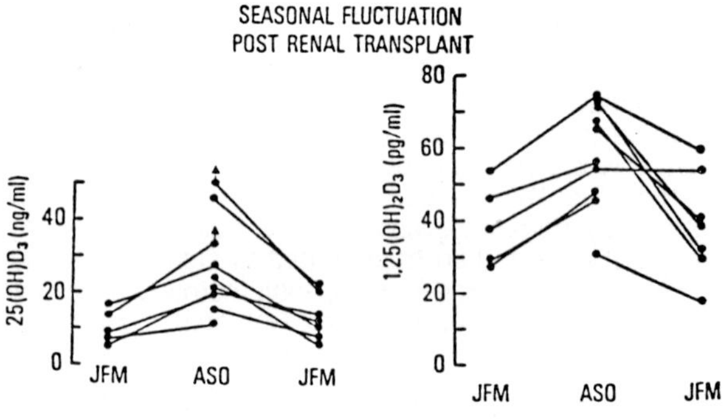

RTX: Fractional calcium absorption was significantly correlated with the level of 1,25(OH)2D3 ($r=0.77$, $p<0.001$). No relation was found with steroid intake and in all but three subjects, calcium absorption was normal. For GFRs 15-90 ml/min, a positive correlation was found between 1,25(OH)2D3 and GFR ($r=0.46$, $p<0.01$), between 1,25(OH)2D3 and 25(OH)D3 ($r=0.69$, $p<0.001$) and between corrected total serum calcium and 1,25(OH)2D3 ($r=0.45$, $p<0.01$). For GFRs 45-75 ml/min, 1,25(OH)2D3 was strongly correlated with 25(OH)D3 ($r=0.77$, $p<0.001$) but not with GFR. For GFRs 15-45 ml/min, 1,25(OH)2D3 was strongly correlated with GFR ($r=0.76$, $p<0.001$) but not with 25(OH)D3. Seasonal variations in 25(OH)D3 and 1,25(OH)2D3 were observed in 10 subjects (GFR 66.9±7.0 ml/min) ($p<0.01$).

RTX vs CRF: 1,25(OH)2D3 for GFRs 45-75 ml/min: 44.1±5.7 (RTX) vs 27.9±2.9 pg/ml (CRF) $p<0.05$. 1,25(OH)2D3 for GFRs15-45 ml/min: 25.3±2.2 (RTX) vs 17.6±2.6 pg/ml (CRF) $p<0.05$. Levels of 25(OH)D3 and iPTH did not differ between RTX and CRF at either level of GFR. iPTH was elevated in both CRF and RTX groups at both levels of GFR ($p<0.002$).

ACUTE CHANGES POST UNILATERAL NEPHRECTOMY

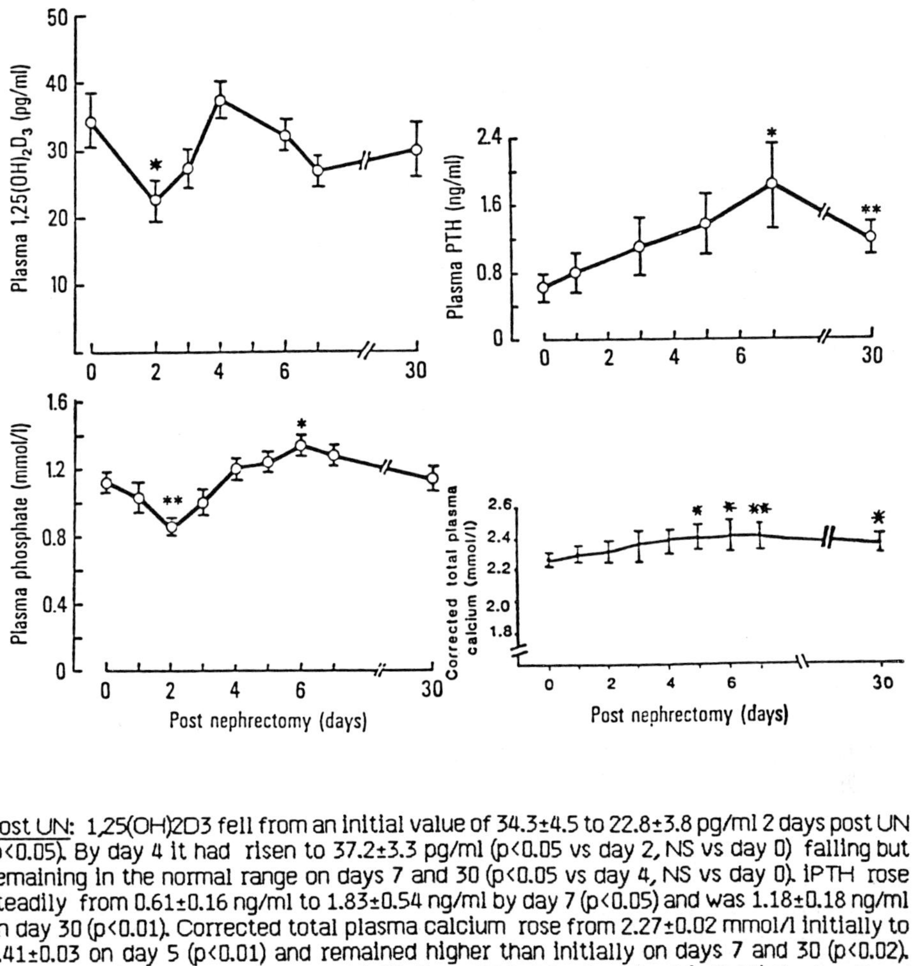

Post UN: 1,25(OH)2D3 fell from an initial value of 34.3±4.5 to 22.8±3.8 pg/ml 2 days post UN ($p<0.05$). By day 4 it had risen to 37.2±3.3 pg/ml ($p<0.05$ vs day 2, NS vs day 0) falling but remaining in the normal range on days 7 and 30 ($p<0.05$ vs day 4, NS vs day 0). iPTH rose steadily from 0.61±0.16 ng/ml to 1.83±0.54 ng/ml by day 7 ($p<0.05$) and was 1.18±0.18 ng/ml on day 30 ($p<0.01$). Corrected total plasma calcium rose from 2.27±0.02 mmol/l initially to 2.41±0.03 on day 5 ($p<0.01$) and remained higher than initially on days 7 and 30 ($p<0.02$). Serum albumin fell from 42.2±1.3 g/l initially to 33.5±1.6 g/l on day 2 ($p<0.01$). By days 7 and 30 it was not differ significantly from day 0 (38.5±2.0 and 42.5±1.0 g/l). Plasma phosphate fell from 1.12±0.06 mmol/l initially to 0.86±0.03 mmol/l on day 2 ($p<0.002$). By day 6 the level had risen to 1.34±0.06 mmol/l, significantly higher than day 0 ($p<0.05$). 25(OH)D3 was within the normal range for all subjects and did not change significantly (day 0: 11.0±1.8 ng/ml).

Discussion:

Our results suggest that the effects of renal insufficiency on circulating 1,25(OH)2D3 differ depending upon the particular clinical situation. In CRF, modest reduction in GFR was associated with significantly lowered 1,25(OH)2D3 levels whereas levels after RTX normal levels were observed at equivalently reduced GFRs. This may in part be explained by the greater renal tubular damage in CRF. The observation of reduced 1,25(OH)2D3 levels early in CRF may be relevant to the pathogenesis of secondary hyperparathyroidism although previous reports addressing this issue have been conflicting (1,2). After UN an acute reduction of GFR was associated with a rapid fall in 1,25(OH)2D3 levels. Restoration of 1,25(OH)2D3 levels to normal occured within 2 days, before any improvement in GFR. In the rat, Taylor et al (6) found 1,25(OH)2D3 levels unchanged 48 hours post-UN but this difference in findings could result from earlier restoration of levels in this species. In any case, the greater ability of the transplanted kidney to maintain 1,25(OH)2D3 levels in the face of a reduction in GFR may correspond to the post-UN response of the single normal kidney.

1,25(OH)2D3 levels after RTX appear to be major determinants of both calcium absorption and serum calcium. Previous reports have suggested that corticosteroid intake may inhibit calcium absorption but we found no evidence for this post RTX, possibly because of the relatively low doses involved. Our data also suggest that above a GFR of approximately 45 ml/min the level of 25(OH)D3 is an important determinant of 1,25(OH)2D3, a finding supported by the observation of seasonal fluctuation in both 25(OH)D3 and 1,25(OH)2D3 levels after RTX.

Post UN, we observed relatively tight control of 1,25(OH)2D3 levels possibly associated with changes in serum phosphate levels. In addition, a steady increase in iPTH associated with a rise in total corrected serum calcium was seen. The stimulus to this increase in iPTH is uncertain but our data from the human situation appear to parallel those obtained by others in the dog (7) and may indicate a change in the set-point for iPTH secretion (8) occurring rapidly after UN. Further study of this phenomenon might contribute to our understanding of the pathogenesis of hyperparathyroidism in CRF.

1. Slatopolsky, E., Gray, R., Adams, N.D., Lewis, J., Hruska, K., Martin, K., Klahr, S., DeLuca, H., Lemann, J. (1978) Kidney Int. 14: 733.
2. Portale, A.A., Booth, B.E., Halloran, B.P., Morris, R.C. (1984) J. Clin. Invest. 73: 1580-1589.
3. Clemens, T., Hendy, G.N., Papapoulos, S.E., Fraher, L.J., Care, A.D., O'Riordan, J.L.H. (1979) Clin. Endocrinol. 11: 225-234.
4. Avioli, L.V., McDonald, J.E., Singer, R.A., Henneman, P.H., Lee, S.W., Hessman, E. (1965) J. Clin. Invest. 44: 128-139.
5. Hales, C.N. and Woodhead, J.S. (1980) In: Methods in Enzymology, Eds. Van Vanukis, H. and Largone, J.J., 70: 334-355.
6. Taylor, C.M., Caverzasio, J., Jung, A., Trechsel, U., Fleisch, H., Bonjour, J-P. (1983) Kidney Int. 24: 37-42.
7. Lopez, S., Galceran, T., Chan, W., Rapp, N., Martin, K., Slatopolsky, E. (1985) Kidney Int. 27: 122.
8. Brown, E.M., Wilson, R.E., Eastman, R.C., Pallotta, J., Marynick, S.P. (1982) J. Clin. Endocrinol. Metab. 54: 172-179.

IMPAIRED VITAMIN D METABOLISM IN THE SPONTANEOUSLY HYPERTENSIVE RAT.

H. KAWASHIMA,
Departments of Medicine, Veterans Administration Wadsworth Medical Center and UCLA School of Medicine, Los Angeles, CA 90073, U.S.A.

Accumulating evidence suggests that calcium homeostasis has a significant role in the development and maintainance of hypertension. Dietary calcium intake is lower in patients with hypertension than in normotensive individuals (1). In epidemiologic studies, low dietary calcium has been associated with hypertension. Low calcium intake increases blood pressure in normotensive Wistar-Kyoto rats (WKY) (2), while high calcium intake lowers it in the spontaneously hypertensive rats (SHR) as well as WKY (3,4). Although total serum calcium is similar in patients with essential hypertension and normotensive controls, serum ionized calcium is decreased in hypertensive patients (5). This is also true in SHR as compared with WKY under comparable feeding condition (6). Serum immunoreactive parathyroid hormone (PTH) is elevated in patients with essential hypertension (7) and SHR (6). Intestinal calcium absorption is reported to be either decreased (8), normal (9), or increased (10) in SHR, in the latter exogenous $1,25(OH)_2D_3$ failed to further stimulate intestinal calcium absorption. Plasma $1,25(OH)_2D$ is reported to be normal in the SHR (8,9). These findings suggest abnormalities in calcium homeostasis in hypertension, particularly vitamin D metabolism, since elevated plasma PTH level seems to fail to raise $1,25(OH)_2D$ above normal. To detect possible defects in the animal model of hypertension, effect of PTH injection on the renal production and serum concentration of $1,25(OH)_2D$ in the SHR before and after development of hypertension has been studied.

SHR and WKY were purchased from the Charles River Company. Blood pressure was monitored with an electrosphygmomanometer on the previous day of the experiment. Rats received S.C. injection of either PTH (50U, bovine 1-34, Beckman) or vehicle at 0, 2, 4 and 6 hr, and blood and urine samples were collected at 8 hr. Kidneys were also removed for the preparation of mitochondria. In another set of experiment creatinine clearance was measured under anesthesia with sodium petobarbital (40 mg/kg i.p.) between 6 and 8 hr. Renal mitochondria were prepared according to the method of Vieth and Fraser (11), and incubated at 25°C for 15 min in the presence of $25(OH)_2D_3$ (1 µg/mg protein). Lipid extraction was performed by the method of Bligh and Dyer, and $1,25(OH)_2D_3$ fractions were obtained by sequential chromatography (LH-20 and HPLC). $1,25(OH)_2D_3$ was measured by a radioreceptor assay using bovine thymic receptor (12).

Vitamin D. A Chemical, Biochemical and Clinical Update

Serum $1,25(OH)_2D$ in the SHR was not different from that in WKY both at 4 and 12 weeks of age. Upon PTH injection, rise in serum $1,25(OH)_2D$ in SHR at 4 weeks of age was also in the normal range. By contrast, at 12 weeks of age, the rise was markedly reduced in SHR, only one third that in WKY despite the similar hypercalcemia caused by PTH. This seems to be due mainly to the impaired production by the kidney of $1,25(OH)_2D$ in response to PTH, since increase in renal production of $1,25(OH)_2D_3$ in response to PTH in SHR was markedly reduced at 12 weeks of age, while it was normal at 4 weeks of age. Creatinine clearance in SHR at 12 weeks of age was not different from that in WKY ruling out the possibility that the reduced response to PTH of renal $1,25(OH)_2D$ production may be due to reduced renal function. Basal $1,25(OH)_2D$ production by the kidney is significantly elevated in the SHR irrespective of the development of hypertension. Thus, there must be hyperparathyroidism or presence of some other agent responsible for the elevated production of $1,25(OH)_2D$, and/or, enhanced catabolism or loss of $1,25(OH)_2D$ in the SHR even before the onset of hypertension. These data suggest that abnormalities in vitamin D metabolism and related calcium disorder may play a role in developing hypertension in SHR.

This study was supported by the American Heart Association.

1. McCarron, D.A., Morris, C.D. and Cole, C. (1982) Science **33**, 2202-2210
2. McCarron, D.A. (1982) Life Sci. **30**, 683-689
3. Ayachi, S. (1979) Metabolism **28**, 1234-1238
4. Schneiderman, R.J., Hann, S.A. and McCarron, D.A. (1984) Intern. Congr. Nephrol., IXth, Los Angeles, 226A (Abstr.)
5. McCarron, D.A. (1982) New Engl. J. Med. **307**, 226-228
6. McCarron, D.A., Yung, N.N., Ugoretz, B.A. and Krutzik, S. (1981) Hypertension **3**(Supple I), I162-I167
7. McCarron, D.A., Pingree, P.A., Rubin, R.J., Gaucher, S.M., Molitch, M. and Krutxik, S. (1980) Hypertension **2**, 162-168
8. Schedl, H.P., Miller, D.L., Page, J.P., Horst, R.L. and Wilson, H.D. (1984) J. Clin. Invest. **73**, 980-986
9. Toraason, M.A. and Wright, G.L. (1981) Am. J. Physiol. **241**, G344-G347
10. Stern, N., Lee, D.B.N., Silis, V., Bech, F.W.J., Deftos, L., Manolagas, S.C. and Sowers, J.R. (1984) Hypertension **6**, 639-646
11. Reinhardt, T.A., Horst, R.L., Orf, J.W. and Hollis, B.W. (1984) J. Clin. Endocrinol. Metab. **58**, 91-98
12. Vieth, R. and Fraser, D. (1979) J. Biol. Chem. **254**, 12455-12460

REGULATION OF 25-HYDROXYVITAMIN D-1-HYDROXYLASE ACTIVITY IN HYP-MICE: A COMPLEX ABNORMALITY.

T. Nesbitt, B. Lobaugh and M.K. Drezner,

Departments of Medicine and Surgery, Division of Metabolism, Endocrinology and Genetics, Duke University Medical Center, Durham, North Carolina.

Hyp-mice exhibit inappropriately low renal 1-hydroxylase activity in the setting of hypophosphatemia. Recently, we examined if this abnormality indeed represents altered enzyme response to phosphate-depletion and/or is indicative of a generalized defect. Initially we discovered that the deranged enzyme function is not due to a phase shift of the response to hypophosphatemia. While renal 1-hydroxylase activity of normal mice (6.1±0.5 fmol/mg/min) increased upon phosphate-depletion (18.3±0.9), enzyme function in Hyp-mice (7.1±0.4) paradoxically declined (2.4±0.3). Subsequently, in studies designed to determine the effects of $1,25(OH)_2D_3$ on enzyme activity we confirmed the absence of phosphate mediated stimulation of 1-hydroxylase in mutants. While enzyme activity of normal and Hyp-mice decreased to similar levels (2.7±0.3, 2.7±0.2) after $1,25(OH)_2D_3$ infusion, 1-hydroxylase activity of phosphate-depleted mice was maintained at supranormal levels (16.8±0.4) in accord with phosphate mediated stimulation (an effect absent in Hyp-mice). In further experiments, we examined if enzyme responsiveness to other stimulants is similarly impaired. While 1-hydroxylase activity in normal and phosphate-depleted mice increased after parathyroid hormone administration (41.3±5.1, 147.4±23.4), enzyme function in Hyp-mice did not change significantly (9.4±0.7). This differential response was not the result of an altered time course or dose response. These data suggest that a generalized enzyme dysfunction is manifest in Hyp-mice.

However, previous studies by Kurokawa et al (1,2) indicate that renal metabolism of 25(OH)D occurs in two cell populations, the proximal convoluted tubules and the proximal straight tubules. Since many of the stimuli used heretofore to characterize the defective vitamin D metabolism of Hyp-mice have been directed at the parathyroid hormone-adenylate cyclase system of the proximal convoluted tubules, we examined the effects of calcitonin on renal 25(OH)D metabolism (in proximal straight tubules) of Hyp-mice to determine if this mechanism governing vitamin D regulation is similarly impaired. Basal levels of 1-hydroxylase in normals and mutants

Vitamin D. A Chemical, Biochemical and Clinical Update

were 3.19±0.45 and 5.69±1.18 fmol/mg/min, respectively. In contrast, after 24 hours of human synthetic calcitonin administration (0.5 u/h S.C., continuously) enzyme activity in _Hyp_-mice increased to levels (20.03±5.24) that were no different from those of normal mice (14.69±2.88). Indeed, time course studies in both animal models revealed a similar pattern of response over 72 hours with maximal activity obtained after 24 hours. Both normal and _Hyp_-mice also exhibited a linear and parallel increase of enzyme activity in response to increasing doses of calcitonin. Furthermore, in _Hyp_-mice the effects of parathyroid hormone (at a maximal stimulatory dose, 0.25 u/h) and calcitonin (0.5 u/h) on 1-hydroxylase activity were additive.

	Basal	PTH	CT	PTH/CT
1-hydroxylase	5.4±1.0	12.3±0.4	16.7±2.9	26.9±2.6

These data indicate that regulation of 1-hydroxylase in _Hyp_-mice occurs by two distinct mechanisms. Moreover, the defective regulation of 1-hydroxylase in _Hyp_-mice is apparently confined to the parathyroid hormone-adenylate cyclase component of enzyme activation, while the calcitonin responsive pathway remains unaffected.

Acknowledgements: This work was supported in part by grants (5 P01 CA11265, 5 T32 AM07012, 5 R01 AM27032) from the National Institutes of Health and a grant (1-852) from the National Foundation.

References:

1. Kawashima, H., Torikai, S. and Kurokawa, K. (1981) Proc Natl Acad Sci. 78, 1199-1203.
2. Kawashima, H., Torikai, S. and Kurokawa, K. (1981) Nature. 291, 327-329.

25-OH-VITAMIN D_3-1α-HYDROXYLASE ACTIVITY IS NOT ACTIVATED IN CULTURED RENAL CORTICAL CELLS AND IN MITOCHONDRIA FROM X-LINKED HYPOPHOSPHATEMIC MICE.

A.B. KORKOR, R.W. GRAY AND R.A. MEYER.
Departments of Medicine and Biochemistry, MEDICAL COLLEGE OF WISCONSIN, Milwaukee, WI 53226 and Department of Basic Sciences, MARQUETTE UNIVERSITY SCHOOL OF DENTISTRY, Milwaukee, WI 53233. USA

We have previously shown that plasma 1,25-$(OH)_2$-D concentrations in x-linked hypophosphatemic mice (Hyp/y) are normal despite the presence of marked hypophosphatemia (1,2). Furthermore when Hyp/y mice ate a low PO_4 diet, plasma 1,25-$(OH)_2$-D levels fell to undetectible levels in contrast to the marked increase observed in response to PO_4 deprivation in their normal littermates (+/y) (2). These observations, as well as studies in patients with x-linked hypophosphatemia (3,4,5,6), raised the possibility that the renal 25-OH-D_3-1α-hydroxylase might be defective in Hyp/y mice. Therefore, we examined the production of 1,25-$(OH)_2$-D_3 by primary cultures of cortical kidney cells in serum free media obtained from Hyp/y or their normal littermates. The methods for the cell isolation and culture have been previously described by others (7,8,9). Briefly, the renal cortex was dissected, minced and then digested in a mixture of collagen and soybean trypsin inhibitor. The isolated cell suspension was removed and washed twice in Hank's balanced salt solution. The cells were then seeded into 25 cm^2 flasks containing 3 ml of serum free medium composed of equal volumes of Dulbecco's modified medium and Ham's F-12 medium containing 2 mM L-glutamine, transferrin 5 μg/ml, insulin 5 μg/ml, prostaglandin E_1 25 ng/ml, 10 mM HEPES and gentamycin 50 μg/ml. Protein content per flask reached a maximum by the 8th day of culture. Protein and DNA content per cell of Hyp/y and +/y were not different. 1,25-$(OH)_2$-D_3 production was measured after two hours of incubation at 37°C with the substrate 25-OH-D_3 at concentrations ranging from 2.5 to 20 μM. The media and the cells were then extracted with acetonitrile and purified by a preprative Sep-Pak and HPLC. 1,25-$(OH)_2$-D_3 content was measured by a competitive binding assay utilizing the calf thymus receptor (10). There was no difference in Km or Vmax between Hyp/y and +/y: 3.0 ± 4.8 SD vs 5.5 ± 6.8 μM and 4.8 ± 6.0 vs 2.3 ± 4.7 pmol/mg protein/hour, respectively. Protein content/flask was also comparable, averaging 900 ± 353 in Hyp/y and 971 ± 419 μg protein/flask in +/y. In view of these negative results, which may have been the result of in vitro changes in cell function, we examined the production of 1,25-$(OH)_2$-D_3 by freshly isolated mitochondria from either Hyp/y or +/y kidneys. The kidneys were decapsulated and dissected from the pelvis and the vessels in the hilus and then minced and homogenized by polytron. After centrifugation at 2000 RPM for 10 minutes the supernatant, enriched in mitochondria, was spun at 5500 RPM for 10 minutes. The mitochondrial pellet was then suspended in a mitochondrial co-factor solution containing either succinate or malate as substrate. 1,25-$(OH)_2$-D_3 production was measured after the addition of 0.1 to 10 μM 25-OH-D_3. Incubation was continued for 20 minutes at 37°C. 1,25-$(OH)_2$-D_3 content was measured as described above in the cell culture. Again, there was no difference in Km or Vmax between Hyp/y or +/y mitochondria: 0.8 ± 0.3 vs 0.5 ± 0.3 μM, and 1.8 ± 0.8 vs 1.7 ± 0.8 pmol/mg protein/20 minutes, respectively. However when we measured the production of 1,25-$(OH)_2$-D_3 by isolated mitochondria in +/y animals fed a low PO_4 diet for 3 days to produce hypophosphatemia comparable to that in Hyp/y, Vmax increased to 4.7 ± 2 pmol/mg protein/20 minutes ($p < 0.02$) and Km remained unchanged at 0.4 ± 0.3 μM. We therefore conclude that despite

Vitamin D. A Chemical, Biochemical and Clinical Update

hypophosphatemia, the renal 25-OH-D-1α-hydroxylase activity in Hyp/y is normal and not activated as expected in the presence of hypophosphatemia.

REFERFNCES

1. Meyer, R.A., Jr., R.W. Gray, B.A. Roos and G.M. Kiebzak. (1982) Endocrinol. 111:174-177.
2. Meyer, R.A., Jr., R.W. Gray and M.H. Meyer. (1980) Endocrinol. 107: 1577-1581.
3. Lyles, K.W., A.G. Clark and M.K. Drezner (1982) Calcif. Tissue Int. 34:125-130.
4. Scriver, C.R., T.M. Reade, H.F. DeLuca and A.J. Hamstra. (1978) N. Eng. J. Med. 299: 976-979.
5. Lyles, K.W. and M.K. Drezner. (1982) J. Clin. Endocrinol. Metab. 54: 638-644.
6. Glorieux, F.H., Marie, P.J., Pettifor, J.M., Ch, B. and Delvin, E.E. (1980). N. Eng. J. Med. 303: 1023-1031.
7. Fukase M., Avioli, L.V., Birge, S.J. and Chase, L.R. (1984) Endocrinol. 114:1203-1207.
8. Taub, M. and Sato, G. (1980) J. Cell Physiol. 105:369-378.
9. Taub, M. and Livingston D. (1981) In Hormonal Regulation of Epithelial Transport of Ions and Water. Scott, W.N. and Goodman, D.B.P., eds. New York Acad. Sci., New York.
10. Reinhardt, T.A., Horst, R.L., Orf, J.W. and Hollis, B.W. (1984) Endocrinol. Metab. 58: 91-98.

URINARY EXCRETION OF D-GLUCARIC ACID IN VITAMIN D_3- COMPARED TO PHENOBARBITAL-TREATED GUINEA PIGS.

L.A. WHEELER and I.C. RADDE.
Research Inst., Hospital for Sick Children, Toronto, Canada.

High doses of vitamin D_3 (VitD) given to vitamin D-replete rats decrease total cytochrome P-450 (Cyt P-450) levels and aniline hydroxylase activity (1). Urinary D-glucaric acid (D-GA), part of the glucuronic acid pathway, is thought to be a quantitative, indirect index of hepatic microsomal enzyme induction/inhibition in guinea pigs and primates. A highly significant correlation was found between total cyt P-450 content and D-GA excretion in the guinea pig after the administration of the classical non-specific enzyme inducer phenobarbital (PB) (2). The aim of this study was to determine, whether (1) the decrease in cyt P-450 content associated with high-dose VitD treatment is reflected in a decrease in urinary D-GA excretion rate, and (2) the correlation between cyt P-450 and D-GA exists after more than one dose of PB or other drugs which may affect hepatic enzymes. We compared the effects of 2 oral doses of VitD (300 µg/kg/day x 6, 3000 µg/kg/day x 6) and 2 oral doses of PB (12.5 mg/kg/day x 6 and 75 mg/kg/day x 6) on D-GA excretion rates in pregnant guinea pigs.

METHODS:

Random bred pregnant guinea pigs (early to late gestation) were divided into 6 groups according to drug treatment (Table I).

Table I: Animal Treatment Groups (No. of animals in group)

Group 1: Control (no drugs) (6); Group 2: Ethanol control (6); Group 3: 300 µg VitD/kg/d (6); Group 4: 3000 µg VitD/kg/d; Group 5: 12.5 mg PB/kg/d (8); Group 6: 75 mg PB/kg/d (8).

Animals were kept in metabolic cages and consecutive, timed 24 h urine collections were made each study day. On day 1 a control urine was collected for each animal. Days 2-7 were drug treatment days. The VitD was dissolved in ethanol. D-GA excretion rates were determined by the method of Colombi et al. (3). On day 8, animals were killed by cervical dislocation and liver microsomes were prepared (4). Protein concentrations (5) and cyt P-450 content (6) were measured.

RESULTS:

Animals of Groups 1-4 all showed a significant decrease in D-GA excretion rate ($p<0.001$) between study days 1 and 2. Excretion rates then remained constant over the duration of the study for the first 3 groups. The D-GA excretion of Group 4 decreased significantly from groups 1-3 ($p<0.01$) after 4 days drug administration. (Fig 1). No difference in cyt P-450 levels was seen between any of the first 4 treatment groups. D-GA excretion increased significantly after 5 days in Group 5, and as early as 2 days in Group 6 ($p<0.001$). (Fig 1). Total cyt P-450 values were significantly increased from control (2.85 ± 0.16 nmol/g liver) (M±SEM) with the low PB-dose (5.93±0.83

Vitamin D. A Chemical, Biochemical and Clinical Update

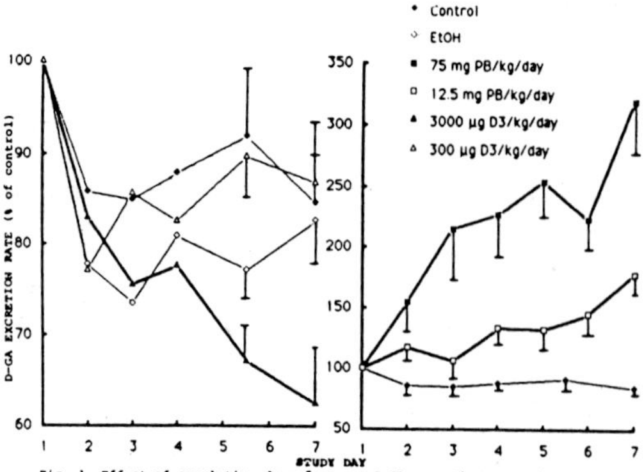

Fig. 1. Effect of cumulative drug doses on D-GA excretion rates (means ± SEM).

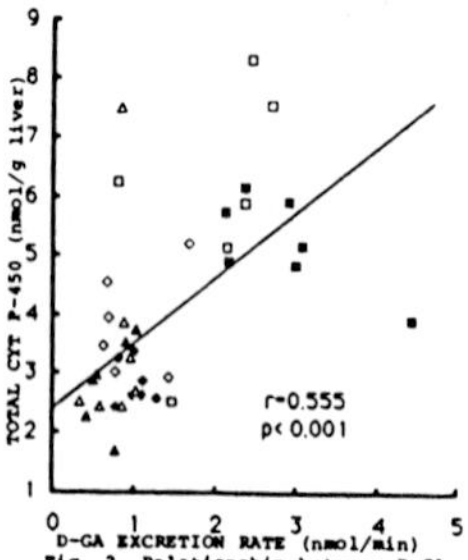

Fig. 2. Relationship between D-GA excretion and Cyt P-450 after various drug treatments.

nmol/g liver, $p<0.005$) and the high dose of PB (5.14 ± 0.33 nmol/g liver, $p<0.001$). A highly significant correlation existed between total cyt P-450 levels and urinary D-GA excretion rates ($p<0.001$) with all treatment groups included. (Fig 2).

DISCUSSION:

The reason for the initial decrease in D-GA excretion rate in the first 4 treatment groups is unknown though it may have been due to stress and/or confinement when animals were first placed in the metabolic cages. Induction with PB masked this initial decrease in Groups 5 and 6. The decrease in D-GA excretion after 4 days of treatment with the higher VitD dose agrees with the results of a previous study (1), yet we found no difference in cyt P-450 levels between groups 1-4. This may indicate that the decrease in D-GA excretion is due to renal damage rather than a change in liver enzyme status though no hypercalcemia was noted. No difference in total cyt P-450 level existed between the 2 doses of PB, which does not agree with the D-GA excretion data. Further investigation may show that the D-GA excretion may be a better index of Phase II conjugation reactions than of Phase I microsomal reactions even though an excellent correlation was found between total cyt P-450 content and D-GA excretion rates after more than one pharmacological treatment of the animals.

REFERENCES:

(1) Gascon-Barre, M., Cote, M.G., and Brodeur, J. (1979) Biochem Pharmacol 28: 313-319.
(2) Hunter, J., Maxwell, J.D., Stewart, D.A. and Williams, R. (1973) Biochem Pharmacol 22: 743-747.
(3) Colombi, A., Maroni, M., Antonini, C., Cassina, T., Gambini, A., and Foa, V. (1983) Clin Chim Acta 128: 337-347.
(4) Cresteil, T.H., Flinois, J.P., Pfister, A., Beroux, J.P. (1979) Biochem Pharmacol 28: 2057-2063.
(5) Lowry, O.H., Rosebrough, N.J., Farr, A.L. and Randall, P.J. (1963) J Biol Chem 193: 265-275.
(6) Omura, T. and Sato, R. (1964) J Biol Chem 239: 2379-2385.

DO PHOSPHOLIPIDS PLAY A ROLE IN 25-HYDROXYVITAMIN D_3 METABOLISM ?

N. S. CUNNINGHAM and H. L. HENRY,
Department of Biochemistry, UNIVERSITY OF CALIFORNIA, Riverside, CA 92521, U.S.A.

Introduction:

PTH is an important regulator of 25-OH-D_3 metabolism in the kidney, stimulating 1-hydroxylase activity and reducing the 24-hydroxylase activity both *in vivo* and *in vitro*, but the mechanism of this effect is presently unknown. In the adrenal cortex, adrenocorticotropin (ACTH) controls steroidogenesis by stimulating the cholesterol side chain cleavage reaction which results in the formation of pregnenolone. Since the 1-hydroxylase and 24-hydroxylase appear to function in a manner analogous to cytochrome P-450scc, and because ACTH and PTH elicit similar responses in their respective target tissues in terms of stimulating cAMP production and stimulating mitochondrial cytochrome P-450-mediated hydroxylations, we were interested in reports which implied that phospholipids (PL) may function as mediators in the steroidogenic action of ACTH in adrenal cells (1,2). The present study was carried out to investigate the possibility of a PL involvement in the renal mitochondrial metabolism of 25-OH-D_3.

Methods:

One week old vitamin D-deficient chicks were divided into two groups, one of which was made vitamin D-replete by oral doses of vitamin D_3 (300 I.U./week for 3 weeks). Control chicks received vehicle. At the time of the experiment, renal mitochondria were prepared by differential centrifugation and resuspension in 0.25 M sucrose. For the enzyme assays, 0.5 ml of mitochondria from D-deficient chicks (-D mito) or D-replete chicks (+D mito) were incubated at 37°C in the presence of 28 mM Tris-HCl (pH 7.4) buffer, 14 mM KCl, 5.6 mM $MgCl_2$, 10 mM malate (pH 7.4), 75 mM sucrose and substrate, 4 x 10^{-8} M 25-OH-[26,27-^{3}H]cholecalciferol (final concentrations) in a total volume of 5 ml. Following the incubation, unconverted [^{3}H]25-OH-D_3 and the two dihydroxylated products, [^{3}H]24,25$(OH)_2D_3$ and [^{3}H]1,25$(OH)_2D_3$ were extracted, separated by HPLC, and quantitated by liquid scintillation counting. To examine the PL composition of the mitochondria, lipids were extracted from the mitochondrial pellet with hexane:IPA (3:2). Following a wash with aqueous Na_2SO_4, the PL's were separated by TLC. After iodine visualization of the spots, the spots were scraped off of the plate, the PL's extracted from the silica gel, and PL phosphorus was quantified.

Results:

Most phospholipids examined had no effect on the 1-hydroxylase and 24-hydroxylase activities. Cardiolipin (CL), however, profoundly altered 1-hydroxylase activity and these effects were dependent on the vitamin D status of the chicks used to obtain the mitochondria (Figure 1). Examination of the PL composition of renal mitochondria from vitamin D-deficient and replete chicks revealed no major differences between the two suggesting that the differential response observed in Fig. 1 is not due to an inherent major difference in PL composition. None of the PL's tested altered the distribution of substrate or products following incubation of +D or -D mitochondria with [^{3}H]25-OH-D_3.

In an effort to determine the mechanism by which cardiolipin exerted such a pronounced inhibitory effect on the 25-OH-D_3-1-hydroxylase activity in -D mitochondria, we investigated the effect of CL on some kinetic parameters of [^{3}H]1,25$(OH)_2D_3$ production. An Eadie-Hofstee plot of the results from these studies is shown in Figure 2. The parallel nature of the lines in the presence or absence of exogenous CL indicates that the apparent K_m for 25-OH-D_3 is not significantly affected by CL but that the V_{max} is dramatically reduced. These results suggest that CL is acting as a noncompetitive inhibitor of the 25-OH-D_3-1-hydroxylase in -D mitochondria. A question which arises is whether the CL effect on the 1-hydroxylase activity is due to the polar head group or the fatty acid component of CL. Investigation of the effect of fatty acid methyl esters on the hydroxylase activities revealed that there was no effect on either hydroxylase activity in +D mitochondria. However, we did observe a significant decrease in the 25-OH-D_3-1-hydroxylase activity in -D mitochondria (Table I) which was dependent on the saturation state of the fatty acid methyl esters tested. The greater the extent of unsaturation, the more effective the fatty acid was as an inhibitor. Interestingly, CL is composed totally of unsaturated fatty acids, whereas, the other PL's have approximately 50:50 ratios of saturated:unsaturated fatty acids. These results suggest that it may be the fatty acid moiety rather than the polar head group of CL which is responsible for its observed effect on the 1-hydroxylase activity.

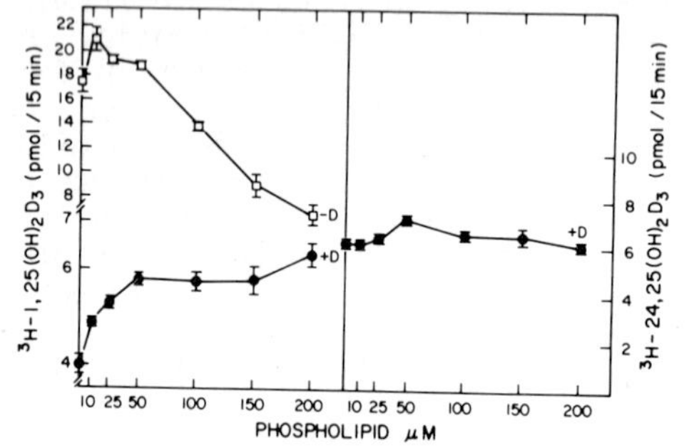

Fig. 1. CL Dose Response.

EFFECT OF FATTY ACID METHYL ESTERS ON 1,25$(OH)_2D_3$ PRODUCTION IN -D MITOCHONDRIA

Fatty Acid Methyl Ester	pmol 1,25$(OH)_2D_3$/10 min rxn
None	18.5 ± 2.95
Methyl Stearate (18:0)	10.3 ± 0.42
Methyl Oleate (18:1^9)	7.8 ± 0.14
Methyl Linoleate (18:2^{9,12})	4.7 ± 0.03

TYPICAL PERCENTAGE COMPOSITION OF FATTY ACIDS OF NATURAL PHOSPHOLIPIDS

Phospholipid	Fatty Acid Composition					
	16:0	16:1	18:0	18:1	18:2	20:0
Cardiolipin	--	2	--	7	90	--
Phosphatidylcholine	44	7	9	32	--	--
Phosphatidylethanolamine	10	--	20	58	--	12

Table I.

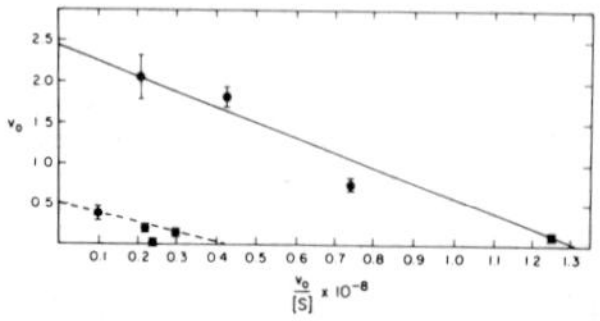

Fig. 2. Eadie-Hofstee plot of kinetic data obtained in the presence (•--•) and absence (•—•) of CL. Slope is equal to $-K_m$, intercept on V_o axis gives value for V_{max}.

1. Farese, R.V., Sabir, A.M., Vandor, S.L. and Larson, R.E. (1980) J. Biol. Chem. 255, 5728-5734.
2. Lambeth, J.D. (1981) J. Biol. Chem. 256, 4757-4762.

CHRONIC INFUSION OF SALMON CALCITONIN ELEVATES PLASMA LEVELS OF CALCIUM IN THYROPARATHYROIDECTOMIZED RATS.

PH. JAEGER, W. JONES, T.L. CLEMENS*, J.P. HAYSLETT
Yale Univ. School of Med., New Haven, Conn., and *Helen Hayes Hosp., West Haverstraw, N.Y. U.S.A.

Introduction:

The existence of a direct effect of calcitonin on vitamin D metabolism remains a matter of controversy. Indeed, whereas Galante et al (1) reported increased production of dihydroxycholecalciferol after administration of salmon calcitonin, contrary results were obtained by two independent groups of investigators (2,3). Recently, however, Horiuchi et al provided new evidence for a calcitonin-induced stimulation of 1α-hydroxylase (4), an effect that Kawashima et al further showed to occur in the proximal straight tubule (5). The present study has been undertaken to see whether this effect can be observed in vivo independently from the pathway calcitonin→hypocalcemia→PTH release→1,25 $(OH)_2D$ synthesis.

Methods:

Male rats weighing 220 to 290 g. underwent thyroparathyroidectomy under ether anesthesia. They were then fed either a regular diet containing 1,2% calcium, or a calcium-free diet. Half of the animals on each diet were infused with salmon calcitonin (Calcimar , Armour Pharmaceutical Co., Kankakee Il.) delivered at a constant rate (0.2 U/h) over 2 weeks via Alzet osmotic minipumps implanted subcutaneously. The remainder of the animals were sham-implanted and taken as controls. Blood was drawn daily and analyzed for calcium,phosphorus. Before sacrifice, (i.e. at the end of the first or of the second week of infusion) the animals were exsanguinated and blood was analyzed for 25-hydroxy-vitamin D [25 (OH) D], and 1,25 dihydroxy-vitamin D [1,25 $(OH)_2$ D].

Results:

On regular diet, chronic calcitonin infusion led to a 37% increment in plasma calcium level ($p < 0.001$) in the absence of change in plasma level of phosphorus. On calcium-free diet, calcitonin led only to a slight rise in plasma calcium (+ 16%, $p < 0.02$), and this also occured in the absence of change in plasma phosphorus. Plasma levels of 25 (OH) D were similar in each of the four groups of animals. Plasma levels of 1,25 $(OH)_2D$ are given in the table.

Table I: plasma levels of 1,25 $(OH)_2D$ in pg/ml

	Controls		Calcitonin	
	1st week	2nd week	1st week	2nd week
	←	$p < 0.05$	→	
Regular diet	38 ± 6 (6)	24 ± 5 (4)	80 ± 17 (5)	28 ± 1 (5)
		$p = 0.025$		$p < 0.001$
Calcium-free diet	-	139±37 (5)	-	460±50 (6)
		←	$p < 0.001$	→

X ± SEM (n)

Vitamin D. A Chemical, Biochemical and Clinical Update

It appears that thyroparathyroidectomized animals fed for 2 weeks the calcium-free diet had much higher 1,25 $(OH)_2D$ levels than those fed the regular diet. Chronic salmon calcitonin infusion into rats fed the regular diet led only to a transient rise in 1,25 $(OH)_2D$ levels whereas that into thyroparathyroidectomized rats fed the calcium-free diet led to a marked rise in this parameter.

Discussion:

This study shows that chronic salmon calcitonin infusion into thyroparathyroidectomized animals fed a regular diet leads to marked increment in plasma level of calcium. This effect is prevented to a large extent by feeding the animals a calcium-free diet, suggesting that stimulation of intestinal absorption of calcium took place during calcitonin treatment. The mechanism governing this association is thought to be a calcitonin-induced activation of 1α-hydroxylase since significantly higher 1,25 $(OH)_2D$ levels were found in calcitonin treated than in untreated animals.

This stimulation is regarded as a direct effect of the hormone since it can be observed in the absence of parathyroid hormone secretion as well as of changes in plasma phosphorus levels. That on regular diet the effect was only transient is interpreted to reflect the depressive action of high plasma calcium on the hydroxylase.

References:

1. Galante L., Colston K.W., MacAuley S.J., MacIntyre I. (1972) Nature 238: 271.273.
2. Rasmussen H., Wong M., Bikle D., Goodman D.B.P. (1972) J. Clin. Invest. 51: 2502-2504.
3. Lorenc R., Tanaka Y., DeLuca H.F., Jones G. (1977) Endocrinology 100: 468-472.
4. Horiuchi N., Takahashi H., Matsumoto T., Takahashi N., Shimazawa E., Suda T., Ogata E. (1979) Biochem. J. 184: 269-275.
5. Kawashima H., Torikai S., Kurokawa K. (1981) Nature 291: 327-329

Supported by USPHSR grants AM 18061 and GE 04724

EFFECT OF MAGNESIUM UPON 25-HYDROXYVITAMIN D 1-ALPHA HYDROXYLASE ACTIVITY.

T.O. Carpenter, D.L. Carnes, and C.S. Anast.
Department of Medicine, Endocrinology Division, Children's Hospital, Boston, MA.

INTRODUCTION

A number of interrelationships exist between magnesium and the calciotropic hormones. Overt hypoparathyroidism (1,2) and rickets have been reported in magnesium deficiency (3). There is evidence in rats and humans to suggest impaired responsiveness to vitamin D in hypomagnesemia (4,5). Furthermore, it is accepted that 25 hydroxyvitamin D 1α hydroxylase (1αOHlase) is a magnesium-dependent enzyme, although minimal data are found in the literature to support this concept (6). These studies examine effects of magnesium depletion upon 1αOHlase activity in vivo and in vitro.

METHODS AND RESULTS

1. The effect of Mg deficiency on the in vivo conversion of 25 OHD to $1,25(OH)_2D$. Weanling rats were placed on a vitamin D-deficient, Mg-replete, or Mg-deplete diets. Vitamin D_3 (100 units 3 times a week) was given by dropper to "+D" animals. After 3 weeks, animals were sacrificed. Animals were sacrificed 16-18 hours after intraperitoneal injection of 25(OH) [26,27-methyl 3H] vitamin D_3. Vitamin D metabolites were extracted from the sera of each animal. Separate and percent conversion was calculated as follows:

$$\% \text{ conversion} = \frac{\text{cpm recovered as } 1,25(OH)_2D_3}{\text{total cpm recovered}}$$

Results:

Group	D+Mg+	D-Mg+	D+Mg-	D-Mg-
N	(8)	(8)	(6)	(8)
% Conversion to $1,25(OH)_2D_3$	0.02 ± 0.01[a]	0.28 ± 0.04	0.02 ± 0.01	0.29 ± 0.04
% Conversion to $24,25(OH)_2D_3$	0.08 ± 0.01	0	0.09 ± 0.03	0

[a] Values represent mean ± standard deviation.

The absence of an effect of Mg deficiency upon in vivo conversion of 25 OHD to either $1,25(OH)_2D_3$ or $24,25(OH)_2D_3$ was demonstrated. Vitamin D-deficient animals showed increased conversion to $1,25(OH)_2D_3$ and decreased conversion to $24,25(OH)_2D_3$, when compared to vitamin D replete animals. No interaction between Mg and vitamin D depletion could be demonstrated by ANOVA, that is, magnesium deficiency does not tend to diminish or exacerbate the vitamin D effects upon this system in vivo.

2. Comparison of 1αOHlase activity in renal mitochondria obtained from Mg-deficient and Mg-replete rats. This assay is performed after isolation of renal mitochondria by standard methods. Hydroxylation is performed by the addition of 25 hydroxyvitamin D_3 in dosages varying from 100 to 3000 pm per flask. Radioactivity is maintained constant at 25,000 cpm per sample. The sample is gassed after addition of substrate with 95% O_2, 5% CO_2, stoppered, and incubated for 20 min. Extraction and separation of vitamin D metabolites follow. Enzyme activity was calculated using the formula:

Vitamin D. A Chemical, Biochemical and Clinical Update

$$V = \frac{\text{\% conversion x substrate added}}{\text{minutes of incubation x mg protein in sample}}$$

Results:

In vitro 1α hydroxylase activity was maintained in magnesium depletion (serum Mg = 0.48 ± 0.03 vs 2.07 ± 0.16 in Mg+ animals). There was no significant difference in Vmax or Km between Mg-deficient and Mg-replete rats. This assay requires stimulation of the enzyme by vitamin D deficiency; there is no detectable activity in the vitamin D-replete animal.

3. 1αOHlase activity in renal mitochondria depleted of Mg in vitro. For studies using Mg-depleted mitochondria, the mitochondrial pellet was recentrifuged twice in media containing 10 mM EDTA. Another centrifugation was performed in the usual buffer (without EDTA). Final pellets were resuspended in media containing between 0 and 2 mM $MgSO_4$. Equal amounts of calcium were added to restore calcium content to pre-EDTA wash levels, determined by atomic absorption (approximately 0.2 mM). Preparations were kept isosmolar with varying concentrations of Na_2SO_4.

Results:

These *in vitro* experiments, using low (500 pmol/ml) and high (3000 pmol/ml) dosages of substrate, demonstrated enzyme activity in 0 mM magnesium media. Activity was biphasic with respect to media magnesium concentrations with a nadir of activity at 0.5 mM magnesium. Enzyme activity at 0 mM magnesium was in the range obtained at 1-2 mM magnesium. Enzyme activity at all Mg concentrations was always greater than any activity seen in a heat denatured control.

CONCLUSION

Our accumulated data from studies assessing the effects of dietary magnesium deprivation upon *in vivo* and *in vitro* metabolism of 25 hydroxyvitamin D are consistent with one another, and support the notion that such dietary effects are not a major factor in the regulation of 1αOHlase activity. Although this enzyme complex is assumed to be magnesium-dependent, there is not consistent support of this notion in previous studies. Our data do not support: 1) the concept that magnesium is a major regulator of enzyme activity; nor 2) the concept that magnesium is an absolute requirement for expression of *in vitro* enzyme activity.

References:

1. Anast, C.S., Mohs, J.M., Kaplan, S.L. and Burns, T.W. (1972) Science 177, 606-608.
2. Suh, S.M., Tashjian, A.H. Jr, Matsuo, N., Parkinson, D.K. and Fraser, D. (1973) J. Clin. Invest. 52, 153-160.
3. Reddy, V. and Sivakumar, B. (1974) Lancet (i), 963-965.
4. Lifshitz, F., Harrison, H.C. and Harrison, H.E. (1967) Proc. Soc. Exp. Biol. Med. 125, 472-476.
5. Medalle, R., Waterhouse, C. and Hahn, T.J. (1976) Am. J. Clin. Nutr. 29, 854-858.
6. Fraser, D.R. and Kodicek, E. (1970) Nature (London) 228, 765-766.

AGE RELATED CHANGES IN CALCIUM HOMEOSTASIS IN RATS WITH CHRONIC VITAMIN D DEFICIENCY.

M. WARNER AND A. TENENHOUSE,
Department of Pharmacology and Therapeutics, McGill University, Montreal, Quebec, Canada.

INTRODUCTION

The conversions of 25-hydroxyvitamin D_3 (25-OH-D_3) to 1,25 dihydroxyvitamin D_3 (1,25 $(OH)_2D_3$) and 24,25-dihydroxyvitamin D_3 are catalysed by renal mitochondrial cytochromes P-450. These enzyme activities are regulated in response to the body's need for calcium and phosphorus. Although the mechanisms by which changes in catalytic activity are brought about are unknown, several mediators have been reported to be involved. These include, parathyroid hormone (PTH), growth hormone, vitamin D and plasma levels of calcium and phosphorus (1-5). The present report is an examination of the ontogeny of the vitamin D hydroxylases in vitamin D deficient rats and presents evidence for two distinct levels of regulation of the enzymes.

METHODS

The animals used in the study were male Sprague Dawley rats born of females who had been weaned on a vitamin D deficient diet (ICN Nutritional Biochemicals, Cleveland, Ohio. Diet AIN 76A) and mated 8 weeks after weaning. The offspring were also maintained on this diet throughout life. Radioimmunoassays were used to measure PTH (Immuno Nuclear Corporation, Stillwater) and cAMP (New England Nuclear). Calcium, Phosphorus and Creatinine were measured with specific diagnostic kits (Lancet division of Sherwood Medical, St. Louis, MO.) and Plasma 1,25 $(OH_2)D_3$ was measured with a calf thymus receptor binding assay (6). The activities of vitamin D hydroxylases were measured in renal mitochondria as described by Vieth and Fraser (7).

RESULTS

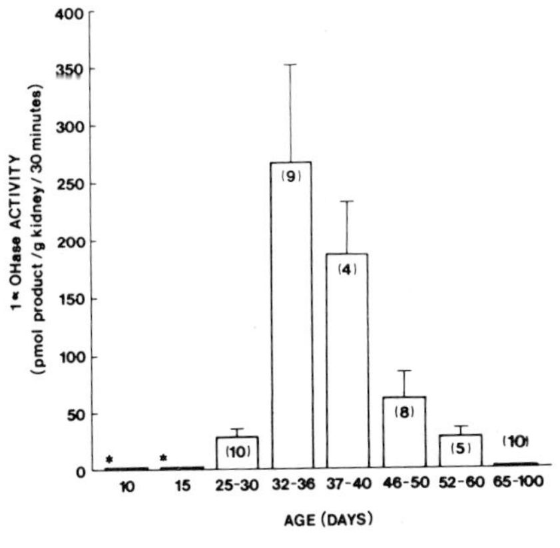

Figure 1: Developmental pattern of renal mitochondrial 1-hydroxylase activity in vitamin D deficient rats. The numbers in parentheses are the number of samples in the age group.
*the result is the mean of two determinations.

Vitamin D. A Chemical, Biochemical and Clinical Update

In the male offspring of vitamin D deficient females, renal mitochondrial 1-hydroxylase activity was undetectable before the 3rd week of life even though the animals were severely hypocalcemic from birth. The 1-hydroxylase activity first became detectable at 26 days of age, rapidly reached a maximum at day 34, then decreased to become undetectable again by 65 days (Fig. 1). Throughout this time serum (Ca) was = 5.0 mg/dl and serum parathyroid hormone (PTH) concentration, measured by a mid-molecule radioimmunoassay was 2-5 fold greater than found in vitamin D replete rats.

1-hydroxylase activity could be restored in the 65+ day old animals by administration of a single dose of 2.6 μg vitamin D_3. Enzyme activity was detected within 24 hours, was maximal at 72 hours and returned to undetectable levels by 96 hours after administration of the vitamin. Serum 1,25-$(OH)_2D$ which was undetectable before administration of the vitamin D_3, was 108 pg/ml 16 hours and 458 pg/ml 40 hours after the injection. The serum concentration of this metabolite then decreased progressively to 80 pg/ml by 6 days. 24-hydroxylase activity first became detectable 48 hours after vitamin D administration, increased to a maximum at 96 hours and thereafter decreased to become undetectable by 7 days.

The urinary excretion of phosphate and cyclic AMP was 10% of control values between 65-90 days of age. These values became normal 4 days after a single dose of 2.5 μg vitamin D_3.

From these data it is concluded that there are two distinct levels of regulation of 1-hydroxylase activity. A vitamin D independent induction of the activity at the time of weaning which is transient and is not associated with any detectable 24-hydroxylase activity. The second is a vitamin D dependent induction of enzyme activity seen in animals which, prior to administration of the vitamin manifest the characteristics of PTH resistance and have no detectable renal hydroxylase activity. The mechanisms of these effects remain to be determined.

REFERENCES

1. Fraser, D.R. and Kodicek, E. (1973) Nature (New Biology) 241, 163-166.
2. Trechsel, U., Eisman, J.A., Bonjour, J.P. and Fleisch, H. (1979). In In Vitamin D: Basic research and its clinical application pp. 511-513 Eds Norman, A.W., Schaefer, K., Von Herrath, D., Grigoleit, H.G., Coburn, J.W., DeLuca, H.F., Mawer, E.B. and Suda, T. Walter de Gruyter, Berlin.
3. Tanaka, Y. and DeLuca, H.F. (1973) Arch. Biochem. Biophys. 154, 566-574.
4. Wongsurawat, N., Armbrecht, H.J., Zenser, T.V, Forte, L.R. and Davis, B.B. (1983) J. Endocr. 101, 333-338.
5. Booth, B.E., Tsai, H.C. and Morris, R.C. Jr. (1985) J. Clin. Invest. 75, 155-161.
6. Reinhardt, T.A., Horst, R.L., Littledyke, E.T. and Beitz, D. (1982) Biochem. Biophys. Res. Commun. 106, 1012-1018.
7. Vieth, R. and Fraser, D. (1979) J. Biol. Chem. 254, 12455-12460.

Vitamin D Nutrition (Human + Animal)

THE ABSORPTION OF VITAMIN D METABOLITES IN BILIARY DUCT LIGATED RATS.

S. Shany, I. Zuili, N. Yankowitz and M. Maislos.

Department of Internal Medicine, Toor Institute and Clinical Biochemistry Unit, Soroka University Hospital, Beer Sheva, Israel.

Introduction

Hypovitaminosis D and osteomalacia are known features of chronic biliary obstruction (1), biliary cirrhosis (2), ileal resection (3) and chronic cholestyramine therapy (4). All these disorders are characterized by a lack of bile salts. It has recently been demonstrated that two different pathways of absorption exist for vitamin D and its metabolites (5). While vitamin D is absorbed almost entirely through the mesenteric lymph, the $1,25(OH)_2D$ is absorbed mainly through the portal system. The 25-OH-D is absorbed through both lymphatic and portal routes (5). In the present study, the effect of the presence or absence of bile salts on the absorption of various vitamin D metabolites was studied in vivo, in the rat. The differential absorption of each vitamin D metabolite into the lymph and the portal blood was carried out in both biliary ligated rats and control rats.

Methods

Four Sprague Dawley male rats (250-300g) were used for each experimental or control group. A day before the experiment took place, the biliary common duct was tied twice and cut behind the ligated portion. On the next day a tubing was introduced into the mesenteric lymph duct. Another tubing was introduced into the duodenum. An intravenous catheter was introduced into the portal vein. The control rats were treated and operated on in the same way as the experimental rats, except for the biliary duct ligation. All the surgical treatments were done while the rats were anesthetized with diethyl ether. However, the rats were kept awake during the experiment. A 1 ml mixture of propylene glycol and Intralipid 10% (1:1), containing 5 nmol of ^{14}C vitamin D_3 or ^3H 25-OH-D_3 or ^3H $1,25(OH)_2D_3$, was introduced into the duodenum. Collection of the mesenteric lymph and portal blood sampling were carried out simultaneously at 0, 30 and 60 min., and at 1 hr intervals thereafter for 3 additional hrs. Radioactivity was assayed on duplicate aliquots of lymph and serum. The amounts absorbed into the mesenteric lymph are expressed in picomoles per total amount of lymph (Mean ± SEM). The amounts absorbed into the portal blood are expressed in pmols/ml serum (Mean + SEM).

Results

The absorption of ^3H $1,25(OH)_2D_3$ into the portal blood was not affected by the biliary duct ligation. Both experimental and control rats showed a rapid absorption with similar peak levels (Fig 1A). The absorption of ^{14}C vitamin D into the portal blood was low in the control and was diminished to zero in the experimental rats (Fig 1C). The ^3H 25-OH-D_3 absorption was affected to some extent by the absence of bile salts (Fig 1B). The absorption of vitamin D, 25-OH-D_3 and $1,25(OH)_2D_3$ into the mesenteric lymph decreased significantly ($P<0.001$) in the biliary duct ligated rats (Fig 2).

Vitamin D. A Chemical, Biochemical and Clinical Update

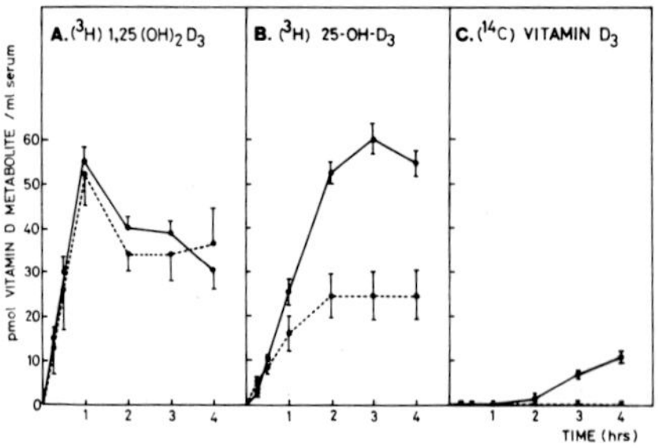

Fig 1: Absorption of vitamin D metabolites into the portal vein. --- in bile duct ligated rats, __ in controls.

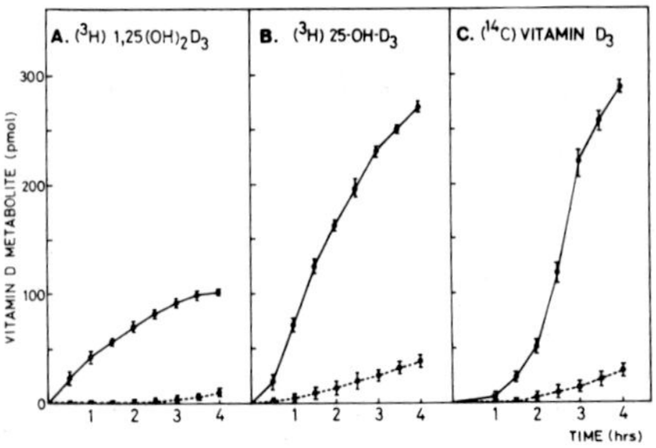

Fig 2: Absorption of vitamin D metabolites into the mesenteric lymph (symbols as in Fig 1).

Conclusions

1. Vitamin D_3 is practically not absorbed in the absence of bile salts.
2. The absorption of the polar vitamin D metabolites is relatively independent of the presence of bile salts.
3. It is recommended that the polar vitamin D metabolites, namely 25-OH-D_3 and 1,25$(OH)_2D_3$, be used in order to prevent osteomalacia in chronic biliary obstruction and similar disorders which cause bile salt deficiency.

References

1. Jung, R.T., Davie, M., Siklos, P., Chalmers, T.M., Hunter, J.O., and Lawson, D.E.M. (1979) Gut 20, 840-847.
2. Compston, J.E., and Thompson, R.P.H. Lancet (1977) 721-724.
3. Compston, J.E., and Horton, L.W.L. Gastroenterology (1978) 74, 900-920.
4. Thompson, W.G., and Thompson, G.R. Gut (1969) 10, 717-722.
5. Maislos, M., Silver, J., and Fainaru, M. Gastroenterology (1981) 80, 1528-1534.

RESTRICTION OF ENTRY OF 1,25(OH)$_2$D$_3$ INTO CEREBROSPINAL FLUID : IMPLICATIONS FOR SUPPRESSION OF FOOD INTAKE.

K.M. SCHNEIDER, D.D. LEAVER, U. TRECHSEL AND H. FLEISCH,
La Trobe University, Bundoora, 3083, Australia, and Institute of Pathophysiology, University of Bern, Switzerland.

Introduction : When sheep are given a pharmacological dose of 1,25(OH)$_2$D$_3$, (250 ng/kg/d) their food intake decreases within 3 days. This response may result from a direct action on appetite control, as the brain contains specific receptors for 1,25(OH)$_2$D$_3$ (1), or it could be an indirect effect due to changes, such as alterations in plasma mineral concentrations, induced by 1,25(OH)$_2$D$_3$. If 1,25(OH)$_2$D$_3$ has a direct effect on the brain then cerebrospinal fluid (CSF) concentrations of 1,25(OH)$_2$D$_3$ should reflect the plasma concentrations. This was examined by feeding rats a low phosphorus (P) diet, to increase their endogenous plasma concentrations of 1,25(OH)$_2$D$_3$, and then comparing plasma and CSF concentrations of 1,25(OH)$_2$D$_3$, P and calcium (Ca). In addition sheep were given graded doses of 1,25(OH)$_2$D$_3$ to test whether lower doses also influence food intake.

Methods : Sheep were fed a diet of 700 g/d of oaten and lucerne chaff (1:1) containing 1.3 g P and 4.5 g Ca. They were treated daily for 5 days with subcutaneous injections of either 1,25(OH)$_2$D$_3$ at dose rates of 25, 50, 75 and 250 ng/kg/d or diluent only. One group was treated for 10 days and were given 50 ng/kg/d for the first 5 days and 75 ng/kg/d for the second 5 days. Pre and post-treatment sampling periods were 5 days and plasma P and Ca concentrations were measured daily. Certain plasma samples were also analysed for 1,25(OH)$_2$D$_3$ (2). Male rats (160 ± 10 g) were fed either a conventional laboratory diet (1.2 % Ca, 0.8 % P) or low P diet (1.2 % Ca, 0.2 % P) for 7 days. They were then anaesthetised with nembutal and blood was collected from the aorta, and CSF from the cisterna magna. Samples from 3 rats were pooled and analysed for Ca, P, and 1,25(OH)$_2$D$_3$.

Results : Food intake was unchanged following treatment with 25 and 50 ng/kg/d, whereas it decreased following treatment with 75 and 250 ng/kg/d, with the latter treatment food intake decreased by 80 %. Plasma Ca and P concentrations increased at the lowest dose (25 ng/kg/d), and they increased even further with higher doses. However the increase was not proportional to dose rate. Concentration of 1,25(OH)$_2$D$_3$ in plasma increased from 20-30 pmol/l during the pretreatment period to 490 pmol/l during the administration of 75 ng/kg/d. Feeding rats a low P diet increased plasma Ca and 1,25(OH)$_2$D$_3$ and decreased plasma P concentrations in the manner reported previously (3). In the case of Ca and 1,25(OH)$_2$D$_3$ the changes in plasma concentration were not reflected in changes in their CSF concentration, but the decline in plasma P concentration was associated with a significant decrease in CSF P concentration (table 1).

Discussion : Relatively modest doses of 1,25(OH)$_2$D$_3$ decreased the food intake of sheep and the changes in plasma concentration of 1,25(OH)$_2$D$_3$ paralleled the changes in food intake over the experimental period. Nevertheless the plasma concentration of 1,25(OH)$_2$D$_3$ increased some 10

Vitamin D. A Chemical, Biochemical and Clinical Update

TABLE 1 : Concentration of Ca, P and $1,25(OH)_2D_3$ in plasma and CSF of rats fed a normal or low P diet (mean ± SD)

	DIET	CSF	PLASMA	CSF : PLASMA
Ca (mmol/l)	NORMAL	1.38 ± 0.01+Δ	2.60 ± 0.23	0.53
	LOW	1.34 ± 0.02	3.15 ± 0.01**	0.42
P (mmol/l)	NORMAL	0.70 ± 0.03	2.89 ± 0.09	0.24
	LOW	0.54 ± 0.01**	1.73 ± 0.12**	0.31
$1,25(OH)_2D_3$ (pmol/l)	NORMAL	52.7 ± 24.3	237.4 ± 50.0	0.24
	LOW	53.9 ± 17.7	479.8 ± 15.0**	0.11

Comparison between normal and low P diets, **, P < 0.01.
Δ, each sample represents pooled plasma or CSF from 3 rats. +, n = 4.

times and the absolute concentration was similar to that found in rapidly growing rats fed a low P diet. Since the sheep were fully grown such an increase is unlikely to occur under physiological conditions and the suppression of food intake probably represents a pharmacological effect of $1,25(OH)_2D_3$. The biological basis of this effect is unlikely to be a direct central action of $1,25(OH)_2D_3$, as in the rat, the brain was protected against the high plasma concentrations of $1,25(OH)_2D_3$. On the other hand in the rats fed the low P diet the CSF P concentration decreased and this decrease could generate a specific appetite, as for example happens with sodium (4), or be responsible for the overall reduction of food intake.

The finding that CSF $1,25(OH)_2D_3$ concentration is independent and lower than the plasma concentration could arise because a transport mechanism in the blood-brain barrier becomes saturated or, since CSF is virtually free of protein, the CSF $1,25(OH)_2D_3$ concentration simply reflects the unbound fraction in plasma. In man, blood and CSF concentrations of $1,25(OH)_2D_3$ are linearly correlated (r=0.5), although the concentrations in CSF were no higher than found in this study, and inspection of the data suggests a curvilinear model may be more appropriate than a linear model (5). Thus the simplest explanation for the restriction of entry of $1,25(OH)_2D_3$ into CSF is that $1,25(OH)_2D_3$ is transported across the blood-brain barrier by a mechanism which is saturated at a relatively low plasma concentration.

We thank Dr. Meier of Hoffmann-La Roche for the gift of $1,25(OH)_2D_3$.

References :

1. Stumpf, W.E., Sar, M., Clark, S.A. and DeLuca, H.F. (1982) Science 215:1403-1405.
2. Reinhardt, T.A., Horst, R.L., Orf, J.W. and Hollis, B.W. (1984) J. Clin. Endocrinology Metab. 58: 91-98.
3. Trechsel, U., Eisman, J.A., Fischer, J.A., Bonjour, J.-P. and Fleisch, H. (1980) Am. J. Physiol. 239:E119-E124.
4. Muller, A.F., Denton, D.A., McKinley, M.J., Tarjan, E. and Weisinger, R.S. (1983) Am. J. Physiol. 244: R810-R814.
5. Balabanova, S., Richter, H.-P., Antoniadis, G., Homoki, J., Kremmer, N., Hanle, J. and Teller, W.M. (1984) Klin. Wochenschr. 62: 1086-1090.

VITAMIN D METABOLISM IN MALNOURISHED CHILDREN WITH RICKETS

N.Raghuramulu and Vinodini Reddy
National Institute of Nutrition, Indian Council of Medical Research, Hyderabad-7, India.

Introduction:

Nutritional rickets is not uncommon in children in India, despite abundant sunshine and is more common in children with protein energy malnutrition than in well-fed children (1,2). It is not clear whether these two conditions merely coexist because of poverty and poor living conditions or malnutrition is causally related to rickets. Attempts were therefore made to evaluate the possible interrelationship between these two deficiency diseases.

Subjects and Methods:

A total of 91 children were investigated. The ages of these children ranged from 1 to 6 years. Fasting blood samples were analysed for serum calcium(3), Phosphorus(4), and alkaline phosphatase(5). Serum 25OHD3 was measured by the competitive protein-binding assay using rat serum(6).

Children with rickets were treated with a single IM dose of 600,000 IU vitamin D_3. Vitamin D_3 was administered orally either as a single massive dose of 600,000 IU or as a daily supplement of 200,000 IU for 20 days to normal and malnourished children. Biochemical studies were repeated 2-3 weeks later.

Results:

Serum Ca., P and 25OHD3 were significantly lower and alkaline phosphatase activity was higher in rachitic children as compared to other children (as shown in the table):

SERUM BIOCHEMICAL PARAMETERS

Group	Serum levels					SBP
	No.	Ca mg/dl	P mg/dl	APTase BU	25 OHD3 ng/ml	n moles 25 OHD3 bound/mg protein
Normals	23	9.5	5.7	7.9	34.7	0.23
Malnourished	46	9.2	4.4	7.0	19.7	0.22
Rickets	(before treatment)					
Wellnourished	4	8.2	2.8	29.3	7.1	-
Malnourished	18	8.9	2.6	20.5	4.8	-
Rickets	(after treatment)					
	22	9.3	4.8	16.0	31.8	-

In malnourished children serum P and 25 OHD3 levels were significantly lower than in normal children. The capacity of serum to bind 25 OHD3 was similar in normal and malnourished

Vitamin D. A Chemical, Biochemical and Clinical Update

children. After vitamin D administration, children with rickets showed improvement in all the biochemical parameters.

Following vitamin D administration, there was a significant increase in serum 25 OHD3 levels with both the dose schedules in normal and malnourished children. The increase with massive dose was similar both in normal children (70 ng/ml) and in malnourished children (62 ng/ml), whereas with small devided doses the increases were small, but similar in normal children (12 ng/ml) and in malnourished children (18 ng/ml).

Discussion:

The cases of rickets investigated are of nutritional origin as evidenced by very low serum 25 OHD3 levels as well as the response to vitamin D treatment.

The lowered initial serum 25 OHD3 levels in malnourished children may not be due to altered metabolism since vitamin D administration resulted in similar increase in both the groups of malnourished and normal children.

It is likely that the vitamin D nutritional status per se is altered in malnourished children.

Summary and conclusions:

Low serum 25 OHD3 levels in malnourished children may be as a result of poor vitamin D nutritional status than the reflection of impaired metabolism. Some of these children may remain indoors for longer times due to some chronic infections which may precipitate vitamin D deficiency resulting in frank clinical signs of rickets.

REFERENCES :

1. Manchanda, S.S. and Lai, H.(1972), Ind.J. Ped. 39, 52-57.
2. Pramanik, A.K., Gupta, S. and Agarwal, P.S.C.(1971), Ind. Ped. 8, 95-99.
3. Raghuramulu, N. and Vinodini Reddy (1982), Br. J. Nutr. 47, 231-234.
4. Chen. P.S. Jr. Tonibara, T.Y. and Warner, H.C.(1956), An. Chem. 28, 1756-1758.
5. Bodansky, A.(1933), J. Biol. Chem. 101, 93-97.
6. Belsey, R.E., Deluca, H.F. and Potts., J.T. Jr.(1974), J. Clin. End. Met. 38, 1046-1051.

CALCIUM, VITAMIN D AND BONE MINERAL STATUS OF PATIENTS ENTERING TPN PROGRAMS

S. EPSTEIN, H. TRABERG, R. McCLINTOCK and G. LEVINE,
Department of Medicine, Albert Einstein Medical Center and Temple University, Philadelphia, Pennsylvania and Indiana University, Indianapolis, Indiana, U.S.A.

INTRODUCTION

Total Parenteral Nutrition (TPN) is commonly used to provide nutrition in seriously ill and debilitated patients. Patients on long term TPN have developed bone disease which histologically resembles osteomalacia despite most cases having no biochemical abnormality of calcium, phosphorus, 25 hydroxyvitamin 25(OH)D and serum immunoreactive parathyroid hormone (PTH) values (1). The TPN formula infusion and/or vitamin D have been blamed for this bone mineralization defect since the withdrawal of vitamin D from these solutions has been associated with improvement in the bone disease (1,2). We were interested to see whether the bone mineral status of patients not on long term TPN but who were just entering TPN programs was already abnormal. If this is the case then the bone problems of TPN could be aggravated.

SUBJECTS

Twenty-five patients suffering from a variety of diseases aged twenty-five to eighty years were studied. Eighteen patients had malignant gastrointestinal disease with or without complicating sepsis. Six patients had sepsis with decubitus ulcers and one patient had sepsis without a diagnosis of the underlying disease ever having been made. No patients had symptoms or signs of osteomalacia or radiographic evidence of fractures or metabolic bone disease.

METHODS

Serum calcium (Ca), phosphate (Pi), bone gla protein (BGP) (3), alkaline phosphatase (AP), 25(OH)D, $1,25(OH)_2D$, and PTH (carboxyl terminal) were measured.

RESULTS

	Calcium mg/dl	Pi mg/dl	AP I.U.	BGP ng/ml	PTH ng/ml	25(OH)D ng/ml	$1,25(OH)_2D$ pg/ml
Norm. subject	9.7±1.2 N = 100	3.5±1.0 N = 100	<140 N = 100	6.6±2.2 N = 82	0.43±.04 N = 20	33.0±1.9 N = 77	31.0±11.5 N = 47
Patients	8.3±0.2 N = 25	3.0±.04 N = 25	136 N = 25	4.8±3.2 N = 12	1.06±.67 N = 25	6.5±1.3 N = 15	31.7±21.4 N = 19
P Value	<.01	<.002	N.S.	N.S.	<.002	<.001	N.S.

N = number subjects ± SEM

The results show that patients entering TPN programs, when compared to normal subjects had significantly lower levels of serum calcium, Pi and 25(OH)D. Serum BGP was not significantly altered but serum PTH was elevated. No difference of $1,25(OH)_2D$ nor AP was observed. From our studies, we conclude that patients by the time that they enter TPN programs have low serum 25(OH)D values with a compensatory increase in PTH secretion to try and maintain serum calcium. The low 25(OH)D presumably

Vitamin D. A Chemical, Biochemical and Clinical Update

reflects their poor nutritional status at the time TPN is instituted. The normal serum BGP values despite the higher serum PTH values may reflect either a resistance of the skeleton to PTH or depressed bone turnover in severly ill patients.

REFERENCES

1. Klein GL, Ament ME, Bluestone R, Norman AW, Targoff CM, Sherrard DS, Young JH and Coburn JW. Bone disease associated with total parenteral nutrition. Lancet (1980) 2:1041-1044.
2. Shike M, Sturbridge WC, Tam CS, Harrison JE, Jones G, Murray TM, Husdan H, Whitwell J, Wilson DR, Jeejeebhoy KN. A possible role of vitamin D in the genesis of parenteral nutrition induced metabolic bone disease. Ann. Inter. Med. (1981) 95:560-568.
3. Epstein S, Poser J, McClintock R, Johnston Jr. CC, Bryce G, and Hui S. Differences in serum bone gla protein with age and sex. Lancet (1984) 1:307-310.

VITAMIN D STATUS AMONG SCHOOL GIRLS IN RIYADH, SAUDI ARABIA, A.T.H. Elidrissy, M.A. Abdullah, S.H. Sedrani, Z.A. Karrar and K.M. Arabi
College of Medicine & Science King Saud University Riyadh Saudi Arabia.

INTRODUCTION:

Vitamin D deficiency was demonstrated among pregnant women and low levels were seen in adult males and females in Saudi Arabia (1, 2,). A definite correlation was found between low levels of 25 hydroxyvitamin D in mothers and the development of rickets in their children (3). Many factors were thought to be as associated with the development of vitamin D deficiency in such a sunny country. Since adult females are at a higher risk of becoming vitamin D deficient during pregnancy and lactation, this study was designed to elucidate the effect of puberty on vitamin D status and to verify the role of changing to the traditional dress of females which takes place at puberty.

MATERIAL AND METHODS:

Serum 25 hydroxivitamin D (25OHD) was measured among 414 school girls from a randomly selected stratified sample of schools in Riyadh. All stages of schooling were represented. Only girls whose parents gave a conscent were subjected to blood sampling. The serum was separated and stored at -20C for analysis at a later date.

25OHD was extracted from serum by chloroform methanol, purified by a 50 cm sephadox LH20 column and quantitated by competitive protein-binding assay using rachitic rat serum (4). The results obtained were analysed by computerized statistical analysis system.

RESULTS:

The levels of 25OHD in different age groups is demonstrated in figure 1. The mean level of 25OHD shows a drop in the ages 10, 11 & 12, years. The school girls were divided into three groups, children (6 to 11 years) adolescents (12 to 15 years)and adults (16 years or more). The mean 25OHD levels in the groups were 19.1 ± 7.9ng, 19.3 ± 8.7 and 21.4 ± 10.3 respectively. Only 13.5, 15.5, and 16.5% of the three study groups showed 25OHD levels below 10 ng/ml. These findings show no significant difference between the three groups.

VITAMIN D LEVELS IN SCHOOL GIRLS

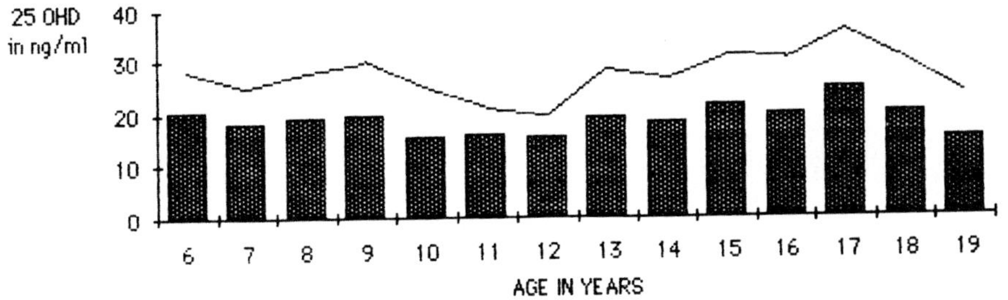

Vitamin D. A Chemical, Biochemical and Clinical Update

DISCUSSION:

This study demonstrates higher levels of 25OHD among school girls compared to the low levels seen in pregnant women (1).The 25 OHD levels in children is comparable to the levels in temperate countries during the summer months (5, 6, 7). Absence of deficiency rickets beyond three years of age in Riyadh is an important indicator of the adequacy of their vitamin D levels through school age. These levels seem to reach a ceiling beyond which it does not rise and it is only 50% of that from a tropical country nearer to the equater. The 25OHD level shows drop during the prepubertal period which confirm the finding of others (9). An interesting finding in this study is that there is no drop in the levels of 25OHD in the third group (adults); During this period girls wear the traditional cover up dressing, a finding which confirms our previous statement that method of female dressing in Saudi Arabia is not a cause of vitamin D deficiency (2)

REFERENCES:

1. Belton NR, Elidrissy ATH, Gaafer TH, Aldrees A, El Swailim AR, Forfar JO, Barr DGD, (1982) Biochemical ana clinical endocrinology of calcium metabolism. Walter de Gruyer 735-737.

2. Sedrani SH, Elidrissy ATH, Arabi KM, (1983) Am J Clin Nutr, 38: 129-132.

3. Elidrissy ATH, Sedrani SH, Lawson DEM (1984) Calcif Tissue Int 36:226-268.

4. Edelstein S, Charmoan M, Lawson DEM, Kodicek E (1974) Competitive binding assay for 25-hydroxycholecalciferol. Clin Sci Mol Med 46:231-236.

5. Poskitt EME, Cole TJ, Lawson DEM. (1979) Br Med J 1979; 1:221-3

6. Ellis G, Woodhead JS, Cooke WT, (1977) Lancet; 1:825-8.

7. Lund B, Sorensen OH. (1979) Scand J Clin Lab Invest; 39:23-30.

8. Linhares ER, Jones DA, Round JM, and Edwards RHT (1984) Am J Clin Nutr; 39:625-630.

9. Fujisawa Y, Kida K and Matsuda H (1984) J Clin Endocrinol Metab 59: 719.

...

25-HYDROXYVITAMIN D (25-OH-D) AND 1,25-DIHYDROXYVITAMIN D_3 (1,25$(OH)_2D_3$) IN PATIENTS WITH FEMORAL NECK FRACTURES (FNF)-- EFFECT OF VITAMIN D SUPPLEMENTATION

H. Schmidt-Gayk, U. Kick, M. Manner, W. Löffler and E. Mayer[Δ]

Chirurgische Klinik and [Δ]Abteilung für Endokrinologie, Medizinische Poliklinik der Universität Heidelberg, D-6900 Heidelberg, F.R.G.

Femoral neck fractures (FNF) often occur in the elderly population in this country. Since foods are not fortified with vitamin D and sunshine exposure is low, we presumed that FNF might be associated with a vitamin D deficient state.

METHODS

Parameters of calcium metabolism were assessed in 22 female patients (mean age 72 years) with FNF occurring within the period from November to April. Blood was withdrawn before and at days 3 and 7 following oral administration of a granulate containing vitamin D_3 (3000 IU/day) and calcium carbonate (1500 mg/day), kindly provided by Dr. Walter, Fa. Dieckmann, Bielefeld, F.R.G. The results are shown in the following table.

	Serum Calcium (Ca) mmol/l	Serum Phosphate (Pi) mmol/l	Calcium x Phosphate	Alkaline Phosphatase (U/l)
day 0	2.15±0.07	0.88±0.08	1.91±0.02	158±40
day 3	2.13±0.05	0.93±0.02	2.00±0.02	142±30
day 7	2.19±0.05	1.01±0.07	2.20±0.02	170±35
normal range:	2.20-2.60	0.8-1.5	1.8-3.9	40-170
P	< 0.20	< 0.05	< 0.005	n.s.

	25-OH-D (nmol/l)	1,25$(OH)_2D_3$ (pmol/l)	hPTH (pmol/l)	U_{cAMP}/U_{Cr} (μmol/g)
day 0	26±20	29±6	12.0±3.5	5.2±0.8
day 3	36±25	44±10	-	5.2±0.8
day 7	49±30	48±15	9.3±2.0	4.5±1
normal range:	25-150	75-175	6-12	2.2-5.1
P	< 0.001	< 0.005	< 0.05	n.s.

Vitamin D. A Chemical, Biochemical and Clinical Update

Before treatment serum calcium and $1,25(OH)_2D_3$ were subnormal with 25-OH-D being in the lower range and PTH and alkaline phosphatase in the upper range of normal. We believe that in these patients a mild secondary hyperparathyroidism (2° HPT) is present as a consequence of hypocalcemia and low $1,25(OH)_2$-D_3. This view is supported by the presence of a low serum phosphate level. Following treatment with vitamin D and calcium, a fall of PTH levels was observed associated with serum phosphate rising and urinary cAMP/Cr decreasing. Remarkably, PTH levels were declining in spite of an unchanged serum calcium level. Further, $1,25(OH)_2D_3$ showed a significant rise. Since a receptor protein specific for $1,25(OH)_2$-D_3 is present in the parathyroids, the decline of PTH might be due to the direct action of $1,25(OH)_2D_3$ on PTH secretion (1). In our patients, after 7 days of treatment, serum $1,25(OH)_2D_3$ had not yet returned to normal. This does not necessarily argue against the direct action of $1,25(OH)_2D_3$ on the parathyroids, since in 2° HPT down-regulation of the $1,25(OH)_2D_3$ receptor may occur (A. Korkor, pers. comm.)

The rise of $1,25(OH)_2D_3$ following 7 days of vitamin D administration was not as pronounced as expected from studies on rachitic children where $1,25(OH)_2D_3$ may well be above the normal range at the beginning of vitamin D treatment. Thus, in our patients with FNF, before vitamin D therapy $1,25(OH)_2D_3$ was low as a consequence of vitamin D deficiency. Further, after initiation of vitamin D therapy, the increase of serum $1,25(OH)_2D_3$ was inappropriate. In accordance with the work of Tsai et al. (2), this finding could well be of importance in the pathogenesis of osteopenia leading to FNF.

To prevent a vitamin D deficient state, we recommend the oral supplementation of vitamin D in elderly people.

1. Au, W.Z.W. (1984) Calcif. Tissue Int. 36, 384-391.

2. Tsai, K., Heath, H. III, Kumar, R. and Riggs, B.L. (1984) J. Clin. Invest. 73, 1668-1672.

VITAMIN D STATUS AND LIVER FUNCTION OF COWS WITH PARTURIENT PARESIS

R. Lappeteläinen, E. Lappeteläinen and P.H. Mäenpää
Department of Biochemistry, University of Kuopio, SF-70211 Kuopio, Finland.

About 10 % of calvings in Finland are complicated with signs of parturient paresis. The therapy consists of parenteral administration of calcium, but the treatment may be affected with different complications. Succesful attempts of prevention have been made with injections of pharmacological doses of active metabolites of vitamin D (1,2). The ultimate reasons for the occurrence of hypocalcemia and hypophosphatemia in some cows and not in others are still largely unknown. The purpose of the present study was to determine the effects of parturient paresis on serum levels of 25(OH)D, selected minerals and other compounds. The effect of season on vitamin D status was also studied.

EXPERIMENTAL

A random sample of Ayrshire and Friesian cows from eastern Finland were studied during the months of April, June and July. Fifteen animals with clinical signs of parturient paresis within one day of calving were utilized as well as eight control cows. One of the control cows calved without signs of parturient paresis and seven were not pregnant. Blood samples were taken by venipuncture from the external jugular vein during clinical investigation. Serum calcium, phosphate, alkaline phosphatase, total protein and protein fractions were determined in a clinical chemistry laboratory (Yhtyneet Laboratoriot, Helsinki, Finland). Serum amino acids were determined by a Kontron amino acid analyzer. Serum levels of allantoin (3) and those of urea (4) were determined as described previously. Serum samples were kept frozen (-20°C) until assayed for 25(OH)D fractions by HPLC (5). The samples were first purified on SEP-PACK C_{18}-columns.

RESULTS AND DISCUSSION

Significant differences were seen in serum calcium and phosphate concentrations comparing paretic and control cows (Table 1). Hypophosphatemia in the paretic cows was generally more severe than reported previously (6). Nearly half of the paretic cows had severe hypophosphatemia with serum concentrations of phosphate less than 0.32 mmol/l. Serum concentrations of albumin were slightly increased in the paretic cows, while those of allantoin and urea were decreased. Serum concentrations of several amino acids were significantly decreased in the paretic cows. The increase in serum glutamine concentration and the decrease in serum arginine, citrulline and urea suggest that the metabolism of amino-N into urea is impaired during parturient paresis. There were no differences in serum 25(OH)D_2 and 25(OH)D_3 concentrations comparing control and paretic animals. Serum concentrations of 25(OH)D_3 increased significantly in June and July. 25(OH)D_2 was always a minor serum 25(OH)D compound and did not show a seasonal variation. These results indicate a pronounced skin synthesis of vitamin D_3 in cows during summer, but no difference in vitamin D status between control and paretic cows. The results also indicate an impaired metabolism of amino-N in cows during parturient paresis. The changes in the concentrations of serum allantoin did not suggest an increased breakdown of adenylates in cells due to low levels of inorganic phosphate (7).

Vitamin D. A Chemical, Biochemical and Clinical Update

Table 1. Serum levels of calcium, phosphate, alkaline phosphatase, total protein, albumin, allantoin, urea and 25(OH)D compounds of control and paretic cows within one day of calving (means ± S.E.).

Compound	Control (n=8)		Paresis (n=15)	
Calcium (mmol/l)	2.19 ± 0.04		0.91 ± 0.07***	
Phosphate (mmol/l)	1.51 ± 0.11		0.44 ± 0.08***	
Alkaline phosphatase (U/l 37°C)	139 ± 33		153 ± 14	
Protein (g/l)	71.5 ± 1.8		71.1 ± 1.5	
Albumin (g/l)	31.1 ± 0.6		35.5 ± 0.9**	
Allantoin (μmol/l)	220 ± 27	(n=6)	153 ± 12	(n=10)*
Urea (mmol/l)	5.87 ± 0.57	(n=4)	3.36 ± 0.39	(n=6)**
$25(OH)D_2$ (ng/ml)	7.9 ± 1.5		7.2 ± 0.9	
$25(OH)D_3$ (ng/ml)	47.1 ± 12.7		43.4 ± 5.8	
Total 25(OH)D (ng/ml)	55.0 ± 12.9		50.6 ± 5.4	

Statistical significances between groups; *p <0.05, **p <0.01, ***p <0.001.

Table 2. Serum concentrations of 25(OH)D compounds of all cows during various months (means ± S.E.).

Month	Compound (ng/ml)		
	$25(OH)D_2$	$25(OH)D_3$	Total 25(OH)D
April (n=5)	9.8 ± 1.8	12.0 ± 3.2	21.9 ± 3.2
June (n=7)	6.3 ± 1.3	34.8 ± 3.2**	41.0 ± 2.7***
July (n=11)	7.1 ± 1.0	65.8 ± 6.5***	73.0 ± 6.7***

Statistical significances (compared to the values in April) as in Table 1.

REFERENCES

1. Gast, D.R., Marquardt, J.P., Jorgensen, N.A., and DeLuca, H.F. (1977) J. Dairy Sci. 60: 1910-1920.
2. Capen, C.C., Hoffsis, G.F., Nagode, L.A., Littledike, E.T., and Norman, A.W. (1982) in Vitamin D: Chemical, Biochemical and Clinical Endocrinology of Calcium Metabolism (Norman, A.W., Schaefer, K., v. Herrath, D. and Grigoleit, H.-G., eds) pp 773-775, de Guyter, Berlin.
3. Young, E.G., and Conway, C.F. (1942) J. Biol. Chem. 142: 839-853.
4. Fawcett, J.K., and Scott, J.E. (1960) J. Clin. Path. 13: 156-159.
5. Parviainen, M.T., Savolainen, K.E., Alhava, E.M., and Mäenpää, P.H. (1981) Ann. Clin. Res. 13: 26-33.
6. Hollis, B.W., Draper, H.H., Burton, J.H., and Etches, R.J. (1981) J. Endocr. 88: 161-171.
7. Raivio, K.O., Kekomäki, M.P., and Mäenpää, P.H. (1969) Biochem. Pharmacol. 18: 2615-2624.

THE EFFECT OF DIET ON BONE MINERAL CONTENT (BMC) AND CALCIUM AND PHOSPHORUS REGULATING HORMONES DURING THE FIRST YEAR OF LIFE: A Longitudinal Prospective Study. J.J. Steichen, R.C. Tsang, P. Lichtenstein, Department of Pediatrics, University of Cincinnati, Cincinnati, Ohio 45267-0541, U.S.A.

INTRODUCTION

Many infants in the United States and other developed countries are fed human milk substitutes as their primary nutritional source. For the most part, these infant formulas are based on cow milk. Multiple studies have shown that the formulas as marketed currently in the United States provide satisfactory growth during early infancy.(1) A large percentage of infants, however, receive formulas based on soy protein. In "underdeveloped" countries the percentage of infants receiving soy protein based formulas is even higher. The question has been raised whether lactose free soy protein isolate formula provides adequate nutrition, especially in regard to mineral and bone homeostasis.(2,3,4)

STUDY DESIGN - METHODS AND POPULATION: The study was designed to compare growth, blood chemical values and bone mineralization in term infants fed various formula regimens and to assess whether diet affects calcium metabolism, mineral regulating hormones and bone mineralization. Three formulas were studied in three groups of healthy term infants. Formula I: Similac 20 calories per ounce (N = 36), Formula II: Similac Whey (N = 18) and Formula III: Isomil, a soy protein based formula (N = 18). All formulas were supplied specifically for the study by Ross Laboratories, Columbus, Ohio. All infants were followed prospectively and longitudinally and were studied repeatedly over the first year of life. In addition, a fourth group of infants (N = 275) were studied between 12 and 18 months in a cross-sectionally designed study.

Calcium, ionized calcium, phosphorus, magnesium, 1,25 dihydroxyvitamin D, 25 hydroxyvitamin D, parathyroid hormone, calcitonin, alkaline phosphatase were measured longitudinally at birth to 2 weeks, 6 weeks, 12 weeks, 6 months, 9 months, and 12 months of age and cross-sectionally from 12 to 18 months.

NUTRITION: Nutrition consisted exclusively of the assigned formula for the first 6 months. After 6 months all infants continued on the original formula and were receiving Gerber infant food. All infants were receiving the same schedule of "beikost" from 6 to 12 months. Infants studied after 12 months were not assigned to any specific baby food and were eating regular infant food and table food.

RESULTS: Summary of results of normative values in infants receiving cow milk based formulas are shown in Table I.

	2 wks	6 wks	12 wks	6 mo	9 mo	12 mo	12-18 mo
25D (ng/ml)	31±11*	41±17	43±17	47±17	46± 9	47±11	45± 3
1,25D (pg/ml)	50±27	66±25	60±25	50±28	60±26	52±20	63± 5
Alk Phos (IU/1)	117±25	167±38	155±29	140±26	148±31	150±22	-----
CT (pg/ml)	39±20	30±21	26±20	30±22	23±22	56±27	64± 8
PTH (ulEq/ml)	62±25	56±30	40±20	45±25	44±14	53±24	-----
Ca (mg/dl)	9.6±.7	9.9±.7	9.9±.6	9.8±.5	10.4±.6	10±.5	9.6±.10
Mg (mg/dl)	2.0±.0	2.1±.2	2.1±.2	2.0±.2	2.2±.2	2.1±.2	2.1±.03
Phos (mg/dl)	8.3±.9	7.2±.7	7.0±.8	6.7±.8	5.9±.9	6.0±.7	5.9±.11
1Ca (mg/dl)	5.1±.1	5.2±.2	5.3±.2	5.3±.2	-----	5.3±.2	5.1±.02

Vitamin D. A Chemical, Biochemical and Clinical Update

*Table I shows mean ± 1 S.D. For calcitonin, all values not detectable (about 20% of patients) were recorded as 10 pg/ml and included in the calculations.

Serum 1,25 dihydroxyvitamin D concentrations were significantly higher in Isomil compared with cow milk formla fed infants at 2 and 6 weeks and 3 months and 6 months of age (p <.005 to p<.02). Serum Ca, P, Mg concentration were not different between groups. Bone mineral content was significantly higher in infants receiving a cow's milk based formula than infants receiving Isomil or human milk, especially over the first 6 months of life. Overall, bone mineralization was decreased in human milk compared to infants receiving cow milk protein formula, and in infants receiving soy protein base formulas compared to cow milk formula.

DISCUSSION: The present project studies the impact of various formulas on mineral homeostasis and bone mineralization in 3 groups of healthy term infants born to healthy middle class mothers. The diet in these infants was signficantly different in carbohydrate, protein and calcium and phosphorus intake. Soy protein has a 1 to 1 ratio of sucrose and corn syrup as carbohydrate source while cow milk based formula has lactose as its sole carbohydrate source. The cow milk formula is lower in protein (1.55% compared to soy milk formula, 2% protein). Protein composition is also significantly different in the three formulas; Similac 20 calories (82% casein, 18% whey) Similac Whey (40% casein, 60% whey). Mineral composition of the three formulas differ as well, soy protein formula having the highest calcium (70 mg/dl) and phosphorus (50 mg/dl) and the Similac whey formula having the lowest calcium (40 mg/dl) and phosphorus (30 mg/dl). Similac 20 cal./oz. contains 51 mg/Ca/dl and 39 mg/P/dl.

CONCLUSION: Our data shows that serum levels of mineral regulating agents may be significantly influenced by infant nutrition, especially during the first six months of life. Normative values during the first year of life vary significantly, especially during the first six months of life. These data will be helpful in the management of young infants with mineral metabolism abnormalities.

REFERENCES:

1. Fomon, S.J.: Infant Nutrition (1974) W.B. Saunders and Company, Philadelphia.

2. Ziegler, E: Calcium and phosphorus balances in term infants fed soy formulas (1979) Ross Clinical Research Conference, LBW Infants Fed Isomil, p. 113-121.

3. Root, A.N. and Harrison, M.E.: Recent advances in calcium metabolism (1976) J. Pediatrics 88:177.

4. Hilman, L.S.: Problems of bone mineralization in low birth weight infants fed soy formulas (1979) Ross Clinical Research Conference, LBW Infants Fed Isomil, p. 93-97.

VITAMIN D DEFICIENCY, INSUFFICIENCY, SUFFICIENCY AND INTOXICATION. WHAT DO THEY MEAN?

M. PEACOCK, P.L. SELBY, R.M. FRANCIS, W.B. BROWN, L. HORDON
MRC Mineral Metabolism Unit, The General Infirmary, Leeds, UK

Introduction:

The term vitamin D deficiency is generally but loosely used to describe a disease state caused by low levels of plasma vitamin D and its metabolites. The best guide to deficiency in an individual is generally thought to be the plasma concentration of 25OHD, the storage form of vitamin D. However, osteomalacia due to vitamin D deficiency may be present at plasma levels of 25OHD which, although less than those of healthy young normal subjects, are measurable. Conversely, subjects with equally low plasma 25OHD levels do not have histological evidence of osteomalacia. The plasma concentration of $1,25(OH)_2D$, the biologically active form of vitamin D, is considered to be irrelevant since it is under tight endocrine control, does not reflect the level of its substrate, plasma 25OHD, and may be in the normal range (1) despite the presence of osteomalacia which heals with physiological amounts of vitamin D. Since we have found that in those in whom the low plasma 25OHD level is causing osteomalacia the plasma parathyroid hormone is elevated we have advocated that vitamin D deficiency should only be applied to subjects where there is clear evidence that the low plasma 25OHD is exerting a clear biological effect on calcium regulation as shown by secondary hyperparathyroidism (2).
In the absence of vitamin D deficiency an individual is considered to have a sufficiency of vitamin D irrespective of the plasma 25OHD levels even though 25OHD, like $1,25(OH)_2D$, can stimulate the vitamin D receptors, albeit at supranormal concentrations of plasma 25OHD. Since we have shown that plasma $1,25(OH)_2D$ levels are not independent of changes in plasma 25OHD (3) we have attempted to define vitamin D deficiency, sufficiency and intoxication in terms of the relationship between the two biologically active vitamin D metabolites, 25OHD and $1,25(OH)_2D$.

Methods and Results:

Data were obtained in various groups of patients with normal renal function including histologically proven vitamin D deficiency osteomalacia, elderly normal subjects, elderly primary osteoporotics - some of whom were treated with long-term $25OHD_3$, primary renal stone formers and patients with primary hyperparathyroidism. Plasma 25OHD and $1,25(OH)_2D$ and radiocalcium absorption were measured before and after 7 days of oral $25OHD_3$, 40 µg/day (3).
The results show (Fig.) that there is a clear inverse relationship between the change in plasma $1,25(OH)_2D$ levels induced by oral $25OHD_3$ and the basal plasma 25OHD, and that these changes in plasma $1,25(OH)_2D$ are biologically important in terms of calcium absorption.

Vitamin D. A Chemical, Biochemical and Clinical Update

Fig. The relationship between initial plasma 25OHD concentration and the change in plasma 1,25(OH)$_2$D concentration (bottom) and the change in radiocalcium absorption (top) in various patient groups given 40 μg 25OHD$_3$ for 7 days.

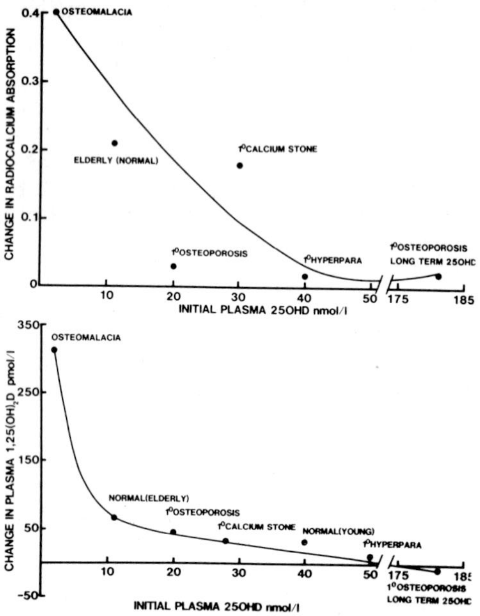

Conclusions:

1. The secretion of 1,25(OH)$_2$D is regulated by plasma 25OHD, at all concentrations.
2. In the presence of normal renal function individual vitamin D status can be accurately defined by the increase in plasma 1,25(OH)$_2$D after 7 days of 40 μg/day of oral 25OHD$_3$:

Deficiency ≡ change in plasma 1,25(OH)$_2$D > Normal range
Sufficiency ≡ change in plasma 1,25(OH)$_2$D = Zero
Intoxication ≡ change in plasma 1,25(OH)$_2$D = Negative

3. The term vitamin D insufficiency should be used to describe that state in which the response is less than deficiency but greater than sufficiency.

References:

1. Peacock,M.,Heyburn,P.J.,Aaron,J.A.,Taylor,G.A.,Brown,W.B., Speed,R., in Vitamin D, Basic Research and its Clinical Application, Ed.Norman e.a., 1979,p1177-1183
2. Peacock,M, in Metabolic Bone and Stone Disease, 2nd Edn. Ed.Nordin, 1984,p71-111
3. Peacock,M.,Francis,R.M.,Selby,P.L.,Taylor,G.A.,Brown,W., Storer,J.,Davies,A.E.J.,in Vitamin D. Chemical, Biochemical, and Clinical Endocrinology, Ed. Norman e.a., 1982,p1057 1059

$1,25(OH)_2D_3$ INCREASES PLASMA MAGNESIUM AND CALCIUM IN MG-DEFICIENT SHEEP.

K.M. SCHNEIDER AND D.D. LEAVER,
La Trobe University, Bundoora, 3083, Australia.

Introduction : Vitamin D increases magnesium (Mg) absorption in the rat, but plasma Mg remains unchanged or decreases, because Mg loss in the urine also increases. However, the net effect of vitamin D on Mg balance could depend on the relative magnitude of these two effects (1) and $1,25(OH)_2D_3$ increases plasma Mg when given to vitamin D-deficient hypomagnesaemic rats (2). Since little Mg is lost in the urine of hypomagnesaemic ruminants (3), administration of vitamin D to these animals should result in a net positive balance for Mg. Hence we examined the effect of $1,25(OH)_2D_3$ on urinary and plasma calcium (Ca), Mg and phosphorus (P) of hypomagnesaemic sheep fed liquid diets and on the Mg, Ca and P balance of sheep fed normally.

Methods : Adult sheep (40 ± 5 kg) fitted with jugular and if necessary abomasal cannulas were housed in metabolism cages and fed 700 g/day of lucerne and oaten chaff 1:1 for 7 days. The diet was then changed to a liquid diet infused into the abomasum and each sheep received 1.5 g P, 250 mg Ca, 35 mg Mg and 420 IU vitamin D daily. After 7 days one group of sheep were treated with either 25 or 250 ng/kg/day $1,25(OH)_2D_3$ and another group with diluent for a period of 7 days. For the higher dose rate the treatments were reversed for a further 7 days. In a second experiment sheep were fed a chaff diet and received 5.1 g Ca, 1.8 g Mg and 1.5 g P daily. They were treated for 7 days with 25 ng/kg/day $1,25(OH)_2D_3$ and a conventional balance trial was conducted over the 5 days prior to and the last 5 days of treatment. Faeces, urine and plasma were analysed for Ca, Mg and P.

Results : When sheep were fed the liquid diet plasma Ca and Mg concentrations decreased progressively, but treatment with $1,25(OH)_2D_3$ at either dose rate reversed this trend for plasma Ca, which increased to 2.5 mmol/l and halted the decline in plasma Mg at 0.6 mmol/l (Fig. 1). Plasma P increased from 2 to 2.5-3.5 mmol/l. For the higher dose rate reversal of the treatment and control groups reversed these changes within 24-48 hours and plasma Mg actually increased from 0.4 to 0.7 mmol/l. For the last 4 days of each treatment period plasma Ca, Mg and P were significantly higher for the treated than untreated groups ($P < 0.01$). Treatment also increased the excretion of Ca, Mg and P in urine, but the increase was small and significant for Mg only. Treatment of sheep fed chaff with 25 ng/kg/day of $1,25(OH)_2D_3$ increased plasma Ca and P. Plasma Mg decreased for the first 4 days but increased to the initial value by the end of the treatment period. Net absorption of Ca, Mg and P and urinary excretion of Mg and Ca increased with treatment, nevertheless there was net retention of Ca, Mg and P (table 1).

Discussion : If sheep are fed liquid diets so they receive a daily intake of 250 mg/day Ca and 1.5 g/day Mg, their plasma Mg is sustained, and plasma Ca declines temporarily and then increases to normal values. Hence the decline in plasma Ca in this experiment must be due to Mg deficiency, and considerable evidence suggests this defect in Ca control is due to

Vitamin D. A Chemical, Biochemical and Clinical Update

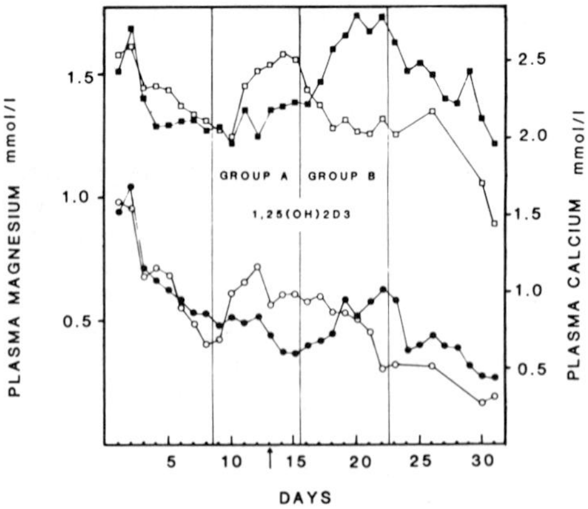

Fig. 1. Plasma concentration of Mg group A, o, B, •, and Ca, group A,□, B,■ during the liquid diet and treatment with 250 ng/kg/day $1,25(OH)_2D_3$. On days 1-12 sheep received 250 mg/day Mg and days 13-31, 35 mg/day Mg.

TABLE 1 : Changes in Mg, Ca and P during two balance trials, control (C) and treatment (T) with 25 ng/kg/day $1,25(OH)_2D_3$ (mean of 5 days, g/day)

MINERAL	INTAKE		FAECAL OUTPUT		URINARY OUTPUT		RETENTION	
	C	T	C	T	C	T	C	T
Mg	1.78	1.81	1.26	0.94	0.23	0.28	0.29	0.59
Ca	5.13	3.85	4.93	2.24	0.04	0.08	0.16	1.53
P	1.51	1.47	0.94	0.26	0.01	0.01	0.56	1.20

parathyroid hormone (4). The results of this experiment indicate the defect also involves vitamin D metabolism or action as low doses of $1,25(OH)_2D_3$ (25 ng/kg/day) restored the plasma Ca to normal values. In the case of Mg, $1,25(OH)_2D_3$ prevented the progressive decline in plasma Mg and at the higher dose rate actually increased plasma Mg, so $1,25(OH)_2D_3$ must have increased the supply of Mg from the gut and/or bone to the plasma pool. However in the sheep fed normally plasma Mg decreased for a short period despite the increased absorption and retention of Mg. Presumably in this situation $1,25(OH)_2D_3$ increases the net loss of Mg from the plasma pool to soft tissue and bone. Although these results for the different physiological states are conflicting, they illustrate that $1,25(OH)_2D_3$ has substantial effects on Mg metabolism in ruminants. Thanks are due to Dr. H. Meier of Hoffmann-La Roche, Basel for the gift of $1,25(OH)_2D_3$ and the AMRC for financial support.

References :

1. Anast, C.S. and Gardner, D.W. (1981) Disorders of Mineral Metabolism, Vol. III, Chapter 7, pp. 423-506, Ed. Bronner, F. and Coburn, J.W., Academic Press, New York.
2. Levine, B.S., Brautbar, N., Walling, M.W., Lee, D.B.N. and Coburn, J.W. (1980) Am. J. Physiol. 239:E515-E523.
3. Rook, J.A.F. and Balch, C.C. (1958) J. Agric. Sci. Camb. 51:199-207.
4. Massry, S.G. (1977) Ann. Rev. Pharmacol. Toxicol. 17:67-82.

SEASONAL VARIATION IN SERUM CONCENTRATION OF 25-HYDROXYVITAMIN D IN RELATION TO VITAMIN D SUPPLEMENTATION IN DAIRY COWS

M. STURÉN
Veterinary Institute, Experimental Station, S-532 00 Skara, Sweden.

Introduction

The effect of season on serum concentration of 25-OH-D is well documented. The UVB irradiation towards the Poles is restricted during the winter and supplementation of feed with vitamin D is more important for animals in these parts of the world.

The purpose of the present investigation was to examine the vitamin D status, assayed as 25-OH-D, in serum of clinically healthy dairy cows.

Material and Methods

Dairy cows (n=182) in eight herds were sampled on three occasions:

1) during winter season 1982 (February)
2) when on pasture 1982 (August)
3) during winter season 1983 (February)

The pasture period was from late May to the end of September.

In two herds (3 and 4) the animals were daily supplemented all the year round with 4,000 IU D_3 through the mineral feed. In two herds (6 and 7) no vitamin D_3 supplementation was given. In the rest of the herds the daily supplementation was given through the concentrates and varied depending on the state of lactation up to 15,000 IU D_3.

Blood samples were centrifuged within one hour after sampling. Serum was kept at -20°C until analysed. 25-OH-D_3 and 25-OH-D_2 were analysed by high performance liquid chromatography (1).

Results and Discussion

The summer values of 25-OH-D_3 were in all herds of the same magnitude, approx. 35-40 ng/ml irrespective of whether vitamin D supplementation was given or not. The winter values of 25-OH-D_3 varied between herds according to the vitamin D_3 supplementation from below 2 ng/ml in the non-supplemented herds to 35 ng/ml in the herds with the highest supplementation.

The seasonal variation in serum concentration of 25-OH-D_3 reported here accords with the results of others (2, 3). The present investigation shows that if the supplementation is adequate the seasonal variation will be small.

This study was financially supported by grants from the Swedish Council for Forestry and Agricultural Research

Table 1. Serum concentration of 25 OH D3 and 25 OH D2 during winter 1982, summer 1982 and winter 1983 (lsmean ± s.e.m.)

Herd	Serum 25 OH D3 ng/ml Winter season 1982	Pasture season 1982	Winter season 1983
1	40.3 ± 4.5	36.1 ± 2.7	34.3 ± 3.0
2	15.5 ± 4.3	39.9 ± 2.8	7.9 ± 3.3
3	18.2 ± 4.4	45.1 ± 3.1	12.5 ± 3.8
4	36.0 ± 4.3	39.2 ± 2.8	46.8 ± 2.9
5	30.7 ± 3.6	33.8 ± 2.0	33.0 ± 2.2
6	5.2 ± 4.4	37.5 ± 4.2	1.9 ± 5.6
7	8.4 ± 4.7	40.4 ± 3.4	2.2 ± 4.0
8	34.8 ± 4.3	35.7 ± 2.8	20.5 ± 3.7

Herd	Serum 25 OH D2 ng/ml Winter season 1982	Pasture season 1982	Winter season 1983
1	18.0 ± 3.2	11.0 ± 1.3	6.9 ± 0.7
2	41.1 ± 3.1	15.6 ± 1.4	16.2 ± 0.8
3	35.1 ± 3.1	9.0 ± 1.5	18.8 ± 0.9
4	28.3 ± 3.0	15.0 ± 1.3	4.5 ± 0.7
5	10.5 ± 2.6	9.5 ± 1.0	5.0 ± 0.5
6	37.7 ± 3.2	16.1 ± 2.1	7.8 ± 1.4
7	21.6 ± 3.3	16.7 ± 1.7	5.8 ± 1.0
8	20.0 ± 3.0	18.8 ± 1.4	5.6 ± 0.9

The 25-OH-D_2 values varied between seasons and between herds. The only important source of vitamin D_2 is roughage (grass, silage, straw and hay). The vitamin D_2 accumulates as the plants approach maturity. Thus fresh grass, early cut silage and early cut hay are fairly poor in vitamin D_2. Herds 6 and 7 had hay as only roughage, while all others had both hay and silage. The marked difference in serum 25-OH-D_2 between the two winter seasons reflects a difference in harvest time, the 1982 year roughage being cut at a considerably later stage than the 1983 year roughage. Animals given an early cut roughage, particularly when kept indoors all the year round, run a risk of vitamin D deficiency if not adequately supplemented.

References

1. Holmberg,I., Kristiansen,T. and Sturén,M. (1984) Scand J. clin. Lab. Invest. 44, 275-282.
2. Hidiroglou,M., Proulx,J.G. and Roubos,D. (1979) J. Dairy Sci. 62, 1076-1080.
3. Smith,B.S.W. and Wright,H. (1984) Vet. Rec. 115, 537-538.

STUDIES ON THE MODE OF ACTION OF 1,25-DIHYDROXYVITAMIN D_3 IN MUSCLE CALCIUM TRANSPORT *IN VITRO*.

A.R. de Boland, L. Drittanti and R.L. Boland

Departamento de Biologia, Universidad Nacional del Sur, 8000 Bahia Blanca, Argentina.

Previous *in vivo* studies have shown that vitamin D_3 affects the activity of transport systems which regulate intracellular Ca^{2+} in skeletal muscle (1, 2). More recent work has indicated a direct involvement of $1,25(OH)_2D_3$ and $25OHD_3$ in cellular Ca in cultured chick soleus muscle and myoblasts (3). These investigations were conducted to further characterize the effects *in vitro* of vitamin D_3 metabolites on muscle Ca uptake and to obtain information about their mode of action.

METHODS:

Soleus muscle and myoblasts were obtained from vitamin D-deficient chicks and 12 day-old chick embryos, respectively, and were cultured as previously described (3). $1,25(OH)_2D_3$ and $25OHD_3$ were used in concentrations of 0.05 ng/ml and 20 ng/ml, respectively. ^{45}Ca uptake by cultures was measured using a 60 min incubation period at 37 °C (3). The kinetics of Ca efflux from ^{45}Ca prelabelled myoblasts was analyzed as described by Uchikawa and Borle (4). To evaluate the effects of protein synthesis inhibitors on $1,25(OH)_2D_3$-dependent Ca uptake myoblast cultures were treated with cycloheximide (50 µM) and actinomycin D (1.6 µM) for 24 h and 12 h, respectively. In addition, soleus muscle cultures were treated with puromycin (50 µM) during 5 h. The phospholipid content and composition of myoblasts were analyzed as reported before (2). Phospholipid synthesis was measured by incubation of the preparations in Krebs-Henseleit-glucose solution containing ^3H-glycerol (0.05 µCi /ml) for 60 min.

RESULTS AND DISCUSSION:

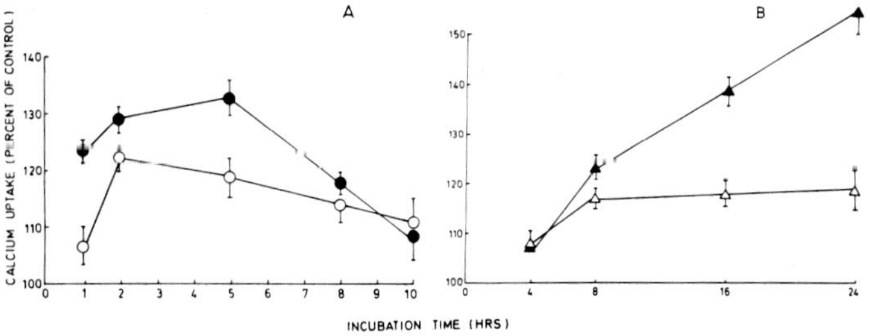

Fig. 1. Time course of changes in Ca uptake in cultured soleus muscle (A) and myoblasts (B) induced by vitamin D_3 metabolites. $25OHD_3$, empty symbols. $1,25(OH)_2D_3$, filled symbols. Values are means ± SD, n=4.

Characterization of the time course of the $1,25(OH)_2D_3$ and $25OHD_3$ responses in Ca uptake by soleus muscle (Fig. 1A) and myoblast (Fig. 1B) cultures

Vitamin D. A Chemical, Biochemical and Clinical Update

showed a greater potency of $1,25(OH)_2D_3$ after various treatment intervals. To obtain information about Ca pools affected by vitamin D_3 metabolites, the kinetics of Ca efflux of myoblasts prelabelled with ^{45}Ca was studied. $1,25(OH)_2D_3$ caused a significant increase in the rate constant of Ca efflux from mitochondria to cytoplasm (3.0 ± 0.12 vs 5.6 ± 0.28 min^{-1}, in control and treated cells, respectively, $p < 0.005$) and in the size of the cytoplasmic Ca pool (29.6 ± 1.5 vs 43.2 ± 2.2 nmol Ca/mg prot, $p < 0.01$). The metabolite increased to a lesser extent the rate constants of Ca efflux from cytoplasm to mitochondria and from cytoplasm to the external medium. The predominant effect of $25OHD_3$ was to increase Ca influx into mitochondria (data not given). The changes in kinetic parameters observed indicate higher Ca turnover in muscle cells treated with $1,25(OH)_2D_3$ than with $25OHD_3$ and, thus, explain their higher labelling with ^{45}Ca.

Puromycin suppressed $1,25(OH)_2D_3$-dependent Ca uptake in soleus muscle cultures (915 ± 75 vs $1,250 \pm 80$ vs 902 ± 49 nmol Ca/g muscle in control, $1,25(OH)_2D_3$ and $1,25(OH)_2D_3$ + puromycin treated preparations, respectivey). Cycloheximide also abolished the response of increased Ca uptake by myoblast cultures exposed to the metabolite (13.4 ± 0.8 vs 17.8 ± 0.8 vs 13.2 ± 0.5 nmol/mg prot in control, $1,25(OH)_2D_3$ and $1,25(OH)_2D_3$ + cycloheximide treated cells, respectively). Treatment of myoblasts with actinomycin D effectively blocked the increase in Ca uptake caused by the sterol (12.2 ± 1.0 vs 18.2 ± 0.4 vs 12.0 ± 0.7 nmol Ca/mg prot in control, $1,25(OH)_2D_3$ and $1,25(OH)_2D_3$ + actinomycin D treated cells, respectively). At the conditions employed the inhibitors did not significantly affect Ca uptake by control cultures. These results indicate that the effects of $1,25(OH)_2D_3$ on muscle Ca transport are mediated by de novo protein and RNA synthesis. In addition the metabolite increased the phospholipid content (63 ± 5 vs 91 ± 4 nmol lipid P/mg prot, in control and treated preparations, respectively, $p < 0.025$) and phosphatidylcholine/phosphatidylethanolamine ratio (1.45 ± 0.1 vs 2.09 ± 0.2, $p < 0.025$) of myoblasts. $1,25(OH)_2D_3$ increased labelling with ^3H-glycerol of the PC fraction whereas a decrease in PE was observed (Fig. 2), indicating that the sterol affects de novo synthesis of both phospholipids.

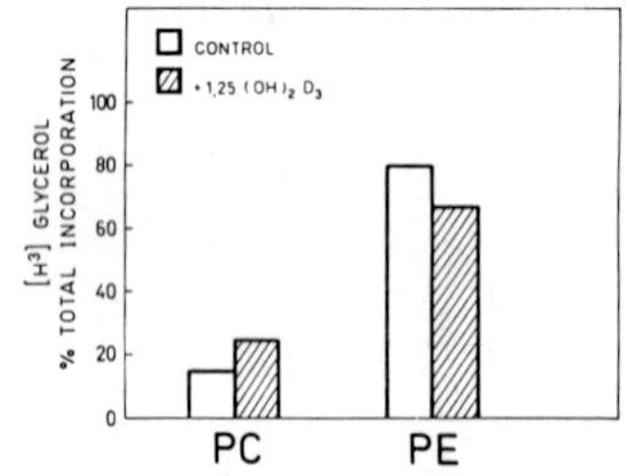

Fig. 2. Effects of $1,25(OH)_2D_3$ on the incorporation of ^3H-glycerol into myoblast phosphatidylcholine (PC) and phosphatidylethanolamine (PE).

The changes in phospholipids may be the consequence of the nuclear action of $1,25(OH)_2D_3$ or, alternatively, represent an independent membrane effect as has been proposed for intestine.

REFERENCES:

1. Curry, D.B., Bastein, J.F. and Smith, R. (1974) Nature 249, 83-84.
2. Boland,A., Gallego,S. and Boland,R. (1983) Biochim.Biophys.Acta 733, 264.
3. Giuliani, D. and Boland, R. (1984) Calcif. Tissue Int. 36, 200-205.
4. Uchikawa, T. and Borle, A. (1978) Am. J. Physiol. 234, R29-R33.

TREATMENT WITH VITAMIN D_3-3B SULFATE DOES NOT CORRECT BONE AND MINERAL ABNORMALITIES IN D-DEFICIENT RATS

L. CANCELA, P.J. MARIE, N. LE BOULCH, L. MIRAVET
Unité 18 INSERM, 6 rue Guy Patin, 75010 Paris-France

Introduction :

A water soluble form of vitamin D has been found in human milk in high amounts (1,2). Studies concerning the antirachitic potency of this derivative, a sulfoconjugated form of vitamin D, led to controversial results. Several works were carried out employing the synthetic vitamin D_3-3B sulfate (SD_3) in order to study its antirachitic activity. Early results had shown an effect of SD_3 upon intestinal absorption of calcium in the male rat (3,4), but more recent reports did not confirm these results (5,6). Since vitamin D sulfate was found in milk, any effect of this vitamin D derivative should be in relation with lactation. We have therefore chosen this physiological stage to examine the activity of synthetic SD_3 upon the calcium metabolism of mother rats and their lactating pups.

Materiel and Methods :

Weaning female rats were fed a D-free diet for 11 weeks. During the lactation period, two groups of D-deficient mothers were orally treated with 650 pmoles/day of either free vitamin D_3 (-D +D) or SD_3(-D+SD), one group was untreated (-D) and one group was vitamin D_3 repleted (650 pmoles/day) from weaning to sacrifice (+D). SD_3 was synthesized in our laboratory, purified by HPLC and its identification achieved by U.V. absorption and mass spectra prior to administration. Mothers and pups were sacrified at day 20 of lactation. Caudal vertebrae from mothers (7th) and pups (7th and 8th) were prepared for quantitative histomorphological determinations after in vivo double labeling with tetracycline. Plasma levels of calcium (Ca and phosphate (P) were determined, as well as plasma concentrations of vitamin D metabolites and immunoreactive parathormone (iPTH) in both mothers and pups.

Results :

At day 20 of lactation -D mothers had reduced body weight (BW) when compared to + D mothers (p 0,001). Plasma levels of Ca, P, 25- hydroxyvitamin D (25(OH)D) and 1,25-dihydroxyvitamin D ($1,25(OH)_2D$) were markedly decreased (Table 1) whereas iPTH was increased above normal levels. Similar results were obtained in pups suckling -D mothers (table 1). After 20 days of SD3 supplemantation, BW and plasma parameters were not different from those in -D non treated mothers, whereas in -D +D mothers they were nearly normal. Pups suckling -D +SD mothers didnot normalize any plasma parameter measured, by contrast with pups from -D +D group that had normal BW and plasma Ca and 25(OH)D levels whereas plasma P, iPTH and $1,25(OH)_2D$ were still abnormal.

	Group	Ca	P	25(OH)D	1,25(OH)2D	iPTH	BW
mothers	-D-D	59[a]	77[a]	< 10	50[a]	186[a]	80[a]
	-D+D	93	92	85[a]	141[a]	118[a]	93[a]
	-D+SD	63[a]	79[a]	< 10	54[a]	138[a]	84[a]
pups	-D-D	84[a]	92[a]	< 10	50[a]	194[a]	82.5[a]
	-D+D	98	95[a]	97	176[a]	137[a]	99
	-D+SD	86[a]	92[a]	< 10	158[a]	169[a]	84[a]

Table 1 : Plasma biochemical parameters and body weight (BW) expressed as percent of values obtained in +D rats. (a: significant at the 5 % level or better level of significance).

Bone histomorphometric data clearly showed defective mineralization and increased resorption in both -D mothers and -D pups (table 2). In -D mother rats treated with SD_3, osteoclastic surface and osteoclast number were nearly normal, while parameters of bone mineralization remained abnormal. By contrast, in -D+D mothers almost all bone parameters were normalized

Vitamin D. A Chemical, Biochemical and Clinical Update

(table 2). Both free and sulfoconjugated vitamin D3 supplementation in mothers did not normalize parameters of bone formation and resorption in lactating pups. However, bone mineralization was improved in pups from -D+D group by contrast with pups from -D+SD group .

	Group	CBV	CR	MOST	OS	NoOCL
mothers	-D-D	49[a]	65[a]	350[a]	167[a]	160[a]
	-D+D	113	79[a]	93	105	119
	-D+SD	49[a]	75[a]	282[a]	113	106
pups	-D-D	101	-	141[a]	154[a]	142[a]
	-D+D	103	-	131[a]	159[a]	131[a]
	-D+SD	98	-	138[a]	148[a]	125[a]

Table 2 : Bone parameters (expressed as percent of values in +D rats. (a:significant at the 5 % level or better level of significance) CBV : calcified bone volume, CR : calcification rate, MOST : osteoid thickness, OS : osteoclastic surface, NoOCl : number of osteoclasts/mm^2.

Conclusion :

Oral treatment with synthetic SD_3 during 20 days of lactation in vitamin D deficient mother rats did not normalize the hormonal, mineral and skeletal abnormalities induced by vitamin D-depletion. By contrast, -D mothers treated with free vitamin D_3 during lactation normalized nearly all the plasmatic and skeletal parameters measured. In pups suckling SD_3-treated mothers, all plasma and bone parameters remained abnormal whereas in pups from -D+D group plasma Ca and 25(OH)D were normalized and histological lesions improved.

In conclusion, synthetic vitamin D_3-3B sulfate is clearly less active than free vitamin D_3 when administered orally at equimolar doses upon mineral homeostasis and bone metabolism during the lactation period in rats.

References :

1 - Sahashi Y., Suzuki T., Higaki M., Asano T. (1967) J. Vitaminol 13, 33-36.

2 - Lakdawala D.R., Widdowson E.M. (1977) Lancet 1, 167-168.

3 - Miravet L., Le Boulch N., Carré M., Marnay-Gulat C., Raoul Y. (1975) IRCS Med. Sci. Lib. Compend, 3, 194.

4 - Le Boulch N., Gulat-Marnay C., Dupuis Y., Carré M., Miravet L. (1977) J. de Physiologie 73, 22-23A.

5 - Reeve L.F., Deluca H.F., Schnoes H.K. (1981) J. Biol. Chem., 256, 823-826.

6 - Nagubandi S., Londowski J.M., Bolloman S., Tietz P., Kumar R. (1981) J. Biol. Chem. 256, 5536-5539.

VITAMIN D DEFICIENCY IN ASIAN CHILDREN IN BRITAIN - A CASE FOR PROPHYLACTIC SUPPLEMENTATION?

N.R. BELTON
Department of Child Life and Health, University of Edinburgh, EH9 1UW, Scotland, U.K.
H. GRINDULIS, P.H. SCOTT, B.A. WHARTON
Sorrento Maternity Hospital, Birmingham, England, U.K.

INTRODUCTION

It is now over 20 years since rickets and osteomalacia were originally described in Asian immigrants in Britain (1). Although there has been an improvement in the vitamin D status of Asian children in Britain (2,3) two official reports in 1980 concluded that Asian infants (4) and adolescents (5) remained at risk of developing rickets.
Studies on the vitamin D status of Asian toddlers in Birmingham and of older Asian children are presented in comparison with a control population of Edinburgh children.

METHODS AND PATIENTS

Plasma 25-hydroxyvitamin D (25-OHD) was measured by a competitive protein-binding assay based on that of Preece (6,7) in 130 Asians (62 boys, 68 girls) in Birmingham aged 21-23 months and in 87 Asians in Edinburgh (37 boys, 50 girls) aged 5, 11 and 14 years. The control group of 221 children in Edinburgh comprised children admitted to a general medical ward.

RESULTS

Plasma 25-OHD in the Edinburgh Asians was 8.3 ng/ml (mean) with an S.D. of 4.2. Boys (9.5 ± 4.4) had a significantly higher 25-OHD ($p<0.05$) than girls (7.5 ± 4.0). All these samples were taken in May and June, and the 25-OHD values in the control group in these months were 24.0 ± 8.0.

Plasma 25-OHD in the Birmingham Asians was 12.5 ± 6.3 ng/ml, boys (14.3 ± 6.8) having significantly higher ($p<0.02$) values than girls (11.5 ± 6.0). By comparison, plasma 25-OHD in the control (Edinburgh) population was 18.0 ± 10.0 (boys 19.2 ± 11.6, girls 16.0 ± 9.3). The seasonal variation of these results is shown in the figure.

It indicates in particular that the Birmingham Asians do not have the summer rise in plasma 25-OHD to the same extent as the Edinburgh children although the latter live 300 miles north in an area which enjoys fewer hours of sunshine. This probably also explains the lower values shown in the Edinburgh Asians by comparison with the Birmingham Asians.

DISCUSSION

These results indicate that Asian toddlers in Birmingham and older children including adolescents in Edinburgh, have an inferior vitamin D status compared to the Caucasian population despite efforts to promote better vitamin D intake. A majority (102 out of 130) of the Birmingham Asian children were in theory receiving vitamin supplements. There was, however, no evidence of poor general health in the Asians although iron deficiency anaemia was an associated finding in the Birmingham Asian toddlers. Two of the 14-year-old Edinburgh Asian girls had biochemical rickets.

Vitamin D. A Chemical, Biochemical and Clinical Update

It is therefore questioned whether fortification of suitable foods with vitamin D should be reviewed again or whether especially in older children a single large oral dose of ergocalciferol should be given in the autumn as a supplement to produce a sustained rise in vitamin D over the winter (8). Such a dose may be worthy of consideration, particularly for adolescent girls who may soon be embarking on child-bearing.

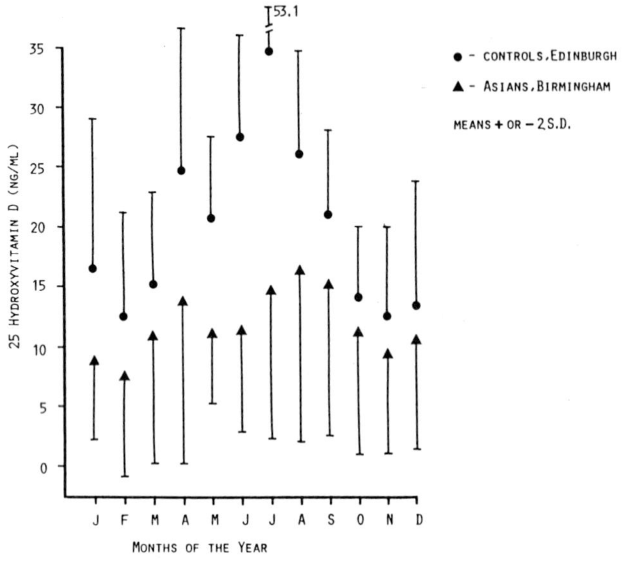

Figure. Seasonal variation in 25-hydroxyvitamin D.

REFERENCES

1. Dunnigan, M.S., Paton, J.P., Hasse, S., McNicol, G., Gardner, M.D. and Smith, C.M. (1962) Scott. Med. J., 7, 159-167.
2. Ford, J.A., Colhoun, E.M., McIntosh, W.B. amd Dunnigan, M.G. (1972) Br. Med. J., 2, 677-80.
3. Stephens, W.P., Klimiuk, P.S., Warrington, S., Taylor, J.L., Berry, J.L. and Mawer, E.B. (1982) Q. J. Med., 51, 171-188.
4. Department of Health and Social Security (1980) Report on Health and Social Subjects No. 20. London, H.M.S.O.
5. Department of Health and Social Security (1980) Report on Health and Social Security No. 19. London, H.M.S.O.
6. Preece, M.A., O'Riordan, J.L.H., Lawson, D.E.M. and Kodicek, E. (1974) Clin. Chim. Acta, 54, 235-242.
7. Belton, N.R. (1985) Proceedings Sixth Vitamin D Workshop. Berlin, de Gruyter.
8. Stephens, W.P., Klimiuk, P.S., Berry, J.L. and Mawer, E.B. (1981) Lancet, 2, 1199-1202.

MICE OSTEOBLAST-LIKE CELLS : EFFECT OF ALUMINUM AND ITS POSSIBLE INTERACTION WITH PTH AND 1,25-$(OH)_2D_3$.

M. LIEBERHERR, B. GROSSE, G. COURNOT-WITMER, S. BALSAN and M.P.M. HERRMANN-ERLEE

Laboratoire des Tissus Calcifiés (CNRS UA.583-INSERM U.30)Hôpital des Enfants-Malades, 75015 Paris, France and Laboratory of Cell Biology and Histology, State University of Leiden, 2333A Leiden, The Netherlands.

It has been shown that aluminum (Al) may interfere with normal bone mineralization (1-3) and formation (4). Furthermore recent data demonstrate that Al deposits are not only found in bone matrix but within the cells, in osteoblasts which synthesize osteoid and regulate mineralization (5). These findings led us to investigate the effects of aluminum on the metabolism of osteoblast-like (OB) cells in culture and to analyze a possible interaction between Al, 1,25-$(OH)_2D_3$ and/or bPTH.

OB-cells were isolated from parietal bones of neonatal mice by sequential enzymatic digestion (6) and cultured in BGJ medium until confluency.These cells are characterized by high alkaline phosphatase activity (ALP), high type I collagen synthesis and cAMP response only to bPTH.

Results show that :

1) Al chloride (10^{-9}-1.5×10^{-6}M) increases ALP activity, ornithine decarboxylase activity (ODC), incorporation of ^{3}H-thymidine into DNA, and has no action on collagen synthesis. At higher concentrations (3×10^{-6}-10^{-5}M) Al inhibits ALP and ODC activities, incorporation of ^{3}H thymidine into DNA, incorporation of ^{3}H proline into DNA and incorporation of ^{3}H proline into collagenase-digestible proteins (CDP). Whatever the concentration used, Al has no effect on cAMP after 5 min incubation.

2) 1,25-$(OH)_2D_3$ (10^{-9}M) decreases ALP and ODC activities, CDP labeling and ^{3}H thymidine incorporation into DNA. bPTH(10^{-9}M) decreases ALP activity and CDP labeling, increases ODC activity, ^{3}H thymidine incorporation into DNA, and cAMP.

3) Preincubation of (OB) cells with Al inhibits in a dose dependent way the cAMP response to bPTH. For cells incubated simultaneously with Al and bPTH (10^{-9}M), only high Al concentrations inhibit ODC activity, whereas bPTH alone increases it. For cells incubated simultaneously with Al and 1,25-$(OH)_2D_3$, the ODC increase induced by Al (10^{-9}-1.5×10^{-6}M) is inhibited by the presence of 1,25-$(OH)_2D_3$ (Table I).

Vitamin D. A Chemical, Biochemical and Clinical Update

Table I

Al Concentrations	ODC activity (nmole CO_2)/mg protein/hour		
	None	+1,25-$(OH)_2D_3$ (10^{-9}M)	+bPTH (10^{-9}M)
Controls (no Al)	5.5 ± 0.3	3.5 ± 0.2	10.9 ± 0.3
10^{-11}M	5.2 ± 0.3	5.1 ± 0.4[a]	10.6 ± 0.1
10^{-10}M	5.9 ± 0.4	5.2 ± 0.6[a]	10.7 ± 0.4
10^{-9}M	7.9 ± 0.1[a]	6.4 ± 0.1[a*]	9.8 ± 0.5
10^{-8}M	8.5 ± 0.2[a]	7.2 ± 0.2[a*]	10.1 ± 0.5
10^{-7}M	9.9 ± 0.5[a]	8.1 ± 0.3[a*]	9.6 ± 0.7
10^{-6}M	9.8 ± 0.5[a]	7.9 ± 0.2[a*]	10.3 ± 0.2
1.5 x 10^{-6}M	8.6 ± 0.5[a]	6.9 ± 0.1[a*]	9.7 ± 0.6
3 x 10^{-6}M	4.5 ± 0.1[c]	4.3 ± 0.1	8.3 ± 0.2[a]
6 x 10^{-6}M	4.1 ± 0.1[b]	4.1 ± 0.05	7.6 ± 0.3[a]
1 x 10^{-5}M	3.8 ± 0.1[b]	3.6 ± 0.2	6.9 ± 0.2[a]

Influence of various concentrations of aluminum chloride on ODC activity of (OB)cells incubated with bPTH, 1,25-$(OH)_2D_3$ or their solvent. Values are the mean ± SEM of 24 groups(8 different experiments with 3 wells for each point). **a,b,c,** values significantly different from their corresponding controls : [a]$p<0.001$, [b]$p<0.05$, [c]$p<0.01$; [*] values significantly different from the values found in cells treated only with Al at various concentrations : ($p<0.001$) (Student's t test).

In conclusion, Aluminum has a biphasic effect on the metabolism of OB-cells, depending on the concentration used. At high doses, Al may interfere with bone matrix formation by inhibiting collagen synthesis and cellular proliferation rate, and with bone mineralization by modulating the alkaline phosphatase activity. In addition, these data suggest a possible interaction between 1,25-$(OH_2D_3$ or bPTH and Al on (OB) cells.

REFERENCES

1. ELLIS HA, MCARTHY JH, HERRINGTON (1979) J Clin Path 32 : 832-44
2. COURNOT-WITMER G, ZINGRAFF J, PLACHOT JJ, ESCAIG F, LEFEVRE R, BOUMATI P, BOURDEAU A, GARABEDIAN M, GALLE P, BOURDON R, DRUEKE T, BALSAN S (1981) Kidney Int 20 : 375-85
3. HODSMAN AB, SHERRARD DJ, ALFREY AC, OTT S, BRICKMAN AS, MILLER NL, MALONEY NA, COBURN JW (1982) J Clin Endocrinol Metab 54 : 539-46
4. OTT SM, MALONEY NA, KLEIN GL, ALFREY AC, AMENT ME, COBURN JW, SHERRARD DJ (1983) Ann Intern Med 98 : 910-4
5. PLACHOT JJ, COURNOT-WITMER G, HALPERN S, MENDES V, BOURDEAU A, FRITSCH J, BOURDON R, DRUEKE T, GALLE P, BALSAN S (1984) Kidney Int 25 : 796-803
6. WONG GL and COHN DV (1974) Nature 252 : 713-5

ESTROGEN TREATMENT OF CHRONIC VITAMIN D DEFICIENCY IN RATS

A. Tenenhouse and M. Warner
Department of Pharmacology and Therapeutics, McGill University, Montreal, Quebec H3G 1Y6, Canada.

In our hands the D-deficient rat model used routinely by many investigators did not predictably produce complete D-deficiency as measured by serum [1,25(OH)$_2$D]. After testing many protocols we chose as our "standard" experimental model Sprague Dawley rats born of mothers who had been fed a D-deficient diet for at least 8 weeks from weaning prior to mating. The pups were maintained on the same D-free diet from weaning. The diet is AIN 76A, ICN Nutritional Biochemicals, Cleveland, Ohio; contents include 20% casein, 50% sucrose, 15% corn starch, 5% fat, 5% fibre, and a standard salt and vitamin D-free vitamin mixture as recommended by the American Institute of Nutrition. By independent analysis the diet has been shown to be free of vitamin D (Hazelton Raltech, Inc., Madison, Wisconsin) and to contain no abnormal concentrations of trace metals (Technitrol Canada Ltd., Dorval, Quebec). The calcium and phosphorus contents of the diet are 0.4% and 0.6% respectively. The rats are housed in a room free of ultraviolet radiation and a 12 hour light/dark cycle. To date this animal model has been used to study the control of renal D hydroxylase activity (1,2) and the role of D in parotid gland function (3).

These animals possess the stigmata of chronic D deficiency; severe hypocalcemia (5.0 $\pm$ 0.2 mg%), elevated serum [PTH] (3-5 times normal) with signs of PTH resistance, retarded growth rate, rickets and decreased survival. Also, there was no detectable serum 1,25(OH)$_2$D. In addition it was noted that male animals have a much poorer survival than females and that this increased mortality occurs at two critical periods in the early life of these rats. The first occurs at about the time of weaning and is survived by about 40% of the males and 90% of the females. The second occurs at 40-50 days of age at which time approximately 50% of the surviving males and less than 1% of the females develop hind limb paralysis and urine retention. If untreated the animals die within 24-48 hours. These survival statistics come from observation of 60 newborn rats from 6 different litters; male:female = 1:1. The early mortality can be prevented and the paralysis prevented or reversed by treatment with either vitamin D_3 (2.5 g, I.P.) or estradiol (E_2). D treatment results in the disappearance of the paralysis and urine retention within 72 hours and is accompanied by a normalization of the serum [Ca] and [PTH]. E_2 is administered continuously by means of a subcutaneous implant made of a polydimethylsiloxane sealed tube containing estradiol-17- (4). Reversal of the clinical syndrome occurs within 3-5 days and is not accompanied by any change in serum [Ca] or [PTH] (n = 6 rats). The plasma concentration of E_2 in male rats with the implant increases from a normal of 60 pg/ml to 645 pg/ml. The plasma [E_2] in age matched female rats is 88 pg/ml.

The cytosolic fraction from various tissues from these animals has been screened for changes in constituent protein using SDS PAGE. When the gels are stained with a nonspecific protein stain such as Coomassie Blue no

Vitamin D. A Chemical, Biochemical and Clinical Update

differences are detected in the electrophoretic pattern from any tissue examined; including duodenal mucosa, kidney, cerebellum, spinal cord, pancreas and parotid gland. When "Stains-All", a stain specific for anionic proteins (5) is used, changes are detected in the cytosolic fraction from spinal cord of male rats (Fig. 1) but not from any other tissues examined.

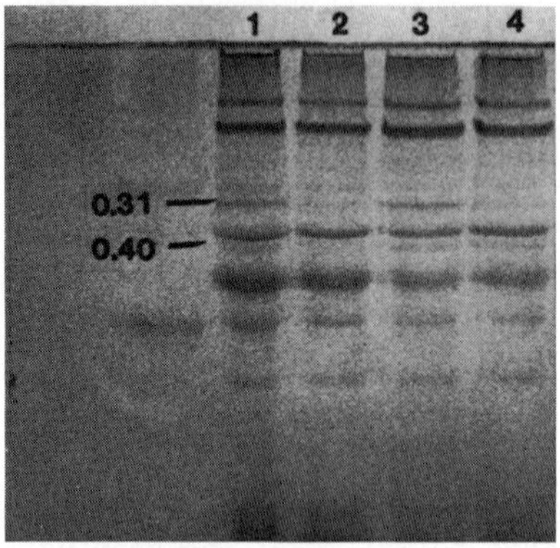

Figure 1. SDS PAGE of male rat spinal cord cytosol stained with "Stains-All". The bands marked with arrows are the major anionic proteins (blue-staining bands), column 1, D+; column 2, D-; column 3, D-,E_2 treated; column 4, D-,E_2 treated but implant removed 6 weeks prior to examination.

As can be seen in Fig. 1 there are several anionic proteins in male rat spinal cord cytosol but the concentration of only the anionic protein of R_f = 0.31 and the doublet of R_f = 0.40 are D-dependent. The concentration of the doublet and the protein of R_f 0.31 are increased upon treatment with E_2 and decrease again after removal of the E_2.

These observations suggest that (1) the consequences of chronic, vitamin D deficiency are severe in males than in females. (2) E_2 can overcome the lethal consequences of this deficiency but does not alter the effects of D deficiency on serum [Ca] or [PTH]. (3) this degree of vitamin D deficiency is associated with the disappearance of anionic proteins from the cytoplasmic fraction of spinal cord. (4) the therapeutic effect of E_2 is associated with the reappearance of these proteins.

References:
1. Warner, M., Tenenhouse, A., (1985). Can. J. Physiol. Pharmacol., in press.
2. Warner, M., Tenenhouse, A., (1985). Sixth Workshop on Vitamin D. in press
3. Glijer, B., Peterfy, C., Tenenhouse, A., (1985) J. Physiol. (London) in press.
4. Robaire, B., Ewing, L.L., Irby, D.C., Desjardins, C., (1979). Biol. Reproduct., 21, 455-463.
5. Campbell, K. P., MacLennan, D.H., Jorgensen, A.O., (1983) J. Biol. Chem., 258, 11267-11272.

IS HYPERVITAMINOSIS D NORMAL IN THE RHESUS MONKEY ?

S.B. Arnaud, D. R. Young, C. Cann, T.A. Reinhardt and R. Henrickson

Departments of Pediatrics and Radiology, University of California, San Francisco, 94143, NASA Ames Research Center, Moffett Field, CA 94035, National Animal Disease Center, Ames, Iowa, 50010, and the California Primate Research Center, Davis, CA 95608.

The rhesus monkey is a valuable asset for the investigation of neuromuscular disorders in man because of similiarities in calcium metabolism (1), parathyroid physiology (2), and the acquired metabolic bone diseases in both species (3). There is, however, little reference data on the nutritional and endocrine status of vitamin D which could be applied to our studies on the evolution of disuse osteoporosis, a model for bone loss during space flight, or, in fact, to the diagnosis and management of clinical disorders in the monkey.

Fasting blood specimens were obtained after ketamine anaesthesia, from healthy animals housed in individual cages at the animal care facilities of 3 institutions. The principal source of vitamin D was a standard monkey chow which contained 6.6IU per gram of diet (1000-1200 IU daily), 0.9% calcium and 0.5% phosphorus. Thirteen of the monkeys at Davis had access to the sun. Serum calcium was determined by atomic absorption or an EGTA titration method, and phosphorus by a modified Fiske Subarrow method. 25-hydroxyvitamin D (25-OH-D) was assayed by a competitive protein binding assay (4), after isolation of the metabolite by Sephadex LH 20 in a mixture of chloroform and hexane or by silicic acid cartridges in ethyl acetate and hexane. 1,25-dihydroxyvitamin D (1,25-$(OH)_2$D) was determined by calf thymus receptor microassay (5). Parathyroid hormone (PTH) was measured by radioimmunoassay which uses an antibody with specificity for the human 1-84 molecule, cross reacts with saline extracts of monkey parathyroid glands and serum, and shows less than 5% displacement of labelled hormone with 100 ul of serum from an hypoparathyroid animal (6) Results of the assays are as follows:

	Ca, mg/dl	PO_4, mg/dl	PTH, pg/ml	25-OH-D ng/ml	1,25$(OH)_2$D pg/ml
Mean	9.59	5.04	134	188	207
±SD	0.74	1.79	78	94	90
n	50	39	20	26	36

There were no sex difference in the 21 females and 29 males tested. The monkeys weighed from 4.8 to 12 kg (average 8±3). Their age range was from 3 to 14 years (average 6 years) in the 29 animals in whom this information was available.

Vitamin D. A Chemical, Biochemical and Clinical Update

The individual variation in this young adult population is striking. Whether this is related to the effects of the anaesthetic, diurnal rhythms from sampling at different times during the day or, is simply characteristic of the species, is unclear. The elevated values for serum 25-OH-D, 4 - 15 times human levels probably reflect the high dietary intake of vitamin D. There was no evidence that this degree of hypervitaminosis was associated with hypercalcemia or hyperphosphatemia, the biochemical features of vitamin D intoxication. The concentrations of $1,25(OH)_2D$ were 3-10 times higher than values reported in other species (rat, chick, man). Our mean level is also greater than the mean value reported by Shinki et al in 6 rhesus monkeys who also had lower levels of 25-OH-D (7). We found no correlation between the two metabolites. Observations of serum 25-OH-D in two monkeys fed a synthetic diet without vitamin D for four weeks revealed decreases from 359 and 454 ng/ml to 40 and 44 ng/ml. Serum $1,25(OH)_2D$ remained high: 259 and 257 pg/ml before and 173 and 213 pg/ml after 4 weeks. There were no differences in the serum $1,25(OH)_2D$ of monkeys housed indoors and outdoors.

The above is consistent with a unique metabolism of vitamin D in the rhesus monkey which may be similiar to that reported in the marmoset, though, less pronounced. As in other species, one-hydroxylase activity appears to be relatively insensitive to changes in circulating 25-OH-D, its substrate. The presence of high circulating levels of $1,25(OH)_2D$ in normocalcemic well animals without evidence of suppressed parathyroid function suggests that hypervitaminosis D is not pathological, but a variation of some aspect of vitamin D metabolism which is normal for this species.

1. Harris RS, Moor JR, Wanner RL. (1961) J Clin Invest 40:1766.
2. Hargis GK, Williams GA, Reynolds WA, Kawahara W, Jackson B, Boswer N, and Pitkin R. (1977) Clin Chem 23:1991.
3. Simon WH and Gorman RA. (1970) Clin Orthop 73:233.
4. Dorantes LM, Arnaud SB, and Arnaud CD. (1978) J Lab Clin Med 91:791.
5. Reinhardt TA, Horst RL, Orf JW and Hollis BW. (1984) J Clin Endo and Metab 58:91.
6. Fleuck JA, DiBella FP, Edis AJ, Kehrwald JM, Arnaud CD. (1977) J Clin Invest 50:1367.
7. Shinki T, Shiina Y, Takahashi N, Tanioka Y, Koizumi H, Suda T. (1983) Biochem and Biophys Res Comm 114:452.

STUDIES ON THE PRESENCE OF VITAMIN D SULPHATE IN HUMAN BREAST MILK

Ruth D. Coldwell, D.A. Seamark, D.J.H. Trafford & H.L.J. Makin

The Steroid Laboratory, Department of Chemical Pathology, The London Hospital Medical College, Turner Street, London E1 2AD, UK

The presence of solvolysable conjugates of vitamin D in human breast milk (HBM) has been a subject of controversy for some years. Modern studies have however been unable to detect the presence of such conjugates in concentrations in excess of 0.5ng/ml (1). However further studies using 3 litres of HBM have claimed to have demonstrated the presence of vitamin D sulphate in HBM, although no values for concentration were given (2).

We have used [^{3}H]vitamin D_3 sulphate, synthesised by the method of Higaki (3), as an internal standard added to HBM at the start of the procedure, thus allowing quantitative estimates of the concentration to be made. Initially we experienced difficulty in obtaining consistent results for the distribution of radiolabel between whey and fat. Initially, this problem was resolved by the addition of human plasma as a source of VDBG, adjustment to pH 9 and addition of antioxidants. Subsequently pH9 was shown to be the optimum pH and it was found that VDBG was not necessary, since addition of VDBG or adjustment to pH9 had the same effect. After incubation of 1 litre of HBM for 1.5 hr at 4°, the whey was obtained by centrifugation. The average recovery of added ^{3}H counts in the whey was 77.5%. Purification on a large Sep-Pak C18 column after extraction with acetonitrile was followed by fractionation on Sep-Pak SIL (4). HPLC of the sulphate on Zorbax ODS was carried out, collecting the appropriate fractions containing radioactivity. Hydrolysis and conversion to the isotachysterol$_3$ isomer was effected using acetyl chloride in methanol. The isotachysterol$_3$ isomer was subjected to HPLC on Zorbax ODS. After correction for recovery and comparison with a standard curve, a concentration of 50ng/litre was calculated. The isotachysterol$_3$ was converted to its trimethylsilyl ether and analysed by mass fragmentography. A peak with the correct retention time was obtained when the ion fragment m/z 456 (M^+) was monitored. Our conclusion is therefore that there is present in human milk a hydrolysable conjugate of vitamin D_3, which behaves like vitamin D_3 sulphate, at concentrations not greater than approximately 50ng/litre.

This study was supported by grants from the Wellcome Trust, Milupa Ltd., the Research Advisory Committee and Special Trustees of the London Hospital.

REFERENCES

1. Makin, H.L.J., Seamark, D.A., and Trafford, D.J.H. (1983) Arch. Dis. Childh. 58, 750-753.
2. Le Boulch, N., Cancela, L., and Miravet, L. (1982) Steroids 39, 391-397.
3. Higaki, M., Takahashi, M., Suzuki, T., and Sahashi, Y. (1965) J. Vitaminol. 15, 1219-1220.
4. Hollis, B.W., Roos, B.A., Draper, H.H. & Lambert, P.W. (1981) J. Nutrit. 111, 384-390.

IDENTIFICATION AND ANALYSIS OF VITAMIN D_3 FORMS IN CHICKEN EGGS

T. Koskinen and P. Valtonen, Department of Clinical Sciences, University of Tampere, P.O. Box 607, SF-33101 Tampere, Finland

Very few constituents of our normal diet contain significant amounts of vitamin D_3. According to nutrition tables, eggs are some of its best sources, containing up to 1750 ng of vitamin D_3 per 100 g (1). This value has, however, been determined by bioassays, which measure the total antirachitic activity of eggs and do not distinguish between the contributions of various vitamin D_3 forms to it. Results from studies on the ability of vitamin D_3 metabolites to support the development of chick embryos suggest that, while vitamin D_3 and $25(OH)D_3$ are transported into eggs, $1,25(OH)_2D_3$ is not (2). Thus, the identification and analysis of vitamin D_3 forms in eggs are required for both nutritional and physiological studies.

Materials and methods

Chicken eggs (55-60 g) were bought from retail dealers. Samples were taken from egg white (10-12 g), yolk (4-6 g) or whole eggs (12-16 g or 30-40 g). Homogenized samples containing the appropriate ^3H-tracers were extracted with dichloromethane followed by treatment of the oily residues (whole egg and yolk samples) with cold methanol and ether (3), alkaline backwash, Sephadex LH-20 chromatography, silica and C18 Sep-Pak purification, preparative reverse phase HPLC and analytical straight phase HPLC. Vitamin D_3 and $25(OH)D_3$ in whole eggs and yolk were determined by HPLC with UV detection, and in egg white by CPB analysis. $24,25(OH)_2D_3$ and $1,25(OH)_2D_3$ were assayed from whole eggs by CPB and radioreceptor assay. Isotachysterol$_3$ (ITS_3) derivatives of vitamin D_3 and $25(OH)D_3$ were formed as described (4).

Results and discussion

Whole eggs and yolk contained two compounds, which comigrated with authentic vitamin D_3 and $25(OH)D_3$ on both reverse and straight phase HPLC. The treatment of these peaks with HCl gas (4) resulted in their cochromatography with corresponding ITS_3 standards on systems capable of separating vitamin D_3 compounds from their ITS_3 derivatives (5). Therefore, we consider the two peaks as vitamin D_3 and $25(OH)D_3$.

Vitamin D. A Chemical, Biochemical and Clinical Update

The following results were obtained from the analyses (ng/100 g):

	whole eggs	yolk	egg white
vitamin D_3	785±129 (n=3)	1992±45 (n=2)	n.d. (< 4)
$25(OH)D_3$	300±61 (n=6)	948±161(n=7)	trace (6.5)
$24,25(OH)_2D_3$	n.d. (< 3)	-	-
$1,25(OH)_2D_3$	see below	-	-

In our initial studies we did not observe $1,25(OH)_2D_3$ in whole egg samples (< 0.1 ng/100 g). Later on, however, displacement of tritiated $1,25(OH)_2D_3$ from the calf thymus receptor by the $1,25(OH)_2D_3$ fraction from whole eggs could be demonstated, corresponding to 6.4 ng/100 g (n=5). This result may be due to the modulation of the receptor by yolk phospholipids (6), which possibility is currently under further investigation.

The lengthy purification procedure of the present work was found necessary for the elimination of the massive amounts of lipid present in eggs. Our assay method for yolk $25(OH)D_3$ was more sensitive than that described earlier (7). In conclusion, vitamin D_3 and $25(OH)D_3$ are present in eggs, mainly in egg yolk, in concentrations which correspond well to the reported antirachitic activity of eggs (1). There seems to be some kind of block that prevents the accumulation of dihydroxylated metabolites in eggs.

References

1. Paul, A.A. and Southgate, D.A.T. (1978) in McCance and Widdowson's the Composition of Foods, H.M. Stationery Office, London

2. Ameenuddin, S., Sunde, M.L., DeLuca, H.F., Ikekewa, N. and Kobayashi, Y. (1983) Arch. Biochem. Biophys. 226, 666-670.

3. Hollis, B.W. (1983) Anal. Biochem. 131, 211-219.

4. Seamark, D.A., Trafford, D.J.H. and Makin, H.L.J. (1980) J. Steroid Biochem. 13, 1057-1063.

5. Koskinen, T. and Valtonen, P (1985) J. Liquid Chromatogr., In Press

6. Chen, T.C., Mullen, J.P. and Meglin, N.J. (1984) J. Lipid Res. 25, 1306-1312.

7. Koshy, K.T. and VanDerSlik, A.L. (1979) J. Agric. Food Chem. 27, 180-183.

IN VITRO MUSCLE PHOSPHATE UPTAKE. CHARACTERISTICS AND ACTION OF VITAMIN D_3 METABOLITES.

T. Bellido and R.L. Boland

Departamento de Biologia, Universidad Nacional del Sur, 8000 Bahia Blanca, Argentina.

INTRODUCTION:

It has been proposed that muscle plays a role in the regulation of P homeostasis (1). In addition, other studies have suggested an action of vitamin D_3 metabolites in muscle phosphate fluxes (2,3). The objective of this work was to characterize in vitro PO_4 transport in muscle cells and the effects of vitamin D_3 metabolites on this process.

METHODS:

Vitamin D-deficient chick soleus muscles and chick embryo skeletal muscle myoblasts were cultured in media supplemented with vitamin D-deficient chick serum as previously described (4). Treatment conditions of cultures with vitamin D_3 metabolites are indicated in Results. Sarcolemma vesicles were isolated from leg muscles of vitamin D-deficient and vitamin D_3-treated chicks by differential centrifugation of homogenates and further purified in sucrose density gradients (3). Phosphate uptake by myoblasts and soleus muscles was measured at 37 °C in Krebs-Henseleit saline solution labelled with ^{32}Pi after preequilibrating the cultures for 60 min. $^{32}PO_4$ transport by sarcolemma vesicles was measured in the presence of a 100 mM NaCl gradient (3).

RESULTS AND DISCUSSION:

The kinetics of PO_4 uptake was characterized in soleus muscle and myoblast cultures. Uptake increased with time and reached equilibrium after 30 min. Saturable responses in PO_4 uptake were observed by increasing PO_4 concentrations from 0.01 to 5.0 mM. Velocity vs log PO_4 concentration plots indicated the presence of two PO_4 uptake systems in soleus muscle cultures and one in myoblast cultures (data not given). Lineweaver-Burk plots showed that the Km of the chick embryo myoblast PO_4 uptake system (0.32 mM) was similar to that of isolated sarcolemma vesicles from chick skeletal muscle (0.33 mM). Replacement of K^+ for Na^+ in equimolar concentration (143 mM) in the uptake medium decreased 50 % PO_4 uptake by myoblasts. AsO_4 (5 mM) and 2,4-dinitrophenol (2 mM) inhibited to the same extent total PO_4 uptake by isolated cells. These results suggest the presence of a specific transport system for PO_4 in the plasma membrane of muscle cells similar to that described for other cell types.

Physiological concentrations of $25OHD_3$ significantly increased PO_4 uptake by vitamin D-deficient chick soleus muscle cultures (% of control values: 111 ± 3 and 120 ± 17 for 25 ng/ml and 40 ng/ml of $25OHD_3$, respectively, $p < 0.0025$ and $p < 0.025$, respectively, N=5 in both cases). $1,25(OH)_2D_3$ in the concentration range of 0.05 to 25 ng/ml had no effects. $24,25(OH)_2D_3$ was also inactive when employed at a concentration of 4.6 ng/ml (data not presented). This suggests a specificity of vitamin D_3 metabolites on differentiated skeletal muscle ionic fluxes as $1,25(OH)_2D_3$ markedly increases Ca uptake in similar preparations (4). $25OHD_3$ was also effective to stimulate PO_4 uptake by myoblast cultures. Maximal effects were observed after 8 h of treatment (Fig. 1A). The dose-dependent response of myoblast cultures to $25OHD_3$

Vitamin D. A Chemical, Biochemical and Clinical Update

increased up to 10-fold the physiological levels of the metabolite (Fig.1B)

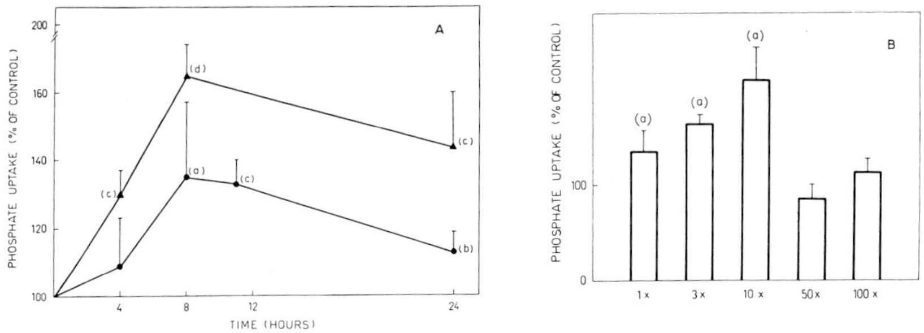

Fig. 1. A. Time course of changes in myoblast PO_4 uptake induced by $25OHD_3$. (●) 20 ng/ml, (▲) 40 ng/ml. B. Effect of $25OHD_3$ concentration on myoblast PO_4 uptake (X=20 ng/ml).

Replacement of K^+ for Na^+ markedly reduced the stimulatory effect of $25OHD_3$ on PO_4 uptake by myoblasts (Fig. 2A). In agreement with this result, Na^+ gradient-dependent PO_4 uptake by sarcolemma vesicles isolated from chick skeletal muscle was increased by previous administration of vitamin D_3 to the animals (Fig. 2B).

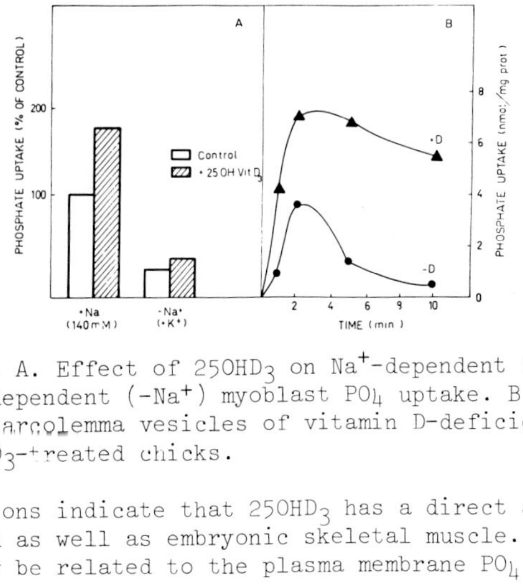

Fig. 2. A. Effect of $25OHD_3$ on Na^+-dependent ($+Na^+$) and Na^+-independent ($-Na^+$) myoblast PO_4 uptake. B. PO_4 uptake by sarcolemma vesicles of vitamin D-deficient and vitamin D_3-treated chicks.

These investigations indicate that $25OHD_3$ has a direct action on PO_4 fluxes in differentiated as well as embryonic skeletal muscle. At least part of these effects may be related to the plasma membrane PO_4 transport system.

REFERENCES:

1. Birge, S. (1978) Mineral Electrolyte Metab. 1, 57-64.
2. Birge, S. and Haddad, J. (1975) J. Clin. Invest. 56, 1100-1107.
3. Boland, A.R. de, Gallego, S. and Boland, R. (1983) Biochim. Biophys. Acta 733, 264-273.
4. Giuliani, D. and Boland, R. (1984) Calcif. Tissue Int. 36, 200-205.

RESPONSIVENESS OF THE 1α HYDROXYLASE SYSTEM IN ELDERLY PATIENTS TREATED WITH VITAMIN D.

E.B. MAWER, M. DAVIES and J.L. TAYLOR,
Department of Medicine, University of Manchester, Manchester M13 9PT, U.K.

INTRODUCTION

An earlier investigation of ours has shown a high incidence of poor vitamin D nutrition in elderly patients in institutions in Rochdale, Lancashire, England (1). The present study monitors the attempt to improve vitamin D nutrition in this group by a form of "stoss-therapie" in in which a large oral dose of vitamin D_2 (2.5mg, 6.5 μmol) was given once or twice yearly. The purpose was to find a regime which would maintain adequate levels of 25-hydroxyvitamin D (10ng/ml or 25 nmol/l) in this elderly population at mimimum administrative expense, and also to investigate the ability of elderly people to hydroxylate vitamin D at the 25- and 1α positions.

PROTOCOL

Patients were divided into 3 groups (n = 60):- controls - received no vitamin D_2 treatment, once-dosed received 2.5mg vitamin D_2 in Dec 82, twice-dosed received 2.5mg vitamin D in Dec 82 and Jun 83. Blood samples were collected at appropriate intervals and sera analysed for calcium, inorganic phosphorus, alkaline phosphatase and vitamin D metabolites. Data for vitamin D metabolites are presented here for a sample of 10 patients from each group.

METHODS

$25(OH)D_2$ and $25(OH)D_3$ were assayed separately by a novel HPLC-UV absorbance method in which an internal u-v absorbing standard is used to monitor recovery, thus permitting a direct printout of final results from automated HPLC equipment. The samples were prepared by extraction of 2ml of serum with 2ml acetonitrile and elution by acetonitrile from C18 Sep-paks (2), $1,25(OH)_2D_2$ and $1,25(OH)_2D_3$ were assayed separately by RIA using antisera of different specificities (gift of Prof. J. O'Riordan) after HPLC separation of an acetonitrile extract of 2-3ml serum cleaned by passage through C18 Sep-paks; normal range (mean + 2sd) 17-60 pg/ml.

RESULTS & DISCUSSION

Assayed concentrations of $25(OH)D_2/D_3$ and $1,25(OH)_2D_2/D_3$ are shown in the table as the means for each group. (data for Mar. and Sep. not shown).

ASSAYED METABOLITES IN SERUM

Patient group	Pretreatment August 82		Post-treatment 1983 Jan		Jun		July		Dec	
25(OH)D ng/ml	D_2	D_3	D_2	D_3	D_2	D_3	D_2	D_3	D_2	D_3
Controls	1.0	5.7	-	-	1.1	9.8	-	-	1.0	10.9
once-dosed	2.0	4.3	23.0	5.6	9.0	5.7	-	-	6.8	6.7
twice-dosed	1.3	5.1	20.3	6.0	7.5	7.2	22.5	7.5	11.7	7.3
1,25(OH) D pg/ml										
Controls	11.3	21.3	-	-	7.0	23.9	-	-	5.3	26.6
once-dosed	7.6	19.3	55.6	11.7	21.0	10.8	-	-	12.8	17.1
twice-dosed	12.6	31.7	44.8	15.7	19.5	27.9	46.0	15.1	19.5	16.5

Vitamin D. A Chemical, Biochemical and Clinical Update

The ratio of D_2/D_3 in the $1,25(OH)_2D$ fraction was plotted against the D_2/D_3 ratio in 25(OH)D. The linear regression for this relationship was strong ($r = 0.97$, $p < 0.001$) but was slightly below the line of equivalence (intercept -0.08).

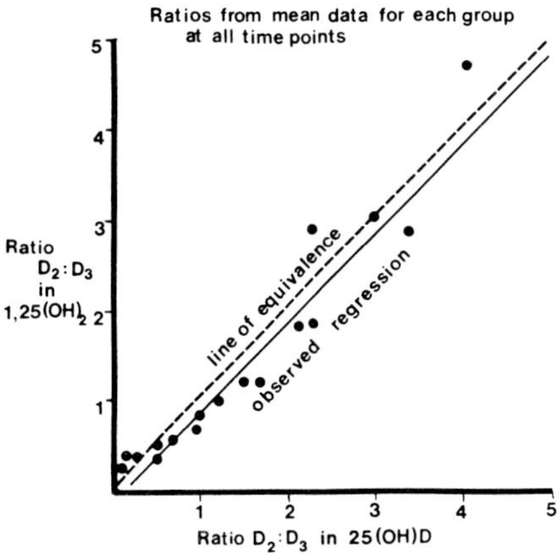

Relationship implies slight discrimination against D_2 at renal level

All the patients treated with vitamin D_2 were able to hydroxylate it at 25- and 1α- positions (except for one patient who was diabetic with poor renal function). As the newly formed $25(OH)D_2$ entered the plasma pool the ratio of D_2/D_3 increased. The ratio of D_2/D_3 in $1,25(OH)_2D$ increased similarly but was slightly lower than in 25(OH)D indicating a possible marginal discrimination by the renal 1α -hydroxylase against $25(OH)D_2$.

At the end of the year in which treatment was given, serum $25(OH)D_2$ was significantly raised in both treatment groups compared to controls ($P < 0.001$). Total serum 25(OH)D was significantly higher in the twice-dosed group compared to controls ($P < 0.005$) but the once-dosed and control groups were not different. Total 25(OH)D was significantly higher after the treatment year in both treatment groups compared to pre-treatment levels, ($P < 0.001$).

Increased $25(OH)D_2$ was accompanied by a rapid rise in $1,25(OH)D_2$ following each dose of vitamin D_2; in several patients this was sufficient to raise the total $1,25(OH)_2D$ out of the normal range. The stimulus to this rise has not yet been identified; no patient was severely hypocalcaemic and serum alkaline phosphatase values were normal in most patients, results of PTH assay are awaited. Some but not all of the patients who made supra-normal concentrations of $1,25(OH)_2D_2$ had very low initial 25(OH)D levels; however, in the twice-dosed group the same patients over-produced $1,25(OH)_2D_2$ from the second dose of vitamin D_2 when they were no longer frankly vitamin D-deficient.

The question thus arises as to whether the exaggerated $1,25(OH)_2D$ response signals some biological need for increased calcium absorption (such as relatively under-mineralised bone). The ability to elicit such a response in individuals whose 25(OH)D level was considerably above the 5 ng/ml conventially regarded as the index of vitamin D deficiency also raises questions as to the definition of vitamin D repletion. Might perhaps vitamin D repletion be defined as the level of 25(OH)D at which no significant perturbation of 1,25(OH) D results when the 25(OH)D pool is increased?

REFERENCES

1. Hann, J.T., Mawer, E.B., Davies, M. and Taylor, J.L. (1985), Metab. Bone Dis. Rel. Res. (in press).
2. Hann, J.T. and Mawer, E.B. (1984), Metab. Bone Dis. Rel. Res., 5, 156.

THE ACTION AND BIOLOGICAL SIGNIFICANCE OF FEMALE AND MALE SEX STEROIDS ON PLASMA TOTAL AND FREE $1,25(OH)_2D$, PARATHYROID HORMONE AND CALCITONIN

M. PEACOCK, P.L. SELBY, R.M. FRANCIS and G.A. TAYLOR
MRC Mineral Metabolism Unit, The General Infirmary, Leeds,UK.

Introduction:

The sex steroids play a fundamental role in normal bone growth and hypogonadism in the adult causes osteoporosis. The mechanisms by which they act on bone are disputed (1). A popular view is that they act through one or other of the calcium regulating hormones (2,3,4). To investigate the mechanism of action of sex steroids on bone and on the calcium regulating hormones we have studied their effects in hypogonadal subjects.

Methods:

Patients were studied in the fasting state before and after 3 weeks of treatment. Oral Ethinyl Oestradiol 30 µg/day or Norethisterone 5 mg/day were given to 18 and 11 healthy post-menopausal women respectively. Testosterone (Sustanon) 250 mg IM every fortnight was given to 8 men with hypogonadism from various causes.

Plasma $1,25(OH)_2D$, 25OHD, DBP, PTH, CT, calcium, FSH and urinary calcium, creatinine, hydroxyproline, and radio-calcium absorption were measured as previously described (5). The dissociation constants of $1,25(OH)_2D$ ($4 \times 10^{-7}M$) and 25OHD ($4 \times 10^{-8}M$) for DBP were established with purified DBP at 4^oC and the bound and free fractions of plasma $1,25(OH)_2D$ calculated from the mass action equation.

Results: (Table)

Ethinyl Oestradiol (EO) significantly reduced urinary calcium and hydroxyproline and plasma calcium and FSH. It significantly increased plasma DBP and total $1,25(OH)_2D$ but not free $1,25(OH)_2D$. It had no effect on plasma PTH and CT, or radio-calcium absorption. Norethisterone (NE) significantly reduced urinary calcium and hydroxyproline. It had no effect on plasma PTH, CT, DBP, total and free $1,25(OH)_2D$ or radio-calcium absorption. Testosterone (T) significantly reduced urinary calcium and plasma FSH. It significantly increased total and free $1,25(OH)_2D$ and radiocalcium absorption. It had no effect on plasma PTH, CT, or urinary hydroxyproline.

Conclusions:

Ethinyl Oestradiol in hypogonadal women reduces bone resorption within three weeks. This is achieved without changing the plasma levels of the calcium regulating hormones. Although Ethinyl Oestradiol causes a rise in $1,25(OH)_2D$ this is completely due to an increase in DBP and is not accompanied by a rise in calcium absorption.

Norethisterone in hypogonadal women also blocks bone resorption without affecting the calcium regulating hormones or calcium absorption.

Vitamin D. A Chemical, Biochemical and Clinical Update

Since the female sex steroids reduce bone resorption and decrease plasma calcium without changing plasma levels of the PTH, 25OHD and $1,25(OH)_2D$ they must also reset the secretion threshold of the calcium regulating hormones.
Testosterone in hypogonadal men causes calcium retention and increases calcium absorption by increasing total and free plasma $1,25(OH)_2D$.

References:

1. Francis,R.M.,Peacock,M.,Taylor,G.A.,Kahn,A.J.,Teitelbaum, S.L. This volume.
2. Heaney,R. (1965) Amer.J.Med.39:877-880
3. Gallagher,J.C.,Riggs,B.L.,DeLuca,H.F.(1980) J.Clin.Endocr. Metab.51:1359-1364
4. Stevenson,J.C.,e.a. (1981) Lancet 1:693-695
5. Peacock,M.,Taylor,G.A.,Brown,W.(1980) Clin.Chim.Acta 101: 93-101

TABLE Blood and urine biochemistry before and after 3 weeks treatment with Ethinyl Oestradiol (EO), Norethisterone (NE) and Testosterone (T)

		Ca^{++} mmol/l	FSH mU/ml	DBP µmol/l	T,1,25D pmol/l	F,1,25D pmol/l
EO	Basal	1.21	38	6.57	103	1.00
	Treated	1.16***	25***	10.18***	158***	0.98
NE	Basal	1.20	28	5.71	86	1.04
	Treated	1.18	27	6.25	73	0.74*
T	Basal	1.17	27	5.38	72	0.78
	Treated	1.18	20*	5.26	96*	1.28*

		PTH pg/ml	CT pg/ml	^{45}Ca Absorp.	Ca/Cr molar	OHPr/Cr molar
EO	Basal	206	10.9	0.58	0.29	0.013
	Treated	193	10.4	0.65	0.14***	0.010*
NE	Basal	152	17.4	0.86	0.35	0.012
	Treated	143	18.6	0.68	0.15**	0.009*
T	Basal	166	-	0.42	0.26	0.014
	Treated	149	-	0.70*	0.15*	0.013

VITAMIN D3-3B SULFATE IN HUMAN MILK : MASS SPECTRUM AND COMPETITIVE BINDING ASSAY

L.CANCELA, N. LE BOULCH, C. LANG, L. MIRAVET
Unité 18 INSERM, 6 rue Guy Patin, 75010 Paris-France

Introduction

The vitamin D content of milk has been a subject of controversial discussions ever since a watersoluble form of vitamin D was found in human and cow's milk (1). At that time, the vitamin D content, of this watersoluble fraction was evaluated to be 950 UI/liter, by contrast with only 17 IU/liter in the liposoluble fraction. This high content of vitamin D was due to the presence of a sulfoconjugated form of vitamin D(1,2). Using similar methodology, comparable results were obtained thereafter (3,4). However,the utilization of new technics allowing a better purification and isolation of the product including HPLC (5,6), did not confirm early data. In this study we have attempted :

1) to identify the vitamin D sulfate (SD) in human milk using desorption chemical ionisation mass spectrometry.
2) to develop a new technic allowing the quantification of small amounts of SD in human milk.

Material and Methods

Human milk was obtained either from lactarium by pooled fractions of 200 ml, or from lactating women during the first month of lactation. In this case, 10 to 30 ml of fresh milk were obtained at the end of early moorning breast-feeding, at day 3,15 and 30 of lactation. Milk was frozen and vitamin D content was determined within three months. Blood samples were obtained from mothers at day 3 and 30 post partum and from paired breast fed infants at day 30 of lactation. Lactarium pooled milk was extracted as previously describbed (7), purified by Seppak and HPLC and then used to physically characterize the SD-like fraction thus obtained by U.V. absorption and mass spectrography using desorption chemical ionization technics (8). Freshly obtained women milk was used to determine the vitamin D content due to free vitamin D and 25-hydroxyvitamin D (25(OH)D) (9) and to vitamin D sulfate. This last compound was extracted by a methylene chlorure/methanol method (5) and after purification was quantified using a competitive binding assay. Vitamin D_3 sulfate either synthetic or from milk extracts was incubated for 2 hours at 4° C with a renal cytosolic protein fraction prepared from normal rats. $25(OH)D_3$-^3H was then added and incubation continued for two additional hours. After separation of free from bound fractions by addition of charcoal/Dextran followed by centrifugation, the supernatant was counted for radioactive determination.Using this technic, we were able to detect as low as 0.8 ng of vitamin D sulfate per assay tube. Serum vitamin D metabolites were determined by competitive binding assay.

Results

The U.V. absorption spectrum of the SD-like fraction obtained from human milk was characteristic of a vitamin D derivative showing a maximum at 265 nm and a minimum at 228 nm, due to the presence of a 5-6-cis triene configuration. We were not able to obtain a full scan mass spectra of SD in the human milk extract because of the poor amount of SD. A selected ion monitoring measurement was then realized with typical ions : 384 for free D3 and 366 for SD3. In this case, the ratio 366/384 is $>$ 1 for SD3 and $<$ 1 for vitamin D3.
The profiles obtained were in accordance with the presence of vitamin D3 sulfate in the natural extract. The determination of vitamin D content in human milk revealed the presence of a SD fraction at a concentration in most cases lower than 1 µg/liter. No correlation was found between the milk content of free vitamin D or 25(OH)D and the amounts of SD found in milk. Accordingly no correlation was found between SD in milk and the plasma 25(OH)D concentration of breast fed infants or lactating women . By contrast, vitamin D and 25(OH)D levels in milk were well correlated with the plasma 25(OH)D levels of paired breast fed infants.

Conclusion

Vitamin D sulfate was found to be present in human milk and was physically characterized by selected ion monitoring technics. However the concentrations determined by competitive protein binding assay were much lower than those early reported and cannot account

Vitamin D. A Chemical, Biochemical and Clinical Update

for the important amounts found previously. The absence of correlation between SD concentration in milk and the plasma 25(OH)D levels of paired breast fed infants or the concentration of free and monohydroxylated vitamin D in paired milk do not support the hypothesis that SD3 represents a preferential derivative of vitamin D during lactation.

References

1 - Sahashi Y., Susuki T., Higaki M., Asano T. (1966) Vitamins (Japan) 34, 467-469.
2 - Le Boulch N., Gulat-Marnay C., Raoul Y. (1974) Int. J. vitamin. Nutr. Res. 44, 167-179.
3 - Lakdawala D.R., Widdowson E.M. (1977) Lancet 1, 167-168.
4 - Antila P., Antila V., Kuujo S. (1979) Meijeritiet Aikak, 37, 1-22.
5 - Hollis B.W., Roos B.A., Draper H.H., Lambert P.W. (1981) J. Nutr. 111, 384-390.
6 - Reeve L.E., Chesney R.W., Deluca H.F. (1982) Am. J. Clin. Nutr., 36, 122-126.
7 - Le Boulch N., Cancela L., Miravet L. (1982) Steroids, 39, 391-
8 - Beaugrand C., Devant G. (1980)"Adv. in Mass spectroscopy", ed. by A. Quayle, 8B, p 1806, Heyden, London.
9 - Hollis B.W. (1983) Anal. Bioch. 131, 211-219.

VITAMIN D ABSORPTION AND 25(OH) D FORMATION IN PATIENTS WITH CHRONIC LIVER DISEASES.

R.Lorenc, J.Ryzko, A.Jurek, K.Kozłowski, J.Łukaszkiewicz. J.Socha. Child's Health Center, Warsaw, Poland.

Introduction: The liver plays an important role in vitamin D metabolism as organ where vitamin D is hydroxylated to 25(OH) D .Instead of several mineral and bone disorders in liver diseases their pathogenesis concerning vitamin D status is not fully understood.In this paper in the aim of evaluating the requirement for vitamin D in liver diseases the Vitamin D absorption and 25(OH) D formation was monitored in 32 children divided in four following groups: chronic hepatitis with (CH + C) n = 10 and without cirrhosis (CH-C) n=7 primary biliary cirrhosis (PBC) n=7 and primary biliary atresia (PBA) n=8.

Material and methods: Liver function was assessed by measurements of serum bilirubin, conjugated bile acids levels (CBA) and prothrombin test.Serum Vitamin D and 25(OH) D levels were measured after preliminary extraction and prepurification by HPLC before and 12 hrs, 1,2,4, and 7 days after an oral dose of 1200 i.u. / kg body weight of Vitamin D_3.Reference control data were obtainned from age matched children with transient diarrhea but with no other posology.

Results: Before dosing with Vitamin D lower serum concentrations of Vitamin D (below detection limits) and of 25(OH)D 2.4-10.1 ng / ml (when normal range was 20-40 ng / ml) were found in all children with cirrhosis. After oral loading with Vitamin D its serum peak increment ($C_p$max) was significantly lower (42.4±10.7 ng ml vs 103.8±6.4 ng ml in controls) in all cirrhotic patients. A negative correlation between $C_p$max 25(OH) D and either serum bilirubin levels ($p < .001$) or CBA ($p < .001$) and positive correlation between $C_p$max 25(OH) D and prothrombin test ($p < 01$) were observed.In the whole group of children with liver diseases, ratios of $C_p$max 25(OH) D over $C_p$max Vitamin D were negatively correlated with in serum bilirubin concentrations ($p < .001$).

Discussion; The data obtained are indicating on multifactorial mechanisms affecting Vitamin D metabolism in liver diseases, The lower bioavailability of Vitamin D after oral dosing together with low 25(OH)D levels observed in cirrhotic patients are indicating on depressed vitamin D absorption form the gut. On the same, our experimental protocol doesn't enable the evaluation of the importance of renal wastage of Vitamin D in liver diseased patients.Whatever the reason,our studies has shown, that the supply and level of 25(OH)D is dropping down parallely with aggrevation of liver function. The analyses of 25(OH)D levels in correlation to Vitamin D supply doesn't indicate on any defects in 25 hydroxylase activity. The enzyme activity parallels the amount of active functionally hepatocytes and even follows the suggestion concerning its stimulation by low Vitamin D levels

Bone changes are present in the majority of studied children (60%) with predominance of osteoporosis in the cirrhotic group and rickets in PBA one. The accompanied changes in protein metabolism invalidate the possibility of the evaluation of the importance of Vitamin D metabolites in the etiopathogenesis of bone changes.

Conclusions: On the basis of data obtained we conclude, that Vitamin D metabolism in liver disease is affected by decreased Vitamin D absorption from the gut and by alterations in the hepatocyte functions. Hence cirrhotic patients are under potential risk for Vitamin D deficiency.

Vitamin D. A Chemical, Biochemical and Clinical Update

PATIENTS – BIOCHEMICAL DATA

Biochemical Test	Normal Range	Chronic Hepatitis Without Cirrhosis /n=7/	Primary Biliary Atresia /n=7/	Chronic Hepatitis With Cirrhosis /n=11/	Primary Biliary Cirrhosis /n=7/
Calcium /mmol/l/	2,3 – 2,5	2,46 ± 0,03	2,28 ± 0,15	2,14 ± 0,07	2,28 ± 0,06
Phosphate /mmol/l/	0,81 – 1,55	1,50 ± 0,08	1,60 ± 0,13	1,31 ± 0,09	1,48 ± 0,09
Alkaline phosphatase /i.u./	175 – 910	755 ± 210	1365 ± 436	1056 ± 205	1600 ± 261
Albumin /g/l/	36 – 49	45,4 ± 1,6	26,8 ± 1,8	36,6 ± 1,7	37,5 ± 2,6
Bilirubin /mg/dl/	1,0	1,6 ± 0,3	5,1 ± 1,5	6,4 ± 2,9	14,7 ± 3,6
CBA /umol/l/	6,0	19,5 ± 8,3	49,2 ± 18,2	23,7 ± 10,0	94,9 ± 24,4
Prothrombin index /%/	80 – 100	96,1 ± 4,0	87,6 ± 7,7	68,6 ± 4,6	59,7 ± 6,6
25-OH-D /ng/ml/	20 – 40	20,5 ± 4,8	14,5 ± 9,0	11,5 ± 3,1	6,6 ± 1,9

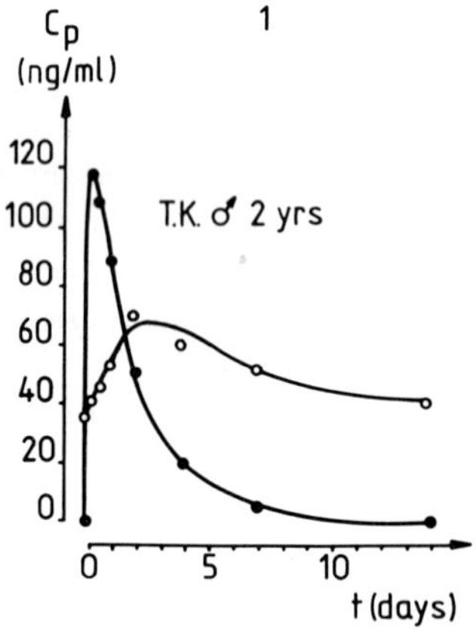

SERUM VITAMIN D (•–•) AND 25(OH)D (○–○) LEVELS IN CONTROL PATIENT (1) (WITHOUT ANY LIVER PROBLEMS) WITH PBA (2) AND PBC (3) DOSED ORALLY AT TIME "0" WITH 30 μg/kg b.w. OF VITAMIN D.

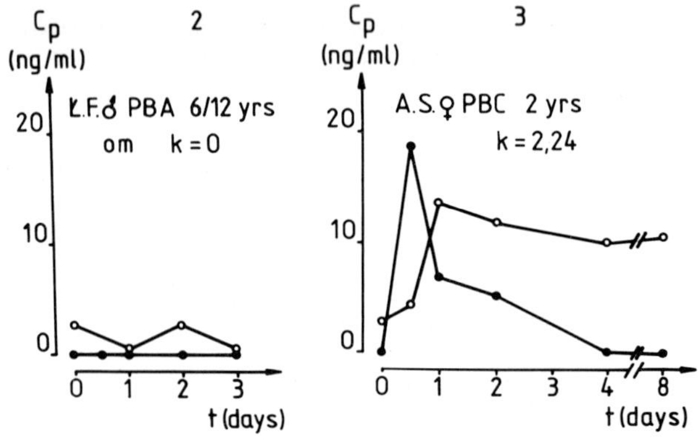

DOES VITAMIN D PERFORM A FUNCTION IN MUSCLE?

R.L. Boland, Departamento de Biologia, Universidad Nacional del Sur, 8000 Bahia Blanca, Argentina.

Vitamin D plays a major role in the regulation of vertebrate calcium and phosphorus metabolism by acting at the level of intestine, bone and kidney. However, recent investigations have implied a function of vitamin D sterols in other non-classical target organs in animals (1,2). Muscle has also been suspected to be a target tissue for vitamin D since early clinical studies describing alterations in skeletal muscle function in vitamin D deficiency. This information will be evaluated together with recent experimental data to assess the role of the sterol in muscle.

Muscle Weakness in Vitamin D Deficiency and Renal Diseases: Clinical observations first suggested a relationship between vitamin D and muscle. These studies have shown that a myopathy characterized by muscle weakness is a common symptom in vitamin deficiency states of various origins and in chronic renal failure (3-7). The main clinical feature of the myopathy associated with osteomalacia consists in predominantly proximal muscle weakness which often gives rise to a waddling gait. Moderate muscle wasting without fasciculation or depression of the tendon reflexes may be observed. Plasma muscle enzyme profiles are generally unaltered and only slight nonspecific histopathological abnormalities may be detected (5,6). Electromyographic evaluation of patients reveals a myopathic pattern as evidenced by a significant reduction in motor unit potential duration and amplitude, and an increased percentage of poliphasicity as compared to controls (4,5). A similar myopathy has been observed in patients with post-gastrectomy vitamin D-deficiency, idiopathic hypophosphataemic osteomalacia and in gluten-sensitive enteropathy (6). Muscle weakness responds to the treatment with vitamin D_3 suggesting that the sterol plays an ethiological role. Moreover, it has been shown that osteomalacic myopathy and neuropathy are not interrelated (5). Patients with end-stage renal failure also develop proximal muscle weakness. The myopathy is demonstrable by quantitative electromyography and its histological characterization reveals selective atrophy of type II muscle fibres. Electron microscopy may show in addition non-specific degenerative changes (7). The myopathy may be considerably improved by the administration of small amounts of $1,25(OH)_2D_3$ (8,9) and renal transplantation (7) whereas treatment with large doses of vitamin D_3 causes only moderate improvement (7). This suggests that impaired synthesis of $1,25(OH)_2D_3$ may play a role in the development of muscle weakness in renal diseases. In disagreement with this interpretation a high incidence of a similar myopathy in patients with primary hyperparathyroidism has been reported (10). However, this observation could not be confirmed in two more recent studies (3,4). It has been proposed that hypophosphataemia may be the basic disorder underlying these

Vitamin D. A Chemical, Biochemical and Clinical Update

myopathies as it is a common feature of primary hyperparathyroidism, osteomalacia and nutritional vitamin D deficiency (11). Contrary to this proposal it has been noted that the myopathy of hypophosphataemic osteomalacia may not resolve with increased phosphate intake, and vitamin D intake is required for recovery. The fact that muscle weakness is absent in x-linked hypophosphataemic rickets has been taken as an indication that mere hypophosphataemia need not to be the ethiological factor involved (6). The myopathy associated with vitamin D deficiency has been electrophysiologically characterized. Using an in situ neuromuscular preparation of the soleus Rodman and Baker (12) found diminished peak tension and prolonged time for recovery halfway to resting tension for single twitches and prolonged relaxation half-life after tetanic contraction in vitamin D deficient rats (Fig. 1).

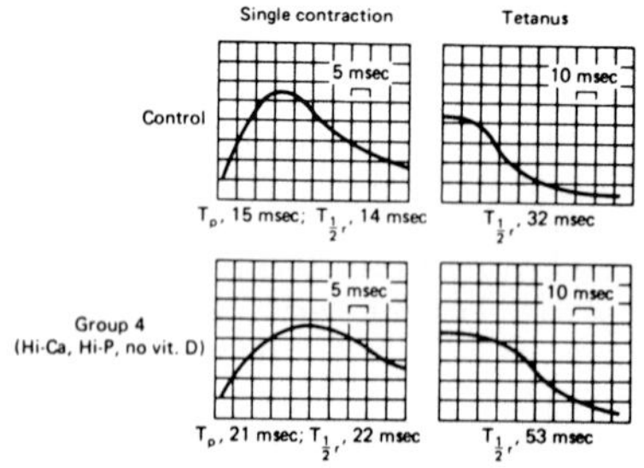

Fig. 1. Kinetics of contraction and relaxation after electrical stimulation of soleus muscle from vitamin D-depleted rats (after Rodman and Baker, ref. 12).

Impaired tension development and slow relaxation after muscle contraction in response to repetitive electrical stimulation were also observed in vitamin D-depleted chicks (13). Interestingly enough both studies clearly showed that these changes were not related to modifications in blood Ca and P levels and could only be reversed to normal by administration of vitamin D_3 (12,13). The data indicate that vitamin D-dependent muscle weakness may be ascribed to a primary disorder of skeletal muscle function. Alterations in muscle Ca and P metabolism have been considered factors responsible for the myopathy. In addition, there is scarce evidence which suggests that alterations in the structure and functional properties of the actomyosin contractile complex may also be involved.

Role of vitamin D in muscle calcium transport:

It is possible that alterations in the mechanisms by which intracellular Ca^{2+} is regulated in the muscle cell play a major role in muscle weakness associated to vitamin D deficiency and renal diseases. Rapid variations in sarcoplasmic Ca^{2+} levels in response to Ca^{2+} release and Ca^{2+} uptake by the sarcoplasmic reticulum (SR) are a key factor in the regulation of skeletal muscle contraction and relaxation, respectively (14). In addition, Ca transport systems located in sarcolemma and mitochondria contribute to the regulation of muscle cytoplasmic Ca^{2+} (15). Several data indicate that vitamin D acts on muscle Ca transport. Ca uptake by SR is diminished in vitamin D-depleted rabbits (16) and chicks (13). $1,25(OH)_2D_3$ may be the active metabolite on SR as nephrectomy and strontium feedin decreased Ca uptake. Dosage of the animal with $1,25(OH)_2D_3$ reversed these changes (17,18). $1,25(OH)_2D_3$ may affect Ca transport across sarcoplasmic reticulum membranes by increasing the number and kinetics of formation of active transport sites of the SR Ca-ATPase. Steady-state levels of phosphoderivative (EP) and phosphorylation velocity of the transport enzyme are decreased in experimental uremia. Administration of $1,25(OH)_2D_3$ restores both parameters to normal (Table 1).

Table 1. Effect of $1,25(OH)_2D_3$ on EP steady-state levels and rate of phosphorylation of SR Ca-ATPase in experimental uremia (after Boland et al., ref. 19).

Experimental group*	EP (nmol/mg prot)	Half-time of EP formation (sec^{-1})
Control	2.05 ± o.25	1.76 ± 0.05
Uremic	1.57 ± 0.23[a]	3.13 ± 0.39[b]
Uremic + $1,25(OH)_2D_3$	2.01 ± 0.29	1.70 ± 0.22

*Control and nephrectomized rabbits were used. a $p < 0.01$; b $p < 0.05$

It has been reported that vitamin D also affects Ca fluxes through mitochondrial membranes from skeletal muscle. Treatment of vitamin D-deficient chicks with the sterol increased the ability of mitochondria to accumulate Ca *in vivo* and markedly stimulated Ca efflux from the organelle preloaded *in vitro* with ^{45}Ca (13). In addition, an action of vitamin D_3 on Ca transport across muscle plasma cell membranes has been reported. Administration of the sterol to vitamin D-deficient chicks markedly increased Ca uptake in subsequently isolated sarcolemma vesicles. This change was accompanied by an increase in Ca-ATPase activity which could in turn be related to increased Vmax and Km (Table 2). Ca efflux from preloaded vesicles was only slightly altered confirming that the effects of vitamin D_3 on sarcolemmal Ca transport are related to the Ca pump and not to the passive permeability properties of the membrane (20). Ca transport by these sarcolemmal preparations probably reflects the Ca-ATPase activity of vesicles with "inside-out" membranes as the physiological function of the pump is to extrude Ca from the cells (15).

Studies with *in vitro* muscle systems have recently provided evidence of a direct action of vitamin D on muscle cellular Ca and made possible identification of active metabolites.

Table. 2. Effect of vitamin D_3 administration on Ca transport and kinetic parameters of Ca-ATPase of chick sarcolemmal membranes (after Boland et al., ref. 20).

	Ca uptake		Ca-ATPase	
	Initial Rate	Total Capacity	Vmax	Km
- vit.D	11.7 ± 0.9	16.4 ± 1.9	1.02	0.45
+ vit.D_3	16.8 ± 1.8[a]	28.5 ± 2.2[b]	1.31	0.32

Rate: nmol/mg prot/min.; Capacity: nmol/mg prot; Vmax: µmol P/mg prot/h; Km: µM. a: $p < 0.05$; b: $p < 0.02$; N=5

Addition of physiological amounts of $1,25(OH)_2D_3$ caused a significant stimulation of ^{45}Ca uptake by cultures of vitamin D-deficient chick soleus muscle and chick embryo skeletal muscle myoblasts. $25OHD_3$ was less potent whereas $24,25(OH)_2D_3$ was without effect in the soleus preparations (Fig. 2).

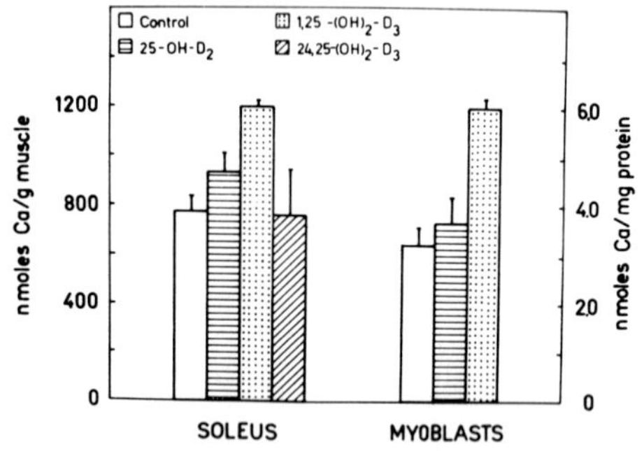

Fig. 2. In vitro effects of vitamin D_3 metabolites on Ca uptake by cultured soleus muscle and myoblasts after 5 h and 16 treatment respectively (after Giulani and Boland, ref. 21).

The greater biological activity of $1,25(OH)_2D_3$ was evident after various treatment intervals (22) and in a wide concentration range (data not given). Increased ^{45}Ca incorporation by myoblasts treated with $1,25(OH)_2D_3$ was accompanied by changes in growth and differentiation of cultures (21). Characterization of kinetic parameters of myoblast Ca pools obtained by desaturation analysis of cells prelabelled with ^{45}Ca indicated, in accord with the previously mentioned in vivo evidence, that $1,25(OH)_2D_3$ stimulates Ca efflux across mitochondrial and plasma cell membranes. The predominant effect of 25OHD3 was to increase Ca influx into mitochondria (22). These data show that the effects of $1,25(OH)_2D_3$ and $25OHD_3$ on muscle Ca metabolism are specific for each metabolite. Both sterols induced similar changes in Ca fluxes in cultures of the fully differentiated soleus muscle although, due to the presence of a well developed sarcoplasmic reticulum system, their effects on a slow-exchangeable Ca pool could be either ascribed to an effect on SR or mitochondrial Ca transport (21). The action of vitamin D on muscle Ca fluxes may contribute to Ca homeostasis in the whole organism. It has been reported that vitamin D depletion of chicks leads to Ca accumulation in muscle tissue (23). Administration of a single dose of $1,25(OH)_2D_3$ quickly reversed this change. The prompt increase in blood Ca which followed administration of the steroid correlated better with the fall in Ca content of muscle tissue than with stimulation of intestinal Ca absorption (Fig. 3).

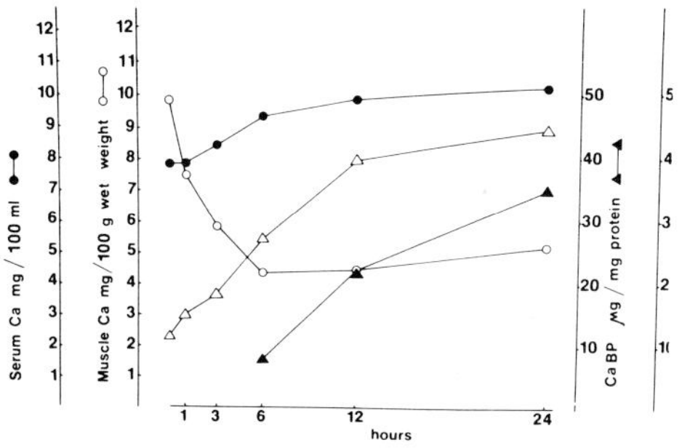

Fig 3. Decrease in muscle Ca in response to $1,25(OH)_2D_3$. Symbols are specified at the ordinates of the figure; intestinal Ca absorption (▲--▲, µg Ca/mm/30 min, right-hand scale).

Increased Ca efflux from mitochondria and cytoplasm in muscle cells treated with $1,25(OH)_2D_3$ observed in the in vitro studies may provide a mechanism of $1,25(OH)_2D_3$ action on Ca mobilization from skeletal muscle of rachitic animals.

Role of vitamin D in muscle phosphate transport:

An action of vitamin D on muscle P fluxes was first suggested by Birge and Haddad (24) who by administration of vitamin D_3 or $25OHD_3$ to vitamin D-deficient, PO_4-depleted rats, detected first a fall in serum P and an increase in in vitro ^{32}P uptake by muscle, followed by an increase in muscle ATP and protein synthesis. Nephrectomy did not obliterate these responses indicating that further conversion of the sterols to $1,25(OH)_2 D_3$ was not required. These changes could be reproduced by treatment in vitro of rat epitrochlear muscle cultures with physiological levels of $25OHD_3$ implying a direct action of this metabolite in muscle PO_4 transport. On the basis of this evidence it was proposed that the osteomalacic myopathy could be attributed to a reduction in muscle intracellular PO4 (11). These observations have been confirmed and further expanded. Measurement of ^{32}P specific activities in serum and skeletal muscle sarcoplasm and intracellular membranes after in vivo $^{32}PO_4$-labelling of vitamin D-deficient and acutely vitamin D_3-treated chicks suggested that the sterol stimulates phosphate transport across muscle plasma membranes (25). This could be confirmed by isolation of highly purified sarcolemma vesicles and evaluation of its phosphate transport properties. Prior treatment of vitamin D-deficient chicks with vitamin D_3 markedly stimulated vesicle PO_4 transport mediated by an externally imposed Na gradient (Fig. 4).

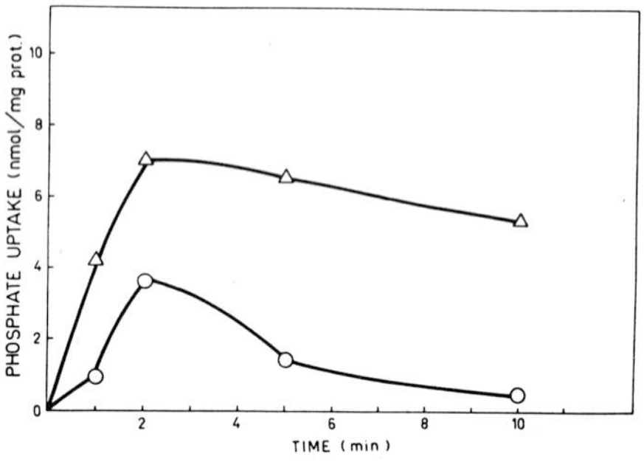

Fig. 4. Time course of PO_4 transport into sarcolemma vesicles isolated from vitamin D-deficient (○) and vitamin D-treated (Δ) chicks (after Boland et al., ref. 20).

Recent evidence obtained employing chick soleus muscle and myoblast cultures indicates that $25OHD_3$ may be the metabolite responsible for the effects of vitamin D on sarcolemmal PO_4 transport (26). A good agreement between the time courses of changes in PO_4 and Ca uptake induced by the metabolite in both preparations could be seen, suggesting that the previously observed effects of $25OHD_3$ on mitochondrial Ca influx may be secondary to the action of the sterol on muscle PO_4 uptake (22, 26).

Effects of vitamin D on muscle contractile proteins:

A few reports have implied vitamin D in the synthesis of skeletal muscle contractile proteins. Ströder and Arensmeyer reported that the content of the actomyosin contractile complex is significantly reduced in skeletal muscle from rats chronically depleted of vitamin D (27). Comparison of electrophoretic patterns of actomyosin isolated from vitamin D-deficient chicks and chicks repleted with vitamin D_3 showed an increase in actin and troponin c as consequence of treatment with sterol (25). Interestingly enough, it has been shown that $1,25(OH)_2D_3$ stimulates the synthesis of an actin-like protein in chick intestinal brush borders (28). A similar reduction in troponin c concentration in muscle from rachitic rabbits was previously reported by Pointon et al. (29). Troponin c is a Ca binding protein with a high degree of homology in its primary structure to other Ca-regulatory proteins, including the intestinal Ca binding protein. The changes observed may also contribute to impaired tension development in vitamin D deficiency. Ca binding to troponin c initiates the mechanism of muscle contraction in vertebrate striated muscle (30).

Mechanism of action of vitamin D in skeletal muscle:

$1,25(OH)_2D_3$-dependent Ca uptake in chick soleus muscle and chick embryo skeletal muscle myoblasts can be suppressed by puromycin (data not given) and cycloheximide (Fig. 5), respectively, indicating that the effects of the metabolite on muscle Ca transport are mediated by de novo protein synthesis. In addition, the increase in myoblast Ca uptake induced by $1,25(OH)_2D_3$ can be effectively blocked by actinomycin D (Fig. 5), suggesting that the metabolite affects protein synthesis via a nuclear mechanism. The nuclear action of $1,25(OH)_2D_3$ in muscle, like in classical target organs, may involve binding to a specific receptor prior to genome activation. Density gradient analysis of the cytosol obtained from myoblasts shows that $1,25(OH)_2D_3$ binds specifically to a 3.7 S macromolecule (Fig. 6). Scatchard analysis indicates that the receptor-like macromolecule binds the sterol with high affinity and low capacity (data not given.

No information is available about possible gene products made in response to $1,25(OH)_2D_3$. Administration of vitamin D to vitamin D-deficient chicks affects the synthesis of troponin c, actin and mitochondrial membrane proteins (25,31). Further studies are required to elucidate if $1,25(OH)_2D_3$ is the metabolite responsible for these changes.

$1,25(OH)_2D_3$ affects, in addition, muscle phospholipids. Treatment of myoblast cultures with the metabolite increases their phosphatidylcholine content (22). These changes are likely to be localized in the plasma membranes of muscle cells, as administration in vivo of vitamin D_3 to vitamin D-depleted chicks results in a similar increase of phosphatidylcholine of subsequently isolated skeletal muscle sarcolemma vesicles (20).

This change may represent part of the mechanism involved in the effects of the sterol on Ca transport across muscle plasma membranes (20-22). Vitamin D_3 increases in vivo the total phospholipid content of sarcoplasmic reticulum and mitochondria

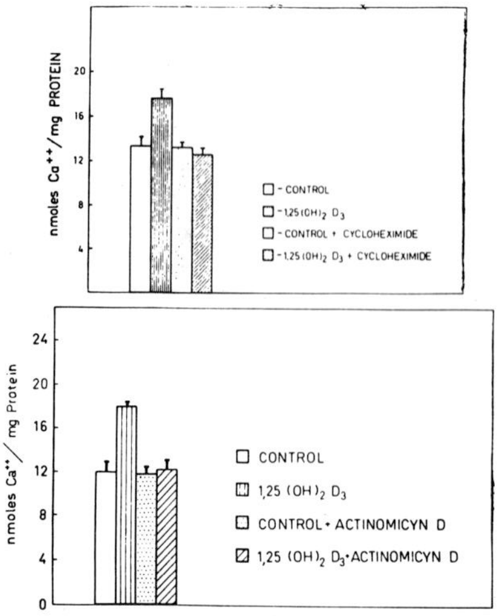

Fig. 5. Effects of protein synthesis inhibitors on $1,25(OH)_2D_3$-dependent Ca uptake by skeletal muscle myoblasts.

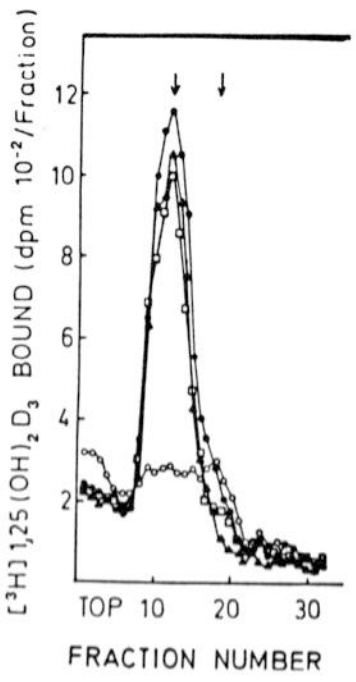

Fig. 6. Sucrose density gradient analysis of (^3H)-$1,25(OH)_2D_3$ binding by chick myoblast cytosol. Binding in the absence (●) and presence of 200-fold molar excess of $1,25(OH)_2D_3$ (o), $25OHD_3$ (▲) or $24,25(OH)_2D_3$ (□). Arrow indicate position of albumin and bovine serum albumin markers (from top to bottom).

without affecting the relative proportions of phospholipid classes (25). This may reflect increased availability of sarcoplasmic PO_4 due to the action of $25OHD_3$ on sarcolemmal PO_4 transport (24-26).

DISCUSSION

S. Massry: The data presented provide evidence of a direct action of $1,25(OH)_2D_3$ on muscle Ca transport. Altered Ca metabolism may be then a factor involved in the myopathy of vitamin D deficiency. However, high levels of PTH as the consequence of secondary hyperparathyroidism might also contribute to muscle disfunction. Receptors for PTH have been found in muscle and the hormone is known to affect the intracellular distribution of Ca. It is important to establish the relative roles of both perturbed vitamin D metabolism and excess PTH in the etiology of this myopathy.

S. Birge: Another effect of $25OHD_3$ on muscle should be taken into consideration. The metabolite has been shown to reduce increased aminoacid release from skeletal muscle in uremic animals.

S. Edelstein: In previous studies low levels of $1,25(OH)_2D_3$ have been found in muscle from experimental animals. In addition, evidence indicating the presence of a receptor for $1,25(OH)_2D_3$ in differentiated skeletal muscle is not yet available. It may be possible that the metabolite affects Ca fluxes in the tissue via a direct membranophilic effect.

R. Simpson: We have found evidence showing that cytosol from cultured skeletal myoblast (G-8) and heart myoblast (H9C2) cells prepared in high salt contain receptors specific for $1,25(OH)_2D_3$. The receptor characteristics were similar to those present in target tissues for the hormone. $1,25(OH)_2D_3$ receptors in both myoblast lines were found to downregulate by 70% when cells were stimulated to differentiate to myotubes. $1,25(OH)_2D_3$ inhibited DNA synthesis and cell proliferation of myoblasts in a dose-dependent manner. We have in addition found that cytosol preparations from cells isolated from skeletal muscle also possess $1,25(OH)_2D_3$ receptors.

CONCLUSIONS:

The discussed data imply that skeletal muscle is a target organ for vitamin D. Electrophysiologically demonstrable abnormalities in muscle contraction and relaxation, independent of changes in blood mineral composition, are observed in vitamin D deficiency. In vivo and in vitro studies clearly suggest that $1,25(OH)_2D_3$ plays a role in the regulation of muscle cell Ca metabolism. The sterol may act on muscle Ca uptake via a nuclear mechanism and through changes in membrane lipids similarly as in intestine. Other work has implied an action of $25OHD_3$ in muscle PO_4 fluxes and protein synthesis. These and future studies may provide an understanding of the etiology of vitamin D-dependent myopathies and may, in addition, prove useful to gain insights into the cellular role of vitamin D in animals.

REFERENCES:

1. De Luca, H.F. and Schnoes, H.K. (1983) Ann.Rev.Biochem. 52, 411-439
2. Norman, A.W., Roth, J. and Orci, L. (1982) Endocrine Rev. 3, 331-366
3. Smith, R. and Stern, G. (1967) Brain 90, 593-602
4. Smith, R. and Stern, G. (1969) J.Neurol.Sci. 8, 511-520
5. Skaria, J., Katiyar, B.C., Srivastava, T.P. and Dube, B. (1975) Acta Neurol.Scandinav. 51, 37-58
6. Schott, G.D. and Wills, M.R. (1976) The Lancet 1, 626-629
7. Floyd, M., Ayyar, D.R., Barwick, D.D., Hudgson, P. and Weightman, D. (1974) Q.J.Med. 43, 509-523
8. Henderson, R.G., Russel, R.G.G., Ledingham, J.G.G., Smith, R., Oliver, D. O., Walton, R.J., Small, D.G., Preston, C., Warner, G.T. and Norman, A. W. (1974) Lancet 1, 379-384
9. Brickman, A.S., Coburn, J.W., Massry, S.G. and Norman, A.W. (1974) Ann. Intern.Med. 80, 161-168
10. Vicale, C.T. (1949) Trans.Am.Neurol.Ass. 74, 143-147
11. Birge, S.J. (1978) Mineral Electrolyte Metab. 1, 57-64
12. Rodman, J.S. and Baker, T. (1978) Kidney Int. 13, 189-193
13. Pleasure, D., Wyszynski, B., Sumner, A., Schotland, D., Feldman, B., Nugent, N. and Hitz, K. (1979) J.Clin.Invest. 64, 1157-1167
14. Ebashi, S. and Endo, M. (1968) Prog.Biophys.Mol.Biol. 18, 123-183
15. Carafoli, E. and Crompton, M. (1978) Curr.Top.Membrane Transp. 10, 151-216
16. Curry, O.B., Bastein, J.F., Francis, M.J.O. and Smith, R. (1974) Nature 249, 83-84
17. Matthews, C., Heimberg, K.W., Ritz, E., Agostini, B., Fritzsche, J. and Hasselbach, W. (1977) Kidney Int. 11, 227-235
18. Boland, R.L., Boland, A.R. de, Ritz, E. and Hasselbach, W. (1983) Calcif.Tissue Int. 35, 190-194
19. Boland, R., Matthews, C., Boland, A.R. de, Ritz, E. and Hasselbach, W. (1983) Calcif.Tissue Int. 35, 195-201
20. Boland, A.R. de, Gallego, S. and Boland, R. (1983) Biochim.Biophys.Acta 733, 264-273
21. Giuliani, D.L. and Boland, R.L. (1984) Calcif.Tissue Int. 36, 200-205
22. Boland, A.R. de, Drittanti, L. and Boland, R.L. (1985) Proc.Sixth Vitamin D Workshop (A.Norman et al., ed.) Walter de Gruyter, Berlin
23. Bauman, V.K., Valinietse, M.Y. and Babarykin, D.A. (1984) Arch.Biochem. Biophys. 231, 211-216
24. Birge, S.J. and Haddad, J.C. (1975) J.Clin.Invest. 56, 1100-1107
25. Boland, A.R. de, Albornoz, L.E. and Boland, R. (1983) Calcif.Tissue Int. 35, 798-805
26. Bellido, T. and Boland, R. (1985) Proc.Sixth Vitamin D Workshop (A.Norman et al., ed.) Walter de Gruyter, Berlin
27. Ströder, J. and Arensmeyer, E. (1965) Klin.Wochenschr. 43, 1201-1202
28. Wilson, P.W. and Lawson, D.E.M. (1978) Biochem.J. 173, 627-631
29. Pointon, J.J., Francis, M.J.O. and Smith, R. (1979) Clin.Sci. 57, 257-263
30. Zot, H.B. and Potter, J.D., in Metal Ions in Biological Systems (H.Sigel, ed.) Marcel Dekker, Inc., New York, 1984, p. 381
31. Boland, A.R. de and Boland, R. (1984) Z.Naturforsch. 39c, 1015-1016

EFFECT OF PLASMA CALCIUM ON BONE IN VITAMIN D DEFICIENT RATS.

W.J. Visser[1], G.J. Schaafsma[2] and S.A. Duursma[1]
[1]Clinical Researchgroup for Bone Metabolism, University Hospital, PO-box 16250, 3500 CG Utrecht, The Netherlands
[2]Department of Nutrition, Netherlands Institute for Dairy Research (NIZO), PO-box 20, 6710 BA Ede, The Netherlands

Introduction

Maternal deprivation of vitamin D causes severe vitamin D deficiency in the offspring of rats at the time of weaning Vitamin D repletion restores bone quality and bone mass.

In the present study we have addressed the question whether the effects of vitamin D on bone are direct ones or mediated by the potency of vitamin D to normalize the plasma calcium concentration.

Therefore we have investigated in detail the relation between plasma calcium and bone in vitamin D deficient rats.

Material and methods

Five groups of male Wistar rats were used. The vitamin D deficient rats were born from vitamin D deficient mothers. Plasma calcium was regulated by dietary manipulation. The experiment started four weeks after birth and was continued for six weeks. At the end of the experiment the femurs were used for chemical and the tibias for histomorphometrical investigation. The rats are subdivided in five groups as follows:

group	n	remarks
D^-	6	D-deficient, D-deficient diet
D^-Ca^+	6	id as D^-, extra Ca (1.0%)
D^-Ca^+Lac	6	id as D^-Ca^+, lactose (15%)
D^+	8	D-deficient, control diet
D^+D^+	6	normal rats, control diet

Results

weight gain, food consumption; a = significantly different from D^+D^+; b = significantly different from D^-; ± SD.

	D^-	D^-Ca^+	D^-Ca^+Lac	D^+	D^+D^+
weight gain (g/6 weeks)	135 ± 20[a]	142 ± 22[a]	147 ± 18[a]	180 ± 31[b]	201 ± 15[b]
consumption (g/6 weeks)	450 ± 31[a]	467 ± 41[a]	500 ± 52[ab]	566 ± 95[b]	604 ± 37[b]

plasma calcium after six weeks; a = significantly different from D^+D^+; b = significantly different from D^-; ± SD.

	D^-	D^-Ca^+	D^-Ca^+Lac	D^+	D^+D^+
plasma Ca(mg/dl)	6.1 ± 0.5[a]	7.0 ± 0.8	9.8 ± 0.7	10.4 ± 0.4	10.5 ± 0.2

Vitamin D. A Chemical, Biochemical and Clinical Update

chemical bone parameters and bone length (femur); a = significantly different from D^+D^+; b = significantly different from D^-; ± SD; dry w. = dry weight (mg); ash% = % dry weight; ash = ash (mg); length = length (mm).

	D^-	D^-Ca^+	D^-Ca^+Lac	D^+	D^+D^+
dry w.	204 ±24a	209 ±24a	282 ±52ab	234 ±24ab	339 ±37b
ash%	57.7± 2.3a	59.5± 1.6a	62.5± 1.4b	63.3± 1.6b	63.5± 1.9b
ash	118 ±17a	125 ±18a	146 ±14ab	178 ±32ab	215 ±29b
length	2.5± 0.1a	2.6± 0.1a	2.7± 0.1ab	2.8± 0.1ab	3.0± 0.1b

histomorphometric parameters (metaphysis, proximal tibia); V_v = volumetric density of trabecular bone (mineralized or not); $V_v os$ = volumetric density of osteoid.

	D^-	D^-Ca^+	D^-Ca^+Lac	D^+	D^+D^+
V_v $^o/oo$	246 ±52a	164 ±25ab	99 ±55b	70 ±21b	73 ±10b
$V_v os$ $^o/oo$	19.5± 7.2a	10.5± 2.3ab	3.3± 3.2ab	< 0.5b	< 0.5b

relation femurlength, ash (% dry weight), V_v $^o/oo$ and $V_v os$ $^o/oo$-in the vitamin D deficient groups (D^-, D^-Ca^+, D^-Ca^+Lac, n = 18) and plasma calcium conc

	r	p
femur length (mm)	0.70	< 0.001
ash $^o/o$	0.81	< 0.001
V_v $^o/oo$	- 0.79	< 0.001
$V_v os$ $^o/oo$	- 0.74	< 0.001

Discussion

It appears that plasma calcium concentrations, which are severely decreased in vitamin D deficient rats, can be brought back to almost normal levels, merely by dietary manipulation. By this measure bone quality parameters like ash $^o/o$, V_v $^o/oo$ and $V_v os$ $^o/oo$ will get almost normal values, whereas the values of the parameters representative for the bone mass (dry weight and bone ash) are only partly restored. The linear correlations which are found between plasma calcium concentrations and bone length, ash $^o/o$, V_v $^o/oo$ and $V_v os$ $^o/oo$ respectively, are at least suggestive for the possibility that these parameters are dependent on the plasma calcium concentration.

Conclusion

Dietary manipulations, resulting in restoration of the plasma calcium concentration of vitamin D deficient rats to nearly normal values, yield almost normal values for bone quality parameters (ash $^o/o$, V_v $^o/oo$, $V_v os$ $^o/oo$), whereas the values for bone mass parameters (dry weight, bone ash) are only partly corrected by this measure.

Pregnancy / Neonatology

HUMAN PLACENTAL 25-HYDROXYVITAMIN D_3-1α-HYDROXYLASE: BIOCHEMICAL CHARACTERIZATION AND ASSESSMENT OF 1α,25-DIHYDROXYVITAMIN D_3 PRODUCTION RATES IN DISORDERS OF MINERAL METABOLISM

J.E. Zerwekh and N.A. Breslau
Department of Internal Medicine, Univerity of Texas Health Science Center at Dallas, Southwestern Medical School, 5323 Harry Hines Blvd., Dallas, TX 75235, U.S.A.

Introduction:

Pregnancy is associated with alterations in calcium (Ca) metabolism and its hormonal regulation, particularly by vitamin D. The serum concentration of 1α, 25-dihydroxyvitamin D [1α,25$(OH)_2$D] has been reported to significantly increase in the mother during pregnancy (1,2) and contributes to the augmented intestinal Ca absorption associated with the pregnant state. Although the kidney is the major site of production of 1,25-$(OH)_2$D in the non-pregnant animal, it has now been well established that the placenta also has the enzymatic capability to produce 1,25-$(OH)_2$D (3-5). In order to understand the placental 25-OHD_3-1α-hydroxylase more fully we have investigated the biochemical nature of this enzyme from normal term placentas obtained at delivery. Furthermore, in order to ascertain whether the placental contribution of 1,25-$(OH)_2D_3$ could be of major significance in pregnant women in whom endogenous renal 1,25-$(OH)_2D_3$ production is deranged, we assessed the in vitro placental 1,25-$(OH)_2D_3$ production rates in two women with PTH-resistant hypoparathyroidism and in one woman with x-linked hypophosphatemic rickets (XLHR).

Methods:

Term human placentas were obtained, with maternal consent, immediately after vaginal delivery and placed on ice. Both amnion and trophoblastic components of the placenta were washed via vigorous squeezing and kneading in ice cold normal saline followed by two washes in 0.25 M sucrose. A 20% (w/v) homogenate of placenta was prepared in 0.25 M sucrose. For studies of subcellular localization, placental mitochondria were prepared as previously described (6). Placental microsomes were obtained after ultra-centrifugation of the mitochondria-free supernatant at 100,00 x g for 1 hour. Placental homogenates were incubated as previously described (4,5). The reaction was initiated by the addition of 200 µg 25-OHD_3 in 20 µl ethanol. Controls were prepared by either boiling the tissue incubation buffer mixture or extracting it with methanol:chloroform (2:1) prior to the addition of 25-OHD_3. The production of 1,25$(OH)_2D_3$ was quantitated by chick intestinal cytosol receptor assay after Sephadex LH-20 and high pressure liquid chromatography. To insure that the putative 1,25-$(OH)_2D_3$ region was authentic, some specimens underwent three additional different HPLC purification steps including the use of a reverse phase systen. In these studies, the putative 1,25-$(OH)_2D_3$ binding activity, as assessed by the cytosol-receptor assay, comigrated with radioactive 1,25-$(OH)_2D_3$ in all HPLC purification steps.

Results:

In all experiments crude homogenates of human placental tropho-

Vitamin D. A Chemical, Biochemical and Clinical Update

blastic tissue were capable of producing $1,25-(OH)_2D_3$ in vitro. The amnion did not demonstrate this activity. The mean production rate for seven normal placentas was 240±61 SE pg/mg protein/hr. An assessment of the sub-cellular localization of the placental $25-OHD_3-1\alpha$-hydroxylase clearly disclosed the enzyme to be of mitochondrial origin. Utilizing mitochondria free of vitamin D binding protein (as assessed by rocket immunoelectrophoresis), the velocity of $1,25-(OH)_2D_3$ formation demonstrated saturation kinetics with an apparent Km of 0.57 μM (Lineweaver-Burk) or 0.44 μM (Eadie-Hofstee).

Table 1 summarizes the $1,25-(OH)_2D_3$ production rates by placental homogenates for seven normal women and for two women with pseudohypoparathyroidism. In addition, a third woman with XLHR was also examined in a similar fashion. Both patients with pseudohypoparathyroidism demonstrated placental $1,25-(OH)_2D_3$ production rates below the mean value for the seven normal subjects. The mean value (161±3) was not significantly different from that of the normal controls. The patient with XLHR demonstrated a placental $1,25-(OH)_2D_3$ production rate of 564 pg/mg protein/hr. This value was significantly different from the normal controls ($p<0.05$) as determined with the 1 sample t-test.

Table 1. Production of $1,25-(OH)_2D_3$ by homogenates of human placenta

Patient	$1,25-(OH)_2D_3$ (pg/mg protein/hr.)
Normal (7)	240±61[a]
Pseudohypopara	165
Pseudohypopara	156
XLHR	564*

[a] Expressed as mean ± SEM. * Significantly different from normals at $p<0.05$ with a 1 sample t-test.

Conclusions:

In the present report, we have demonstrated that the human placenta is capable of synthesizing $1,25-(OH)_2D_3$. The enzymatic activity is principally in the trophoblasts and is localized to the mitochondria. The production rates, while less than those reported for the kidney, are of sufficient magnitude to conceivably supply the mothers' requirements for $1,25-(OH)_2D_3$ and ensure a normal calcium supply for the fetus. Additional studies will be required to fully delineate the role of placental $1,25-(OH)_2D_3$ synthesis in pregnancy and what metabolic and endocrine factors regulate its production.

References:

1. Steichen, J.J., Tsang, R.C., Gratton, T.L., Hamstra, A. and DeLuca, H.F. (1980) N. Engl. J. Med. 302, 315-319.
2. Kumar, R., Cohen, W.R., Silva, P. and Epstein, F.H. (1979) J. Clin. Invest. 63, 342-344.
3. Gray, T.K., Lester, G.E. and Lorenc, R.S. (1979) Science 204, 1311-1312.
4. Tanaka, Y., Halloran, B., Schnoes, H.K. and DeLuca, H.F. (1979) Proc. Natl. Acad. Sci. U.S.A. 76, 5033-5035.
5. Whitsett, J.A., Ho, M., Tsang, R.C., Norman, E.J. and Adams, K.G. (1981) J. Clin. Endocrinol. Metab. 53, 484-488.
6. Simpson, E.R. and Miller, D.A. (1978) Arch. Biochem. Biophys. 190, 800-808.

VITAMIN D IN THE RAT FETUS AND NEONATE; INTRAUTERINE TRANSFER AND MILK SUPPLY

M.R. CLEMENTS and D.R. FRASER,
University Department of Medicine, Manchester Royal Infirmary, Manchester M13 9WL, and University of Cambridge and Medical Research Council, Dunn Nutritional Laboratory, Cambridge CB4 1XJ, England.

Vitamin D-deficient female Norwegian hooded rats were given depot injections of ^{3}H-vitamin D_3 or ^{14}C-vitamin D_3 both subcutaneously (in propylene glycol) and intramuscularly (in arachis oil) prior to mating. The ^{3}H-dosed rats were sacrificed during gestation on days 14,17,19 and 21. Total lipid was extracted from individual fetuses with chloroform: methanol (1:2 v/v) and chromatographed on Silica Sep-paks and Sephadex LH20 to determine the distribution of metabolites.

Results

The fetuses increased in weight from 127.6 ± 3.5 mg (mean ± s.e.m.) on day 14 to 4.82 ± 0.14 g at birth on day 22. The total vitamin D content of individual fetuses increased rapidly during the last third of gestation to 62.2 ± 3.3 pmol/pup at birth. There was a linear increase in the concentration of $25(OH)D_3$, $24,25(OH)_2D_3$, and D_3 itself from days 14-19. During this period, $t_{\frac{1}{2}}$ of ^{3}H in maternal plasma fell by a factor of 17-fold, suggesting that a specific mechanism was transferring vitamin D molecules into the fetuses.

At birth the major metabolite in the pups was $25(OH)D_3$ (58.3 ± 1.2%) with significant amounts of $24,25(OH)_2D_3$ (29.0 ± 1.2%) and unchanged D_3 (3.0 ± 0.2%). The highest tissue concentration of vitamin D was found in the hind limbs (16.72 ± 0.54 pmol/g) where it was equally distributed between muscle and skin. Lower concentrations were found in the carcass (14.35 ± 0.57 pmol/g), stomach (9.37 ± 2.5 pmol/g), intestine (8.99 ± 0.45 pmol/g), and liver (5.67 ± 0.30 pmol/g). The predominant metabolites in muscle were $25(OH)D_3$ (46%), D_3 itself (14%) and $24,25(OH)_2D_3$ (9%).

Vitamin D levels in the gut reflected those in the rat milk. Immediately after birth, the pups from ^{3}H- and from ^{14}C-labelled mothers were exchanged and later sacrificed after 1-3 weeks of suckling. Total lipid extracts were chromatographed and analysed for ^{3}H and ^{14}C content to determine the relative contribution of vitamin D supplied before birth via the placenta and after birth in the milk. The vitamin D content of the rat milk was relatively high (1.1-3.3 µg/l) becuase of its high fat content (17-21%) and the vitamin, was present mainly as D_3 itself (70.6 ± 7.4%) during the first week of lactation. Nevertheless the supply of vitamin D in utero, rather than from milk, was the main determinant of vitamin D status in early neonatal life.

These results are the first demonstration in a mammal of the existence of a specific transfer mechanism which allows the fetus to accumulate vitamin D from the mother during the last third of gestation. The vitamin is widely distributed within the fetus in multiple extrahepatic tissue sites.

25-HYDROXYVITAMIN D LEVELS IN PREFEEDING AND POSTFEEDING HUMAN MILK.

M. Ala-Houhala and T. Koskinen

Department of Pediatrics, University Central Hospital of Tampere, Department of Clinical Sciences, University of Tampere, P.O. Box 607, SF-33520 Tampere, Finland.

Breast milk, the sole source of energy of newborn, contains adequate amounts of most nutritients, but not of vitamin D (1-2). Factors influencing the excretion of antirachitic sterols into milk in breast tissue have not, however, been identified. We attempted to elucidate the factors affecting the antirachitic value of human milk by measuring 25-hydroxyvitamin D (25(OH)D) levels in prefeeding and postfeeding breast milk obtained from mothers with and without vitamin D supplementation.

MATERIALS AND METHODS

We obtained milk (prefeeding and postfeeding) and serum samples from healthy women (n=40) after 20 weeks' lactation in May and in December. The samples were stored at -70°C until analysed. Half of the mothers were supplemented with 1000 IU of vitamin D_2 daily.

25(OH)D consentrations in breast milk were determined by the competitive protein-binding method after purification described by Parviainen et al (3). Serum 25(OH)D levels were determined by the competitive protein-binding method after C_{18} Sep-Pak chromatography and high-performance liquid chromatography. Statistically significant differences were tested by non-paired Student's t-test.

RESULTS

25(OH)D (mean ± SEM) levels in human milk and serum samples collected in May and in December are presented in the supplemented (1000 IU D_2/day) and nonsupplemented mother groups in Table:

	Supplemented mothers 25(OH)D (ng/ml)	Nonsupplemented mothers 25(OH)D (ng/ml)
May (n=12)		
Milk		
-prefeeding	$0.24^a \pm 0.04$	$0.13^a \pm 0.01$
- postfeeding	$0.35^b \pm 0.04$	$0.19^b \pm 0.03$
Serum	$28^c \pm 3.5$	$16^c \pm 2.3$
December (n=8)		
Milk		
-prefeeding	0.41 ± 0.07	0.21 ± 0.07
-postfeeding	0.45 ± 0.07	0.31 ± 0.08
Serum	15 ± 1.1	12 ± 1.4

a: $p < 0.01$, b: $p < 0.05$, c: $p < 0.02$

Vitamin D. A Chemical, Biochemical and Clinical Update

The 25(OH)D levels in human milk were affected according to the supplementation and the season, but the 25(OH)D levels in human milk did not correlate to the serum levels of the mothers or infants. In postfeeding breast milk samples, which reportedly have higher lipid concentration than in prefeeding milk (4), the levels of 25(OH)D tended to be higher.

COMMENTS

The present study suggests that the antirachitic activity of breast milk is dependent on the mother's exposure to sunlight and vitamin D intake.

References

1. Jennes, R. (1979) Seminares in Perinatology 3, 225-239.
2. Ala-Houhala, M. J. Pediatr. Gastroenterol. Nutr. in press.
3. Parviainen, M.T., Koskinen T., Ala-Houhala, M and Visakorpi, J.K. (1984) Acta Vitaminol. Enzymol. 6, 211-219.
4. Dorea, J.D., Horner, M.R., Bezerra, V.L.V.A. (1982) J. Pediatr. 101, 80-83.

THE PATTERN OF PLASMA IONIZED CALCIUM, CALCITONIN AND VITAMIN D METABOLITES IN DEVELOPING CHICK EMBRYOS

S.K. Abbas, J. Fox and A.D. Care, Department of Animal Physiology and Nutrition, University of Leeds, Leeds LS2 9JT, United Kingdom.

INTRODUCTION: Parathyroid hormone (PTH) and calcitonin (CT) influence calcium homeostasis during the last quarter of incubation in chick embryos (1-3) and it is known that chick embryonic kidney is capable of metabolising 25-(OH)D to 1,25-$(OH)_2D$ (4,5) from day 9 onwards. Ichikawa et al. (6) found detectable serum levels of vitamin D metabolites in 15 day old chick embryos. Generally the secretion of CT is not associated with conditions favouring the secretion of 1,25-$(OH)_2D$ although there are reports of 1-hydroxylase stimulation in rat kidney by CT (7,8). In contrast, CT has been found to inhibit the conversion of 25-(OH)D to 1,25-$(OH)_2D$ in isolated renal tubules from vitamin D-deficient chicks (9) but this has not been confirmed. This study was designed to investigate the relationships between ionized calcium (Ca^{++}), CT and vitamin D metabolites and their effects on calcium homeostasis during the last phase of incubation in chick embryos.

MATERIALS AND METHODS: Blood samples were collected from chick embryos from day 16 of incubation until hatching (day 20/21) and from newly-hatched (NH) and 1,2 and 7 day-old (DO) chicks. Equal volumes of plasma were pooled to give a sample of 3ml for assay (n=5/day). Plasma Ca^{++} concentrations were determined by an ionized calcium electrode. Chick plasma CT levels were measured by radioimmunoassay using a rabbit anti-salmon CT (sCT) antiserum (a gift from Professor T.G. Taylor). Assay sensitivity was 250 pg/ml when synthetic sCT (Armour Pharmaceutical Co., U.K.) was used both as standard and tracer in a non-equilibrium assay. Vitamin D metabolites were extracted from 2 ml of plasma (10) and were measured by radioimmunoassay (11). Data were subjected to analysis of variance or Student's t-test where appropriate.

RESULTS: As incubation proceeded, plasma Ca^{++} concentration increased from 0.91 ± 0.02 (SEM) mmol/l at day 16 to 1.28 ± 0.03 mmol/l ($P<0.001$) at pipping (day 20B). IT then decreased in NH chicks before rising again in 1, 2 and 7 DO chicks. Plasma CT levels increased from 1.1 ± 0.1 ng/ml on day 16, peaking at 2.7 ± 0.1 ng/ml at pipping ($P<0.001$) and decreased in all hatched chicks. There is a positive correlation between CT and Ca^{++} (Fig.1) during the last quarter of incubation ($n = 30$; $r = 0.73$; $P<0.001$). Plasma 1,25-$(OH)_2D$ gradually decreased from day 16 (59.1 ± 2.9) to 42.9 ± 2.6 pg/ml ($P<0.01$) until pipping but increased afterwards in hatched chicks. There is a negative correlation between 1,25-$(OH)_2D$ and CT ($n = 29$; $r = -0.59$; $P<0.001$) (Fig.2) and Ca^{++} and 1,25-$(OH)_2D$ ($n = 29$; $r = -0.46$; $P<0.05$) (Fig.3) during incubation. 25-$(OH)D_3$ and 25,26-$(OH)_2D_3$ showed only minor changes while 24,25-$(OH)_2D_3$ did not change throughout the period of study (Fig.4).

DISCUSSION: The increase in plasma CT levels as the incubation proceeded presumably resulted from the increase in Ca^{++} concentrations seen during that period and accords with the findings of Baimbridge and Taylor (3). The decrease in 1,25-$(OH)_2D$ also seen during that period may be a normal homeostatic responce to hypercalcaemia, similar to that observed in chicks after hatching (12). The significant negative correlation between CT and 1,25-$(OH)_2D$ in embryonic chick plasma suggests that CT has no stimulatory effect on 25-(OH)-1-hydroxylase activity. The rise in plasma 1,25-$(OH)_2D$ at hatching correlates with a fall in Ca^{++} concentration which presumably resulted from the delay between cessation of influx of shell calcium and the onset of absorption of dietary calcium. The plasma CT concentration at this time falls along with Ca^{++} and further negates a positive correlation

Vitamin D. A Chemical, Biochemical and Clinical Update

between CT and 1,25-(OH)$_2$D secretion. The reason for the changes seen in other vitamin D metabolites are not clear.

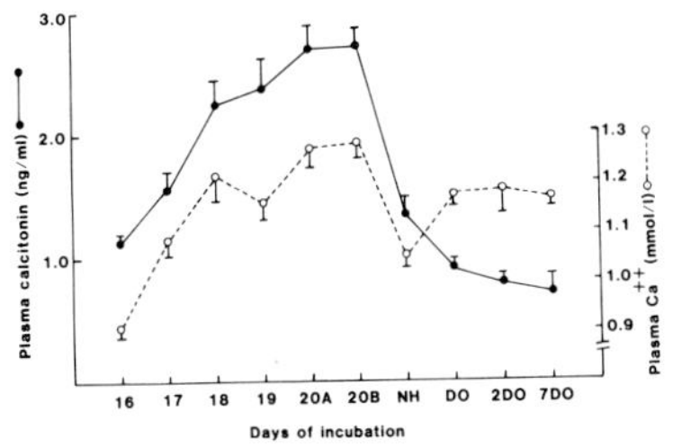

Fig.1. Plasma calcitonin (ng eq. sCT) and ionized calcium in chick embryos before and after hatching.

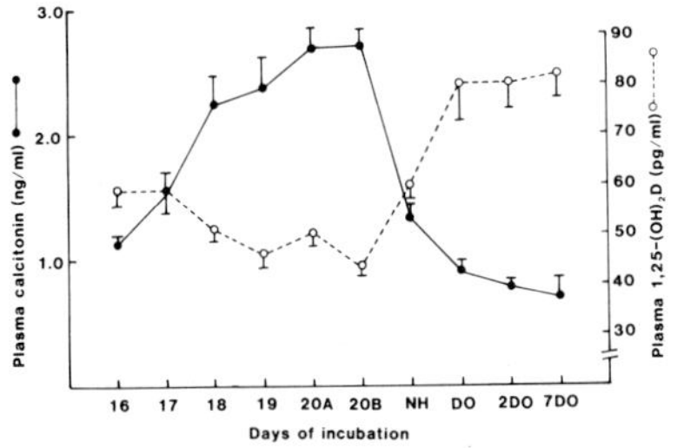

Fig.2. Plasma calcitonin and 1,25-(OH)$_2$D in chick embryos before and after hatching.

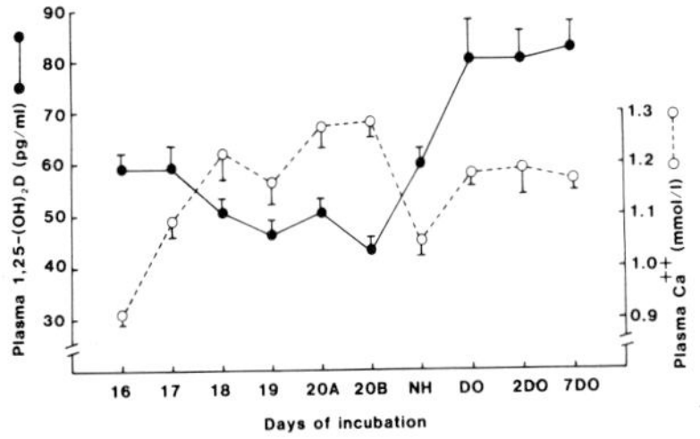

Fig.3. Plasma ionized calcium and 1,25-(OH)$_2$D in chick embryos before and after hatching.

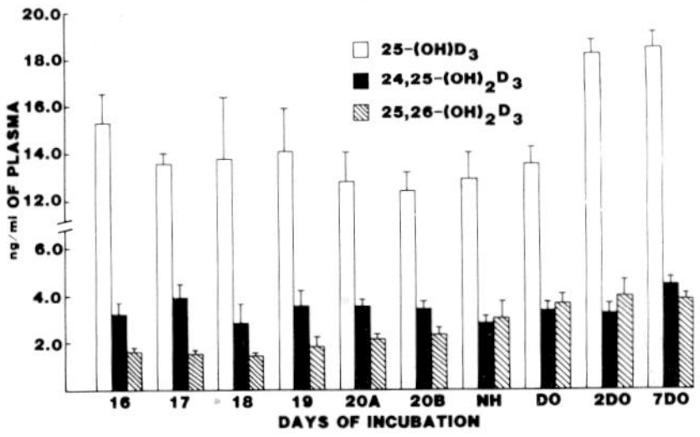

Fig.4. Plasma 25-(OH)D$_3$, 24,25-(OH)$_2$ D$_3$ and 25,26-(OH)$_2$D$_3$ in chick embryos before and after hatching.

20A, Lung respiration; 20B, Pipping; NH, Newly hatched chick; DO, Day-old; 2DO, 2 days old and 7DO, 7 days old chicks.

REFERENCES

1. Narbaitz, R. (1975) Gen. Comp. Endocrinol. 27, 122-124.
2. Clark, N.B. and Mok, L.L.S. (1982) Gen. Comp. Endocrinol. 48, 14-19.
3. Baimbridge, K.G. and Taylor, T.G. (1980) J. Endocrinol. 85, 171-185.
4. Moriuchi, S. and DeLuca, H.F. (1974) Arch. Biochem. Biophys. 164, 165-167.
5. Bishop, J.E. and Norman, A.W. (1975) Arch. Biochem. Biophys. 167, 769-773.
6. Ichikawa, M., Ishige, H., Yoshino, H., Yamaoka, K., Ishida, M., Yabuuchi, M. and Avioli, L.V. (1982) In: "Vitamin D Chemical, Biochemical and Clinical Endocrinology of Calcium Metabolism" Eds: Norman, A.W., Schaefer, K., Herrath, D.V. and Grigoleit, H.G. Walter de Gruyter & Co., Berlin, New York. pp. 97-99.
7. Horiuchi, N., Takahashi, H., Matsumoto, T., Takahashi, N., Shimazawa, E., Suda, T. and Ogata, E. (1979) Biochem. J. 184, 269-275.
8. Kawashima, H., Torikai, S. and Kurokawa, K. (1981) Nature 291, 365-370.
9. Rasmussen, H., Wong, M., Bikle, D. and Goodman, D.B.P. (1972) J. Clin. Invest. 51, 2502-2504.
10. Fraher, L.J., Adami, S., Clemens, T.L., Jones, G. and O'Riordan, J.L.H. (1983) Clin. Endocrinol. 19, 151-165.
11. Clemens,T.L., Hendy, G.N., Papapoulos, S.E., Fraher, L.G., Care, A.D. and O'Riordan, J.L.H. (1979) Clin. Endocrinol. 11, 225-234.
12. Fox, J and Care, A.D. (1978) Calcif. Tiss. Res. 26, 243-245.

CLINICAL & BIOCHEMICAL STUDIES IN INFANTILE HYPERCALCAEMIA

N.D.T. Martin, G.J.A.I. Snodgrass, R.D. Cohen, Caroline E. Porteous, Ruth D. Coldwell, D.J.H. Trafford & H.L.J. Makin.
Medical Unit and Departments of Child Health & Chemical Pathology, The London Hospital Medical College, London E1 2AD, UK.

139 cases of 'The Elfin Facies Syndrome' (1) have been studied and the results obtained extend our previously reported findings (2). Males and females were equally affected and their age ranged from 1 - 31 years. We estimate that the incidence in the United Kingdom is 1:25,000 total live births, given that 50% of cases have been identified. We compared the clinical features of 87 cases who had proven hypercalcaemia of infancy (Group 1) with 52 cases for whom such evidence was lacking (Group 2) and confirmed that the phenotype was identical. However we found that, in general, feeding problems and developmental delay were more marked in Group 1. Therefore we suggest that hypercalcaemia is linked to this phenotype but is expressed with variable frequency and penetration. For 31 cases in whom IQ data were available, a negative correlation was found between the age of diagnosis and the subsequent IQ. These data were not standardised but do suggest that earlier diagnosis could improve eventual intelligence.

Concentrations of metabolites of vitamin D_3 and 25-hydroxyvitamin D_2 (25-OHD_2) were estimated in plasma from 52 cases from Group 1 and 31 cases from Group 2 and compared with values obtained from 33 age matched controls of normal intelligence (Table 1). Metabolites were assayed by

Table 1. Plasma concentrations of vitamin D metabolites in the 'elfin facies syndrome'.

	GROUP 1	GROUP 2	CONTROLS
25-OHD_2	3.3 ± 0.7 (46)	2.0 ± 0.3 (27)	2.6 ± 0.6 (27)
25-OHD_3	14.7 ± 0.9 (52)*	14.0 ± 1.4 (30)*	21.0 ± 2.4 (30)
1,25$(OH)_2D$	51.7 ± 7.1 (38)	53.7 ± 17.7 (20)	58.5 ± 12.2 (17)
24,25$(OH)_2D_3$	0.75 ± 0.10 (40)	0.84 ± 0.14 (22)	1.14 ± 0.24 (20)
25,26$(OH)_2D_3$	0.19 ± 0.02 (31)*	0.20 ± 0.03 (19)*	0.35 ± 0.07 (10)

All values are expressed as Mean + 1SEM (n) and the units are in ng/ml except for 1,25(OH)D which is in pg/ml. * indicates a significant difference from control values ($P < 0.05$).

mass fragmentography, HPLC and radioreceptor assay. No difference was found between cases with or without proven hypercalcaemia of infancy. The plasma concentration of 25-OHD_3 was significantly less in cases than controls but no difference was found in the levels of 1,25-dihydroxyvitamin D (1,25$(OH)_2D$). We suggest this difference may be due to the mental handicap in the patients, leading to a more sedentary life-style and hence less sunlight exposure. Two infants were seen during the hypercalcaemic phase, before treatment had been started. The plasma concentrations of 25-OHD_2 appeared to be elevated (8.0 and 33.1 ng/ml) but the concentrations of 25-OHD_3, 1,25$(OH)_2D$ and 24,25-dihydroxyvitamin D_3 (24,25$(OH)_2D_3$) were normal. However the range of

Vitamin D. A Chemical, Biochemical and Clinical Update

plasma 25-OHD_2 concentrations associated with vitamin D intoxication is much higher than the values observed here, and similar levels of 25-OHD_2 were seen in 2 normocalcaemic cases, and thus the relevance of these observations to the presence of hypercalcaemia in these infants remains obscure.

We have also studied the metabolism of an intravenous bolus injection of tritiated vitamin D_3 in 5 adolescents with the elfin facies syndrome, their mothers', and 5 controls of normal intelligence who were matched for age with the cases. It had previously been suggested that there might be some abnormality of 25-OHD metabolism in this syndrome, since after administration of pharmacological doses of vitamin D, higher plasma concentrations of 25-OHD were found in cases than in normals (3). However in our study,there appeared to be no difference in the metabolism of 25-OHD_3, since we were unable to show any difference in the rate at which radiolabel appeared in or was removed from the 25OHD fraction between any of the groups studied (Figure 1). The results of

Figure 1. Clearance of tritium from the 25-OHD fraction. Mean ± SEM

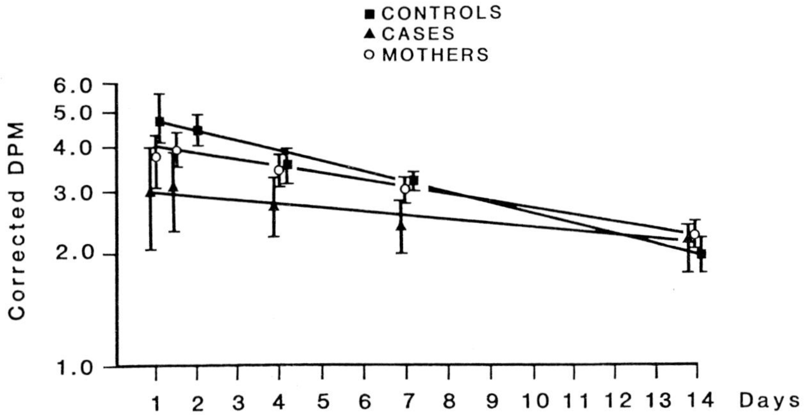

the studies reported here therefore provide no evidence to suggest that an abnormality in vitamin D metabolism is involved in the pathogenesis of hypercalcaemia associated with the 'elfin facies syndrome'. However we consider that if there is some disturbance in vitamin D metabolism in these children, it is more likely to involve vitamin D_2 rather than vitamin D_3.

These studies were directly supported by grants from The Infantile Hypercalcaemia Foundation and Action Research for the Crippled Child to whom we are very grateful.

REFERENCES

1. Jones, K.L., and Smith, D.W. (1975) J. Pediatr. 86, 718-723
2. Martin, N.D.T., Snodgrass, G.J.A.I., and Cohen, R.D. (1984) Arch. Dis. Childh. 59, 605-613
3. Taylor, A.B., Stern, P.H., and Bell, N.H. (1982) New Eng. J. Med. 306, 972-975

EFFECTS OF 24,24-F_2-1α,25-[OH]$_2$-VITAMIN D (F_2-VD) ON SERUM ELECTROLYTES, CIRCULATING LEVELS OF VITAMIN D (VD) METABOLITES, AND SERUM PARATHYROID HORMONE (iPTH) IN PARTURIENT DAIRY COWS.

C.C. CAPEN, K. KERSTING, R.L. HORST,* G.F. HOFFSIS, E.T. LITTLEDIKE,*
Depts. Veterinary Pathobiology & Clinical Sciences, THE OHIO STATE UNIVERSITY, Columbus, Ohio; National Animal Disease Center,* Ames, Iowa, U.S.A.

Introduction:

Dairy cows have active and responsive mineral homeostatic mechanisms because of the profound drain of calcium (CA) into the milk. The failure of these control mechanisms at parturition results in the development of a disease (termed parturient hypocalcemia (PH) or "milk fever") characterized by rapidly developing hypocalcemia, hypophosphatemia, and muscle paresis.

The objectives of this investigation were: (1) To determine the effects of a single (100 µg) intramuscular (IM) dose of F_2-VD on serum CA, phosphorus (P), and magnesium (MG); (2) to correlate circulating levels of selected VD metabolites with changes in serum electrolytes and iPTH, and ultrastructural changes in parathyroid glands; and (3) to evaluate potential toxic effects of F_2-VD in pregnant dairy cows.

Methods and Experimental Design:

Serum CA was determined by atomic absorption spectrophotometry. Serum P (1) and VD metabolites (2) were determined by methods described. F_2-VD was separated from 1α,25-(OH)$_2$-VD by HPLC on a Zorbax Sil column developed with 97:3 methylene chloride:isopropanol. 1α,25-(OH)$_2$-VD migrated at the 29 ml region whereas F_2-VD migrated at 20 ml. Serum iPTH was determined by radioimmunoassay using an N-terminal antibody, ^{125}I-labeled bovine PTH (1-84), and bovine PTH (1-34) for the standard (3). Urinary total hydroxyproline (HOP) was determined by the method of Kivirriko et al. (4) and creatinine (CR) by the method of Clarke (5).

Experimental (exp.) cows - Seven pregnant, PH-susceptible Jersey cows (mean body wt. 468 kg) were injected IM with a 100 µg dose (mean 0.21 µg/kg) of F_2-VD on day (da.) 8 (mean) (range 1-16) prior to the actual date of parturition. Controls - Parturient Jersey cows (n=6) were injected with placebo 3.25 da. (range 1 to 5) prepartum. Both groups of cows were fed an identical grain-corn cob mix supplemented with $CACO_3$ to provide 80 gm CA/da. but no hay.

Results:

Serum CA (mg/dl) in pregnant cows administered F_2-VD was elevated above baseline after 1 da., attained peak values by da. 3 (10.6 $\pm$ 0.5), and remained above baseline levels for 6 da. post-injection (PI). Serum CA in exp. cows on da. 3 PI was increased 2.4 mg/dl above controls (Fig. 1). Serum MG in exp. cows had declined by da. 1 PI and remained below baseline values and control cows for 6 da. PI. PH-susceptible cows given F_2-VD did not develop clinical signs of hypocalcemia near parturition. Serum P (mg/dl) in cows administered F_2-VD were elevated above baseline at da. 1 PI (6.9 $\pm$ 0.5), attained peak levels at 4.5 da. PI (8.3 $\pm$ 0.9), and remained increased above baseline and controls for 7 da. PI.

Serum F_2-VD (pg/ml) in exp. cows was increased markedly (70 $\pm$ 12) by da. 1 PI of difluorinated metabolite compared to baseline and controls (<2), had declined progressively to 6.0 $\pm$ 4 on da. 6 PI, and returned to baseline by PI da. 7 (Fig. 2). There was a reciprocal decline in serum 1α,25-(OH)$_2$-VD in exp. cows as the F_2-VD and serum CA concentrations increased after injection of the difluorinated metabolite. Serum 1α,25-(OH)$_2$-VD levels at PI da. 3 (peak serum CA) were 30.5 $\pm$ 6 compared to baseline (64.2 $\pm$ 14). Serum 1α,25-(OH)$_2$-VD in controls increased with

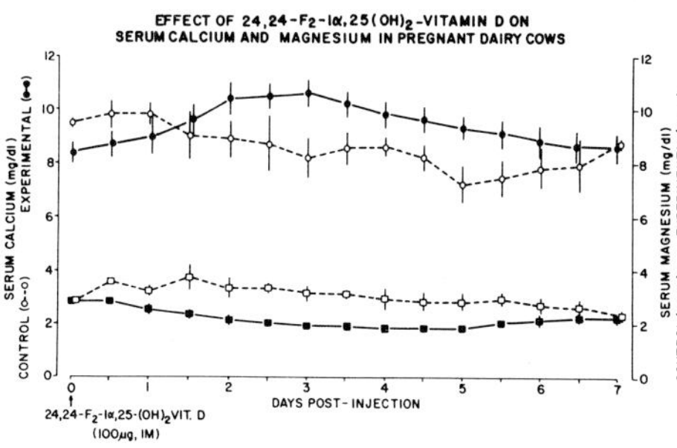

Fig. 1

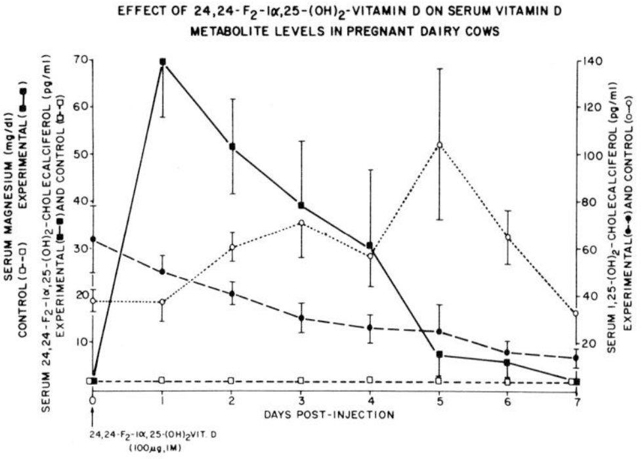

Fig. 2

the approach of parturition (baseline - 38 $\pm$ 5; da. 5 PI = 105 $\pm$ 32) in response to the greater decline in serum CA than in exp. cows that received the F_2-VD (Fig. 2).

Serum iPTH (ng/ml) in cows administered F_2-VD was decreased on PI da. 2 (0.3 $\pm$ .06) and da. 3 (0.25 $\pm$ .06) ($p<0.05$) compared to controls (PI da. 2 = 0.93 $\pm$ .14; da. 3 - 0.94 $\pm$ 0.3). The decline in serum iPTH correlated with the increase in serum CA on da. 2 and 3 PI in exp. cows whereas the increase in circulating iPTH levels corresponded to the decrease in serum CA from da. 1 to 4 PI in controls (Fig. 1).

Urinary excretion of CA, P, MG, and HOP:CR was evaluated as % change between pre- and post-injection of F_2-VD. Urinary P (51%), CA (16%), and HOP (1.8%) were increased in cows receiving F_2-VD. The decreased serum MG in exp. cows was accompanied by a lesser increase in urinary MG excretion (1.6%) than in controls (5%). Urine samples were collected 1 (control) or 2 (exp.) da. pre-injection and 5 (control) or 5.7 da. (exp.) PI (mean intervals).

Active chief cells with well-developed organelles predominated in parathyroid glands from cows administered F_2-VD. There often was a peripheral accumulation of PTH-containing secretory granules near the plasma membrane in response to the increased serum CA in cows receiving F_2-VD. There were no gross or microscopic lesions of soft tissue mineralization or other evidence of toxicity in pregnant cows administered 100 μg F_2-VD.

Summary:

(1) PH-susceptible Jersey cows administered F_2-VD (100 μg) had elevated serum CA and P, decreased serum MG, and more stable circulating electrolyte levels in the immediate postpartal period than control parturient cows; (2) Circulating F_2-VD increased rapidly (peak on day 1 PI) following IM injection of the difluorinated metabolite but progressively declined to baseline levels by day 7 PI. The increased serum CA in experimental cows was associated with a progressive decline in circulating 1α,25-$(OH)_2$-VD and iPTH levels, accumulation of secretory granules in parathyroid chief cells, and increased urinary CA (and P) excretion; (3) Parturient dairy cows administered F_2-VD did not develop soft tissue mineralization in response to the moderately increased serum CA and P.

References:

1. Fiske, C.H., Subbarow, Y., (1925) J. Biol. Chem. 66:375-400.
2. Horst, R.L., et al. (1981) Anal. Biochem. 116:189-203.
3. Arnaud, C.D., Tsao, H.S., Littledike, E.T. (1971) J. Clin. Invest. 50:21-33.
4. Kivirikko, K.I., Laitinen, O., Prockop, D.J. (1967) Anal. Biochem. 19:249-255.
5. Clarke, J.T. (1961) Clin. Chem. 7:371-383.

25-HYDROXYVITAMIN D IN HUMAN BREAST MILK

N.R. BELTON
Department of Child Life and Health, University of Edinburgh, Edinburgh EH9 1UW, Scotland, U.K.
F. COCKBURN
Department of Child Health, University of Glasgow.

INTRODUCTION

Despite reportedly low concentrations of biologically active vitamin D in human breast milk (< 20 I.U./l), breast-fed babies rarely suffer from neonatal hypocalcaemia and are not regarded as being particularly susceptible to rickets. In 1977 it was suggested (1) that water-soluble vitamin D sulphate in human milk might be an important anti-rachitic factor. More recent studies have shown that it is unlikely to be so (2). It seemed possible, however, that other vitamin D metabolites were present in human milk in significant amounts.

We have measured 25-hydroxyvitamin D in breast milk obtained from mothers during the first week after delivery of their infants and compared the values with the plasma 25-OHD results obtained from blood collected at the same time.

METHOD

5 or 10 ml of breast milk was extracted with chloroform/methanol (1:1) and the extract thereafter treated as described for plasma extracts. Plasma 25-hydroxyvitamin D was measured by a competitive protein-binding assay based on that of Preece (3). The method was chloroform/methanol (1:1) extraction, silicic acid chromatography (Sigma LC-325 mesh) and the assay used serum from vitamin D-deficient rats, high specific activity ^{3}H 25-hydroxycholecalciferol (22Ci/umol - Amersham) and dextran (Pharmacia T20) coated charcoal (Norit GSX) to separate bound from free 25-OHD. The coefficient of variation between assays was 10.2% (n = 20).

RESULTS

Mean 25-OHD concentration in breast milk was 224 pg/ml (S.D. ± 226) and the range 34 - 730. Plasma 25-OHD (ng/ml) was 12.1 (mean) ± 5.3 (S.D.) with a range 6.9 - 24.9. As can be seen from the figure there is no significant correlation between plasma and breast milk 25-OHD concentrations (r = 0.12).

Vitamin D. A Chemical, Biochemical and Clinical Update

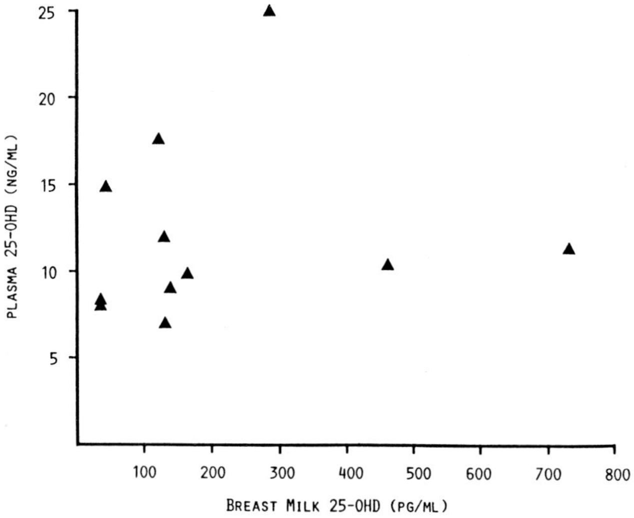

Figure. Comparison of 25-hydroxyvitamin D (25-OHD) in human breast milk and plasma.

DISCUSSION

It seems clear from these studies that 25-OHD in human breast milk is only present in a concentration equivalent to less than 10% of its concentration in plasma. The possibility must be considered that as our estimation only measures free 25-OHD in the lipid fraction our results might not necessarily reflect the total 25-OHD if, for example, in human milk a significantly higher proportion of the total than in the plasma was protein-bound and not extracted. However, as the total protein in human milk (just over 1 g/100 ml) is significantly less than that in plasma (7 g/100 ml), this seems unlikely. Greer et al (4) in a recent study agreed that there was no significant correlation between the serum concentration of 25-hydroxyvitamin D_3 and its concentration in human milk but gave no actual values. They also found no correlation between the fat content of human milk and the concentrations of vitamin D_3, vitamin D_2, 25-hydroxyvitamin D_3, 25-hydroxyvitamin D_2 or total vitamin D.

From our study, therefore, 25-OHD in human breast milk does not appear to be a significant source of vitamin D intake in the breast-fed infant.

REFERENCES

1. Lakdawala, D.R., Widdowson, E.M. (1977) Lancet, 1, 167-8.
2. Greer, F.R., Reeve, L.E., Chesney, R.W. and De Luca, H.F. (1982) Pediatrics, 69, 238.
3. Preece, M.A., O'Riordan, J.L.H., Lawson, D.E.M. and Kodicek, E. (1974) Clin. Chim. Acta, 54. 235-242.
4. Greer, F.R., Hollis, B.W., Cripps, D.J. and Tsang, R.C. (1984) J. Pediatr., 105, 431-3.

BONE MINERAL CONTENT (BMC) OF INFANTS OF DIABETIC MOTHERS (IDM's)

F. Mimouni, M.D.; J. Steichen, M.D.; W. Brazerol, B.S.; V. Hertzberg, Ph.D.; R.C. Tsang, M.D.
Department of Pediatrics, University of Cincinnati Medical Center, 231 Bethesda Avenue, Cincinnati, Ohio 45267-0541, USA

Introduction:

The mechanism of hypocalcemia in IDM's is poorly understood. Hypomagnesemia, due to maternal magnesium losses, has been suggested as a cause of functional hypoparathyroidism in IDM's, and subsequent hypocalcemia (1,2). Decreased BMC has been reported in diabetic patients (3). Bone mineralization of IDM's has not been systematically evaluated. The present study was done to test the hypothesis that IDM's have decreased BMC at birth, correlating with poor control of diabetes during pregnancy and with the development of neonatal hypocalcemia.

Patients and methods:

54 full term IDM's and 55 normal full term controls, infants of non-diabetic mothers (InDM's) were prospectively studied. Mothers of the IDM's enrolled prior to 9 weeks of gestation were randomly assigned to one of two groups; I: "Strict management", to achieve euglycemia (fasting blood sugar (FBS) < 80 mg/dl; 1.5 hour post prandial blood sugar (PPBS) < 120 mg/d; II: "customary management", to provide diabetic and obstetric care as practiced in the community (FBS $\leq$ 100 mg/dl, PPBS < 140 mg/dl). A group enrolled after the first trimester (III) was managed identically to group II.

Bone mineral content (by photon absorptiometry) and glycosylated hemoglobin (HbA_1C) were measured in the mothers prior to delivery. Infant serum calcium was measured at age 24 and 72 hours, infant serum glucose at age 1/2 hr, 1 hr, 2 hr, 24 hr, and 3 days, and infant BMC at age 3 days (4). Hypocalcemia was defined as a serum total calcium less than 8 mg/dl on at least one of the samples, and hypoglycemia as a serum glucose less than 40 mg/dl on at least one of the samples. Infant weight percentile was calculated from the intrauterine curves of Lubchenco (5).

Results:

Multiple regression analysis showed that infant's BMC in IDM's is

Vitamin D. A Chemical, Biochemical and Clinical Update

not correlated with maternal BMC, neonatal hypoglycemia, neonatal hypocalcemia, and infant weight percentile, but correlates with the management group: IDM's from groups II and III have significantly lower BMC (respectively 87.3 $\pm$ 15.0 mg/cm (mean $\pm$ SD) and 84.3 $\pm$ 14.7) than IDM's from group I (108.3 $\pm$ 63.7) ($p < 0.02$). IDM's from group I and control InDM's (106.0 $\pm$ 27.0) had similar BMC.

Discussion:

Decreased BMC is observed in IDM's and may be prevented by strict control of diabetes during pregnancy. Decreased BMC in IDM's does not seem to play a role in the pathogenesis of neonatal hypocalcemia. The mechanism of decreased BMC in IDM's remains to be explained. Insulin deficiency may lead to decreased BMC, but IDM's theoretically have fetal hyperinsulinism (6). We have demonstrated elevated cord blood concentrations of 1,25 $(OH)_2$ D in IDM's (7), but it appears unlikely that these concentrations are high enough to enhance bone resorption. We speculate that decreased BMC in IDM's is due to an imbalance between increased bone matrix formation (due to fetal hyperinsulinism) and relatively inappropriate calcium supply through the placenta; alternatively decreased BMC could be due to maternal and fetal subclinical acidosis (8).

References:

1. Tsang R.C., Kleinman L., Sutherland J.M., Light I.J. (1972) J. Pediatr., 80, 384-395.
2. Tsang R.C., Strub R., Steichen J.J., Brown D.R., Hartman C., Chen I.W. (1976) J. Pediatr. 83, 115-119
3. Levin M.E., Boisseau V.C., Avioli L.V. (1976) N. Engl. J. Med. 294, 241-245.
4. Steichen J.J., Kaplan B., Edwards N., Tsang R.C. (1976) Am. J. Roentgenol. 126, 1283-1285.
5. Lubchenco L.O., Hansman C., Dressler M. (1963) Pediatrics 32, 793-800.
6. Sosenko I.R., Kitzmiller J.L., Loo S.W., Blix P., Rubenstein A.H., Gabbay K.H. (1979) N. Engl. J. Med. 301, 859-863.
7. Steichen J.J., Ho M., Hug G., Tsang R.C. (1980) Pediatr. Res. 14, 581.
8. Griffiths H.J., Zimmerman R.E. (1978) Skeletal Radiol. 3, 1-9.

ABNORMALITIES IN THE REGULATION OF VITAMIN D METABOLISM ASSOCIATED WITH BOVINE PARTURIENT PARESIS (MILK FEVER).

P.N. Smith and F.A. Kallfelz.
New York State College of Veterinary Medicine, Cornell University, Ithaca, New York 14853, U.S.A.

INTRODUCTION

Previous evaluations of dairy cows revealed that animals exhibiting signs of parturient paresis had abnormally high serum 1,25(OH)$_2$D levels (1). A preliminary study also showed an elevation in circulating 24,25(OH)$_2$D in the serum of affected animals (2). Since these animals are unable to correct the severe parturient hypocalcemia despite elevated circulating 1,25(OH)$_2$D, further evaluation of circulating vitamin D metabolites of both the dam and neonate was undertaken to better define the vitamin D profile of animals affected with this metabolic disorder.

METHODS

The experimental animals consisted of 22 parturient paretic Holstein cows and 14 normal parturient Holstein cows. In addition, the calves from each group were also sampled. Blood samples were obtained on the day of parturition or on Day 1 postpartum. Serum calcium was determined with atomic absorption spectrophotometry.

Serum lipids were extracted with methanol:methylene chloride and subjected to serial chromatographic separation. Separation with Silica Sep-Pak® (Waters Associates) (3) was followed by HPLC (hexane:isopropanol [97:3] or hexane: isopropanol [89:11] and methylene chloride:isopropanol [98:2]). Competitive protein binding assays (rat plasma or rachitic chick intestinal cytosol) and UV absorbance were used to quantify the metabolites.

RESULTS

When maternal and neonatal parameters were analyzed with linear regression and correlation, significant differences were apparent between the two groups. Maternal and neonatal 25,26(OH)$_2$D were well-correlated in both groups (controls: r^2=0.928; paretics: r^2=0.754; $P < 0.02$). The remaining metabolites showed no maternal-neonatal correlation in the controls, however, there were significant correlations in the affected group (25(OH)D: r^2=0.506; 24,25(OH)$_2$D: r^2=0.706; 1,25(OH)$_2$D:r^2=0.687; $P < 0.02$).

Comparison of the two groups revealed that mean calcium, 25(OH)D, 25,26(OH)$_2$D, 24,25(OH)$_2$D and 1,25(OH)$_2$D of the paretic cows were higher than and significantly different from that of control cows. However, only 24,25(OH)$_2$D and 25,26(OH)$_2$D of calves from paretic cows were higher than and significantly different from control calves (Table 1).

TABLE 1

Calcium and vitamin D metabolites in control and paretic cows and calves ($\bar{x}$ ± SEM).

	Control	Paretic
Serum Levels (Cows)		
Calcium (mg/dl)	9.19 ± 0.28	5.11 ± 0.29*
25(OH)D (ng/ml)	27.36 ± 1.73	36.46 ± 2.22*
25,26(OH)$_2$D (ng/ml)	1.12 ± 0.32	3.59 ± 0.44*
24,25(OH)$_2$D (ng/ml)	1.25 ± 0.28	2.11 ± 0.28*
1,25(OH)$_2$D (pg/ml)	98.21 ± 20.26	270.59 ± 30.70*
Serum Levels (Neonatal Calves)		
Calcium (mg/dl)	12.03 ± 0.29	11.97 ± 0.20
25(OH)D (ng/ml)	10.62 ± 1.48	12.30 ± 1.16
25,26(OH)$_2$D (ng/ml)	1.67 ± 0.29	3.05 ± 0.28**
24,25(OH)$_2$ (ng/ml)	1.98 ± 0.38	4.17 ± 0.43**
1,25(OH)$_2$D (pg/ml)	98.96 ± 26.03	117.27 ± 17.29

*, ** Significantly different from the control group; $P < 0.05$ (cows and neonatal calves, respectively).

DISCUSSION

The elevations in circulating metabolites seen in parturient paretic animals may be the result of enhanced hydroxylation or of reduced degradation and removal of the metabolites. The differences in neonatal-maternal correlations of the two groups may indicate a failure of the paretic animals to maintain neonatal (fetal)-maternal independence of vitamin D hydroxylation. This may be due to placental alterations resulting in increased permeability to the metabolites or mutually increased hydroxylation of the metabolites. Such a fetal-maternal interdependence of vitamin D hydroxylation may allow an unregulated hydroxylation cascade and elevations in circulating metabolites similar to those seen in the affected animals in this study.

We suggest that the reduced independence in maternal-fetal vitamin D hydroxylation associated with parturient paresis may contribute to the hypocalcemia seen in this metabolic disorder. Metabolites other than 1,25(OH)$_2$D (a) may compete for binding sites reducing the ability of 1,25(OH)$_2$D to correct hypocalcemia or (b) may specifically reduce bone calcium availability by stimulating bone mineralization.

This work was supported by a grant from the Harold Wetterberg Foundation.

REFERENCES

1. Horst, R.L., Eisman, J.A., Jorgensen, N.A. and DeLuca, H.F. (1977) Science 196: 662-663.
2. Smith, P.N., Padilla, M., Wasserman, R.H. and Kallfelz, F.A. (1982) Calcif. Tissue Int. 34: 564-566.
3. Adams, J.S., Clemens, T.L. and Holick, M.F. (1981) J.Chromatogr. 226: 198-201.

MATERNAL AND FETAL PLASMA VITAMIN D METABOLITES IN THE RAT BETWEEN DAYS 16 AND 21 OF GESTATION.

A. HALHALI, T.M.NGUYEN, H. GUILLOZO, M. GARABEDIAN and S. BALSAN.
CNRS UA.583, Hôpital des Enfants-Malades, 75015 Paris, France.

Concentrations of vitamin D metabolites have been assayed in the plasma of rat fetuses and of their mothers, fed a normal vitamin D diet, from day 16 to 21 of gestation.

METHODS

2-3 month old female Wistar rats had been thyroparathyroidectomized (TPTX) or not on day 12.5 of pregnancy. They were anesthetized, uterus horns were opened,care being taken not to interrupt placental circulation. Each fetus was separately excised and weighted after blood collection from axillary vessels. Maternal blood was collected after aortic puncture. Vitamin D metabolites were measured with competitive protein binding assays, after methanol-chloroform extraction of plasma samples, and purification of the chloroform extracts by Sephadex LH20 and straight phase HPLC chromatographies.

RESULTS

In intact pregnant rats, plasma 25-(OH)D and 24,25-$(OH)_2$D concentrations were not significantly different between days 16 and 21 of gestation but plasma 1,25-$(OH)_2$D concentrations were higher on days 20 ($p<0.01$) and 21 (165 $\pm$ 21 pg/ml, $p<0.001$) than before (54 $\pm$ 9 pg /ml on day 19). This increase occurred also in TPTX rats (38 $\pm$ 6 pg /ml on day 19, 125 $\pm$ 20 pg/ml on day 21).

In fetuses from intact rats, the evolution of plasma vitamin D metabolite concentrations paralleled that observed in mothers with one exception, plasma 1,25-$(OH)_2$D concentrations were elevated on days 16 and 17, lower on days 18 and 19, and again elevated on days 20 and 21 in the plasma of fetuses. Maternal thyroparathyroidectomy did not significantly influence

Vitamin D. A Chemical, Biochemical and Clinical Update

fetal plasma 1,25-$(OH)_2D$ concentrations.

Fetal plasma 25-(OH)D and 24,25-$(OH)_2D$ were positively correlated with respective maternal plasma concentrations in intact rats ($r=0.80$, $p<0.01$ for 25-(OH)D ; $r=0.50$, $p<0.05$ for 24,25-$(OH)_2D$) as well as in TPTX rats ($r=0.70$, $p<0.02$ for 25-(OH)D ; $r=0.75$, $p<0.01$ for 24,25-$(OH)_2D$). In contrast, for 1,25-$(OH)_2D$, a positive correlation between maternal and fetal plasma concentrations was found in TPTX rats ($r=0.78$, $p<0.01$), but not in intact rats.

CONCLUSIONS

The different evolutions of plasma 1,25-$(OH)_2D$ concentrations in mothers and their fetuses and the absence of correlation between these two concentrations in intact rats suggest that rat fetuses may regulate their own circulating 1,25-$(OH)_2D$ concentrations. Factors other than maternal thyroid and parathyroid hormones are responsible for the elevation of fetal and maternal plasma 1,25-$(OH)_2D$ at the end of gestation, but thyroid and/or parathyroid hormones may modulate the placental transfer of 1,25-$(OH)_2D$.

EFFECT OF HIGH MINERAL AND PROTEIN INTAKES ON VITAMIN D METABOLISM AND MINERAL HOMEOSTASIS IN PREMATURE INFANTS, L. Hillman, S. Salmons, M. Erickson, J. Hansen, R. Hillman, Department of Pediatrics, Washington University School of Medicine, St. Louis, Missouri, U.S.A.

INTRODUCTION

Premature infants fed standard formula designed for term infants develop frequent moderate-severe osteopenia with occasional fractures and rickets if 25-hydroxy vitamin D (25-OHD) is also low (1). Increasing vitamin D supplementation improves mineralization and serum calcium (2). However, since standard formula cannot provide adequate minerals to match a calculated in utero accretion even with absorption improved, a new generation of higher mineral formlae has been created. Using a formula containing 1326 mg/L calcium, 662 mg/L phosphorus, serum 25-OHD was unchanged, remaining low (<15 ng/ml) in half of infants (3). Study was thus undertaken of a formula (EPF) containing 900 mg calcium, 450 mg phosphorus and 3.0 gm/100 kcal protein with infants supplemented with either 400 IU vitamin D, 800 IU vitamin D or 2 μg 25-OHD_3. On this formula serum calcium and phosphorus were normalized. Moderate-severe osteopenia was essentially never seen, however, bone densitometry measurements failed to consistently parallel in utero curves regardless of the type of vitamin D supplementation (4). Urine calcium/urine creatinine was noted to be increased over both standard formulae and the previously studied high mineral formulae suggesting an increased calcium absorption with incomplete retention. It was also noted that the great majority of infants fed this formula developed a generalized aminoaciduria which had been infrequently seen on standard formula or the first high mineral formula. An explanation for the aminoaciduria and calciuria in the face of incomplete mineralization was sought. Possibilities considered were 1) inadequate vitamin D and metabolites, 2) elevation of PTH, 3) an effect of high protein on renal tubular resorption of calcium, 4) renal tubular damage secondary to high mineral, and 5) a developmental limitation on use of increased minerals for bone accretion.

METHODS:

Three high mineral formulae which were the same as EPF except for variation of protein content were created. Protein contents were A) 3.0 gm/100 kcal, same as EPF, B) 2.7 gm/100 kcal, and C) 2.2 gm/100 kcal, the same as standard formula. Measurements were made of calcium, magnesium, phosphorus, PTH, vitamin D, 25-OHD, 1,25$(OH)_2$D, bone mineral content (BMC), urine N-acetyl-glucosamidase (NAG) and β_2 microglobulins (B_2M).

RESULTS:

Serum vitamin D, 25-OHD, 1,25-OHD, and PTH were the same as previously seen with standard formula plus 400-800 IU D/day (2) (Table 1). Serum D was high, 25-OHD normal, 1,25$(OH)_2$D high normal, and PTH normal.

Table 1: Serum D,25-OHD, 1,25$(OH)_2$D and PTH (mean $\pm$ S.E.)

	High Mineral[5] (n=4)	Standard Mineral[5] (n=5)	Normal Adult[5]
D, ng/ml	7.8 $\pm$ 2.5	20.3 $\pm$ 4.8	1.1 $\pm$ 0.1 (10)
25-OHD, ng/ml	22.3 $\pm$ 3.2	20.4 $\pm$ 3.2	23 $\pm$ 7 (22)
1,25$(OH)_2$D, pg/ml	44.3 $\pm$ 8.7	60.0 $\pm$ 6.7	37 $\pm$ 0.5 (22)
PTH, mEq/ml	4.7 $\pm$ 1.5	6.2 $\pm$ 2.1	2 - 10

Serum, urine and BMC values at four weeks of age can be seen in Table 2. Values at two and six weeks of age were similar. Generalized aminoaciduria (GAA) was seen on all high mineral formulae. Calciuria increased on the lowest protein formula and serum calcium fell. Serum and urine phosphorus and magnesium remained normal. Serum albumin was lower on high mineral formula with 2.2 gm/100 kcal protein (C) or 2.7 gm/100 kcal (B) than on 3.0 gm/100 kcal (A) (or commercial EPF) or standard mineral formula with 2.2 gm/100 kcal. BMC was similar on all high mineral formula.

Table 2: Mean ± S.D. values at four weeks of age by study formula

	n	S Ca mg/dl	Alb g/dl	U Ca / U Cr	%c̄ GAA	BMC g/cm
STD	13	9.4 ± .6	3.3 ± .3	0.16 ± .1*	38	--
EPF	23	9.6 ± .8	3.4 ± .5	0.31 ± .2+	63+	0.10 ± .03
A	8	9.6 ± .4	3.3 ± .3	0.14 ± .2	60+	0.11 ± .04
B	9	9.4 ± .5	3.0 ± .5*+	0.34 ± .2+	71+	0.11 ± .03
C	9	8.9 ± .4*+	3.0 ± .4*+	0.49 ± .2*+	75+	0.10 ± .02

$p<.05$ different from STD (+) or EPF (5)

Markers of renal tubular injury, N-acetyl glucosamidase and β_2 microglobulins did not differ between infants fed any of the high mineral formula and standard mineral formula. Four week values were standard formula: NAG 61 ± 40 mmol/mg creatinine and β_2M .27 ± .18 mg/L/mg creatinine; high mineral formula: NAG 87 ± 47 and β_2M .41 ± .23.

DISCUSSION:

The generalized aminoaciduria remains unexplained. It did not appear to be due to vitamin D deficiency, parathyroid elevation, a protein effect or renal tubular damage. Urinary calcium losses in the face of incomplete mineralization were not due to an effect of high protein intake and indeed losses increased with a lower protein intake. An unexpected finding was that protein intakes which sustained normal serum albumin on standard mineral intakes were unable to do so at high mineral intakes. Thus concommitant increases in mineral and protein intakes are needed either to a) meet the needs of increased growth and retention, or b) compensate for an interaction of protein and mineral gastrointestinal absorption. Developmental factors may partially limit utilization of high mineral intakes for bone mineralization. While no evidence of renal tubular damage was seen on high mineral formula, study of the effects of intermediate mineral intakes on aminoaciduria, calciuria, and bone mineralization are indicated.

REFERENCES:

1. Hillman, L., Hoff, N., Salmons, S., Martin, L., McAlister, W., Haddad, J. (In Press) J. Pediatrics.
2. Hillman, L., Hollis, B., Salmons, S., Martin, L., Slatopolsky, E., McAlister, W., Haddad, J. (In Press) J. Pediatrics.
3. Hillman, L., Martin, L., Salmons, S., Fiore, B., McAlister, W. (1982) Pediatric Research, 16:258A.
4. Hillman, L., Erickson, M., Salmons, S. (1984) Calcified Tissue International, 36:515.
5. D,25-OHD, $1,25(OH)_2D$ on high minerals were run in Dr. Laura Hillman's laboratory. Samples on standard minerals and adults were previously run by Dr. Bruce Hollis. The methodology used was that of Dr. Bruce Hollis in both laboratories.

INTESTINAL CALCIUM ABSORPTION IN SUCKLING PIGLETS WITH PSEUDO VITAMIN D DEFICIENCY RICKETS; TYPE I

J. Harmeyer*, Lachenmaier-Currle, U. and R. Kaune
Institute of Physiology, School of Vet. Med., 3000 Hannover, FRG

Introduction:

The "Hannover Pig Strain" which has been described earlier suffers from pseudo vitamin D-deficiency rickets, type I(1). The inherited rachitic trait develops rickets in offspring by an autosomal recessive gene(2). First clinical symptoms of rickets appear at an age of four to six weeks (3). Rachitic lesions can successfully be treated by massive doses of vitamin D_3 or by physiological amounts of 0.5mg/d of 1,25-$(OH)_2D_3$ (4). Renal 1-hydroxylase and 24-hydroxylase activities are absent in renal cortex and mitochondrial preparations from rachitic piglets (5). Homozygote piglets appear clinically normal at birth and grow normally during the first three weeks after birth. It is investigated why rachitic piglets develop no rachitic symptoms during the first four weeks of live.

Animals and methods:

Homozygote and heterozygote (normal) litter mates 1/2 to 8 weeks old equipped with permanent catheters in the int. jugular veins were orally administered appr. 3.7 GBq $^{45}CaCl_2$ in 1.5ml of saline through an esophageal tube. Thirty to fourty 0.5ml blood samples were collected during 24 hours. Blood samples were also collected at four days intervals over 8 weeks. Plasma Ca, Pi and alkaline Pase were estimated by colorimetric procedures, ^{45}Ca by liquid scintillation, vitamin D and vitamin D-metabolites by HPLC-chromatography and radioimmuno assay for 1,25-$(OH)_2D_3$ (6).

Results:

Concentrations of plasma Ca, Pi and the activity of alkal. Pase are normal in newborn homozygote piglets and remain in a normal range during the following two or four weeks of life (fig.1). Body weights rise with the same rate in homozygotes and heterozygotes from 1.5 to 4.4 kg during the first 5 weeks. One to three weeks old homozygote piglets absorb Ca from the intestine at the same rate as heterozygote litter mates (fig.2). Absorption of Ca declines significantly in homozygotes with age. At an age of 6 weeks Ca absorption is only 55% the value of the corresponding heterozygote litter mate. Mean concentrations of 25-OHD_3, 24,25-$(OH)_2D_3$ and 1,25-$(OH)_2D_3$ differ significantly between both genotypes (Table 1) but remain unchanged in homozygotes during transition from the state of absorbing to non-absorbing Ca.

Discussion:

1,25-$(OH)_2D_3$ in plasma of homozygote piglets which is in the range of 20 to 30 pg/ml appears to be too low to maintain plasma Ca and Pi normal. However, homozygote piglets under 5 to 6 weeks absorb Ca from the intestine to maintain normocalcemia. Do the intestines of newborn piglets possess a mechanism for Ca absorption which is independent of vitamin D? Or is the 1,25-$(OH)_2D_3$ receptor affinity increased which allows exertion to vitamin D-hormon effects with subnormal 1,25-$(OH)_2D_3$ concentrations? Vitamin D independent processes during the reproductive cycle appear more likely (7).

*Supported by the Deutsche Forschungsgemeinschaft, Sonderforschungsbereich 146 "Versuchstierforschung"

Table 1:
Vitamin D and vitamin D-metabolites in plasma ($\pm$SD) of control piglets (heterozygotes) and piglets with pseudo vitamin D-deficiency rickets, type I (homozygotes) at an age of 1 to 2 and 6 to 8 weeks (*different from rachitic animals with $p < 0.01$)

Animal	Age weeks	vitamin D_3 (ng/ml)	25-OHD$_3$ (ng/ml)	1,25-(OH)$_2$D$_3$ (pg/ml)	24,25-(OH)$_2$D$_3$ (ng/ml)	25,26-(OH)$_2$D$_3$
Normal	1-2	0.1	4.9*	161*	3.3	1.1
control	6-8	5.1	1.0*	88*	6.8	2.3
Rachit.	1-2	3.8	43	29	4.1	1.8
animal	6-8	3.5	47	24	9.2	2.3

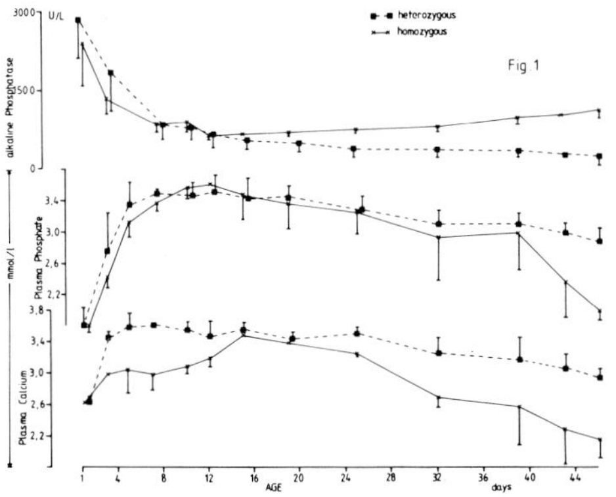

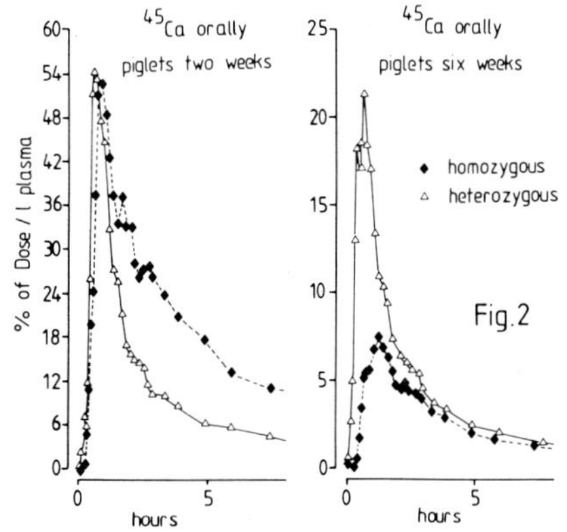

Fig.1: Ca, Pi and alkal. Pase in plasma of rachitic and normal piglets during the first 8 weeks of life.

Fig.2: Appearance of ^{45}Ca in plasma after an oral dose of 3.7 GBq $^{45}CaCl_2$ in 1.5 ml saline, two litter mates at an age of 2 and 6 weeks

1.) Plonait, H. (1969) Zbl. Vet. Med. A. 16, 271-316

2.) Meyer, H. and Plonait, H. (1967) Zbl. Vet. Med. A. 15, 482-493

3.) Harmever. H., v. Grabe, C. and Winkler, J. (1982) Exper. Biol. Med. (Basel) 7, 117-125

4.) Harmeyer, J., v. Grabe, C. and Martens, H. (1977) Proc. 3rd Workshop on vitamin D p. 784-788

5.) Winkler, J., Schreiner, F. and Harmeyer, J. (1985) Zbl. Vet. Med. A. (in press)

6.) Kaune, R. and Harmeyer, J. (1984) Königsteiner Chromatographietage, Edit. H. Aigner Waters GmbH p. 225-236

7.) Halloran, B.P. and DeLuca, H.F. (1983) In: Perinatal Calcium and Phosphorus Metabolism. Edit. Hollick, M.F., Gray, T.K. and Anast, C.S. p. 105-124

SERUM CONCENTRATIONS OF VITAMIN D METABOLITES, CALCIUM AND ALKALINE PHOSPHATASE IN EPILEPTIC MOTHERS AND IN THEIR NEWBORNS.

T. Kuoppala , R. Tuimala and T. Koskinen.
Departments of Clinical Sciences and Obstetrics and Gynecology, University of Tampere , 33520 Tampere , Finland .

Introduction:

Epileptic patients on anticonvulsant therapy have quite often disturbed mineral metabolism such as hypocalcemia, elevated alkaline phosphatase levels and decreased bone mineral content (1). It has been suggested that altered vitamin D metabolism might be important in the etiology of these changes(2). Anticonvulsant drugs influence hepatic vitamin D metabolism and they also modify the synthesis of dihydroxylated metabolites in the kidney. (3) During pregnancy the increased fetal calcium and phosphorus requirements demand elevated maternal mineral absorption, which is mediated by increased synthesis of active vitamin D metabolites. Therefore we have studied the effect of anticonvulsant therapy on vitamin D and calcium metabolism in pregnant epileptic women and in their newborns.

Materials and methods:

Our material comprised 21 epileptic women who delivered in Tampere University Hospital. Ten mothers delivered in winter and 11 in summer. Ten mothers received vitamin D supplementation with 100 units per day in the first trimester. Two mothers had convulsions during pregnancy and their treatment had to alter, while all others were in good balance. Seven mothers were treated with diphenylhydantoin or in different combinations with phenobarbital, primidone, carbamazepin and clonazepam: this group was referred to as the diphenylhydantoin group (DPH). A total of 14 patients were treated with carbamazepin alone or in combination with sodiumvalproate and were defined as the carbamazepin group (CARB). Serum concentrations of these drugs were controlled at every trimester and values were in the suggested ranges. Control mothers were healthy and they delivered in the same season as epileptics. They received no vitamin D supplementation. All mothers in both groups delivered a normal-weight full-term baby. Blood samples were drawn in the third trimester and just after delivery, when also mixed blood samples from umbilical cord were collected. Samples were centrifuged and serum frozen at $-20^{o}C$ until analyzed. We measured 25(OH)D , $24,25(OH)_2D$, $1,25(OH)_2D$, calcium and alkaline phosphatase. Our vitamin D analysis method included HPLC purifications and competitive protein-binding assay. Calcium and ALP (Alk.phos.)were analyzed by routine methods.

Results:

There was no significant difference in 25(OH)D values between epileptic and control mothers. Epileptic mothers who received negligible vitamin D supplementation in the first trimester had 25(OH)D values similar to those of mothers without supplementation. Also the DPH and CARB groups had similar 25(OH)D values borh during pregnancy and at delivery. There was little change in dihydroxylated vitamin D metabolites. $24,25(OH)_2D$ concentrations were lower and $1,25(OH)_2D$ values higher in epileptic than in controlmothers. These changes were almost significant. Within the epileptic groups there was no difference between DPH and CARB. Calcium concentrations were higher in controls than in epileptics. The difference was almost significant at the third trimester and significant at delivery ($p<0.001$). Concentrations of ALP were higher in epileptics than in the control group. The difference was significant in cord blood ($p<0.05$) and almost significant at delivery. Though there were differences in maternal values between epileptics and

Vitamin D. A Chemical, Biochemical and Clinical Update

controls, the fetal concentrations of vitamin D and calcium were quite similar in both groups.

Table Vitamin D metabolites, calcium and ALP concentrations in control mothers and epileptics with different anticonvulsant therapy (Mean± SD). Statistical analysis was performed by student's t-test .

	25(OH)D ng/ml	24,25(OH)$_2$D ng/ml	1,25(OH)$_2$D pg/ml	S-calcium mmol/l	ALP IU/l
3rd trimester					
Controls	10,9±3,6	1,75±1,10	77±30	2,29±0,07	209±60
Epileptics	12,6±5,3	1,49±0,79	95±49	2,24±0,11	225±85
-DPH	13,2±4,3	1,07±0,17	92±46	2,25±0,09	245±90
-CARB	12,3±5,9	1,81±0,76	97±51	2,23±0,09	214±89
Delivery					
Controls	15,7±6,0	1,65±1,05	69±32	2,31±0,05	310±69
Epileptics	13,5±6,8	1,46±0,63	95±54	2,22±0,06**	370±123
-DPH	12,8±5,7	1,55±0,88	100±53	2,22±0,02**	368±141
-CARB	13,9±7,6	1,41±0,46	85±31	2,23±0,06**	371±120
Cord blood					
Controls	9,7±4,0	1,69±1,04	69±43	2,69±0,16	258±67
Epileptics	9,5±4,0	1,74±1,16	68±48	2,67±0,20	328±128*
-DPH	10,3±5,0	1,58±0,76	60±13	2,74±0,09	321±144*
-CARB	9,2±3,4	1,93±1,29	73±53	2,65±0,20	331±126*

* $p<0.05$ ** $p<0.001$

Comments:

25(OH)D illustrates vitamin D nutritional status. It has been concluded in many studies that anticonvulsants tend to lower 25-hydroxyvitamin D (4). We could not confirm this. 25(OH)D concentrations were similar in both groups and different anticonvulsant drugs had no influence on values. 24,25(OH)$_2$D concentrations tended to be low in epileptic mothers. Similar results have been reported by Zerwekh et al. (5). 1,25(OH)$_2$D values were higher in epileptics than in the control group, agreeing with earlier reports (3 ,6). It has long been known that patients treated with anticonvulsant drugs have low serum calcium concentrations (4). Also in our study calcium values were in the low normal range. However, only three mothers were slightly hypocalcemic and none received calcium therapy. All control mothers and babies were normocalcemic.

We may conclude that there were only slight alterations in vitamin D metabolites, and serum calcium concentrations were in the low normal range in the patients treated with anticonvulsant drugs, and these changes cannot explain hypocalcemia and osteopenia found in these patients.

References:

1. Hahn,T.J. (1980) Clin Endocrinol Metab 9:107-125 .
2. Hahn,T.J.,Hendin,B.A.,Scharp,C.R.,Boisseau,V.C. and Haddad,J.G. (1975) N Engl J Med 292:550-554 .
3. Levison,J.C.,Kent,G.N.,Worth,G.K.and Retallack,R.W.(1977) Endocrinol 101:1898-1901 .
4. Markestad,T.,Ulstein,M.,Strandfjord,R.E.,Aksnes,L. and Aarskog,D.(1984) Am J Obstet Gynecol 150:254-258 .
5. Zerwekh,J.E.,Homan,R.,Tindall,R. and Pak,C.Y.C.(1982) Ann Neurol 12:184-186 .
6. Jubiz,W.,Haussler,M.R.,McCain,T.A. and Tolman,K.G. (1977) J Clin Endocrinol Metab 44:617-621 .

VITAMIN D METABOLITES IN AMNIOTIC FLUID

G. Kidroni, Ph.D., J. Menczel, M.D., L. Schwartz, M.Sc., Z. Palti, M.D. and M. Ron, M.D.

Res. Lab., Depts. of Medicine and Obstetrics and Gynecology, Hadassah University Hospital, Mt. Scopus, Jerusalem, Israel.

Concentrations of 25-hydroxyvitamin D_3 [25(OH)D_3], 24,25-dihydroxyvitamin D_3 [24,25(OH)$_2D_3$] and 1,25-dihydroxyvitamin D_3 [1,25(OH)$_2D_3$] were determined in amniotic fluid, fetal cord and maternal sera. The respective levels ($\pm$ S.D.) of 25(OH)D_3, 24,25(OH)$_2D_3$ and 1,25(OH)$_2D_3$ in maternal serum were 18.03$\pm$10.8 ng/ml, 1.473$\pm$1.562 ng/ml and 36.5$\pm$21.5 pg/ml; fetal cord serum levels were 13.15$\pm$8.3 ng/ml, 0.90$\pm$0.76 ng/ml, 29.2$\pm$18.55 pg/ml and amniotic fluid levels were 0.732$\pm$0.508 ng/ml, 0.121$\pm$0.104 ng/ml and 14.3$\pm$10.0 pg/ml. Levels of the three metabolites in maternal and fetal cord sera were not statistically different. A significant difference was found between the levels of the three metabolites in maternal serum and amniotic fluid. Significant differences were also found between the levels of 25(OH)D_3 and 24,25(OH)$_2D_3$ but not 1,25(OH)$_2D_3$ levels in fetal cord serum and amniotic fluid. Only 25(OH)D_3 levels in both maternal serum and fetal cord serum correlated well with the respective amniotic fluid levels. This significant correlation suggests the possibility of evaluating fetal 25(OH)D_3 status by measuring amniotic fluid level.

The source of the unconjugated vitamin D metabolites determined in amniotic fluid is most probably not from fetal urinary excretions but from maternal to fetal transplacental tranfer.

Vitamin D. A Chemical, Biochemical and Clinical Update

THE EFFECTIVENESS OF INTRAVENEOUS PHOSPHATE FOR THE PREVENTION OF RICKETS IN VERY LOW BIRTH WEIGHT INFANTS

T.Tüschen, A.Westfechtel,A.Otten,H.Wolf

Department of Pediatrics, Justus-Liebig-University,Giessen-W.-Germany

Purpose of the investigation:

Previous studies had shown HYPOPHOSPHATEMIA to be an early sign and possibly the cause of rickets in very low birth weight infants (VLBW) who had received prolonged total parenteral nutrition (TPN).

This study was conducted to evaluate the effectiveness of i.v.phosphate supplementation in the prevention of rickets.

Patients and Methods:

29 VLBW infants (gestational age : 27 - 32 weeks,birth weight: 860-1580 g) were examined.

In 15 babies receiving TPN for more than 4 weeks, sodium phosphate was supplemented intraveneously at a dosage of 60 mg/kg daily.

The TPN solution contained glucose,amino acids,and lipid emulsion.

Additional supplementation: calcium according to serum levels (30 - 80 mg/kg), multivitamin preparation, Vit.D_3 (400 I.U.).
The increase of the phosphate supplementation was the only change in the TPN regimen compared with our previous study (1).
The other 14 babies received early oral feedings with breast milk or an adapted formula providing up to 90 mg calcium/kg and 70 mg phosphate/kg. Additional Vitamin D supplementation : 1000 I.U.daily.

Parameters measured:

serum: calcium
phosphate
alkaline phosphatase activity
25-(OH)-Vitamin D_3
1,25-$(OH)_2$-Vitamin D_3

urine: amino acid excretion

Blood samples were taken between the 2nd and 12th weeks of life at intervals of 2-3 weeks.
Criteria for the diagnosis of rickets:
- clinical symptoms
- rise of alkaline phosphatase avtivity over 650 U/l
- bone demineralisation (x-ray)
- hyperaminoaciduria

Vitamin D. A Chemical, Biochemical and Clinical Update

Results:

I.

In the group of VLBW infants receiving TPN with i.v. phosphate supplementation, 13 out of 15 infants showed no signs of bone demineralisation.

II.

The remaining two developed rickets according to the criteria mentioned above. This is an evident decrease in the incidence of rickets: 15% compared with 78% in our previous study.

III.

In the group of VLBW infants receiving early oral feeding, 9 out of 14 infants showed normal bone mineralisation.

IV.

The other 5 babies developed clinical symptoms of rickets; 2 of whom had received their mother's milk.

Serum calcium levels remained normal throughout the observation period in all infants.
Vitamin D deficiency could be excluded in all cases:

25-(OH)-Vitamin D_3 : 25-266 nmol/l

1,25-$(OH)_2$- Vitamin D_3: 201-800 pmol/l.

Conclusions

I.v. supplementation of phosphate at a dosage of at least 60 mg/kg daily can prevent the development of rickets in VLBW infants.
This observation once again shows that this type of rickets is caused by a lack of phosphate and not by Vitamin D deficiency. Thus, phosphate supplementation should be considered as a necessary adjunct in the nutrition of VLBW infants.

References:

1. Westfechtel,A.,Tüschen,T.,Otten,A.,Wolf,H.
Monatsschr.Kinderheilkunde 132: 212-216 (1984)

2. Brewer,E.D.,Winslow,C.S.,Dell,L.,Conley,S.B.,Morris,F.H.
Abstracts Fifth Workshop on Vit.D,Williamsburg 216 (1982)

3. Steichen,J.J.,Gratton,T.L.,Tsang,R.C.
J. Pediatr. 96 : 528-534 (1982)

VITAMIN D METABOLITES IN HUMAN AMNIOTIC FLUID. CORRELATION WITH CORD SERUM VALUES.

S. Bertelloni, G. Cesaretti, G. Federico, U. Bottone and G. Saggese
Department of Pediatrics, University of Pisa, Pisa, Italy.

Introduction.

In the last years there has been a great deal of interest about fetal and maternal calcium metabolism. However little is known about the origin, metabolism and physiological role of vitamin D active metabolites in the fetus and placenta. Recent studies showed that there is an indipendent vitamin D metabolism in the feto-placental unit (1,2). In fact only 25-hydroxycholecalciferol (25-OH-D3), seems to pass across the placenta (3). The 1,25-dihydroxycholecalciferol (1,25(OH)2D), synthetized in non-pregnant mainly in the kidney, do not pass from the mother to the fetus (3,4) and fetal 1,25(OH)2D comes out from a placental synthesis (4). On the other hand, fetal liver P-450 cytocrome is not active before birth and no placental 25-hydroxylase activity has been reported. These findings show that the unique source of 25-OH-D for the fetus is the mother pool. 25-OH-D and 1,25(OH)2D levels in amnios, even if may provide an indices of vitamin D status of the fetus and vitamin D metabolism of the placenta, are poorly studied (5,6). In the present study we measured the concentrations of 25-OH-D and 1,25(OH)2D in human amniotic fluid and in cord blood in normal pregnancy at term.

Patients and methods.

Amniotic fluid samples were obtained from a total of 16 women at 37-42 gestation weeks by artificial rupture of the amniotic sac. None of the women was receiving vitamin D supplements or drugs known to alter vitamin D metabolism. All mothers had a satisfactory physical activity and exposure to sun-light in the last trimester of pregnancy. Nutritional status was good. No examined amniotic fluid samples were visibly contaminated with blood. Cord blood samples of respective newborns were collected at delivery.

All the samples were centrifuged at 3000 rpm and the cell-free supernatant was frozen immediately and stored at -20 C until just before analysis. 25-OH-D and 1,25(OH)2D values were determined by competitive radioreceptor assay, as previously described (7,8). Detection limit of the methods was 0.5 ng/ml for 25-OH-D and 2 pg/ml for 1,25(OH)2D. All the study was performed in October. Results are expressed as the mean + SEM and analyzed using standard statistical methods: Student's "t" test and linear regression analysis.

Results.

25-OH-D and 1,25(OH)2D were detected in amniotic fluid of each women. Levels ranged from 0.5 to 5.7 ng/ml (mean 2.7 ± 0.6 ng/ml) for 25-OH-D and 3 to 17 pg/ml (mean 8.3 ± 2.1 pg/ml) for 1,25(OH)2D. Cord serum values were as follows: 25-OH-D 23.3 ± 1.3 ng/ml (range 17.4 - 31.9

Vitamin D. A Chemical, Biochemical and Clinical Update

ng/ml); 1,25(OH)2D 19.8 ± 3.0 pg/ml (range 21.1 - 29.7 pg/ml). Vitamin D metabolites levels in amniotic fluid were significantly lower than values in cord serum ($p < 0.001$). A significant positive correlation was found between amniotic and cord serum concentration: 25-OH-D: $r = 0.973$, p 0.001; 1,25(OH)2D: $r = 0.758$, $p < 0.001$.

Discussion.

In this study we showed, in agreement with Ron (5) and Lazebnik (6), the presence of vitamin D metabolites in human amniotic fluid. The presence of 25-OH-D and 1,25,(OH)2D in this compartment raises the question of their origin and metabolism. Placental transfer of 25-OH-D from maternal circulation into the fetal compartment has been reported in humans, rat and sheep (3,9). It may be possible that 25-OH-D present in human amniotic fluid derive from mother by a passage into this compartment trought the placental structures. Experimental works have showed that human and rat placenta (1,2) are capable to synthetize 1,25(OH)2 in vitro. Amnios levels of this metabolite can derive by a direct secretion of placenta in amniotic fluid. Indipendently of vitamin D metabolites source, we have showed a clear correlation between cord serum and amniotic fluid levels, suggesting that 25-OH-D and 1,25(OH)2D concentrations in amnios may reflect, thought indirectly, the fetal vitamin D status. The clinical significance of vitamin D metabolites in amniotic fluid awaits further studies, even if their presence may suggest an important role in mineral homeostasis regulation of uterine annexes.

References:

1) Tanaka, Y., Halloran, B., Schoenes, H.K., De Luca, H.F., (1979) Proc. Natl. Acad. Sci. USA 76 : 5033-5035.
2) Weisman, A., Harell, A., Edelstein, S., David, M., Spirer, Z., Golander, A., (1979) Nature 281 : 317-319.
3) Hollis, B.W., Pittard, W.B. (1984) J. Clin. Endocrinol. Metab. 59 : 652-657.
4) Gray, T.K. (1984) in "Vitamin D", Kumar R. ed., Martinus N. Pub., Boston, pp. 217-232.
5) Ron, M., Kidroni, G., Schwartz, L., Scherer, D., Menczel, J., Palti., Z. (1982) Am. J. Obstet. Gynecol. 142 : 113-114.
6) Lazebnik, R., Eisemberg, Z., Spirer, Z., Weisman ,J. (1983) J. Clin. Endocrinol. Metab. 56 : 632-634.
7) Saggese G., Bertelloni S., Federico G., Baroncelli G.I., Bottone E. Proceedings "RIA '84" Albertini A. ed., Milan, May 15-16 1984, p. 58.
8) Eisman, J.A., Hamstra, A.J, Kream, B.E., DeLuca, H.F. (1976) Arch. Bioch. Bioph. 176 : 235-243.
9) Lester, G.E., Gray, T.K., Lorenc R.S. (1981) Biol. Neonate 39 : 232-238.

IS VITAMIN D (VitD) AN ETIOLOGICAL FACTOR FOR THE HYPERCALCIURIA IN PREMATURE INFANTS?

I.C.RADDE, S.A.ATKINSON, C.F.CIFUENTES, A.MOORE, J.SHEEPERS.
Research Inst., Hospital for Sick Children, Toronto, Canada.

Recent reports (1,2) indicate a high incidence of elevated Ca excretion rates in very low birthweight (VLBW) infants. In this retrospective study we report the results of serial measurements of urinary Ca in thriving VLBW infants subjected to dietary manipulations (Ca, Na, or PO_4 supplementation, variations in VitD intake, and feeding formula or expressed breastmilk). The study aim was to assess the role of VitD intake as a pathogenetic factor for hypercalciuria.

PATIENTS:

131 infants of birthweight <1.3 kg are included in the study, starting at 10-14 days postnatal age and ending when the weight reached 1.8 kg, 2-6 weeks later. In each of the successive phases outlined in Table I, infants were pair-matched according to birthweight and gestational age. All infants received 180-200 ml/kg/24 h of formula or breastmilk.

Table I: Study Phases (A=Group A; B=Group B)

Phase I:	Ca supplementation: 2.5 (A) vs 6.25 mmol/kg/24 h (B)
" II:	Na supplementation: 1.5 (A) vs 3 mmol/kg/24 h (B)
III:	PO_4-supplementation: 2.6 (A) vs 3.9 mmol/kg/24 h (B)
IV:	VitD-free formula + 12.5 µg VitD (A) vs 2.5 µg/kg/24 h (B)
V:	Formula as in I-IV + 12.5 µg VitD/kg/24 h vs Own mother's milk + 12.5 µg VitD/kg/24 h (B).

RESULTS:

The incidence of hypercalciuria (urinary Ca excretion >0.15 mmol/kg/24 h) (3) is summarized in Table II and the urinary Ca excretion rate in Fig 1. None of the infants were hypercalcemic at any time during the study. Changes in Ca- or Na-supplementation or in VitD dosage did not change the incidence of severity of hypercalciuria. However, in Phase IV infants there was an inverse relationship between urinary Ca excretion and plasma 25-hydroxyvitD level ($p<0.15$). On the other hand, increasing the PO_4-intake from 2.6 to 3.9 mmol/kg/24 h, significantly reduced the incidence and degree of hypercalciuria. Infants fed their own mother's milk showed a significant increase in hypercalciuria which could be reduced by giving breastmilk and formula alternately. In Phases I-III urinary Ca

Table II: INCIDENCE OF HYPERCALCIURIA (<0.15 mmol/kg/24 h)

	Control (A)		Experimental (B)		
Phase I	7/66	(10.6%)	5/28	(17.9%)	NS
Phase II	10/100	(10.0%)	20/134	(14.9%)	NS
Phase III	19/96	(19.8%)	3/50	(6 %)	$p<0.05$
Phase IV	23/99	(23.2%)	21/60	(31.8%)	NS
Phase V	F 1/14	(7.1%)	BM 7/14	(50 %)	$p<0.05$

Vitamin D. A Chemical, Biochemical and Clinical Update

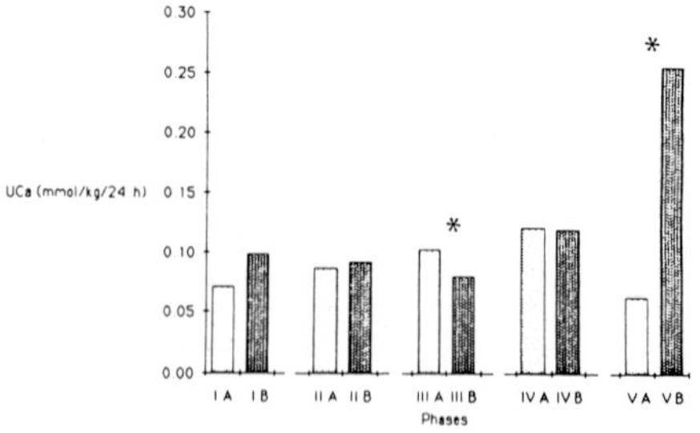

FIG. 1

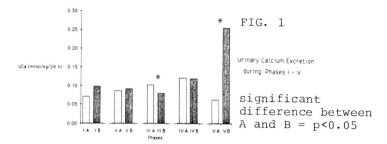

Urinary Calcium Excretion during Phases I - V

* significant difference between A and B = $p<0.05$

concentrations were correlated with Ca excretion rates ($p<0.001$), during both normo- and hypercalciuria.

DISCUSSION:

Of the nutritional factors tested, VitD dosage did not affect the incidence or severity of hypercalciuria in VLBW infants. There was even a decrease in calciuria with increasing plasma 25-OH-VitD levels. The greater growth rate observed in infants given the higher dosage of VitD might be in part responsible for this phenomenon. Hypercalciuria after VitD administration can occur in the absence of hypercalcemia (4). PO_4-intake affected the renal handling of Ca in Phase III and, presumably, in Phase V, in which formula supplements given to breastfed infants led to a 50% decrease in urinary Ca excretion. PO_4 depletion has been described in breastfed infants (5), and this may be the basis of the increased hypercalciuria in our study infants fed breastmilk. As to pathogenetic mechanisms for hypercalciuria, all infants except those of Phase 1A absorbed Ca from the intestine at 40-75% of intake and growth rates proceeded at or above intrauterine rates in Phases II-IV. The greatest hypercalciuria was seen during weeks 34-36 postconceptional age, when various nephron segments mature rapidly. Thus, the hypercalciuria of VitD-replete VLBW infants is multifactorial in origin. The findings suggest that PO_4 intake, rather than VitD status, is a major pathogenetic factor.

REFERENCES:

(1) Hufnagle,K.G., Khan, S.N., Penn, D., Cacciarelli, A., Williams, P. (1982) Pediatrics, 70: 360-363.
(2) Goldsmith, M.A., Bhatia, S.S., Kanto, W.P., Jr., Kutner, M.D., Rudman, D. (1981) Am J Dis Child, 135: 538-543.
(3) Ghazali, S., Barratt, T.M. (1974) Arch Dis Child, 40: 97-101.
(4) Lemann, J., Jr., Adams, N.D., Gray, R.W. (1979) N Engl J Med, 301: 535-541.
(5) Rowe, J.C., Wood, D.H., Rowe, D.W., Raisz, L.G. (1979) N Engl J Med 300: 293-296.

CHANGES IN LEVELS OF CALCIUM-BINDING PROTEIN (CaBP) AND VITAMIN D METABOLITES IN RESPONSE TO PARTURITION IN THE NORMAL DAIRY COW

P.N. Smith, J.P. McCann, T.J. Reimers, R.H. Wasserman and F.A. Kallfelz
New York State College of Veterinary Medicine, Cornell University
Ithaca, New York 14853, U.S.A.

INTRODUCTION

Dairy cows affected with parturient paresis (milk fever) develop severe hypocalcemia at parturition despite elevations in circulating $1,25(OH)_2D$ (1). To provide a more complete profile of the periparturient vitamin D-calcium regulatory system, serum metabolites, CaBP and calcium as well as duodenal CaBP were evaluated in 3 normal cows from 40 days prepartum (Day -40) to 22 days postpartum (Day +22).

METHODS

Duodenal mucosa was obtained through preplaced duodenal cannulae. Serum and mucosa were evaluated for CaBP with a radioimmunoassay (2). Serum calcium was determined with atomic absorption spectrophotometry.

Vitamin D metabolites were quantified by competitive protein binding assays (rat plasma or rachitic chick intestinal cytosol) following lipid extraction, low pressure chromatography (Silica Sep-Pak®, Waters Associates) and HPLC (hexane:isopropanol [97:3] or hexane:isopropanol [89:11] and methylene chloride:isopropanol [98:2]).

RESULTS

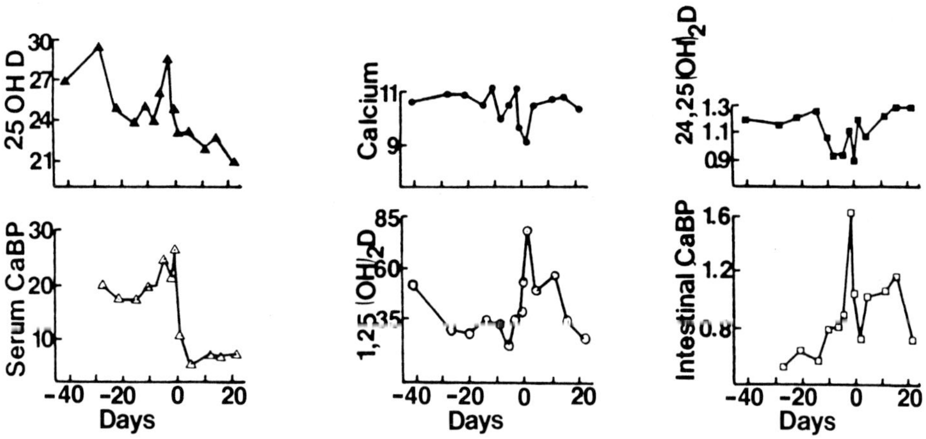

Figure 1. In normal Holstein cows, serum 25(OH)D (ng/ml), $1,25(OH)_2D$ (pg/ml), CaBP (ng/ml) and intestinal CaBP (ng/mg protein) rose sharply with parturition. In contrast, serum calcium (mg/dl) and $24,25(OH)_2D$ (ng/ml) declined in the immediate periparturient period. Serum $1,25(OH)_2D$ and intestinal CaBP esponded similarly in the periparturient period. Serum CaBP declined rapidly following parturition and placental expulsion.

Vitamin D. A Chemical, Biochemical and Clinical Update

In the normal parturient cow, circulating $24,25(OH)_2D$ decreased transiently with the hypocalcemia of parturition. Elevated prepartal serum CaBP levels declined immediately following parturition and lower levels were maintained postpartum. Duodenal mucosal CaBP tended to be higher postpartum than prepartum, a trend similar to that of $1,25(OH)_2D$.

DISCUSSION

The relative hypocalcemia normally associated with the immediate periparturient period is accompanied by an increase in $1,25(OH)_2D$ and a slight decline in circulating $24,25(OH)_2D$. This finding is of interest since it may support our previous work that showed an association between bovine parturient hypocalcemia and elevations in serum $24,25(OH)_2D$.

The reciprocal responses in serum and duodenal mucosal CaBP reflect the predominance of circulating CaBP prepartum in contrast to that of intestinal CaBP postpartum. The rapid decline in circulating levels at parturition suggests that the placenta may be a major source of serum CaBP or that the placenta may provide a stimulus for CaBP synthesis (e.g. estrogens). The relative increase in duodenal CaBP during the immediate postpartum period may reflect a response to elevated serum $1,25(OH)_2D$ in order to meet the increased calcium demands associated with the onset of lactation.

This work was supported by a grant from the Harold Wetterberg Foundation.

REFERENCES

1. Horst, R.L., Eisman, J.A., Jorgensen, N.A. and DeLuca, H.F. (1977) Science 196: 662-663.
2. McCann, J.P., Cowan, R.G. and Reimers, T.J. (1983) J. Anim. Sci. 57: 966-977.
3. Smith, P.N., Padilla, M., Wasserman, R.H. and Kallfelz, F.A. (1982) Calcif. Tissue Int. 34: 564-566.

RICKETS PROPHYLAXIS FOR PREMATURE INFANTS WITH FORMULA ENRICHED WITH VITAMIN D_3 OR 25-OH-VITAMIN D_3

A. Otten, S. Rentschler, H. Wolf and H. Schmidt-Gayk
Dept. of Pediatrics, Justus-Liebig-University Giessen; Clin. Chem. Lab., Dept. of Surgery, University Heidelberg (F.R.G.)

Introduction

In addition to calcium and phosphate which are sometimes inadequately supplied by the commonly used premature formulas and mother's milk, premature infants also require an exogenous supply of vitamin D_3. Nutritional formulas currently offered premature infants contain various amounts of vitamin D_3: from 400 I.U./l in the F.R.G. to 2800 I.U./l in Italy and some socialist countries. Absorption studies (3) have revealed gestational age (GA) - related differences for both vitamin D_3 and 25-OH-vitamin D_3. Continuous rickets prophylaxis requires administration of about 3 times more vitamin D_3 than 25-OH-vitamin D_3 in order to achieve the same protective effect (2). 5 mcg of 25-OH-vitamin D_3 given once daily result in a somewhat higher steady state level in a shorter period of time than the daily administration of 25 mcg vitamin D_3.

Recent investigations measuring the vitamin D_3 content breast milk revealed a relatively low total amount of vitamin D_3 and its metabolites. However, the major component was constituted by the apparently better absorbable 25-OH-vitamin D_3 (1). The goal of our study was to determine the bioavailability of vitamin D_3 and 25-OH-vitamin D_3 incorporated in milk formulas given premature infants using a feeding schedule evenly divided over 24 hours.

Patients and methods

Premature infants, the majority of whom born in the period from late fall to early spring, were entered into the study. The infants were divided into 6 groups on the following basis:

Control group:	9 premature infants (GA 32-36 weeks, 1750-2230 g birth weight (BW))were given meb-Milupa without vitamin D_3 supplementation
Group I:	5 premature infants (GA 33-34 weeks, 1970-2100 g BW):Humana 0, supplemented with 10 mcg vit. D_3/l

Vitamin D. A Chemical, Biochemical and Clinical Update

Group 2: 5 premature infants (GA 32-34 weeks, 1500-1710 g BW): Humana 0, supplemented with 70 mcg vitamin D_3/l

Group 3: 6 premature infants (GA 32-34 weeks, 1560-2170 g BW): meb-Milupa without vitamin D_3 but additionally up to 200 ml breast milk daily,2of those almost exclusively mother's milk

Group 4: 3 premature infants (GA 33-37 weeks, 1500-1810 g BW): Humana 1 supplemented with 5 mcg 25-OH-vitamin D_3/l (Dedrogyl$^{(R)}$)

Dedrogyl$^{(R)}$-group: 9 premature or hypotrophic infants (GA 30-40 weeks, 1460-2280 g BW): 5 mcg 25-OH-vitamin D_3 once daily (Dedrogly$^{(R)}$ drops) in addition to vitamin D_3-free formula.

Blood levels were obtained once a week for the determination of 25-OH-vitamin D_3. The planned total observation period was 4 weeks.

Results

The basal values of serum 25-OH-vitamin D_3 prior to beginning of the study (at 3 to 7 days of age) averaged 21 ng/ ml (range: 6-69 ng/ml). In the control group as well as in Group 3 (vitamin D_3-free formula plus breast milk) the blood levels did not significantly decrease from the beginning to and of the study. The average blood level of 25-OH-vitamin D_3 in Group 1 (10 mcg vitamin D_3/l) demonstrated a slight, but not significant increase over the study period. In contrast to Group 1, Group 2 (70 mcg vitamin D_3/l) exhibited a steep linear increase in average blood level of 25-OH-vitamin D_3. A steady state condition could not be achieved. The 25-OH-vitamin D_3levels of infants in Group 4 rose rapidly, achieving a steady state within one week. In the course of the 4-week observation period, the premature infants received maximally 2.5 mcg 25-OH-vitamin D_3 daily. The results of the Dedrogyl$^{(R)}$ Group has been in partpreviously reported (3). In all groups, the alkaline phosphatase values remained within the normal range.

Conclusions

The addition of breast milk to formula feedings did not supply the premature infant with an adequate amount of vitamin D_3. 400 I.U. vitamin D_3 = 10 mcg/l incorporated in an adapted formula was also not adequate. On the other hand, 2800 I.U. vitamin D_3 = 70 mcg/l resulted in very high blood levels of 25-OH-vitamin D_3. 5 mcg of 25-OH-vitamin D_3/l formula provided an constant supply of the metabolite predominantly found in breast milk. The fact that 25-OH-vitamin D_3 is quantitatively the predominat form of vitamin D_3 in both breast milk and cow's milk suggests that this metabolite is the basis of the natural supply of vitamin D_3. Our investigations showed that premature infants absorb 25-OH-vitamin D_3 much better than vitamin D_3. The supplementation of formulas with 10 mcg vitamin D_3/l, the advocated daily allowance in the F.R.G., is useless and urgently requires revision.

References

1. Kunz, O., Niesen, M., Lilienfeld-Toal, H. C., Burmeister, W. (1984) Int. J. Vit. Nutr. Res. 54, 141-148
2. Wolf, H., Kerstan, D., Kerstan, J. (1975) Klin. Pädiat. 187, 331-341
3. Wolf, H., Rentschler, S., Schmidt-Gayk, H. (1982) in: Vitamin D. Chemical, Biochemical und Clinical Endocrinology of Calcium Metabolism. W. de. Gruyter, Berlin-New-York, p. 591-593

VITAMIN D DEFICIENCY IN PRETERM INFANTS

L. Silvestro - M. Zaffaroni

Department of Puericulture (Head: Prof. G.C. Mussa) University of Turin - Italy.

Introduction. Transient hypocalcemia occurs frequently in preterm infant. During pregnancy the fetus has a high Calcium requirement because of its rapid growth. The serum calcium levels are higher in the umbilical vein than in maternal blood and this indicates that there is an active transport of Calcium through the placenta to the fetus. After birth the main factor underlying hypocalcemia is the interruption of the transplacental mineral supply at a time when the needs of the fetus are high. Furthermore transient hypoparathyroidism, hypercalcitoninemia, Vitamin D deficiency, defects in Vitamin D metabolism, and end-organ resistance to hormonal effects have all advocated to explain the inadeguate Calcium homeostasis in preterm newborns and their conseguent hypocalcemia. The role of Vitamin D in preventing or reducing the severity and duration of neonatal hypocalcemia in preterm infant is still discussed.

Patients and Methods. This study was carried out on 222 newborn infants with a gestational age of 37 weeks or less. The gestational age was assessed according to the last mestruation or, when necessary, by the score of Dubowitz. The subjects were divided into two groups. Whereas the first, considered as controls, received no vitamin supplementation, the second received a daily oral dose of 10 µg of 25 OH D3 during the first ten days of life. (Tab.1). For all the infants the feeding started during the first 24 hours of life. The feed consisted of commercially available adapted formulas reconstituited in water. Venous samples of blood were routinarely taken at 1, 2, 3, 5, 7, and 10 days for determination of calcemia. Serum Calcium concentrations below 3.5mEq/L were considered as hypocalcemic values. These newborns received Calcium-gluconate as a 10% solution lowly i.v.

Tab. 1 subjects :	n° 222		gestational age (weeks)	birth weight (gms)
Control group :	n° 121	M±SD	34.2 ± 2.4	1990 ± 497
		range	27 - 37	1050 - 3000
25 OH D3 group :	n° 101	M±SD	33.4 ± 2.8	1882 ± 391
		range	27 - 37	890 - 3110

Results. There were no significant differences in gestational age or birth weight between the two study groups. During the first 3 days of life the frequency of early-onset hypocalcemia was 40.5%(control group) and 39.6%(25 OH D3 group). Table 2 represents the frequency of hypocalcemia in preterm newborns with different gestational age. The observed incidence

Vitamin D. A Chemical, Biochemical and Clinical Update

of hypocalcemia was inversely proportional to gestational age and birth weight.Therefore 25 OH D3 failed in preventing early hypocalcemia in preterm infants.After the third day of life the frequency of hypocalcemia was 11.6%(controls)and 4%(25 OH D3 group).No differences vere found between infants receiving various adapted formulas.

Tab. 2 - Frequency of hypocalcemia in preterm infants.

gestational age (weeks)	subjects n°	normal serum Ca		hypocalcemia early-onset		hypocalcemia after 3rd day	
Control group:							
≤ 32	33	11	33.3 %	22	66.7 %	5	15.1 %
33 - 35	38	25	65.8 %	13	34.2 %	4	10.5 %
36 - 37	50	36	72 %	14	28 %	5	10 %
total	121	72	59.5 %	49	40.5 %	14	11.6 %
25 OH D3 group:							
≤ 32	38	19	50 %	19	50 %	2	5.3 %
33 - 35	36	22	61.1 %	14	38.9 %	2	5.6 %
36 - 37	27	20	74.1 %	7	25.9 %	-	-
total	101	61	60.4 %	40	39.6 %	4	4 %

Discussion. It has been shown that neonatal hypocalcemia is caused by a transient phisiologic hypoparathyroidism of the newborn infants.This relative hypoparathyroidism has been attributed to the increased serum calcium of the fetus,which reflects a calcium gradient across the placenta.During the first days of life inactive parathyroid glands fail to respond normally to low serum calcium concentrations.Furthermore in smaller infants (less than 32 weeks of gestation)Vitamin D is not adeguantely adsorbed and hydroxylated in liver and kidney.This study confirm the findings of previous reports which showed poor effects on early neonatal hypocalcemia by 25 OH D3 in preterm infant.Early hypocalcemia in preterm newborn is unlikely to be caused by an umpairment of Vitamin D activation in fact after 32 weeks of gestation,renal 25-hydroxyvitamin D-1alfa-hydroxylase activity is present.However 25 OH D3 is effective in treatment of late hypocalcemia and in preventing rickets in preterm infant.Further work needs to determine the absorption and metabolism of Vitamin D and to evaluate the role of 25 OH D3 on calcium homeostasis in newborn infant during the first days of life.

References. Glorieux F.H.,Salle B.L.,Delvin E.E.,David L. 1981 J.Ped. 99: 640-643. Mussa G.C.,Bona G.,Silvestro L.,Barberis L 1983 Atti III Giornate Pediatriche di Noli. Ed.Tipo Lito Tecnografica - Parma: 77-92. Huston R.K.,Reynolds J.W.,Jensen C., Buist N.R.M. 1983 Pediatrics 72: 44-48. Duvina P.L. and Simoni M.R. 1982 Riv. Ital. Ped. 8: 536.

FETAL AND NEONATAL UPTAKE AND MICROSOMAL C-25 HYDROXYLATION OF (^{3}H)-VITAMIN D_3 BY THE RAT LIVER.

MARIELLE GASCON-BARRE, VICTOR PLOURDE, PIERRE HADDAD AND JOHANNE MARTIAL, DEPT. PHARMACOLOGIE, FAC. MED. AND CENTRE DE RECHERCHES CLINIQUES, HOPITAL ST-LUC, UNIVERSITE DE MONTREAL, MONTREAL, QUEBEC, CANADA.

It is generally accepted that 25(OH)D is most likely passively transferred to the fetus across the placenta and that the fetus can rely on the maternal 25(OH)D to meet his needs in vitamin D (D) (1,2). Some studies have shown that unmetabolized D could also be transferred across the placenta (3,4). This raises the question of the ability of the fetal liver to take up D and to transform it into 25(OH)D. The purpose of the present studies was to evaluate 1) the uptake of ^{3}H-D_3 and 2) the activity of the D_3-25 hydroxylase in fetuses and newborn rats.

MATERIALS AND METHODS

A) *Uptake Studies*: The liver ^{3}H-D_3 uptake was studied in 19-21 day old fetuses and in neonates at days 3, 7, 14, 22, and 60. In fetuses, 0.01 μCi ^{3}H-D_3 (25 μCi/mmol) as well as 0.01 μCi ^{14}C-sucrose (used as extracellular marker) were injected into the umbilical vein. The livers were immediately homogenized in isotonic saline and evaluated for ^{14}C activity. Aliquots of homogenates were extracted and ^{3}H-D_3 uptake was evaluated. In neonates, the ^{3}H-D_3-^{14}C-sucrose solution was injected into the portal vein; the livers were immediately processed as described above.
B) *^{3}H-D_3-25 Hydroxylation Studies*: All animals were born on day 22 of gestation. They were studied on days 1, 2, 3, 14, 30 and 60. Fetuses were studied on days 19 and 22 of gestation. The ^{3}H-D_3-25 hydroxylase was evaluated using 15 mg microsomal protein, 26 pmol ^{3}H-D_3 and an NADPH generating system. After 40 min incubation, the mixture was extracted; ^{3}H-D_3 and ^{3}H-25(OH)D_3 were separated by HPLC. All data are expressed as means ± S.E.M. Statistically significant differences between groups were analyzed by ANOVA.

RESULTS AND DISCUSSION

There were highly significant differences in the liver ^{3}H-D_3 uptake during the period of time studied ($p<0.0001$) (Fig 1A) ^{3}H-D_3 uptake was highest after weaning with an uptake of 42±1.9% ($p<0.0001$) of the dose injected. The fetuses had significantly higher ^{3}H-D_3 uptake (11.3±1.1%) than the 3,7, and 14 day old pups ($p<0.0001$). The liver ^{3}H-D_3 uptake did not change significantly from day 3 to 14 after birth. HPLC analysis of the liver extracts showed only unmetabolized ^{3}H-D_3. The presence of detectable D_3-25 hydroxylase activity was already present in microsomes obtained from 19 day old fetuses (Fig 1B) and the activity of the 22 days old fetuses was found to be similar to that of rats of the same conceptual age (one day old pups). The enzymatic activity increased on days 2 and 3 after birth where it reached a plateau for the remaining period of time studied.
These results indicate that D_3 can be taken up by the fetal rat liver. Indeed the uptake of D_3 during the neonatal period was found to be significantly lower to that observed in the late fetal period and remained low for the first two weeks after birth. Between days 14 and 22 after birth, a six fold increase in the uptake of D_3 was observed suggesting that the liver uptake mechanisms had undergone transformations

Vitamin D. A Chemical, Biochemical and Clinical Update

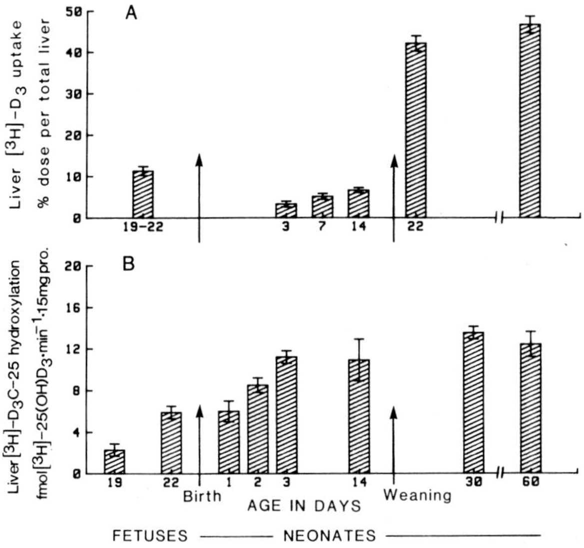

Fig. 1: Rat liver ^3H-D_3 uptake and C-25 hydroxylation

which allowed D_3 to be taken up in quantities similar to the one observed in older animals (5).

The data also illustrate that the liver C-25 hydroxylation of D_3 is present during the fetal period. Contrary to its uptake capacity, the C-25 hydroxylation reaches maximum activity as early as day 3 after birth, to remain unchanged for the next 2 months. The progressive increase in enzyme activity during the perinatal period supports the observation, made in human infants, that the D_3 C-25 hydroxylation capacity might be more related to the post conceptual age than to the *post-partum* age (6). This is further supported by the similarity in enzymatic activity observed between 22 day old fetuses and 1 day old pups who, in fact, were of the same conceptual age. These results illustrate that during the perinatal period, the total liver capacity to form $25(OH)D_3$ must take into consideration its uptake capacity for D_3. Integration of these two phenomena is of paramount importance in the interpretation of the homeostatic mechanisms involved in the hepatic metabolism of D_3 during the developmental period.

REFERENCES

1. Paunier, L., Lacourt, G., Pilloud, P., Schlaeppi, P., Sizonenko, P.C. (1978) Helv. Paediat. Acta 33, 95-103.
2. Wieland, P., Fisher, J.A., Trechsel, U., Roth, H.-R., Vetter, K., Schneider, H., Huch, A. (1980) Am. J. Physiol. 239, E385-E390.
3. Haddad Jr, J.G., Boisseau, V., Avioli, L.V. (1971) J. Lab. Clin. Med. 77, 908-915.
4. Chan, G.M., Buchino, J.J., Mehlhorn, D., Bove, K.E., Steichen, J.J., Tsang, R.C. (1979) Pediat. Res. 13, 121-126.
5. Gascon-Barré, M., Elbaz, H. (in press) Metabolism.
6. Hillman, L., Haddad, J.G. (1975) J. Pediatr. 6, 928-935.

VITAMIN D STATUS OF INFANTS IN THE FIRST SIX MONTHS OF LIFE

N.R. BELTON
Department of Child Life and Health, University of Edinburgh, Edinburgh EH9 1UW, Scotland, U.K.

INTRODUCTION

Although plasma 25-hydroxyvitamin D (25-OHD) concentrations at birth (cord blood) are directly related to but lower than those in the maternal plasma, previous studies (1) have shown that breast-milk-fed infants have lower plasma 25-OHD values than those fed on artificial formulae at 6 days of age. As part of infant feeding studies 16 breast-fed infants and 52 bottle-fed infants who had received one of four different artificial low solute milks had their plasma 25-OHD concentrations measured at 6 days, 6 weeks and 3 months of age. All of the artificial formulae were given in the liquid, ready-to-feed form in the first week of life in the maternity hospital. Thereafter the infants fed Osterfeed (Farley Health Products Ltd), Premium (Cow & Gate) and Gold Cap (SMA) received feeds made up from powder by the mother, but one group received Osterfeed RTF liquid ready-to-feed formula (Farley Health Products Ltd) up to 3 months of age. Plasma 25-OHD was also measured in a further group of 33 bottle-fed infants at 6 months, 7 of whom were receiving cow's milk instead of formula when the blood samples were obtained.

METHOD

Plasma 25-hydroxyvitamin D was measured by a competitive protein-binding assay based on that of Preece (2). The method was chloroform/methanol (1:1) extraction, silicic acid chromatography (Sigma LC-325 mesh) and the assay used serum from vitamin D-deficient rats, high specific activity ^3H 25-hydroxycholecalciferol (22Ci/umol - Amersham) and dextran (Pharmacia T20) coated charcoal (Norit GSX) to separate bound from free 25-OHD. The co-efficient of variation between assays was 10.2% (n = 20).

RESULTS

These are shown in detail in the Table for the infants up to 3 months of age. Plasma 25-OHD in the 33 bottle-fed infants at 6 months of age showed a mean of 18.8 ng/ml (S.D. $\pm$ 5.9). Values in the 7 infants on cow's milk alone were 15.4 $\pm$ 6.0.

DISCUSSION

These studies indicate that artificial milk formulae with a vitamin D content of about 1 µg (40 I.U.)/100 ml substantially improve the vitamin D status of young infants. We have previously shown that mothers in Edinburgh and hence their newborn infants have a relatively poor vitamin D status as a group (1). The breast-fed infants at 6 days in this study reflect this with a mean plasma 25-OHD of only 10.0 ng/ml. This was lower than that of the bottle-fed group. At 6 weeks the difference was more marked, the breast-fed infants having a significantly lower plasma 25-OHD than all of the other formula-fed groups ($p<0.01$ in all cases). At 3 months the difference between breast-fed and bottle-fed was less than at 3 weeks. Our information indicates that by 3 months only about 10% of the mothers in all groups were also giving their infants some supplementary vitamin D in the form of drops of liquid multivitamin preparations.

Table Plasma 25-hydroxyvitamin D (ng/ml) in infants during the first 3 months. Means ± S.D. are shown with n (no. of samples) in parentheses.

Milk or Formula	Age 6 days	Age 6 weeks	Age 3 months
Breast milk	10.0 ± 4.5 (17)	9.2 ± 4.4 (6)	20.3 ± 11.0 (5)
Premium	12.2 ± 6.1 (6)	26.7 ± 8.6 (15)	31.7 ± 5.8 (14)
Osterfeed	11.6 ± 7.3 (11)	20.7 ± 4.2 (14)	25.9 ± 4.9 (14)
Osterfeed RTF	15.6 ± 9.0 (6)	24.4 ± 5.6 (11)	27.3 ± 10.8 (7)
Gold Cap	19.1 ± 11.3 (8)	38.7 ± 10.2 (12)	44.4 ± 15.8 (12)

These findings show that formula-fed infants receive appropriate vitamin D supplementation in their feeds. Our calculations suggest that the bottle-fed infants received a daily average of 5.3 µg (212 I.U.) at 6 days, 8.5 µg (340 I.U.) at 6 weeks and 8.7 µg (350 I.U.) at 3 months of vitamin D in their feeds. The vitamin D status of most breast-fed infants, although poorer than that in the formula-fed infants, is probably adequate to prevent rickets. However, some infants in groups such as the Asians in our community when breast-fed remain at risk of developing vitamin D deficiency and rickets, particularly if no supplementary vitamin D is given (3).

ACKNOWLEDGEMENT
This study was supported by Farley Health Products Ltd.

REFERENCES

1. Cockburn, F. Belton, N.R., Purvis, R.J., Giles, M.M., Brown, J.K., Turner, T.L., Wilkinson, E.M., Forfar, J.O., Barrie, W.J.M., McKay, G.S. and Pocock S.J. (1980) Brit. Med. J., 281, 11-14.
2. Preece, M.A., O'Riordan, J.L.H., Lawson, D.E.M. and Kodicek, E. (1974) Clin. Chim. Acta, 54, 235-242.
3. Belton, N.R., Grindulis, H., Scott, P.H. and Wharton, B.A. (1985) in Proceedings Sixth Vitamin D Workshop, ed. Norman, A.W. Berlin, de Gruyter.

25-HYDROXYCHOLECALCIFEROL PROPHYLAXIS IN EARLY NEONATAL HYPOCALCEMIA.

G. Saggese, S. Bertelloni, G.I. Baroncelli and E. Bottone.
Department of Pediatrics, University of Pisa, Pisa, Italy.

Introduction:

Early neonatal hypocalcemia (ENH) is one of the most common complication in preterm infants (PI) occurring approximately in 30-50 % of these subjects (1).An alteration in perinatal vitamin D metabolism appear to be an important pathogenetic factor (2). Hepatic 25-hydroxylase is depressed in PI, who did not appear to increase their low 25-hydroxy cholecalciferol (25-OH-D) levels until a postconceptual age of 35-37 weeks (3). Serum 1,25-dihydroxy cholecalciferol (1,25(OH)2D) levels are low in cord-serum (4) but can increase also in PI (5). Hence hepatic synthesis of 25-OH-D seems to be the limiting metabolic step to substain ENH. We evaluate the use of this compound in the prophylaxis and therapy of ENH.

Patents and Methods:

Thyrty PI were studied: group A (n=15,body weight 1921±103,gestational age 31.4±1.1 wks) was supplemented with 25-OH-D (Didrogyl, Roussel Maestretti) at 5 ug/Kg/daily for 7 days; group B (n=15, body weight 2014±91, gestational age 32.1±0.8 wks) was not prophylaxed.

All the neonates were feeded with standard humanized formula containg 400 IU/vitamin D/L. The group B PI who showed hypocalcemia were treated with Didrogyl (50 ug/daily for 5 days) plus calcium gluconate (2-3 ml/Kg/daily), the hypocalcemic group A were treated with calcium gluconate only. Calcium salts were administrated by mouth to the normalization of the calcemia.

In each PI were determined calcium (Ca), phosphorus (P), magnesium (Mg), by standard laboratory methods, parathyroid hormone (PTH), calcitonin (CT), by RIA, and 25-OH-D, by radio protein binding assay (6), in 1°,2°,3°,7°,14° day of life. 1,25(OH)2D levels were measured (7) only at delivery in cord blood.

Results:

Hypocalcemia come out in 2° day of life in 2 PI group A (13.3%) and in 9 PI group B (60%). P and Mg were in all the neonates in normal range. PTH levels increased during the study, CT values (509±132 pg/ml) were higher than in older children (46.7±19.3 pg/ml, n=141). 25-OH-D levels (15.8±1.5 ng/ml) were significantly lower ($p<0.001$) in 1° day than normal values at term (23.3±1.3 ng/ml). 1,25(OH)2D concentrations in cord blood (21.6±5.1 pg/ml) were significantly lower ($p < 0.001$) than in older normal children (38.2±7.5 pg/ml) but in the same range of term infants (19.8±3.0 pg/ml). The group A showed during the study a significantly ($p < 0.001$) increase of 25-OH-D levels (from 16 ng/ml at day 1 to 35 ng/ml at day 14).In the normocalcemic PI of group B we detected only a slight increase (from 15.7 ng/ml to 19.4 ng/ml). The associated calcium salts and 25-OH-D therapy is

Vitamin D. A Chemical, Biochemical and Clinical Update

capaple to normalize calcemia in all the hypocalcemic PI.

Discussion:

Our study provides further data on the effectiveness of 25-OH-D prophylaxis and therapy in ENH. The exact pathogenesis of ENH is unknown. An alteration of vitamin D endocrine system may play an important patogenetic factor (1,2). In our PI we found, in agreeement with other AA (1,3,8), low 25-OH-D levels at birth, and no significat increase in postnatal period in group B PI, suggesting a defective function of hepatic 25-hydroxylase. Mouth therapy was able to increase quickly 25-OH-D levels showing a good absorption of this vitamin D metabolite in the gut also in PI. The exact mode of action of 25-OH-D in preventing ENH is unknown. Some AA (10) substained a pharmacologic action of this compound. We do not think it. In fact 25-OH-D supplementation in our doses increase 25-OH-D to normal levels, while pharmacologic effect require much high values that we never found. 25-OH-D may act extending available body pool to provide sufficient substrate for 1,25(OH)2D synthesis. The increased 1,25-OH-D levels augment the intestinal absorption and bone mobilization of calcium with restoration of normcalcemia. Other AA (10) substained a more specific action of 25-OH-D suggesting its permessive role on 1,25(OH)2D action at level of target cells.

R eferences:

1) Saggese, G., Biagioni, M., D'Accavio, L., Lenzoni, N., Boldrini, A. (1983) Ped. Oggi 3 : 458-464.
2) Fleishman, A.R., Rosen, J.F., Natheson, G. (1978) Am. J. Dis. Child. 132 :973-977.
3) Hillman, L.S., Haddad, J.G. (1983) J. Clin. Endocrinol. Metab. 56 : 189-191.
4) Steichen, J.J., Tsang, R.C., Gratton, T.L., Hamstra, A.J., DeLuca, H.F. (1980) N. Engl. J. Med. 302 : 315-319.
5) Markestad, T., Aksnes, L., Finne, P.H., Aarskog, D. (1984) Ped. Res. 18 :269-272.
6) Saggese, G., Bertelloni, S., Federico, G., Baroncelli, G.I., Bottone, E., Proc. "RIA '84", Albertini A. ed., Milano, May 15-16, 1984, p.31.
7) Eisman, J.A., Hamstra, A.J., Kream, B.E., DeLuca, H.F. (1976) Arch. Bioch. Bioph. 176 : 235-243.
8) Hillman, L.S., Haddad, J.G. (1975) J. Ped. 86 : 928-935.
9) Glorieux, F.H., Salle, B.L., Delvin, E.E., David, L. (1981) J. Ped. 99 : 640-643.
10) Bordier, P., Rasmussen, H., Marie, P., Miravet, L., Gueris, J., Ryckwaert, A. (1978) J. Clin. Endocrinol. Metab. 46: 289-295.

DISTRIBUTION AND INTERACTIONS OF D-BINDING PROTEIN (Gc) AND ACTIN IN HUMAN PLACENTAL TISSUE.

D.L. EMERSON, P.A. WERNER, M.H. CHENG and R.M. GALBRAITH,
Departments of Basic and Clinical Immunology and Microbiology, and Medicine, Medical University of South Carolina, Charleston, S.C. 29425, U.S.A.

Introduction:

The regulation of calcium and phosphate metabolism in the developing fetus is dependent in part upon Vitamin D metabolites supplied by the mother, and hydroxylase enzyme activity in the placenta (1). In view of the facts that; a) Gc (Vitamin D-binding protein) is the major serum protein responsible for transport and storage of Vitamin D metabolites (2,3), b) Gc binds G-actin and Vitamin D metabolites contemporaneously (4,5), and c) that both actin and Gc have been consistently found in trophoblast membrane preparations (6,7), the present study was undertaken to examine the distribution of these two proteins and their possible interactions in the normal human full-term placenta.

Materials and Methods:

Term placenta and matched maternal and cord serum were obtained immediately after vaginal delivery. Serum was also obtained from a patient with chronic active hepatitis who showed high titers of smooth muscle autoantibodies. The sera were stored at -20°C. Purified actin was obtained from Sigma, and Gc was purified from normal human serum as previously described (8). Cryostat sections (3um) were prepared from snap-frozen central cotyledon tissue, and syncytiotrophoblast membranes were purified as previously described (8). Sections were examined immunocytochemically with rabbit anti-Gc and rabbit and human anti-actin, using sheep anti-rabbit Ig FITC or goat anti-human Ig FITC as appropriate (10). Isolated trophoblast membranes were washed with either 3M KCl, 3M ammonium thiocyanate (NH_4SCN) 6M urea, or 0.05M glycine-HCl pH 3.8 before or after reaction with Gc protein. The trophoblast membrane washes were analyzed by SDS-PAGE, and Gc was detected by immunoperoxidase staining of nitrocellulose transblots (11). Identically prepared material, and matched maternal and fetal cord sera, were also subjected to analytical isoelectric focusing in conjunction with print immunofixation (IEF-PIF) (12).

Results and Discussion:

Immunofluorescence of native placental sections showed that both Gc and actin shared a similar geographical distribution on smooth muscle cells lining the fetal stem vessels, intervillous fibrin, villous fibrinoid, trophoblast membrane, and cytoplasm of villous stromal cells. Binding of Gc was demonstrated by prior incubation of sections with purified Gc which led to a striking increase in intensity of Gc fluorescence, but actin fluorescence was unaffected by this procedure and by preincubation with actin. Endogenous Gc and actin could also be removed by pre-washing of tissue sections as judged by fluorescence and SDS-PAGE immunoblots of the wash supernatants. In constrast to native sections, binding of exogenously added Gc on such treated sections was undetectable, but could be restored if the latter were first exposed to purified actin. These results indicated the presence of endogenous Gc and also of binding sites capable of binding exogenous Gc at several sites within the chorionic

Vitamin D. A Chemical, Biochemical and Clinical Update

villus. Experiments were then performed with purified trophoblast membranes to further examine endogenous Gc and in particular to attempt to establish if this Gc was of maternal or fetal origin. Initially IEF-PIF screening was perfomred on the maternal and cord serum pairs to select potentially informative pairs which demonstrated Gc phenotypic disparity. Comparison of the Gc bands in membrane washed with matched maternal and fetal cord serum indicated that the trophoblast membrane associated Gc was predominantly of maternal origin (Fig. 1).

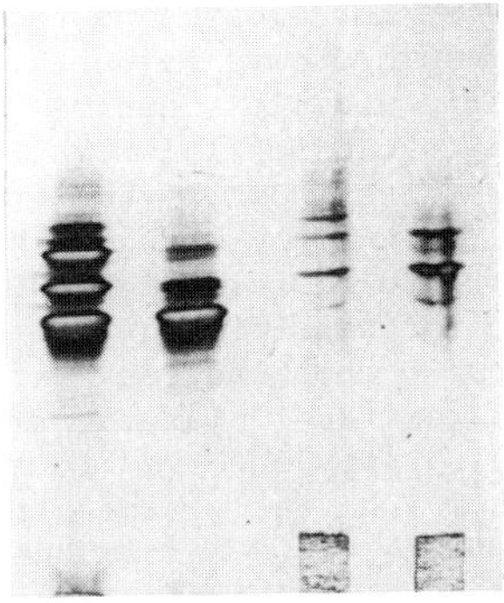

Fig. 1: IEF-PIF of matched maternal and fetal cord sera, and corresponding trophoblast membrane washes. From left to right the lanes contain maternal sera diluted 1:8 (Gc 1,2 phenotype), fetal cord serum diluted 1:8 (Gc2 phenotype), glycine-HCl wash and 3M NH_4SCN wash of trophoblast membranes. Note the major bands of Gc 1,2 phenotype in all washes, and the presence of additional anodal bands correspnding to Gc-actin and Gc:D_3 complexes.

These results indicated that Gc is bound to the trophoblast membrane in vivo, and may interact with placental actin. Such binding of Gc may represent the first step in the transport of Vitamin D metabolites from the maternal circulation through the placenta for distribution to the fetus.

Acknowledgments. Research supported in part by NIH Grant CA-27062, Institutional Award CR-17, and Labcatal Laboratories, France. RMG was recipient of NIH Research Career Development Award CA-00611.

References:

1. Fraser, D.R. (1980) Phys. Rev. 60, 551-613.
2. Daiger, S.P., Schanfield, M.S., Cavalli-Sforza, L.L. (1975) Proc. Nat. Acad. Sci. USA 72, 2076-2080.
3. Putnam, F.W., in The Plasma Proteins, Ed. Putnam, F.W., London: Academic Press, 1977, p334-354.
4. Van Baelen, H., Bouillon, R., DeMoor, P. (1980) J. Biol. Chem. 255, 2270-2272.
5. Haddad, J.G. (1982) Arch. Biochem. Biophys. 213, 538-544.
6. Ogbimi, A.O., Johnson, P.M., Brown, P.J., Fox, H. (1979) J. Reprod. Immunol. 1, 127-140.
7. Okamura, K., Powell, J.E., Lee, A.C., Stevens, V.C. (1981) Placenta 2, 117-128.
8. Chapuis-Cellier, C., Gianazza, E., Arnaud, P. (1982) Biochim. Biophys. Acta. 709, 353-357.
9. Emerson, D.L., Kantor, R., Arnaud, P., Galbraith, R.M. (1983) Am. J. Reprod. Immunol. 3, 32-42.
10. Galbraith, G.M.P., Galbraith, R.M., Faulk, W.P. (1980) Placenta 1, 33-46.
11. Towbin, H., Staehelin, T., Gordon, J. (1979) Proc. Nat. Acad. Sci. USA 76, 4350-4354.
12. Emerson, D.L., Galbraith, R.M., Arnaud, P. (1984) Electrophoresis 5, 22-26.

MITOCHONDRIAL CALCIUM AND BONE MINERALIZATION IN RAT FETUS.

J.J. PLACHOT, C.L. THIL, S. HALPERN*, G. COURNOT-WITMER and S. BALSAN
CNRS UA.583-INSERM U.30, Hôpital des Enfants-Malades, Paris, 75015, France.
*UNIVERSITE PARIS-VAL DE MARNE, Créteil, 94010, France.

Introduction:

It is generally admitted that in cartilage and bone, membrane surrounded bodies, i.e., matrix vesicles, represent the earliest loci of calcification, because the first hydroxyapatite cristals are found within them or in their immediate vicinity (1,2). However, recent studies using techniques which allow to detect labile mineral (ultracryomicrotomy, pyroantimonate fixation) have shown that, in addition to matrix vesicles, not membrane-bound electron dense deposits may be observed in extracellular matrix (3). Moreover, the diffraction pattern of these deposits indicate the presence of a mineral phase other than hydroxyapatite (4). Although the mechanism of calcification is largely unknown, it appears to be related to mitochondrial calcium metabolism. Indeed, the presence of calcified granules has been demonstrated in mitochondria of hypertrophic chondrocytes, and there is a progressive decrease of these deposits as extracellular matrix calcifications begins (5). Similar granules have also been observed in mitochondria of osteoblast. Our purpose was to study the early mineralization in rat fetal perichondral ossification ring of the tibia before the vascular invasion (17th day of gestation). Mitochondrial and extracellular mineral deposits were analyzed after conventional processing and after pyroantimonate treatment and their Ca/P ratios were evaluated by quantitative X-ray microanalysis.

Materials and Methods:

-Electron microscopy : Small pieces of tibial periosteum of normal 17 day old rat fetuses were dissected in tris maleate buffer. Half of the samples were fixed for 3 hours in a cacodylate buffered 2.4 % solution of glutaraldehyde and paraformaldehyde and post-fixed in 1 % osmium tetroxyde. The remaining samples were fixed for 24 hours in 2 % K pyroantimonate (PAO) and post-fixed in a fresh solution of 5 % formaldehyde in 2 % PAO. Thereafter, the samples were dehydrated and embedded in epon 812. Ultrathin sections were obtained with an L.K.B. ultratome III microtome with a diamond knife, spread flat on tris maleate buffer and mounted on copper or titanium grids. They were examined (Siemens Elmiskop 101) unstained or after staining with uranyl acetate and lead citrate.

-X-Ray microanalysis was performed on 600 Å thick unstained sections, mounted on titanium grids and carbon coated, with a CAMECA MBX microprobe (Voltage 45 kV, beam current intensity 150 nA ; incident electron beam diameter, 1000-2000 Å). L α line for antimony, K α line for calcium and phosphorus were chosen for analysis. Values for Ca/P ratios obtained in the different mineralized deposits were compared to the theoretical value for hydroxyapatite (1.67) and to the values obtained on the cristallites associated with matrix vesicles.

Results:

After conventional processing, osteoblasts showed an irregular outline. In contact with osteoid their plasmalemma extended in protoplasmic processes, but in several areas it was indistinct or interrupted. Rough endoplasmic reticulum was abundant. Mitochondria were numerous and contained a few electron dense granules. Within the osteoid homogenous dense matrix vesicles (600-2000 Å) contained or were surrounded by small hydroxyapatite

Vitamin D. A Chemical, Biochemical and Clinical Update

needles. Other deposits had the aspect of roundish cristallite clusters, with no orientation nor definite relationship with collagen fibres. Moreover, lying free in the organic matrix, numerous isolated mitochondria with clearly recognizable cristae were observed. In some cases mitochondrial membranes had a coiled aspect.

After PAO treatment the intra and extracellular mineral deposits were more abundant than after conventional processing. Within the mitochondria of osteoblasts small granules (300 Å) were numerous, isolated or assembled to form large clusters (2000-3000 Å). Outside the cells similar granules and clusters were observed within the mitochondria, or free in the organic matrix. All these deposits had an amorphous aspect, in contrast to the mineral associated with matrix vesicles, which was cristalline. The Ca/P ratios measured in the different deposits varied greatly. The highest values were observed in intramitochondrial deposits, either within or outside the osteoblasts (11.5 $\pm$ 2.54). In the granules lying free in the matrix the Ca/P ratio was 4.8 $\pm$ 0.75, it was 2.54 $\pm$ 0.09 in the clusters and 1.52 $\pm$ 0.07 in mineralized matrix vesicles.

Discussion:

Our results show that during early fetal ossification, in addition to hydroxyapatite cristallites, numerous amorphous mineral deposits with variable Ca/P ratios are observed in the organic matrix. Moreover the presence of calcium phosphate loaded mitochondria within but also outside the osteoblasts suggest that, at the developmental stage studied, mitochondria are directly involved in mineral deposition.

The presence of amorphous calcium phosphate (ACP) preceeding the cristalline phase during bone mineralization has been observed by others, using morphological or biochemical technique (6), and it has been suggested that there is not just one sort of ACP but a whole range of salts. This hypothesis is supported by our data showing that the amorphous material has variable Ca/P ratios.

It is generally admitted that mitochondrial calcium plays an essential role in biological calcification, but the mechanism by which the ion is transferred to the extracellular environment is not clear. Our results show that at the first stage of perichondral ossification, the mitochondria of osteoblasts, rich in calcified granules, are directly exported into the organic matrix. It may be that subsequently the inorganic material is released by degradation of mitochondrial membranes. Furthermore, the decrease of the Ca/P ratios, from intracellular granules to extracellular clusters may be due to a progressive phosphate enrichment of the mineral deposits, the phosphate supply depending on matrix vesicles alkaline phosphatase.

References

1. Bonucci, E., (1967) J. Ultrastruct. Res. 20 : 33-50.
2. Anderson, H.C., (1969) J. Cell. Biol. 41 : 59-72.
3. Brighton, C.L., Hunt, R.M., (1974) Clin. Orthop. Rel. Res. 100 : 406-416.
4. Landis, J.W., Glimeher, J.M. (1982) J. Ultrastruct. Res. 78 : 227-268.
5. Brighton, C.L., Hunt, R.M., (1978) J. Bone, Joint Surgery 60 : 630-639.
6. Posner, A.S., (1969) Physiol. Rev. 49 : 760-792.

MATERNAL VITAMIN D SUPPLEMENTATION DURING LACTATION - EFFECT ON INFANT AND MOTHER.

C.Lamberg-Allardt, L.Salmenperä, J.Perheentupa and M.A.Siimes. Children's Hospital,University of Helsinki; Endocrine Research Laboratory, University of Helsinki, Minerva Foundation, P.O.Box 819, 00101 Helsinki, Finland.

Introduction

In recent years the duration of exclusive breast-feeding has gradually increased. The aim of this study was to find out whether the maternal route of supplementation would meet the infant's need for vitamin D , as this route could be considered more physiological than direct supplementation of the infant.

Subjects and methods

We studied infants born in June through December, and their mothers.In regard to daily vitamin D3 supplementation the subjects were randomized at delivery in three groups : 1) the infant received 400 IU(10 ug) (according to RDA) and the mother 100IU(2.5 ug) (N=26); 2) the mother received 2100 IU(52.5 ug)(N=46); 3) the mother received 900 IU(22.5ug)(N =21).Blood was drawn from the mother and from the umbilical cord at delivery and thereafter from the mother and the infant at 2,4 and 6 months after delivery.

The serum 25-hydroxy-vitamin D (25-OH-D) concentration was determined by a competitive protein binding assay using human vitamin-D deficient serum as binder and purification of the samples on small,open silicic acid columns. Serum alkaline phosphatase activity and calcium concentration were measured by routine assays.

Results

None of the infants developed clinical rickets during the study. The maternal and infantile serum alkaline phosphatase activity and calcium concentration were normal and similar in all three groups.The mean infant 25-OH-D concentration increased in the same manner in groups 1 and 2.In contrast, the mean concentration in group 3 was lower than in the two other groups at 2 and 4 months. At 6 months the concentration was the same in all three groups of infants.In the mothers,the mean 25-OH-D concentration was significantly lower in group 1 than in the other groups all through the study (Fig.). The mean concentration was significantly lower in group 2 than in group 3 at 2 months but thereafter it was similar in these groups.

Discussion

The results indicate that the vitamin D status of the infant is affected by the supplementation of the mother during exclusive breast-feeding.We found that the serum 25-OH-D concentration of the infants gradually increased in the group where

Vitamin D. A Chemical, Biochemical and Clinical Update

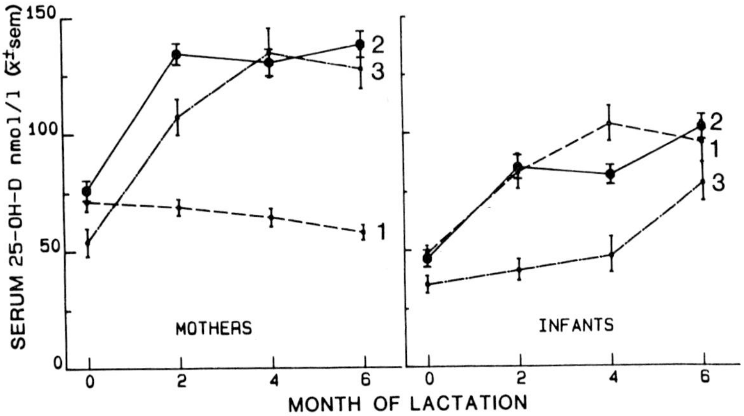

FIGURE The serum 25-OH-D concentration of the mothers and the infants in the different supplementation groups during 6 months of lactation.

the mother received 2100 IU of vitamin D daily during lactation and that the level equalled that of the infants receiving 400 IU of vitamin D daily. Thus, vitamin D or 25-OH-D is transferred in sufficient amounts from the mother to the infant during lactation if the vitamin D status of the mother is good enough. There was also a slow but significant increase in the 25-OH-D-concentration of the infants whose only supplement was 900 IU of vitamin D given daily to the mother.Our finding is in contrast to earlier reports of no effect on the infantile serum 25-OH-D concentration by maternal vitamin D supplementation(1,2).This is probably due to the smaller dosages given to the mothers in the other studies and to shorter study periods.High vitamin D dosages could,however, entail a risk for hypercalcaemia in the mother. The 2100 IU supplementation increased the maternal serum 25-OH-D concentration significantly as compared to the initial concentration,but a plateau was reached at 2 months after delivery and the concentration stayed at this level for the remaining study period.The mean plateau concentration (160 nmol/l) was high as compared to the reference range of our laboratory (25-124 nmol/l).The maternal serum calcium concentration in this supplementation group was similar to that in group 1 (mothers receiving 100 IU). The daily 900 IU supplement also increased the maternal serum 25-OH-D concentration significantly but the plateau was reached later than in the 2100 IU group. In conclusion, our results indicate that adequate vitamin D supplementation of the infant may be carried out via the mother, without any detectable risk.

Litterature

1.Markestad T.(1983) Eur.J.Pediatr.141,77-80.
2.Rothberg A.D.,Pettifor J.M., Cohen D.F,Sonnendecker E.W.W.and Ross F.P.(1982) J.Pediatr.101,500-503.

D-Binding Proteins

VITAMIN D-BINDING PROTEIN AND FREE 1,25-DIHYDROXYVITAMIN D IN ANIMALS AND CLINICAL MEDICINE

R. Bouillon, B. Nyomba , W. Decleer and H. Van Baelen,
Laboratorium voor Experimentele Geneeskunde en Endocrinologie and Laboratorium voor Experimentele Heelkunde, Gasthuisberg, B-3000 Leuven, Belgium.

The serum transport system for vitamin D metabolites certainly functions as a storage system for 25-hydroxyvitamin D but the role of DBP in the bioavailability of 1,25-$(OH)_2D$ is more disputed. From previously described experiments we believe that only 1,25-$(OH)_2D$ not bound to DBP is available for cellular entry and therefore of physiological importance (1,2). The present paper will try to summarize the arguments for and against this concept.

Sexual difference in DBP and 1,25-$(OH)_2D$ in man, rat and chick

In the three species from which we isolated DBP, a sexual difference in DBP concentration is known, but associated changes in 1,25-$(OH)_2D$ are less well documented. In normal adult man DBP concentrations are similar in males and females but estrogen treatment increases both the DBP and 1,25-$(OH)_2D$ concentrations without a significant change in calculated free 1,25-$(OH)_2D$ (3,4) and without significant change in intestinal calcium absorption (5).

In the rat, however, DBP levels are higher in males than in females and this is due to a stimulatory effect of androgens on DBP concentrations (6). Whether 1,25-$(OH)_2D$ levels would change in concert with DBP levels was analyzed in 3 groups of male rats, which were either gonadectomized, sham-gonadectomized or gonadectomized with subsequent androgen treatment. As expected, serum DBP decreased significantly by castration and could be restored by androgen therapy. Total 1,25-$(OH)_2D$ also decreased after gonadectomy and could be nearly normalized by androgen therapy. The molar ratio of 1,25-$(OH)_2D$ over DBP used as an index for 1,25-$(OH)_2D$ levels therefore remained unchanged (Fig. 1). This constitutes another example of changes in total 1,25$(OH)_2D$ due to changes in DBP, similar to the estrogen effect in women.

In the chick, sexual maturation is also associated with an increase in serum DBP, but higher values are now observed in hens than in roosters and this effect can be reproduced by estrogen therapy of immature chicks (7,8). Hens, however, also need higher amounts of calcium for egg shell calcification. To dissociate the effect of DBP levels from the effect of increasing calcium demands on 1,25-$(OH)_2D$ levels, several groups of chick and hens were compared as to their DBP and 1,25$(OH)_2D$ levels. This work was performed in collaboration with Dr. Y. NYS from Tours, France (8). DBP concentrations markedly increased in immature chicks treated with estrogens but still higher levels were observed in mature hens whether laying eggs with hard shells or laying soft eggs without calcification due to the presence of a thread in utero. Total 1,25-$(OH)_2D$ markedly increased due to estrogen therapy or sexual maturation. The values were however much higher in hens laying hard eggs than in soft-egg laying hens, which could be explained by their different calcium needs for egg shell calcification. The free 1,25-$(OH)_2D$ ratio, therefore, was slightly increased by estrogen therapy alone, probably due to its acute effect on new

Vitamin D. A Chemical, Biochemical and Clinical Update

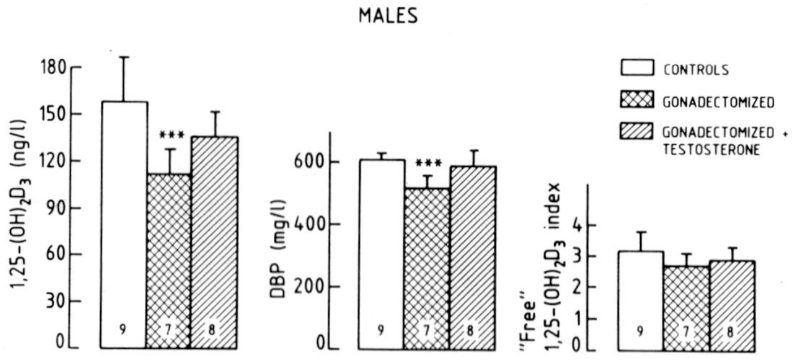

Fig. 1. Effect of gonadectomy with or without androgen therapy on serum concentrations of DBP, 1,25-$(OH)_2$D and free 1,25-$(OH)_2$D index in male Wistar rats.

bone formation. Hens without extra need for calcium, however, had free 1,25-$(OH)_2$D similar to those of immature chicks although their serum estrogen levels were identical to those of hens laying calcified eggs. The normal hens needing extra calcium for egg shell calcification had markedly increased free 1,25-$(OH)_2$D concentrations (8). This situation can be compared to human pregnancy which also involves the combined effect of estrogens and extra calcium needs. Simple increase in DBP without increased calcium demands e.g. due to estrogen therapy in women or by blocking the calcium needs in adult hens leaves the free 1,25-$(OH)_2$D index unchanged. In association with increased calcium demands the free index increases as is observed at the end of human pregnancy or during normal egg shell formation.

Influence of DBP on 1,25-$(OH)_2$D concentrations in human diseases

Many diseases with abnormal vitamin D concentrations are associated or due to abnormal DBP levels. A first possibility is abnormal liver synthesis of proteins such as can be found in *liver cirrhosis*. The serum concentrations of albumin and DBP were markedly decreased. 25-OHD concentrations remained normal in most patients.Total 1,25-$(OH)_2$D concentrations were significantly lower but when corrected for DBP a normal free 1,25-$(OH)_2$D ratio could be calculated which is further reflected by normal ionized calcium concentrations (9). Similar observations have now been made by Haddad's group using ultrafiltration measurements of free 1,25$(OH)_2$D (10). Vitamin D abnormalities in liver cirrhosis are thus mainly secondary adaptations to lower protein synthesis and only exceptionally a truly disturbed vitamin D metabolism can be found. A second example of DBP-associated vitamin D disturbances is to be found in *nephrotic syndrome*, a disease characterized by an abnormal loss of serum proteins in the urine. In a selected group of such patients with normal glomerular filtration rate, serum albumin was markedly decreased but serum DBP levels were only slightly below normal, indicating a better homeostasis for DBP than for albumin, an observation which could also have been made in liver cirrhosis. Total 25-OHD levels were decreased, which is now well known and due to the excessive urinary loss of 25OHD (11). Since 1,25-$(OH)_2$D was also decreased and more than could be explained by the decrease in DBP, the free 1,25-$(OH)_2$D index was below normal. Nephrotic syndrome is thus characterized by low 1,25-$(OH)_2$D partly due to low DBP levels but aggravated by substrate deficiency of 25-OHD due to urinary loss of DBP (12).

Another difficult example of possible vitamin D disturbance is to be found in *diabetes mellitus*. Several previous reports mentioned low levels of 1,25-$(OH)_2$D in streptozotocin-induced diabetic male rats whereas in human diabetes both normal and decreased concentrations were reported. DBP and 1,25-$(OH)_2$D were therefore measured in Wistar rats after streptozotocin-induced diabetes.

A marked decrease in DBP was observed, associated with a decrease in serum 1,25-$(OH)_2$D. This phenomenon was most marked in adult male rats. On sequential analysis the DBP decrease preceeded the decrease in 1,25-$(OH)_2$D. The free 1,25-$(OH)_2$D as well as their protein-corrected serum calcium, however, did not decrease (13). Similar observations were made in another strain of rats, called BB rats, which develops a genetically autoimmune form of diabetes which in many aspects is similar to the human type I diabetes (14).

Concerning human diabetes, normal DBP and 1,25-$(OH)_2$D levels were observed in insulin-treated caucasians, whereas DBP and 1,25-$(OH)_2$D levels were significantly decreased in less-well insulin-treated Bantu diabetics from Zaire (14).

Influence of additional vitamin D-binding proteins on serum 1,25-$(OH)_2$D concentrations

The role of endogenous binding proteins for vitamin D can also be studied by acute or chronic modification of the vitamin D-binding capacity of serum. Total 1,25-$(OH)_2$D concentrations were, therefore, measured in rabbits previously immunized with vitamin D analogues.

A 100-fold increase in total 1,25-$(OH)_2$D was observed in rabbits with the highest titer of antibodies whereas in general a good correlation was observed between antibody titer and total 1,25-$(OH)_2$D concentration (Table 1). This indicates that the circulating concentration of 1,25-$(OH)_2$D is adapted according to the chronic serum binding capacity.

To test the in vivo effect of DBP on vitamin D action, the short term effect of large amounts of exogenous DBP on calcium metabolism was investigated in rats. About 1 g of human DBP was isolated by immuno-affinity chromatography from several liters of human blood. The protein was then further purified by chromatofocusing which also eliminated endogenous vitamin D metabolites (1). The half-life of human DBP in rabbits and rats

$1,25-(OH)_2D$ IN VITAMIN D-IMMUNIZED RABBITS

	total $1,25-(OH)_2D$ (pg/ml)	serum dilution to bind 40% of 20 pg $[^3H]1,25-(OH)_2D$
Control rabbits (n = 19)	62 ± 13	-
rabbits immunized with $1,25-(OH)_2D$-3-HS-BSA		
rabbit H	6000	1 : 40,000
rabbit Q	2430	1 : 15,000
rabbit T	1680	1 : 12,500
rabbit S	1105	1 : 2,000
rabbits immunized with 1α-cholecalcioic acid-BSA		
rabbit N	770	1 : 8,000
rabbit M	960	1 : 8,000

Table 1. Serum concentrations of total $1,25-(OH)_2D$ in adult rabbits, previously immunized against $1,25-(OH)_2D$-3-hemissucinate-BSA or against 1α-cholecalcioic acid-BSA, compared with their binding capacity for $1,25-(OH)_2D$ in a radioimmunoassay system.

was found to be about 4 and 3 hours respectively, so that continuous infusion was necessary to obtain stable levels. Three groups of 6 male rats were studied after (temporary) hypnorm anesthesia for insertion of an i.v. and i.a. canula by microsurgery. Thereafter an infusion was started with either 145 mg of human serum albumin, 150 mg of hDBP or the gammaglobulins isolated from 1.5 ml of a potent rabbit antiserum against $1,25-(OH)_2D$. One fifth of this dose was given as a priming dose and the remaining amount infused over the next 24 h. At the end a calcium absorption test and terminal blood sampling was performed. Since about 4 ml of blood was taken at the start and replaced by a sodium chloride solution a decrease in rat serum albumin was not unexpected. This decrease of about 20% was similar in all groups of rats. The serum calcium concentration also decreased by about 17% so that the protein-corrected calcium concentration remained constant. The serum concentration of 25-OHD decreased in all groups by 20% without any significant difference between subgroups. This decrease corresponds to the observed decrease in serum albumin and can be explained by the amount of blood taken for the initial analysis at the start of the infusion. It does, however, indicate that restoration of 25-OHD concentration does not occur within 24 h. The serum concentration of $1,25-(OH)_2D$ fell in the rats infused with human albumin nearly in proportion to the observed decrease in serum 25-OHD and serum rat albumin concentrations. In the rats infused with hDBP or anti-$1,25-(OH)_2D$ antibodies, restoration or even a slight increase in $1,25-(OH)_2D$ concentration was observed. This increase however was small when compared to the amount of binding proteins infused over 24 h. The combined human and rat DBP concentration in the hDBP-infused rats was five times higher than before the start of the experiment, whereas the binding capacity was increased two-fold in the anti-1,25-$(OH)_2D$ infused rats. The five-fold increase in DBP was only compensated by a significant but small increase in 1,25-$(OH)_2D$ after 24 h (+ 10%), in the same order as the increase in rats infused with gamma globulins. The intestinal calcium absorption was only slightly but not even significantly lower in the DBP- infused group and unchanged in the antibody-infused rats. Similarly no difference on serum calcium levels were observed.

We therefore conclude that an acute increase in serum specific vitamin D binding capacity either by DBP or antibody infusion does not significantly alter serum calcium homeostasis within 24 h suggesting that circulating 1,25-$(OH)_2D$ are not critical for the acute calcium homeostasis. Moreover it demonstrates that adaptation of 1,25-$(OH)_2D$ to circulating levels of binding proteins requires more than 24 h of adapatation.

References

1. Bouillon, R. and Van Baelen, H. in Vitamin D chemical, biochemical and clinical endocrinology of calcium metabolism, Ed. A.W. Norman et al., W. de Gruyter, 1982, p 1181-1186.
2. Bouillon, R. and Van Baelen, H. (1981) Calcif. Tissue Intern. 33: 451-453.
3. Bouillon, R., Van Assche, F.A., Van Baelen, H., Heyns, W., De Moor, P. (1981) J. Clin. Invest. 67: 589-596.
4. Aarskog, D., Aksnes, L., Markestad, T., Rodland, O. (1983) J. Clin. Endocr. Metab. 57: 1155-1158.
5. Crilly, R.G., Marshall, D.H., Horsman, A., Nordin, B.E.C., Bouillon, R. in Osteoporosis: Recent advances in pathogenesis and treatment. Ed. H.F. DeLuca et al., Park Press Baltimore, 1981, p 425-432.
6. Bouillon, R., Van Baelen, H., Rombauts, W., De Moor, P. (1978) J. Biol. Chem. 253: 4426-4431.
7. Bouillon, R., Van Baelen, H., Biauw, K.T., De Moor, P. (1980) J. Biol. Chem. 255: 10925-10930.
8. Nys, Y., Bouillon, R., Williams, J. submitted for publication.
9. Bouillon, R., Auwerx, J., De Keyser, L., Fevery, J., Lissens, W., De Moor, P. (1984) J. Clin. Endocrin. Metab. 59: 86-89.
10. Bikle, D.D., Gee, E., Halloran, B., Haddad, J.G. (1984) J. Clin. Invest. 74: 1966-1971.
11. Schmidt-Gayk, H., Schmitt, W., Grawunder, C., Ritz, E., Tschöpe, W., Pietsch, V., Andrassay, K., Bouillon, R. (1977) Lancet ii: 105-108.
12. Auwerx, J., De Keyser, L., Bouillon, R., De Moor, P. submitted for publication.
13. Nyomba, B.L., Bouillon, R., Lissens, L., Van Baelen, H., De Moor, P. Endocrinology in press.
14. Nyomba, B.L., Bouillon, R., Bidingija, M., Kandjingu, K., De Moor, P. submitted for publication.

THE INTERACTION OF D-BINDING PROTEIN (Gc) WITH LYMPHOCYTES AND ITS POSSIBLE BIOLOGICAL FUNCTION.

ROBERT M. GALBRAITH AND PHILIPPE ARNAUD, Departments of Basic and Clinical Immunology and Microbiology, and Medicine, Medical University of South Carolina, Charleston, SC 29425

INTRODUCTION: Group-specific component (Gc) or Vitamin D-binding protein (DBP) was first described in human plasma in 1959 (1), but knowledge of its biological relevance has been slow to develop. For many years, the main focus of interest concerned its extensive polymorphism (2) and possible use as a genetic tool. The realization that Gc interacts with, and constitutes the major serum carrier for, D3 metabolites came only in 1975 (3). This observation led to several studies of Gc levels and phenotype or allele frequencies in various disorders (4-6). Parallel studies in a wide variety of nucleated cells showed a ubiquitous DBP which appeared to be similar to serum Gc, although generally present in the form of a 5.8S complex with another unidentified cell component (7-9). The latter was found to be G-actin (10,11), and this protein is now known to undergo a specific high affinity ($Ka=1.5-1.9 \times 10^8\ M^{-1}$) with Gc (12). These twin interactions, with vitamin D3 metabolites and with G-actin, have led to renewed interest in Gc, and certain findings will now be summarized prior to further consideration of functional properties. It should be noted that detailed discussions of the relevance of Gc to vitamin D3 metabolism and clinical disease, and to the biological function of actin respectively are included elsewhere in this volume (13,14), and will not be considered further here. Another point of some importance is that the piecemeal nature of discoveries in this area has resulted in a variety of designations for this protein, including Gc, DBP and even actin-binding protein (ABP). For convenience, we will use Gc throughout, with the understanding that this term is interchangeable with DBP.

BASIC PROPERTIES OF Gc AND INTERACTIONS WITH OTHER LIGANDS: Interactions of Gc with D3 metabolites and G-actin (see also 13,14) result in modification of the isoelectric point (pI) as shown by progressively anodal migration - in the order of 25-(OH) D3:Gc, Gc:G-actin and 25-(OH) D3:Gc:G-actin complexes - in comparison with native Gc (15,16). Electrophoretic mobility is also increased (15,17,18). Indirect association between Gc and proteins which bind to G-actin is also possible, and Deoxyribonuclease I (E.C.3.1.21.1., DNase) has been shown to form a ternary complex with Gc: G-actin by a combination of methods, including polyacrylamide gel electrophoresis (PAGE) in the absence of SDS (12), two dimensional (2d) electrophoresis and gel filtration (12). This complex, in contrast, does not exhibit changes in pI (Table I), and will also bind 25-(OH) D3 to yield the quaternary complex - 25-(OH) D3:Gc:G-actin:DNase (12). It should be noted that the affinity (Ka) of interaction between Gc and 25-(OH) D3 is not significantly altered by additional complexing with G-actin or G-actin:DNase (19); neither is the Ka of Gc binding to G-actin noticeably affected by complexing of the latter with DNase (12). In other respects however, additional interaction of G-actin with DNase may cause major changes. Thus, phospholipid/$Ca2^+$-dependent phosphorylation of Gc (see below) is unaffected by G-actin complexing but apparently abrogated by ternary interaction with Gc:G-actin (unpublished results). The precise

Vitamin D. A Chemical, Biochemical and Clinical Update

Table 1: Alteration of the isoelectric point(s) of Gc following complex formation with specific ligands

Sucrose gels		Urea gels (2.0M)	(6.0M)	Triton 1%
Gc 1	F 4.83	4.79		4.84
	S 4.88	4.83		4.92
Gc 1 + 25(OH) D3				
	F 4.76	4.71		4.84
	S 4.82	4.76		4.92
Gc 1 + Actin				
	F 4.72	4.60		4.67
	S 4.74	4.63		4.68
Gc 1 + Actin + DNase				
	F 4.72			
	S 4.74			
Gc 1 + Actin + 25(OH) D3				
	F 4.70			4.67
	S 4.72			4.68
Gc2	5.0	4.86	5.55	4.94
Gc2 + 25(OH)D3				
	4.97	4.80	5.55	4.94
Gc2 + Actin	4.83	4.67	5.55	4.72
Gc2 + Actin + DNase				
	4.83			
Gc + Actin + 25(OH)D3				
	4.80	4.62	5.55	4.72

The gels were run as in (15), and measurement of the pI was performed by cutting slices out of the gel. Gc and its complexes were revealed by print immunofixation (15). The pI values are given for the two bands (F and S) of the Gc1 phenotype and the single band of Gc2. Note that, in sucrose gels, all ligand binding to Gc is followed by a change in the pI of the protein towards more acidic values, except for DNase I which does not change the pI of the Gc-actin complex. Similar findings are found in 2.0 M urea gels. In contrast, when the urea concentration is raised to 6.0 M, dissociation of the complexes occur and Gc has in all cases a similar value, shifted by about 0.5 pH units towards the basic values as often observed with urea. In addition, Triton X-100 does not influence the binding of Gc to actin, but apparently dissociates the complex between Gc and 25(OH)D3. From Ref. 12 and 15, and unpublished data.

biological relevance of these complex interactions is unclear. However, certain concepts of possible physiological function have begun to emerge, and recent key findings will now be considered in relation to the cell biology of peripheral blood lymphocytes (PBL) and monocytes.

BIOLOGICAL RELEVANCE OF Gc IN LYMPHOCYTES: The finding of Gc in the cytoplasm of cells (9-11), as well as in the circulation (1,2), raises the possibility of expression of Gc on the cell membrane. It has been known for some years (see 20,21) that peripheral blood mononuclear cells (MNC) may display at least one protein on the cell membrane of molecular weight (MW) identical to that of Gc (54-56 K). In addition, Constans and co-workers reported apparent interaction between serum Gc and the surface membrane of unfractionated MNC (22). More recently, we have demonstrated evidence of endogenous membrane Gc on a proportion of MNC, as detected by immunocytochemistry and physicochemical methods such as SDS-PAGE and analytical isoelectric focusing (IEF) with transblotting (21,22). As judged by immunofluorescence, membrane expression appears to be heterogeneous, with >90% of B cells and monocytes positive, but less than 10% native T cells positive, irrespective of populations or subsets (21), although physicochemical methods indicated evidence of association with T cell membrane as assessed by radioiodination and immunoprecipitation (see below). In the cytoplasm, on the other hand, Gc is clearly present in small amounts in all cell types, and binding studies performed with purified Gc indicate the presence of a substantial number of unoccupied binding sites. Taken together with the fact that large amounts of Gc are present in the plasma, these findings are compatible with the possibility that Gc associated with lymphocytes is taken up from the circulation. However, to date no evidence of binding to the membrane of intact lymphocytes has been obtained (21), and recent studies have indicated that lymphocytes can synthesize Gc (unpublished results).

Normal B Cells: The finding of clear positivity for Gc in normal B cells (20,21) (Fig. 1A) was of particular interest. The integral membrane immunogloblin (mIg) of B cells demonstrates clonal specificity and is thought to function as a specific receptor for the appropriate homologous antigen (23). Stimulation with ligand, either oligoclonally with antigen, or polyclonally with anti-Ig, is known to result in transduction intracellularly of a signal which under optimal conditions results in activation and proliferation (23). Ligand occupation has been shown both by immunocytochemical and physicochemical methods to lead to attachment of mIg to actin, and possibly other components of the cytoskeleton (23,24). One major protein which was postulated on the basis of experiments with bifunctional cross-linkers to be involved (25,26) was also of MW 55-56 K. We have demonstrated that this protein is a homologue of serum Gc, based on immunoprecipitation and transblotting of detergent-solubilized membrane preparations with antiserum to Gc, and by these methods, Gc also appears to be capable of interacting with ligand-crosslinked mIg and actin contemporaneously (20). These findings were further confirmed by two color fluorescence protocols. Since reaction of B cells with anti-Ig resulted not only in patching and capping of mIg as expected (24), but also in co-mobility of Gc (20), these results therefore indicated that Gc might play an important role in signal transduction and activation of B cells through the mIg receptor.

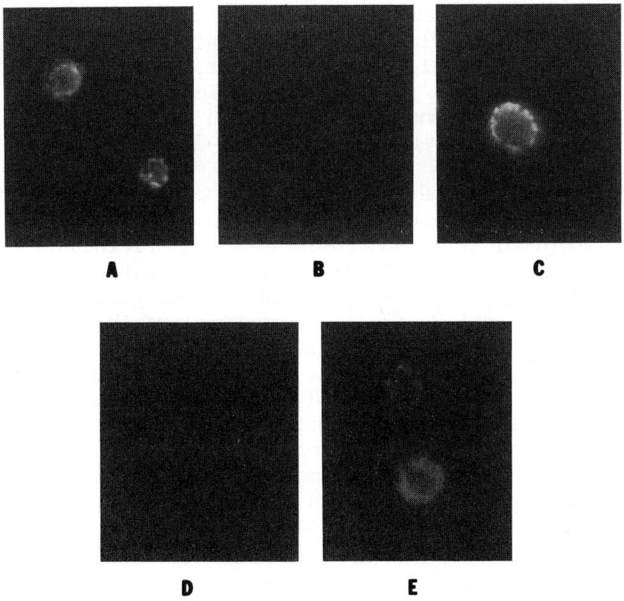

Fig. 1.: Membrane Gc fluorescence of human lymphocytes. A = native B lymphocytes, B = malignant B cells obtained from a patient with chronic lymphocytic leukemia, C = as B but reacted first with antiserum recognizing membrane immunoglobulins, D = native normal T-cells and E = as D, after primary reaction with Leu 1 antiserum.

Abnormal B Cells: Further information relevant to this question has also been obtained by examination of abnormal B cells, particularly in certain malignant cells obtained from patients with chronic lymphocytic leukemia (CLL) and to a lesser extent in transformed B lymphoblastoid cell lines (LCL). In contrast to normal B cells, transformed and malignant B cells respond only partially to standard stimuli such as anti-Ig (27). This deficiency appears to be associated with abnormalities in the membrane expression and mobility of mIg (28), although the reasons for that are unknown. Recent experiments have therefore focussed on the membrane expression of mIg and Gc on both CLL and LCL cells (29). By fluorescence, the quantity of mIg and Gc was indeed variable (Fig. 1B), and patching and capping of both antigens with anti-Ig were greatly reduced in comparison with normal B cells (29). On the other hand, protocols in which surface radioiodination was followed by detergent solubilization, immunoprecipitation with antiserum to Gc, and SDS-PAGE with autoradiography, showed essentially a single radiolabeled protein MW 56 K. This protein was also reactive upon transblotting with antiserum to Gc (29). However, cross-linking of such cells with anti-Ig was found to lead to a consistent increase in the intensity of Gc fluorescence (Fig. 1C) as confirmed in a fluorescence-activated cell sorter (29). In addition, examination of such cross-linked cells by SDS-PAGE showed that radiolabeling of immunoprecipitated Gc was substantially increased (29). The explanation for these rather unusual findings is unclear at this point, but may involve alteration of the topographical relationship of Gc with the lipid bilayer (T cells, see below). In practical terms however, they may provide one possible explanation for the poor or negligible membrane expression of mIg, and the deficient response of transformed or malignant B cells to activating signals such as reaction with anti-Ig.

T Lymphocytes: Expression of Gc on native T cells appears to be limited as judged by immunofluorescence (Fig. 1D). However, analysis by SDS-PAGE after surface radioiodination and specific immunoprecipitation has shown radiolabeled material of MW 56 K, as was the case with certain of the abnormal cells tested (see above) and this species also reacts positively on transblotting with anti-Gc (30). These findings thus indicated that Gc is associated with the native T cell membrane, although in a form not detectable by immunofluorescence (30). Further evidence that the finding of Gc associated with the membrane did not simply represent an artefact was obtained by studies of the Fc gamma receptors present on 20-25% of T cells. These structures bind complexed IgG (30) and interactions between Gc and Ig in relation to the membrane might occur under appropriate conditions, as noted earlier in B cells (20,21). The possible association of Gc with IgG bound to T cells was tested by affinity chromatography of radioiodinated, detergent-solubilized T-cell extracts, using a column on which soluble immune complexes of Ig:anti-Ig were generated. SDS-PAGE analysis of the eluate demonstrated evidence of immunoreactive Gc which was radiolabeled and derived, therefore, in part from the membrane (30). At least some of this material appeared to be present in the form of complexes with a 42K component presumed to be G-actin (30). In addition, fluorescence studies in which T cells were incubated with EA to complex membrane Fc gamma and then reacted with anti-Gc showed a consistent increase in the proportion of cells positive (Fig. 1E), from less than 10% to 20-25% (30). This effect appeared similar to that noted for abnormal B cells (see above).

The precise significance of this finding is unclear. In particular, it is not known if Gc is primarily involved in binding of cytophilic IgG, or becomes associated secondarily with IgG after the latter has bound. In favor of the former is the fact that, despite some disagreement, the major Fc-binding structure visualized by this approach has been found in the majority of relevant studies to be in the same MW range viz. 56-60 K, although transblotting with antiserum to Gc has not been performed previously (see 30). On the other hand, spatial association of Gc with two different membrane structures, mIg of B cells and Fc gamma of T cells, and the observed phenomenon of fluorescence enhancement raises the possibility that similar interactions might occur with other membrane proteins upon appropriate manipulation. This hypothesis has been tested more recently in studies of normal T cells reacted with antisera recognizing membrane structures distinct from Fc gamma.

The main reagent used (Leu 1) reacts with >95% of native human peripheral blood lymphocytes (anti-pan-T) (31). The other two - 5E9 which recognizes transferrin receptors (32) and anti-DR - react only with stimulated T cells, since membrane expression of homologous antigens requires activation (33,34). Fluorescence protocols in which native unstimulated cells were reacted with Leu 1 followed by anti-Gc demonstrated a substantial increase in Gc fluorescence, both qualitatively and quantitatively, and warming of such cells to 37°C demonstrated patching of Leu 1 antigen and co-patching of Gc (35). The use of 5E9 and anti-DR, and T cells activated by phytohemagglutinin showed similar co-mobility of Gc with the primary antigen. Thus, fluorescence enhancement was obtained in each case, and, although the rate of patching with these three antisera varied, each induced co-distribution of membrane Gc upon warming to 37°C. Moreover, reaction of native unstimulated T cells with 5E9 or anti-DR provided a useful negative control in that such cells were essentially negative both with the primary antiserum and with anti-Gc.

The phenomenon of fluorescence enhancement is currently unexplained, but can tentatively be considered to represent an altered topographical relationship of Gc in the membrane, possibly due to vertical movement in a direction perpendicular to the surface, rather than in the plane of the lipid bilayer as with lateral mobility. The findings of parallel studies using physicochemical methods lend some support to this hypothesis. Surface radioiodination followed by detergent solubilization and immuno-precipitation with anti-Gc allow an estimate to be made of the relative labeling of membrane Gc. Reaction of T or B cells with primary antisera noted to induce fluorescence enhancement prior to radioiodination, and preadsorption with Staphylococcus Aureus Cowan I of soluble extracts to remove any radioiodinated primary antiserum IgG consistently led to increased radiolabeling of labeled Gc (28,30,35). This evidence of increased "exposure" of membrane Gc to detection both by immunofluores-cence and radioiodination is consistent with translocation of Gc within or through the lipid bilayer. However, although the biological consequences of this interesting phenomenon remain unclear, it is important to note that the results of co-distribution studies indicate that association of Gc with membrane glycoproteins and subsequent movement upon warming may be a more general phenomenon than hitherto anticipated (30,35).

PHOSPHORYLATION REACTIONS: Recently, there has been substantial interest in the role of kinases and phosphorylation reactions in cellular activa-tion (36), and an unidentified 56K protein has been noted to be a substrate, both for tyrosine kinase (37) and phospholipid-Ca^{++}-dependent kinase (C-kinase) (38). Current studies of C-kinase have demonstrated that the phosphorylated 56K protein exhibits physicochemical properties (MW 56K; pI 4.8-5.2) indistinguishable from Gc, binds ^{125}I-G-actin and also reacts positively on transblotting with anti-Gc (38). Moreover, experiments with partially purified C-kinase and homogeneous Gc have confirmed that the latter is a substrate for C-kinase. The significance of this finding for the basic properties of Gc and its biological function remains to be determined, but, as noted above, interactions of Gc with other proteins (G-actin with or without DNase) may influence the extent of phosphorylation and vice-versa.

IN SUMMARY, Gc exhibits a number of interesting properties, and the dual interaction with G-actin and vitamin D3 metabolites poses some tantalizing possibilities for its biological function. However, the overall biological role(s) of Gc in lymphocytes and other cells remains to be established. Although its association with the membrane of all cells tested, and its presence in the cytoplasm of all nucleated cells, indicate possible involvement of Gc in cellular vitamin D3 metabolism, there is to date little direct evidence to support this concept and membrane-associated Gc can apparently become spacially related to several other membrane glycoproteins, including certain receptor structures, and can undergo extensive movement in relation to the lipid bilayer. In view of this, and the observation that Gc may be a major substrate for C-kinase, it is not unreasonable to speculate that this protein may play an hitherto unrecognized and important role in stimulus-response coupling. In this regard, the lymphocyte will represent a useful model cell for further studies of the involvement of Gc in signal transduction.

ACKNOWLEDGEMENTS: The work discussed has involved a large number of colleagues and collaborators, including Dr. Robert C. Allen, Dr. Bernard Boutin, Dr. H. Ming Cheng, Dr. David L. Emerson, Dr. Pascal J. Goldschmidt-Clermont, Dr. Joe W. Krayer, Dr. William M. Lee, Dr. Andre E. Nel, Dr. Mario Petrini, Philip A. Werner and Dr. Marie W. Wooten. Without their industry and enthusiasm this review could not have been written. Supported in part by NIH grant CA-27062 and Institutional research awards GR25 and GR45, and Labcatal Laboratories, Paris, France. RMG was the recipient of a NIH Research Career Development Award CA-00611.

REFERENCES:

1. Hirschfeld, J. (1959) Acta Pathol. Microbiol. Scand. 47, 160-168.
2. Putnam, F.W. (1977) in: The Plasma Proteins (Putnam, F.W., ed.) vol. III, Academic Press, New York, pp. 333-357.
3. Daiger, S.P., Schanfield, M.S., and Cavalli-Sforza, L.L. (1975) Proc. Nat. Acad. Sci. USA 72, 2076-2080.
4. Brissenden, J.E. and Cox, D.W. (1978) J. Lab. Clin. Med. 91, 455-462.
5. Bouillon, R., Van Assche, F.A., Van Baelen, H., Heins, W., and DeMoor, P. (1981) J. Clin. Invest. 67, 589-596.
6. Constans, J., Arlet, P., Viau, M., and Bouissou, C. (1983) Clin. Chim. Acta 130, 219-230.
7. Van Baelen, M., Bouillon, R., and de Moor, P. (1977) J. Biol. Chem. 252, 2515-2518.
8. Cooke, N.E., Walgate, J., and Haddad, J.G. Jr. (1979) J. Biol. Chem. 254, 5958-5964.
9. Cooke, N.E., Walgate, J., and Haddad, J.G. Jr. (1979) J. Biol. Chem. 254, 5965-5971.
10. Van Baelen, H., Bouillon, R., and de Moor, P. (1980) J. Biol. Chem. 255, 2270-2272.
11. Haddad, J.G. (1982) Arch. Biochem. Biophys. 213, 538-544.
12. Goldschmidt-Clermont, P., Galbraith, R.M., Emerson, D.L., Nel, A.E., and Arnaud, P. (1985) Biochem. J. (in press).
13. Bouillon, R. (1985) This proceedings.
14. Haddad, J.G. (1985) This proceedings.
15. Emerson, D.L., Galbraith, R.M., and Arnaud, P. (1984) Electrophoresis 5, 22-26.
16. Emerson, D.L., Arnaud, P., and Galbraith, R.M. (1983) Amer. J. Reprod. Immunol. 4, 185-189.
17. Goldschmidt-Clermont, P.J., Galbraith, R.M., Emerson, D.L., Nel, A.E., and Lee, W.M. (1985) Electrophoresis (in press).

18. Goldschmidt-Clermont, P.J., Galbraith, R.M., Emerson, D.L., Werner, P.A.M., Nel, A.E., and Lee, W.M. (1985) Clin. Chim. Acta (in press).
19. Boutin, B., Galbraith, R.M., and Arnaud, P. (1985) This proceedings.
20. Petrini, M., Emerson, D.L., and Galbraith, R.M. (1983) Nature 306, 73-74.
21. Petrini, M., Galbraith, R.M., Werner, P.A.M., Emerson, D.L., and Arnaud, P. (1983) Clin. Immunol. Immunopathol. 31, 282-295.
22. Constans, J., Oksman, F., and Viau, M. (1981) Immunol. Lett. 3, 159-162.
23. Kehrl, J.M., Muraguchi, A., Butler, J.L., Falkoff, R.J.M., and Fauci, A.S. (1984) Immunol. Rev. 78, 75-96.
24. Flanagan, J., and Koch, G.L.E. (1978) Nature 273, 278-281.
25. Koch, N. and Haustein, D. (1983) Mol. Immunol. 20, 33-37.
26. Rosenspire, A.J. and Choi, Y.S. (1982) Mol. Immunol. 19, 1515-1526.
27. Fu, S.M., Chiorazzi, M., and Kunkel, H.G. (1979) Immunol. Rev. 48, 23-44.
28. Cohen, H.J. and Gilbertsen, B.B. (1975) J. Clin. Invest. 55, 84-93.
29. Nel, A.E., Navailles, M., Emerson, D.L., Goldschmidt-Clermont, P., Pathak, S.K., Tsang, K.Y., and Galbraith, R.M. (1985) This proceedings.
30. Petrini, M., Galbraith, R.M., Emerson, D.L., Nel, A.E., and Arnaud, P. (1985) J. Biol. Chem. 260, 1804-1810.
31. Becton-Dickinson: Data Information Sheet, 1985.
32. Haynes, B.F., Hemler, M., Cotner, T., Mann, D.L., Eisenbarth, G.S., Strominger, J.L., and Fauci, A.S. (1981) J. Immunol. 127, 347-351.
33. Russo, C., Quantara, V., Indiveri, F., Pellegrino, M.A., and Ferrone, S. (1980) Immunogenetics 11, 413-416.
34. Galbraith, R.M., Werner, P., Arnaud, P., and Galbraith, G.M.P. (1980) J. Clin. Invest. 66, 1135-1143.
35. Galbraith, R.M. (1985) This proceedings.
36. Nishizuka, Y. (1984) Nature 308, 693-698.
37. Nel, A.E., Landreth, G.E., Goldschmidt-Clermont, P.J., Tung, H.E., and Galbraith, R.M. (1984) Biochem. Biophys. Res. Comm. 125, 859-866.
38. Wooten, M.W., Galbraith, R.M., Nel, A.E., and Wrenn, R.W. (1985) This Proceedings.

PLASMA VITAMIN D BINDING PROTEIN - ACTIN INTERACTIONS: FACT AND ARTIFACT

John G. Haddad
Endocrine Section, Department of Medicine, University of Pennsylvania School of Medicine, Philadelphia, Pennsylvania, 19104

Historical Notes

Initially identified as group-specific component or Gc globulin (1,2), the plasma binding protein for vitamin D and its metabolites (DBP) is now recognized to be a major plasma protein in most species examined to date (3). The protein has been isolated from the plasma of man, rabbit, rat and chicken, and DBP gene deletion is thought to be a lethal mutation since Gc protein has always been detected in over 100,000 human sera examined.

The protein is made in the liver, and is a single chain polypeptide, 56-58 K daltons, with approximately 1-2% carbohydrate, and a pI of 4.6 - 4.9. It sediments at 3.5S in the analytical ultracentrifuge. Each DBP molecule binds one molecule of vitamin D sterol, with a preference for 25-OHD> $1,25-(OH)_2D$ and the parent vitamin (4). Plasma concentrations are approximately 5μM in man, and do not vary with vitamin D sufficiency and deficiency (3). In fact, little mechanistic insight was gained from DBP levels in blood, unlike the information gained for the mechanism for vitamin A transport.

Compared to its sterol ligands, the molar excess of DBP in blood is very large at 50-100 to 1, and the reason for such an abundancy of this protein is not known. Some have considered this to be a huge circulating reservoir or a buffer against toxicity. Neither of these speculations seem attractive for a passive transport system since sterol storage can be effected in adipose tissue, and vitamin D toxicity, as we know it, is a true artifact occuring long after the DBP system was put into place.

Table I lists the chronology of some of the work related to DBP and introduces another fact about DBP - that of its high-affinity and species-independent association with monomeric or G-actin. The last 15 years of work in this area has suggested other roles for DBP than plasma vitamin D sterol transport, and some of the recent studies are quite interesting.

Vitamin D. A Chemical, Biochemical and Clinical Update

Table 1

Events Related to the DBP-Actin Story

1959	-	Gc protein isolated (2) Human plasma anti-rachitic activity in α-globulins (5)
1970	-	Plasma or Tissue Extract as Binders in 25-OHD CPB assays (6)
1971	-	Tissue Binder of 25-OHD is larger than Plasma Binder (6)
1974	-	25-OHD-1αhydroxylase inhibitor in plasma and tissue is DBP (7,8)
1975	-	Big DBP found in all nucleated tissues (9) and is a nuisance to 1,25-$(OH)_2$D "receptorologists"
1976	-	Human DBP isolated (3) Plasma DBP levels seem constitutive (3)
1977	-	Tissue DBP = DBP + heat-labile component (10)
1979	-	High-affinity selective association of DBP and Tissue DBP Binder (11)
1980	-	Actin is the heat labile component (12)
1981	-	Rapid DBP Turnover in Man & Rabbit (13)
Recent	-	DBP "expressed" on cells (14,15) DBP migrates with mIgG (14,15) DBP sequesters actin monomers (16)

DBP-Actin as Artifact

The early evidence for an interaction between DBP and a tissue component came from the observations of (5-6S) faster sedimentation of 3H-sterols in linear sucrose gradients than could be explained by the sedimentation behavior of DBP alone or of the 1,25-$(OH)_2$D receptor. "Big" or "tissue DBP" was a nettlesome aspect of dealing with tissue extracts if 1,25-$(OH)_2$D receptor activity was the main objective.

Another major area of interest was the 25-OHD-1α hydroxylase activity in kidney, and early studies of this enzyme in mammals was thwarted by an inhibitor of the enzyme in rat plasma and tissues. It is striking that rat plasma DBP was first purified as a 25-OHD-1 hydroxylase inhibitor (7). It is also important that this inhibitor was found in well-washed organelles from well-perfused tissues (8), arguing against its origin in the plasma. Others found the "tissue DBP" in relatively non-vascular tissues such as cartilage (9) and cultured mouse bone cells (17), also suggesting a tissue origin of the DBP.

However, the binding activity of tissue DBP and plasma DBP were strikingly similar for vitamin D sterols. Furthermore, most workers did not show an affinity of "tissue DBP" for nuclei or chromatin, although the 5-6S binder could be extracted from nuclei. When cells were cultured in the absence of plasma, the 5-6S binder was difficult to demonstrate in cell extracts. The possibility of an interionic bond between DBP and a cell component was explored in 0.5MKCl buffers, but no dissociation to 3.5S DBP was demonstrated (9). Eventually, heat produced the plasma form of DBP from "tissue DBP" (10), and a high-affinity association of DBP with a 43K dalton protease-sensitive material found in all cell extracts was shown (11). The cellular protein was shown to be actin (12), and such an association was found in human skeletal muscle (18).

The prevailing view was that when plasma (heavily endowed with DBP) contaminated cell or tissue extractions, an artificial exposure of the intracellular protein, actin, to plasma DBP occurred, creating the 5-6S binder. Although the force of attraction between these two proteins was strong, most observers felt that this interaction between a blood protein and a cytoskeletal component had no physiological meaning.

Studies of sterol access into cells, furthermore, revealed that external DBP had an inhibitory effect on cellular entry of sterols (19). Similar results were found in perfused organ experiments (20). If DBP facilitated sterol transfer, these studies did not find evidence for it. Many experiments (unpublished) to detect specific binding of DBP by cells and plasma membranes were negative. At this juncture, therefore, DBP was considered to be a plasma protein of hepatic origin whose role was extracellular. Since apparent depolymerization of polymeric or fibrous (F-actin) actin was seen with DBP, an actin "scavenger" role for DBP in the circulation was suggested (12). Some roles for DBP are listed in Table II.

Table II

DBP Function(s)

1) PLASMA TRANSPORT OF VITAMIN D STEROLS

2) CIRCULATING RESERVOIR OF STEROLS

3) CELLULAR ACCESS OF STEROLS (+/-)

4) ACTIN-BINDING

a) "SCAVENGER" ?

b) LINK TO CYTOSKELETON ?

Nature of DBP-Actin Association

Actin depolymerizing activity in plasma can be attributed to plasma gelsolin (21) and DBP (16). Gelsolin severs preformed filaments of F-actin, as assessed by a cytochalasin binding assay, and rapid reductions of the viscosity of F-actin are seen. Although DBP can also reduce the viscosity of F-actin in high-shear and low-shear viscometers, it is required at higher concentrations. DBP appears to sequester actin monomers and prevent them from participating in the polymerization process (16).

Most of the experiments carried out to date have involved muscle or erythrocyte actin. The association of the two proteins does not appear to be influenced by calcium ions, unlike the gelsolin-actin association. This feature has been useful in designing an affinity (actin-agarose) support capable of extracting gelsolin and/or DBP from the plasma of several species (22). Preliminary studies do not show a preference by G-actin for holo (vitamin D sterols) DBP over apo-DBP.

For those attracted to the "scavenger" hypothesis, the dual effects of gelsolin (sever filaments) and DBP(bind monomers) afford a powerful system for dealing with extracellular actin. Little is known of the disposition of actin extracellularly. This is an interesting pathophysiological area, and the roles of DBP and gelsolin would be of interest.

Cellular DBP

Recently, studies have been carried out to demonstrate

the "expression" of DBP on/in human circulating mononuclear cells (14,15). Immunofluorescence studies have revealed DBP antigenicity on/in monocytes and in lymphocytes. Results with monocytes revealed that most of these cells exhibited the antigen. Although antibody interaction with DBP did not initiate capping and patching, the DBP-antibody complex did co-migrate with mIgG-antibody complex in lymphocytes. These provocative findings suggested a close association of DBP with the mechanism whereby clonal amplification and IgG secretion are stimulated at the cell plasma membrane. Furthermore, a binding of DBP and DBP-actin to Fc portions of IgG (or Fc clusters) was shown on affinity supports.

Attempts at extracting DBP from cells revealed that harsh conditions were required, suggesting an integral placement of DBP in the membrane (15). No positive information, to date, has been obtained to support the hypothesis that DBP can be biosynthesized by blood cells. It is therefore possible that membranous DBP can be acquired from plasma at some stage in the ontogenesis of circulating mononuclear cells. Additional studies are needed to determine whether DBP synthesis and DBP mRNA can be found in non-liver cells.

Preliminary work in my laboratory has revealed that a murine monoclonal antibody to human DBP may be directed toward an epitope hidden from the surface of circulating mononuclear cells, cytotrophoblasts and several transformed lymphocyte and monocyte cell lines. In viable cells, consistently negative immunofluorescent results were obtained with the monoclonal antibody, although polyclonal rabbit anti-DBP gave positive membrane fluorescence. Fixation of cells and non-ionic detergent treatment, however, resulted in positive monoclonal antibody adherence to the cell plasma membrane.

Could DBP be acquired from plasma to serve a transducer function in certain cells? Or is there a DBP, unlike the hepatic one destined for plasma transport function, that is synthesized and incorporated in plasma membranes to link surface signals to the cytoskeleton? Finally, where does the vitamin D sterol fit into these schemes?

There are a large number of cellular actin-binding proteins (23,24) that are thought to modify the motile processes effected by stress fibers and microfilaments. As an initial step toward finding a role for DBP in the disposition of actin, we are directing efforts to search for shared actin binding sites with other proteins, using a labeled actin-DBP-anti-DBP system. DNase I has been confirmed not to share a binding site on actin with DBP. Other studies shall involve EM with immunoprobes and microinjection of cells with fluorescent probes. It is hoped that a high fact: artifact ratio can be achieved and maintained.

Acknowledgments

I thank Drs. E. Lange, J. McLeod and J. Nestler for allowing me to cite their preliminary studies, and J. Dubbs for help in preparing the manuscript. Portions of work cited were supported by grant AM28292 from the PHS.

References

1. Daiger, S.P., Schanfield, M.D., Cavalli-Sforza, L.L. (1975) Proc. Nat. Acad. Sci. USA 72L:2076-2080.

2. Bearn, A.G., Cleve, H. (1966) In: The Metabolic Basis of Inherited Disease, Stanbury, J.B., Wyngaarden, J.B., Frederickson, D.S. (eds), McGraw-Hill, New York, p 1321-1342.

3. Haddad, J.G. (1982) In: Advances in Nutritional Research, vol. 4, Draper, H.H. (ed), Plenum, New York and London, p 35-58.

4. Haddad, J.G. (1984) In: Vitamin D-Basic and Clinical Aspects, Kumar, R. (ed), Martinus Nijhoff, Boston/The Hague/Dardrecht, Lancaster, p 383-396.

5. Thomas, W.C., Morgan, H.F., Connor, T.F., Haddock, L., Bills, C.E. and Howard, J.E. (1959) J. Clin. Invest. 38:1078-1085.

6. Haddad, J.G. and Birge, S.J. (1971) Biochem. Biophys. Res. Comm. 45:829-832.

7. Botham, K.M., Tanaka, Y. and DeLuca, H.F. (1974) Biochemistry 13:4961-4966.

8. Botham, K.M., Ghazarian, Kream, B. and DeLuca, H.F. (1976) Biochemistry 15:2130-2135.

9. Haddad, J.G. and Birge, S.J. (1975) J. Biol. Chem. 250:299-304.

10. Van Baelen, H., Bouillon, R., DeMoor, P. (1977) J. Biol. Chem. 252:2515-2518.

11. Cooke, N.E., Walgate, J. and Haddad, J.G. (1979) J. Biol. Chem. 254:5965-5971.

12. Van Baelen, H., Bouillon, R., DeMoor, P. (1980) J. Biol. Chem. 255:2270-2272.

13. Haddad, J., Fraser, D.R. and Lawson, D.E.M. (1981) J. Clin. Invest. 67:1550-1560.

14. Petrini, M., Emerson, D.L. and Galbraith, R.M. (1983) Nature 306:73-74.

15. Petrini, M., Galbraith, R.M., Werner, P.A.M., Emerson, D.L. and Arnaud, P. (1984) Clin. Immunol. & Immunopathol. 31:282-295.

16. Lees, A., Haddad, J.G. and Lin, S. (1984) Biochemistry 23:3038-3047.

17. Chen, T-C., Hirst, M.A. and Feldman, D. (1979) J. Biol. Chem. 254:7491-7494.

18. Haddad, J.G. (1982) Archives of Biochem. & Biophysics 213:538-544.

19. Manolagas, S.C. and Deftos, L.J. (1980) Lancet 2:401-402.

20. Olgaard, K., Schwartz, J., Finco, D., Arbelaey, M., Haddad, J., Avioli, L., Klahr, S. and Slatopolsky, E. (1982) J. Clin. Invest. 69:684-690.

21. Yin, H.L., Albrecht, J.H. and Fattoum, A. (1981) J. Cell Biol. 91:901-906.

22. Haddad, J.G., Sanger, J.W. and Kowalski, M.A. (1984) Biochem. J. 218:805-810.

23. Craig, S.W. and Pollard, T.D. (1982) TIBS 7:88-92.

24. Weeds, A. (1982) Nature 296:811-816.

THE CLONING AND DNA SEQUENCE ANALYSIS OF RAT SERUM VITAMIN D BINDING PROTEIN cDNA

N.E. COOKE
Departments of Medicine and Human Genetics, University of Pennsylvania, Philadelphia, PA 19104 USA

Vitamin D binding protein (DBP) (1) is an abundant serum glycoprotein secreted by the liver. It serves as the major transport protein for the 25(OH)D metabolite of vitamin D. The fact that only 5% of the potential sterol binding sites appear to be occupied suggests that the molecule may have additional functions. These additional functions may be related to the binding of DBP to G-actin with high specificity and affinity (2,3) and its association with membranous immunoglobulin on the B lymphocyte surface (4). As an initial step in identifying the functional domains of this molecule and their possible interrelationships, we have cloned and sequenced a cDNA copy of rat DBP mRNA.

Since there was no available rat DBP sequence data on which to base the synthesis of an oligonucleotide probe, we chose an immunological approach (5) to identify the DBP cDNA. A polyclonal anti-rat DBP antiserum was raised in rabbits to actin affinity-purified rat serum DBP (6). This antiserum was made RNase-free by chromatography on Staph A Sepharose CL-4B and the purified antibody fraction was incubated with rat liver polysomes. The immune complexes that formed between the DBP antibody and polysomes containing nascent DBP protein chains were selected by chromatography over Staph A Sepharose CL-4B. Polyadenylated mRNA encoding DBP was released from the polysomes by addition of EDTA, and the mRNA was subsequently purified by oligo(dT) cellulose chromatography. A labelled DNA copy of this DBP-enriched mRNA was synthesized and used as an in situ hybridization probe to screen a rat liver cDNA library (7) cloned in the bacteriophage expression vector lambda gt11. Clones positive by hybridization were rescreened for direct expression of a β-galactosidase-DBP fusion protein by protein blotting with affinity-purified anti-DBP and iodinated protein A. Two DBP-expressing clones were identified. The cloned DNA was confirmed to encode DBP by translation of hybrid-selected mRNA into a 56,000 dalton protein specifically recognized by anti-DBP.

The larger DNA insert of the two expressing clones was subcloned and sequenced. The nucleotide sequence translated into a single open reading frame. The molecular weight of the encoded protein was 43,100, not the expected 56,000, indicating that part of the 5' end of the mRNA was missing from the cDNA clone. This was confirmed by primer extension analysis (8) which demonstrated that the full-length DBP mRNA was 1650 nucleotides, 305 nucleotides longer at the 5' end than were encoded by the sequenced clone.

The most striking feature of the amino acid sequence of rat DBP was the high number of cysteine residues, 24 of the 384 amino acids, and the periodicity of their placement. When compared to the sequences of albumin and alpha-feoprotein (AFP), the placement of cysteine residues was identical. More careful alignment of the rat DBP and rat albumin (9) or rat AFP (10) mRNAs indicated an overall amino acid homology of about

Vitamin D. A Chemical, Biochemical and Clinical Update

21% and a nucleotide homology of about 38%. There is a higher degree of homology between albumin and AFP, 33% amino acid homology and 48% nucleotide homology. Rat DBP terminated 123 amino acids sooner than albumin accounting for the difference in their molecular weights. The rat DBP sequence contains two potential N-linked glycosylation sites (Asn-X-Ser or Thr). There are no glycoslyation sites in rat albumin, and the two sites in rat AFP are in different positions.

The rat DBP cDNA cross-hybridized to human DBP on Northern blots. This finding was exploited to select a human DBP cDNA by cross-hybridization to a human liver cDNA library. The selected human DBP clone was sequenced and found to have 72% amino acid homology to rat DBP. It terminates one amino acid residue earlier than rat DBP. Two short DBP peptide fragments sequenced by Svasti et al. (11) were located in our sequence, further confirming this clone's identity as human DBP. The human DBP cDNA clone was used as a hybridization probe to directly confirm the chromosomal localization of DBP on chromosome 4.

Based on these results we conclude that DBP is a member of a multigene family clustered on human chromosome 4 also encoding the abundant serum proteins albumin and AFP. Since in most multigene families, intron position and number are conserved, it can be predicted that the DBP gene will have 12 exons, based on the gene structures of albumin and AFP. If mutational rates in each gene were equivalent, based upon their homology, it can be predicted that DBP existed before the albumin/AFP gene duplication, more than 300-500 million years ago (12).

REFERENCES

1. Haddad, J.G., and Walgate, J. (1976). J. Biol. Chem. 251, 4803-4809.
2. Van Baelen, H., Bouillon, R., and DeMoor, P., (1980). J. Biol. Chem. 255, 2270-2272.
3. Cooke, N.E., Walgate, J., and Haddad, J.G. (1979). J. Biol. Chem. 254, 5965-5971.
4. Petrini, M., Emerson, D.L., and Galbraith, R.M., (1983) Nature 306, 73-74.
5. Kraus, J.P., and Rosenberg, L.E., (1982) Proc. Natl. Acad. Sci. U.S.A. 79, 4015-4109.
6. Haddad, J.G., Kowalski, M.A., and Sanger, J.W., (1984) Biochem. J. 218, 805-810.
7. Schwarzbauer, J.E., Tamkun, J.W., Lemischka, I.R., and Hynes, R.O., (1983) Cell 35, 421-431.
8. Liebhaber, S.A., and Kan, Y.W., (1981) J. Clin. Invest. 68, 439-446.
9. Sargent, T.D., Yang, M., and Bonner, J., (1981) Proc. Natl. Acad. Sci. U.S.A. 78, 243-246.
10. Jagodzinski, L.L., Sargent, T.D., Yang, M., Glackin, C., and Bonner, J., (1981) Proc. Natl. Acad. Sci. U.S.A. 78, 3521-3525.
11. Svasti, J., Kurosky, A., Bennet, A., and Bowman, B.H., (1979) Biochemistry 18, 1611-1617.
12. Eiferman, F.A., Young, P.R., Scott, R.W., and Tilghman, S.M. (1981). Nature 294, 713-718.

ALTERED CONFIGURATION OF D-BINDING PROTEIN (Gc) ON MEMBRANES OF ABNORMAL AND MALIGNANT B LYMPHOCYTES.

ANDRE E. NEL, MARIO PETRINI, DAVID L. EMERSON, PASCAL J. GOLDSCHMIDT-CLERMONT, and ROBERT M. GALBRAITH, Departments of Basic and Clinical Immunology and Microbiology, and Medicine, Medical University of South Carolina, Charleston, S.C. 29425, U.S.A.

Introduction: A membrane homologue of the serum vitamin D-binding protein (Gc) is detectable on normal B cells, and is closely related spatially to the membrane immunoglobulin (mIg) antigen receptor in that it co-distributes with this protein during patch and cap reaction and is co-eluted with mIg during affinity chromatography (1). Abnormal B cells, such as lymphoblastoid cell lines (LCL) and B cells from patients with chronic lymphocytic leukemia (CLL) exhibit a sparcity or absence of mIg (2). It was therefore of interest to examine the membrane expression of Gc on such abnormal cells and the possible spatial relationship of this protein to mIg.

Materials and Methods: B cell populations were obtained from peripheral blood of normal and CLL patients (3), and certain B lymphoblastoid cell lines (Table I) grown in culture (4). The presence of membrane Ig and Gc was determined by indirect one and two color fluorescence protocols performed at 4°C with appropriate controls, and mobility of mIg and co-mobility of Gc was assessed by warming to 37°C (1). The intensity of fluorescence was quantitated in a fluorescence-activated cell sorter (5). The presence of Gc on cell surfaces was also examined after surface radioiodination by detergent-solublilization and specific immune precipitation (5). These procedures were performed both on resting B cells, and cells treated with a crosslinking antibody. The presence of membrane Gc and labeling were assessed by SDS-PAGE followed by immune transblotting and autoradiography (5). Aliquots of labeled material were counted to reveal differences in the accessibility of Gc protein to radioiodination in native and anti-Ig crosslinked samples.

Results: In comparison with normal B cells, all abnormal cells showed reduced or negligible expression of mIg and this was associated with decreased or absent fluorescence of Gc protein (Table I).

Table I: mIg and Gc Fluorescence

Cell Type	% positive and intensity mIg	% positive and intensity Gc
1. Normal	75-80 / 4+	80-83 / 4+
2. CLL cells (3)	>90 / 2+	>80 / 1-2+
3. RPMI 6410	>90 / 1-2+	>90 / 1-2+
4. RPMI 8226	0 / -	± / ±
5. IMK 101	0 / -	± / ±
6. Raji	0 / -	± / ±

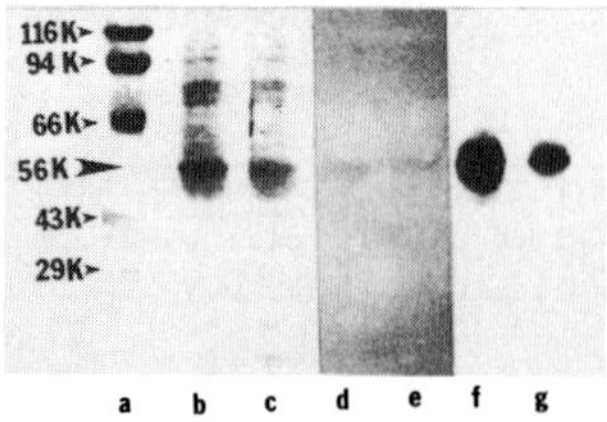

Fig. 1: SDS-PAGE showing immune precipitates from crosslinked (lane b) and native cells (lane c), Immunoblotting (lanes d,e) and autoradiography (f,g). Lane b corresponds to d and f and lane c=e and g.

Rapid patching and capping of mIg with co-mobility of Gc was seen with normal cells but was poor for both antigens in the case of CLL cells and mIg-positive LCL (RPMI 6410). During the course of the latter studies, it was noted that the intensity of Gc fluorescence was enhanced on CLL cells and LCL by incubating cells with anti-Ig prior to anti-Gc. These differences were quantitatively confirmed by cell sorter (FACS) analysis. Prior mIg crosslinked samples revealed enhanced fluorescence intensity as compared to native cells reacted for Gc before or without subsequent reaction for mIg. A similar phenomenon was demonstrated upon comparison of crosslinked and control cells after radioiodination. This showed an apparent increase of 70-150% in the amount of Na-^{125}I incorporated into cell surface Gc protein. Thus, an equal amount of a 56K protein reactive with anti-Gc in immunoblots could be immune-precipitated from Triton X-100 soluble material of both samples, but Gc from radioiodinated crosslinked cells clearly incorporated more label (Fig. 1). This phenomenon of Gc fluorescence enhancement was not observed with normal B cells, but it should be noted that these cells were already brightly positive for Gc in this native state.

Discussion: Abnormal B cells reveal a parallel paucity of mIg and Gc. The close spatial relationship with Gc in a horizontal plane (co-mobility) in normal B cells seems to be lost in these cell types, but crosslinking of mIg in such samples results in greater availability of this protein as judged by fluorescence and surface radioiodination. This may reflect differences in membrane fluidity between normal and abnormal cells. Furthermore, it is possible that Gc may play a stabilizing role for mIg expression in B cells and may therefore be associated with sparcity of mIg and reduced lateral mobility in malignant or transformed B cells. Finally, it is important to note that similar enhancement of detectable membrane Gc has recently been found in normal T cells upon occupation of the Fc gamma receptor (5), and the ability of Gc to move in both lateral and vertical planes may be of wider cell biological significance.

Acknowledgment: We are grateful to Dr. K.Y. Tsang for provision of certain LCL. Research supported in part by NIH Grant CA-27062, MUSC Award CR-17, and Labcatal Laboratories.

References:

1. Petrini, M., Emerson, D.L., Galbraith, R.M. (1983) Nature 305, 73-74.
2. Fu, S.M., Chiorazzi, N., and Kunkel, H.G. (1979) Immunol. Rev. 48, 24.
3. Petrini, M., Galbraith, R.M., Werner, P.A.M., Emerson, D.L., Arnaud, P. (1984) Clin. Immunol. Immunopathol. 31, 282-295.
4. Galbraith, G.M.P., Galbraith, R.M. and Faulk, W.P. (1980) Cell. Immunol. 49, 215.
5. Petrini, M., Galbraith, R.M., Emerson, D.L., Nel, A.E., Arnaud, P. (1985) J. Biol Chem. 260, 1804.

IDENTIFICATION OF Gc (VITAMIN D-BINDING PROTEIN) AS A SUBSTRATE FOR PHOSPHOLIPID/Ca^{2+}-DEPENDENT PROTEIN KINASE IN ISOLATED PANCREATIC ACINI.

MARIE W. WOOTEN, ANDRE E. NEL*, ROBERT M. GALBRAITH* and ROBERT W. WRENN
Department of Anatomy, Medical College of Georgia, Augusta, GA 30912 and Departments of Basic and Clinical Immunology and Microbiology, and Medicine, Medical University of South Carolina, Charleston, SC 29425

Introduction: Phosphorylation reactions involving phospholipid/Ca^{2+}-dependent kinase (C-kinase) have been implicated in an increasing number of potential biological processes (1), but the identity of the major biological substrates for this enzyme are as yet unknown. C-kinase appears to contribute to stimulus-response coupling in exocrine pancreatic cells (2,3), and previous studies have shown a 56K protein to be a particularly prominent substrate (2). This study further investigated the possibility that this substrate might represent Gc (Vitamin D-binding protein).

Materials and Methods: Endogenous proteins phosphorylated by C-kinase were examined in detergent-solubilized extracts of rat pancreatic acinar cells as previously described (2,3). After stopping the reactions, samples were then analysed by SDS-PAGE with autoradiography (2,3), transblotting with a monospecific antiserum to Gc (4,5), and also by two dimensional electrophoresis (6). In view of the considerable cross-species specificity of antisera to human Gc (7), immunoprecipitation of soluble phosphorylated rat pancreas extracts was performed (8) with this antiserum. Partially-purified C-kinase was obtained as previously described (3), and Gc was purified from normal human serum (6). Immunocytochemical detection of Gc was undertaken with antiserum to Gc (4-6), using either cryostat sections of normal snap-frozen pancreatic tissue or small clumps of viable cells.

Results: Brilliant specific Gc fluorescence was seen in the cytoplasm of pancreatic cells, and also on the membrane of whole viable cells (Fig. 1), indicating the widespread presence of Gc in pancreatic acinar cells. SDS-PAGE and autoradiography of phosphorylated soluble extracts showed a 56K protein with enhanced labeling upon addition of Ca^{2+} and phosphatidyl serine (2,3), and this substrate reacted strongly upon transblotting with antiserun to Gc. Two dimensional electrophoresis then confirmed that this substrate was the only protein recognized upon transblotting, and showed an isoelectric point (pI-4.8-5.2) corresponding to that of purified Gc (9,10). Specific immunoprecipitation with anti-Gc yielded a single radiolabeled band (MW=56K) which was not obtained with non-immune rabbit serum. Finally, experiments with purified Gc and C-kinase provided direct evidence that Gc is a substrate for this enzyme.

Discussion: Ca^{2+} is closely involved in the modulation of pancreatic exocrine function (11,12), and this effect appears to be mediated in part via activity of phospholipid/Ca^{2+}-dependent kinase (C-kinase) (3,4). The present study demonstrates that Gc is a major substrate for C-kinase, and more recent preliminary experiments have indicated that this is also the case under more physiological conditions, such as with stimulation of intact pancreatic acinar cells with carbachol (2,3). These results have

Vitamin D. A Chemical, Biochemical and Clinical Update

several interesting implications. In terms specificially of pancreatic exocrine function, phospholipid/Ca^{2+}-dependent phosphorylation of Gc may represent a hitherto undescribed mechanism of stimulus-response coupling. However, Gc is also widely distributed in other tissues (13,14) undergoes a high affinity interaction with G-actin (8,15,16), and has been implicated in signal transduction in B lymphocytes (4). These observations suggest that cellular interaction with biologically-active ligands may induce C-kinase-mediated phosphorylation of Gc and possibly other proteins of the membrane or cytoskeleton, and that this process might represent an important general phenomenon in cell signaling.

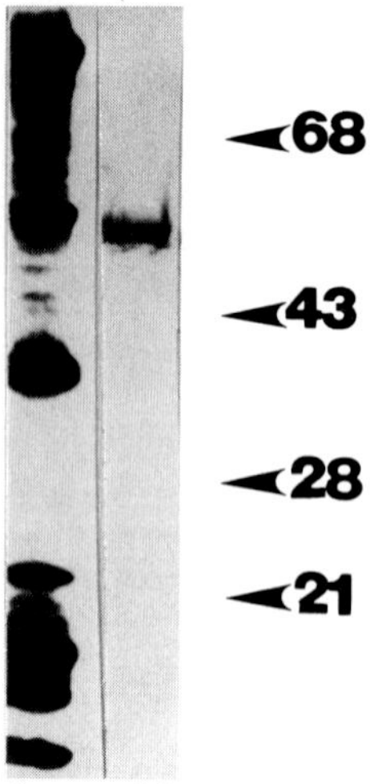

Fig. 1. Endogeneous substrates for C-kinase in soluble rat pancreatic acinar extracts. Lane a is an autoradiogram showing the range of substrates phosphorlylated in a Ca^{++}/phosphatidylserine dependent fashion. Lane b is an immunoblot of Lane a reacted with anti-Gc antibody and a peroxidase coupled secondary. The 56K substrate is homologous with Gc protein.

Acknowledgements. NIH grant CA 27062, Labcatal Laboratories, and MUSC GR25/GR45. A.E.N. and R.M.G. were supported by MUSC NIH RCDA CA 00611.

References:

1. Nishizuka, Y. (1984) Nature 308, 693-698.
2. Wrenn, R.W. and Wooten, M.W. (1984) Life Sciences 35, 73-102.
3. Wrenn, R.W. and Wooten, M.W. (1984) Biochim. Biophys. Acta 775, 1-6.
4. Petrini, M., Emerson, D.L. and Galbraith, R.M. (1983) Nature 306,73-74.
5. Petrini, M., Galbraith, R.M., Werner, P.A.M., Emerson, D.L. and Arnaud, P. (1984) Clin. Immunol. Immunopathol. 31, 282-295.
6. Petrini, M., Galbraith, R.M., Emerson, D.L., Nel, A.E. and Arnaud, P. (1985) J. Biol. Chem. 260, 1804-1810.
7. Daiger, S.P., Schanfield, M.S. and Cavalli-Sforza, L.L. (1975) Proc. Natl. Acad. Sci. U.S.A. 72, 2076-2080.
8. Kessler, S.W. (1976). J. Immunol. 117, 1482-1489.
9. Emerson, D.L., Galbraith, R.M. and Arnaud, P. (1984) Electrophoresis 1,159-163.
10. Bouillon, R., Van Baelen, H., Rombauts, W. and De Moor, P. (1978) J. Biol. Chem. 253, 4426-4431.
11. Case, R.M. and Clausen, J. (1973) J. Physiol. (Lond) 235, 75-102.
12. Gardner, J.D. (1979) Ann. Rev. Physiol. 41, 55-66.
13. Van Baelen, H., Bouillon, R. and De Moor, P. (1977) J. Biol. Chem. 252, 2515-2518.
14. Cooke, N.E., Walgate, J. and Haddad, J.G. (1979) J. Biol. Chem. 254, 5958-5964.
15. Van Baelen, H., Bouillon, R. and De Moor, P. (1980) J. Biol. Chem. 255, 2270-2272.
16. Haddad, J.G. (1982) Arch. Biochem. Biophys. 213, 538-544.

D-BINDING PROTEIN CONCENTRATION IN SERUM

Relations to age, sex, malnutrition, inflammation and 25-OH-D levels

G Toss and B Sörbo
Depts of Internal Medicine and Clinical Chemistry, University Hospital, Linköping, Sweden

The serum concentrations of liver synthesized transport proteins are in different manners influenced by the concentration of its ligand, by malnutrition, inflammation, estrogens, sex and age. The serum concentration of vitamin D binding protein (DBP) has been reported to be low in sick elderly people, but the role of age and disease is not clear.

Subjects and methods

In a health screening of 263 randomly selected people 75 or 80 years old 86 were found to be healthy and living in their own homes (Group A). In order to examine the relationship between serum 25-OH-D and DBP 28 people institutionalized in homes for the elderly but with minor or no disease were examined (Group B). A group of healthy young adults (age 32±7 years) was recruited among the staff of the hospital (Group C). Patients with protein energy malnutrition (Group D) or acute inflammation (Group E) were found in the health screening mentioned above and among patients admitted to the hospital. Sex ratio was similar in all groups. Malnutrition was defined as having subnormal value for at least three of the following measures: weight index (body weight divided by reference weight for height and age), triceps skin fold, arm muscle circumference, serum albumin and prealbumin and delayed cutaneous hypersensitivity reaction.
DBP was determined by radial immunodiffusion technique.

Results

Serum concentration of DBP in healthy elderly people did not differ from that in young adults (Table 1). Not only young females but also elderly females had slightly higher DBG level than males (0.32 vs 0.30±0.04 mg/l). Institutionalized elderly people with low serum 25-OH-D levels had normal DBP concentration (Table 1).

Table 1. Serum concentrations of DBP and 25-OH-D in elderly and young controls and in institutionalized elderly people (mean±SEM). Difference from elderly controls is marked by * ($p<0.05$), ** ($p<0.01$) or *** ($p<0.001$)

Subjects	n	DBP mg/l	25-OH-D nmol/l
A. Elderly non-institutionalized controls	86	0.30±0.01	59±2
B. Institutionalized elderly people	28	0.30±0.01	28±1
C. Healthy young adults	20	0.31±0.01	74±3

Vitamin D. A Chemical, Biochemical and Clinical Update

In people with protein energy malnutrition a slight reduction in serum DBP was found (Table 2). The reduction of DBP in malnutrition was less pronounced than that of albumin, prealbumin and retinol binding protein but comparable to that of transferrin.

People with acute inflammation (mainly acute bacterial infections) expressed in an elevation of serum haptoglobin had normal serum concentration of DBP as well as 25-OH-D.

Table 2. Serum concentration of DBP, 25-OH-D, albumin and some other proteins in elderly people with protein energy malnutrition, acute inflammatory disease compared with elderly controls (mean±SEM). Difference from elderly controls is marked as in Table 1. (N.d. = not determined).

		Group D Malnourished elderly people n=16	Group E Elderly people with acute inflammatory disease n=20	Group A Elderly controls n=86
DBP	mg/l	0.28±0.01*	0.32±0.02	0.31±0.004
25-OH-D	nmol/l	44±4**	N.d.	59±2
Albumin	g/l	36.3±1.0***	32.2±1.0***	40.4±0.04
Prealbumin	mg/l	0.21±0.02***	N.d.	0.29±0.01
Haptoglobin	g/l	N.d.	4.8 0.5***	1.6 0.1
Retinol binding protein	mg/l	50±4**	N.d.	62±1
Transferrin	g/l	2.6±0.01*	N.d.	2.9±0.1

Discussion

The reduction in serum DBP that may be seen in sick elderly people (1,2) is in view of the present results not dependent on age per se. Effect of age was neither seen in young and middle-aged subjects in a previous study (3). Neither was the concentration of 25-OH-D related to the DBP level, which is in accordance with previous reports (3). Furthermore we found no evidence that DBG behave as an acute phase reactant. However, in protein energy malnutrition a small but significant reduction in serum DBP was seen, that is not reported before. This reduction is too small to be useful in the diagnosis of malnutrition. In conclusion the concentration of DBP is remarkably stable.

References:

1. Imawari M, Kozawa K, Akanuma Y et al (1980) Gastroenterology 79, 255-258
2. MacLennan WJ and Hamilton JC (1979) J Clin Pathol 32, 240-243
3. Bouillon R, van Asche FA and DeMoor P (1977) J Clin Endocrinol Metab 45, 225-231

APPARENT VERTICAL DISPLACEMENT OF Gc PROTEIN IN THE MEMBRANE OF NORMAL T LYMPHOCYTES

ROBERT M. GALBRAITH, ANDRE E. NEL and DAVID L. EMERSON. Departments of Basic and Clinical Immunology and Microbiology, and Medicine, Medical University of South Carolina, Charleston, SC 29425

INTRODUCTION: In contrast to normal human B cells which express membrane Gc (Vitamin D-binding protein) easily detectable by immunofluorescence, <5% T cells are similarly positive (1,2). However, recent experiments with surface radioiodination have indicated that Gc may be associated with the T cell membrane (3), and that the ability to detect this protein may be related to vertical as well as lateral mobility of Gc in the plane of the lipid bilayer. This possibility was further investigated in the present study.

MATERIALS AND METHODS: Enriched T cells were separated from normal human peripheral blood, radioiodinated, extracted with non-ionic detergent and submitted to SDS-PAGE in one and two dimensions with autoradiography as previously described (3). Gc was recognized by reactivity of transblots with specific antiserum (1). Membrane expression of Gc was examined immunocytochemically with anti-Gc and fluorescein isothiocyanate (FITC)-labeled conjugate (1-3). T cells were also reacted with antisera recognizing other membrane determinants present on native cells, or on cells stimulated with phytohemagglutinin (PHA) as described (4). These included monoclonal anti-pan T (Leu 1), anti-transferrin receptor (5E9) and anti-DR (DR), and also sheep erythrocytes coated with anti-red cell antibody (EA) (3).

RESULTS: Examination of native cells confirmed the lack of detectable Gc fluorescence noted previously (3). However, parallel SDS-PAGE of soluble extracts after specific immunoprecipitation clearly showed the presence of 56K material which reacted positively with anti-Gc on transblotting, and was radiolabeled (Fig. 1).

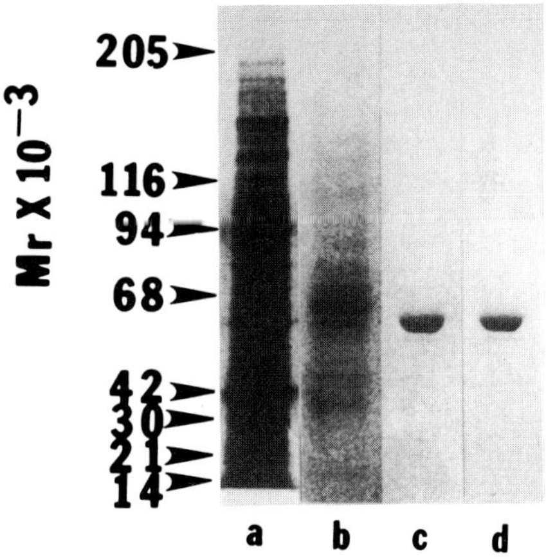

Fig. 1. SDS-PAGE of soluble T cell extracts before (a,c) and after (b,d) immunoprecipitation with anti-Gc. Lane a. is an autoradiogram, lane b. is stained with silver, lane c. is a transblot of a., and lane d. is an autoradiogram of c.

Vitamin D. A Chemical, Biochemical and Clinical Update

Reaction of native T cells with Leu 1 prior to anti-Gc showed obvious qualitative enhancement of fluorescence and this was confirmed by quantitative studies in a fluorescence cell sorter. Heating of cells to 37°C during the fluorescence protocol resulted in patching and capping not only of Leu 1 antigen but also co-mobility of Gc, and EA rosetting revealed comparable phenomena as shown previously (3). Similar primary reaction with 5E9 or anti-DR gave essentially negative results with native unstimulated cells, but showed both fluorescence enhancement and evidence of co-distribution of Gc when cells were activated by PHA. Finally, primary reaction with Leu 1 caused increased specific activity of labeled Gc as determined after specific immunoprecipitation with anti-Gc.

DISCUSSION: Although Gc cannot apparently be detected in relation to the plasma membrane by standard immunocytochemical means on native T cells, it is clearly visulaized by physicochemical means. Moreover, primary incubation of such cells with antisera known to recognize surface components of resting or stimulated T cells results in enhancement of fluorescence intensity to a level comparable to that obtained with native B cells, and a parallel increase in lactoperoxidase-induced radioiodination (see also 3). These results suggest that Gc is associated with the membrane of native cells, but in a relatively cryptic form. A similar phenomenon has been reported previously in cells reacted with antisera to Rh antigens, and the suggestion was made that this was due to changes in lipid composition of the cell membrane (5), but the precise mechanisms involved remain obscure. In summary, the finding of apparent vertical translocation of Gc within or through the lipid bilayer in additon to lateral mobility (2), and the ability of several distinct antisera to promote these phenomena argue for a more general role of Gc in mobility of membrane glycoproteins.

ACKNOWLEDGEMENTS: Research supported in part by NIH Grant CA-27062, Institutional Award CR-17, and Labcatal Laboratories, France. RMG was recipient of NIH RCDA CA-00611.

REFERENCES:

1. Petrini, M., Galbraith, R.M., Werner, P.A.M., Emerson, D.L., Arnaud, P. (1984) Clin. Immunol. Immunopathol. 31, 282-295.

2. Petrini, M., Emerson, D.L., Galbraith, R.M. (1983) Nature 305, 73-74.

3. Petrini, M. Galbraith, R.M., Emerson, D.L., Nel, A.E., Arnaud, P. (1985) J. Biol. Chem. 260, 1804.

4. Galbraith, R.M., Werner, P., Arnaud, P. and Galbraith, G.M.P. (1981) J. Clin. Invest. 66, 1135.

5. Shinitsky, M., and Sourojon, M. (1979) Proc. Natl. Acad. Sci. U.S.A. 76, 4438.

Photobiology

Serum levels of vitamin D and 25(OH)D are shown in the Table.

		IRRADIATED			NON-IRRADIATED		
Dosed	Day	Vitamin D ng/ml	$25(OH)D_3$ ng/ml	$25(OH)D_2$ ng/ml	Vitamin D ng/ml	$25(OH)D_3$ ng/ml	$25(OH)D_2$ ng/ml
	0	12.7	7.5	30.6	19.1	1.4	32.0
	2	16.6	1.1	30.2	17.1	3.4	31.1
	5	32.8	2.0	39.9	16.7	2.3	39.2
	8	15.0	0	37.0	19.0	0	24.1
Undosed	0	4.0	0	0	0	0	0
	2	2.2	6.3	0	lost	0	0
	5	4.1	10.0	0	4.9	0	0
	8	5.4	4.9	0	2.6	0	0

In the D/I group high serum vitamin D on day 5 must represent D_3 released from skin, however, little of this is converted to $25(OH)D_3$; in the UD/I group little vitamin D remains in circulation but the decay of skin D_3 is reflected in increased serum $25(OH)D_3$. The results suggest that the control of serum $25(OH)D_3$ after a single dose of UVR is exerted at the hepatic rather than the cutaneous level. High serum $25(OH)D_2$ in the dosed animals probably reflects a high hepatic level of vitamin D_2 thus inhibiting hydroxylation of incoming vitamin D_3 (6) with consequent retention of D_3 in circulation. D-deficient animals metabolised the new vitamin D_3 efficiently.

REFERENCES

1. Haddad, J.G. and Chyu, K.G. (1971), J. Clin. Endocrinol. 33, 992-995.
2. Holick, M.F. (1981), J. Invest. Dermatol. 74, 51-58.
3. Stanbury, S.W., Mawer, E.B., Taylor, C.M. and de Silva, P. (1980), Min. and Elect. Metab. 3, 51-60.
4. Takada, K., Takashima, A. and Yasuko, S. (1981), J. Steroid Biochem. 14, 1361-1367.
5. Shepard, R.M. and DeLuca, H.F. (1980), Methods in Enzymol. 67, 522-528.
6. Mawer, E.B. and Reeve, A. (1977), Calc. Tiss. Res. 22s, 24-28.

EFFECTS OF ULTRAVIOLET IRRADIATION ON SERUM VITAMIN D METABOLITES IN HEALTHY SUBJECTS AND IN PATHOLOGICAL CONDITIONS

LORE', F., DI CAIRANO G., MARCHETTI F., BATTISTELLI S. and MANASSE G.
Clinica Medica (Head: Prof. A. Caniggia), University of Siena, Italy

Although the role of ultraviolet irradiation (UVI) in vitamin D physiology has been recognized for decades, only few reports are available concerning its effects on vit. D metabolites in man.

We have studied the changes induced by whole-body artificial UVI in 28 normal subjects and in 22 patients with liver cirrhosis (7), diabetes (8) or postmenopausal (p.m.) osteoporosis (7). A mercury arc Hanovia 7A prescription lamp of known spectrum and energy was placed at 50 cm from the front and back of subjects. Low total energies were administered with progressively increasing irradiation times, a total of 13.5 min being delivered over 5 days; eight subjects underwent UVI for 10 min; 2 were irradiated after seaside holidays. Blood samples were obtained before and, at various intervals, up to 21 days after the initiation of UVI. Vit. D metabolites were measured, after lipid extraction of samples and column chromatography followed by HPLC, by competitive protein binding assay, using rat serum as the source of binding protein for 25OHD and 24,25(OH)2D and a cytosol of intestinal mucosa from rachitic chicks for 1,25(OH)2D.

Serum 25OHD increased in normal subjects (from a mean basal value of 15.9 ng/ml $\pm$ 6.6 SD, with a maximum increase of 22.8 $\pm$ 11.2 ng/ml on the 11-th day after initiation of the study). Subjects who received only 10 min of UVI showed a much smaller response (maximum increase 6.6 $\pm$ 3.2 ng/ml). A significant correlation was found between areas below the response curves and basal 25OHD values. Sex and age-related differences were not significant. 24,25(OH)2D levels almost paralleled 25OHD response (maximum increase 0.8 $\pm$ 0.4 ng/ml), but decreased more slowly after the peak value. 1,25(OH)2D response varied widely in different subjects, but in most cases showed some rise (mean basal value 37.9 $\pm$ 9.2 pg/ml, maximum increase 24.2 $\pm$ 22.8 pg/ml). Cirrhotic patients showed a slightly lower response of 25OHD and a higher response of 1,25(OH)2D. P.m. osteoporotic women showed a higher 25OHD and lower 1,25(OH)2D response. 25OHD response of diabetic patients was similar to that of normal subjects, but the increase in 1,25(OH)2D was lower. However, due to the variability of responses, almost none of the differences between patients and normal subjects was statistically significant.

Our results indicate that serum 25OHD increases remarkably in response to UVI, despite the low energy levels used. The response was influenced by the dose administered, but the dose-response relationship was probably not linear, since a small decrease in UVI time resulted in a much lower rise in 25OHD. The magnitude of 25OHD response was related to the initial 25OHD value, so that subjects with low serum 25OHD showed a greater response. This finding is consistent with previous reports, indicating that vit. D-

Vitamin D. A Chemical, Biochemical and Clinical Update

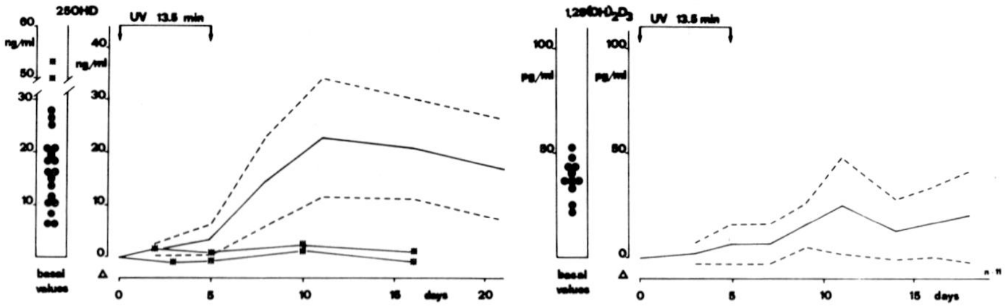

Fig. 1. Changes in 25OHD (left) and 1,25(OH)2D (right) after artificial ultraviolet irradiation in normal subjects (means $\pm$ SD are indicated, asterisks refer to subjects irradiated after seaside holidays).

deficient subjects convert vit. D to 25OHD better than vit. D-replete subjects; it is likely that a further regulation occurs in skin, since only minor responses were observed in normal subjects exposed to UVI after seaside holidays. On the other hand, in our experience oral 25OHD does not prevent 25OHD to rise after UVI to such extent. Our finding of a similar response of young and elderly subjects to UVI seems to indicate that the low serum 25OHD of the elderly is not due to an impairment of cutaneous synthesis or liver hydroxylation of vit. D. Serum 24,25(OH)2D increased after UVI, as in our earlier results (1). The subsequent decrease was slower than that of 25OHD, according to the longer half-life of the former metabolite. The behaviour of 24,25(OH)2D is a good confirmation of the view that its synthesis is mainly dependent on the availability of 25OHD, and is not consistent with the hypothesis of an important physiological role for 24,25(OH)2D. The increase in 1,25(OH)2D we observed in most subjects confirms our earlier reports (1) and indicates that a rise in precursor compounds may promote the synthesis of the final vitamin D metabolite, despite the regulatory mechanisms of 1α-hydroxylase (1α-OHase), at least in the conditions of the present study. The responses of 25OHD, 24,25(OH)2D and 1,25(OH)2D in patients with liver cirrhosis, p.m. osteoporosis or diabetes did not differ significantly form those of normal subjects. However, the only slightly impaired 25OHD response in cirrhotic patients is in agreement with the view that hepatic hydroxylation is not remarkably impaired in these patients, except in the most severe cases. The higher 25OHD and lower 1,25(OH)2D responses in osteoporotic patients are consistent with the hypothesis of an impairment of 1α-OHase in these patients with consequent increase in 25-hydroxylase activity.

REFERENCE

1. Loré, F., Di Cairano, G. and Marchetti, F. (1983) in Mineral Metabolism Research in Italy, pp. 175-178, Wichtig Editore, Milan.

PATHOGENESIS OF RICKETS IN A SUNNY COUNTRY

A.T.H. ELIDRISSY DEPARTMENT OF PAEDIATRICS COLLEGE OF MEDICINE, RIYADH.

INTRODUCTION:

The sunshine in Riyadh did not prevent the occurance of vitamin D deficiency rickets as expected (1). The disease is commonly seen in the age range from 6 to 18 months among breast fed town dewellers. Mothers of rachitic infants were found to be vitamin D deficient as well. (2) Factors associated with the development of vitamin D deficiency in such a sunny country is discussed.

VITAMIN D STATUS:

Different sectors of the community were found to have low levels of vitamin D according to european standards (3,4,5). The low levels of 25OHD noticed in such a place might be enough to stimulate formation of adequate 1,25OHD necessary to maintain normal bone calcification. It is during periods of stress or increased demand that the balance is tipped to the extent of mane-festing as rickets or osteomalacia.

FACTORS ASSOCIATED WITH RICKETS IN RIYADH

FEEDING	:	BREAST
HOUSING	:	FLATS
NUTRITIONAL STATUS	:	GOOD
MATERNAL VIT D	:	LOW
EXPOSURE TO SUN	:	NONE
CUSTOMS	:	WRAPPING

ALTHOUGH IT IS SUNNY A FORM OF AN UMBERELLA IS PREVENTING PEOPLE FROM HAVING DIRECT EXPOSURE TO THE SUN WHICH IS TOO HOT IN SUMMER.

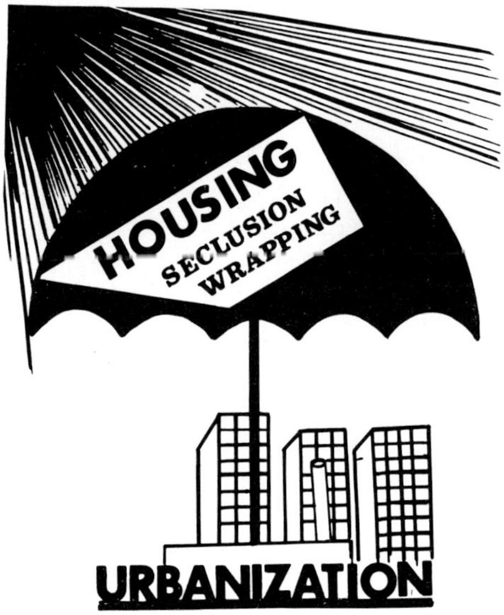

Vitamin D. A Chemical, Biochemical and Clinical Update

DISCUSSION:

The environmental factors prevailing in Riyadh simulates what was prevailing in Europe following the industrial revolution (6). Many people are moving from rural areas to Riyadh and live in poorly illuminated flats with no access to direct sunlight. Saudi diet is poor in vitamin D content (7). Although the mean levels of 25OHD in normal adults is 12.8 ng/ml for males and 11.5 ng/ml for females (4) it falls sharply during pregnancy and cord blood levels correlate with maternal levels (8). The calcium levels are maintained in the prenatal period (8) but drops in the postnatal (9). Our finding of very low levels of 25OHD mothers of rachitic infants ties up the strings (2) and proves our original hypothesis (1) that maternal vitamin D deficiency is a major cause of rickets in their infants. From the available evidence it can be stated that rickets occurs among infants born to vitamin D deficient mothers and being reared under the same umbrella with his mother in avoidance to the too hot sun while being breast fed. Breast feeding does not supply enough vitamin D even if maternal levels were normal but adequate antinatal stores might prevent rickets in the first year of life. Accordingly infantile rickets can be prevented through maintaining normal vitamin D status during pregnancy.

REFERENCES:

1. Elidrissy ATH, Taha SA. (1980) Proceeding of 5th Saudi Medical Meeting 409-418.

2. Elidrissy ATH, Sedrani SH, Lawson DEM (1984) Calcif. Tissue Int. 36:226-268.

3. Belton NR, Elidrissy ATH, Gaafer TH, Aldrees A, El Swailim AR, Forfar JO, Barr DGD, (1982) Biochemical and Clinical Endocrinology of Calcium Metabolism. Walter de Gruyter 735-737.

4. Sedrani SH, Elidrissy ATH, Arabi KM, (1983) Am J Clin Nutr 38: 129-132.

5. Arabi KM, Sedrani SH, Elidrissy ATH (1984) Journal of Tropical and Geographical Medicine.

6. Harrison EH and Harrison Helen C (1979) Disorders of Calcium and phosphate metabolism in childhood and adolescence 143.

7. Woodhouse NYJ, Norton WL, (1982) King Faisal Sp Hosp. Med J 2: 127-131.

8. Elidrissy ATH, Serinius S and Swailem AR (Proceeding of 8th Saudi Medical Conference (in press).

9. Taha S, Dost S and Sedrani S (1984) Paediatric Res. 38.

INCREASE IN SKIN 7-DEHYDROCHOLESTEROL INDUCED BY AN HYPOCHOLESTEROLEMIC AGENT ASSOCIATED WITH ELEVATED 25-HYDROXYVITAMIN D_3 PLASMA LEVEL

J.-PH. BONJOUR, U. TRECHSEL, K. MULLER and D. SCHOLER,
Department of Pathophysiology, University of Berne, Division of Physiopathology, Department of Medicine, University of Geneva and Ciba-Geigy Limited, Basel, Switzerland.

Introduction:

Vitamin D_3 is generated in skin by UV irradiation of 7-dehydrocholesterol (7-DEHC). It is not known whether the 7-DEHC amount in skin may influences the formation of vitamin D_3 and thereby plasma level of 25-hydroxyvitamin D_3 (25(OH) D_3). HCG 917 (0-[2-Hydroxy-3-[N'-(2-chloro-phenyl)-N-piperazinyl]-1-propyl]-4-chloro-benzaldoxim-hydrochlorid) is a new hypocholesterolemic agent which inhibits 7-DEHC reductase and thereby increases skin 7-DEHC. In the present work we report on the influence in rats of HCG 917 on vitamin D_3, calcium and phosphorus metabolism.

Methods

Rats were treated orally with HCG 917 for 13 days at daily doses of 0.3 and 5.0 mg/kg b.w.. Calcium and phosphorus balance were determined from day 10 to 13 as previously described (1). On day 13th, rats were bled by aortic puncture. The liver, and a piece of skin were removed and frozen on dry ice. Total cholesterol and 7-DEHC were determined in plasma, liver and in skin by the method of Curtis and Burgi (2) and Folch et al (3) respectively. 25(OH)D_3 level in plasma was determined by competitive binding assay (4). Plasma 1,25-dihydroxyvitamin D_3 (1,25(OH)$_2D_3$) was measured by competitive radioreceptor assay using D-deficient chick intestinal cytosol as binding protein source (5,6).

Results and discussion

HCG 917 caused a dose dependent-decrease in cholesterol and a concomittant accumulation of 7-DEHC in plasma, liver and skin. In skin 7-DEHC content ($\bar{x}$ ± SE) was: control, 1.05 ± 0.20; HCG 917, 0.3 mg/kg: 1.41 ± 0.22; HCG 917, 5.0 mg/kg: 2.35 ± 0.35 mg/g). At 0.3 mg/kg HCG 917 had not no significant influence on the plasma level of neither 25(OH) D_3 nor 1,25(OH)$_2D_3$, whereas at 5.0 mg/kg HCG 917 increased significantly the 25(OH)$_2D_3$ plasma level (control: 44.2 ± 3.5; HCG 917, 0.3 mg/kg: 48.8 ± 4.0; HCG 917, 5.0 mg/kg: 67.6 ± 4.2 nmol/l. This was accompanied by a slight but not significant rise in plasma 1,25(OH)$_2D_3$. (control: 1.62 ± 18; HCG 917, 0.3: 167 ± 15; HCG 917, 5.0: 196 ± 25 pmol/l). Calcium balance studies indicated that HCG 917 did not influence the intestinal or urinary Ca

Vitamin D. A Chemical, Biochemical and Clinical Update

excretion. The phosphorus balance was not affected by treatment with the hypocholesterolemic agent. At 5.0 mg/kg HCG 917 decreased slightly both the total protein and total Ca concentrations in plasma.

In conclusion, the hypocholesterolemic agent HCG 917 induces a significant rise in skin 7-dehydrocholesterol which is accompanied by an increase in the plasma 25-hydroxyvitamin D_3 level. These results suggest that variations in skin 7-dehydrocholesterol could directly influence the skin production of vitamin D_3 and thereby affect the 25-hydroxyvitamin D_3 status of the organism.

References

1. Bonjour, J.-P., Trechsel, U., Fleisch, H., Schenk, R., DeLuca, H.F. and Baxter, L.A. (1975) Am.J.Physiol. 229, 402-408.

2. Curtis, H.-Ch. and Burgi, W. (1966) Z.klin.Chem. 4, 38

3. Folch, J., Lees, M. and Sloane-Stanley, G.H. (1957) J.Biol.Chem. 226, 497-509

4. Preece, M.A., O'Riordan, J.L.H., Lawson, D.E.M. and Kodicek, E. (1974) Clin.Chim.Acta 54, 235-242

5. Trechsel, U., Eisman, J.A., Fischer, J.A., Bonjour, J.-P. and Fleisch, H. (1980) Am.J.Physiol. 239, E119-E124

6. Eisman, J.A., Hamstra, A.J., Kream, B.E. and DeLuca, H.F. (1976) Arch.Biochem.Biophys. 176, 235-243

SERUM VITAMIN D IN RESPONSE TO ULTRAVIOLET IRRADIATION IN ASIANS

by Clifford W. Lo, M.D., M.P.H., Philippe W. Paris, M.D., and Michael F. Holick, Ph.D., M.D. Vitamin D Laboratory, Endocrine Unit, Massachusetts General Hospital, Harvard Medical School, Boston, Massachusetts 02114, U.S.A.

Osteomalacia and rickets, due to deficiency of vitamin D, are a particularly prevalent and persistent problem among Asians in Great Britain (1,2). Many factors have been suggested to contribute to the development of vitamin-D deficiency, including differences in diet, cultural habits, amount of exposure to sunlight, skin pigmentation, and impaired production of vitamin D in the skin (3). Although skin pigmentation may be a factor affecting vitamin D production in the skin, no similar occurrence of rickets has been reported among Blacks in Great Britain (4). We previously demonstrated that melanin did reduce the amount of vitamin D produced in response to UV-radiation exposure, but that it was not an absolute inhibitor of vitamin D synthesis, as black subjects exposed to proportionately larger doses of UV radiation did produce similar amounts of vitamin D (5). To investigate whether the capacity to produce vitamin D in the skin of Asians is impaired independent of skin pigmentation, we determined the serum vitamin-D concentrations of Asian subjects in response to a measured dose of UV radiation.

PATIENTS AND METHODS

6 Asian subjects (Indian and Pakistani immigrants), aged 18-30 years, were recruited from an university community. 4 age-matched Caucasian subjects served as controls. All subjects were told to avoid excessive sun exposure or oral vitamin D supplements for 2 weeks before the study. The minimal erythemal dose (MED) for each subject was determined by exposing 9 small patches of skin on the back to increasing amounts of radiation from a bank of 12 fluorescent sunlamps (Elder Pharmaceuticals FS36T12 UVB:HO, power 0.77 mW/cm^2), timed to range from 15.6 to 93.1 mJ/cm^2 in 25% increments. The dose that gave a definite erythemal response with distinct borders when observed 24 hours later was designated the MED.

The subjects were then exposed to a whole body dose of UV radiation calculated at 1.5 x MED in a walk-in irradiation chamber (National Biological Corporation, Cleveland, Ohio) equipped with 16 vertically arranged fluorescent sunlamps (National Biological FSX72T12 UVB:HO, power 0.66 mW/cm^2). Serial blood samples were obtained at 0, 1, 2, 3, 6, and 9 days after UV exposure and serum was stored in glass vials at 20°C under argon. Serum samples were assayed for vitamin-D concentration by HPLC (6).

Vitamin D. A Chemical, Biochemical and Clinical Update

RESULTS AND DISCUSSION

The MED for the 6 Asian subjects ranged from 49 to 133 mJ/cm^2, with a mean of 76 ± 13 mJ/cm^2. In contrast, the MED for the Caucasian subjects were much lower, with a mean of 41 ± 4 mJ/cm^2 and a range of 31 to 48 mJ/cm^2, an indication of lighter skin pigmentation. All subjects had baseline serum vitamin-D concentrations of less than 6 ng/ml. The mean serum vitamin-D concentration was 2 ± 1 ng/ml for the Asian subjects and undetectable (less than 1 ng/ml) for the Caucasian subjects. Maximum serum vitamin D concentrations were seen at 1 day after UV irradiation, and were slightly but not significantly higher in Asian subjects, 38 ± 5 ng/ml, than in Caucasians, 27 ± 3 ng/ml. Serum vitamin-D concentrations declined gradually back to baseline over the next 9 days (see fig. 1).

As results in this report show, Asians have no impairment of vitamin-D synthesis from 7-dehydrocholesterol in their skin. However, they do require somewhat longer exposure to UV radiation to produce a MED. Thus, Asians may need longer exposure to sunlight than Caucasians do to give a similar response in vitamin D production, but the capacity to produce vitamin D is no different in Asian skin than in Caucasian skin.

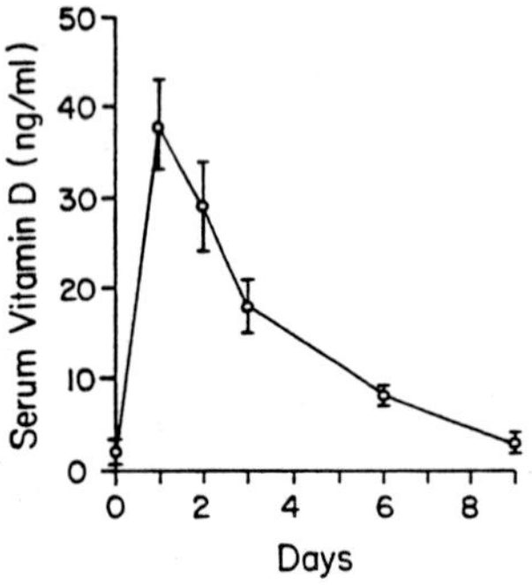

Fig. 1. Serum vitamin D concentrations in Asian subjects after 1.5 x MED whole body UV exposure. Means ± standard error.

REFERENCES

1. Dunnigan MG, Paton JPJ, Haase S, McNicol GW, Gardner MD, Smith CM (1962). Scot Med J 7:159-167.
2. Stephens WP, Klimiuk PS, Warrington S, Taylor JL, Berry JL, Mawer EB (1982). Quart J Med 51:171-188.
3. What is the link: Asians, osteomalacia and the United Kingdom? (1982) Hum Nutr: Appl Nutr 36A:493.
4. Stamp TCB, Walker PG, Perry W, Jenkins MV (1980). Clin Endocr Metab 9:81-105.
5. Clemens TL, Adams JS, Henderson SL, Holick MF (1982). Lancet i:74-76.
6. Adams JS, Clemens TL, Parrish JA, Holick MF (1982). N Engl J Med 306:722-725.

This work was supported by U.S. Public Health Service grants AM27334 and AG04616 from the National Institutes of Health.

PRODUCTION OF VITAMIN D_3 IN SHEEP IN RESPONSE TO ARTIFICIAL ULTRAVIOLET LIGHT EXPOSURE. M.S. Chaudhary and A.D. Care, Department of Animal Physiology and Nutrition, University of Leeds, Leeds LS2 9JT, U.K.

INTRODUCTION

The fluctuations in the serum levels of vitamin D_3 and $25OHD_3$ in response to solar irradiation have been reported in men, sheep, cows and pigs (1-3) but the effect of exposure to an ultraviolet (u.v.) lamp have only been investigated in humans, rats and pigs. We have studied the response of plasma concentrations of vitamin D, $25OHD_3$ and $1,25(OH)_2D$ to the graded exposure of sheep to u.v. irradiation. The effect on the fleece in this respect was also investigated.

METHODS

The sheep were exposed to irradiation from a u.v. lamp at a distance of 50 cm, for varying periods of time. A Phillips u.v. lamp, emitting 1.33 mw/cm^2 at a Wavelength of 365 nm, was used in these studies. Daily blood samples were taken prior to u.v. treatment. Initially, six sheep were exposed to u.v. light for two weeks. In the second experiment, three sheep were given u.v. light treatment for three weeks. After four weeks they were shorn and again subjected to the same procedure. Vitamin D was estimated by a non-equilibrium binding assay and $25OHD_3$ and $1,25(OH)_2D$ were estimated by radioimmunoassays.

RESULTS

The concentration of $25OHD_3$ in the plasma of six sheep was unchanged after two weeks exposure to u.v. light but there was a significant ($P<0.05$) increase in vitamin D concentration (Fig 1). In the second experiment there was an increase in vitamin D concentration in shorn and unshorn sheep but it was significantly ($P<0.05$) higher in the former group. The plasma $25OHD_3$ and $1,25(OH)_2D$ levels were unaffected in both groups (Fig 2).

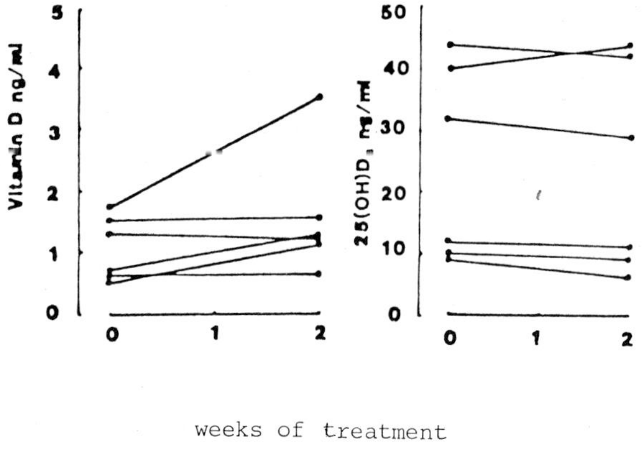

Fig.1.

Effect of u.v. light treatment on plasma concentrations of vitamin D and $25(OH)D_3$

Vitamin D. A Chemical, Biochemical and Clinical Update

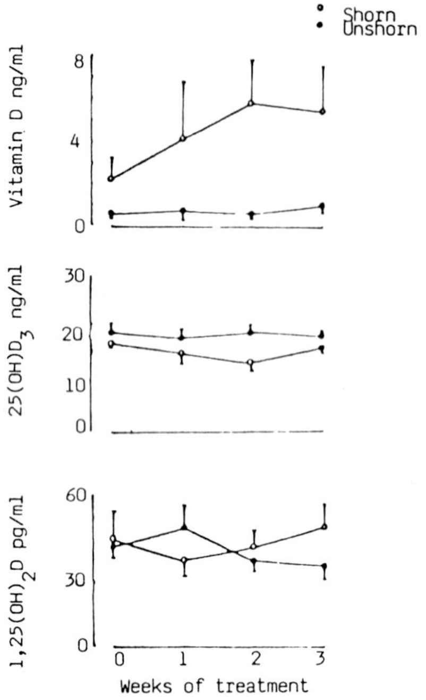

Fig 2. Effect of u.v. light treatment on plasma concentration of vitamin D, $25(OH)D_3$ and $1,25(OH)_2D$ in sheep.

DISCUSSION

The results of both these experiments demonstrate a significant increase in plasma vitamin D concentration and no change in $25OHD_3$ and $1,25(OH)_2D$ concentrations. Thus, it appears that exposure to u.v. light can lead to significant synthesis of vitamin D_3 in the skin of sheep, especially when shorn. The lack of change in plasma $25OHD_3$ concentrations, despite an increase in vitamin D levels, indicates the possibility of some constraint during vitamin D sufficiency on hepatic 25-hydroxylation of vitamin D as reported by others (4-5).

REFERENCES

1. McLaughlin, M., Fairney, A. and Lester, E. (1974) The Lancet I, 536-538.
2. Smith, B.S.W. and Wright, H. (1981) Vet. Record 109, 139-141.
3. Ross, R. (1978) Ph.D. Thesis, University of Leeds.
4. Mawer, E.B. and Reeve, A. (1977) Calcified Tissue Res. 22 (suppl.), 24-28.
5. Stanbury, S.W., Mawer, E.B., Taylor, C.M. and DeSilva, P. (1980) Mineral Electrolyte Metab. 3, 51-60.

Evolutionary Aspects of Vitamin D

EFFECT OF ACTIVE VITAMIN D_3 ON HUMAN IMMUNE FUNCTION IN VIVO

K. Okano, S. Kou, M. Shimizu, Y. Nozawa, T. Kato, Y. Yamada, C. Nawa, K. Ohira, N. Shinagawa, M. Yajima and K. Someya
Third Department of Internal Medicine, St. Marianna University School of Medicine, Kawasaki 213, Japan

In the recent years, evolutionary aspects of vitamin D - its effect on cell differentiation and immune function have been drawing attention. In the present report, we studied the effect of 1α-hydroxyvitamin D_3 (1α-OHD_3) on human immune function in vivo.

Materials and Methods

The study population consisted of 51 normal aged human subjects and the patients with senile osteoporosis, some of whom were orally administered 1.5 μg/day 1α-OHD_3 for up to 12 months. Peripheral mononuclear cells were separated from heparinized blood by Ficoll-Hypaque. T lymphocytes were determined by E rosette method and B lymphocytes by surface marker immunoglobulin method. IgG-FcR^+T cells and IgM-FcR^+T cells were determined by double rosette method using microplates. The incorporation of [^{3}H]-thymidine into mononuclear cells was expressed as a stimulation index, a parameter for lymphocyte blasttransformation, after the incubation of these cells with PHA, Con A or PWM at 37 C for 48 h and subsequently with [^{3}H]-thymidine for 24 h at 37 C. $OKT3^+$ cell (pan T cell), $OKT4^+$ cell (helper/inducer T cell), $OKT8^+$ cell (suppressor/cytotoxic T cell), $Leu7^+$ cell (natural killer cell) and $OKM1^+$ cell (null cell, monocyte) were determined by a flow cell sorter (Japan Spectroscopic Co., Ltd., FCS-1), after hemolization of whole blood and subsequent incubations with monoclonal antibody and with FITC-labeled antimouse immunoglobulin. 1α-OHD_3 was kindly supplied from Chugai Pharmaceutical Co., Ltd. Statistical analyses were carried out by Student t test and paired comparison t test.

Results

Serum calcium levels showed no significant alterations after 1α-OHD_3 administration in normal group and osteoporotic group. Peripheral white blood cell count significantly increased at 8 weeks in the normal group ($p < 0.05$) and at 8 and 16 weeks in the osteoporotic group ($p<0.01$, respectively) after 1α-OHD_3 administration. Lymphocyte count significantly increased at 8 and 16 weeks of 1α-OHD_3 administration in the normal group ($p < 0.05$, respectively), while it remained unaltered in the osteoporotic group. T lymphocyte remained unaltered after 1α-OHD_3 administration in these groups. B lymphocyte was significantly increased at 8 weeks ($p<0.01$) and significantly decreased at 16 weeks ($p<0.05$) after 1α-OHD_3 administration in the osteoporotic group, while it remained unaltered in the normal group. As shown in Fig. 1, IgG-FcR^+T cells significantly increased at 8 weeks of 1α-OHD_3 administration in these groups. Percentage of IgM-FcR^+T cells in the normal group was significantly higher than that of the osteoporotic group and significantly decreased at 16 weeks of 1α-OHD_3 administration. Serum IgG, IgA and IgM levels remained unaltered after 1α-OHD_3 administration in these groups. As shown in Fig. 2, tuberculin reaction was enhanced in these two groups after 1α-OHD_3 administration for 8 weeks. Stimulation index tended to increase after 1α-OHD_3 administration to the aged for 8 weeks, when PHA, Con A or PWM was used. After the administration of 1α-

Vitamin D. A Chemical, Biochemical and Clinical Update

OHD_3 to the aged for 12 months, the percentage of $OKT3^+$ cells remained unaltered, $OKT4^+$ cells tended to increase, $OKT8^+$ cells tended to decrease, and $OKT4^+$ cell/$OKT8^+$ cell ratio tended to increase, while $Leu7^+$ cells and $OKM1^+$ cells remained unaltered.

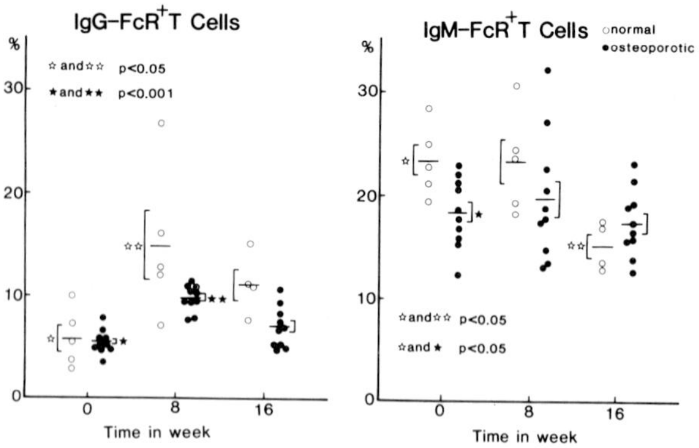

Fig. 1. Alteration of IgG-FcR^+T cells and IgM-FcR^+T cells after oral administration of 1.5 µg/day 1α-OHD_3 to the aged.

Discussion

A significant increase of peripheral white blood cell count after 1α-OHD_3 administration in this study, might reflect an increase of null cells and /or granulocytes, in view of a significant increase of lymphocyte count and no significant or steady increase in T cells and B cells and a report on the promotion of cell differentiation by 1,25-dihydroxyvitamin D_3 [1,25$(OH)_2D_3$] (1). A significant increase of IgG-FcR^+T cell after 1α-OHD_3 administration might explain for such an increase, in view of a recent report that it is null cell or activated T cell (2). Administration of 1.5 µg/day 1α-OHD_3 to the aged caused a tendency to increase $OKT4^+$ cell/$OKT8^+$ cell ratio in this study, and some other group reported that it was decreased by 0.5 µg/day 1α-OHD_3, suggesting that this ratio is influenced by the dose of 1α-OHD_3 and probably by the duration of its administration. The fact that 1α-OHD_3 enhanced tuberculin reaction and lymphocyte blasttransformation <u>in vivo</u>, suggests that 1,25$(OH)_2D_3$ converted from 1α-OHD_3 in the liver influences on immunoregulatory system.

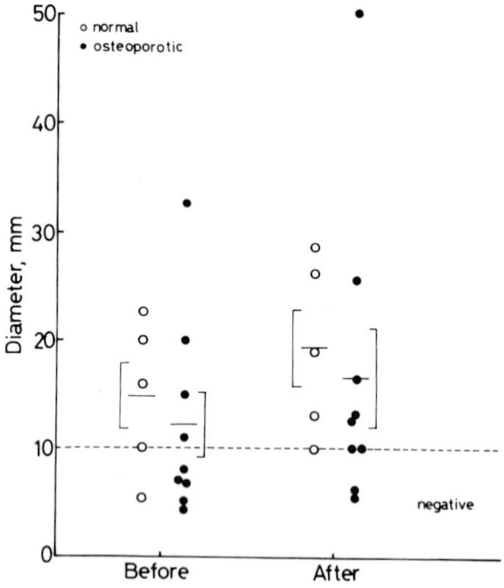

Fig. 2. Alteration of tuberculin reaction after oral administration of 1.5 µg/day 1α-OHD_3 to the aged.

References

1. Abe, E., Miyaura, C., Sakagami, H., Takeda, M., Konno, K., Yamazaki, T., Yoshiki, S. and Suda, T. (1981) Proc. Natl. Acad. Sci. USA <u>78</u>, 4990-4994.
2. Pichler, W. J. and Broder, S. (1981) Immunological Rev. <u>56</u>, 163-191.

IS VITAMIN D A CALCIUM REGULATING HORMONE IN INVERTABRATES?

S. Edelstein, N. Fine, S. Shine and S. Weiner,
Departments of Biochemistry and Isotopes, The Weizmann Institute of Science, Rehovot 76100, Israel.

There are two main lines of evolutionary pressures impinging upon Ca metabolism in animals. The first evolutionary influence which can be identified is the need to regulate the internal environment of Ca as animals have colonized increasingly hostile environments such as fresh water and dry land. The second evolutionary influence affecting Ca metabolism concerns the development of mineralized skeletons. The most primitive of multicellular animals, the coelenterates and sponges, have a skeletal system based on an elevated turgor pressure within stiffened compartments. In these hydrostatic skeletons a limited capacity for tissue contractility and movement is available. In their need to move in search for food or as means of self-defence, many species have developed more effective skeletons which are hardened by impregnation with mineral salts. These serve as a rigid support upon which contractile tissues may be anchored and protection against carnovorous predators. In many species the mineralized tissues are located externally like in the Arthropoda and Mollusca.

In the majority of animals the major Ca salt in mineralized tissues is carbonate, reflecting the abundance of bicabonate in the environment. Only in vertebrates and few invertebrates is phosphate important. It is in the class Amphibia that parathyroid glands make their first phylogenic appearance and perhaps therefore the metabolism of vitamin D and its involvement in a Ca metabolism was considered only in vertebrates.

Wagge (1) in 1952 showed for the first time that cholecalciferol or ergocalciferol are essential nutrients for the terrestrial snail Helix aspersa, as their absence in the diet results in the death of the snails. On the other hand, increased concentrations of these sterols in the diet results in increased Ca absorption from the food and increased ability to utilize Ca reserves in the shell and digestive-gland. H. aspersa fed on an increased cholecalciferol diet regernated pieces of damaged shall with a richer organic matrix surrounding the inorganic crystals (1).

These observations of Wagge (1) together with the more recent findings on the metabolism of vitamin D raise the question as to whether molluscs, and in particular land snails, possess a functional metabolism of the vitamin.

Weiner et al. (2) in 1979 showed that when radioactively labelled cholecalciferol was injected into the land snails Levantina hiersolima and Theba pisana, three metabolites (C, D and E, Fig, 1), more polar than cholecalciferol were formed.

Vitamin D. A Chemical, Biochemical and Clinical Update

Figure 1: Sephadex LH-20 chromatographic profile of lipid extracts from <u>L. hiersolyma</u> 10 days after an injection of (1,2-^{3}H)cholecalciferol.

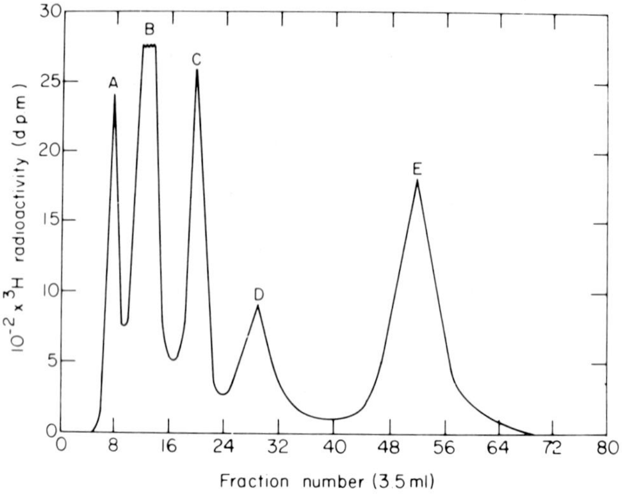

Peaks B, C and E co-chromatographed with cholecalciferol, 25(OH)D_3 and 24,25$(OH)_2D_3$ respectively. An injection of 25-hydroxy(26,27-^{3}H)cholecalciferol into these terrestrial snails resulted in peak E being predominantly formed. Co-chromatography of peaks B, C and E with synthetic cholecalciferol, 25(OH)D_3 and 24R,25$(OH)_2D_3$ on HPLC indicated that peaks B and C indeed co-eluted with cholecalciferol and 25(OH)D_3 respectively, whereas peak E was found to be more polar than 24R,25$(OH)_2D_3$. This was confirmed by the periodate cleavage test in which the control 24,25-dihydroxy(26,27-^{3}H)cholecalciferol was cleaved and lost its radioactive labelling, whereas metabolite E was unaffected.

After injection of ^{3}H-labelled cholecalciferol or 25(OH)D_3, the major portion of radioactivity was localized in the digestive gland (Table 1).

Table 1: Distribution of cholecalciferol in the tissues of <u>L. hiersolyma</u> after an injection of (1,2-^{3}H)cholecalciferol.

Tissue	Distribution of radioactivity (%)
Digestive gland	62.4
Intestine	9.4
Mantle	4.3
Muscle	17.3
Sexual organs	6.6

Analysis of the lipid extracts from this tissue showed that this radioactivity is composed mainly of $25(OH)D_3$ and metabolite E. The digestive gland in land snails is thus probably one of the sites at which cholecalciferol acts.

The site of the formation of metabolite E was found to be the intestine. When tissue homogenates of L. hiersolyma were incubated in vitro for 5 h at 27°C with 25-hydroxy(26,27-^{3}H)cholecalciferol about 5 times more metabolite E was formed in the intestine than in the other tissues (Table 2)

Table 2: $25(OH)D_3$ hydroxylase in L. hiersolyma tissues

Tissue	Formation of peak E (%)′
Digestive gland	2.0
Intestine	11.2
Mantle	2,0
Muscle	2.0
Sexual organs	None

The above findings show that land snails do metabolize vitamin D. The metabolic pathway partially resembles that of vertebrates such as mammals and birds in which cholecalciferol is hydroxylated at C-25 to form $25(OH)D_3$. Whereas in mammals and birds, the latter compound is further metabolized into $1,25(OH)_2D_3$ and $24,25(OH)_2D_3$, in land snails $25(OH)D_3$ is predominantly metabolized into as yet unidentified polar metabolite E.

Metabolite D, on the other hand, is predominantly formed from cholecalciferol itself.

Molluscs live in many diverse environments which can be very variable in Ca content. Terrestrial molluscs are faced with extreme shortage of Ca while marine molluscs living in sea water represent the upper extreme of salinity. We therefore studied the metabolism of vitamin D in marine gastropods (Testus dentatus, Trochus sp. and Lambis truncata sebae) and in marine bivalves (Chlamys squamosa and Crassostrea gigas). Fig. 2 summarizes the metabolic pathways of vitamin D in land molluscs as compared to marine molluscs

Considering the above differences in the metabolism of vitamin D between land and marine molluscs and the availability of Ca in sea water compared with terrestrial environments it would seem most likely that the function of metabolite E in land snails is related to Ca absorption, either from the food or the removal from the digestive-gland (3).

Sails are known to mobilize Ca minerals by specialized transporting cells called amoebocytes. When snails were injected with radiolabelled $25(OH)D_3$, autoradiographic studies of digestive-gland tissue preparations and mantle preparations showed an accumulation of the vitamin in the amoebocytes (Fig. 3, 4).

Figure 2: The metabolic pathway of cholecalciferol in land and marine molluscs.

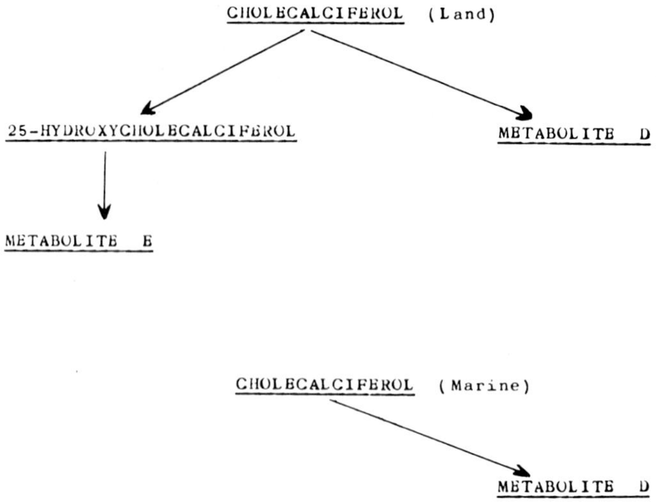

Figure 3: Autoradiographic localization of ^{3}H-25(OH)D_3 in amoebocytes in the digestive-gland.

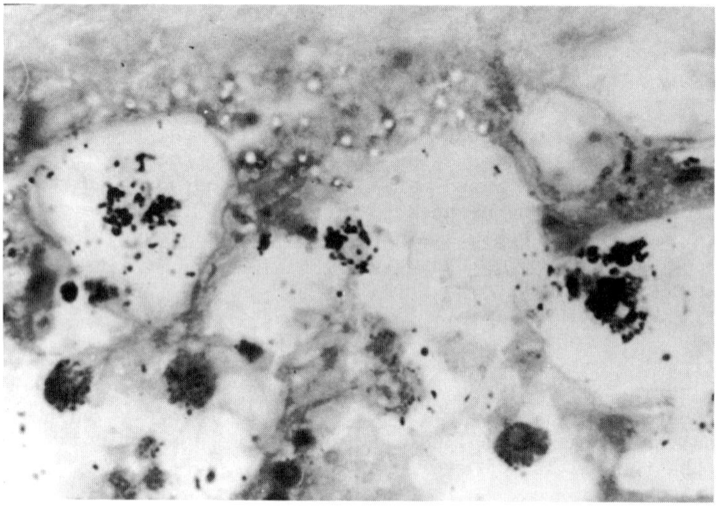

Figure 4: Autoradiographic localization of ^{3}H-25(OH)D_3 in amoebocyte in the mantle

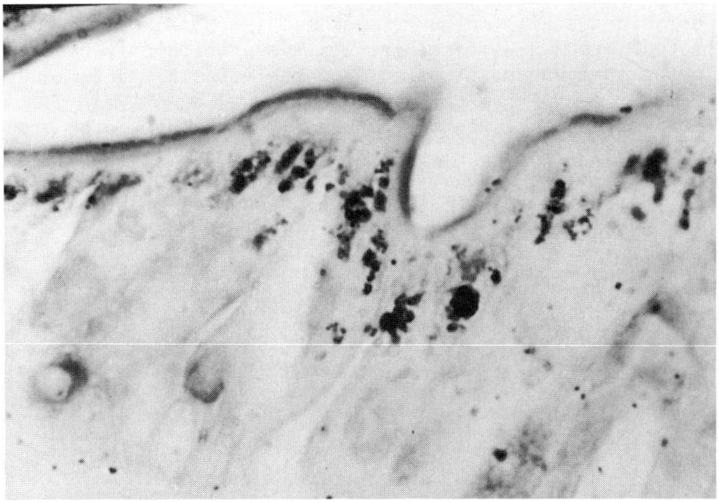

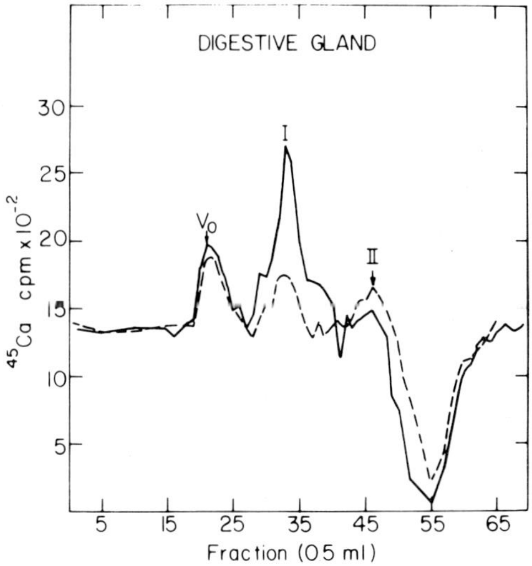

Figure 5: Elution profile of digestive-gland homogenates chromatographed on ^{45}Ca equilibrated Sephadex column (—— control snails; ---- vitamin D-deficient snails).

Further support to the notion that vitamin D is functional in Ca-metabolism in land snails comes from the presence of CaBP in the digestive gland. When snails were made vitamin D-deficient by feeding them paper and their digestive-gland homogenates were analysed for ^{45}Ca binding in comparison to non-deficient snails, a CaBP (peak I, Fig. 5) was detected in ^{45}Ca equilibrated Sephadex G-75 column, while significalntly reduced content was noted in the homogenates prepared from the vitamin D-deficient snails.

The molecular weight of the CaBP in snails was found to be around 14,000 daltons (Fig. 6).

Figure 6: Molecular weight estimation of snail's CaBP on calibrated Sepahdex G-100 column

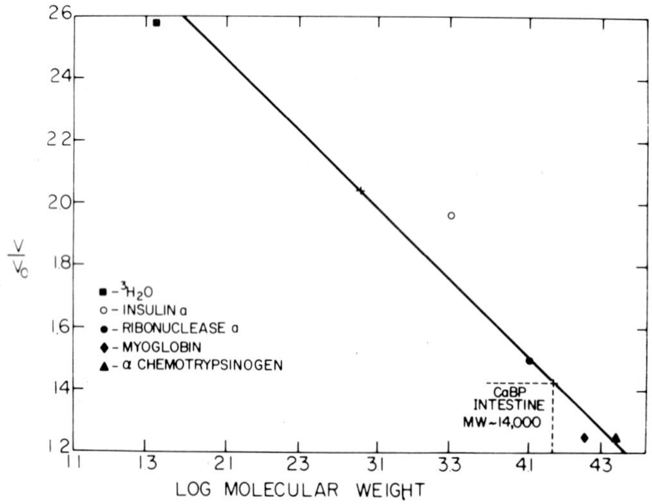

In almost all phylogenetic schemes of the animal kingdom, the molluscs and the chordates are at opposite extremes (4) and their common ancester probably dates back to the very late Precambrian period soon after the metazaons evolved, but before the onset of biomineralization. The finding of vitamin D in molluscs is most easily understood by assuming that the vitamin or a close analogue was also required by the common ancester. In this case, vitamin D is presumable present in many other invertebrates and can be identified as a hormone which has evolved primarily as a regulator of Ca metabolism in many classes of invertebrates.

References:

1. Wagge, L-E- (1952) J. Exp. Zool. 126, 311-342.
2. Weiner, S., Noff, D., Meyer, M.S., Weisman, Y. and Edelstein, S. (1979) Biochem. J. 184, 157-161.
3. Burton, R.F. (1972) Comp. Biochem. Physiol. 434, 655-663.
4. Valentyne, J.W. (1977) in Patterns of Evolution as Illustrated by the Fossil Record (Hallam, A., ed) p. 591, Elsevier Scientific Publ. Co. Amsterdam, Oxford and New York.

VITAMIN D_3 ACTIVITY IN *IN VITRO* CALCIUM UPTAKE AND GROWTH OF *PHASEOLUS VULGARIS* ROOTS.

M.A. Vega and R.L. Boland

Departamento de Biologia, Universidad Nacional del Sur, 8000 Bahia Blanca, Argentina.

The presence of vitamin D_3 sterols has been demonstrated in several plant species (1-4). These studies were performed to investigate a possible role of these compounds in plant cell function.

METHODS:

Root tips of 1 cm length obtained from 2 day-old *Phaseolus vulgaris* seedlings were cultured in Shenk-Hildebrandt medium (5) at 28 °C under darkness. Root growth was measured by root elongation and ^3H-leucine incorporation into protein. Length measurements were made after 14 h culture in the absence (control) or presence of vitamin D_3 (10^{-9} M) or Ca ionophore X-537 A (10^{-5} M). To evaluate ^3H-leucine incorporation into protein, roots cultured for a similar period in the absence of sterol were incubated with vitamin D_3 (10^{-9} M) and ^3H-leucine (1 μCi/ml) for 2 h. Roots were washed, dissolved in hot 0.1 N NaOH and labelled proteins precipitated with 10 % TCA. Ca uptake by 14 h-root cultures was measured during a 2 h-interval in the presen- of vitamin D_3 or ionophore using 0.5 μCi/ml $^{45}CaCl_2$. To evaluate the effects of protein synthesis inhibitors on Ca uptake, cycloheximide and puromycin (10^{-5} M) were added to the medium simultaneously with vitamin D_3 or ionophore and $^{45}CaCl_2$. For double labelling experiments, roots cultured 14 h in basal medium were incubated 2 h with ^3H-leucine in the presence of vitamin D_3 or with ^{14}C-leucine in the absence of sterol. The tissues were homogenized in 50 mM Tris-HCl pH 7.4, 3 mM $MgSO_4$, 3 mM EGTA, 400 mM NaCl, 10 mM ß-mercapthoethanol, 0.5 mM phenylmethylsulfonylfluoride, followed by heating at 100 °C 5 min and centrifugation. The supernatant was treated with 10 % TCA and the precipitate was extracted with 50 mM Tris-HCl pH 7.4, 150 mM NaCl, 10 mM ß-mercapthoethanol. Polyacrylamide (10 %) gel electrophoresis of soluble proteins was made in 200 mM Tris-Bicine pH 8.2, 0.2 % SDS. Gels were sliced, dissolved in H_2O_2 at 70 °C and counted for ^3H and ^{14}C. Corrections for quenching were made.

RESULTS AND DISCUSSION:

Roots treated with vitamin D_3 or the Ca ionophore X-537 A grew significantly less than control roots ($p < 0.0125$ and $p < 0.01$, respectively, by Wilcoxons non parametric test applied to frequency-distribution histograms of length, data not shown). The effects of the sterol on root elongation could be correlated with an inhibition of ^3H-leucine incorporation into proteins (661 ± 148 dpm/μg prot vs 296 ± 92 dpm/μg prot in control and treated roots, respectively, $p < 0.0025$, Student's t test). Both vitamin D_3 and the ionophore significantly increased root ^{45}Ca uptake respect to controls, as shown in Table 1. This suggests that a causal relationship may exist between the effects of the sterol on root Ca uptake and growth. Cycloheximide and puromycin at a concentration which inhibited ^3H-leucine incorporation into protein by 70 %, blocked the stimulation of Ca uptake produced by vitamin D_3 without significantly affecting the corresponding controls (data not given). This suggests that the action of vitamin D_3 on root Ca uptake is mediated

Vitamin D. A Chemical, Biochemical and Clinical Update

by *de novo* protein synthesis.

Table 1. Effects of vitamin D_3 (10^{-9} M) and Ca ionophore X-537 A (10^{-5} M) on Ca uptake by *Phaseolus vulgaris* roots.

	Ca uptake, umol Ca/mg protein	
	Vitamin D_3	Ionophore X-537 A
Control	5.71 ± 1.20 (6)	3.11 ± 0.91 (13)
Treated	7.33 ± 1.47 (9)[a]	4.10 ± 1.81 (13)[b]

[a] $p < 0.025$, [b] $p < 0.05$, Students t test

In addition, double labelling experiments indicate that the sterol induces the synthesis of heat and acid stable low molecular weight proteins (Fig.1)

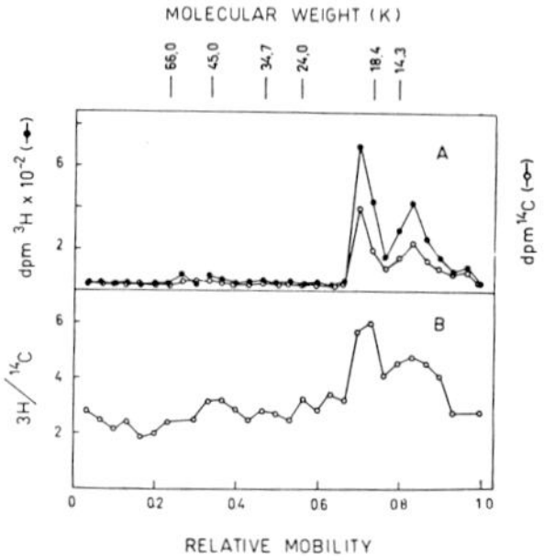

Fig. 1. SDS-PAGE of proteins labelled with ^{3}H-leucine (vit. D_3) or ^{14}C-leucine (control). A. Heat and acid stable proteins. B. dpm ^{3}H (vit. D_3)/dpm ^{14}C (control).

Further characterization of one of the proteins synthetized in response to vitamin D_3 revealed a MW of 14,300 ± 800 and an isoelectric point of 4.11, as determined by SDS-PAGE and polyacrylamide gel electrofocusing, respectively.

REFERENCES:

1. Haussler, M.R., Wasserman, R.H., Mc Cain, T.A., Peterlik, M., Bursac, K. M. and Hughes, M.R. (1976) Life Sciences 18, 1049-1056.
2. Wasserman, R.H., Corradino, R.A. and Krook, L. (1975) Biochem. Biophys. Res. Commun. 62, 85-91.
3. Rambeck, W.A., Kreutzberg, O., Bruns-Droste, C. and Zucker, H. (1981) Z. Pflanzenphysiol. Bd. 104, 9-16.
4. Horst, R.L., Reinhardt, T.A., Rusell, R.J. and Napoli, J.L. (1984) Arch. Biochem. Biophys. 231, 67-71.
5. Shenk, R.U. and Hildebrandt, A.C. (1972) Can. J. Bot. 50, 199.

METABOLISM OF ^3H-$25OHD_3$ AND ITS RELATIONSHIP TO CALCIUM IN THE RAINBOW TROUT *SALMO GAIRDNERI*

M.E. HAYES*, D.F. GUILLAND-CUMMING, R.G.G. RUSSELL AND I.W. HENDERSON.
*Department of Medicine, University of Manchester, Manchester M13 9PT.
Departments of Human Metabolism and Zoology, University of Sheffield, Sheffield S10 2TN, U.K.

INTRODUCTION

Many teleosts, particularly marine, have large hepatic stores of vitamin D_3; its source, metabolism and functional significance are poorly defined, however. In the rainbow trout there is a growth-related dietary requirement for vitamin D_3 (1), although this species can form limited amounts of pre-vitamin D_3 from epidermal 7-dehydrocholesterol during exposure to U-V light (2). The formation and hepatic storage of $25OHD_3$ has also been demonstrated (3), although production of more polar metabolites particularly the renal synthesis of $1,25(OH)_2D_3$ has not been shown unequivocally (4,5). The present study examines the metabolism of $25OHD_3$ to more polar metabolites in trout adapted to varying calcium regimes.

EXPERIMENTAL METHODS AND RESULTS

Unfed freshwater and seawater adapted trout, with arterial catheters implanted, were adapted to waters of varying calcium concentrations (0.25-20 mmol/l). ^3H-25OHD (2-5 µCi, 0.05 µCi/nmol) was administered intraarterially, and blood collected 6 hours later. Vitamin D_3 metabolites were extracted from plasma in hexane: isopropanol: butanol (92:4:3) and analysed by straight phase HPLC (Zorbax sil, 6mm x 25cm), with a hexane: isopropanol: methanol (95:6:4) mobile phase, for the formation of dihydroxy metabolites of vitamin D_3.

Trout metabolised $25OHD_3$ to a series of more polar metabolites:- product A chromatographed between $25OHD_3$ and $24,25(OH)_2D_3$; product B with $24,25(OH)_2D_3$; product C with $25,26(OH)_2D_3$; product D between $25,26(OH)_2D_3$ and $1,25(OH)_2D_3$ and product E with $1,25(OH)_2D_3$. In addition, the latter metabolite co-chromatographed with authentic $1,25(OH)_2D_3$ on Zorbax sil with a dichloromethane: isopropanol (95:5) mobile phase. With decreasing environmental or plasma calcium concentrations fish formed more "$1,25(OH)_2D_3$" (Fig 1), whilst with increasing concentrations products A and C predominated. Of these the major metabolite formed was product C (Fig 1) which co-chromatographed with authentic $25,26(OH)_2D_3$, but product C does not represent $25,26(OH)_2D_3$ as it is insensitive to periodic acid. $24,25(OH)_2D_3$ (product B), occurred in minimal amounts. The ability of trout tissues (liver, kidney, gut mucosa, gill filaments, scales and corpuscles of Stannius) to metabolise $25OHD_3$ was assessed *in vitro* by incubation with ^3H-$25OHD_3$ (0.25 µCi, 0.5µCi/nmol) for 6 hours. Of these only liver significantly metabolised this substrate.

SUMMARY

The metabolism of $25OHD_3$ in trout appears to be predominantly hepatic and not renal as in some species of fish (5), with plasma calcium concentration, reflecting environmental calcium availability, exerting major influences (Fig 2). In normocalcaemic trout a number of as yet unidentified metabolites are formed, whilst in hypocalcaemic (<2.4 mmol/l) fish $1,25(OH)_2D_3$ appears to be formed. In such unfed trout $1,25(OH)_2D_3$ may influence the rate of branchial uptake of calcium by interacting with specific $1,25(OH)_2D_3$ recep-

Vitamin D. A Chemical, Biochemical and Clinical Update

tor-like proteins that are present in the gill (6).

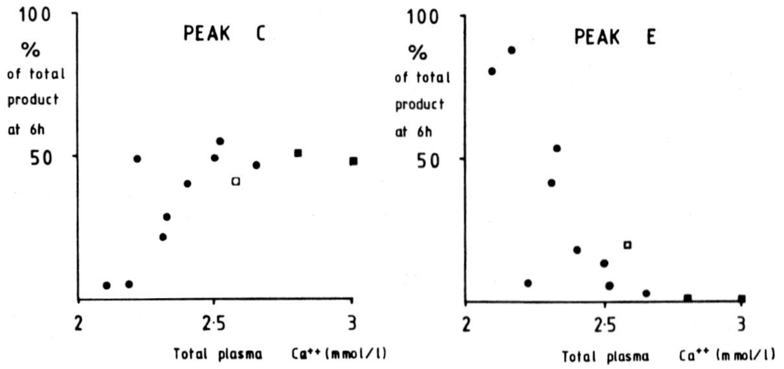

Figure 1: Formation of products C and E ($1,25(OH)_2D_3$) in relation to the plasma calcium concentration in freshwater (●), seawater (■) and low calcium artificial seawater adapted (□) trout.

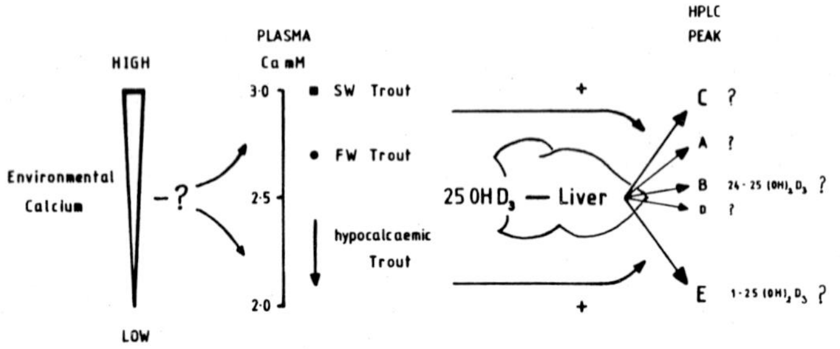

Figure 2: Hypothetical modulation of hepatic metabolism of $25OHD_3$ in rainbow trout.

REFERENCES

1 Barnett, B.J., Cho, C.Y. & Slinger, S.J. (1979) Comp. Biochem. Physiol. 63A, 291 - 297.

2 Holick, M.F., Holick, S.A. & Guillard, R.L. (1982) In "Comparative Endocrinology of Calcium Regulation". Japan Sci. Soc. Press, Tokyo 85 - 92.

3 Fraser, D.R. (1979) In "Paediatric disease related to calcium". Elsevier, North Holland, New York. 59 - 73.

4 Yanda, D.M. & Ghazarian, J.G. (1981) Comp. Biochem. Physiol. 96B, 183 - 188.

5 Henry, H.L. & Norman, A.W. (1975) Comp. Biochem. Physiol. 50B, 431 - 434.

6 Guilland-Cumming, D.F., Clayton, J., Hayes, M.E., Henderson, I.W., Johnson, S. & Russell, R.G.G. (1982) Proc. 1st Joint Meet. Brit. Endocr. Soc. Abstr. 114.

This work was funded by the Natural Environmental Research Council U.K.

EFFECT OF 1,25-DIHYDROXYVITAMIN D_3 ON HUMAN IMMUNE FUNCTION IN VITRO

K. Okano, S. Kou, M. Shimizu, Y. Nozawa, Y. Yamada, T. Kato, C. Nawa, K. Ohira, N. Shinagawa, M. Yajima, S. Fujibayashi and K. Someya
Third Department of Internal Medicine, St. Marianna University School of Medicine, Kawasaki 213, Japan

In the present report, we studied the effects of various vitamin D_3 metabolites on human peripheral lymphocyte subsets, interleukin 2 receptor, transferrin receptor and lymphocyte blasttransformation *in vitro*, in an attempt to elucidate the mechanisms of actions of vitamin D_3 metabolites on immune function.

Materials and Methods

Peripheral blood mononuclear cells from 29 normal young men were separated by Ficoll-Hypaque. 10^6 cells suspended in RPMI 1640 containing 10% fetal calf serum and PHA, were incubated *in vitro* with 10^{-7}-10^{-10}M 1,25-dihydroxyvitamin D_3 [$1,25(OH)_2D_3$] for 48 h at 37 C under 5% CO_2 and 95% air. The number of intact mononuclear cells was counted using trypan blue and a hemocytometer under a microscope. $OKT3^+$ cell (pan T cell), $OKT4^+$ cell (helper/inducer T cell), $OKT8^+$ cell (suppressor/cytotoxic T cell), $OKIa1^+$ cell (B cell, activated T cell), $Leu7^+$ cell (natural killer cell), Tac^+ cell (interleukin 2 receptor) and $OKT9^+$ cell (transferrin receptor), were determined by a flow cell sorter (Japan Spectroscopic Co., Ltd., FCS-1), after the incubation of the cells with these monoclonal antibodies and subsequently with FITC-labeled anti-mouse immunoglobulin. The incorporation of [^3H]-thymidine into mononuclear cells was expressed as a stimulation index, a parameter for lymphocyte blasttransformation, after the incubation of 10^5 cells with 10^{-7}-10^{-12}M $1,25(OH)_2D_3$, 10^{-7}-10^{-11}M 24,25-dihydroxyvitamin D_3 [$24,25(OH)_2D_3$], 10^{-6}-10^{-10}M 25-hydroxyvitamin D_3 (25-OHD_3) and 10^{-7}-10^{-11}M 1α-hydroxyvitamin D_3 (1α-OHD_3) as well as PHA, Con A or PWM for 48 h at 37 C and subsequently with [^3H]-thymidine for 24 h at 37 C. Tac monoclonal antibody was a kind gift of Dr. T. Uchiyama, Kyoto University. 1α-OHD_3 was kindly supplied from Chugai Pharmaceutical Co., Ltd. Statistical analyses were carried out by paired comparison *t* test.

Results

Number of the mononuclear cells incubated with PHA and various doses of $1,25(OH)_2D_3$, showed no significant alterations compared to that incubated only with PHA. After incubation of the cells with various doses of 1,25-$(OH)_2D_3$, the percentage of $OKT4^+$ cells showed no significant alteration, $OKT8^+$ cells tended to increase, and $OKT4^+$ cell/$OKT8^+$ cell ratio tended to decrease. $Leu7^+$ cells showed no significant alteration by $1,25(OH)_2D_3$. $OKIa1^+$ cells significantly decreased by 10^{-9}M $1,25(OH)_2D_3$ ($p < 0.05$). As shown in Fig. 1, Tac^+ cells significantly decreased by 10^{-10} and 10^{-9}M $1,25(OH)_2D_3$ ($p < 0.05$, respectively). As shown in Fig. 2, $OKT9^+$ cells tended to decrease along with an increase of $1,25(OH)_2D_3$ concentration and significantly decreased at 10^{-7}M $1,25(OH)_2D_3$ ($p < 0.05$). Stimulation index was significantly increased by 10^{-12}M ($p < 0.01$) and 10^{-11}-10^{-8}M ($p < 0.05$, respectively) $1,25(OH)_2D_3$, when PHA was used as a mitogen. It was significantly increased by 10^{-12}, 10^{-11} and 10^{-9}M $1,25(OH)_2D_3$ ($p < 0.05$, respec-

Vitamin D. A Chemical, Biochemical and Clinical Update

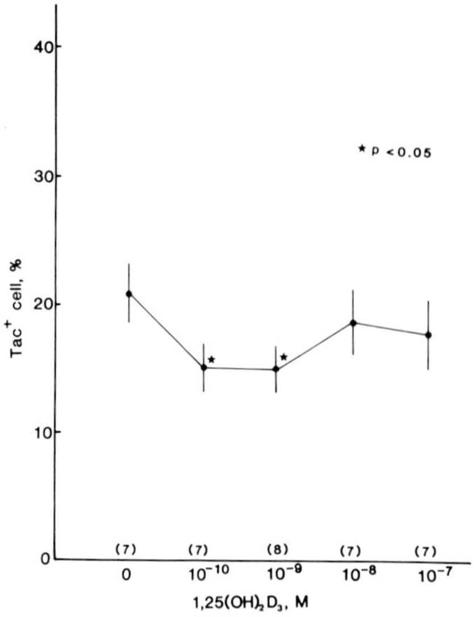

Fig. 1. Effect of $1,25(OH)_2D_3$ on human PHA-induced Tac^+ cells *in vitro*.

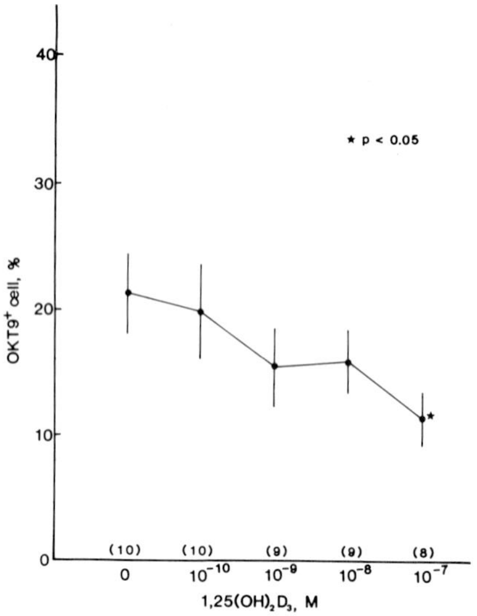

Fig. 2. Effect of $1,25(OH)_2D_3$ on human PHA-induced $OKT9^+$ cells *in vitro*.

tively) when Con A was used. 10^{-12}, 10^{-11} and 10^{-9}M $1,25(OH)_2D_3$ also significantly increased stimulation index ($p < 0.05$, respectively) when PWM was used. $24,25(OH)_2D_3$, $25\text{-}OHD_3$ and $1\alpha\text{-}OHD_3$ caused no significant alterations in stimulation index.

Discussion

Our results that $1,25(OH)_2D_3$ significantly decreased interleukin 2 receptor and transferrin receptor in human peripheral mononuclear cells *in vitro*, suggest that $1,25(OH)_2D_3$ influences on the induction of interleukin 2 receptor and transferrin receptor. Neckers et al. (1) reported that the presence of interleukin 2 receptor was necessary for transferrin receptor induction and subsequent initiation of DNA synthesis and cell division. Tsoukas et al. (2) reported that $1,25(OH)_2D_3$ decreased interleukin 2 production *in vitro*. Our data that $1,25(OH)_2D_3$ significantly increased lymphocyte blasttransformation, do not necessarily coincide with a decrease of transferrin receptor, in view that they alterate almost in a parallel fashion. Further investigation including the changes in incubation time of the cells with vitamin D metabolites, is needed in order to elucidate the mechanisms of actions of $1,25(OH)_2D_3$ on immune function.

References

1. Neckers, L. M. and Cossman, J. (1983) Proc. Natl. Acad. Sci. USA 80, 3494-3498.
2. Tsoukas, C. D., Provvedini, D. M. and Manolagas, S. C. (1984) Science 224, 1438-1439.

VITAMIN D_3 AND $25(OH)D_3$ METABOLISM IN THE MUSSEL M. EDULIS

I. Lehtovaara and T. Koskinen. University of Tampere, Department of Clinical Sciences, P.O. Box 607, SF-33520 Tampere, Finland

While the metabolism of vitamin D_3 is well documented in mammals and avian species, very little is known about the occurrence of corresponding reactions in nonvertebrates. There are several species of nonvertebrates which may obtain vitamin D_3 from their diet or synthetize it from endogenous 7-dehydrocholesterol. Of special interest is the question whether they, especially those with shells or other calcified tissues, can metabolize or utilize it. In the present study we investigated the existence of metabolic pathways for vitamin D_3 and $25(OH)D_3$ in the common mussel, Mytilus edulis.

Materials and methods

M. eduli were collected near Blåbergsholm, The Baltic Sea, and maintained in our laboratory in sea water at +4°C. 40 % (w/v) homogenates of M. edulis tissue (without shells and feet) were prepared in 15 mM Tris-acetate buffer, pH 7.7, containing 190 mM sucrose and 1.9 mM magnesium acetate. Into incubation flasks were pipetted 2 ml of homogenate, 1 ml of cocactor solution (25 mM sodium succinate, 7.5 mM glucose-6-phosphate, 1.5 mM NADP and 0.5 unit glucose-6-phosphate dehydrogenase in Tris buffer), and the purified substrate, (^3H)vitamin D_3 or (^3H)$25(OH)D_3$, was added. After a 3-h incubation at +25°C with shaking, lipids were extracted with dichloromethane followed by analysis of the residues by Sephadex LH-20 chromatography and HPLC.

Results

From control incubations, which were stopped immediately, only unreacted substrates were recovered. During the three-hour incubation, both vitamin D_3 and $25(OH)D_3$ were converted to polar metabolites (Figures 1 and 2).

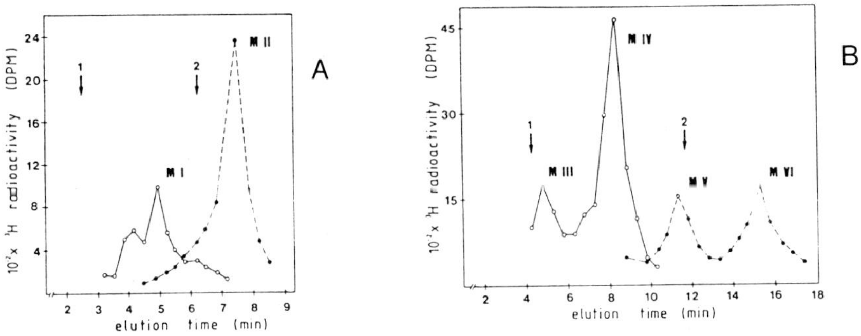

Fig. 1. HPLC analysis of (^3H)vitamin D_3 metabolism. A) Zorbax-Sil eluted with hexane-isopropanol (96:4); 1 = vitamin D_3, 2 = $25(OH)D_3$. B) same column, hexane-isopropanol (90:10); 1 = $24,25(OH)_2D_3$, 2 = $1,25(OH)_2D_3$.

Vitamin D. A Chemical, Biochemical and Clinical Update

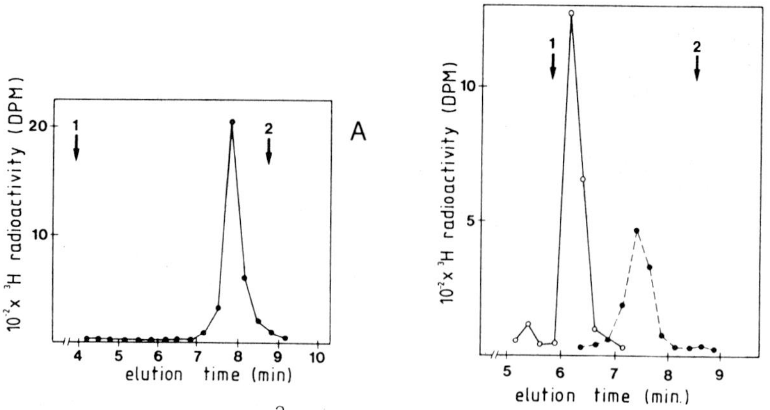

Fig. 2. HPLC analysis of (^{3}H)25(OH)D_3 metabolism. A) Zorbax-Sil, hexane-isopropanol (94:6); 1 = 25(OH)D_3, 2 = 24,25$(OH)_2D_3$. B) Zorbax-CN, hexane-isopropanol-methanol (96:8:1); 1 = 24,25$(OH)_2D_3$, 2 = 1,25$(OH)_2D_3$.

The present work demonstrates that mussels are capable of vitamin D_3 and 25(OH)D_3 metabolism. For the mussel metabolites we observed chromatographic properties different from those of known standards (Figs. 1 and 2), and accordingly, we conclude that the reaction pathways present in M. edulis are not similar to the well-known vertebrate systems. As no 25(OH)D_3 was formed from vitamin D_3 nor 1,25$(OH)_2D_3$ from 25(OH)D_3, the observed reactions may not represent an activation of the molecule.

Early studies on vitamin D_3 already suggested its possible significance to a group of nonvertebrates, land snails (1,2). Later on it was demonstrated that land snails convert (^{3}H)vitamin D_3 and (^{3}H)25(OH)D_3 into unknown polar products (3). In one study (4), vitamin D_3 metabolism occurred in the sea urchin. Our results thus confirm earlier findings about vitamin D_3 metabolism in nonvertebrates. The necessity of vitamin D_3 to M. edulis cannot be proved by the present work, but it is likely that mussels obtain small amounts of vitamin D_3 from the food chain and metabolize it even in vivo.

This study was supported by The Magnus Ehrnrooth Foundation.

References

1. Howes, N.H. (1937) Biochem. J. 8, 187
2. Wagge, L.E. (1952) J. Exp. Zool. 120, 311-342.
3. Weiner, S., Noff, D., Meyer, M.S., Weisman, Y. and Edelstein, S.(1979) Biochem. J. 184, 157-161.
4. Hobbs, R.N. and Pennock, J.F. (1977) Biochem. Soc. Trans. 5, 1713-1714.

Chemistry of Vitamin D Seco-Steroids

SYNTHESIS OF 24R,25-DIHYDROXYCHOLECALCIFEROL. A STEREOSELECTIVE SYNTHESIS OF 24R,25-DIHYDROXYCHOLESTEROL.

A. Fürst, L. Labler and W. Meier
Pharmaceutical Research Department, F. Hoffmann-La Roche & Co., Ltd., 4002 Basle, Switzerland

Since its discovery [1] and structural elucidation [2] 24R,25-dihydroxyvitamin D_3 (1) has become of increasing biologic importance [3]. This motivated us to look for efficient methods of synthesis. The abundant plant sterol stigmasterol (2) is an attractive starting material for large scale preparations of vitamin D metabolites. It is readily transformed by a 5-step sequence in almost 60% yield into the 3,5-cyclo-20-methylpregnane-21-tosylate 3 [4] already chosen by Roche chemists as a building block in the synthesis of precursors such as 25-hydroxycholesterol [4,5], 24R,25- [6,7], 25S,26- [8] as well as 23S,25-dihydroxycholesterol [9]. We have now used the same building block 3 for a novel stereoselective synthesis of 24R,25-dihydroxycholesterol (4) which was then converted to the title compound 1.

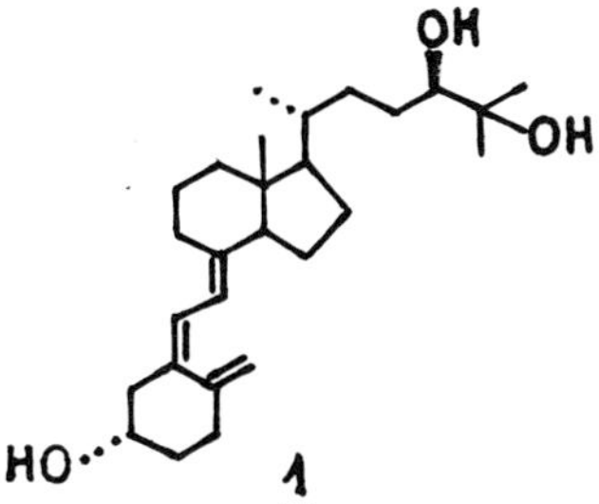

1

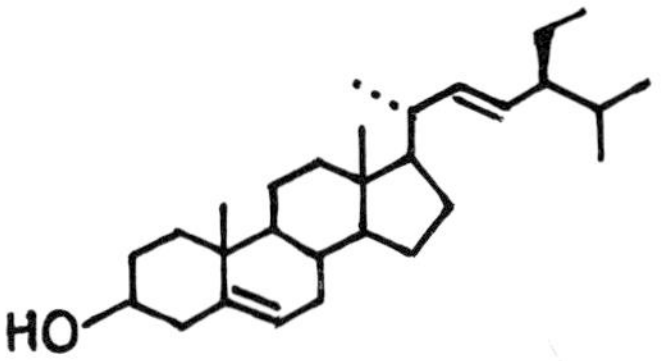

2

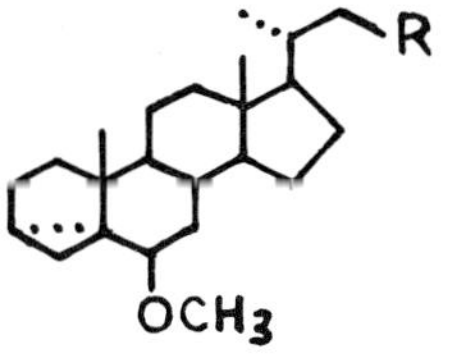

3 R = OTS

7 R = I

8 R = 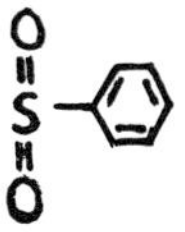 = SO_2Ph

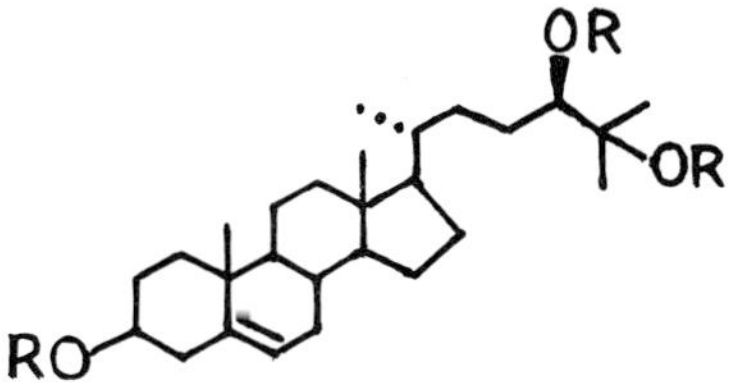

4 R = H

5 R = Ac

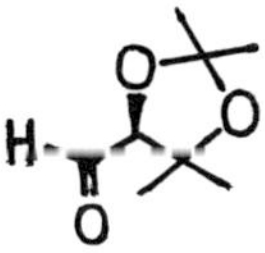

6

TS = 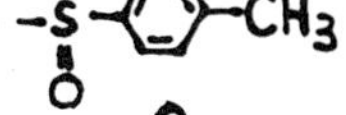

Ac = 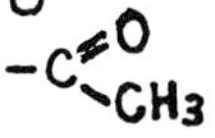

Vitamin D. A Chemical, Biochemical and Clinical Update

The key step of this synthesis is the combining of the C-21 phenyl sulfone 8 [10] with ß,ß-dimethyl-S-glyceraldehyde acetonide (6) which introduces the 24R chirality of the end product.

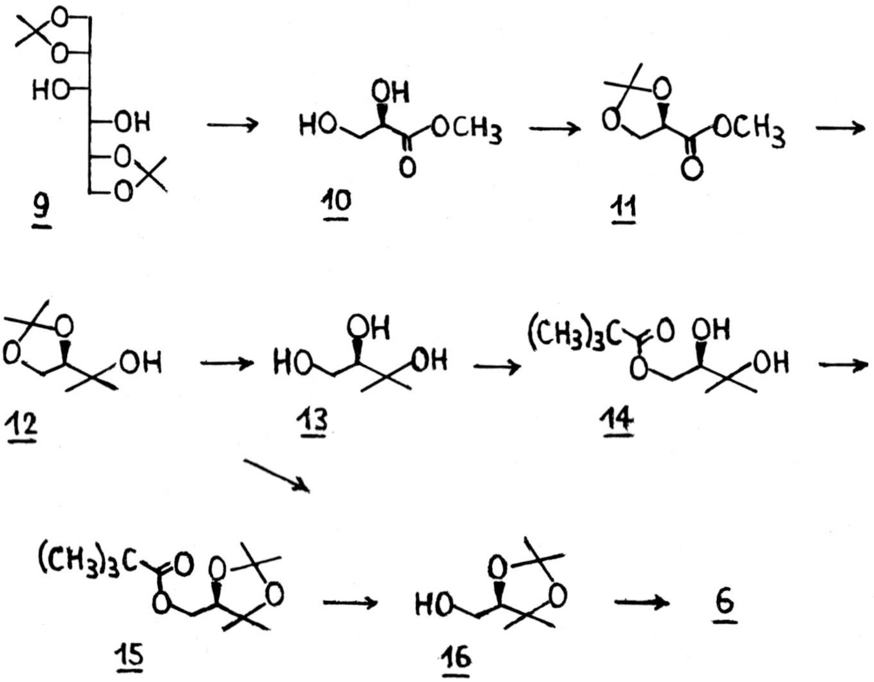

The phenyl sulfone 8 was obtained from the 21-tosylate 3 in 65% yield via the iodide 7 [4] using essentially the conditions described recently [10]. For preparation of the aldehyde 6 the inexpensive D-mannitol diacetonide 9 was converted according to [11,12] to R-glyceric acid methylester (10) which upon acetalization furnished the derivative 11 in 31% overall yield from 9. Reaction with methylmagnesium bromide as recently published [13] transformed the derivative 11 into the tert. carbinol 12 (83% yield). Acidic treatment of this product and reaction of the triol 13 [14] formed with one equiv. of pivaloyl chloride in pyridine led to the ester 14 (72% yield). Subsequent acetalization to compound 15 followed by alkaline hydrolysis furnished the alcohol 16 (82% yield) which was then oxidized to the target aldehyde 6 using pyridinium chlorochromate in methylene chloride (50% yield). As shown in the racemic series the tert. carbinol 12 on standing in acetone under acidic catalysis equilibrates to a 1:1 mixture of the compounds 12 and 16 separable by distillation, thus offering a shorter access to the alcohol 16.

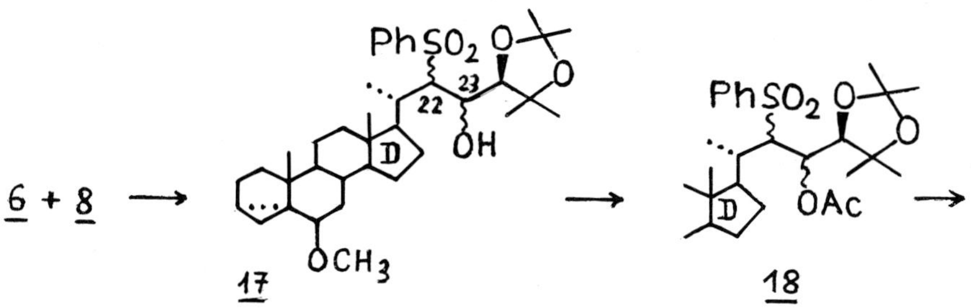

17 18

a 22R 23R b 22S 23R
c 22S 23S d 22R 23S

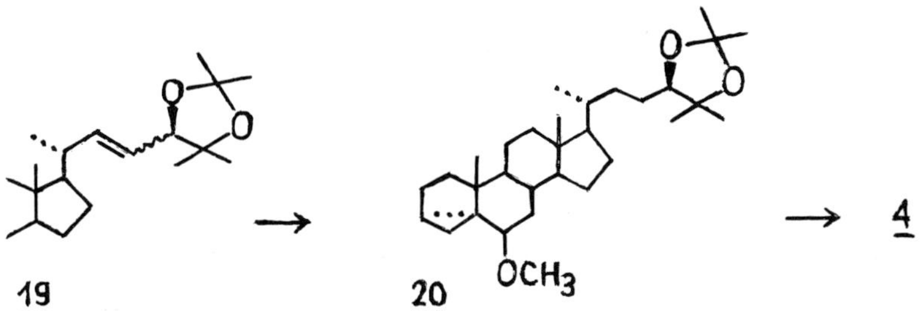

19 20

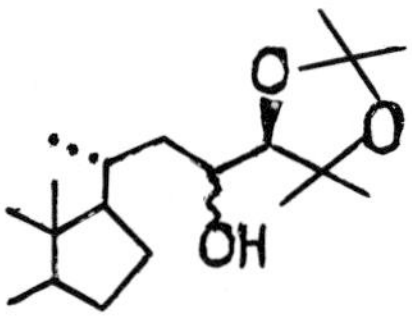

21 23R
22 23S

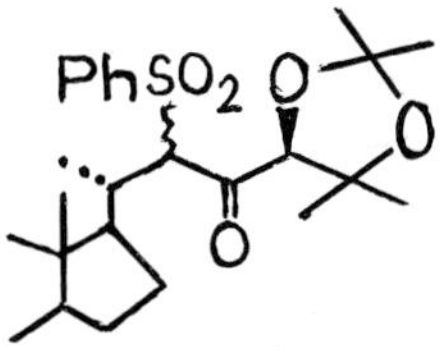

23 22R
24 22S

Connection of the building blocks 8 and 6 was achieved by reaction of the magnesium bromide derivative [15] of the sulfone with 1.2 equiv. of the aldehyde in benzene to give the mixture of diastereoisomers 17 in 67% yield along with ca. 30% of the starting sulfone. All four possible diastereoisomers were found in the mixture 17. Upon direct separation the isomer 17a was shown by X-ray analysis to possess the 22R,23R configuration. The three other components 17b, 17c and 17d were obtained by alkaline hydrolysis of the corresponding pure acetates isolated from the mixture of the acetates 18. This was prepared by heating the mixture 17 with acetic anhydride-triethyl amine in presence of p-dimethylaminopyridine. Their structures indicated in the scheme were deduced from that of the isomer 17a. The C-23 assignments resulted from reductions with lithium in ammonia yielding the 23R alcohol 21 from the compounds 17a (23R) and 17b, the 23S alcohol 22 from the two other isomers. The C-22 assignments followed from oxidations with pyridinium dichromate in dimethylformamide in which remarkable differences in velocity were observed due to distinct sterical hindrance. The compounds 17a (22R) and 17d yielded the 22R ketosulfone 23, the two other isomers the 22S epimer 24. Under the conditions used only slow and negligible epimerization of the ketosulfones occurred. An X-ray analysis of the acetyl derivative of the isomer 17b gave additional evidence for the structural assignments made. The product ratio of the components 17a, 17b, 17c, 17d formed in the key step proved to be approximately 1.5:1:3.6:2.5.

The mixture of the acetates 18 was treated with sodium amalgam in methanol-ethyl acetate to give the olefin 19 as the *trans*/*cis* 3:1 mixture in 66% yield. When subjected individually to this reductive elimination the highest *trans*/*cis* ratio (7:1) was monitored with the acetate of the isomer 17b and the lowest (11:9) with that of the isomer 17d. This preferred formation of the *trans* olefin accords with published work [16].

Hydrogenation over Raney nickel catalyst in ethanol converted the mixture of olefins 19 to the saturated steroid 20 which upon acidic treatment underwent retro-i-rearrangement and acetal cleavage to furnish 24R,25-dihydroxycholesterol (4) [7,17,18] in 88% yield. Acetylation of the product to the triacetyl derivative 5 revealed the presence of less than 1% of the 24S diastereoisomer. This was isolated from mother liquors. The stereoselective construction of the 24R,25-dihydroxycholesterol side chain described here represents an alternative to that recently reported by Japanese workers [19]. They connected a C-21 sulfone with the primary tosylate of the triol 13.

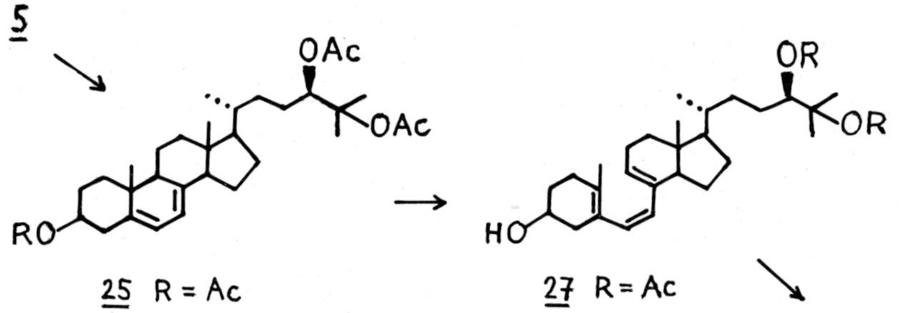

25 R = Ac
26 R = H

27 R = Ac
28 R = H

The transformation into the title metabolite 1 was accomplished in the classical manner using the triacetyl derivative 5 as starting substrate. Usual allylic bromination with N-bromosuccinimide in hexane and subsequent heating with s-collidine in xylene yielded a mixture consisting essentially of the 5,7-diene 25 and the isomeric 4,6-diene as a byproduct from which the desired compound 25 was isolated in 49% yield. Partial saponification of this with one equiv. of potassium hydroxide in methanol-tetrahydrofuran gave the 3-hydroxy 24R,25-diacetate 26 (78% yield) which was irradiated in dioxane to 50% conversion. The precholecalciferol derivative 27 isolated, upon deacetylation with lithium aluminium hydride in tetrahydrofuran, furnished the triol 28 which was then thermally isomerized to give 24R,25-dihydroxycholecalciferol (1) [17,20] in 52% yield related to reacted 5,7-diene 26.

REFERENCES

[1] Holick, M.F., Schnoes, H.K., DeLuca, H.F., Gray, R.W., Boyle, T.T. and Suda, T. (1972) Biochemistry 11, 4251-4255.

[2] Tanaka, Y. DeLuca, H.F., Ikekawa, N., Morisaki, M. and Koizumi, N. (1975) Arch. Biochem. Biophys. 170, 620 626. Partridge, J.J., Baggiolini, E.G., Mahgoub, A., Shiuey, S.-J. and Uskoković, M.R. (1975) Abstr. of the 169th Meeting of Amer. Chem. Soc., Philadelphia, Pa, April 6-11, MEDI 36.

[3] Norman, A.W., Roth, J. and Orci, L. (1982) Endocrine Reviews 3, 331-366.

[4] Partridge, J.J., Faber, S. and Uskoković, M.R. (1974) Helv. Chim. Acta 57, 764-771.

[5] Fürst, A., Labler, L. and Meier, W. (1982) Helv. Chim. Acta 65, 1499-1521.
[6] Uskoković, M.R., Partridge, J.J., Narwid, T.A. and Baggiolini E.G. (1980) Vitamin D: Molecular Biology and Clinical Nutrition, ed. A.W. Norman, Marcel Dekker Inc., New York and Basel, 1-57.
[7] Partridge, J.J., Toome, V. and Uskoković, M.R. (1976) J. Amer. Chem. Soc. 98, 3739-3740.
[8] Barner, R., Hübscher, J., Daly, J.J. and Schönholzer, P. (1981) Helv. Chim. Acta 64, 915-938.
[9] Partridge, J.J., Chadha, N.K., Shiuey, S.-J., Wovkulich, P.M., Uskoković, M.R., Napoli, J.L. and Horst, R.L. (1982) Vitamin D, Chemical, Biochemical and Clinical Endocrinology of Calcium Metabolism, Walter de Gruyter & Co., Berlin-New York, 1073-1078.
[10] Koch, P., Nakatani, Y., Luu, B. and Ourisson, G. (1983) Bull. Soc. Chim. France II, 189-194.
[11] Baer, E., Grosheintz, J.M. and Fischer, H.O.L. (1939) J. Amer. Chem. Soc. 61, 2607-2609.
[12] Wulff, G., Sarhan, A., Gimpel, J. and Lohmar, E. (1974) Chem. Ber. 107, 3364-3367.
[13] Dumont, R. and Pfander, H. (1983) Helv. Chim. Acta 66, 814-823.
[14] Nielsen, B.E., Larsen, P.K. and Lemmich, J. (1969) Acta. Chim. Scand. 23, 967-970.
[15] Kocienski, P.J., Lythgoe, B. and Ruston, S. (1978) J. Chem. Soc. Perkin I, 829-834.
[16] Kocienski, P.J., Lythgoe, B. and Waterhouse, I. (1980) J. Chem. Soc. Perkin I, 1045-1050.
[17] Seki, M., Koizumi, N., Morisaki, M. and Ikekawa, N. (1975) Tetrahedron Letters, 15-18.
[18] Koizumi, N., Ishiguro, M., Yasuda, M. and Ikekawa, N. (1983) J. Chem. Soc. Perkin I, 1401-1410.
[19] Takayama, H., Ohmori, M. and Yamada, S. (1980) Tetrahedron Letters 21, 5027-5028.
[20] Redel, J., Bazely, M., Delbarre, F. and Calando, Y. (1976) Compt. Rend. Acad. Sc. Paris, t. 283, Série D, 857-860.

SYNTHESIS OF SELECTED VITAMIN D_3-METABOLITES.

M. VANDEWALLE, P.J. DE CLERCQ+, L. VANMAELE, J. VAN DER EYCKEN, N.A. RABI, L. VAN WABEEKE,
State University of Ghent, Department of Organic Chemistry, Laboratory for Organic Synthesis, Krijgslaan, 281 (S. 4), B-9000 Gent (Belgium)

S.J. HALKES, W.R.M. OVERBEEK,
Duphar BV, P.O. Box 2, 1380 AA Weesp (Holland)

I. SYNTHESIS OF 1α,25-DIHYDROXY VITAMIN D_3

1α,25-Dihydroxy vitamin D_3 1a is considered as the most important and active natural metabolite of vitamin D_3 (1). Recently we have described a novel synthesis (2) of the 1α-hydroxy vitamin D_3 analogue 1b, via a route essentially based on the C-1 functionalization of a previtamin D_3 derivative. We now report the application of this general plan to the synthesis of the title compound (3).

Our strategy is based on structural properties of the previtamin triene system; it has been shown that the 6,8-diene exists as a s-cis diene with the 5,10 double bond diverging from that plane (4). Therefore a selective reaction of a dienophile on the 6,8-diene could be anticipated. This would leave the cyclohexene ring A untouched, an ideal situation for selective introduction of the requisite 1α-hydroxyl function. Finally, concerted cycloreversion and subsequent thermal isomerization should lead to a 1α-hydroxylated vitamin D_3.

Treatment of crude 25-hydroxy previtamin D_3 2c (obtained upon low temperature irradiation of 25-hydroxy-7-dehydrocholesterol with a high-pressure Hg-lamp) (5) with phenyl-1,2,4-tri-

Vitamin D. A Chemical, Biochemical and Clinical Update

azoline-3,5-dione in CH_2Cl_2 (0°C, N_2, 2 min) led with complete regio- and stereoselectivity (α-attack) to the adduct 3 in 49 % yield, calculated on consumed 25-hydroxy-7-dehydrocholesterol. After selective protection of the 3-hydroxyl function as the tert-butyldimethylsilyl ether (4; 92 % yield), allylic bromination with 1,3-dibromo-5,5-dimethylhydantoin in hexane-CH_2Cl_2 (collidine, AIBN, 20 min reflux) led with high regioselectivity to the diastereoisomeric bromides at C-1 (crude yield > 80 %). Immediate oxidation of the allylic bromides with bis-tetrabutyl-ammoniumdichromate (6) in $CHCl_3$ (reflux, 3 h) led to enone 5 in 56 % overall yield (from 4) after column chromatography on silica gel. This two-step C-1 functionalization is a modification superior to the three-step procedure previously described (2), for the synthesis of the 1α-hydroxy vitamin D_3 analogue 1b.

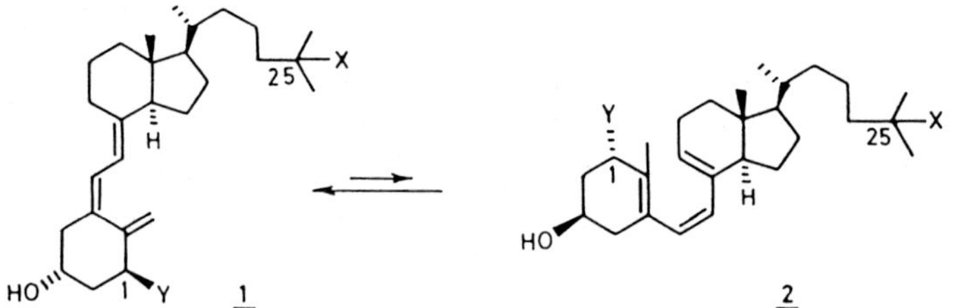

1 2

a X = OH ; Y = OH
b X = H ; Y = OH
c X = OH ; Y = H

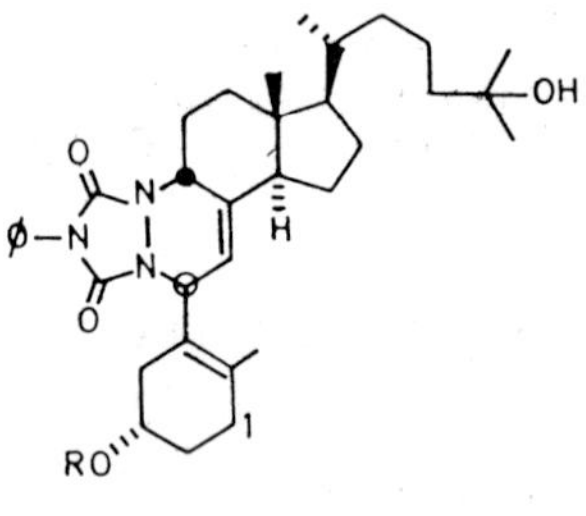

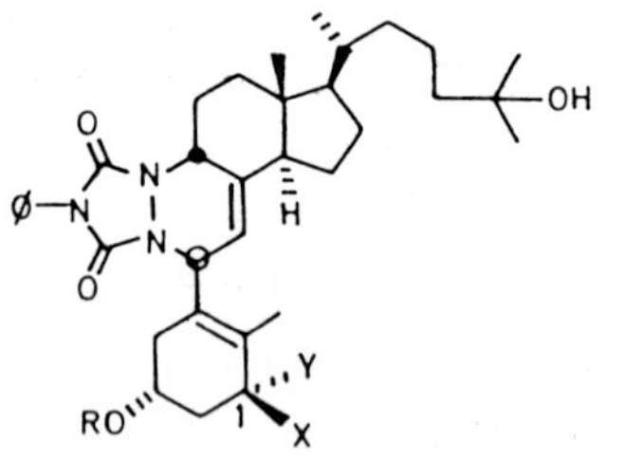

3 R = H
4 R = Si(t-Bu)Me_2

5 R = Si(t-Bu)Me_2; X,Y = O
6 R = H; X,Y = O
7 R = H; X = OH; Y = H

After cleavage of the silyl ether in 5 (n-butyric acid, $(n.Bu)_4NF$, THF, 2 h, 20°C; 84 % yield), the reduction of 6 with aluminumhydride in THF at -70°C afforded with high stereoselectivity the triol 7 (yield 87 % after HPLC purification). The stereochemical result is rationalized by an intramolecular hydride transfer after reaction of the reducing agent with the 3-hydroxyl group. Deprotection of the 6,8-diene system upon refluxing 7 at 85°C in carefully degassed methanol - 15 N KOH under Ar for 70 h afforded after HPLC purification 1(S),25-dihydroxy vitamin D_3 (1a) next to 1(S),25-dihydroxy previtamin D_3 (2a) in a 5.7:1 ratio (61 % yield). The mechanism of this cycloreversion step is discussed in more detail in section II (vide infra).

Heating of 2a for 2 h at 70°C in order to establish equilibration gave 1a which after crystallization from benzene-ethyl acetate (m.p. 95-96°C) showed spectral properties in accord with previous reports (7). The overall yield of crystalline 1a starting from the adduct 3 is 20 %.

II. 1α-HYDROXY PREVITAMIN D_3 AND ITS SELECTIVE FORMATION OF 1-KETO PREVITAMIN D_3

Little attention has been devoted so far to practical syntheses of 1α-hydroxylated previtamin D_3 (2b), the fundamentally important minor isomer in the natural equilibrium vitamin D $\rightleftarrows$ previtamin D (20 % previtamin at 36°C). Among the existing methods leading to 1α-hydroxy vitamin D_3, only the classical photochemical-thermal isomerization of 1α-hydroxy provitamin D_3 provides a direct access to 1α-hydroxy previtamin D_3 (7).

We presently want to describe a modification of our previously described synthesis of 1b which leads conveniently to crystalline 1α-hydroxy previtamin D_3 2b (8). The one-pot generation of the vitamin triene system, i.e. 7 → 1a (vide supra; section I) or 10 → 1b (scheme 2) (2), almost necessarily has to involve four discrete transformations : (a) saponification to the cyclic hydrazine 11; (b) oxidation to the elusive unsaturated azo derivative (9); (c) facile stereospecific cycloreversion to the original previtamin skeleton 2; (d) thermal isomerization to 1b under the conditions used. In view of this scheme, however, the direct obtention of 1b merely implies that either the oxidation step (b) occurs in spite of the "inert" atmosphere or that another pathway is in fact involved (9,10). If the above cited sequence is operative it is obvious that when the reaction at higher temperature can be stopped at the stage of 11, subsequent low temperature oxidation would lead exclusively to 1α-hydroxy previtamin D_3 2b. Reinvestigation of the reaction conditions carried out as a model study, on 8, has revealed that indeed traces of oxygen were present.

We have now found that when the hydrolysis is carried out under enforced oxygen-free conditions (vigorous reflux in carefully degassed 15 N KOH-MeOH, under fast Ar flow) the hydrazine 12 is indeed an intermediate which can be detected after rapid work-up. The highly air sensitive 12 was difficult to isolate; it was characterized as the dibenzoyl derivative 13.

Consequently, treatment of 10 (as described for 8) followed by aerial oxidation of crude 11 (diethyl ether, air flow, 0°C) leads after recrystallization (diethyl ether) to 2b in 74 % yield (m.p. 120-122°C). To the best of our knowledge this is the first time a non-derivated previtamin D_3 has been obtained in crystalline form.

One important reason for having good access to 1α-hydroxy previtamin D_3 2b is related to the observation of Mazur et al. (11) indicating that of the two isomers 1b and 2b the latter is the better substrate for allylic oxidation (11,12) to 1-keto previtamin D_3 15. The reduction of 15 has been reported to yield predominantly (vide infra) 1β-hydroxy vitamin D_3 (after thermal isomerization), which is a serious drawback with regard to eventual preparation of radiolabelled 1α-hydroxy vitamin D_3.

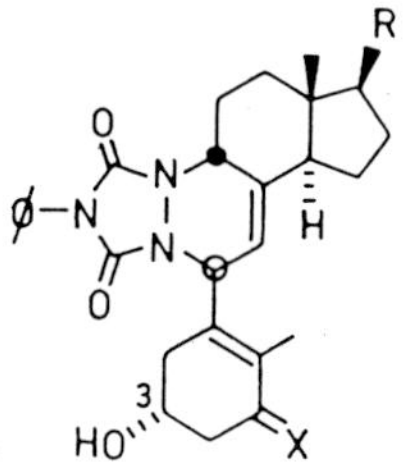

8 X = H
9 X = O
10 X = H, OH

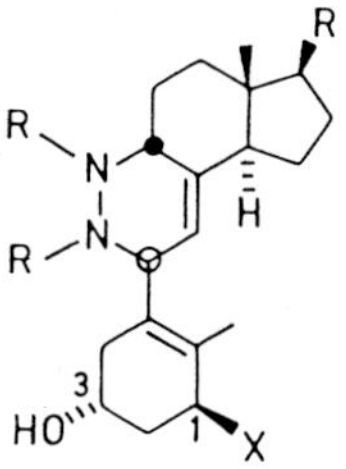

11 R = H; X = OH
12 R = H; X = H
13 R = COϕ; X = H

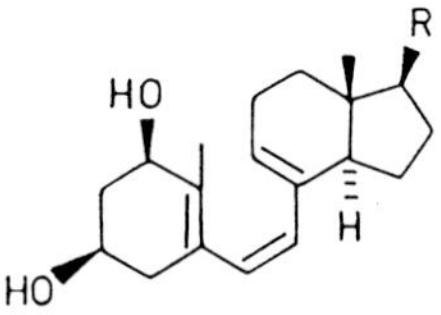

14

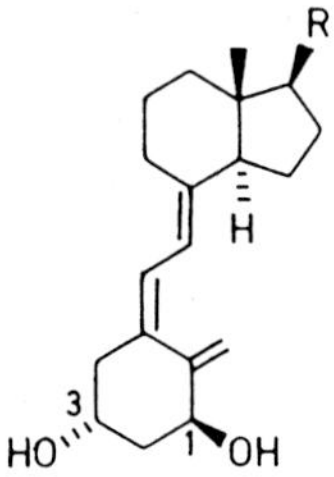

1b

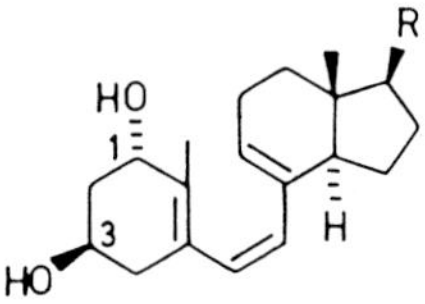

2b

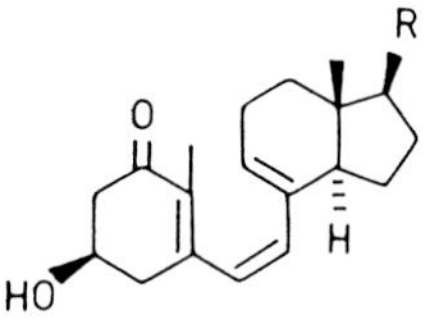

15

R = 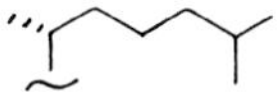

Oxidation of 2b (commercial MnO_2 in diethyl ether, Argon, ultrasonic bath) gave (67 %) 1-keto previtamin 15. With 15 in hand we investigated the possibility for the stereoselective reduction to 2b using internal hydride delivery which proved successful in the transformation of 6 to 7 and 9 to 10 (2). Treatment of 15 with aluminum hydride (prepared in situ) in THF at -60°C yielded a mixture of 2b and 14 (ratio 4:1; 91 % total yield) from which 2b was obtained in 72 % yield by preparative HPLC (Waters Model : 6000 A Solvent Delivery System HPLC; hexane/aceton; 9:1). This stands in contrast with previously described results which have shown the opposite stereoselectivity; a comparison is given in the table.

TABLE : Observed stereoselectivity upon reduction of 15

Reagent	2b (1α-OH)	14 (1β-OH)	Yield %	Ref.
$NaBH_4$, CH_3OH, 0°C	0	1	70	(11)
$LiAlH_4$, ether, 0°C	1	2.8	60	(11)
$LiAlH_4$[x], ether, -20°C	1	4	100	(12)
AlH_3, THF, -60°C	4	1	91	

[x] inverse addition

Thus, when aluminum hydride is the reducing agent, faster interaction between the 3-hydroxyl group and the aluminum atom assures internal hydride introduction at C-1.

Because of the obvious advantage of introducing the label in the last step in the synthesis of a radioactive compound our result offers the possibility for a suitable preparation of 1β-tritium labelled 1α-hydroxylated vitamin D_3.

III. AN APPROACH TO 24(R),25-DIHYDROXYCHOLESTEROL

Some preliminary results of our study for stereocontrol at C-24 via relative asymmetric induction from the C-20 chiral center are presented. Our strategy is based on the potential of a carboxyl group to direct epoxidation of an olefin via the iodolactonization process. Stereoselective alkylation of the known ester 16 is well documented (13); accordingly trapping of the enolate anion (LiCa, THF, HMPA, -78°) gave 17 as the only isomer. Ester cleavage was affected with MeSLi in HMPA (86 %) (14). No epimerization at C-20 was observed as was proven by esterification (CH_2N_2) of 18 back to solely 17.

Bartlett (15) has demonstrated that using I_2 in MeCN, the thermodynamically favored iodolactone is formed with excellent selectivity. Unfortunately this procedure failed on 18 : possibly this is due to the tri-substituted nature of the 24,25 double bond as all high yield examples reported (15) involve terminal double bonds. Therefore iodolactonization was carried out in basic medium ($NaHCO_3$; Kl, I_2, CH_2Cl_2-H_2O; 65 %); indeed low selectivity was observed as 19 and 20 were formed in a 2:1 ratio. At this stage the structures were tentatively assigned. As DBU mediated elimination of both 19 and 20 led to 21, epimerization at C-20, on the lactone stage, can be excluded.

Despite the low stereoselectivity some subsequent classical transformations have been investigated. Treatment of 19 with sodium carbonate in MeOH (15) led to 22 which upon epoxide ring opening (5 % $HClO_4$, THF, H_2O)(16) gave only one diol ester 23. On the other hand dibah reduction of 19 to 24 and subsequent treatment with $NaBH_4$ gave 25 (30 % overall). Substantial amounts of 26 arising from internal attack are formed during purification of 25 and during the subsequent tosylation to 27. Perchloric acid mediated epoxide opening gave 28. The same sequences have been carried out on the epimeric iodolactone 20.

Although this approach opens a route to the title compound 29, presently the low selectivity of the idolactonization makes it unefficient. Further work is in progress.

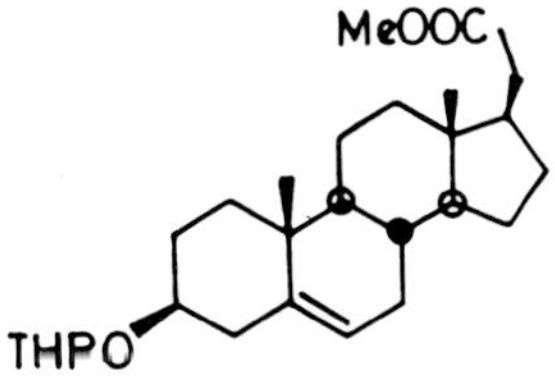

16

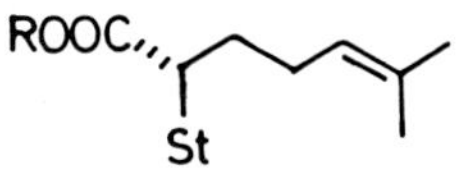

17 R = Me
18 R = H

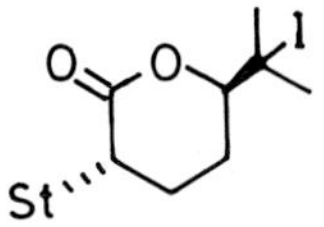

19 (24,R)

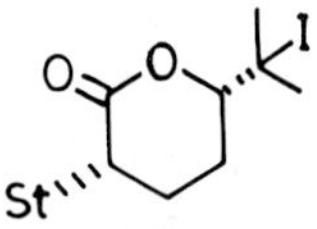

20 (24,S)

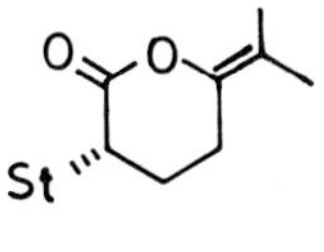

21

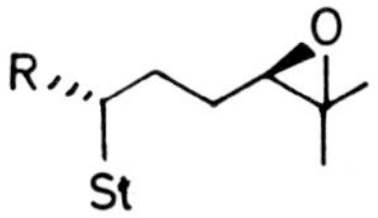

22 R=COOMe
25 R=CH_2OH
27 R=CH_2OTos

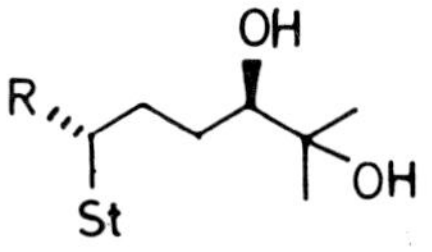

23 R=COOMe
28 R=CH_2OTos
29 R=CH_3

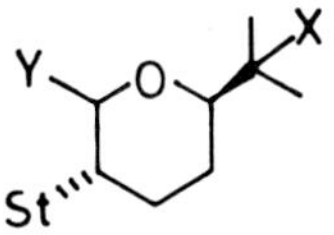

24 Y=OH, X = I
26 Y= H, X=OH

Acknowledgement - Financial support of the NFWO and the "Ministerie voor Wetenschapsbeleid" is gratefully acknowledged.

References

1. Vitamin D. Chemical, Biochemical and Clinical Endocrinology of Calcium Metabolism. Ed. A.W. Norman, K. Schaefer, D.v. Herrath and H.G. Grigoleit in W. De Gruyter Berlin - New York, 1982.
2. L.J. Vanmaele, P.J. De Clercq and M. Vandewalle (1982), Tetrahedron Lett., 995-998.
3. L.J. Vanmaele, P.J. De Clercq and M. Vandewalle,(1985), Tetrahedron, 41, 141-144.
4. (a) L. Velluz, G. Amiard and A. Petit (1949), Bull. Soc. Chim. Fr., 501-507; (b) J.L.M.A. Schlatmann, J. Pot, E. Havinga, (1964), Rec. Trav., 83, 1173-1184; (c) A. Verloop, A.L. Koevoet, E. Havinga, (1957), Rec. Trav. Chim. Pays-Bas, 76, 689-702.
5. S.J. Halkes and N.P. Van Vliet, (1969), Rec. Trav. Chim. Pays-Bas, 88, 1080-1083.
6. F. Rolla and D. Landini, (1979), Chem. & Ind., 213.
7. For other syntheses, see : (a) E.J. Semmler, M.F. Holick, H.K. Schnoes and H.F. DeLuca, (1972), Tetrah. Lett., 4147-4150; (b) D.H.R. Barton, R.H. Hesse, M.M. Pechet and E. Rizzardo, (1974), J.C.S. Chem. Comm., 203-204; (c) Z. Cohen, E. Keinan, Y. Mazur and A. Ulman, (1976), J. Org. C Chem., 41, 2651-2652; (d) T. Sato, H. Yamauchi, Y. Ogata, M. Tsujii, T. Kunii, K. Kagei, S. Toyoshima, T. Kobayashi, (1978), Chem. Pharm. Bull., 26, 2933-2940; (e) W.G. Dauben, R.B. Phillips and P. Jefferies, (1982), 79, 5115-5116.
8. L.J. Vanmaele, P.J. De Clercq, M. Vandewalle, S.J. Halkes and W.R.M. Overbeek, (1984), Tetrahedron, 40, 1179-1182.
9. This step is assumed in view of the much higher reactivity for cycloreversion of unsaturated azo compounds compared to the corresponding unsaturated hydrazo compounds; see : B.T. Gillis and P.E. Beck, (1963), J. Org. Chem., 28, 3177; J.A. Berson, S.S. Olin, E.W. Petrillo, Jr., P. Bickart, (1974), Tetrahedron, 30, 1639-1649.
10. W. Reischl, E. Zbiral, (1978), Liebigs Ann. Chem., 745-746; D.J. Aberhart, A. Chi-Tung Hsu, (1976), J. Org. Chem. 41, 2098-2102.
11. M. Sheves, N. Friedman, Y. Mazur, (1977), J. Org. Chem., 42, 3597-3599.
12. H.E. Paaren, H.K. Schnoes, H.F. DeLuca, (1977), J.C.S. Chem. Comm., 890-892.
13. J. Wicha and K. Ball, (1975), Chem. Comm., 968-970; J.J. Partride, S.J. Shiuey, N.K. Chadha, E.G. Baggiolini, J.F. Blount and M.R. Uskokovic, (1981), J. Am. Chem. Soc., 103, 1253-1255.
14. T.R. Kelly, H.M. Dali and W.G. Tsang, (1977), Tetrah. Lett., 3859-3860.
15. P.A. Bartlett and J. Myerson, (1978), J. Am. Chem. Soc., 100, 3950-3952.
16. C.H. Behrens, K.B. Sharpless, (1983), Aldrichimica Acta, 16, 67-79.

SYNTHESIS AND BIOLOGICAL ACTIVITY OF 1β-THIOVITAMIN D_3 AND 1β-THIO-25-HYDROXYVITAMIN D_3

Brian de Costa, Sally Ann Holick, and Michael F. Holick, Vitamin D Laboratory, Endocrine Unit, Massachusetts General Hospital, Harvard Medical School, Boston, MA, 02114 U.S.A.

1α,25-Dihydroxyvitamin D_3 (1,25-$(OH)_2$-D_3) has been established as the hormonally active form of vitamin D_3 (1). It is known that the 1α-hydroxy group is important in the binding of 1,25-$(OH)_2$-D_3 with its intestinal cytosolic receptor and in the expression of its calcium transport activity (2).

It has previously been shown that replacement of the 3β-OH group of vitamin D_3 with an -SH made the vitamin biologically inert (3). 1α-Fluorovitamin D_3 has been synthesized and shown to possess biological activity possibly as a result of 25-hydroxylation (4). However, 1α,25-difluoro vitamin D_3 was found to be biologically inert (5).

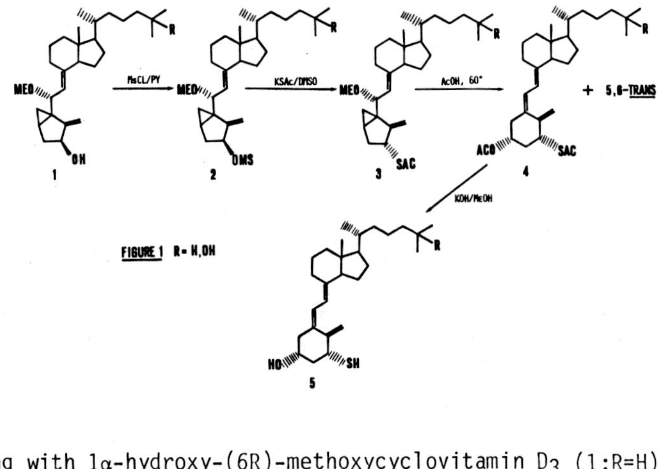

FIGURE 1 R= H,OH

Starting with 1α-hydroxy-(6R)-methoxycyclovitamin D_3 (1:R=H) (6) and 1α,25-dihydroxy-(6R)-methoxycyclovitamin D_3 (1:R=OH) (Fig. 1) (6), the sequence of mesylation (MsCL, pyridine 0°) followed by S_N2 displacement of the mesyloxy group with potassium thiolacetate (KSAc) in DMSO (10 min. at 20°C) gave 1β-thiolacetoxy-(6R)-methoxycyclovitamin D_3 (3:R=H) (48% yield from 1, R=H) and 1β-thiolacetoxy-25-hydroxycyclovit D_3 (3:R=H) (26% yield from 1:R=OH). It is interesting that neither 19-thiolacetoxy nor 1α-thiolacetoxy isomers of (3:R=H, OH) were formed.

Cycloreversion (6) of (3:R=H, OH) in acetic acid (55°, 15 min) gave the corresponding 1β-thiolacetoxyvitamin D_3-3-acetates (4:R=H,OH) which on careful hydrolysis (4%, KOH; MeOH at 20°C) and HPLC purification gave 1β-thiovitamin D_3 (5:R=H) and 1β-thio-25-hydroxyvitamin D_3 (5:R=OH).

Vitamin D. A Chemical, Biochemical and Clinical Update

Preliminary bioassays (7) on (5:R=H, OH) with vitamin D and calcium deficient rats indicated that they were biologically inactive in stimulating intestinal calcium transport and bone calcium mobilization. However, binding studies of (5:R = OH) using chick intestinal cytosolic receptor showed that it was capable of competing with 1,25-$(OH)_2$-D_3 (7). Because 1β-SH-25-(OH)-D_3 was about 5 times more effective than 25-OH-D in displacing 1,25-$(OH)_2$-D_3 from its receptors, it was evaluated in vitro in cultured human fibroblasts (8). Cells (2.5×10^5) in quadruplicate were exposed to one of the following for 7-days (a) 95% ETOH, (b) 1α,25-$(OH)_2$-D_3 (10^{-8}M), (c) 1β-SH-25-OH-D_3 (10^{-6}M), or (d) 1β,SH-25-OH-D_3 (10^{-6}M) for two days followed by 1α,25-$(OH)_2$-D_3 (10^{-8}M) + 1β-SH-25-OH-D_3 (10^{-6}M). After 7 days, the cells were recovered and counted. 1α,25-$(OH)_2$-D_3 increased by about 30% the cell generation time of the fibroblasts when compared to the control group. The cell generation time of the cells that received 1β-SH-25-OH-D_3 or 1β,SH-25-OH-D_3 with 1α,25-$(OH)_2$-D_3 were no different from the control group. These data suggest that 1β-SH-25-OH-D_3 completely antagonized the action of 1α,25-$(OH)_2$-D_3. If these preliminary data are confirmed, this would be the first synthetic analog of 1α,25-$(OH)_2$-D_3 that is a pure antagonist and could have wide ranging therapeutic application.

REFERENCES

1. DeLuca, H.F. and Schnoes, H.K. (1976) Annu. Rev. Biochem. 45, 631; Norman, A.W., Roth, J. and Orci, L. (1982) Endocrine Rev. 3, 331.
2. Norman, A.W. (1980) Vitamin D, Basic and Clinical Nutrition, Marcel Dekker, Inc. 2, 224-231; Franceschi, R.T., Simpson, R.U. and DeLuca, H.F. (1981) Arch. Biochem. Biophys. 210 1.
3. Bernstein, S. and Sax, K.L. (1951) J. Org. Chem. 16, 685.
4. Napoli, J.L., Fivizzani, M.A., Schnoes, H.K. and DeLuca H.F. (1979) Biochemistry 18, 1641.
5. Paaren, H.E., Fivizzani, Schnoes, H.K. and DeLuca, (1981) Arch. Biochem. Biophys. 209, 579.
6. These compounds were prepared by selenium dioxide oxidation of 3,5-cyclo-(6R)-methoxy-vitamin D_3 and 25-hydroxy-3,5-cyclo-(6R)-methoxy-vitamin D_3 by the procedure of H.E. Paaren, D.E. Hamer, H.K. Schnoes, and H.F. DeLuca (1978) Proc. Natl. Acad. Sci. USA 75, 2080.
7. Holick, M.F., Garabedian M. and DeLuca H.F. (1972) Biochemistry 11, 2715.
8. Clemens, T.L. Adams, J.S., Horiuchi, N., Gilchrest, B.A., Cho, H., Tsuchiya Y., Matsuo, N., Suda, T. and Holick, M.F. (1983) J. Clin. Endocrinol. Metab. 56, 824-830.
9. This work was supported in part by NIH grant AM32324.

STEREOSELECTIVE SYNTHESIS OF SELECTED VITAMIN D METABOLITES

Stephen R. Wilson, A. M. Venkatesan, Linda Jacob and M. Serajul Haque
Department of Chemistry, New York University, Washington Square,New York, NY 10003

Recently we have reported (1,2) our intramolecular Diels-Alder approach to the synthesis of vitamin D_2 (eq 1.)

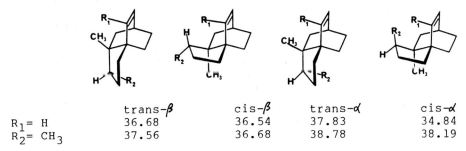

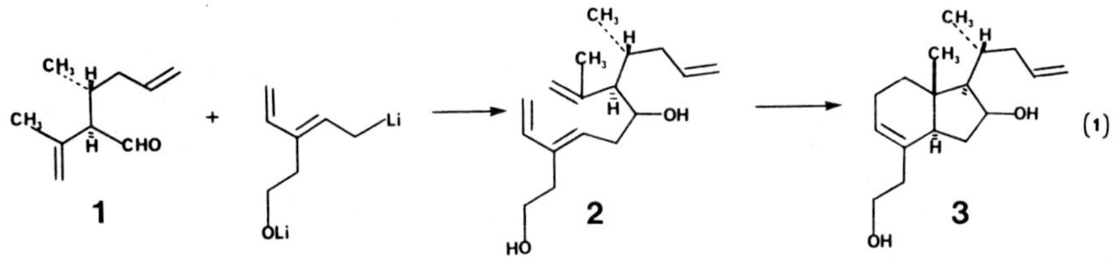

The key cyclization reaction **2** → **3** forms all the critical stereochemistry of the steroid C/D ring <u>and the side chain</u> in one step! In other words, one stereoisomer (out of four possible) is formed selectively in the Diels-Alder cyclization. We have extensively explored this cyclization reaction and the reasons for its selectivity. Figure 1 shows models for the four possible intramolecular Diels-Alder reaction transition states. We have carried out energy minimization calculations using Allinger's MM2 force-field(2) where both R_1 and R_2 = H or CH_3. The results show the relative energy differences of the four possible cyclization modes. Substituents are fortuitously needed exactly where they are required for the vitamin D series.

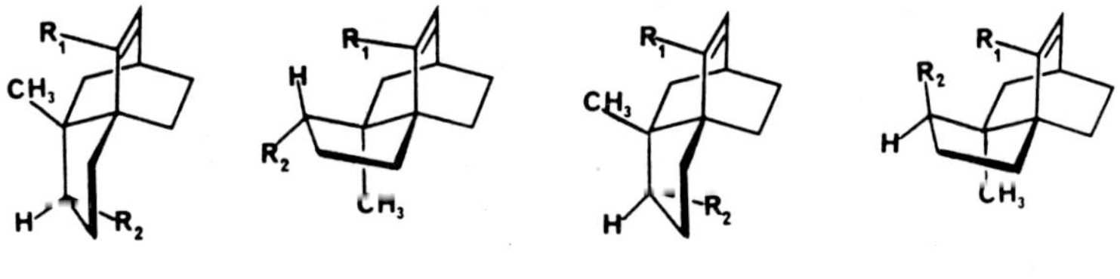

	trans-β	cis-β	trans-α	cis-α
R_1 = H	36.68	36.54	37.83	34.84
R_2 = CH_3	37.56	36.68	38.78	38.19

<u>Figure 1.</u> MM2 ENERGIES FOR INTRAMOLECULAR DIELS-ALDER TRANSITION STATE MODELS (KCAL/MOL)

Vitamin D. A Chemical, Biochemical and Clinical Update

Our overall strategy for the vitamins is based on our development of a one step diene construction using 3-substituted pentadienyl lithium reagents (eq 2.) We have been able to produce E-1,3-dienes by reaction of

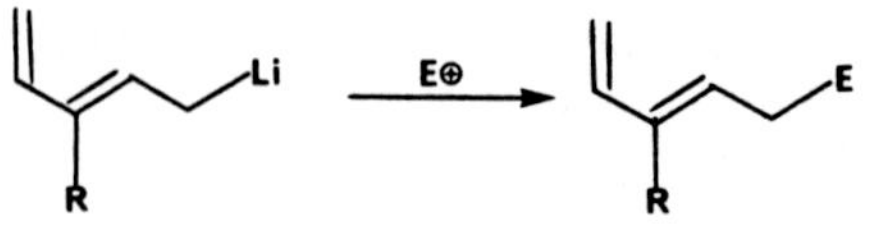

(2)

a wide variety of these reagents with suitable electrophiles (E+).

Thus the stage was set for a much more convergent approach to vitamin D and its metabolites. Our original synthesis involved the use side-chain synthon 1 (5) followed by construction of the steroid side chain. If we could synthesize the completely elaborated electrophilic "side-chain synthons" such as 4 or 5, they could be coupled to the diene precursur carrying the A-ring. Both "pieces" would have to be available in optically active form.

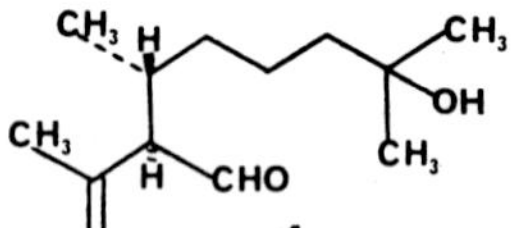

4

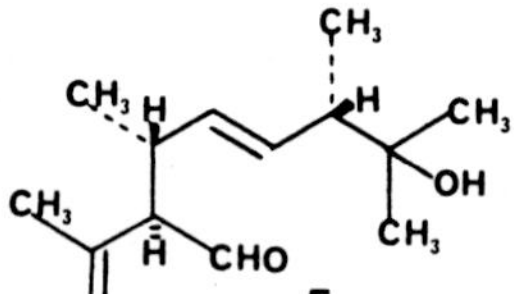

5

The side chains of the well known D2 and D3 metabolites which are hydroxylated at C-25 were logical synthetic targets. We began our synthesis of 4 by the stereospecific construction of key intermediate 6 via an ester enolate Claisen rearrangement (6).

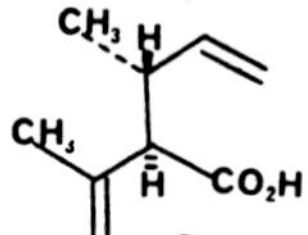

6

The acyclic stereocenter at the eventual C-17 and C-20 carbons are produced in the proper relative relationship because of the chair transition state in the Claisen rearrangement:

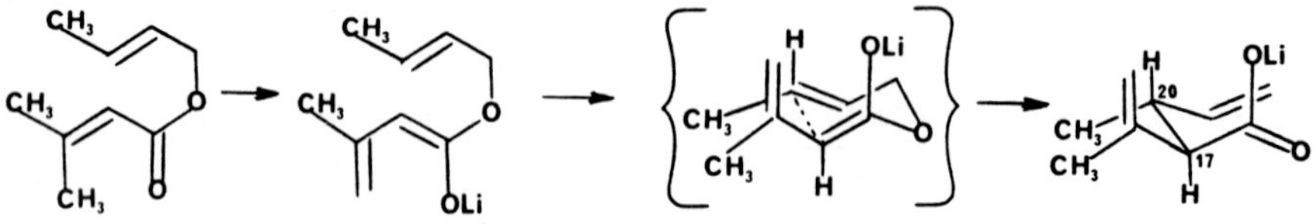

Acid 6 is formed in 95% yield and may be recrystallized to remove minor isomeric impurities. Resolution could be accomplished by formation (7) of its diastereomeric phenylglycinol

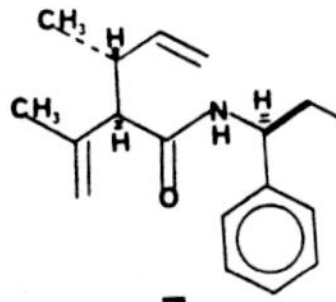
7

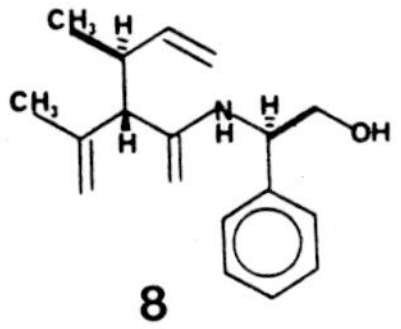
8

amides 7 and 8, although the experiments described here were carried out on the racemate. Acid 6 could be reduced (LAH) and protected (TBDMSCl/imidazole) leading to compound 9. Selective hydroboration (disiamyborane/H_2O_2) of the terminal olefin gave alcohol 10.

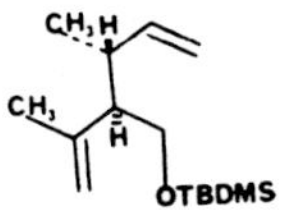
9

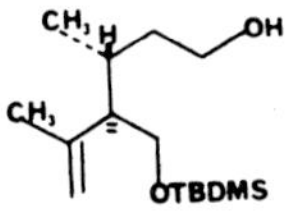
10

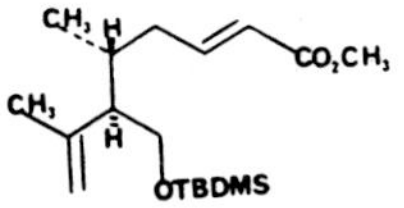
11

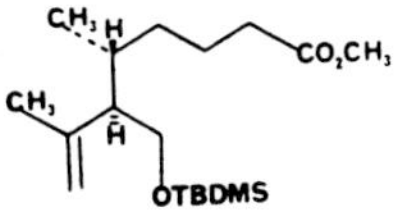
12

Oxidation (PCC) of 10 and Wittig reaction with $Ph_3PCH_2COOCH_3$ produces unsaturated ester 11. The conjugated double bond of 11 was reduced with Li/NH_3 to give 12. When 12 was treated with MeLi, deprotected with $Bu_4N^+F^-$, then oxidized with PCC, hydroxy-aldehyde 4, the side-chain synthon for 25-hydroxy vitamin D_3 was produced. This alcohol is being used in a 25-hydroxy-vitamin D_2 total synthesis now in progress.

Our approach to the side chain of 25-hydroxy vitamin D_2 begins with commercially available ester 13. Addition of methyl lithium gave diol 14 (75%). Swern oxidation (8) of 14 gave a sensitive aldehyde (52%) which was not purified but reacted immediately with trans-propenyl lithium (9) to give a diastereomeric mixture of two alcohols in a ratio of 2:1 (39% yield.)

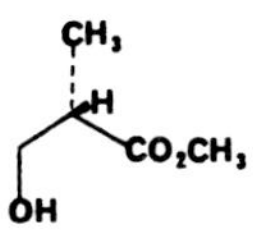
13

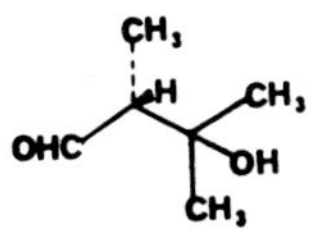
14

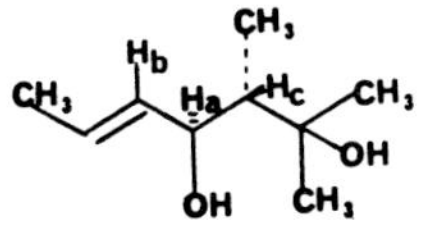
15

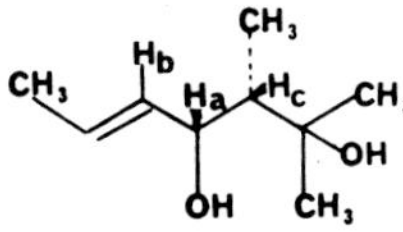
16

These alcohols could be separated readily by chromatography on silica gel (50/50 ether-hexane). One diol (Rf= .14, $[\alpha]_D$= -5.5°) was crystalline, mp = 67-69° , while the other (Rf=.18. $[\alpha]_D$= +2.6°) was an oil. The 300 MHz NMR spectra of these diols , although similar, showed several interesting differences. In particular, the methine hydrogen H_a for the crystalline isomer showed a triplet ($J_{ab}=J_{ac}$=5 Hz) whereas the second isomer showed only a broadened doublett (J_{ab}=5 Hz) Decoupling experiments indicated that the 5 Hz coupling was due to coupling with the vinylic hydrogen shown. Thus significant conformational differences must exist between the isomers. Fortunately the crystalline isomer yielded to single crystal X-ray analysis (fig 2).

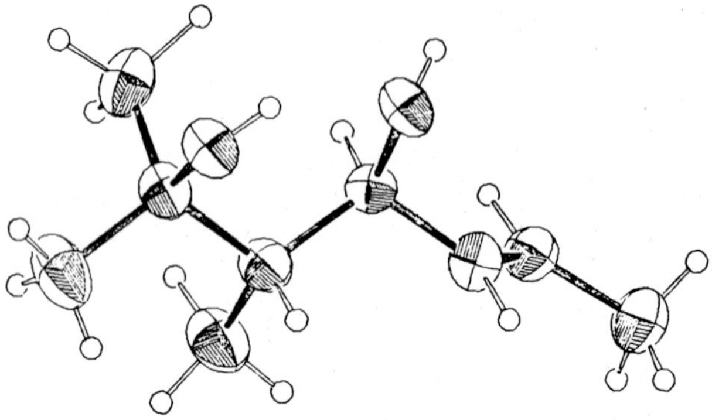

Figure 2. ORTEP DRAWING OF MOLECULE 16.

This allowed us to assign structure 15 to the non-crystalline isomer (minor product.) The minor isomer is the one required for the synthesis of natural vitamin D_2 since the chirality at C-23 of diol 15 will be "transferred" to C-20 to produce the correct absolute configuration via the Claisen rearrangement. Esterification of diol 15 by the method of Mukaiyama (10) gave

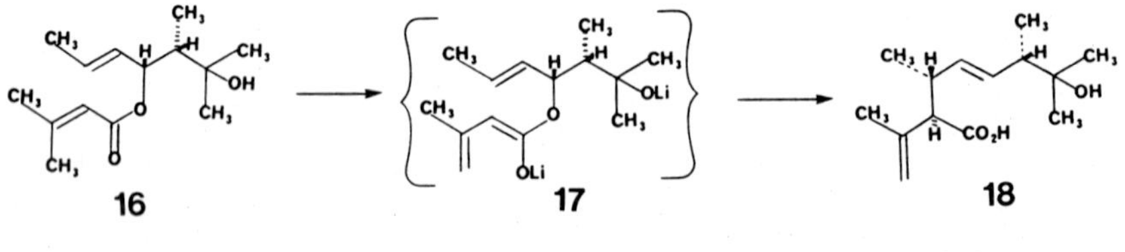

ester 16 (46 %). Deprotonation of 16 with two equivalents of LDA gave dianion 17, the intermediate required for the ester enolate Claisen rearrangement. The rearrangement proceeded satisfactorily to produce 18. Acid 18 could be reduced with LAH, then oxidized with PCC to provide our optically active vitamin D_2 side-chain synthon 5.

With both 25-hydroxylated precursers 4 and 5 in hand, we turn our attention to ring-A. We have already published(2) our approach to the application of a new chiral ring-A reagent 19. We now plan to make the entire strategy more convergent by incorporation of ring-A into the pentadienyl-lithium reagent. Bromide 20(2), the precurser of ring-A synthon 19, can be oxidized at C-1 using SeO_2 to produce alcohol 21(68%). Assignment of the desired alpha-hydoxy configuration was based on literature precedent(11). The 300 MHz NMR spectrum of 21 showed a multiplet at 4.21 ppm for the proton adjacent to oxygen. Protection (TBDMSCl/imidazole) of alcohol 21 gives synthon 22(72%) for 1- hydroxy-ring A construction.

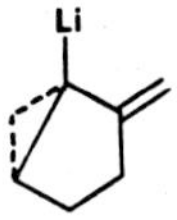

19

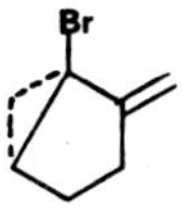

20

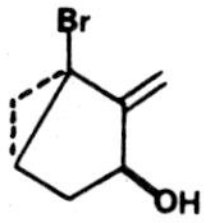

21

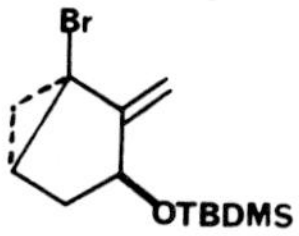

22

We can transmetallate either 20 or 22 and react them with aldehyde 23 to produce alcohols 24 or 25. Thus we have available suitable fragments for the convergent synthesis of several combinations of hydroxylated vitamin derivatives. We are presently bringing up more material in order to realize this enhanced and convergent intramolecular Diels-Alder approach to both vitamin D_2 and D_3.

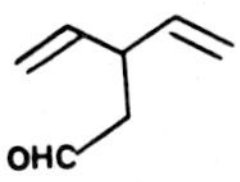

23

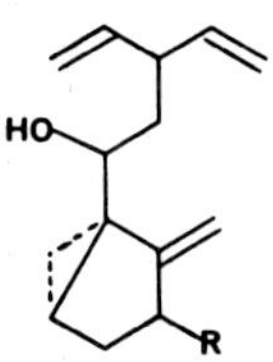

24 R = H
25 R = OTBDMS

References:

1. Wilson, S. R., Haque, M. S. (1984) Tetrahedron Lett. 3147-3150.

2. Wilson, S. R., Haque, M. S., Venkatesan, A. M., Zucker, P. A., (1984) Tetrahedron Lett. 3151-3154.

3. Burkert, U., Allinger, N. L. (1982) "Molecular Mechanics", ACS Monograph 177.

4. Wilson, S. R., Jernberg, K. M., Mao. D. T. (1976) J. Org. Chem. 40, 3209-3210.

5. Wilson, S. R., Haque. M. S. (1982) J. Org. Chem. 47, 5411-5413.

6. Wilson, S. R., Myers, R. S. (1975) J. Org. Chem. 40, 3309-3311.

7. Helmchen, G., Nill, G., Flockerzi, Youssef, M. S. K. (1979) Angew. Chem. Intl., Ed. Eng. 18, 63-65.

8. Nagaoka, H., Kishi, Y. (1981) Tetrahedron 37, 3873-3888.

9. Linstrumelle, G., Krieger, J. K., Whitesides, G. M. (1975) Organic Synthesis 55, 103-113.

10. Mukaiyama, T., Usui, M., Shimada, E. (1975) Chemistry Letters 1045-1048.

SYNTHESIS OF 1α,25S,26-TRIHYDROXY-Δ^{22}-CHOLECALCIFEROL, A POTENT INDUCER OF CELL DIFFERENTIATION.

P.M. Wovkulich, A.D. Batcho, E.G. Baggiolini, A. Boris, G. Truitt, and M.R. Uskoković
Roche Research Center, Hoffmann-La Roche Inc., Nutley, NJ 07110

Vitamin D_3 metabolites serve a vital role in regulating calcium and phosphorous levels in serum and calcium absorption in the intestine. Certainly, the development and maintenance of bone are critically dependent on this role. However, bone growth and remodeling processes may also depend in part, on the ability of vitamin D_3 metabolites to participate in the regulation of proliferation of different stem cells, thereby promoting, for example, the biosynthesis of bone matrix proteins. For specific pharmacologic exploitation of these latter effects, it is necessary to identify analogs which exhibit separation of their activity to regulate cellular proliferation and differentiation from their potentially dose-limiting impact on calcium metabolism. As a model, one of the recently isolated and fully characterized metabolites, 1α,25S,26-trihydroxycholecalciferol (2)[1,2], is of particular interest since in rat it exerts an inhibitory effect on the biosynthesis of 1α,25-dihydroxycholecalciferol (1) despite the fact that it is nearly equipotent to 1 in the HL-60 cell differentiation activity. In normal cows, 1α,25S,26-trihydroxycholecalciferol (2) is approximately one-tenth as potent as 1α,25-dihydroxycholecalciferol in causing hypercalcemia, as judged from the magnitude and duration of the response.[3] With this as background, we were especially interested in the influence of the Δ^{22}-double bond on the stimulation of intestinal calcium absorption, bone mineralization and cell differentiation-inducing activities. We have, therefore, synthesized 1α,25S,26-trihydroxy-Δ^{22}-cholecalciferol (3) and investigated its properties in comparison to 1 and 2.

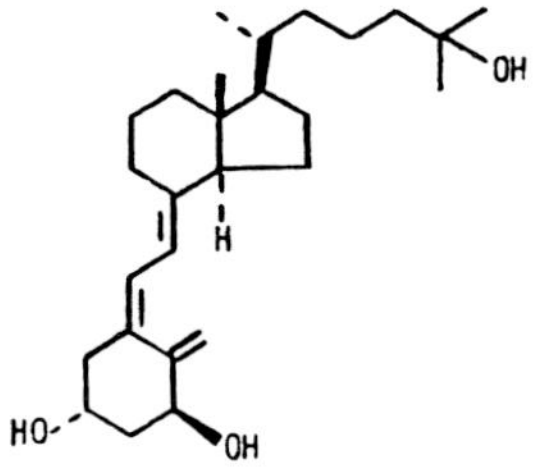

1

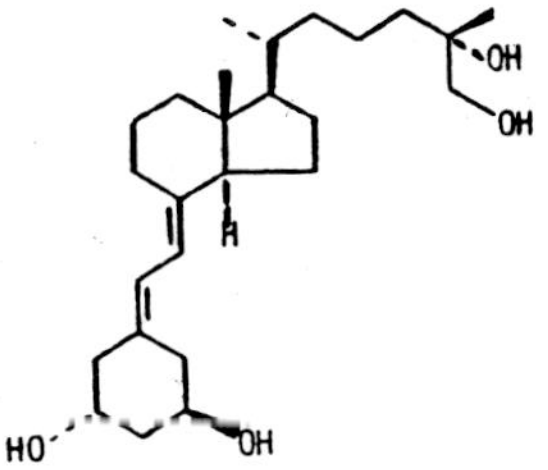

2

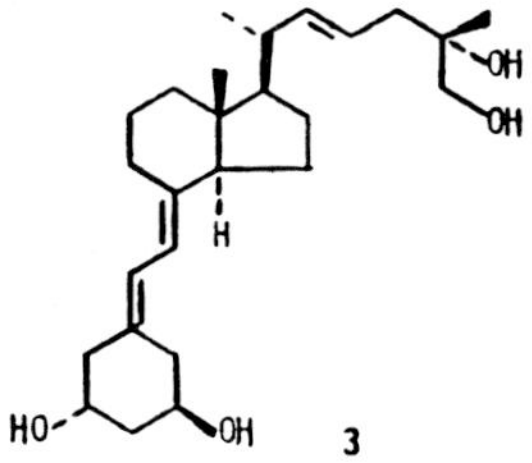

3

pages in wrong order 80 to 762 & work backwards!

At Roche, vitamin D metabolites and analogs are routinely evaluated for binding to chick intestinal cytosol $1,25-(OH)_2D_3$ binding protein, in the antirachitogenic test in chicks, and for kidney ^{45}Ca levels in rats as indication for hypercalciuria. The comparative results for $1\alpha,25$-dihydroxy-, $1\alpha,25S,26$-trihydroxy-, and $1\alpha,25S,26$-trihydroxy-Δ^{22}-cholecalciferol are shown in the following tables:

Ratio Relative to $1\alpha,25-(OH)_2D_3$ Binding to Chick Intestinal Cytosol $1,25-(OH)_2D_3$ Binding Protein

$1\alpha,25-(OH)_2D_3$	1
$1\alpha,25S,26-(OH)_3D_3$	11
$1\alpha,25S,26-(OH)_3,\ ^{22}-D_3$	18

Anti-Rachitogenic Activity

Dose/Day	Mean Tibia Ash mgs.		
ng/chick, p.o.	$1\alpha,25-(OH)_2D_3$	$1\alpha,25S,26-(OH)_3D_3$	$1\alpha,25S,26-(OH)_3-\Delta^{22}D_3$
0	120.7	112.1	152.5
30	244.7	124.9	135.6
100		159.4	164.1
300		187.0	168.8
1000		210.4	175.6

^{45}Ca Retention in Kidney in Rats

Dose/Day	Mean Renal ^{45}Ca (CPM/0.2mL, Digest)		
ng/rat, s.c.	$1\alpha,25-(OH)_2D_3$	$1\alpha,25S,26-(OH)_3D_3$	$1\alpha,25S,26-(OH)_3-\Delta^{22}D_3$
0	76	95	109
100	415	95	102
200	3178	96	101
500	6630	104	109
1000	11,191	113	115

In the inhibition of the EHDP-induced mineralization block in rats, 1α,25S,26-trihydroxy- and 1α,25S,26-trihydroxy-Δ^{22}-cholecalciferol have shown no activity in doses up to 10 mg/day, p.o., while 1α,25-dihydroxycholecalciferol is fully active at 100 ng/day, p.o. (data not shown).

Testing the anti-proliferative and differentiation-inducing efficacy of vitamin D compounds was done using human promyelocytic (HL-60) tumor cells. Triplicate culture flasks containing HL-60 cells were incubated for four days in the presence of tissue culture medium only (medium control), a final concentration of 0.001%, v/v, of ethanol in tissue culture medium (vehicle control), or varying concentrations of experimental compounds in tissue culture medium with a constant vehicle concentration of 0.001%. At assay the number of HL-60 cells per ml of tissue culture medium in each flask was determined and the anti-proliferative effect of the experimental compounds was assessed as the reduction of cell density relative to vehicle control cultures. Undifferentiated and differentiated cells were enumerated using cells pooled from replicate flasks by reaction with nitroblue tetrazolium (NBT). Differentiated cells were thus judged to have acquired an enzymatic oxidative function in response to stimulation by 12-O-tetradecanoylphorbol-13-acetate.

As shown in the following table, 1α,25-dihydroxycholecalciferol (1) inhibited the proliferation and induced the differentiation of HL-60 cells in a dose-dependent fashion. The addition of a hydroxylation group at carbon 26 (ie 1α,25S,26-trihydroxycholecalciferol) reduced this activity slightly. In the experiment shown 1α,25S,26-trihydroxycholecalciferol was approximately one-half as potent as 1α,25-dihydroxycholecalciferol which was confirmed in four additional experiments. The efficacy of 1α,25S,26-trihydroxy-Δ^{22}-cholecalciferol (3) was nearly equipotent to 1α,25-dihydroxycholecalciferol (1) as shown in the representative experiment and confirmed in three additional experiments. Furthermore, the relative potencies of these three compounds was identical when cellular differentiation was assessed functionally as the ability to phagocytize particulate material (data not shown). Clearly, then both 1α,25S,26-trihydroxycholecalciferol and 1α,25S,26-trihydroxy-Δ^{22}-cholecalciferol are potent inducers of HL-60 cell differentiation, *in vitro*.

Having fulfilled their role in controlling the C-25 stereochemistry, the oxygen and nitrogen groups now had to be excised. Treatment of 23 with sodium methoxide in methanol gave 25 (Scheme 6). Mesylation of the free hydroxyl (26) followed directly by displacement with bromide generated the bromoisoxazolidine 27. Reductive elimination of 27 with zinc in acetic acid proceeded rapidly (15-20 min) to olefin 28 followed more slowly (5 hr) by N-O bond cleavage to 29. Reduction of the carbomethoxy group (30) and then desilylation with aqueous HF gave triol 31 which, on treatment with 2,2-dimethoxypropane in the presence of acid, produced acetonide 7 in high overall yield.

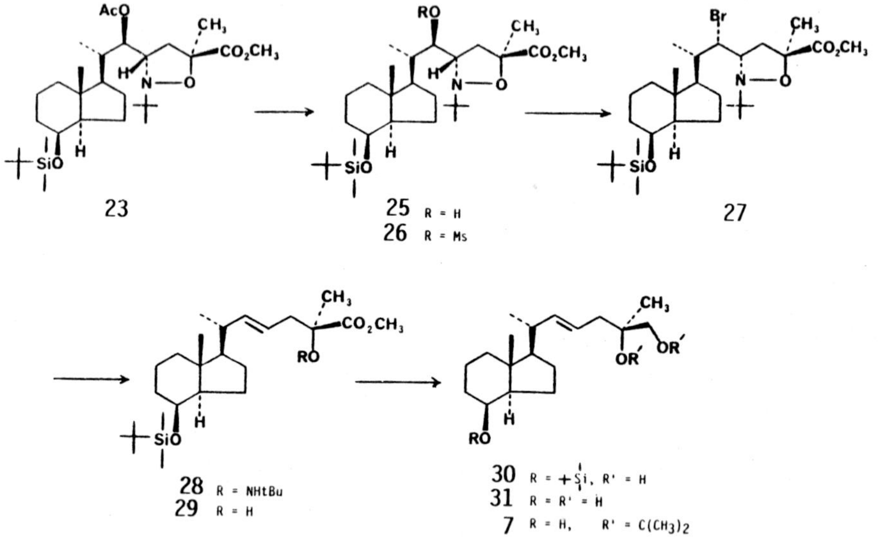

Scheme 6

The last stage of the synthesis followed in exactly the same manner as the previously described protocol for the preparation of 1α,25-dihydroxycholecalciferol (1)[4], 1α,25S,26-trihydroxycholecalciferol (2)[5] and calcitriol lactone[6]. Oxidation of 7 with 2,2'-bipyridinium chlorochromate produced the ketone 4. Then, reaction of 4 with the anion 5 at -78°C gave the coupled product 6 (Scheme 1) which on removal of the protecting groups generated 1α,25S,26-trihydroxy-Δ^{22}-cholecalciferol (3).

the rotational orientation of the nitrone when an alpha proton is replaced by oxygen but it was not apparent that the dramatic shift from exo to endo as observed here would occur. The benzyl analog of nitrone 22 produced

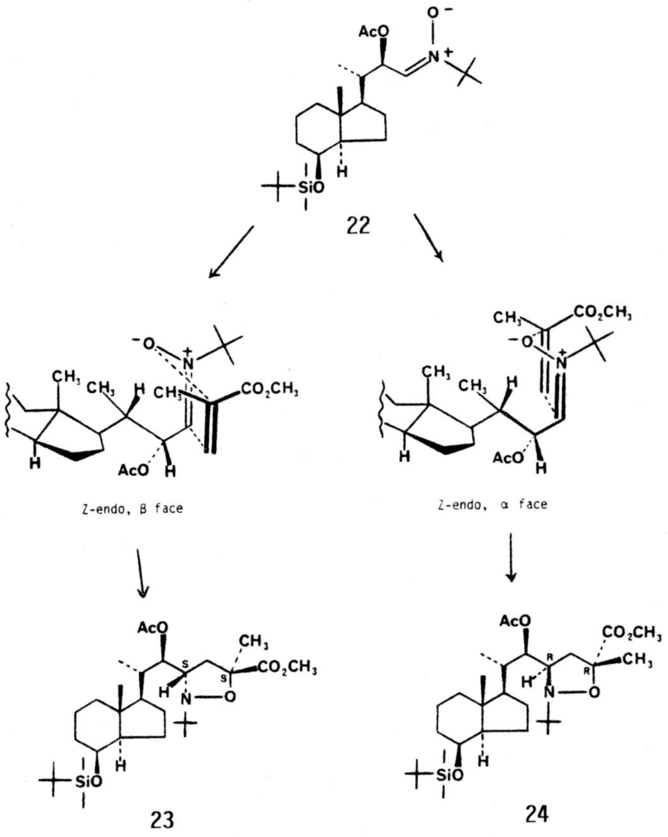

Scheme 5

an 82:1:7:10 mixture of isomers where the major adduct bears the same absolute configuration as 23. The drop in the endo/exo ratio from 99% endo in the t-butyl case to 92:8 in the N-benzyl suggests that the steric bulk of the substituent on nitrogen may in part govern the endo/exo selectivity. While other factors, such as substituents on the carbon end of the nitrone undoubtedly make contributions as well, it appears that whatever the endo/exo ratio is, it will be increased when the bulk of the nitrogen substituent is increased.

The previously described diol 14[5] on treatment with a slight excess of benzoyl chloride in pyridine gave the mono benzoate 15 which was silylated (16) and then debenzoylated to give the crystalline silyl ether 17 (Scheme 4). Oxidation with pyridinium chlorochromate led to aldehyde 18 which on exposure to vinyl magnesium bromide gave alcohol 19 in 63% yield from 17 as well as 12% of the epimeric alcohol. Acetylation of 19 followed by ozonolysis in methanol at -78° and dimethylsulfide work up gave the α-acetoxy aldehyde 21 which with t-butylhydroxylamine produced the desired nitrone 22. Heating 22 at 50° with methyl methacrylate for 42 hr gave an 81:18.7:0.3 mixture of isomers in 99% yield. An X-ray crystallographic analysis of the major isomer revealed it to be the SS adduct 23 and not the expected RS isomer 13 as portrayed in Scheme 3. The near identity of the proton NMR signals of the next most predominant isomer, particularly of the isoxazolidine ring protons, suggested that the relative stereochemistry at C-23 and C-25 was the same as in 23 (i.e. trans) but of the opposite absolute configuration. The RR configuration of 24 was also confirmed by an X-ray crystallographic analysis. This result is especially intriguing since the mode of cycloaddition is 99% from the endo transition state and not the exo mode as experienced with nitrone 9 (Scheme 5). From the work of Vasella[7], one might expect a change in

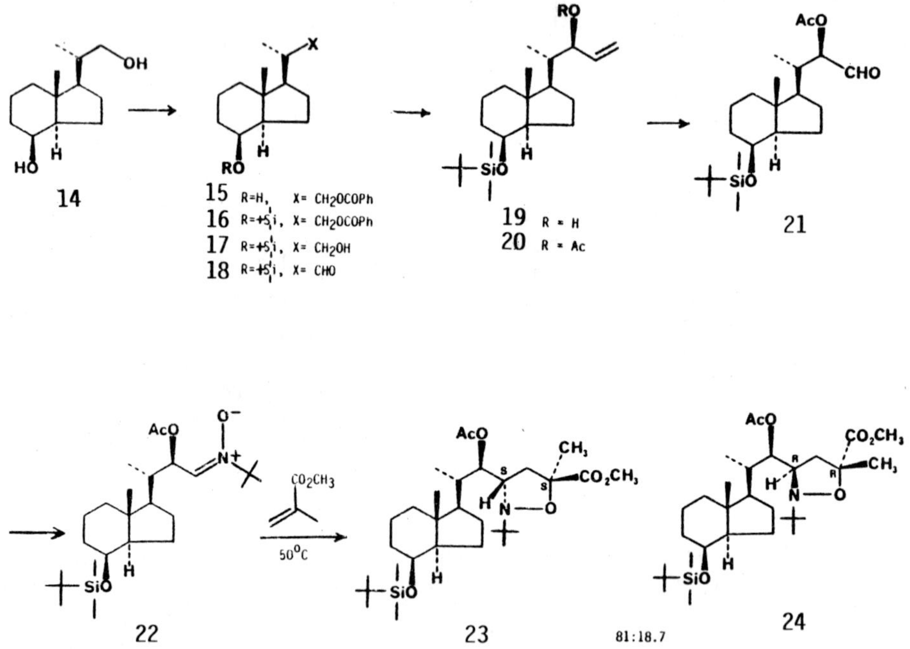

Scheme 4

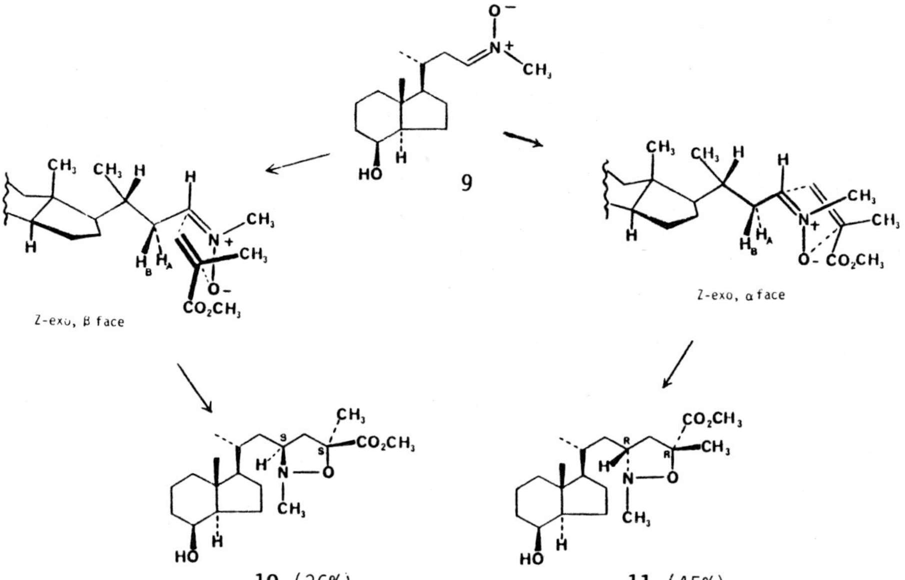

10 (36%) 11 (45%)

Scheme 2

The key cycloaddition reaction with methyl methacrylate proceeded smoothly at room temperature. To our disappointment, this reaction, though regiospecific, produced in high yield diastereomeric 23S;25S, 23R;25R, 23S;25R, and 23R;25S isoxazolidines corresponding to 8 in a ratio of 36:45:7:12[5]. While the diastereoselectivity of the 1,3-dipolar cycloaddition was low, the mode of cycloaddition (i.e. exo vs endo) is significant. As illustrated in Scheme 2, where the Z-nitrone 9 is shown in the extended form, the two predominant diastereomers 10 and 11 arise from the exo transition state in which approach of the methacrylate from the same face as H_B (β face) produces 10 and approach from the H_A (α) face gives 11. Consequently, the proportion of 11 would be expected to decrease if approach from the H_A face were made less favorable. To test this hypothesis, a system where H_A is replaced by a removable "steric protecting" function (R_2O-) was considered. For example, a nitrone such as 12 might be expected to form preferentially the isoxazolidine 13 via the Z-exo transition state (Scheme 3). Its synthesis was undertaken next[5].

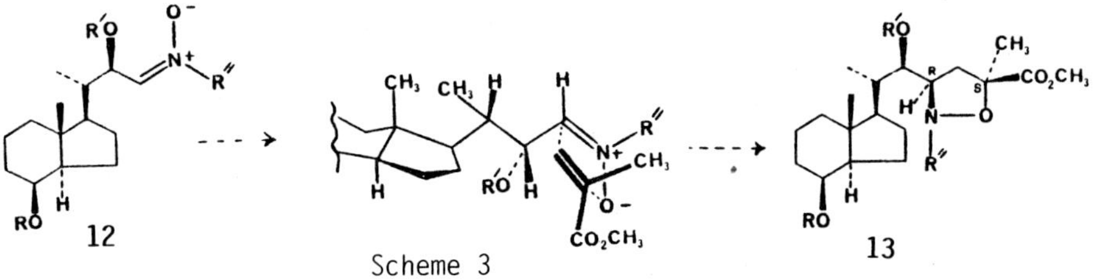

12 13

Scheme 3

We based the synthesis of 3 on a convergent approach in which a CD ring synthon 4 would be coupled with the phosphinoxy anion 5 to give 6 which on removal of the protecting groups would yield 3 (Scheme 1). Such an approach has already been successful in the total synthesis of 1[4], 2[5], and calcitriol lactone[6]. The major portion of the synthetic effort was therefore directed at the preparation of the CD ring synthon 4.

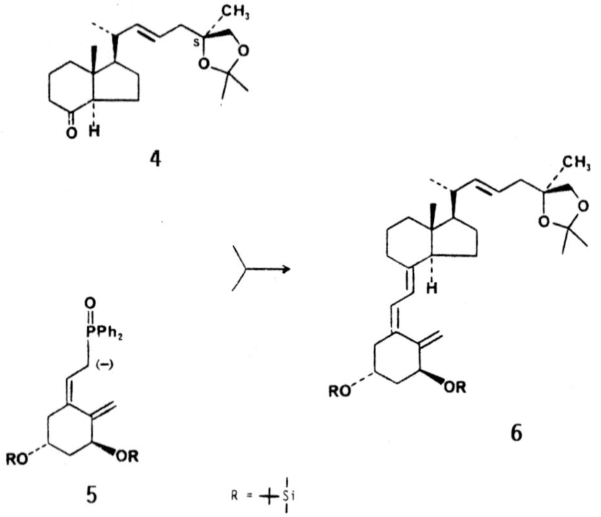

Scheme 1

One of the objectives in the synthesis of 4 was to generate the isolated chiral functionality at the C-25 position without resorting to the use of additional chiral pieces. For this purpose, we wished to explore methods which would utilize the existing asymmetry in the bicyclic ring portion of the CD synthon. Specifically, the concept was to take advantage of the chirality at C-20 to influence the diastereoselectivity of a 1,3-dipolar cycloaddition of the previously described C-23 nitrone 9[5] with methyl methacrylate. Synthon 7 would then be accessible from the resulting isoxazolidine 8.

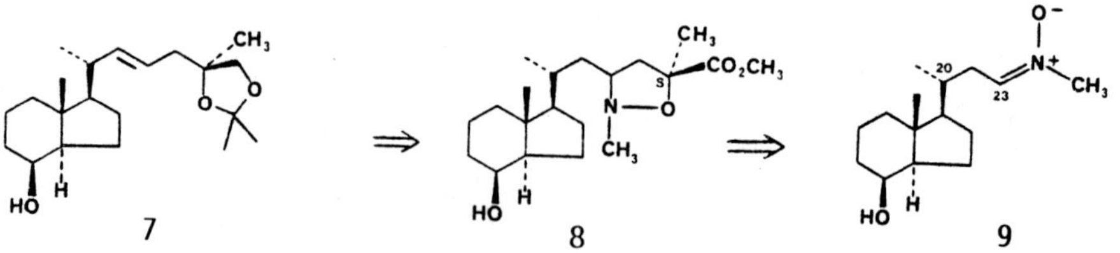

ANTI-PROLIFERATIVE AND DIFFERENTIATION-INDUCING EFFECTS OF 1α,25-DIHYDROXYCHOLECALCIFEROL, 1α,25S,26-TRIHYDROXYCHOLECALCIFEROL, and 1α,25S,-26-TRIHYDROXY-Δ22-CHOLECALCIFEROL ON HL-60 CELLS, *IN VITRO*.

Compound and concentration ($x10^{-9}$ molar)		Proliferation		Differentiation	
		HL-60 cells per mL $x\ 10^{-4}$	Inhibition of proliferation %	formazan "+" cells Tot.cells counted	%"+"
Medium control		68.5 ± 4.8	---	2/277	1
Vehicle control		66.3 ± 3.2	0	2/241	1
1α,25-$(OH)_2D_3$	3	65.3 ± 4.6	2	82/289	28
	10	45.1 ± 2.3	32	176/274	64
	30	33.1 ± 1.3	50	236/256	92
	100	26.9 ± 1.6	59	235/239	98
1α,25S,26-$(OH)_3D_3$	3	68.3 ± 4.0	0	12/278	4
	10	70.0 ± 2.2	0	80/266	30
	30	43.3 ± 3.9	35	194/244	80
	100	29.3 ± 1.7	56	258/265	98
1α,25S,26-$(OH)_3$,Δ^{22}-D_3	3	59.3 ± 1.6	11	78/272	29
	10	50.4 ± 1.1	24	165/270	61
	30	35.6 ± 1.6	46	228/257	89
	100	28.9 ± 0.6	56	241/252	96

Taken together, the data presented here suggest the possible separation of the potentially dose-limiting calcium effects of select vitamin D derivatives from their capacity to restrict the proliferation and promote the differentiation of certain cells. Continued and more extensive efforts along the lines reported here may thus provide for the development of compounds with diverse pharmacologic applications.

References

1) T.A. Reinhardt, J.L. Napoli, D.C. Beitz, E.T. Littledike and R.L. Horst, Biochem. Biophys. Res. Commun., 99, 302 (1981).

2) J.J. Partridge, S.-J. Shiuey, N.K. Chadha, E.G. Baggiolini, B.M. Hennessy, M.R. Usković, J.L. Napoli, T.A. Reinhardt, and R.L. Horst, Helv. Chim. Acta, 64, 2138 (1981).

3) K. Hove, R.L. Horst, and E.T. Littledike, J. Dairy Science, 66, 59 (1983).

4) E.G. Baggiolini, J.A. Iacobelli, B.M. Hennessy and M.R. Usković, J. Am. Chem. Soc., 104, 2945 (1982).

5) P.M. Wovkulich, F. Barcelos, A.D. Batcho, J.F. Sereno, E.G. Baggiolini, B.M. Hennessy, and M.R. Usković, Tetrahedron, 40, 2283 (1984).

6) P.M. Wovkulich, E.G. Baggiolini, B.M. Hennessy, M.R. Usković, E. Mayer, and A.W. Norman, J. Org. Chem., 48, 4433 (1983).

7) B. Bernet and A. Vasella, Helv. Chim. Acta, 62, 2411 (1979).

STEREOSPECIFIC SYNTHESIS OF 1α,25-DIHYDROXY-24R-FLUOROCHOLECALCIFEROL (Ro 23-0233).

Shian-Jan Shiuey, John J. Partridge, Naresh K. Chadha, Alfred Boris, and Milan R. Uskokovic
Roche Research Center, Department of Chemistry, Hoffmann-La Roche Inc., Nutley, New Jersey 07110

Since the discovery of the principal physiologically active vitamin D_3 metabolite, 1α,25-dihydroxycholecalciferol (calcitriol), substances have been sought that exhibit a longer half-life and possess increased anti-rachitogenic activity. With these goals in mind, 1α,25-dihydroxy-24R-fluorocholecalciferol (Ro 23-0233) was stereospecifically prepared. By placing a fluoro group at one of the principal sites of calcitriol catabolism, a potent long lasting anti-rachitogenic analog was obtained.

Our strategy involved a convergent synthesis using as starting materials commercially available l-malic acid and dehydroepiandrosterone (Scheme 1). These substances were converted to the side chain synthon a and the suitably functionalized steroid b. Using the key Wicha alkylation sequence[1,2], the protected cholesterol c was formed and this substance was then converted to 1α,25-dihydroxy-24R-fluorocholecalciferol d.

Scheme 1
Synthesis Outline

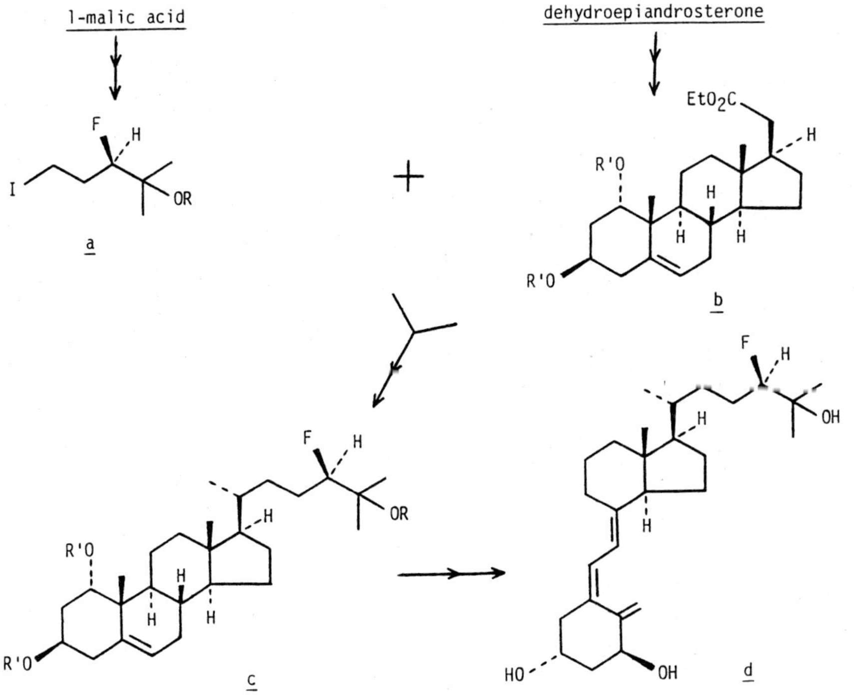

Vitamin D. A Chemical, Biochemical and Clinical Update

1α,25-Dihydroxy-24R-fluorocholecalciferol [24R-F-1α,25-$(OH)_2$-D_3] was submitted to a variety of biological evaluations. The plasma half-life of this subtance after i.v. administration in dogs was 14.4 hr, compared to 3.6 hr for calcitriol. Potent anti-rachitogenic activity was also demonstrated. An oral dose of 30 ng/day in six week old vitamin D deficient chicks increased the tibia ash weights to 338 mg compared to 245 mg for an equivalent dose of calcitriol. Thus, placement of a fluorine moiety at the 24R-position leads to a potent long-lasting analog of calcitriol.

At Roche vitamin D_3 metabolites and analogs are routinely evaluated for binding to the chick intestinal cytosol 1α,25-$(OH)_2D_3$ binding protein and for anti-rachitogenicity in chicks. Analysis for kidney ^{45}Ca levels in rats is used as an indication for hypercalcuria. The comparative results for 24R-F-1α,25-$(OH)_2$-D_3 and 1α,25-$(OH)_2$-D_3 (calcitriol) are shown in the following tables.

Ratio Relative to 1α,25-$(OH)_2$-D_3. Binding to Chick Intestinal Cytosol 1α,25-$(OH)_2$-D_3 Binding Protein

1α,25-$(OH)_2$-D_3	1.0
24R-F-1α,25-$(OH)_2$-D_3	1.4

Anti-Rachitogenic Activity

Dose/Day ng/chick, p.o.	Mean Tibia Ash Weights (mg) 1α,25-$(OH)_2$-D_3	24R-F-1α,25-$(OH)_2$-D_3
0	120.7	120.9
3	128.7	293.3
10	177.9	330.4
30	244.5	337.9

^{45}Ca Retention in Kidney in Rats

Dose/Day ng/rat, s.c.	Mean Renal ^{45}Ca (CPM/0.2 ml, digest) 1α,25-$(OH)_2$-D_3	24R-F-1α,25-$(OH)_2$-D_3
0	76	76
50	158	142
100	415	296
200	3178	1894
500	6630	13,121
1000	11,191	12,795

In the inhibition of the EHDP-induced mineralization block in rats, 24R-F-1α,25-$(OH)_2$-D_3 was approximately equivalent to 1α,25-$(OH)_2$-D_3.

SYNTHESIS OF 6-FLUOROVITAMIN D_3

William G. Dauben, Boris Kohler (1), and Alex Roesle
Department of Chemistry, University of California, Berkeley, California 94720 U.S.A.

Vitamin D_3 is an important biological regulator of calcium and phosphorus metabolism (2). It is now established that the parent vitamin D_3 is sequentially metabolized in various tissues to the steroid hormone 1,25-(OH_2-D_3 (calcitriol) which exerts the highest biological activity of all vitamin D_3 metabolites. This hormonal derivative stimulates the intestinal absorption of calcium (ICA) and phosphorus (3), and the mobilization of bone calcium (BCM) (2) through a target organ receptor mediated mechanism (4). All the metabolites so far isolated are polar derivatives, bearing extra hydroxyl, carboxyl, or lactone groups at C-1 or near the extremity of the sidechain. In addition to the synthesis of the metabolites, a great amount of synthetic effort has been directed towards the preparation of new derivatives bearing polar groups on the periphery of the molecule. For example, fluorine-substituted vitamin D_3 metabolites have been synthesized in order to evaluate metabolic events obligatory to the vitamin activity (5). It has been found that 24,24-difluoro-1α,25-dihydroxyvitamin D_3 shows 5-10 times more _in vivo_ activity than the parent 1,25-$(OH)_2$-D_3 steroid hormone (6).

By contrast, little attention has been directed to the role of the triene portion of the vitamin D_3 molecule in relation to the biological activities. Is the role of this portion of the molecule limited solely to geometric requirements or does the π-system interact with the bioreceptors?

Vitamin D. A Chemical, Biochemical and Clinical Update

With these concerns in mind, coupled with our continuing interest in the role of dipolar excited states in polyene photochemistry (7), the synthesis of 6-fluorovitamin D_3 (6-F-D_3) was undertaken.

6-Fluorocholesteryl acetate (2a) was first prepared by Boswell (8) by allowing 6-ketocholestanyl acetate (1a) to react with diethylaminosulfur trifluoride (DAST). Although a slightly higher yield of 2a can be obtained using DAST, the use of piperidinosulfur trifluoride (9) simplifies the

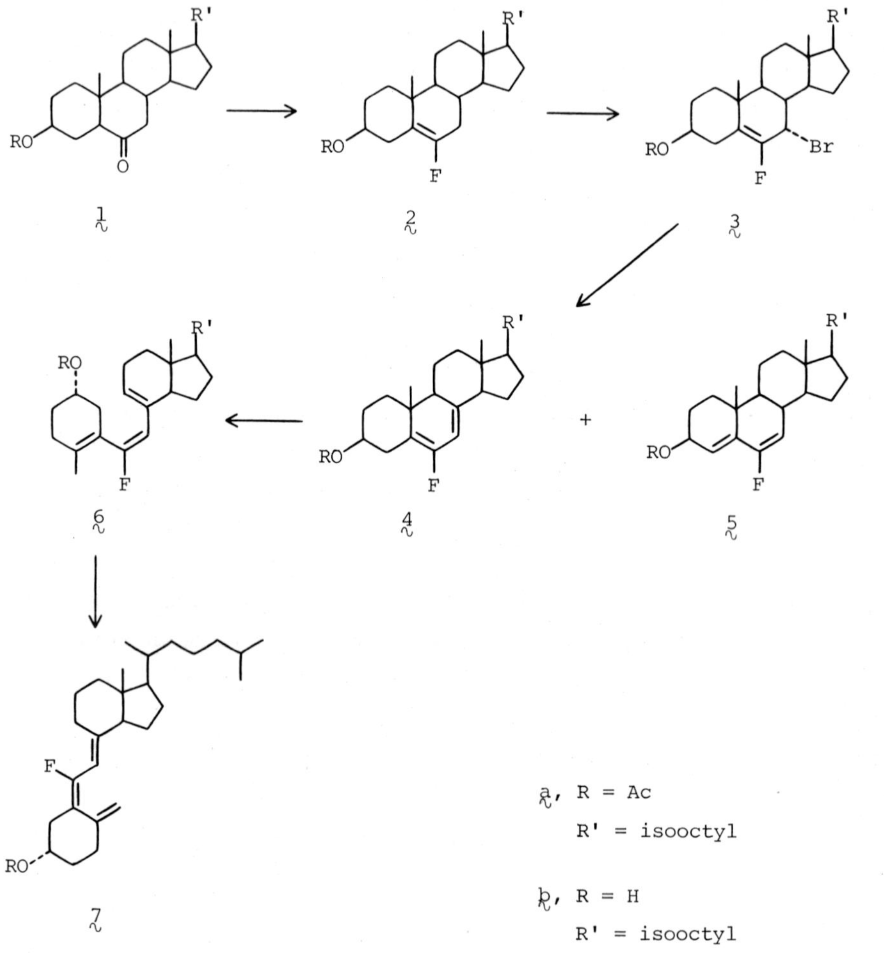

a, R = Ac
R' = isooctyl

b, R = H
R' = isooctyl

synthetic operation and gives 2a in 55% yield. The desired 7-allylic-bromination of the fluoro-ene was readily achieved using N-bromosuccinimide (peroxide catalyst plus light) and the crystalline 7α-bromo-derivative 3a was obtained in a 44% yield. The dehydrobromination of 3a to give in good yield the desired 6-fluoro-7-dehydrocholesteryl acetate (4a) proved to be a difficult reaction, clearly showing that the fluorine substituent had affected the process. Many common amine bases employed in the synthesis of the non-fluorinated provitamin gave complex mixtures of numerous products and with s-collidine, in particular, there was no indication (by UV spectroscopy) of any of the desired 5,7-diene derivative. The use of trimethyl phosphite in refluxing xylene gave a clean reaction product (84% yield), however, the product was a 2:1 mixture of the 4,6-diene 5a and the 5,7-diene 4a (analysis by HPLC). Compared with the corresponding elimination reaction using the non-fluorinated derivative, the trimethyl phosphite elimination with 3a was very slow, five days compared to four hours.

During this latter study, the use of tetra(n-butyl)-ammonium fluoride at 25 °C was shown to be the most effective agent to produce the provitamin in good yield (10). Further studies also showed that 1,3-dibromo-5,5-dimethylhydantoin was a more effective halogenating agent than N-bromosuccinimide. From the preparative standpoint, the finding that standard silica gel column chromatography readily separated the two isomeric diene alcohols 4b and 5b was of key importance. Starting with 6-fluorocholesteryl acetate (2a) and not purifying any intermediate materials until after the removal of the acetate group by LAH reduction, the desired diene 4b was obtained in an overall yield of 48% and the isomeric 4,6-diene 5b in 11% yield. The ultraviolet spectra of 4b and 5b showed less pronounced structure and the molecular extinction coefficients are about 30% less than their non-fluorinated counterparts.

The 6-fluoro-7-dehydrocholesterol (4b, 6-F-Pro-D_3) was irradiated in a degassed ethereal solution at ∿0 °C in a Rayonet reactor using 300 nm light. The reaction was followed by analytical HPLC and stopped when a maximum buildup of the previtamin was observed. The irradiation reaction mixture, using HPLC analysis, showed a 90:10 ratio of 6-fluoroprevitamin D_3 (6b) to starting 6-fluoroprovitamin D_3 (4a). The two products were readily separated by flash chromatography (11) in an isolated yield of 43% of 6-F-Pre-D_3 and 12% of the 6-F-Pro-D_3, indicating that some decomposition of the previtamin had occurred during the work-up and chromatography. Besides these two products, analytical HPLC showed the presence of two very minor ultraviolet-active products which were not isolated. This is an interesting result since in the non-fluorinated series, using 300 nm light, the quasi-photostationary state has the composition of 5% Pro-D_3, 68% Pre-D_3, 19% of tachysterol$_3$, and 8% lumisterol$_3$ (12). The apparent inefficient formation of the C-6:C-7 trans isomer 6-fluorotachysterol$_3$ indicates that the fluoro-substituent has an effect on the photochemical cis-trans olefin isomerization.

The [1,7] sigmatropic hydrogen rearrangement to convert the previtamin to the vitamin is normally readily achieved at 80 °C over a period of no longer than 18 h. At this temperature, the 6-F-Pre-D_3 was stable for a period of 24 h. It was found that when an n-isooctane solution of 6b was heated in a sealed tube at 120 °C for 4-5 h, the hydrogen rearrangement did occur and yielded a mixture, as analyzed by HPLC, of 6-F-Pre-D_3 to 6-F-D_3 in a ratio of 15:85. The vitamin 7b was isolated by preparative TLC as a colorless oil in a yield of 30%. TLC of the crude reaction product showed the presence of some polar material which did not move from the origin upon development of the plate. The isolated 6-F-D_3 has a UV max at 268 nm (ε 10,300) and was shown to be a single compound by analytical HPLC.

The 6-F-D_3 is very sensitive to air. The decomposition was detected by the broadening of the UV absorption peak, accompanied by a hypsochromic shift and diminution of the molar extinction coefficient when the material was allowed to stand in non-degassed cyclohexane solution. The mass spectra of several decomposition products each showed a peak at M+16 or M+17, indicating the uptake of oxygen. The 6-F-D_3 can be repurified from the polar products by chromatography with the recovery of 60-70% of the vitamin. Interestingly, the mass spectrum of 6-F-D_3 does not show the characteristic fragmentation of other vitamin D derivatives with the cleavage of the C-7:C-8 double bond (13).

A complete inhibition of the [1,7] sigmatropic hydrogen rearrangement has been reported for 19,19-difluoroprevitamin D_3 (14). That this retardation of the reaction may be due to changes in the electron distribution in the triene system is the finding of the non-reversible formation of 19-acetoxy-vitamin D_3 from the previtamin (14). The retardation of the rate of rearrangement in the 6-F-D_3 formation supports this suggestion but the finding that the equilibrium composition is similar to other vitamin D_3 derivatives suggests that the problem is more complex than previously thought.

In the course of our synthetic studies, the presence of the fluorine substituent created many problems. One of the more interesting was the finding that 6-fluorocholesteryl acetate was highly deactivated towards allylic oxidation.

Photooxidation (15), aqueous N-bromosuccinimide (HOBr) oxidation (16), and Collins oxidation (17) are reported to give high yields of the non-fluorinated 7-ketocholesteryl acetate. When applied to the fluorinated material **2**, these procedures were impractical. Even under forcing conditions and prolonged reaction times, the reactions remained incomplete and afforded complex mixtures of products. The best isolated yield of 6-fluoro-7-ketocholesteryl acetate was 10%, obtained with the Collins oxidation. A dramatic improvement in yield was obtained by using a 20-fold excess of the more reactive 3,5-dimethylpyrazole-chromium trioxide reagent (18), which has been shown to be a superior reagent in the oxidation of cholesteryl benzoate (19), and extending the reaction time to 48 h (vs. 30 min with the non-fluorinated derivative). The desired keto derivative was obtained in 84% yield.

With the availability of the 7-keto derivative, two other synthetic approaches to the 7-dehydro derivative were studied. First, reduction of the methoxymethyl ether with DIBAL afforded the 7β-hydroxy derivative in 80% yield. Various pyrolytic reactions, based upon literature precedence, were investigated but only trace amounts of the desired diene were obtained. Second, the Bamford Stevens procedure developed by Cagliotti (20) was evaluated. The low reactivity of the 7-keto grouping made preparation of the intermediate tosylhydrazone difficult, the reaction requiring a large excess of tosylhydrazine and a prolonged reaction period (24 h). The crude product was obtained in 50% yield but could not be readily purified on a preparative scale; analysis of the mixture indicated about equal amounts of the *E*- and *Z*-isomers and an unidentified impurity. This crude product when allowed to react with lithium hydride in refluxing toluene yielded the desired 6-fluoro-7-dehydrocholesteryl acetate in an overall crude yield of 40% but the product was difficult to purify. All in all, this process is inferior to the approach discussed earlier.

Preliminary studies (21) of the *in vivo* biological activity of 6-F-D_3 (**7**) assessed with vitamin D deficient ducks revealed no agonist intestinal (ICA) or bone (BCM) activity. However, when 6-F-D_3 is administered with the steroid hormone, 1,25-$(OH)_2$-D_3, it serves as an ICA and BCM antagonist. This is the first vitamin D analog found to be an *in vivo* antagonist which also shows competitive *in vitro* binding to the 1,25-dihydroxy-vitamin D_3 receptor.

Acknowledgement. This study was supported by Grant No. 00709, National Institute of Arthritis, Diabetes, Digestive, and Kidney Diseases. The authors wish to express their appreciation to Dr. G. A. Boswell of the du Pont Company for all his aid, advice, and encouragement.

References and Notes

1. Recipient of Swiss National Foundation Grant No. 82-611-0-78.
2. Norman, A. W. (1979) in Vitamin D: The Calcium Homeostatic Steroid Hormone, Academic Press, New York, p. 1-490.
3. Adams, T. H., Norman, A. W. (1970) J. Biol. Chem. 245, 4421-4431.
4. Norman, A. W., Roth, J., Orci, L. (1982) Endocrine Rev. 3, 331-366.
5. For a general survey, see: (a) Ikekawa, N. (1983) Steroid Biochem. 19, 907-911. (b) Kobayashi, Y., Taguchi, T (1982) in Biomed. Aspects in Fluorine Chem., Filler, R., Kobayashi, Y., eds., Kodansha, Tokyo, Japan, p. 33-53 (Eng) (C.A. 1983, 99, 158707).
6. (a) Corrandino, R. A., DeLuca, H. F., Tanaka, Y., Ikekawa, N., Kobayashi, Y. (1980) Biochem. Biophys. Res. Commun. 96, 1800-1803. (b) Okamoto, S., Tanaka, Y., DeLuca, H. F., Kobayashi, Y., Ikekawa (1983) Am. J. Physiol. 244, E159-E163.
7. For a general review of the photochemistry in the vitamin system, see Dauben, W. G., McInnis, E. L., Michno, D. M. (1980) in Rearrangements in Ground and Excited States, deMayo, P., Ed., Academic Press, New York, Vol. 3, p. 91-129.
8. Boswell, G. A., Jr., U. S. Patent 4,212,815, 15 July, 1980 (C.A. 1980, 93, 239789).

9. Markovskij, L. N., Pashinnik, V. E., Kirsanov, A. V. (1973) Synthesis, 787-789.

10. Rappoldt, M. P., Hoogendoorn, J., Pauli, L. F. (1982) in Vitam. D: Chem., Biochem. Clin. Endocrinol. Calcium Metab., Proc. 5th Workshop Vitamin D, p. 1133-1135 (C.A. 1982, 97, 216563).

11. Still, W. C., Kahn, M., Mitra, A. (1978) J. Org. Chem. 43, 2923-2925.

12. Dauben, W. G., Phillips, R. B. (1982) J. Am. Chem. Soc. 104, 355-356.

13. Okamura, W. H., Hammond, M. L., Jacobs, H. J. C., van Thuijl, J. (1976) Tetrahedron Lett., 4807-4810.

14. Sialom, B., Mazur, Y. (1980) J. Org. Chem. 45, 2201-2204.

15. Friedman, N., Gorodetsky, M., Mazur, Y. (1971) J. Chem. Soc. Chem. Comm., 874.

16. Finucane, B. W., Thomson, J. B. (1969) J. Chem. Soc. Chem. Comm., 1220.

17. Dauben, W. G., Lorber, M., Fullerton, D. S. (1969) J. Org. Chem. 34, 3587-3592.

18. Corey, E. J., Fleet, G. W. J. (1973) Tetrahedron Lett. 45, 4499-4501.

19. Salmond, W. G., Barta, M. A., Havens, J. L. (1978) J. Org. Chem. 43, 2057-2059.

20. Caglioti, L., Grasselli, P., Maina, G. (1963) Chim. Ind. 45, 559-560.

21. Wilhelm, F., Dauben, W. G., Kohler, B., Roesle, A., Norman, A. W. (1984) Arch. Biochem. Biophys. 233, 127-132.

SYNTHESIS OF DIASTEREOMERIC 24,25-DIHYDROXYVITAMIN D_2 AND SEPARATION OF ITS (24R)- AND (24S)-ISOMERS BY A PREPARATIVE HPLC METHOD

T.Kobayashi, K.Katsumi, T.Okano, O.Miyata*, T.Naito* and I.Ninomiya*

Department of Hygienic Sciences and *Medicinal Chemistry, Kobe Women's College of Pharmacy, Higashinada-ku, Kobe 658, Japan

Diastereomeric 24,25-dihydroxyvitamin D_2 [24,25-$(OH)_2$-D_2] (I) was synthesized and its (24R)- and (24S)-isomers (Ia and Ib) was separated by a HPLC method. As shown in Chart 1, ergosterol (II) was converted into the known 20-aldehyde (IV) *via* the route involving the protection of the 5,7-diene and ozonolysis according to Barton *et al.*[1] The aldehyde (IV) was then converted to the enone (V) by the aldol condensation according to Eyley and Williams [2] in 36% yield. Methylation of (V) with MeLi afforded the methylated 24,25-glycol (VI) as a mixture of diastereomers in 60% yield, which without separation was refluxed with $LiAlH_4$ in tetrahydrofuran to afford the desired 24,25-$(OH)_2$-pro-D_2 (VII) also a mixture of diastereomers in 70% yield. UV λ_{max}: 272, 281 and 292 nm (in EtOH).

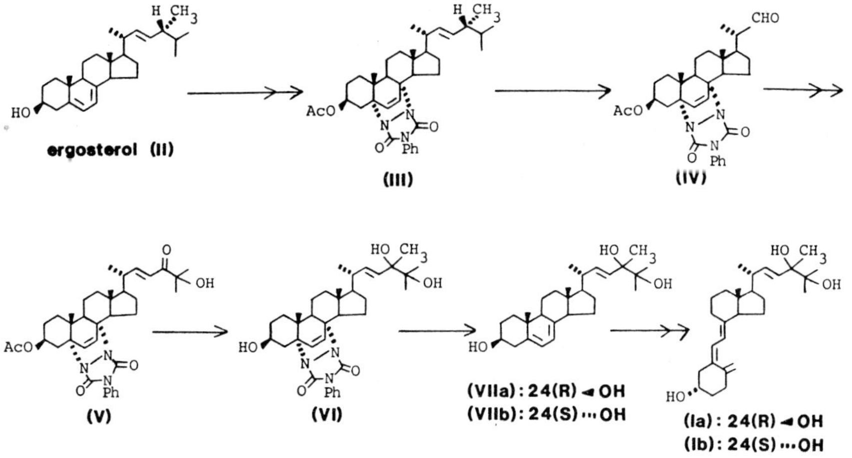

Chart 1. Our Synthetic Course of 24,25-$(OH)_2$-D_2

Vitamin D. A Chemical, Biochemical and Clinical Update

The diastereomers (VIIa and VIIb) were successfully separated one another by a HPLC method as follows: Apparatus, Shimadzu LC-3A with a UV detector (254 nm); Column, Zorbax SIL (4.6 x 250 mm); Mobile phase, 2.5% iso-PrOH in n-hexane; Flow rate, 2 ml/min. The first peak was confirmed as (24S)-24,25-$(OH)_2$-pro-D_2 (VIIb) and the second as (24R)-24,25-$(OH)_2$-pro-D_2(VIIa) by converting the respective fractions into the corresponding 24,25-$(OH)_2$-D_2 (Ib and Ia) upon UV irradiation followed by thermal isomerization. UV (in EtOH) λ_{max}: 265nm, λ_{min}: 228nm.

Synthesis of 24,25-$(OH)_2$-D_2(I) and determination of the absolute configuration of its (24R)- and (24S)-isomers (Ia and Ib) were first performed by Jones, Mazur and others.[3] The absolute configuration of our synthesized and isolated isomers was determined by co-chromatography with the respective authentic specimens kindly donated by Dr. Jones and Dr. Mazur as shown in Fig. 1. The condition of HPLC were the same as described above.

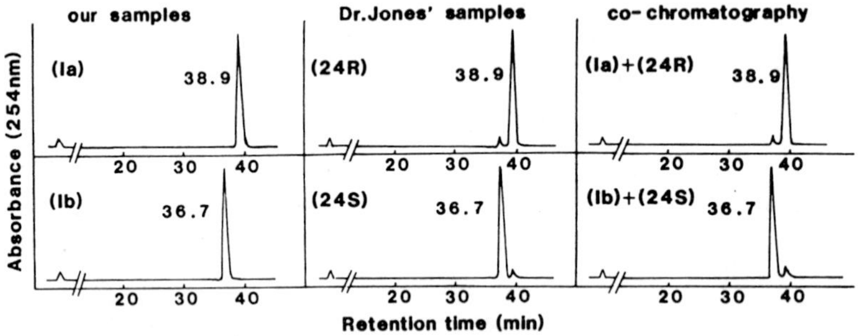

Fig. 1. Co-chromatography of Our Synthesized and Isolated Compounds (Ia and Ib) with the Authentic Samples

ACKNOWLEDGEMENT We wish to thank Dr. G. Jones of Queen's University, Canada, and Dr. Y. Mazur of the Weizmann Institute of Sciences, Israel, for their kind gift of the authentic samples and valuable advice.

REFERENCES

1) Barton,D.H.R., Shioiri,T. and Widdowson,D.A. (1971) *J. Chem. Soc. (C)*, 1971, 1968-1974.
2) Eyley,S.C. and Williams,D.H. (1976) *J. Chem. Soc., Perkin Trans. I*, 1976, 727-731.
3) Jones,G., Rosenthal,A., Segev,D., Mazur,Y., Frolow,F., Halfon, Rabinovich,D. and Shakked,Z. (1979) *Biochemistry*, 18, 1094-1101.

RECENT ADVANCES IN VITAMIN D CHEMISTRY: [1,7]-SIGMATROPIC HYDROGEN SHIFTS AND tert-BUTYL SUBSTITUTED VITAMIN D ANALOGUES.

William H. Okamura, Carl A. Hoeger, Allen D. Johnston and Antonio Mouriño
Department of Chemistry, University of California, Riverside, California 92521, USA

The current understanding (1) of the principal metabolic route leading from 7-dehydrocholesterol to 1α,25-dihydroxyvitamin D_3 [1α,25-$(OH)_2$-D_3], the active calcium regulating form of vitamin D_3, is summarized in FIG 1.

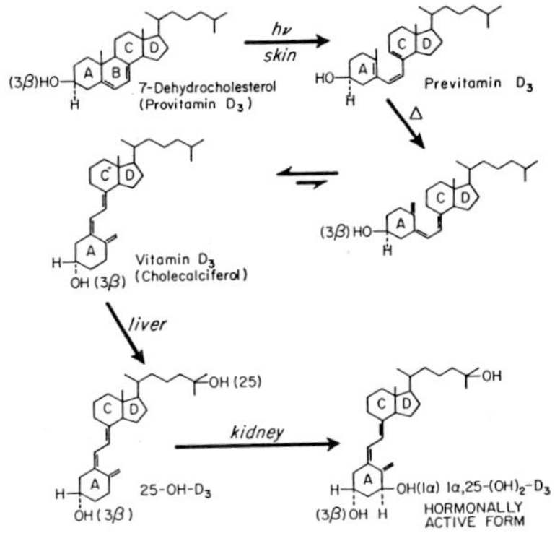

FIGURE 1. Vitamin D. Metabolism

Of great interest is the emergence of the concept that this active form of vitamin D should be considered to be a steroid hormone, analogous in terms of structure and function to the more classical systems such as estradiol, testosterone, cortisol, and aldosterone. Also of interest has been the notion that in terms of structure-function correlations, the 1α-hydroxyl group in 1α,25-$(OH)_2$-D_3 is of unusual importance (2). In this regard, our chemical synthetic studies have led to the development of the vinylallene strategy (3,4) to vitamin D (see FIG 2) wherein a

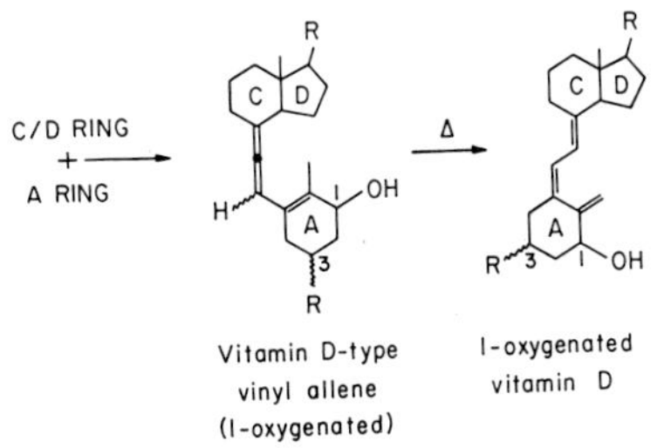

FIGURE 2. Vinylallene Synthetic Strategy

Vitamin D. A Chemical, Biochemical and Clinical Update

preformed CD fragment is coupled with a suitable A-ring fragment to afford a vinylallene, which may be thermally rearranged to the 1-hydroxylated vitamin D system.

Since the introduction of the vinylallene technology in 1978 (4a), a variety of A-ring analogues of vitamin D possessing a 1α-OH group have been synthesized (4) and these are shown in FIG 3. The most recent

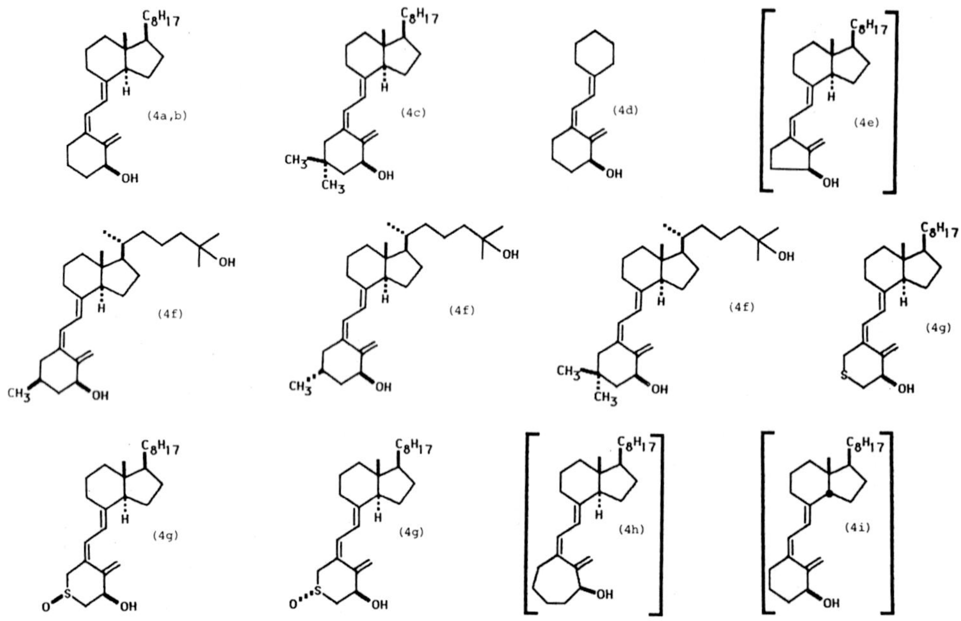

FIGURE 3. Analogues Synthesized by the Vinylallene Strategy of FIG 2. Numbers under each structure refer to literature citations at the end of this article. Structures in brackets indicate that the substance has yet to be successfully synthesized by the vinylallene scheme, although attempts were made.

application of the vinylallene scheme has led to the synthesis of several 3-tert-butyl analogues of 1-OH vitamins (FIG 4) wherein the presence of the bulky tert-butyl groups essentially locks the A-ring of the vitamin D into one chair form or the other (5). Although we cannot predict whether these analogues will possess significant biological activity, these substances will serve as stereochemical probes for further studies of the chemistry of vitamin D.

[1,7]-SIGMATROPIC SHIFTS. A more recent venture in the Riverside vitamin D efforts concerns the development of an understanding of the stereochem-

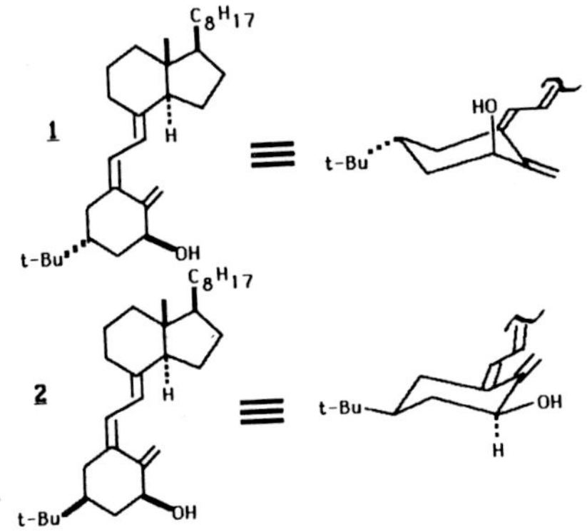

FIGURE 4. A-Ring Analogues Recently Synthesized Via Vinyl-allenes. The t-Bu group virtually locks the A-ring into a single chair form. In isomer **1**, the 1α-OH group is axial; in **2** it is equatorial.

ical details of [1,7]-sigmatropic shifts (6,7). The prototype of this process is illustrated in FIG 5 and it is important to point out that not only had the stereochemical course of this thermal reaction not been established to occur antarafacially, but this process has been of long-standing interest in the vitamin D field. Namely, the metabolic transformation of previtamin D_3 to vitamin D_3, the formal final step in the

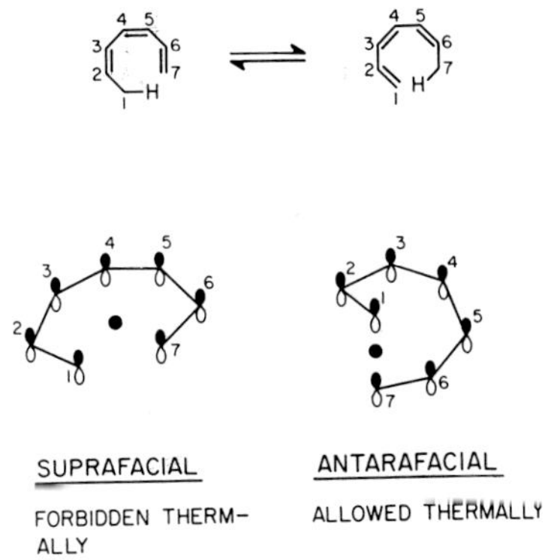

FIGURE 5. [1,7]-Sigmatropic Hydrogen Shifts

formation of vitamin D_3 in vivo, is considered to be a biological example of the [1,7]-hydrogen shift process (1d). It is not known whether this metabolic step is enzyme mediated or whether it occurs thermochemically in the absence of protein.

An imperfection in our vinylallene route (3,4) to the 1-hydroxyvitamin D system was in fact directly responsible for the emergence of our interest in delving further into [1,7]-shifts. As shown for one selected example in FIG 6, when a vinylallene of the vitamin D type (e.g., **3**) is heated at 100°C (refluxing iso-octane), two competing [1,5]-sigmatropic shifts

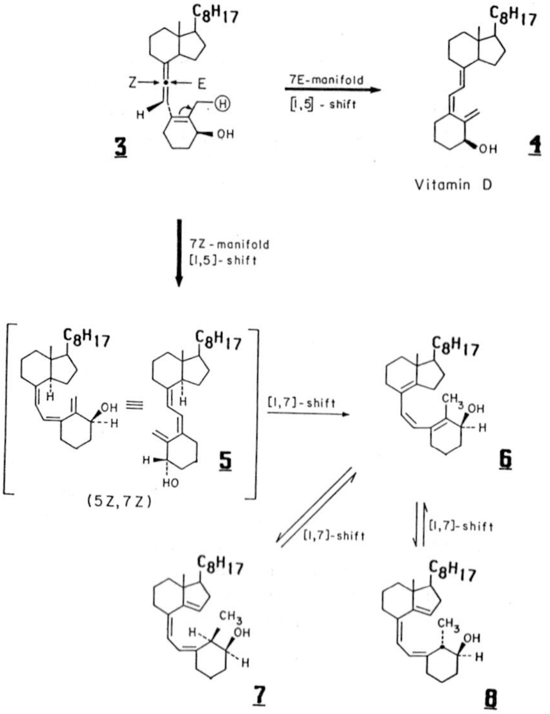

FIGURE 6. The Complete Thermal Reaction Surface During Thermolysis of a Typical Vinylallene of the Vitamin D Type. Reaction condition: refluxing isooctane, 10^{-3} M, ~10 hours.

occur. One leads to the desired vitamin D analogue **4** and this pathway is termed the E-manifold. The other pathway leads to a mixture of three vitamin D-type double bond isomers (**6**, **7** and **8**) which are believed to be formed through the intermediacy of the 7Z-geometric isomer of vitamin D (**5**) (4a,b). Although we have yet to detect the primary intermediate **5**, it was easy to show that **6**, **7** and **8** could be thermally interconverted in an equilibrium fashion via [1,7]-sigmatropic shifts. It became immediately apparent that with suitable isotopic labeling, we had serendipitously uncovered a mechanistic tool by which we could demonstrate for the first time the stereochemical course of the thermal [1,7]-shift process. Before delving into this topic, it should be mentioned that this imperfection in the vinylallene scheme, namely the occurrence of the 7Z-manifold, could be partially overcome by proper choice of stereochemistry in the vinylallene itself. FIG 7 depicts this succinctly; by utilizing the 1S,6S or 1R,6R stereoisomers of the vinylallenol, one can optimize production of the desired vitamin D chromophore (i.e., the 7E geometric isomer) during the [1,5]-sigmatropic shift of the vinylallene (4a,b).

Returning to the matter of the stereochemical course of the [1,7]-shift, an analysis of the ternary equilibrium, **7** ⇄ **6** ⇄ **8** (FIG 6), suggested, for example, a study of the corresponding stereospecifically labeled 15α-deuterio variant shown in FIG 8. If **12** were available, its thermolysis

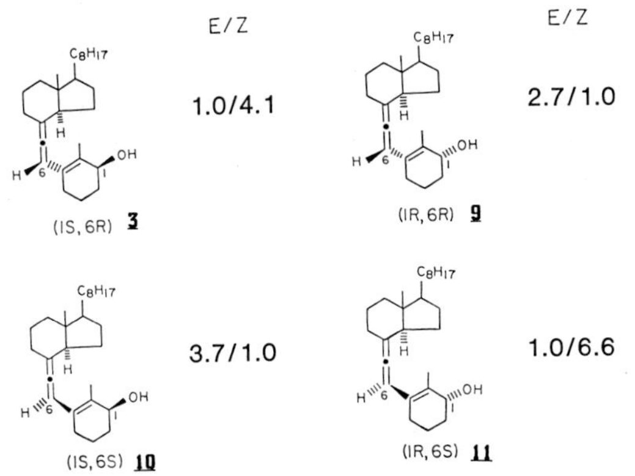

FIGURE 7. 7E vs. 7Z Manifold Ratios. The rearrangement pathway for (1S,6R)-vinyl-allene is shown in FIG 6. The E/Z ratio of 1.0/4.1 for **3** represents the ratio of products **4** to **6** + **7** + **8**. For **10**, the ratio is 3.7/1.0 for the same set of products. The corresponding products resulting from **9** and **11** are not shown, but would correspond to those shown in FIG 6 with the opposite C-1 configurations.

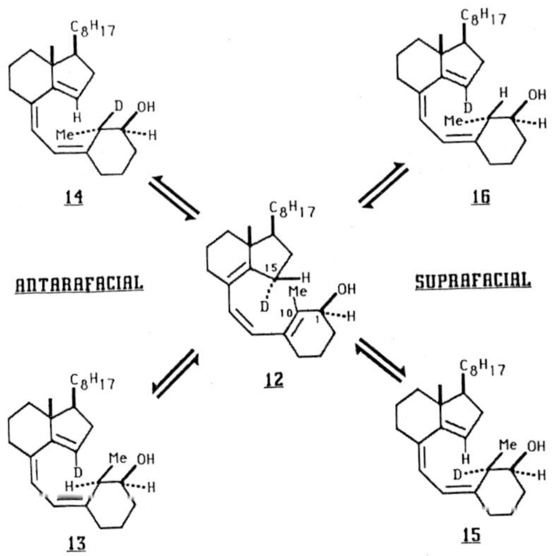

FIGURE 8. Antarafacial vs. Suprafacial Modes of Rearrangement: for the 15α-deuterated derivative of **6** (FIG 6), numbered here as **12**.

would yield only **13** and **14** for the predicted antarafacial pathway; production of **15** and **16** should result from the suprafacial pathway; a mixture of all four isomers **13** - **16** could obtain from a more complex pathway. Thus, the goal was the synthesis of **12** and its C-1-OH stereoisomer.

The strategy for synthesizing **12** (referred to below as a 6,7-<u>cis</u>-isotachysterol derivative) is depicted in FIG 9. The idea was to transform Grundmann's ketone (**21**, vide supra), the ozonolysis product of vitamin D_3, to the unsaturated ketone **17** and then to the 15α-deuterated Grund-

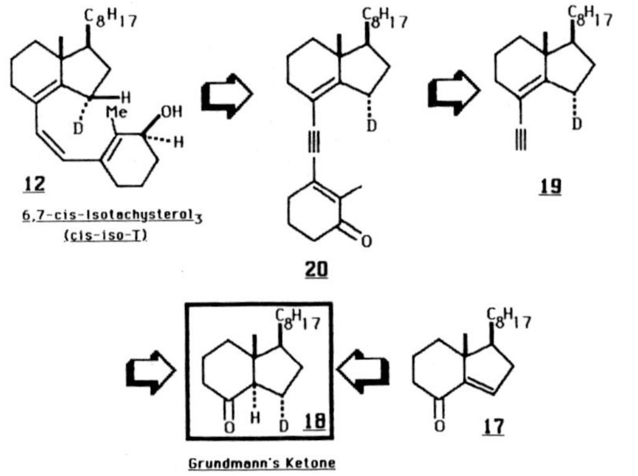

FIGURE 9. Synthetic Strategy Leading to Stereospecifically Labeled 6,7-<u>cis</u>-Isotachysterol.

mann's ketone **18** shown in FIG 9. With **18** in hand, it could be transformed by a procedure previously developed in this laboratory (4i, 5) to the labeled enyne **19** and then to the final 15α-deuterated cis-isotachysterol **12** via dienyone **20**. The transformation of Grundmann's ketone to enone **17** proceeded in a straightforward fashion as depicted in FIG 10. Of

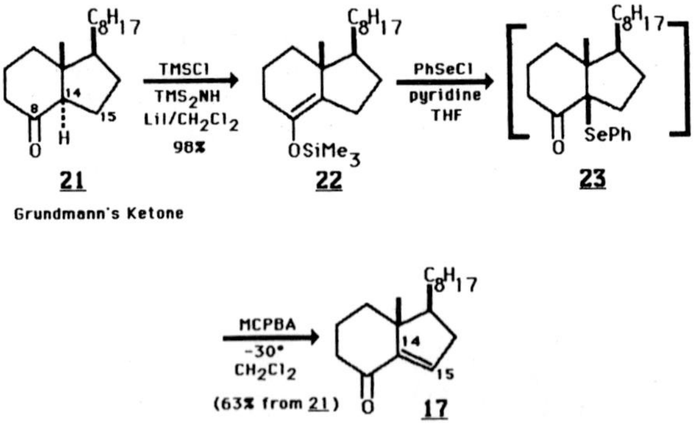

FIGURE 10. Transformation of Grundmann's Ketone 21 to Enone 17.

particular utility was a variant of Miller's trimethylsilyl iodide approach (8a) for synthesizing the thermodynamic enol silyl ether **22**. This was followed by Reich's enone sequence (8b) leading to **17**. FIG 11 outlines the first successful scheme leading to the desired 15α-deuterated enyne **19**. Because of the low yield encountered in the transformation of dihydroxyacetylene **27** to **19**, we sought an alternative procedure. Attempts to directly catalytically reduce the enone **17** with deuterium gas over a suitable catalyst not surprisingly failed. Not only did hydrogenation occur competitively from both the alpha and beta face of the double bond in **17**, but epimerization at the bridgehead C-14 occurred under the conditions of the hydrogenation. The ultimately successful route is sum-

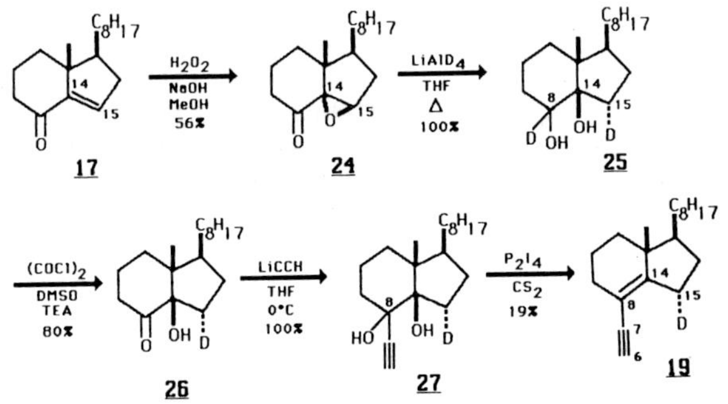

FIGURE 11. First Transformation of Enone 17 to Enyne 19.

marized in FIG 12. In two very stereochemically exceptional results, it was determined that the enone **17** could be reduced with sodium borohydride

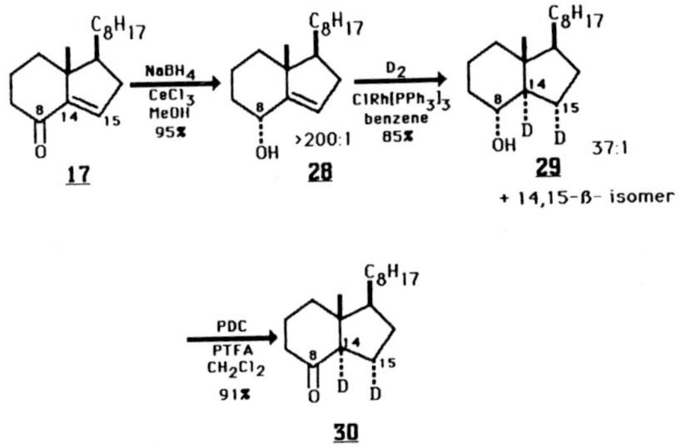

FIGURE 12. An Exceptionally Stereoselective Conversion of 17 to 14α,15α-Dideuterio-Grundmann's Ketone 30.

in the presence or absence of cerium chloride to the 8α-alcohol **28** with greater than 200:1 stereoselectivity and that the hydrogenation of **28** using deuterium gas could be directed with high selectivity from the alpha face to afford the 14α,15α-dideuterio alcohol **29**. Only a small amount of the β,β-isomer was detected. Finally, PDC oxidation afforded the desired bis-deuterated ketone **30**. As shown in FIG 13, the ketone **30** was transformed to enyne **19** (see also FIG 11) by modification of a previous procedure and then the latter was converted without incident to the penultimate trienone **32**. FIG 14 shows the completion of the desired synthetic goal, namely, the production of the easily separated mixture of the 1R and 1S <u>cis</u>-isotachysterols (**33** and **12**, respectively).

In the crucial thermolysis experiment, a 10^{-3} molar solution of the labeled 1S-isomer **12** was heated at 98.4°C in a sealed tube for 26 hours.

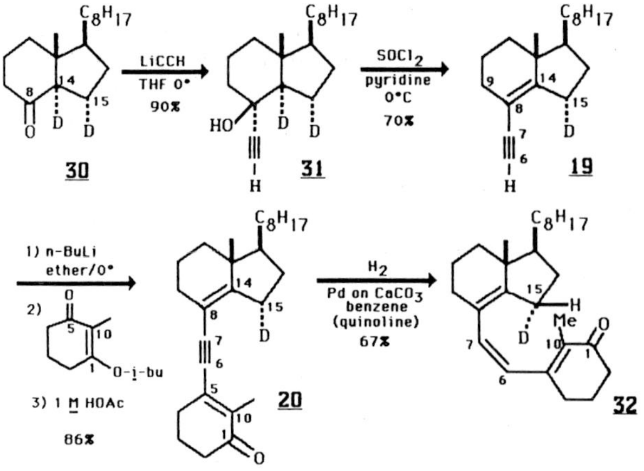

FIGURE 13. Transformation of Di-deuterated Grundmann's Ketone to 15α-Deuterated-6,7cis-isotachysterone 32.

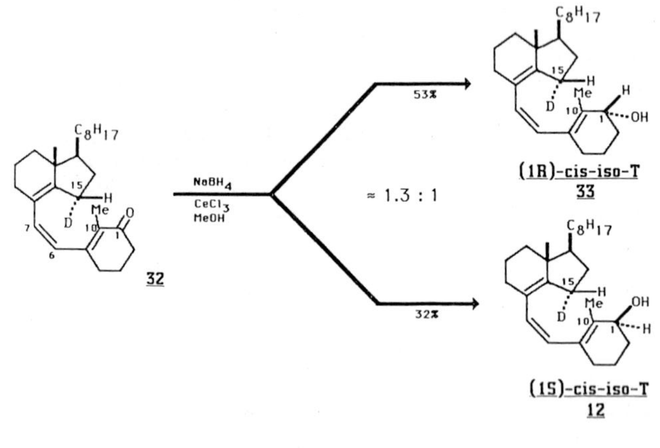

FIGURE 14. Preparation of Stereospecifically Labeled Epimeric Alcohols 12 and 33.

With respect to FIG 8, the sole products consisted of 22% **12**, 47% **14**, and 31% **13**. In short, this experiment indicates that the sole stereochemical pathway of the [1,7]-sigmatropic shift is antarafacial as predicted by the Woodward-Hoffmann rules (6). The analogous result (antarafacial path) was obtained with the corresponding 1R-epimer of compound **12**, namely **33**.

KINETIC STUDIES. With the antarafacial stereochemical pathway for the thermolysis of cis-isotacysterol systems **12** and **33** established, kinetic investigations were commenced. Such studies were of great interest in light of earlier direct investigations of the parent vitamin D_3-previtamin D_3 equilibrium pioneered by Velluz and Havinga (9), who were responsible for the characterization of the thermally labile previtamin D_3.

Akhtar and Gibbons (7d) showed through radio-labeling experiments that the [1,7]-shift of previtamin D_3 to vitamin D_3 occurs intramolecularly. More recently, in 1979, Mazur synthesized 19,19-dideutero-vitamin D_3 (FIG 15) and investigated the kinetics as well as new stereochemical details

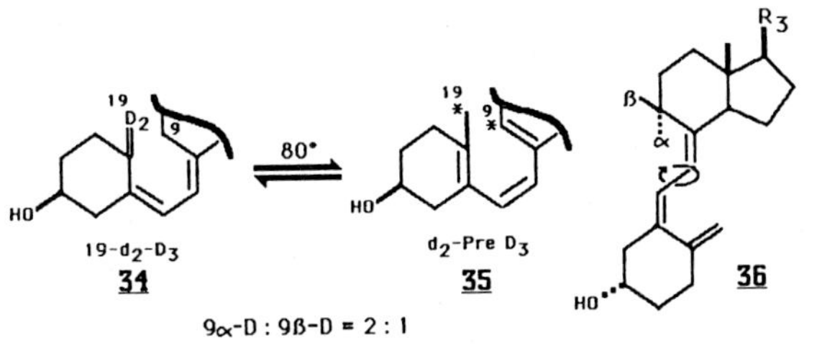

FIGURE 15. Mazur's 1979 Studies of the Vitamin D_3-Previtamin D_3 Equilibrium.

of this transformation (7c). First, they determined that the [1,7]-sigmatropic shift occurred with a k_H/k_D ratio of 45! Second, they determined that of the two helical antarafacial modes of rearrangement, migration of a 19-deuterium in previtamin D_3 to the 9α-position in vitamin D_3 occurred twice as fast as to its 9β-position.

FIGS 16 and 17 summarize the results of our preliminary kinetic investigations of the 15α-deuterated **12**, its alcohol epimer **33** and also the corresponding undeuterated materials **6** and **39**, respectively. FIG 16 reveals

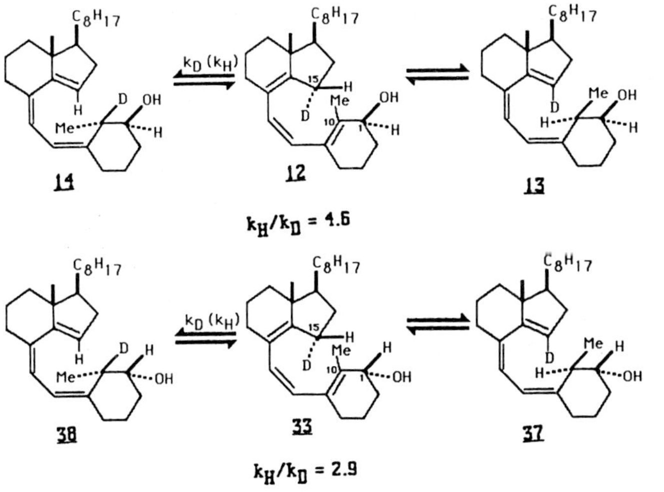

FIGURE 16. Kinetics of Rearrangement of Deuterated Cis-Isotachysterols 12 and 33. Conditions: 10^{-3} M isooctane, 98.4°± 0.1° C. Data: k, **33→37**=1.87x10^{-4}; k, **33→38**=1.25x10^{-5}; k, **12→13**=3.03x10^{-5}; k, **12→14**=3.63x10^{-5}. All rate constants are first order.

that in our case, the k_H/k_D ratio is significant (2.9 and 4.6 versus 45), but an order of magnitude smaller than that observed by Mazur for the parent previtamin D_3 case (FIG 15). FIG 17 reveals that of the two helical antarafacial modes of rearrangement of the [1,7]-sigmatropic shift,

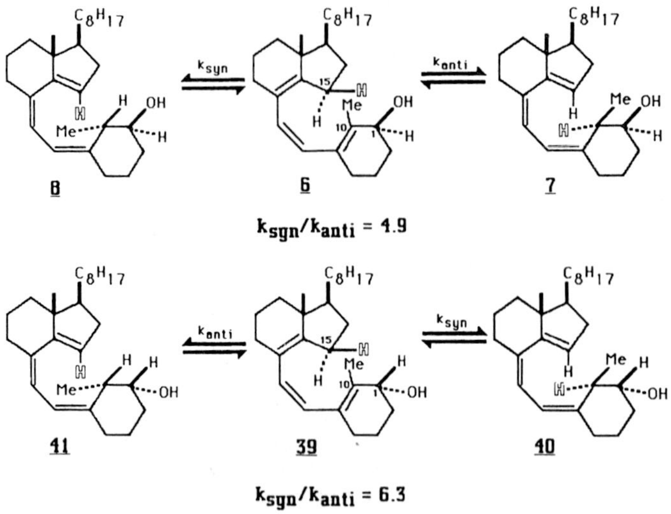

FIGURE 17. Kinetics of Rearrangement of Unlabeled Isotachysterols 6 and 39. Conditions: Same as described in the caption to FIG 16. Data: k, **39**→**40**= 2.26×10^{-4}; k, **40**→**39**=8.90×10^{-5}; k, **39**→**41**=3.61×10^{-5}; k, **41**→**39**=1.15×10^{-5}; k, **6**→**7**=3.42×10^{-5}; k, **7**→**6**=1.60×10^{-5}; k, **6**→**8**=1.68×10^{-4}; k, **8**→**6**=7.98×10^{-5}. All rate constants are first order.

the allylic hydroxyl influences the preferred helicity of rearrangement. That is, the hydrogen which leaves C-15 (in either **39** or **6**) is that which terminates at C-10 with a syn orientation with respect to the C-1 OH group. The syn/anti kinetic preference ranges from 4.9 to 6.3. By contrast, in the parent vitamin D system, Mazur's helical selectivity was smaller, approximately a factor of two (FIG 15). A more detailed analysis is in progress.

SUMMARY. In conclusion, we have demonstrated directly for the first time the antarafacial stereochemical nature of the thermal [1,7]-sigmatropic shift, consistent with theory. Preliminary kinetic studies have revealed that the primary deuterium kinetic isotope effect for the [1,7]-shift is significant for the cis-isotachysterol system, but modest compared to the value of 45 reported for the parent previtamin D-vitamin D system. Moreover, the kinetic studies reveal a significant helical preference for one of the two possible antarafacial modes of rearrangement. It remains for future experiments to develop a better understanding of the finer details of [1,7]-sigmatropic shifts, particularly in the parent vitamin D system (10).

Acknowledgment. The National Institutes of Health (USPHS Grant AM-16595) and the Intramural Committee on Resarch (UC Riverside) provided the financial support for this project. We are grateful to Dr. M. Rappoldt of Philips-Duphar (Weesp, the Netherlands) for generous gifts of the vitamins D_2 and D_3 utilized in this study.

References

(1) Reviews: (a) Norman, A.W., "Vitamin D, the Calcium Homeostatic Steroid Hormone"; Academic Press: New York, 1979; (b) DeLuca, H.F., Paaren, H.E., Schnoes, H.K., (1979) Top. Curr. Chem., 83, 1; (c) Georghiou, P.E., (1977) Chem. Soc. Rev., 6, 83; (d) Fieser, L.F., Fieser, M., "Steroids"; Reinhold: New York, 1959.

(2) For references, see: Okamura, W.H., Norman, A.W., Wing, R.M., (1974) Proc. Natl. Acad. Sci. U.S., 71, 4194-4197.

(3) Okamura, W.H., (1983) Acc. Chem. Res., 16, 81-88.

(4) (a) Hammond, M.L., Mouriño, A., Okamura, W.H., (1978) J. Am. Chem. Soc., 100, 4907-4908; (b) Condran, P., Jr., Hammond, M.L., Mouriño, A., Okamura, W.H., (1980) J. Am. Chem. Soc., 102, 6259-6267; (c) Mouriño, A., Lewicka-Piekut, S., Norman, A.W., Okamura, W.H., (1980) J. Org. Chem., 45, 4015-4020; (d) Condran, P., Jr., Okamura, W.H., (1980), J. Org. Chem., 45, 4011-4015; (e) Gerdes, J.M., Lewicka-Piekut, S., Condran, P., Jr., Okamura, W.H., (1981) J. Org. Chem., 46, 5197-5200; (f) Leyes, G.A., Okamura, W.H., (1982) J. Am. Chem. Soc., 104, 6099-6105; (g) Haces, A., Okamura, W.H., (1982) J. Am. Chem. Soc., 104, 6105-6109; (h) Gerdes, J.M., Okamura, W.H., (1983) J. Org. Chem., 48, 4030-4035; (i) Jeganathan, S., Johnston, A.D., Kuenzel, E.A., Norman, A.W., Okamura, W.H., (1984) J. Org. Chem., 49, 2152-2158.

(5) Johnston, A.D., (1983) Ph.D. Thesis, University of California, Riverside; Enas, J.D., unpublished observations.

(6) Woodward, R.B., Hoffmann, R., (1965) J. Am. Chem. Soc., 87, 2511.

(7) (a) Hoeger, C.A., Okamura, W.H., (1985) J. Am. Chem. Soc., 107, 268-270; (b) Moriarty, R.M., Paaren, H.E., (1980) Tetrahedron Lett., 21, 2389-2392; (c) Sheves, M., Berman, E., Mazur, Y., Zaretskii, Z.V.I., (1979) J. Am. Chem. Soc., 101, 1882-1883; (d) Akhtar, M., Gibbons, C.J., (1965) Tetrahedron Lett., 509-512; (e) see also, Onisko, B.L.; Schnoes, H.K.; DeLuca, H.F., (1978) J. Org. Chem., 43, 3441-3444.

(8) (a) Miller, R.D., McKean, D.R., (1979) Synthesis, 730; (b) Reich, H.J., (1979) Acc. Chem. Res., 12, 22.

(9) (a) Velluz, L., Amiard, G., Goffinet, B., (1957) Bull. Soc. Chim. Fr., 882-886; (b) Havinga, E., (1973) Experientia, 29, 1181 and references cited.

(10) For an insightful study with leading references, see: Cassis, E.G., Weiss, R.G., (1982) Photochem. Photobiol., 35, 439-444.

AN STEREOCONTROLLED SYNTHESIS OF 25-HYDROXYVITAMIN D_2 (1)

J. Sardina, A. Mouriño and L. Castedo.
Department of Organic Chemistry. Faculty of Chemistry and C.S.I.C. (Organic Chemistry Section).
R. Tojo.
Department of Pediatrics. Faculty of Medicine.
Santiago de Compostela. Spain.

Despite the many metabolic and biochemical similarities between vitamin D_2 and D_3 there are several subtle differences. One difference is the biological activity in chicks (2), which justifies a closer attention to the biological significance and metabolism vitamin D_2. A detailed and systematic study of the biochemistry of vitamin D_2 has been thwarted by the lack of significant amounts of its metabolites, especially those hydroxylated at C-25: 25-OH-D_2 (1) and 1 ,25-(OH)-D_2 (2). Thus, the need for short, stereselective and convergent syntheses of these metabolites was obvious. Herein we report on our synthesis of 25-OH-D_2.

Diol 3 was selectively tosilated (3) and then benzoylated to yield 4 which was oxidized by Kornblum's method (4) to give aldehyde 5 without noticeable epimerization at C-20 (steroidal numbering). Treatment of 5 with LiC≡C$(CH_3)_2$OMOM afforded a 1:1 mixture of 6a,b (epimers at C-22). Because only the 22R isomer was needed, we proceeded to oxidize the mixture 6a,b with PDC. Reduction of the resulting ketone 7 with a chiral reducing agent afforded 6a (selectivity 17:1). Semihydrogenation of 6a and carbamoylation of the resulting allylic alcohol gave carbamate 8. Cuprate displacement of the carbamate group of 8 transcurred stereospecifically (5) in a syn fashion to yield 9, in which the side chain of 25-OH-D_2 is fully assembled. Deprotection of the benzoate group of 9 with LAH and oxidation of the resulting alcohol gave ketone 10 which was coupled with the lithium phosphinoxycarbanion of 11 in a Wittig-Horner reaction (6). The resulting deprotected form of 25-OH-D_2 was shown to be stereochemically pure and was converted into 1 by means of a cation exchange resin.

Vitamin D. A Chemical, Biochemical and Clinical Update

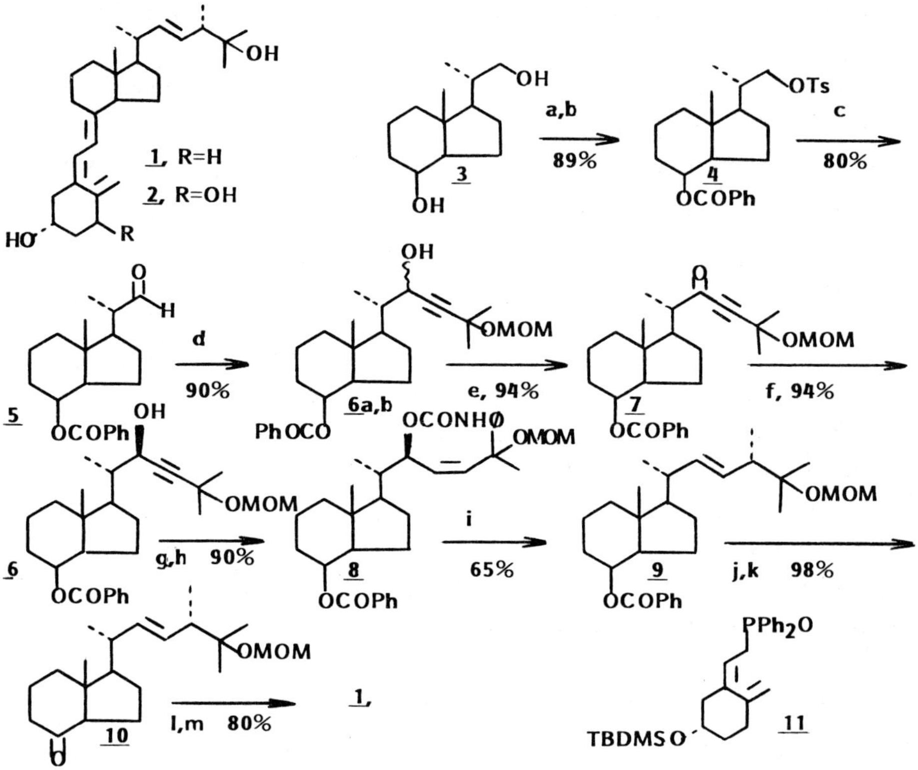

a) TsCl/Py; b) PhCOCl/DMAP-Py; c)DMSO/s-Collidine; d) LiC≡C(CH_3)$_2$OMOM,-78º/THF; e) PDC/CH_2Cl_2; f)LiAlH_4-(l-(-)-methylephedrine)-(3,5-dimethylphenol)$_2$/ether; g) H_2/Pd-BaSO_4; h) PhNCO/DMAP-Py; i) $Li_2Cu_3(CH_3)_5$; j) LiAlH_4; k) PDC; l)Anion of 11; m)AG-50W-X_4.

REFERENCES AND ACKNOWLEDGEMENTS

(1) We thank the Spanish Comisión Asesora for financial support and Hoffmann-La Roche for the generous gifts of vitamin D_2.

(2) (a) Jones, G., Schnoes, H.K., DeLuca, H.F., (1976) Biochemistry, 15, 713; (b) Hunt, R.D., García, F.G., Hedsted, D.M., (1967) Lab. Animal Care, 17, 222.

(3) Lythgoe, B., Roberts, D.A., Waterhouse, I., (1977) J.C.S. Perkin I, 2608-2612.

(4) Kornblum, N., (1959) J. Am. Chem. Soc., 81, 4113.

(5) Sardina, F.J., Mouriño, A., Castedo, L., (1983) Tetrahedron Lett., 4477-4480.

(6) Lythgoe, B., Moran, T.A., Nambudiry, M.E.N., Tideswell, J., (1978) J.C.S. Perkin I., 590-595.

ON SELECTIVE OXIDATIONS OF THE VITAMIN D_3 TRIENE SYSTEME

Wolfgang Reischl and Erich Zbiral
Department of Organic Chemistry, University of Vienna
A-1090 Vienna, Austria.

Efforts, in our laboratory, have been directed towards modifying the triene part of vitamin D_3 by reacting it with 4-phenyl-1,2,4-triazoline-3,5-dione (PTAD) (1) and SO_2 (2). In search for additional selective transformations of the triene we undertook a systematic reinvestigation of the behavior of vitamin D_3 1 towards m-chloroperbenzoic acid (MCPBA) (3) and Payne's reagent (PhCN, H_2O_2, $KHCO_3$, MeOH) (3) with the goal to establish the stereochemistry of the reaction products. The present paper discloses these results along with an additional oxidative modification method of 1 by means of N-bromo-succinimide (NBS).

Oxidation with MCPBA:
Treatment of 1 with MCPBA in chloroform results in the exclusive formation of the 7,8-mono-oxirane 2 in excellent yield. Blocking the 3-hydroxyl in 1 by an ester- or a silylgroup has no influence of the stereochemical outcome on this reaction. The 7R8R stereochemistry of the oxirane ring was established by single crystal X-ray analysis of PTAD-derivative of 2.

Oxidation with Payne's reagent:
In contrast to the method discribed above epoxidation of 1 with Payne's reagent yields exclusively the 5,6-mono-oxirane 3. Further epoxidation with the same reagent gives the 5,6-7,8-bis-oxirane 4 and the 5,6-7,8-10,19-tris-oxirane 5. The order of oxidation of the double bonds in 1 is first $\triangle$ 5, then $\triangle$7 and at last the exomethylengroup in a remarkable way. No regio- and stereoisomeres could be dedected. The stereochemistry of the oxiranes were established by X-ray analysis of the p-bromo-benzoate derivatives of 4 and 5 and is for 3 5S6R, for 4 5S6R-7R8R, and for 5 5R6R-7R8R-10S. When the 3-OH in 1 is blocked by a silylgroup the reaction looses completely regio- and stereoselectivity. Therefore we conclude a directing effect of the homoallylic C-3 hydroxyl during the epoxidation of the $\triangle$ 5 double bond with Payne's reagent. On the basis of this assumption we conclude the 5S6S stereochemistry for the epoxy isomer 6 when 5,6-trans vitamin D_3 is used as starting material in this reaction.

Oxidation with NBS:
N-bromo-succinimide adds in a stereoselective manner across the triene systeme of 1 to give 8S-hydroxy-19-bromo-9,10-seco-5,6(10)-cholestadiene-3β -ol 7a. Displacement of the C-19 bromine in this highly reactive bromohydrine with NaOAc or NaN_3 results in the clean formation of 7b and 7c respectively. The triol 7e could be generated by LAH-saponification of 7b.

Vitamin D. A Chemical, Biochemical and Clinical Update

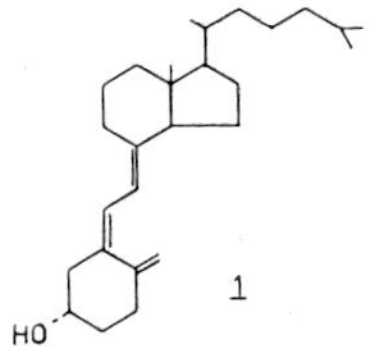
1

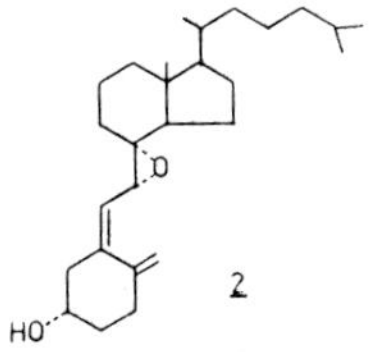
2

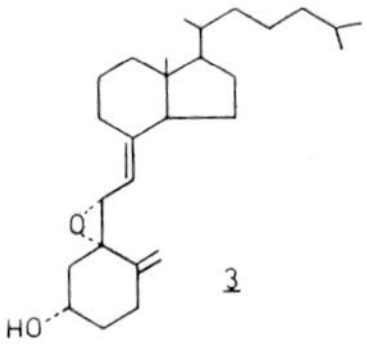
3

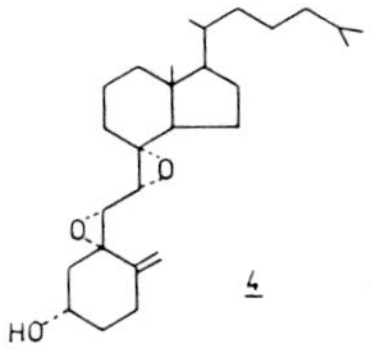
4

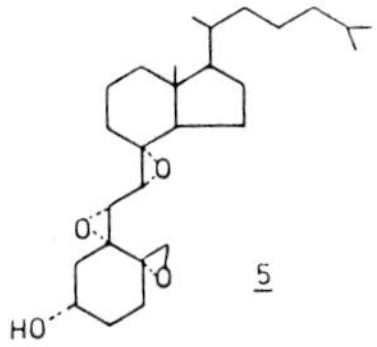
5

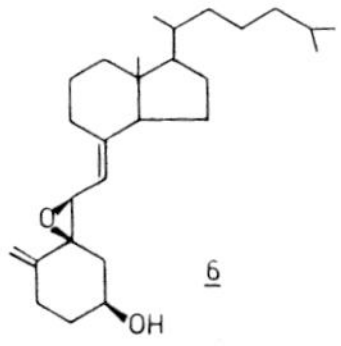
6

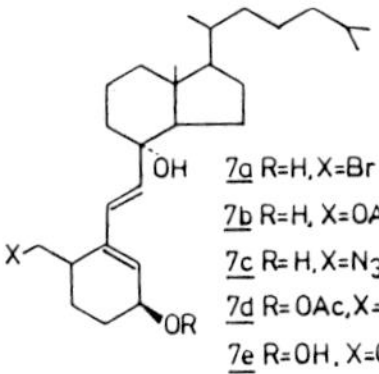
7a R=H, X=Br
7b R=H, X=OAc
7c R=H, X=N_3
7d R=OAc, X=N_3
7e R=OH, X=OH

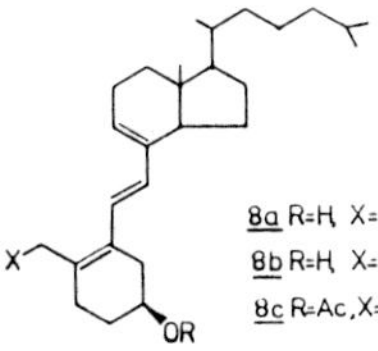
8a R=H, X=N_3
8b R=H, X=NH_2
8c R=Ac, X=NHAc

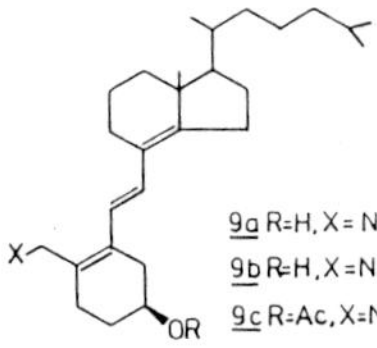
9a R=H, X=N_3
9b R=H, X=NH_2
9c R=Ac, X=NHAc

Acidic elimination of the C-8 hydroxyl results in the formation of C-19 functionalized tachysterol- and isotachysterol derivatives 8a and 9a. The utility of this method was demonstrated by synthesizing 19-acetamidotachysterol 8c and 19-acetamidoisotachysterol 9c via LAH reduction of 8a and 9a and subsequent acetylation.

Acknowledgement: Financial support to this project was provided by the Hochschuljubilaeumsstiftung der Stadt Wien. We are indebted to Drs. H.Bernhard and C.Kratky, Department of Physical Chemistry, University of Graz for the X-ray structure determinations and Hoffmann-La Roche AG, Basel for generous gifts of vitamin D_3.

References:

(1) Reischl,W. and Zbiral,E. Liebigs Ann.Chem. 1978, 745
Reischl,W. and Zbiral,E. Helv.Chim.Acta 63, 860 (1980)
(2) Reischl,W. and Zbiral,E. Helv.Chim.Acta 62, 1763 (1979)
Reischl,W. and Zbiral,E. Monatsh.Chem. 110, 1463 (1979)
(3) Velluz,L., Amiard,G. and Goffinet,B. Bull.Soc.Chim. 1955, 1341
Baron,Ch. and Didallier,J. Bull.Soc.Chim. 1959, 1330
Le Boulch,N., Raoul,Y. and Ourisson,G. Bull.Soc.Chim. 1964, 647
Le Boulch,N., Raoul,Y. and Ourisson,G. Bull.Soc.Chim. 1967, 2413

A SIMPLE ENTRY TO 25-KETODERIVATIVES OF VITAMIN D. A NEW ROUTE TO RADIO-LABELLED VITAMIN D METABOLITES AND ANALOGUES(1)

B. Fernandez, J.L. Mascareñas, M.C. Pumar, M.J. Vila, A. Mouriño, and L. Castedo.

Department of Organic Chemistry. Faculty of Chemistry and C.S.I.C. (Organic Chemistry Section). Santiago. Spain.

The chemistry and biochemistry of vitamin D have advanced considerably since the discovery of 1,25-dihydroxyvitamin D_3 as the hormonally active form of vitamin D_3. In fact, this metabolite and 25-hydroxyvitamin D_3 are now currently used clinically in the treatment of several bone diseases (2). Our efforts in this area have centered on developing both an effective and a general approach to isotopically unlabelled and labelled vitamin D metabolites and several other analogues.

In this work we selected 25-ketoderivatives as key compounds since they may be easily labelled and also converted into derivatives variously hydroxylated on the side chain at several carbon atoms. Our synthesis (Fig. 1), starts from vitamin D_2 (1). Hydroxylation of 1 according to published procedures ($KMnO_4$/EtOH,-20º)(3), produced the triol 2 (65%), which was subjected to selective protection (ClTIPS/Imidazole-DMF), to give the diol 3 (85%). Lead tetraacetate cleavage in dry methylene chloride (4), followed by reduction with Red-Al afforded cleanly 4 (96%) and 5 (95%). Side chain cleavage of the protected alcohol 4 when treated with ozone in methanol-pyridine followed by in situ sodium borohydride reduction gave the alcohol 6 (87%) which was converted into the iodide 7 following standard procedures (p-TsCl/Py; NaI/Acetone, 94%). The key coupling between the latter and the silylated unsaturated ketone 8 was accomplished in one pot reaction as follows: metallation of iodide 7 (t-BuLi/ether/-78º, 2 equiv) followed by the addition of Corey's copper-I reagent (5) led to the formation of the mixed copper intermediate 9 (6) which in turn was treated with the silylated ketone 8 to generate finally 10. One pot removal of the silyl groups (HF/Acetonitrile) followed by carbonyl protection (MED/p-TsOH) gave 11 (60% overall yield from 7) which was oxidized with pyridinium dichromate (7) to afford the key ketone 12 (90%). Introduction of the triene system was achieved using the well documented Wittig Horner reaction between the carbanion of 14 and 12 (8). The alcohol 5 was converted into the chloride 13 and this into 14 by known procedures (NCS/SMe_2/CH_2Cl_2-DMF, 94%; Ph_2PLi/THF/H_2O_2, 65%) (8). Dropwise addition of ketone 12 to a slight excess of the lithium phosphinoxycarbanion obtained from 14 on treatment with n-BuLi, afforded the desired protected 25-ketoderivative 15 (93%). As an example of the versatility of this approach, 15 was easily transformed into 25-hydroxyvitamin D_3 (FH/MeCN, cation exchange resin (9), MeLi, 75%). (The overall yield from vitamin D_2 was 16%).

Fig.1

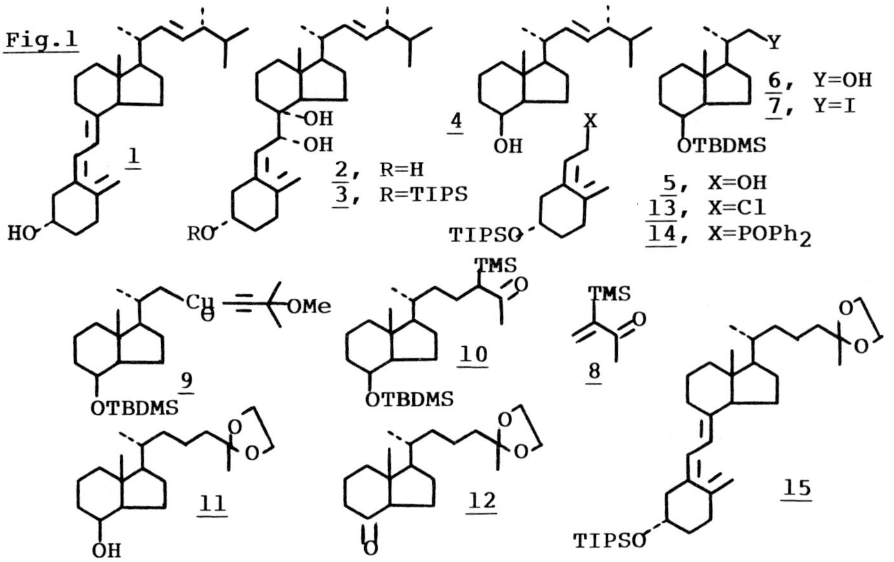

(1) We thank the Spanish Comisión Asesora for financial support and Hoffmann-La Roche (Basel) for the generous gift of vitamin D_2.

(2) For general reviews on vitamin D, see: (a) Norman, A.W., "Vitamin D, the Calcium Homeostatic Steroid Hormone"; Academic Press: New York, 1979; (b) Norman, A.W., "Vitamin D, Molecular Biology and Clinical Nutrition"; Marcel Dekker: New York, 1980; (c) DeLuca, H.F., Paaren, H.E., Schnoes, H.K., (1979) Top. Curr. Chem., 83, 1; (d) Jones, H., Rasmusson, G.H., (1980) Progress in the Chemistry of Organic Natural Products, 39, 63-121; (e) Georghiou, P.E., (1977) Chem. Soc. Rev., 6, 83-107; (f) Lythgoe, B.,(1980) Chem. Soc. Rev., 9, 449-474.

(3) Toh, H.T., Okamura, W.H., (1983) J. Org. Chem., 48, 1414-1417 and references therein.

(4) Corey, E.J., Iguchi, S., Albright, J.O., Do, B., (1983) Tetrahedron Lett.,24, 37-40.

(5) Corey, E.J., Floyd, D., Lipshutz, B.H., (1978) J. Org. Chem., 43, 3418-3420.

(6) The structure in solution of mixed copper reagents has not been fully established.

(7) Corey, E.J., Schmidt, G., (1979) Tetrahedron Lett., 399-402.

(8) Baggiolini, E.G., Iacobelli, J.A., Hennessy, B.M., Uskoković, M.R., (1982) J. Am. Chem. Soc., 104, 2945-2948 and references therein.

(9) Wovkulich, P.M., Barcelos, F., Batcho, A.D., Sereno, J.F., Baggiolini, E.G., Hennessy, B.M., Uskoković, M.R., (1984) Tetrahedron, 48, 2283-2296

HYDROTITANATION-PROTONATION OF VITAMIN D_2 A SIMPLE ENTRY TO DIHYDROVITAMINS D_2(1)

L. Castedo, J.G. Cota, M.C. Meilán, A. Mouriño and R. Tojo.

Departments of Organic Chemistry and Pediatrics, and C.S.I.C.(Organic Chesmistry Section).

University of Santiago de Compostela. Spain.

Among several dihydrovitamins D_2 (3,4,Fig.1), dihydrotachystero$_2$ (4b,DHT_2) has attracted much attention due to its high biological activity. In fact, this compound is used clinically in many countries to treat a variety of vitamin D related diseases (2). In the past, much effort has been put into the syntheses of DHT_2 and related dihydrovitamins D although without much success due in part to the sensitivity of the triene system of starting materials and also to complicated reaction mixtures (2c). In fact, it was not until 1978 that their definitive stereochemistries were fully established (3). In spite of recent work in this area, yields in DHT from 5,6-trans-D_2 are still low: (i) hydroboration-protonation (6%)(5); (ii) rhodium-catalyzed hydrogenation (34%)(3,5) and (iii) hydrozirconation-protonation (36%)(6). The possibility of improving yields in DHT_2 and other recent features (7), led us to consider this area an issue of major concern.

Titanocene dichloride (Cp_2TiCl_2) was chosen for this study because it works well in the catalytic hydrometallation of simple alkenes (8). Table I, shows the most representative results of vitamin D_2 and 5,6-trans-D_2 with Cp_2TiCl_2-LAH or Cp_2TiCl_2-Red-Al, in THF. In all cases overall yields higher than 95% were obtained. Under catalytic conditions (entry 5), the reaction was very slow. The reaction rate was substantially increased however by increasing the amount of transitium metal halide. Interestingly, the stereoselectivity is reversed on changing from Red-Al to LAH. In an attempt to understand these results, protected-D_2 and 5,6-trans-D_2 were subjected to the same reaction conditions (entries 8,9,10), but no appreciable stereoselectivity was observed. These results are explained in terms of a hydroxy-assisted pathway by coordination with Ti or Al when LAH is used as the hydride source. However, this pathway may be blocked to some extent when Red-Al is used. In order to extend this procedure to the preparation of labelled dihydrovitamins D and other 19-derivatives, and to study the reaction mechanism further we proceeded to carry out deuteration experiments. Some preliminary results are presented in Table I (entries 3,4,5,7). When the catalytic hydrometallation reaction was quenched with D_2O, the reaction products contained low percent deuterium according to mass spectral analysis. Under usual conditions, the deuterium incorporation rose to approximately 70%. Longer reaction times (entry 4), showed substantial decrease in deuteration, but approximately the same reaction product ratio. These results indicate that no equilibration occurs between hydrometallated intermediates during the reaction course. The substantial amount of reduction products noted at the initial stages of the reaction after deuteration may be due to hydrogenolysis of C-Metal bonds or reaction of them with hydride species.

Although these studies are currently under investigation to increase the percent deuterium incorporation, it is clear that an operationally simple route to various dihydrovitamins D is now available. This method is highly recommended for the rapid preparation of DHT_2 (9).

Vitamin D. A Chemical, Biochemical and Clinical Update

FIG.1

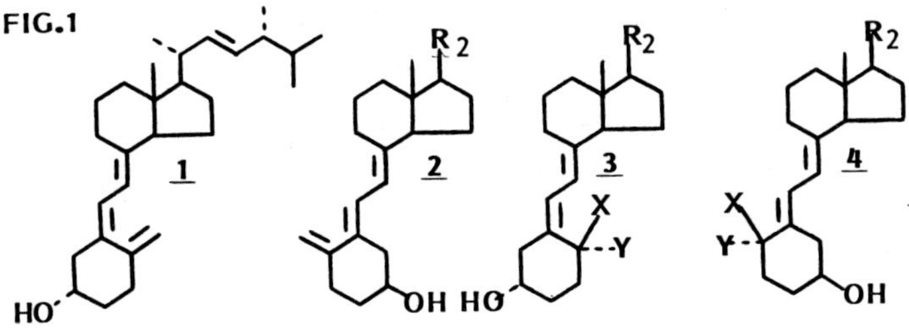

a, X=Me, Y=H
b, X=H, Y=Me

TABLE I

	S:Ti:H-Al	Molar ratio (Time, hrs)	% Yield (Deuteration) 3a	3b	4a	4b	No.Exp.
1)	1:Ti:Red-Al	1:2:4 (1½)	20	80	—	—	4
2)	1:Ti:Red-Al	1:2:4 (4½)	40	60	—	—	2
3)	1:Ti:LAH	1:2:2 (2½)	85(72)	15(68)	—	—	5
4)	1:Ti:LAH	1:2:2 (50)	80(45)	20(40)	—	—	1
5)	1:Ti:LAH	1:0.5:2 (55)	50(20)	50(13)	—	—	3
6)	2:Ti:Red-Al	1:2:4 (1½)	—	—	30	70	2
7)	2:Ti:LAH	1:2:2 (2)	—	—	10(40)	90(50)	5
8)	1-OR:Ti:Red-Al	1:2:3 (2)	40	60	—	—	2
9)	1-OR:Ti:LAH	1:2:1.7 (2)	40	60	—	—	2
10)	2-OR:Ti:LAH	1:2:1.7 (2)	—	—	60	40	1

S:D_2 or 5,6-t-D_2. H-Al: Aluminum hydride. LAH: $LiAlH_4$. Ti:Cp_2TiCl_2, R=TBDMS, Red-Al=$NaAlH_2(OCH_2CH_2OCH_3)_2$."Ti" was added to a solution of substrate/H-Al.

REFERENCES AND ACKOWLEDGEMENTS

(1) We thank the Spanish Comisión Asesora for financial support and Hoffmann-La Roche (Basel) for generous gifts of vitamin D_2.

(2) (a) Norman,A.W.,(1979)"Vitamin D, the Calcium Homeostatic Steroid Hormone"; Academic Press; (b) Holick,M.F., DeLuca,H.F.,(1974)Advances in Steroid Biochemistry",4; (c) Lawson,D.E.M., (1978)"VitaminD", Academic Press; (d) Bosch,R., Duursma,S.A.,(1982)"Vitamin D, Chemical, Biochemical and Clinical Endocrinology of Calcium Metabolism", Walter de Gruyter & Co, 1141-1143; (e) Kage,M., Chatterjee,G., Cohen,G.F.,(1970)Ann. Intern. Med., 4194-4197.

(3) Mouriño,A., Okamura,W.H.,(1978) J. Org. Chem., 43, 1653-1655.

(4) Okamura,W.H., Hammond,M.L., Rego,A., Norman.,A.W. Wing,R.M., (1977) J. Org. Chem., 42, 2284-2291.

(5) Barret,A.G.M., Barton,D.H.R., Russell,R.A., Widdwson,D.A.,(1977) J.C.S. Perkin I, 631-643.

(6) Messing,A.W., Ross,F.P., Norman,A.W., Okamura,W.H.,(1978) Tetrahedron Lett., 3635-3636.

(7) (X=CH_2OH) in the vitamin D_3 series, has shown antivitamin D_3 properties (2a). 19-vitamin D derivatives have been recently prepared to generate anti-bodies for radioimmunoassay (Yamada,S., Suzuki,T., Takayama,H., (1983) J.Org.Chem., 48, 3483-3488). The physiological mode of action was reported to be unknown (2d).

(8) (a) Ashby,E.C., Noding,A., (1980)J.Org.Chem., 45, 1035-1041; (b) Isasawa,K., Tatsumi,K., Otsuji,Y., (1977)Chem. Lett., 1117-1120, and ref. therein.

(9) When 1g. of 5,6-trans-D_2 was used a 65% yield in DHT_2 could be obtained by crystallization of the crude reaction mixture.

IS FLUORINE A BIOLOGICALLY BENIGN REPLACEMENT FOR HYDROGEN IN VITAMIN D ANALOGS

F. P. Ross, Dept. Biochem., Univ. Calif., Riverside, CA 92521, USA.

The use of fluorine insertion to alter selectively the biological activity of steroid hormones is a subject about twenty-five years old which has produced drugs of major clinical importance. Vitamin D analogs labelled with fluorine have been synthesized only during the last seven years. In contrast to the other steroid hormones the explicit purpose of the fluoro-vitamin D derivatives was to block hydroxylation at strategic sites. During these studies interesting results appeared as to the biological activity of these compounds. The interpretation of these results assumed that (i) fluorine behaves like hydrogen, (ii) the C-F bond is stable, and (iii) that the presence of fluorine has no effect on the biological properties of the molecule into which it is inserted. It is the purpose of this paper to review very briefly the chemistry of organic fluorine, to highlight some recent findings on the metabolism of organofluorine compounds and to assess critically the results obtained using fluorine containing vitamin D analogs. An excellent monograph covering many aspects of carbon-fluorine bio-organic chemistry has been published(1).

Some salient physico-chemical features of fluorine and related elements and functional groups are given in Table 1. On the one hand its small size and the strength of the C-F bond has led this element to be considered close to H in its reactivity. However its high electronegativity and electronic structure (it is iso-electronic with -OH) means that, unlike other halogens, it has the potential for acting as an acceptor in hydrogen bonding as shown in Fig. 1. It cannot exhibit the possible dual functions in this regard as shown for -OH. Direct evidence for such bond formation is limited but has been deduced from ^{19}F NMR analysis of the binding of trifluoroacetylated chitotriose to lysozyme (2) and from the x-ray structures of erythyritol and 2-deoxy-2-fluoroerythritol (3). More indirectly, glucose containing fluorine at C-3 in place of -OH appears to be actively transported when the 3-deoxy derivative is not (4).

Table 1

Selected Properties of Elements/Groups Related to Fluorine

	Bond Length	Vander Waals Radius	Electronegativity
H	1.09	1.20	2.1
F	1.39	1.35	4.0
OH	1.43	1.40	3.5
CF_3	-	2.44	-

Vitamin D. A Chemical, Biochemical and Clinical Update

```
PROTEIN —— X-H - - - - - - - - - - F ———
                                   H
PROTEIN —— XH  - - - - - - - - - - O ———

PROTEIN —— X - - - - - - - - - H — O ——
```

Fig. 1. Model of possible hydrogen bonding by fluorine and oxygen.

In a like manner the belief that C-F bonds are not readily cleavable is without both theoretical and experimental support. A consideration of thermodynamic parameters shows that the C-F bond, although of high bond energy, is thermodynamically unstable to hydrolysis (5). This reaction has been shown to occur in a variety of bacterial systems (6). Recently rodent liver has been shown to de-active the poison fluoroacetate (7,8). The mechanism probably involves displacement F via a thiol intermediate, which is itself subsequently reduced.

The Biological Activity of Fluoro Steroids

This area is the subject of an excellent review (9). Once again the picture is not as simple as first seems. In summary fluorine has been inserted at a number of positions in the steroid ring, usually vicinal to an oxygen function, most often -OH. In the case of the glucocorticoids, a given fluorine analog often produced differential augmentation of the three major effects; glycogenesis, anti-inflammation and sodium retention.

The suggested mode of action of fluorine is largely via its inductive effect. This increases the acidity and putatively the binding to the receptor of the adjacent oxygen function. However this cannot be the full explanation since, for example, 9α fluoro cortexone acetate which does not contain the usual C-11 OH, has much enhanced mineralocorticoid but not glucocorticoid activity (9). Such results speak of more complex mechanisms including one in which fluorine may be behaving like oxygen. Full understanding awaits the isolation and comparison of receptors from different tissues in the same animal. Even this may not give the answer since such experiments remove the receptor from the possible influence of possible local regulators.

In the absence of both purified receptor and suitable radio-labelled photoaffinity probes the nature of the receptor binding site for 1,25-dihydroxyvitamin D_3 is totally unknown. As a model it can be envisaged that attachment is directed largely by the three hydroxyl groups situated at the terminal ends of the molecule (Fig. 2). The role of fluorine would thus depend on (i) the position of insertion and (ii) the ability of the inserted molecule to modulate binding. From a steric standpoint the size of the atom (Table 1) would ensure minimal interference. The main feature is therefore likely to be the ability of fluorine to act like hydrogen or hydroxyl. The only other direct evidence in this regard apart from that reviewed below concerns studies on a range of side chain hydroxylated analogs of cholesterol as substrates for the adrenal side chain cleavage system (10). Of 34 substrates tested the three shown in Figure 3 were among the best. Both 25-hydroxy- and 25-fluoro-cholesterol were about 40% as effective as the natural precursor for cleavage. This suggests that fluorine is acting here like a hydroxyl group.

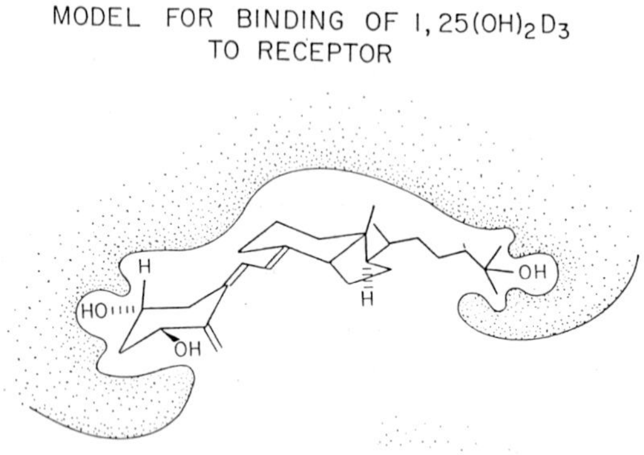

Fig. 2.

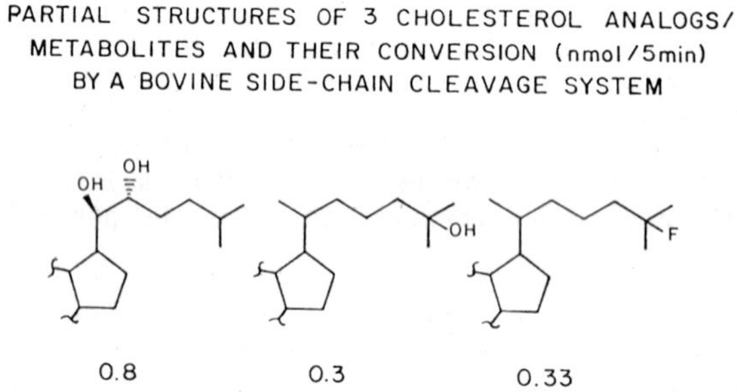

Fig. 3.

Fluorinated Vitamin D Analogs

Fluorine has been introduced at six different positions in the vitamin D molecule viz. 1,2, 6, 24, 25 and 26/27 as seen in Fig. 4. An examination of the activity of the various derivatives allows no simple conclusion as to the effects of fluorine substitution. In summary, as with other steroid hormones, the effect is somewhat site dependent. A brief summary of the reactivity of the various fluoro compounds follows. A review of some aspects of this work has been published (11).

25 Fluoro Compounds

In these compounds fluorine appears to be indistinguishable from hydrogen. Both 1α-hydroxy-25-fluorovitamin D_3 and 24R-hydroxy-25-fluorovitamin D_3 have been tested *in vivo* and *in vitro* for biological activity (12-14). The compounds were between 300 and 500 fold less effective than 1,25-dihydroxyvitamin D_3 in binding to chick intestinal receptor, values similar to that obtained for their non-fluorinated analogs. *In vivo* their activity as measured in several assays in the rat was considerably higher. Evidence has been presented that both compounds can undergo hydroxylation at the appropriate position to give 1α,24R-dihydroxy-25-fluorovitamin D_3 (15), a compound with binding ability for the chick intestinal receptor similar to that of 1,25-dihydroxyvitamin D_3.

24,24 Difluoro Compounds

In contrast the introduction of fluorine at C24 alters both the chemical and biological properties of the relevant molecules. The original report on the biological activity of 24,24-F_2-25-hydroxyvitamin D_3 suggested that it was equal to or better than 25-hydroxyvitamin D_3 *in vivo* studies in the rat (16,17). These authors also converted the same analog *in vitro* to the 1α-hydroxylated form. Both compounds are less polar on HPLC than their non-fluorinated analogs (18). This is particularly true for 24,24-F_2-25-hydroxyvitamin D (29 vs 41 ml on Zorbax-sil 4.6 X 250 mm column eluted with 3% isopropanol in hexane). One possible explanation is that the vicinal fluorine atoms are forming hydrogen bonds with the 25 hydroxyl group, decreasing its interaction with the column matrix. A precedent is found in the lower polarity of 24,25-dihydroxyvitamin D_3 as compared with 1,25-dihydroxyvitamin D_3.

In binding to chick intestinal receptor the parent compound 24,24-difluoro-25-hydroxyvitamin D_3 is about 6 fold more potent than 25-hydroxyvitamin D_3 and about 25 fold more so than 24,25-dihydroxyvitamin D_3. Both 1,25-dihydroxyvitamin D_3 and its 24,24-difluoro analog are equipotent in this assay and about 10 fold more active than 1,24,25-trihydroxyvitamin D_3 (19). Clearly the fluoro atoms are having effects which defy simple explanaton. However, as a generalization the presence of the 1α-hydroxyl group is dominant in controlling binding to the receptor and thus may mask more subtle effects of fluorine. The *in vivo* results for both difluoro compounds demonstrate a greater potency than 1,25-dihydroxyvitamin D_3. This represents the first report of a compound in the vitamin D series more active than the natural hormone.

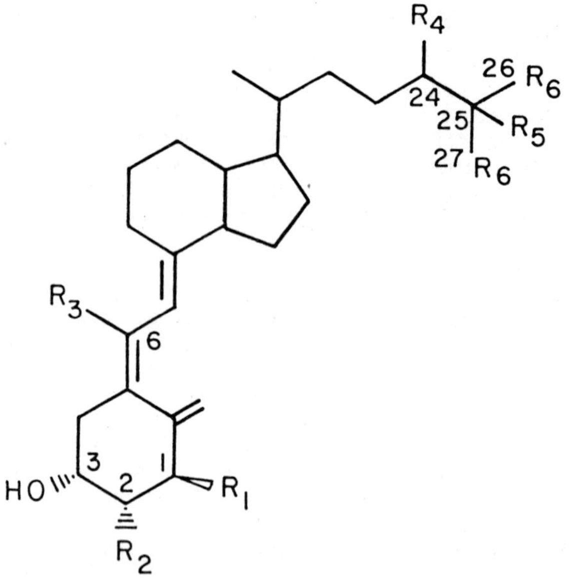

COMPOUND	R_1	R_2	R_3	R_4	R_5	R_6
I	OH	H	H	H	OH	CH_3
II	F	H	H	H	H	CH_3
III	F	H	H	H	F	CH_3
IV	H	H	H	H	F	CH_3
V	H	H	H	OH(<u>R</u>)	F	CH_3
VI	H	H	H	F_2	OH	CH_3
VII	OH	H	H	F_2	OH	CH_3
VIII	H	H	H	H	OH	CF_3
IX	OH	H	H	H	OH	CF_3
X	H	H	F	H	H	CH_3
XI	OH	F	H	H	H	CH_3

Although it is tempting to suggest altered pharmacokinetics as the mechanism, this hypothesis remains to be tested, e.g. by measuring serum levels of the hormone following a single dose.

Hexafluoro Derivatives

As an extension of earlier work the same group synthesized and assayed 25-hydroxy-26,26,26,27,27,27-hexafluorovitamin D_3. This compound was again equipotent with 25-hydroxyvitamin D_3 in *in vivo* assays in the rat (20). Once metabolized to the 1α-hydroxy derivative it once again showed altered chemical and biological properties. On Sephadex LH-20 chromatography the dihydroxy analog behaved as a molecule more polar than all other dihydroxy metabolites, being retained. Here it is possible that the two trifluoromethyl groups act somewhat in an hydroxyl-like manner, but now interact more with the column matrix. The compound binds less avidly to the chick intestinal receptor but once again displays increased biopotency in assays in the rat. Significantly the activity of synthetic 26,26,26,27,27,27-hexafluoro-1,25-dihydroxyvitamin D_3 is about 10 times greater than that of 1,25-dihydroxyvitamin D_3 and is also more long lasting, suggesting that altered pharmacokinetics may indeed play a role (21). If this is so it suggests that 26-hydroxylation may be a major pathway of inactivation of 1,25-dihydroxyvitamin D_3.

A-Ring Analogs

Three compounds with fluorine in the A-ring have been synthesized and tested. In concordance with other work in the steroid field 2β-fluoro-1α-hydroxyvitamin D_3 is more potent that the parent compound, presumably after hydroxylation at C-25 (22).

The picture of 1-fluoro-substitution is less clear. 1α,25-difluorovitamin D_3 is a compound completely inert in the rat, displaying neither hormone nor anti-hormone activities (23). In contrast 1-fluorovitamin D_3 is surprisingly active being only 15 fold less active than vitamin D_3 in BCM and 100 fold less active in ICA when measured in the rat (24). Since the active form is presumably 25 hydroxylated the question arises as to whether or not hydroxylation has occurred at C1. It has been suggested that, since the time course of activity of this compound is similar to that of vitamin D, hydroxylation has occurred both at C-25 and possibly elsewhere. An alternative hypothesis is that the 1-fluoro compound is a poor substrate for the 25-hydroxylase and that the fluorine is behaving as a 'weak' hydroxyl group.

Two problems arise with all the above results: Firstly, there is the species difference between the *in vitro* bioassay system (chick intestinal mucosa) and that used for *in vivo* studies (the rat). These species show significantly different sensitivity to vitamin D_2 and D_3. This can be ascribed to differences in receptor binding and/or metabolism of the two forms. In this regard it has been shown that the rat, when presented with equimolar amounts of vitamins D_2 and D_3 preferentially metabolizes vitamin D_2 as undexed by serum levels of the two 25 hydroxy derivations (25); Secondly, the failure to use as a control the appropriate levels of 24,25-dihydroxyvitamin D_3 renders direct, meaningful comparison very difficult, if not impossible.

Undoubtedly the most interesting compound to be synthesized is 6-fluorovitamin D_3. This compound shows in vitro binding to the chick intestinal receptor somewhat greater than that of 25-hydroxyvitamin D_3 but less than 1α-hydroxyvitamin D_3. Following administration to chicks the compound blocks the biological activity of both physiological and pharmacological doses of vitamin D_3 and 1α-25-dihydroxyvitamin D_3 (26). The molecular basis for this activity can only be speculated upon. Either the mesomeric effect of fluorine has altered the nature of the interaction of the triene system with the receptor or else fluorine is acting like hydroxyl and binding to some appropriate group on the receptor.

In summary, the use of fluoro analogs of vitamin D has produced results which are tantalizing but incomplete. I suggest that to help clarify the issue several approaches, involving both the chemists and biochemists in the field, will have to be followed. The availability of radio-labelled fluoro analogs would allow the unambiguous determination of the metabolism of these compounds and eventually the structure of active metabolites. In order to remove ambiguities in the results obtained when using different species of animals and even between different organs in the same species it will be necessary to use purified receptors to study ligand receptor interaction. At another level the pursuit of the molecular biology approach will allow for the elucidation of the nature and significance of post-receptor events on the expression of hormone function.

At this stage each of the above approaches is at best in the embryonic phase. I feel confident that we will be kept busy in the years ahead.

References:

1. Elliott, K. and J. Birch. (1972) (eds) Carbon Fluorine Compounds. Chem. Biochem. and Biol. Act. Elsevier, Amsterdam.
2. Raftery, M. A., Heustis, W. H. and Millet, F. (1971) Codd Spring Harbour Symp. Quant. Biol., 36, 541-550.
3. Bekoe, A. and Powell, H. M. (1959) Proc. Royal. Soc. A. 250, 301-315.
4. Barnett, J. E. G. (1972) in Carbon Fluorine Compounds (Elliott, K. and Birch, J., eds). Chem. Biochem. and Biol. Act., Elsevier, Amsterdam, pp. 95-110.
5. Sharpe, A. G. (1972) in Carbon Fluorine Compounds (Elliott, K. and Birch, J., eds). Chem. Biochem. and Biol. Act., Elsevier, Amsterdam, pp. 33-49.

6a. Goldman, P. (1972) in Carbon Fluorine Compounds (Elliott, K. and Birch, J., eds). Chem. Biochem. and Biol. Act., Elsevier, Amsterdam, pp. 335-349.

6b. Taylor, N. F. (1972) in Carbon Fluorine Compounds (Elliott, K. and Birch, J., eds). Chem. Biochem. and Biol. Act., Elsevier, Amsterdam, pp. 215-235.

7. Kostyniak, P.J., Bosmann, H. B. and Smith, F. A. (1978) Toxical. Appl. Pharmacol. 44, 89-97.
8. Soiefer, A. I. and Kostymiak, J. P. (1984) J. Biol. Chem. 259, 10787-10792.
9. Wettstein, A. (1972) in Carbon Fluorine Compounds (Elliott, K. and Birch, J., eds). Chem. Biochem. and Biol. Act., Elsevier, Amsterdam, pp. 281-297.
10. Morisaki, M., Dugne, C., Ikekawa, N. and Shikita, M. (1980) J. Steroid. Biochem. 13, 545-550.
11. Ikekawa, N. (1983) J. Steroid. Biochem. 19, 907-911.
12. Napoli, J. L., Fivizzani, M. A., Schnoes, H. K. and DeLuca, H. F. (1978) Biochemistry 17, 2387-2392.
13. Napoli, J. L. Fivizzani, M. A., Hamstra, A. H., Schnoes, H. K., DeLuca, H. F. and Stern, P. H. (1978) Steroids 32, 453-466.
14. Napoli, J. L., Mellon, W. S., Fivizzani, M. A., Schnoes, H. K. and DeLuca, H. F. (1979) J. Biol. Chem. 254, 2017-2022.
15. Napoli, J. L., Mellon, W. S., Schnoes, H. K. and DeLuca, H. F. (1979) Arch. Biochem. Biophys. 197, 193-198.
16. Tanaka, Y., DeLuca, H. F., Kobayashi, Y., Taguchi, P., Ikekawa, N. and Morisaki, M. (1979) J. Biol. Chem. 254, 7163-7167.
17. Tanaka, Y., Wichmann, J. K., DeLuca, H. F., Kobayashi, Y. and Ikekawa, N. (1983) Arch. Biochem. Biophys. 225, 649-655.
18. Tanaka, Y., DeLuca, H. F., Schnoes, H. K., Ikekawa, N. and Kobayashi, Y. (1980) Arch. Biochem. Biophys. 199, 473-478.
19. Okamoto, S., Tanaka, Y., DeLuca, H. F., Kobayashi, Y. and Ikekawa, N. (1983) Am. J. Physiol., 244E, 159-163.
20. Tanaka, Y., Pahnja, D. N., Wichmann, J. K., DeLuca, H. F., Kobayashi, Y., Taguchi, T. and Ikekawa, N. (1982) Arch. Biochem. Biophys., 218, 134-141.
21. Tanak, Y., DeLuca, H. F., Kobayashi, Y. and Ikekawa, N. (1984) Arch. Biochem. Biophys. 229, 348-354.
22. DeLuca, H. F., Ikekawa, N., Tanaka, Y., Morisaki, M. and Oshida, J. (1981) United States Patent 4,254,045.
23. Paaren, H. A., Fivizzani, M. A., Schnoes, H. K. and DeLuca, H. F. (1981) Arch. Biochem. Biophys. 209, 579-583.
24. Napoli, J. L., Fivizzani, M. A., Schnoes, H. K. and DeLuca, H. F. (1979) Biochemistry 18, 1641-1646.
25. Horst, R. L., Napoli, J. L. and Littledike, E. T. (1982) Biochem. J. 204, 185-189.
26. Wilhelm, F. E., Dauben, W. G., Kohler, B., Roesle, A. and Norman, A.W. (1984) Arch. Biochem. Biophys. 233, 127-132.

FPR was supported while on sabbatical leave by the South Africa Medical Research Council.

Assay Methodology: Vitamin D + Metabolites

RECENT DEVELOPMENTS IN QUANTITATION OF VITAMIN D_2 AND VITAMIN D_3 AND THEIR METABOLITES IN BIOLOGIC FLUIDS.

R.L. HORST,* T.A. REINHARDT,* B.W. HOLLIS,[†] and J.L. NAPOLI[‡]
National Animal Disease Center, ARS, USDA, Ames, IA 50010;* Case Western Reserve University, Cleveland, OH 44106;[†] and The University of Texas Health Science Center, Dallas, TX 75235,[‡] U.S.A.

I. Introduction

To date, radioligand binding, spectral assays, and bioassays have been described for the quantitation of some of the physiologically important vitamin D metabolites (1-3). Accurate quantitation of the vitamin D metabolites requires extensive and time-consuming chromatographic techniques. With few exceptions during the development of these techniques, little attention has been given to the migration of vitamin D_2 metabolites in relation to the migration of vitamin D_3 metabolites. This problem has resulted mainly from the lack of vitamin D_2 metabolite standards. Horst et al. (1) and others (2,4) have described methods for the separation and individual quantitation of vitamin D_2, vitamin D_3, 25-hydroxyvitamin D_2 (25-OHD_2) and 25-OHD_3 by high-pressure liquid chromatography (HPLC). Heretofore, no techniques have been described for the complete resolution and individual quantitation of dihydroxylated vitamin D_2 metabolites. Most of the multiple assay techniques described assume very near migration or comigration of the D_2 and D_3 metabolites on HPLC and other chromatographic procedures and also assume their equal potency on radioligand binding assays (1,2). In this report we will describe HPLC methods for the quantitation of vitamin D_2, vitamin D_3, and several of their mono-, di-, and trihydroxylated metabolites and a non-HPLC method for 1,25-$(OH)_2$D analysis (5).

II. Assays Using HPLC Purification

A. Materials and Methods

1. Apparatus -- All HPLC was carried out with a Waters Associates Model LC-204 chromatograph fitted with a Model 6000-A pumping system and a Model 440 UV fixed wavelength (254 nm) detector. The samples and standards were automatically introduced onto the HPLC columns with a No. 710A Waters "intelligent" sampling processor (WISP 710A) or manually using a U6K injector.

2. Solvents -- Diethylether was purchased from J. T. Baker, Inc., Phillipsburg, NJ. All other solvents used in the extraction, conventional chromatography, and HPLC were purchased from Burdick and Jackson, Muskegon, MI.

3. Assay Procedures -- A well-mixed plasma sample was placed in a 50-ml screwcap tube. To each plasma sample (3-5 ml) and to counting vials (in duplicate) was added 1000 cpm of the following radioactive standards for monitoring of the analytical recoveries of the assay: [^{3}H]-vitamin D_3, [^{3}H]-25-OHD_3, [^{3}H]-25-OHD_2, [^{3}H]-24,25-$(OH)_2D_3$, [^{3}H]-24,25-$(OH)_2D_2$, [^{3}H]-25,26-$(OH)_2D_3$, [^{3}H]-25-OHD_3-26,23 lactone, and [^{3}H]-1,25-$(OH)_2D_3$. After vortex mixing of the plasma samples, the lipids were extracted by adding 3.0 volumes of peroxide-free ether, capping the tube, and shaking it horizontally for 5 min at 120 oscillations/min. After shaking, the aqueous layer was allowed to separate for 1-2 min and was frozen in a dry ice/acetone bath. The ether layer was poured into a 25 x 150-cm tube for drying. The aqueous layer was thawed and the above procedure repeated. The final extraction involved denaturing the plasma proteins by adding 4 volumes of 1:3 methanol:methylene chloride and shaking for 3-5 min. This step generally resulted in an emulsion, which was broken by adding 1 volume of methanol. The tube was shaken again for 15 sec. The upper aqueous layer was removed by aspiration and the lower methylene chloride layer was washed twice with 0.1 M phosphate (pH 10.5). The washed methylene chloride layer was combined with the ether fraction and dried under N_2. This final 1:3 methanol:methylene chloride extraction was needed to facilitate the removal of 25-OHD_3-26,23 lactone and 25-OHD. The resulting lipid extract was chromatographed on a 0.6 x 15.5-cm Sephadex LH-20 column developed in H_2O-saturated 1:1:9 chloroform:methanol: hexane. As described in Figure 1, the column eluant was divided into 3 fractions (vitamin D, 25-OHD, and dihydroxyvitamin D). After the lipid residue was applied with two 0.5-ml washes, 2.5 ml of solvent was added to the column and collected as fraction 1 (vitamin D). The next 4.5 ml (2.5-7.0 ml fraction) was collected as fraction 2 (25-OHD); and finally, the next 12.0 ml (7.0-19.0 ml fraction) was collected as fraction 3 (the dihydroxylated metabolites of vitamin D and 25-OHD_3-26,23 lactone).

4. Resolution and Quantitation of the 3 Vitamin D and Vitamin D Metabolite Fractions -- Fraction 1 (vitamin D). The Sephadex LH-20 fraction containing the vitamin D was dried under N_2 and chromatographed on a Lipidex 5000 (Packard) column (0.6 x 14.5 cm) in 5:95 chloroform:hexane. The sample was applied in 0.5 ml of column solvent, which was followed by a 0.5-ml wash. Thereafter, the first 6.0 ml was discarded. The next 4.0 ml of column eluant was collected, and it contained the vitamin D.

The eluant from the Lipidex 5000 column containing the vitamin D was dried under N_2 and prepared for HPLC by the

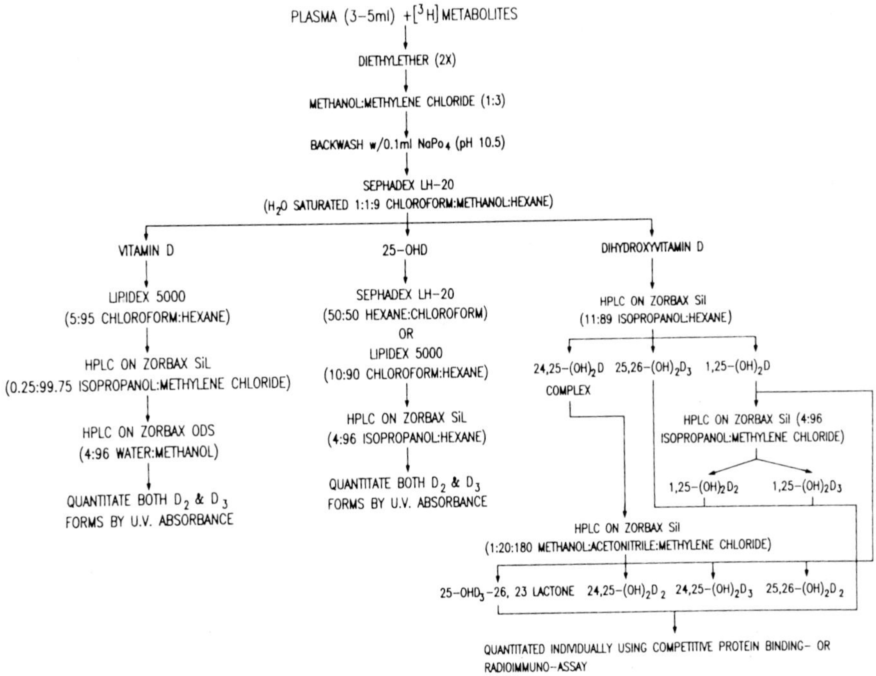

Figure 1. Flow diagram representing the methods used for separating vitamin D and vitamin D metabolite fractions for analysis.

addition of 150 µl of 0.25:99.75 isopropanol:methylene chloride. The sample was chromatographed on a Zorbax Sil column (0.45 x 25 cm) developed in 0.25:99.75 isopropanol:methylene chloride with a flow rate of 2.0 ml/min. Vitamin D_2 and vitamin D_3 comigrated in this system and eluted in the 14- to 18-ml fraction. The vitamin D fraction was dried under N_2, and the vitamin D_2 and vitamin D_3 were quantitated individually by reverse-phase chromatography as previously described (2,5).

Fraction 2 (25-OHD). The 25-OHD fraction was further purified by a Sephadex LH-20 column developed in 1:1 chloroform:hexane. The sample was applied in 0.5 ml of column solvent followed by a 0.5 ml wash. Thereafter, the first 2.5 ml were discarded and the next 5.5 ml collected as 25-OHD. To affect absolute removal of UV contaminating material, the 25-OHD fraction frequently requires further purification on a Lipidex 5000 (Packard) column developed in 10:90 chloroform:hexane. After applying the sample in column solvent as above, the first 9 ml were discarded and the next 13 ml collected as 25-OHD. After drying, the 25-OHD_2 and 25-OHD_3 can be quantitated individually on a HPLC column developed in 4:96 isopropanol:hexane.

Fraction 3 (dihydroxyvitamin D metabolites and 25-OHD_3-26,23 lactone. As shown in Figure 1, the dihydroxyvitamin D metabolite-containing fraction from the initial Sephadex LH-20 column was subjected to HPLC on a Zorbax Sil column developed in 11:89 isopropanol:hexane at a flow rate of 2.0 ml/min. The 24,25-$(OH)_2D$ complex, consisting of 24,25-$(OH)_2D_2$, 24,25-$(OH)_2D_3$, 25,26-$(OH)_2D_2$, and 25-OHD_3-26,23 lactone, migrated in the 8.0-11.5 ml region of this column, whereas 25,26-$(OH)_2D_3$ and 1,25-$(OH)_2D_3$ migrated in the 16-18 ml and 26-30 ml regions, respectively. For complete resolution of the 4 metabolites in the 24,25-$(OH)_2D$ complex, the fraction was collected and resubjected to HPLC on a Zorbax Sil column (0.45 x 25 cm) developed in 1:20:180 methanol: acetonitrile:methylene chloride at a flow rate of 2.0 ml/min. This HPLC system resolved the 24,25-$(OH)_2D$ complex into its component parts (Figure 2). Table 1 compares the relative migration of these metabolites with others using several chemically distinct HPLC systems.

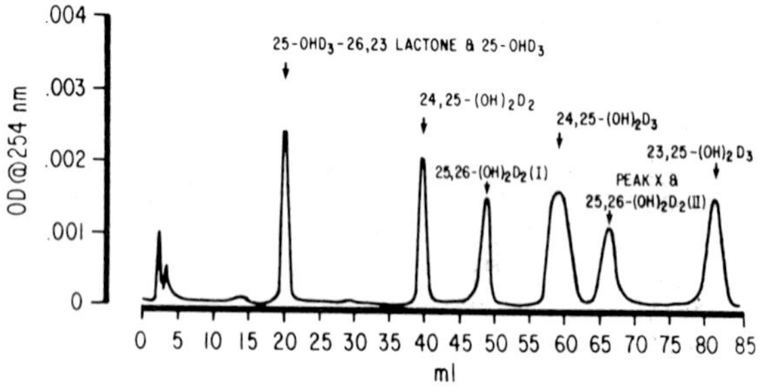

Figure 2. Separation of the 24,25 complex by HPLC using a Zorbax Sil column developed in 1:20:180 methanol:acetonitrile:methylene chloride.

Final analysis of the 1,25-$(OH)_2D$ is done by competitive protein binding assays using the 1,25-$(OH)_2D$ receptor prepared from calf thymus (as described in the non-HPLC assay for 1,25-$(OH)_2D$ section). The other metabolites from fraction 3 can be quantitated by competitive protein binding assay using diluted rat plasma (1) or by radioimmunoassay. The latter offers the advantage of little or no

TABLE 1. Elution Positions of 25-OHD Derivatives Relative to $25\text{-}OHD_3$ in HPLC[a]

Substance	HPLC System[b]				
	Silica			Cyano	ODS
	I	II	III	IV	V
			α[c]		
$25\text{-}OHD_2$	0.84	0.73	0.76	0.80	1.09
$25\text{-}OHD_3$[d]	1.00	1.00	1.00	1.00	1.00
23*S*,25-$(OH)_2D_3$	1.92	3.77	3.51	2.52	0.24
24*R*,25-$(OH)_2D_2$	2.31	2.23	2.18	2.12	0.31
Lactone	2.65	1.00	1.00	4.27	0.13
24*R*,25-$(OH)_2D_3$	2.65	3.06	2.90	2.60	0.23
X[e]	2.65	3.47	3.30	3.17	0.28
25,26-$(OH)_2D_2$ (I)[f]	3.10	2.68	2.50	2.60	0.37
25,26-$(OH)_2D_2$ (II)[f]	3.14	3.39	3.07	2.86	0.37
25,26-$(OH)_2D_3$	4.80	4.11	4.06	3.90	0.31
10-oxo-$25\text{-}OHD_3$ (I)[g]	5.28	3.34	3.68	3.96	0.24
10-oxo-$25\text{-}OHD_3$ (II)[g]	6.01	4.62	4.62	4.50	0.23
1,25-$(OH)_2D_2$	7.31	6.02	6.41	5.00	0.39
1,25-$(OH)_2D_3$	8.33	8.00	8.60	6.40	0.32

[a]Columns used were Dupont Zorbax (0.46 x 25 cm). The mobile phase volumes (Vm) were 3.5 ml.

[b]Mobile phases used were: I, methanol:2-propanol:hexane (1:3:96); II, methanol:acetonitrile:dichloromethane (1:20:180); III, methanol:1,2-dichloroethane (1:79); IV, acetonitrile:ethanol:dichloromethane:hexane (1:1.5:6:11.5); V, water:methanol (1:3).

[c]$\alpha = k\ (\text{substance})/k\ (25\text{-}OHD_3)$; $k = Vr - Vm$.

[d]Elution volumes for $25\text{-}OHD_3$ range from: I, 17-20 ml; II, 10-13 ml; III, 15-18 ml; IV, 11-14 ml; V, 155-165 ml.

[e]This $25\text{-}OHD_2$ metabolite has not yet been positively identified, but preliminary evidence suggests it is 25,28-$(OH)_2D_2$.

[f]C(25) stereochemistry unknown.

[g]C(5) stereochemistry unknown.

discrimination between 24,25-$(OH)_2D_2$ and 24,25-$(OH)_2D_3$ (Figure 3). The radioimmunoassay is conducted using a 1/8500 dilution of antibody (prepared in rabbits using a side-chain acid conjugate as antigen) in 50 mM KPO_4 (pH 7.4) buffer containing 0.04% gelatin. After 90 min at 4 C, the bound hormone is separated from free using 0.1% dextran 1% charcoal suspended in the same buffer.

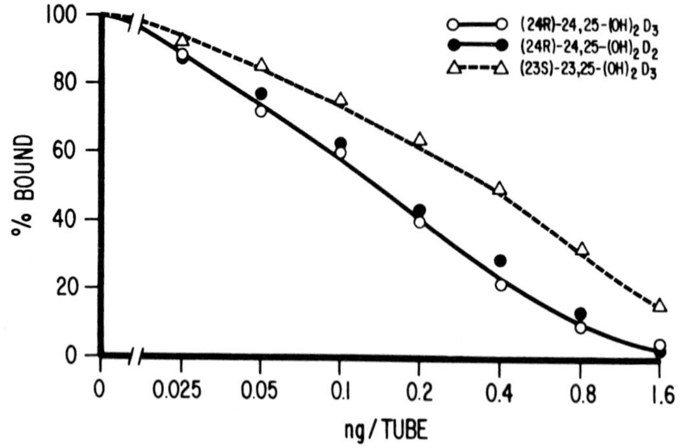

Figure 3. Competitive displacement of $[^3H]$-25-OHD by metabolites in the radioimmunoassay for 24,25-$(OH)_2D$.

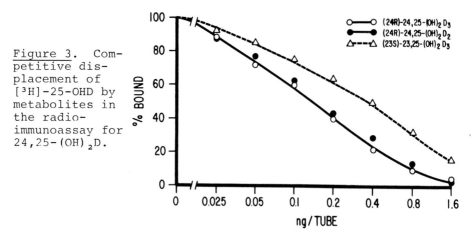

Trihydroxyvitamin D metabolites. These metabolites generally circulate in plasma at very low values (<10 pg/ml). However, there are some pharmacologic states where plasma levels are elevated, such as during 1,25-$(OH)_2D_3$ therapy. Table 2 demonstrates several means whereby separation of the trihydroxy metabolites can be achieved. Final quantitation was by competitive protein binding using 1,25-$(OH)_2D$ receptor isolated from calf thymus, as described in the section dealing with non-HPLC assay for 1,25-$(OH)_2D$ section.

III. Non-HPLC Assay for 1,25-$(OH)_2D$ As Described by Reinhardt et al. (5)

A. Materials and Methods

1. Preparation of thymic cytosol -- Thymus gland cytosol was prepared as previously described (6) with slight modifications. Thymus glands were removed from 5- to 20-week-old Jersey calves. The glands were washed in ice-cold saline and cut into small cubes (approx. 2 cm^3). They were then frozen in liquid nitrogen and stored in a freezer at -56 C until used. Under these storage conditions, there was no loss of 1,25-$(OH)_2D$ receptor activity for at least 1 yr. Frozen or fresh glands were prepared as follows (all steps were carried out at 4 C): thymus glands were homogenized (25%, wt/vol) in a buffer containing 50 mM Tris-HCl, 500 mM KCl, 5 mM dithiothreitol, 10 mM for at

TABLE 2. Elution positions of 1,25-$(OH)_2D$ Derivatives Relative to 1,25-$(OH)_2D_3$ in Normal-Phase HPLC[a]

Substance	Mobile Phase[b]		
	VI	VII	VIII
		α	
1,25-$(OH)_2D_2$	0.90	0.83	0.90
10-oxo-25-OHD_3	0.96	0.43	-
1,25-$(OH)_2D_3$	1.00	1.00	1.00
24-oxo-1,25-$(OH)_2D_3$	1.20	0.71	-
23-oxo-1,25-$(OH)_2D_3$	1.53	0.83	-
24-oxo-1,23,25-$(OH)_3D_3$	1.57	1.17	1.06
1,23,25-$(OH)_3D_3$	1.60	2.25	1.42
1,24,25-$(OH)_3D_2$	1.88	1.81	1.67
1,24,25-$(OH)_3D_3$	2.07[c]	2.60	1.85
1α-OH-lactone	2.29[c]	1.06-1.16[c]	1.68
1,25,28-$(OH)_3D_2$	2.41	3.60	2.20
1,25,26-$(OH)_3D_2$	2.47	2.60	2.23
1,25,26-$(OH)_3D_3$	3.10	4.25	2.70

[a]Data was obtained with a Dupont Zorbax-Sil column (0.46 x 25 cm). The mobile phase volume (Vm) was 3.5 ml. Formulae used were α = k substance/k 1,25-$(OH)_2D_3$; k = Vr - Vm. Differences of 0.1 indicate noticeable separation, if not complete resolution.

[b]Mobile phases used were: VI, 10% 2-propanol:hexane; VII, 5-7% 2-propanol:dichloromethane; VIII, 12-15% 2-propanol in (hexane:dichloromethane; 8:1). Elution volumes for 1,25-$(OH)_2D_3$ were: VI, 25-30 ml; VII, 19-22 ml; VIII, 13-17 ml.

[c]These values depend on the individual column used; the relative elution positions in hexane of 1α-OH-lactone and 1,24,25-$(OH)_3D_3$ can be the reverse of that shown here.

$Na_2MoO_4 \cdot 2H_2O$, and 1.5 mM EDTA, pH 7.5, by four 20-sec bursts of a Polytron PT-20 tissue disrupter (Brinkmann Instruments, Westbury, NY) at setting 7. Homogenates were centrifuged for 1 h at 300,000 x g, and the cytosol (minus the pellet and floating lipid layer) was removed and fractionated by the slow addition of solid $(NH_4)_2SO_4$ (enzyme grade, Schwarz-Mann, Orangeburg, NY) to 35% saturation. The cytosol was then stirred slowly for 30-60 min. Cytosol was aliquoted into 15-ml centrifuge tubes (10 ml) and centrifuged at 20,000 x g for 20 min. The supernatant was discarded, and the pellets were stored under nitrogen at -20 C. Before use in the assay, the pellets were redissolved in 10 ml of the buffer described above. This buffer should be prepared fresh biweekly. An aliquot of this stock receptor solution was diluted 1:7 with buffer and used in the assay, and the remainder of the stock receptor solution was immediately re-frozen for use in later assays. The stock receptor solution may be thawed and refrozen at least 2 times without loss of receptor activity. The correct dilution of stock receptor for the assay should be determined empirically for each new batch of $(NH_4)_2SO_4$ pellets prepared; however, we have found very little batch to batch variability.

2. Preparation of dextran-coated charcoal -- Six grams of charcoal (Norit-A, Sigma Chemical Co., St. Louis, MO) and 0.6 g Dextran T-70 (Pharmacia Fine Chemicals, Piscataway, NJ) were suspended in 500 ml of a buffer containing 0.1 M boric acid and 0.05% BSA, pH 8.6, and stirred overnight at 4 C. The next morning, the suspension was centrifuged at 1500 x g for 15-20 min, and the supernatant was carefully decanted and discarded. The pelleted dextran-coated charcoal was resuspended in 500 ml of the buffer described. This charcoal suspension was stable for at least 2 weeks at 4 C.

3. Sep-Pak washing procedure -- Both new and used Sep-Paks (Waters Associates, Inc., Milford, MA) were prepared as follows before use. C-18 Sep-Paks were washed by the sequential addition of 5 ml hexane, 5 ml chloroform, 5 ml methanol, and 5 ml distilled water. Silica Sep-Paks were washed by sequential additions of 5 ml methanol, 5 ml chloroform, 5 ml hexane, and 5 ml hexane:isopropanol (96:4). This conditioning procedure allowed reuse of Sep-Pak cartridges at least 4 times without significant loss of capacity or changes in elution patterns.

4. Sample preparation -- The method of sample extraction and preparation is demonstrated in Figure 4. Plasma (0.2-1.0 ml) was added to 12 x 75-mm borosilicate glass tubes and brought up to 1 ml with saline. Eight hundred counts per min of $[^3H]$-1,25-$(OH)_2D_3$ in 20 μl ethanol were

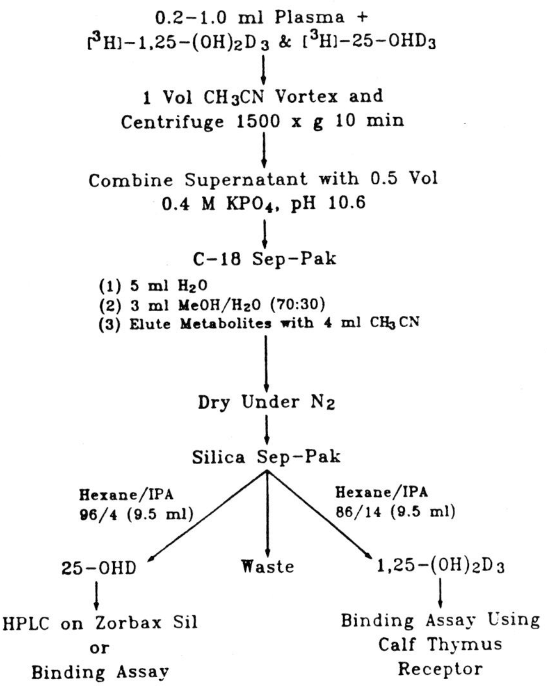

Figure 4. Flow diagram represents the methods used for the non-HPLC assay for 1,25-$(OH)_2D$. IPA = isopropanol. CH_3CN = acetonitrile. MeOH = methanol.

added to each plasma sample and to a counting vial for monitoring of recoveries. The samples were then vortexed and allowed to stand for 10 min. The solid phase extraction of vitamin D metabolites was done using a modified version of a previously described method (7). One volume of acetonitrile was added to each plasma sample. The samples were vortexed vigorously for 20 sec, followed by centrifugation for 10 min at 1500 x g. After centrifugation, the supernatant was decanted into a tube containing 0.5 vol 0.4 M K_2HPO_4, pH 10.6, and vortexed. This extract was applied directly to a prewashed C-18 Sep-Pak (Waters Associates, Inc., Milford, MA). Excess salt was removed by washing the cartridge with 5 ml distilled water, and polar lipids were removed by washing the cartridge with 3 ml methanol:water (70:30). The vitamin D metabolites were then eluted with 4 ml acetonitrile, and this fraction was dried under a stream of nitrogen. The vitamin D metabolite extract was applied to a silica Sep-Pak cartridge in 0.5 ml hexane:isopropanol (99:1), and the tube was washed with an additional 0.5 ml solvent, which was applied to the cartridge. The cartridge was washed with 10 ml of the starting solvent, followed by 9.5 ml of (96:4) hexane:isopropanol, resulting in the elution of 25-OHD. Next, the cartridge was washed with 8 ml hexane:isopropanol (94:6), which removed 60% of the 24,25-$(OH)_2D$. The

1,25-$(OH)_2D$ was then eluted with 9.5 ml hexane:isopropanol (86:14) and dried under a stream of nitrogen. The 25-OHD fraction was prepared for analysis by HPLC as described in the previous section. The 1,25-$(OH)_2D$ fraction was redissolved in 100 µl absolute ethanol. From this volume, 30 µl purified sample were used to determine the recovery of tracer, and two 30-µl aliquots were used for assay.

5. Nonequilibrium radio receptor assay -- Standards (1-64 and 800 pg for nonspecific binding determination) and samples were added to either 12 x 75-mm glass tubes on ice. An aliquot of stock receptor sufficient for the number of tubes to be assayed was diluted as described above, and 450 µl receptor solution (approx. 0.7 mg protein/tube) were added to the standards and samples on ice and vortexed. The samples and standards were incubated in a 25 C water bath for 45 min with gentle shaking. At the end of 45 min, the tubes were transferred to an ice bath and allowed to cool for 5 min, and then each tube received 5000 cpm [^{3}H]-1,25-$(OH)_2D$ (90 Ci/mmol) in 25 µl ethanol. The tubes were vortexed, and the incubation was continued for 15 min in a 25 C water bath with shaking. The tubes were allowed to cool for 5 min in an ice bath, and 200 µl dextran-coated charcoal suspension were added to each, followed by vortexing. The tubes were vortexed again after 10 min, and after 20 min of charcoal treatment, bound and free hormones were separated by centrifugation. Glass tubes were centrifuged at 2000 x g for 10 min, and microcentrifuge tubes were centrifuged at 12,000 x g for 45 sec. The supernatant containing bound hormone was decanted into a scintillation vial and counted (counting efficiency, 40%).

Conclusion. Both the HPLC and non-HPLC methods are being used extensively in our laboratory. We are currently modifying the non-HPLC method to accommodate the analysis of 24,25-$(OH)_2D_2$, 24,25-$(OH)_2D_3$ and 25-OHD_3-26,23 lactone.

References

1. Horst, R. L., Littledike, E. T., Riley, J. L., and Napoli, J. L. (1981) Anal. Biochem. 116:189-203.
2. Shepard, R. M., Horst, R. L., Hamstra, A. J., and DeLuca, H. F. (1979) Biochem. J. 182:52-64.
3. Eisman, J. A., Hamstra, A. J., Kream, B. E., and DeLuca, H. F. (1976) Science 193:1021-1023.
4. Jones, G. (1978) Clin. Chem. 24:287-298.
5. Reinhardt, T. A., Horst, R. L., Orf, J. W., and Hollis, B. W. (1984) J. Clin. Endo. Met. 58:91-98.
6. Reinhardt, T. A., Horst, R. L., Littledike, E. T., and Beitz, D. C. (1982) Biochem. Biophys. Res. Commun. 106:1012-1018.
7. Turnbull, H., Trafford, D. J. H., and Makin, H. L. J. (1982) Clin. Chim. Acta 120:65-70.

AN EASY METHOD TO DETERMINE THE TWO MOST IMPORTANT VITAMIN D METABOLITES, 25(OH)D and 1,25$(OH)_2$D, IN HUMAN SERUM

L. Hummer, D. Hartwell and C. Christiansen
Department of Clinical Chemistry, Glostrup Hospital, Denmark

Introduction:

The determination of 25-hydroxyvitamin D (25(OH)D) and 1,25-dihydroxyvitamin D (1,25$(OH)_2$D) has become increasingly important in the diagnosis and management of patients with a wide range of mineral and skeletal disorders (1,2). Several methods to measure these two metabolites have been described (3-6). They are generally time consuming and involve several extraction and chromatography steps. We present a rapid microassay for 25(OH)D and 1,25$(OH)_2$D. The extraction and purification is based on Sep-pak cartridges and quantitation by competitive protein binding assay CPBA).

Materials and methods:

Samples were obtained from 40 healthy postmenopausal women during one year. The serum samples (0.5 ml)were deproteinated by addition of acetonitrile and purified over Sep-pak C_{18}. After removal of salts and lipid excess the vitamin D metabolites were eluated by acetonitrile (7). Further purification and separation were performed on Silica Sep-pak (8). The 25(OH)D metabolite was eluated by hexane/isopropanol (96/4, v/v) and the 1,25$(OH)_2$D metabolite by hexane/isopropanol (85/15, v/v). In the purified extract 25(OH)D was measured by CPBA using vitamin D binding protein from rachitic rat serum (9). The quantitation of 1,25$(OH)_2$D was performed by a minor modification of the procedure described by Reinhardt et al. (8) employing 1,25$(OH)_2$D cytosol receptor from calf thymus.

Results:

Extraction of 25(OH)D and 1,25$(OH)_2$D from serum by the Sep-pak procedure was found to be 62.3% ± 4.1% (mean ± SD) of the labelled 25(OH)D and 58.4% ± 4.1% of the labelled 1,25$(OH)_2$D. Detection limit for the 25(OH)D assay was 25 pg/tube and the useful range of the assay was 25-400 pg/tube. For the 1,25$(OH)_2$-D assay the detection limit was 1.5 pg/tube and the useful range 1.5-35 pg/tube.
The specificity of the vitamin D binding protein and the receptor from the calf thymus are summarized in the Table. The specificity for the D_2 and D_3 forms of the metabolites was equal. The intra- and interassay coefficient of variation for the 25(OH)D and 1,25$(OH)_2$D assays were found to be 6%/13% and 8%/19%, respectively.

Vitamin D. A Chemical, Biochemical and Clinical Update

Metabolite Binder Dilution	25(OH)D rachitic rat serum 1:10,000	$1,25(OH)_2D$ calf thymus receptor 1:12
$25(OH)D_3$	1	>400
$25(OH)D_2$	1	>400
$1,25(OH)_2D_3$		1
$1,25(OH)_2D_2$		1
$24R,25(OH)_2D_3$	1	>450
$25S,26(OH)_3D_3$	1	>120
$1,24R,25(OH)_3D_3$		1.6

The 25(OH)D and $1,25(OH)_2D$ measured by the microassay were compared to the results obtained by the extraction/purification procedure described by Shepard et al. (3), using cytosol receptor from calf thymus in the $1,25(OH)_2D$ assay (8). A highly significant linear correlation was found, r=0.89, SEE=19% in the 25(OH)D assay and r=0.89, SEE=21% in the $1,25(OH)_2D$ assay.

Conclusion:

The present assay performed on a small sample volume, 0.5 ml serum have low time/labour and cost requirements. The precision is acceptable and the biologically most important metabolite $1,25(OH)_2D$ is quantitated by the highly specific cytosol receptor protein from calf thymus. The measurements of 25(OH)D using vitamin D binding protein will include some $25,26(OH)_2D$ and $24,25(OH)_2D$. Even so, we conclude that the data indicate that this microassay is an easy and acceptable alternative to the assay procedures, which involve Sephadex LH 20 and HPLC for purification of the individual metabolites.

References:

1. Kumar R. Physiol Rev 1984; 64: 478-504.
2. Avioli LV, Haddad JG. N Engl J Med 1984; 311: 47-49.
3. Shepard RM, Horst RL, Hamstra AJ, DeLuca HF. Biochem J 1979; 182: 55-69.
4. Gray TK, Eisman J, Forman DT. Clin Chem 1983; 29: 196-200.
5. Horst RL, Littledike ET, Riley JL, Napoli JL. Anal Biochem 1981; 116: 189-203.
6. Manolagas SC, Culler FL, Howard JE, Brickman AS, Deftos LJ. J Clin Endocrinol Metab 1983; 56: 751-760.
7. Hummer L, Nilas L, Tjellesen L, Christiansen C. Scand J Clin Lab Invest 1984; 44: 163-167.
8. Reinhardt TA, Horst RL, Orf JW, Hollis BW. J Clin Endocrinol Metab 1984; 580 91-98.
9. Hummer L, Tjellesen L, Rickers H, Christiansen C. Scand J Clin Lab Invest 1984; 44: 595-601.

SPECIFIC MONOCLONAL ANTIBODIES FOR THE IMMUNOASSAY OF 1,25-DIHYDROXYVITAMIN D

J.L. BERRY, A. WHITE* and E.B. MAWER
Department of Medicine, University of Manchester, Manchester, M13 9PT, U.K.
* Department of Chemical Pathology, Hope Hospital, Salford, M6 8HD, U.K.

INTRODUCTION

Methods for the measurement of 1,25-dihydroxyvitamin D ($1,25(OH)_2D$) include radioimmunoassays and receptor binding assays. Both methods require extensive extraction and chromatographic procedures to purify the metabolite prior to assay, the whole process being highly labour intensive. Our aim was to produce monoclonal antibodies (MAb) with high sensitivity and specificity for $1,25(OH)_2D$ with the ultimate intention of improving and simplifying the existing purification and assay procedures.

METHODS

We have assessed two different antigens 1α hydroxyvitamin D_3-24 calcioic acid - BSA conjugate (24-calcioic acid) and 1 α hydroxyvitamin D_3-25 oxime-BSA conjugate (25 oxime) for their ability to produce MAbs for the immunoassay of $1,25(OH)_2D$. Both conjugates contained 30-36 steroid residues per mole BSA as indicated by uv analysis. Six fusions to produce hybridomas were performed (1) three with each conjugate. Cultures were screened for Ab activity using a pre-precipitated 2nd Ab method (2). Positive cultures were cloned by limiting dilution and recloned at least once to establish stable Ab secreting hybrids.

RESULTS AND DISCUSSION

We have been successful in raising several MAb for the assay of $1,25(OH)_2D$ using two different antigens. A large number of hybrids were produced with both conjugates, although after immunisation with 25-oxime few hybrids secreted Ab and most were unstable and required repeated cloning (see table 1).

TABLE 1 FUSION DETAILS

IMMUNOGEN	24-calcioic acid			25-oxime		
FUSION	1	2	6	3	4	5
AB TITRE AT FUSION*	1:450	1:3000	1:15000	1:6000	1:2000	1:2500
NO. HYBRIDS	533	399	576	478	574	572
(% Total 576)	(93%)	(60%)	(100%)	(83%)	(99%)	(99%)
NO. AB SECRETING	42	104	520	5	3	2
HYBRIDS (%)	(8%)	(26%)	(90%)	(1%)	(0.5%)	(0.3%)
NO. STABLE AB CHARACTERISED	9	2	5	0	1	2

* Titre (dilution of Ab binding 50% $^3H-1,25(OH)_2D_3$) of polyclonal antiserum from mouse at time of fusion.

All the MAb produced, irrespective of antigen, were of higher specificity than the polyclonal Ab currently in use in our laboratory (3), but with the exception of 5F2 (fusion 5) none were as sensitive (see table 2). 5F2 secreted a MAb of high affinity which did not seem to discriminate between $1,25(OH)_2D_2$ and $1,25(OH)_2D_3$ suggesting that in future assays it may be possible to measure these two forms together.

Vitamin D. A Chemical, Biochemical and Clinical Update

TABLE 2

MAb CHARACTERISTICS

IMMUNOGEN	24-calcioic acid			25-oxime	
FUSION	1	2	6	4	5
MAb	3E11	2D8	1G7[1]	3A8	5F2[1]
TITRE[2]	1:25000	1:45000	1:15	1:2000	1:150
DISPLACEMENT[3]	40	80	60	100	25
SPECIFICITY[4]					
1,25$(OH)_2D_3$	100	100	100	100	100
1,25$(OH)_2D_2$	13	45	20	29	95
25(OH)D_3	6	15	0	15	10
24,25$(OH)_2D_3$	11	27	0	43	19
25,26$(OH)_2D_3$	25	-	0	43	43
1 (OH)D_3	0.6	0.5	1	3	2

1. Data from MAb in supernatant medium.
2. Titre as in table 1.
3. Displacement: concentration (pg) of 1,25$(OH)_2D_3$ displacing 50% radioligand.
4. Cross-reactivity with 1,25$(OH)_2D_3$.

MAb IG7 (fusion 6) is highly specific and does not cross-react with 25(OH)D_3, 24,25$(OH)_2D_3$ or 25,26$(OH)_2D_3$ at the concentrations found in normal human serum (see figure 1). Using this MAb the lengthy extraction and chromatographic separation could be eliminated and a non-chromatographic assay system is currently being investigated.

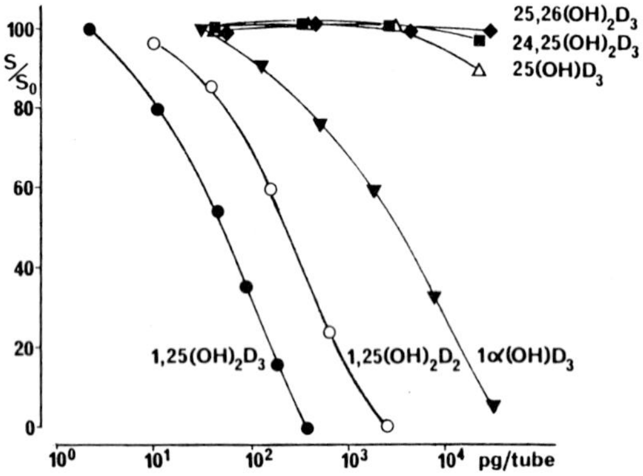

Fig 1. Displacement curves to vit. D metabolites using MAb IG7.

REFERENCES

1. White, A., Gray, C. & Corrie, J.E.T. (1985), J. Steroid Biochem., 22, (in press)
2. White, A., Anderson, D.C. & Daly, J.R. (1982), J. Clin. Endocr. Metab. 54, 205-207.
3. Clemens, T.L., Hendy, G.N., Papapoulos, S.E., Fraher, L.J., Care, A.D. & O'Riordan, J.L.H. (1979), Clin. Endocr. 11, 225-234.

A METHOD FOR DETERMINATION OF 25-HYDROXYVITAMIN D_3 BOUND TO VITAMIN D BINDING PROTEIN IN HUMAN PLASMA

S.Masuda, T.Okano and T.Kobayashi

Department of Hygienic Sciences, Kobe Women's College of Pharmacy, Higashinada-ku, Kobe 658, Japan

Vitamin D and metabolites are circulating in human plasma as the forms bound to vitamin D binding protein (DBP). Significance of free and bound forms of the metabolites has been discussed.[1] In order to clarify the significance more detail, we established a method for the determination of 25-hydroxyvitamin D_3 (25-OH-D_3) bound to DBP in human plasma.

Procedure for assay of 25-OH-D_3 bound to DBP in human plasma

Exactly 1 ml of plasma is applied to a DEAE Affi-gel blue column (5.5 ml, 15 x 32 mm) and the column is eluted in steps by 40 ml of 0.01M-K_2HPO_4 buffer solution (pH 8.0), 25 ml of 0.02M-K_2HPO_4 buffer solution (pH 8.0 containing 0.05M-NaCl) and 40 ml of 0.02M-K_2HPO_4 buffer solution (pH 8.0 containing 1.4M-NaCl). Immunoglobulin G (IgG), DBP and albumin are eluted in the 1st, 2nd and 3rd eluates, respectively. The 2nd eluate corresponding to a DBP fraction is collected, saponified with ethanolic KOH and extracted the unsaponifiable matter. The unsaponifiable matter is first subjected to preparative HPLC using a Nucleosil $5C_{18}$ column (8.0 x 300 mm)with 20% MeOH in acetonitrile as a mobile phase and a 25-OH-D_3 fraction is collected. The fraction is subsequently subjected to analytical HPLC using a Zorbax SIL column (4.6 x 250 mm) with 5.5% iso-PrOH in n-hexane as a mobile phase and 25-OH-D_3 is assayed by estimating the peak height. On the other hand, total 25-OH-D_3 concentrations are determined by applying the lipid extract of a plasma sample to the same two steps of the HPLC.

Profiles of chromatography at each step of the procedure

Figure 1 shows the profiles of chromatography at each step

Vitamin D. A Chemical, Biochemical and Clinical Update

included in the proposed method. The shadow parts represent those including 25-OH-D_3. As shown in the profile of analytical HPLC, the peak due to 25-OH-D_3 was clearly separated from other interfering peaks and gave a single peak.

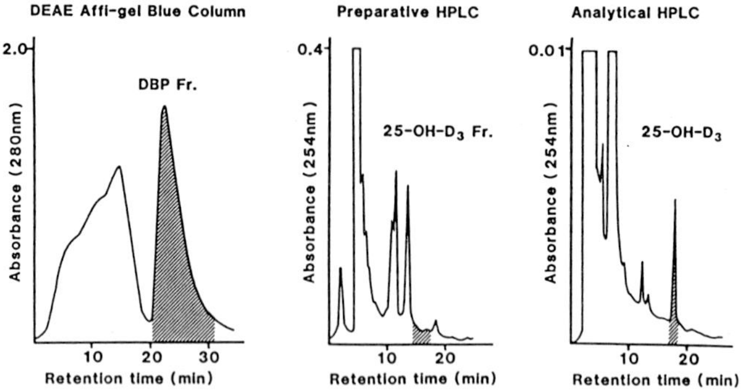

Column :	DEAE Affi-gel blue (15x32mm)	Nucleosil $5C_{18}$ (8.0x300mm)	Zorbax SIL (4.6x250mm)
Eluant or Mobile phase :	0.02M K_2HPO_4 buffer, containing 0.05M NaCl	20% MeOH/Acetonitrile	5.5% iso-PrOH/Hexane
Flow rate :	2.0 ml/min	1.8ml/min (39kg/cm^2)	0.6ml/min (20kg/cm^2)

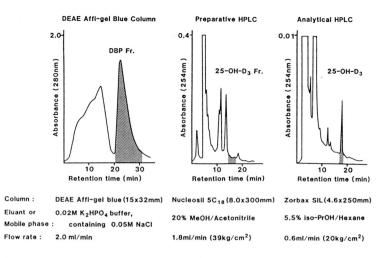

Fig. 1. Profiles of Chromatography at Each Step

Assayed values of total and bound forms of 25-OH-D_3 in plasma

As shown in Fig. 2, more than 90% of 25-OH-D_3 (average : 94.1%) in healthy human plasma was assayed as bound forms.

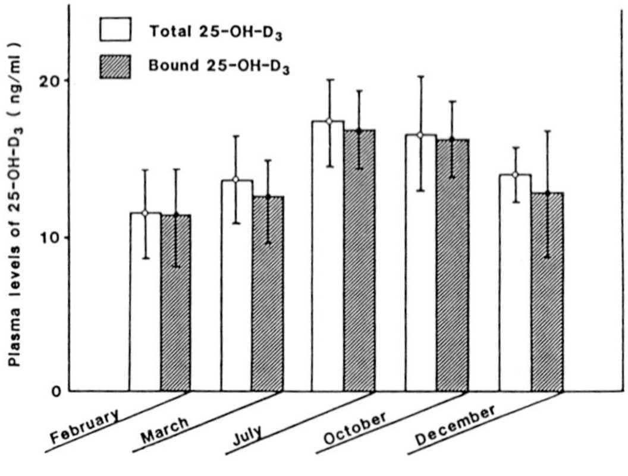

Fig. 2. Assayed Values of Total and Bound Forms of 25-OH-D_3

REFERENCE 1) Bouillon,R., van Assche,F.A., van Baelen,H., Heyns,W. and De Moor,P. (1981) *J. Clin. Invest.*, 67, 589-596.

GAS CHROMATOGRAPHY-MASS SPECTROMETRY OF VITAMIN D METABOLITES - THE DEFINITIVE ASSAY SYSTEM?

H.L.J. Makin & D.J.H. Trafford,

The Steroid Laboratory, Department of Chemical Pathology, The London Hospital Medical College, Turner Street, London E1 2AD, UK.

Gas chromatography-mass spectrometry (GC-MS) is widely accepted as providing a definitive assay system against which the specificity of other assays can be evaluated. Recent inter-laboratory studies of the specificity and precision of plasma assays for 25-hydroxyvitamin D (25-OHD), 24,25-dihydroxyvitamin D (24,25$(OH)_2$D) and 1,25-dihydroxyvitamin D (1,25$(OH)_2$D) have clearly shown that many of these assays, using protein binding methods for quantitation, are imprecise and lack specificity (1,2). Indeed in one of these studies (1), it was pointed out that a majority of the laboratories taking part could not distinguish major physiological changes in the concentration of metabolites, particularly 1,25$(OH)_2$D. It is clear that a considerable degree of purification , usually carried out by high-performance liquid chromatography (HPLC), is required before quantitation in order to achieve satisfactory specificity. In addition to non-specific interference, the increasing awareness of the presence of other metabolites in fractions previously thought to be pure, has led to increasing efforts to improve purification prior to quantitation (i.e. 3).

Gas chromatography-mass spectrometry provides the ideal solution to this analytical problem since it has the necessary sensitivity to measure the majority of vitamin D metabolites, for which standards are available. In addition, GC-MS provides a high degree of specificity.

Table 1. Mass chromatography of 25-OHD_3 in human plasma: demonstration of specificity by monitoring 5 ions simultaneously.

m/z	ion	Peak height ratios found	Peak height ratios standard
413	$(M-131)^+$	0.769	0.727
439	$(M-90-15)^+$	1.000	1.000
454	$(M-90)^+$	0.105	0.091
529	$(M-15)^+$	0.091	0.100
544	M^+	0.337	0.290

The analysis was carried out on a VG 12250 quadrapole mass spectrometer. The concentration of 25-OHD_3 was calculated from the ratio of the intensities of the ions m/z439/m/z445 (the equivalent ion from hexadeuterated 25-OHD_3) and was found to be 22.4ng/ml.

Vitamin D. A Chemical, Biochemical and Clinical Update

We have described GC-MS assays for D_3, 25-OHD_3, 25-OHD_2, and 24,25$(OH)_2D_3$ (4) using tritiated internal standards prior to GC. Deuterated standards have been synthesised and used in developing more precise assays for 24,25$(OH)_2D_3$ (5) and 25,26$(OH)_2D_3$ (6). These assays were developed using a single focussing magnetic sector instrument with no data handling facilities using conventional packed columns and electron impact ionisation. Modern mass spectrometers with associated data handling equipment offer considerable advantages, such as the facility of mass chromatography which allows the collection and storage of complete mass spectra at regular intervals throughout the chromatographic run. Peaks of interest can thus be shown to be homogenous by obtaining mass spectra at various points on the peak which should all be the same as that obtained from a pure standard. A further check on specificity can be carried out using mass chromatography or multiple ion detection by monitoring a number of mass fragments simultaneously. The demonstration that the ratio of these mass fragment peaks is the same as that obtained in the mass spectrum of the pure standard is an indication of specificity (Table 1). In addition the peak of interest can be quantified. The provision of multiple channels enables a number of metabolites to be measured, and their specificity checked in a single chromatographic run. With modern mass spectrometers sensitivity is adequate for the measurement of 1,25$(OH)_2D$ in 1ml of plasma. Figure 1 shows a mass fragmentogram obtained after injection of

Figure 1. Mass fragmentogram of the n-butyl boronate-3-trimethylsilyl ether derivative of 24,25$(OH)_2D_3$ (10pg on column)

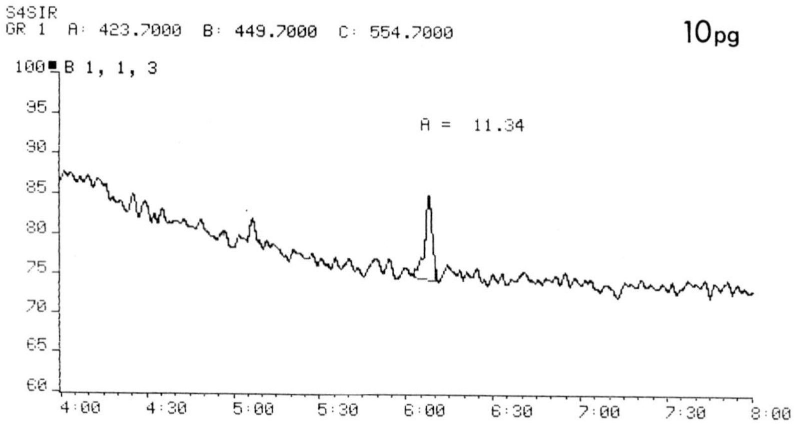

The analysis was carried out on a VG 12250 quadrapole mass spectrometer, monitoring three ions. Only the m/z449 trace is illustrated here.

10pg of the n-butyl-boronate-3-trimethylsilyl ether of $24,25(OH)_2D_3$ monitoring the peak at m/z 449 $(M-90-15)^+$ and thus illustrates how sensitive mass fragmentography can be. Even 1-2pg injected can also be clearly distinguished from the background. A further increase in sensitivity can be expected by the use of negative ion chemical ionisation mass spectrometry provided that sufficiently stable electron capturing derivatives can be obtained. Although high resolution mass spectrometry is inherently less sensitive than low resolution, the increase in signal to noise ratio more than compensates for this sensitivity loss. Further increase in sensitivity may be obtained if daughter ions formed in field free regions are monitored or if tandem mass spectrometry is used. The availability of satisfactory HPLC-MS interfaces, particularly the thermospray offer the possibility of extending the use of mass spectrometry as a highly specific and sensitive detector for HPLC.

While GC-MS is not recommended as a routine procedure for the measurement of vitamin D and its metabolites, it is of importance in our view to continue to develop this methodology if only as a means of providing definitive assays against which other less rigorous procedures can be evaluated.

THe work reported here has been supported by grants, for which we are grateful, from the Wellcome Trust, The Medical Research Council, and The Research Advisory Committee of the London Hospital. The London Hospital Special Trustees kindly provided assistance in the purchase of the LKB 2091 mass spectrometer. We are grateful to VG Masslab and Nermag SN for providing mass spectrometric facilities.

REFERENCES

1. Jongen, M.J.M., Van Ginkel, F.C., van der Vijgh, J.F., Kuiper, S., Netelebos, J.C., and Lips, P. (1984) Clin. Chem. 30, 399-403.
2. Mayer, E., and Schmidt-Gayk, H. (1984) Clin. Chem. 30, 1199-1204
3. Jones, G. (1983) J. Chromatogr. 276, 69-75
4. Seamark, D.A., Trafford, D.J.H., and Makin, H.L.J. (1980) Clin. Chim. Acta 106, 51-62.
5. Coldwell, R.D., Trafford, D.J.H., Makin, H.L.J., Varley, M.J., and Kirk, D.N. (1984) Clin. Chem. 30, 1193-1198.
6 Coldwell, R.D., Trafford, D.J.H., Makin, H.L.J., Varley, M.J., and Kirk, D.N. (1985) J. Chromatogr. 328, 289-302.

TROUBLESHOOTING AND ERROR SOURCES IN ASSAYS OF SERUM VITAMIN D AND ITS METABOLITES

T. Koskinen, Department of Clinical Sciences, University of Tampere, Teiskontie 35, SF-33520 Tampere, Finland

There is a plethora of published methods for the analysis of serum vitamin D and its metabolites, but it is likely that almost every laboratory performing these assays has its own variation of the basic themes. None of the publications have been universally accepted as a reference method, and interlaboratory comparisons have indicated large variations between individual laboratories and methods. This suggests that even minor modifications in methods may greatly influence the results obtained. There is usually a large number of preparative steps within a method, and each of these contains potential sources of error. The following presentation lists some of the factors which may cause erroneous results in the assays of vitamin D compounds. A brief troubleshooting chart is also given.

1. Materials. The purity of standards and tracers will have an effect on the results, and they should be checked periodically. Stock solutions should be stored in a deep-feezer, and working solutions prepared when appropriate. New standards and tracers should be compared with old ones to observe possible shifts in results. Also buffers, charcoal suspensions etc. are not always stable for long, and they are easily replaced.

2. Equipment. Often very small volumes are pipetted during the course of the assays. The accuracy and reproducibility of all pipets are therefore crucial. Liquid chromatographs require constant and trouble-free operation to ensure reproducible separation within an assay series.

3. Human factors. The assay of serum vitamin D compunds is more complicated than most routine laboratory methods, and it takes time to learn to perform it. Sufficient practice and a thorough knowledge of the method are needed to avoid errors caused by human factors. There should not, but may be, differences in results obtained by different persons, due to e.g. different working habits or to different drawing and reading of standard curves.

Troubleshooting (symptom + possible causes)

General

low recovery of added radioactivity: incomplete extraction; losses during chromatography or dissolving; impure tracer

variation in recovery of radioactivity: varying extraction; inconsistent performance of chromatograph or fraction collector; errors in manual fraction collecting; varying amounts of tracer added

low or high recovery of added nonradioactive compounds: performance of method dependent on sample concentration; interference from sample constituents

results "too high": standard concentrations too low; contaminated tubes, syringes or injector (especially after standardization); interference

Vitamin D. A Chemical, Biochemical and Clinical Update

from sample constituents; adsorption of tracers into scintillation vials (during determination of recovery)

results "too low": standard concentrations too high; interference from sample constituents; adsorption of tracer into scintillation vials (totals)

high intra-assay variation: probably a combination of several causes: varying amounts of tracer added; wrong measuring range; high scintillation counting error; wrong working habits; poor standard curve; contaminated materials; interference from sample constituents; low recovery

high interassay variation: high intra-assay variation, systematic errors; standards or tracers changed between series; errors in standardization; results dependent on analyst

CPB methods

low total binding: dilution of tracer too high; dilution of binding protein too high; inactive binding protein; wrong pH of buffer; wrong incubation temperature; sample and tracer not soluble into incubation mixture; errors in separation of free and bound tracer

low sensitivity: low recovery; low total binding; dilution of binding protein too low; low specific activity of tracer

high nonspecific binding: inactive binding protein; impure tracer; wrong separation of free and bound tracer

HPLC methods

low sensitivity: low recovery; interference from sample constituents; wrong detector or recorder settings or wavelength; poor column performance

nonlinear standard curve: wrong injection technique; varying injection volume; errors in dilution of standards

THE CONCENTRATIONS OF VITAMIN D METABOLITES AND THE VITAMIN D_3 BIOLOGICAL ACTIVITY OF MILK OF CONTROL OR 1αHYDROXYVITAMIN D_3 INJECTED COWS.

R. PERLMAN*, M. SACHS** and A. BAR*

Institute of Animal Science, ARO, The Volcani Center, Bet Dagan*, and The "Haklait" Veterinary Clinical Services, Netanya**, Israel.

Introduction:

Parenteral administration of 1αhydroxyvitamin D_3 (1αOH D_3) prevents parturient paresis in dairy cows (1,2,3). The purpose of the present study was to determine the content of vitamin D metabolites and the vitamin D_3 biological activity of milk obtained from 1α(OH)D_3-treated or non-treated cows.

Methods:

Experiment 1: The concentrations of vitamin D metabolites were determined in the milk of non-injected (control) and 1α(OH)D_3-injected (700 μg, i.m. in PG) Israeli-Friesian cows that calved 36-43 h after the treatment. Milk samples were taken 60 h after calving and radiolabeled vitamin D_3 metabolites were added. The samples were lyophilized and extracted by chloroform:methanol, dried, dissolved in hexane:diethylether and filtered through 10 x 65 mm silica columns. The retained vitamin D metabolites were eluted with 5% methanol in diethylether. The eluted samples were chromatographed by HPLC through a Radial pak uPorasil cartridge using an isocratic-gradient combination of solvents from 2.5 to 20% isopropanol in hexane. The eluted D metabolites were rechromatographed by HPLC through a C-18 uBondopak Radial pak cartridge using an isocratic-gradient combination of H_2O in methanol (3,4). Vitamin D (Perlman et al., in preparation), 25(OH)D, 24,25$(OH)_2$D (5), 1α(OH)D_3 (6) and 1,25$(OH)_2$D (4) were determined by competitive binding assays. Vitamin D and 1α(OH)D_3 were estimated by nonequilibrium assays (linear between 0.1 to 30 ng and 0.03 to 10 ng, respectively).

Experiment 2: Cows of the same breed were injected twice, at 72 h intervals, with 350 μg 1α(OH)D_3. Five liters of milk were taken 60 h after calving from cows that calved 37-60 h after the second injection. The milk samples were lyophilized and extracted. For the determination of vitamin D_3 activity, light breed male chicks were fed vitamin D deficient diets, containing 30, 60, 120 or 240 IU D_3/kg diet, or milk extracts equivalent to 1 or 2 l/kg diet. Body weight, blood Ca, mg ash and ash percentage in the tibia were determined (7).

Results and Discussion:

The results obtained in the first experiment are shown in Table 1. The values given in the table for the colostrum-like milk are slightly different from those obtained in other studies conducted with normal milk (8,9). No significant differences were found in the milk of treated and non-treated cows. 1α(OH)D_3 concentration in treated cows' milk was less than 10 ng/l.

The biological activity of the milk examined in the second experiment was 40±3 IU/l. Such activity is within the range of normal cow's milk (10-12), considering the similarity of the examined cow's milk to colostrum.

Vitamin D. A Chemical, Biochemical and Clinical Update

Table 1. The concentrations of vitamin D derivatives in cow milk

	Vitamin D	25(OH)D	$24,25(OH)_2D$	$1(OH)D_3$*	$1,25(OH)_2D$
			ng/liter		
Non-treated	372±24**	264±68	68±26	-	21±3
Treated	385±98	329±49	59±31	<10	22±3

*Standards were diluted in a normal milk extract (HPLC purified)
**Means±SE of 4-8 milk samples.

The results suggest that the vitamin D_3 biological activity and/or vitamin D metabolites content of milk obtained (60 h after calving) from cows injected with $1\alpha(OH)D_3$ (42-36 h before calving) did not differ significantly from the milk of non-treated cows.

Acknowledgements:
Supported by a grant from the U.S.-Israel Binational Agricultural Research and Development Fund (BARD #352-81). The technical assistance of Mrs. S. Strym and M. Cotter is gratefully acknowledged.

References:
1. Sachs, M., Bar, A., Cohen, R., Mazur, Y., Mayer, E., Hurwitz, S. (1977) J. Vet. Res. 38, 2039-2041.
2. Bar, A., Sachs, M., Hurwitz, S. (1980) Vet. Rec. 106, 529-532.
3. Bar, A., Sachs, M. (1983) Proc. 5th Int. Conf. on production diseases in farm animals, Upsala, pp. 19-21.
4. Bar, A., Rosenberg, J., Hurwitz, S. (1984) Comp. Biochem. Physiol. 78B, 75-79.
5. Bishop, J.E., Norman, A.W., Coburan, J.W., Roberts, P.A., Henry, H.L. (1980) J. Min. Elect. Metab. 3, 181-189.
6. Bar, A., Perlman, R., Sachs, M. (1985) J. Dairy Sci. in press.
7. Bar, A., Edelstein, S., Eisner, U., Ben-Gal, I., Hurwitz, S. (1982) J. Nutr. 112, 1779-1786.
8. Reeve, L.E., Jorgensen, N.A., De Luca, H.F. (1982) J. Nutr. 112, 667-672.
9. Kunz, C., Niesen, M., Lilienfeld-Toal, H., Burmeister, W. (1984) Internat. J. Vit. Nutr. Res. 54, 141-148.
10. Gast, D.R., Marquardt, J.P., Jorgensen, N.A., De Luca, H.F. (1977) J. Dairy Sci. 60, 1910-1920.
11. Leerbeck, E., Sondergaard, H. (1980) Br. J. Nutr. 44, 7-12.
12. Eaton, H.D., Spielman, A.A., Loosli, J.K., Thomas, J.W., Norton, C.L., Turk, K.L. (1947) J. Dairy Sci. 30, 787-794.

RADIOIMMUNOASSAY FOR SERUM 25,26(OH)$_2$D$_3$

L. Hummer, J.S. Johansen and C. Christiansen
Department of Clinical Chemistry, Glostrup Hospital, Denmark

Introduction:

A selective radioimmunoassay (RIA) for 25,26-dihydroxycholecalciferol (25,26(OH)$_2$D$_3$) has been developed. High titer antibodies were generated in rabbits immunized with 1-alpha-hydroxycholacalcioic acid coupled to bovine serum albumin. One antiserum recognized 25,26(OH)$_2$D$_3$ and a RIA has been established with tritiated 1,25-dihydroxycholecalciferol (1,25(OH)$_2$D$_3$) as tracer and synthetic 25,26(OH)$_2$D$_3$ as standard.

Materials and methods:

1-alpha-cholacalcioic acid, 25S,26(OH)$_2$D$_3$ was kindly donated by Dr. M.R. Uskokovic, the Hoffman-La Roche Company, Nutley, New Jersey, USA. (26,27-methyl-^{3}H)-1,25(OH)$_2$D$_3$, specific activity 130-180 Ci/mmol was purchased from the Radiochemical Centre, Amersham, UK.

Extraction and purification of serum samples:

Serum samples (3-5 ml) were extracted by methanol/dichloromethane following a modification (1) of the procedure described by Shepard et al. (2). The lipid extracts were purified by Sephadex LH 20 and the dihydroxyvitamin D fraction was further purified by high pressure liquid chromatography (HPLC) on a Lichrosorb Si 60 (7 um) column developed by hexane/isopropanol (9/1, v/v), flow 2 ml/min. The fraction co-eluting with 24,25-(OH)$_2$D$_3$, (8-13 ml) 25,26(OH)$_2$D$_3$ (17-22 ml) and the 1,25(OH)$_2$D fraction (27-33 ml), respectively, were collected for final assays (1-4).

Radioimmunoassay of 25,26(OH)$_2$D$_3$:

Standard solutions (50 ul) of 25,26(OH)$_2$D$_3$, ranging from 4-1000 pg 25,26(OH)$_2$D$_3$/tube, or 50 ul sample eluate were taken to dryness under nitrogen, and 50 ul of the radiolabelled 1,25(OH)$_2$D$_3$ 3000 cpm (10 pg) diluted in 50% ethanol was added to all tubes. 500 ul antiserum diluted 1:100,000 in 0.1 mol/l sodium phosphate buffer (0.1% (w/v) bovine serum albumin, 0.25% phenyl mercuri acetate) pH 7.2 was added to each tube. The tubes were incubated for 48 h at 4°C. The free sterol was separated from the antibody bound fraction by 200 ul dextran-coated charcoal (2.5% Norite A, 0.25% Dextran T-80 in 0.1 mol/l phosphate buffer, pH 7.2). After incubation for 10 min. at 4°C and centrifugation (4°C) at 2,500 g the radioactivity was measured in 400 ul of the supernatant.

Results:

The specificity of the antiserum was tested by determining the extent to which related sterols would displace the ^{3}H-1,25(OH)$_2$-D$_3$ tracer. The amount of 25,26(OH)$_2$D$_3$ which results in 50%

displacement of the maximal binding is defined as 1. The results from the selected antiserum are shown in Table 1. The displacement pattern of vitamin D-binding protein in rabbit serum (CPBA) is also shown in the table for comparison. The antiserum is not specific for $25,26(OH)_2D_3$. However, this has no significance as $25,26(OH)_2D_3$ can be separated from these metabolites.

Binder Dilution Tracer	Antiserum 7633 1:100,000 ^3H-1,25(OH)2D3	Rabbit serum 1:100,000 ^3H-25(OH)D3
$25,26(OH)_2D_3$	1	1
$25(OH)D_3$	2	0.3
$25(OH)D_2$	3	0.2
$1,25(OH)_2D_3$	0.1	40
$1,25(OH)_2D_2$	0.2	18
$24,25(OH)_2D_3$	0.8	0.2
$1,24,25(OH)_3D_3$	0.3	39

The detection limit was 4 pg/tube using the RIA and 16 pg/tube using CPBA with rabbit serum. The interassay variation determined on a control sample assayed in 10 assays over a period of two months was 12% (RIA) compared to 17% (CPBA). The intra-assay variation was 8% (n=10) and 12% in the two assays, respectively.

Serum samples (n=39) from thirteen healthy postmenopausal women, aged 45-55 years, were obtained during one year. The samples were assayed by RIA 0.49 0.19 (mean SD) and by CPBA 0.59 0.25 (mean SD). A linear correlation was found between the results obtained by the two methods, r=0.78, SEE=26%, $(25,26\text{-}(OH)_2D_{CPBA} = 1.0 \times 25,26(OH)_2D_{RIA} + 0.1)$. The intercept was not significantly different from zero.

Conclusion:

The present data indicate that the radioimmunoassay for determination of $25,26(OH)_2D_3$ is a reliable alternative to the competitive protein binding assay.

References:

1. Hummer L, Riis BJ, Christiansen C, Rickers H. Scand J Clin Lab Invest 1985. (In press).
2. Shepard RM, Horst RL, Hamstra AJ, DeLuca HF. Biochem J 1979; 182: 55-69.
3. Hummer L, Christiansen C. Clin Endocrinol 1984; 21: 71-79.
4. Fraher LJ, Clemens TL, Papapoulos SE, Redel J, O'Riordan JLH. Clin Sci 1980; 59: 257-263.

ESTIMATION OF 1,25 DIHYDROXYVITAMIN D BY CYTORECEPTOR AND COMPETITIVE PROTEIN BINDING ASSAYS WITHOUT HIGH PRESSURE LIQUID CHROMATOGRAPHY (HPLC)

RW Retallack, JC Kent, GC Nicholson and DH Gutteridge
Department of Endocrinology and Diabetes, Sir Charles Gairdner Hospital, Nedlands, Western Australia.

Using two different rat osteosarcoma cell lines (UMR 106 and ROS 17/2.8) we have investigated the cytoreceptor assay (CR) for $1,25(OH)_2D$ (1). With both cell lines we obtained a standard curve with a sensitivity of 2.4 fmole/tube. Measurement of $1,25(OH)_2D$ levels in serum extracted by Clin Elut columns (1) gave variable results and usually higher than expected values for all samples. Addition of 73nmol/L $25OHD_3$ to serum samples significantly increased the assayed level of $1,25(OH)_2D$, even in the presence of α-globulin. Solvent blanks were undetectable, but assay of benzene or benzene plus water which had passed through the column showed that some Clin Eluts contained impurities which interfered with the assay and had not been removed by the recommended 10ml benzene pre-wash (1).

A 3.5x0.5cm silicic acid (SA) (Sigma SIL-LC) column attached directly to the Clin Elut adsorbs the vitamin D metabolites eluted by the benzene. Washing the detached SA column with ether:hexane (1:1,v/v) then ether removes the vitamin D, 25OHD and $24,25(OH)_2D$. The $1,25(OH)_2D$ can then be eluted separately with methanol:ether (1:19,v/v)(2). Assay values obtained using this extraction method and the first batch of SA were high. However subsequent batches of SA eliminated all contaminants and the CR assay of these extracts was not changed by further purification on HPLC. We have applied this extraction method to the calf thymus cytosol competitive protein binding assay (CTC) (3) for normals, patients with chronic renal failure (CRF) or primary hyperparathyroidism (HPT), and vitamin D deficient chicks (DDC) and the results correlate well with those obtained using the CR (Table 1, Fig 1, slope = 0.77, intercept = 9.5, r = 0.91, n = 97)

Table 1

ASSAY	Normal	CRF	HPT	DDC	Intra-assay CV (%)	Inter-assay CV (%)	DL* fmole/tube
CR	94±25 (34)	45±15 (7)	129±35 (6)	12±6 (8)	21.3	23.7	2.4
CTC	85±15 (23)	31±13 (8)	107±50 (7)	7±4 (9)	15.9	22.1	1.2

$1,25(OH)_2D$ results are pmol/L [mean±1SD (n)]
* DL = Detection Limit

Vitamin D. A Chemical, Biochemical and Clinical Update

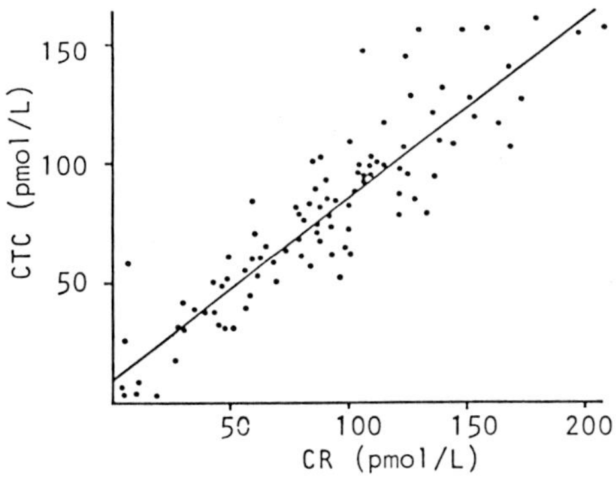

Fig 1.
Comparison of assay values for $1,25(OH)_2D$ obtained using the CR and CTC. Samples extracted on Clin Elut plus SA.

This extraction method allow omission of α-globulin from the incubation medium and allows simultaneous preparation of 50 samples. The CTC method is preferred since no tissue culture is required, the binding protein is very stable, its preparation is simple and yields sufficient reagent for a large number of assays, the assay is more sensitive (samples as small as 0.25ml can be assayed) and more reproducible than the CR (Table 1).

This assay has been applied to a longitudinal study of $1,25(OH)_2D$ levels in human pregnancy and lactation. In late pregnancy the levels were very high and decreased rapidly after parturition to normal levels at 3 weeks of lactation. They then rose again and at 16 weeks of lactation were significantly different from normals.

Analysis of frequent samples taken during the menstrual cycle revealed no change in serum levels of ionized calcium, immunoreactive PTH or $1,25(OH)_2D$ (Fig 2).

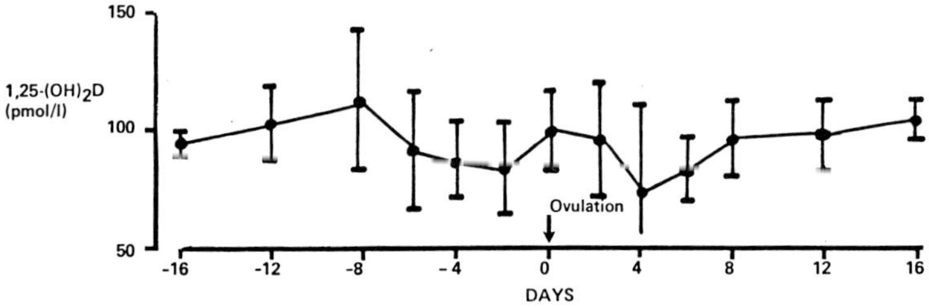

Fig 2. 6 Subjects studied throughout the menstrual cycle. Ovulation determined as day of peak LH. Results mean SD.

1. Manolagas,SC, Culler,FL, Howard,JE, Brickman,AS, Deftos, LJ(1983) J Clin Endocrinol Metab,56,751-760.
2. Nicholson,GN, Kent,JC, Gutteridge,DH, Retallack,RW(1985) Clin Endocrinology,22,in press.
3. Reinhardt,TA, Horst,RL, Orf,JW, Hollis,BW(1984) J Clin Endocrinol Metab,58,91-98.

OPTIMISATION OF A BINDING ASSAY FOR 25-HYDROXY VITAMIN D

S Whateley, M J O'Sullivan, C A Spensley, J R Bullock, P J Nott and G L Guilford. Tritium Products Department, Amersham International plc, Forest Farm, Whitchurch, Cardiff, United Kingdom CF4 7YT

INTRODUCTION

Although 25-Hydroxy vitamin D (25OHD) binding assays have been used for a number of years, there is no single accepted standard protocol. Indeed two recent studies have highlighted the wide inter-laboratory variation in 25OHD measurements. This paper outlines our attempts to define the optimal format for a 25OHD assay. We concentrated our efforts on two areas. Firstly, we aimed to develop a simple, reproducible and reliable purification technique which removed potential interfering compounds from the sample prior to the binding assay. Secondly, we wished to develop a convenient robust assay with maximum precision over the required analyte concentration range.

METHODS

Sample Purification. A 0.5ml aliquot of serum was vortex mixed for 15 sec with 0.5ml of distilled water and 1.0ml of acetonitrile. The tubes were centrifuged for 10 minutes at 1000xg. The supernatant was then decanted into glass tubes containing 0.5ml of 0.4M phosphate buffer pH 10.5. After mixing the samples were applied to Sep-Pak C_{18} cartridges which were then washed with 10ml of distilled water followed by 5ml of methanol:water. The samples were finally eluted into glass tubes with 3ml of acetonitrile. The eluates were blown down under nitrogen at 37°C and stored at -20°C until required for the binding assay.

The Binding Assay. The purified sample extract was reconstituted with 1.0ml of ethanol. A 50µl aliquot of tracer in ethanol was incubated with 50µl of standard or sample and 500µl of binding protein solution. The samples were mixed and then incubated for 2h at 4°C. At the end of this period 500µl of ice cold dextran coated charcoal was added to each tube. The tubes were mixed and allowed to stand at 4°C for 20 min, then centrifuged at 2000xg for 15 min at 4°C. The supernatants were decanted into 10ml of scintillant, mixed and counted for 4 minutes.

RESULTS AND DISCUSSION

Purification of the sample by straight solvent extraction was unsatisfactory. It resulted in high and variable 25OHD serum values. We adapted a very straightforward Sep-Pak procedure to isolate a fraction containing the total vitamin D metabolites. The between-assay recovery of [^{3}H]25OHD$_3$ was determined to be 80 ± 6% (n=20) with this technique. By extending the methanol:water wash from 5ml to 25ml it proved possible to remove >90% of the 24,25(OH)$_2$D$_3$ whilst retaining >90% of the 25OHD$_3$. This provides a method of measuring 25OHD with slightly greater accuracy if so desired.

Sephadex LH-20 column chromatography with a hexane:chloroform:methanol (9:1:1) mixture gave superior resolution of the vitamin D metabolites, but the procedure was more cumbersome than this single step Sep-Pak

Vitamin D. A Chemical, Biochemical and Clinical Update

procedure. However, 25OHD serum levels determined after purification by either the Sep-Pak or Sephadex LH-20 procedures were identical.

The standard curve covers the range 1 to 32ng/ml with a mid-point of ~10ng/ml. Approximately 1.5ng/ml (75pg/tube) of 25OHD is required to reduce the zero dose binding by two standard deviations. The 25OHD binding protein has approximately equivalent cross-reactivity with a number of vitamin D metabolites. It recognises both D_2 and D_3 derivatives, but discriminates against the parent vitamins.[2] The precision of the assay was determined using a number of pure 25OHD controls and pooled human serum. Both within and between-assay precision for the 25OHD controls was 10% or less. Within and between-assay precisions were 7% and 14% for pooled normal human serum.

Quantitative recovery of both $25OHD_2$ and $25OHD_3$ was obtained with this protocol. The measured 25OHD serum concentration was independent of the sample size over the range 100µl to 1000µl. Further analysis by Sephadex LH-20 column (16 x 1cm) chromatography of the total vitamin D metabolite fraction obtained from the Sep-Pak indicated that >90% of the activity in the binding assay co-eluted with $[^3H]25OHD_3$ and <10% with $24,25(OH)_2D_3$. This is strong evidence to substantiate the lack of non-specific interference in this assay.

In summary, serum samples can be purified by either reverse phase Sep-Pak cartridges or Sephadex LH-20 columns. Cartridges are more convenient if only 25OHD measurements are required. Sephadex LH-20 column chromatography is the method of choice for measuring both 25OHD and $1\alpha,25(OH)_2D$ in the same sample extract. The results indicate that a reliable 25OHD assay can be developed when attention is given to careful optimisation of the assay parameter.

Data for a typical 25OHD standard curve is shown in Table I below :

TABLE I

Standard (ng/ml)	CPM
Totals	6259, 6301
Non-specific binding	180, 199
Zero standard	3270, 3354
1	3223, 3235
2	3132, 3130
4	2671, 2594
8	1758, 1661
16	1039, 991
32	685, 795

1,25-DIHYDROXYVITAMIN D_3 RADIOMMUNOASSAY: MODIFICATIONS HAVE OPTIMIZED SENSITIVITY AND REPRODUCIBILITY.

N. HANAFIN, L. PALMER, AND M.F. HOLICK,
Harvard Medical School, Massachusetts General Hospital, Boston, MA, 02114, USA.

Advances in the early seventies allowed the chemical identification of the major vitamin D metabolites and elucidated the metabolic sequence of hydroxylations necessary to produce the biologically active form of the vitamin 1,25-$(OH)_2$- D_3. In 1974, Brumbaugh first reported a clinically functional radioreceptor assay for 1,25-$(OH)_2$-D_3 using the cytoplasmic chick receptor (1). Because of a number of problems inherent in the receptor-type assay, particularly the relative instability of receptor preparations, several radioimmunoassays for this metabolite have been developed in the past several years (2-5).

A major problem in developing a RIA for 1,25-$(OH)_2$-D_3, as with other steroid hormones, has been its low molecular weight. To be immunogenic, this hapten must be covalently coupled to a macromolecule. We previously reported a RIA that utilized an antisera with high specificity and affinity for 1,25-$(OH)_2$-D (2). Since both the position of conjugation and the type of chemical bridge ultimately affect antibody specificity and affinity, the conjugate's design was crucial. 1α-OH-D_3-24-oic-acid (6), which has a reactive functional group in the side chain, was synthesized and coupled directly to BSA by formation of the mixed-acid anhydride (7). The rationale was that this coupling at the C_{24} position would confer immunodominance to the A ring and 1-hydroxy group in the hapten, reducing the significance of the side chain as an antigenic determinant. Previous conjugates, with hemisuccinate coupling groups on the A ring itself produced only moderately specific antisera.

Since then, a number of RIA parameters have been closely evaluated to improve assay sensitivity and reproducibility. Of crucial importance in any RIA is the buffer. It maintains ionic concentration and pH in the assay system; factors which strongly affect the affinity and avidity of the antigen-antibody bond. Optimal sensitivity of R_8 antiserum was achieved using 0.05 M PO_4 in 0.1 M KCl (pH 7.4) as the assay buffer. In contrast to the previous assay diluent which was 0.07 M KH_2 PO_4 (pH 7.4), this acid-base pair system of both monobasic and dibasic phosphates in conjunction with higher ionic concentration increased buffering capacity and stability. Additionally, since immunizations with a hapten protein conjugate can often produce antibodies with specificity for the carrier protein itself, 1% gamma-globulin free horse serum was substituted for BSA in the assay buffer to eliminate any potential for such antibodies to cross react and actually bind to the BSA interfering with hapten-specific binding. With these buffer modifications, final antisera titer doubled to 1:60,000, maximal specific binding increased from 24% to 42%, and nonspecific binding was consistently <5% of total tracer added.

Providing the antigen-antibody complex has a slow dissociation constant it is theoretically possible to increase sensitivity in the

Vitamin D. A Chemical, Biochemical and Clinical Update

reversible A_g-Ab reaction by incubating in 2 steps. The high affinity R_8 antiserum suggested high avidity, or a low tendency to dissociate. First incubation time studies empirically determined 4 hours as the optimal tracer addition delay time. With over night incubation at 4°C, these disequilibrium conditions decreased Bo midpoint sensitivity from 48 pg/tube to 32 pg/tube. (Most importantly, assay sensitivity was optimized to 2 pg/tube) two to four time greater than the previous assay (Fig. 1). This consistently reproducible sensitivity improved detection limits and reduced sample requirements by one third. Based on quality control data the assay demonstrated 5% intra- and 6% interassay variation. This assay should be a valuable diagnostic tool in accessing clinical disorders caused by disturbances in the metabolism of 25-OH-D_3 to 1,25-$(OH)_2$-D_3.

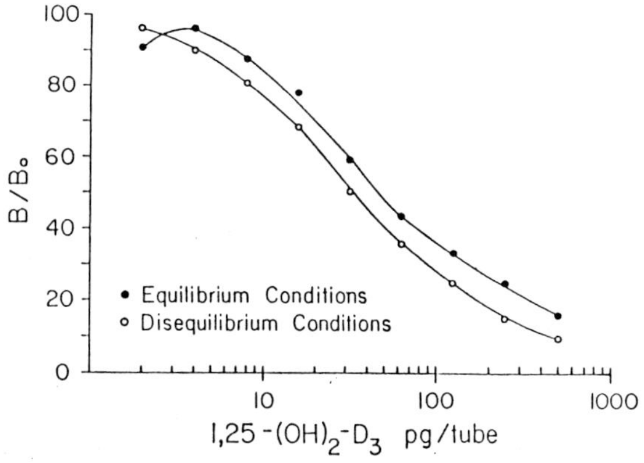

REFERENCES

1. Brumbaugh, P.F., Haussler, D.H., Bressler, R. and Haussler, M.F. (1974) Science 183, 1089-1091.
2. Clemens, T.L., Henderson, S., Meng, X., Baggiolini, E.G., Uskokovic, M.R., Holick, S.A. and Holick, M.F. (1983) Steroids 42, 503-509.
3. Gray, T.K., McAdoo, T., Pool, D., Lester, G.E., Williams, M.E. and Jones, G. (1981) Clin. Chem. 27, 458-463.
4. Bouillon R., DeMoor, P., Baggiolini, E.G. and Uskokovic, M.R. (1980) Clin. Chem. 26, 562 567.
5. Sharla, S., Schmidt-Gayk, H., Reichel, H. and Mayer, E. (1984) Clinica Chimica Acta 142, 325-338.
6. Koizum, N., Morisaki, M., Ikekawa, N. Tanaka, Y. and DeLuca, H.F. (1979) J. Steroid Biochem. 10, 261-267.
7. Erlanger, B.F., Borek, F., Berser, S.M. and Luberman, S. (1959) J. Biol. Chem. 234, 1090-1094.
8. This work was supported in part by NIH grants AM27334 and AM32324.

A SIMPLIFIED HPLC-METHOD FOR THE DETECTION OF 25-HYDROXY-VITAMIN D_3 IN HUMAN SERUM USING ELECTROCHEMICAL OR UV DETECTION.

Jan Wilske, Barbro Hulthe, Depts of Nephrology and Analytical and Marine Chemistry, University of Göteborg, Göteborg, Sweden.

Vitamin D_2 and D_3 have been detected by a voltammetric technique (1). However, no application has been reported in a chromatographic context. The aim of this work was to use electrochemical detection in combination with HPLC, which enhances sensitivity and selectivity compared to UV detection. Sample pretreatment can be simplified and the increased sensitivity makes it possible to study vitamin D_3 metabolites which occur in very low concentrations.

METHODS

For the normal phase system a Waters 45-A pump with an U6K variable loop injector and a 250 x 4.6 mm Lichrospher II Si-100 5 µ column (Merck) was used. The mobile phase was 4% isopropanol in heptane, flowrate 1.5 ml per min. The UV-detector was a Waters 480 Lambda-Max variable wave length detector set at 264 nm with a range of 0.01 absorbance units fullscale.

In the reversed phase system a LKB 2150 HPLC pump, an external pulse dampener (LKB), and a Rheodyne 7125 injection valve equipped with a sample loop of 24 µl was used. The column, 70 x 4.6 mm with Shandon Hypersil ODS 3 µm particles, was packed upwards with isopropanol as a slurry solvent and hexane as the pumping medium. For the mobile phase 35% of 50 mM H_3PO_4 in acetonitrile was used with a flow rate of 1.5 ml/min. For electrochemical detection a Bioanalytical System LC-4B controller was used in connection with a thin-layer detector cell of our own construction. The potential of the working electrode was maintained at + 1.10 V vs. Ag/AgCl (with an inner solution of 1 M NaCl). The R/C filter time constant of the amplifier was chosen as 2 s.

The design of the electrolytic cell: The thin layer cavity was constructed of two polyvinylidendifluorid (PVDF) blocks separated by a fluorocarbon sheet (Tefzel, Du Pont), 0.13 mm thick and with a 3.3 mm wide channel. The working electrode was made of a glassy-carbon disk of 3 mm diameter contained in the center of one of the blocks. The reference electrode and the auxiliary electrode (stainless steel) were held in a cylindrical chamber, filled with 1 M NaCl, in the other block. A porous plug, 1.6 mm in diameter, (zirconiumoxide) coinstituted the liquid junction between the electrolyte chamber and the working electrode. The amperometric detector cell presented in this investigation is of a construction similar to that of the coulometric detector presented by Hagihara et al (13). The advantage of this construction is the use of a separate electrolyte chamber, containing the reference electrode and the auxiliary electrode, which shields the reference electrode chemically from the mobile phase but provides good conductivity.

To a 1 ml aliquot of serum sample 4000 dpm of radioactive 25-OH-D_3 in 20 µl of ethanol was added. After equilibration at room temperature for 30 minutes, one ml of acetonitrile was added slowly. The sample was vortex mixed and then allowed to stand for 15 min. A 4 ml aliquot of hexane

Vitamin D. A Chemical, Biochemical and Clinical Update

was added and the tube was shaken for 3 minutes. Of the hexane phase 3 ml was transferred to unother test tube and after evaporation under nitrogen to dryness the residue was immediately reconstituted for either reversed or normal phase HPLC.

When the separation was performed with the normal phase column, the residue was reconstituted with 100 µl of the isopropanol/heptane mobile phase and 70 µl was injected into the HPLC system.

For use in the reverse phase system, 100 µl of 65% acetonitrile in water was added and the solution was filtered (Millex-HV4, Millipore) prior to injection.

RESULTS AND DISCUSSION

There has been rapid progress in the use of electrochemical detectors in HPLC because of their selectivity in combination with good sensitivity and linear response over a wide concentration range (2, 3, 4).

The detection limit of the system is dependent on the flow characteristics of the HPLC pump used. Pulsations will give rise to noise, which affects this limit. With electrochemical detector it was 0.2 ng injected amount (signal to noise ratio 2:1). Twelve repeated injections of a 0.2 ng/µl solution of 25-OH-D_3 showed a C V of 1.8%. Duplicate determinations for each amount were performed in the range 0.75 - 24 ng. The amperometric response is linear with respect to concentration with a regression (r^2) coefficient of 0.999 and an intercept of 0.05 ng, which is well below the detection limit. In the normal phase system the limit was 1 ng injected amount of 25-OH-D_3.

The sample pretreatment described in this work is fast and convenient. Acetonitrile was found to be an effective deproteinizing agent when added in an amount equal to the serum volume. The recovery experiment with labelled 25-OH-D_3 resulted in an extraction efficiency of 53% with a C V of 5.1% (n=12). In the normal phase system, lipids in high content will interfere with 25-OH-D_3. With serum samples taken from donors, who have been fasting for four hours, however, no interferences have been observed which is a normal value for humans.

Results in this work indicate that other metabolites of vitamin D_3 can be determined in serum by HPLC and electrochemical detection, and an analysis method for 1.25-$(OH)_2$-D_3 is under investigation.

REFERENCES

1. Atuma, S.S., Lundström, K. and Lindquist, J. (1975) Analyst 100, 827-834.
2. Stulík, K. and Pacáková, V. (1981) J. Electroanal Chem. 129, 1-24.
3. Hanekamp, H.B., Bos, P. and Frei, R.B. (1982) Trends. Anal. Chem. 1, 135-139.
4. Surmann, P., Fresenius, Z. (1983) Anal. Chem. 316, 373-381.
5. Hagihara, B. (1983) J. Chromatogr. 281, 59-72.

MEASUREMENT OF VITAMIN D METABOLITES

L. Hummer and C. Christiansen
Department of Clinical Chemistry, Glostrup Hospital, Denmark

Recent studies have shown that vitamin D_3 is metabolized differently in chick, rat and pigs, and we have demonstrated that treatment with equal doses of vitamin D_2 and vitamin D_3 has different effect on bone mineral content in man. Several multiple assay systems have been published (1) for measuring vitamin D, 25(OH)D, 24,25$(OH)_2$D, 25,26$(OH)_2$D and 1,25$(OH)_2$D. Some of them do include the capacity to determine individually vitamin D_2 and D_3 metabolites. In our laboratory we have established two multiple assay systems. One, requiring 5 ml serum (2) and one quick assay requiring 0.5 ml serum.

A: "5 ml" VITAMIN D ASSAY

This method includes a 3-step dichloromethane/methanol extraction, purification by chromatography on Sephadex LH 20, resulting in three fractions containing vitmain D, monohydroxylated vitamin D and dihydroxylated vitamin D, respectively.

Vitamin D: After purification on Lipidex 5000 followed by a 2-step HPLC purification D_2 and D_3 can be separated and quantitated by UV detection.

25(OH)D: The monohydroxylated fraction is purified on Lipidex 5000 and separated in 25(OH)D_2 and 25(OH)D_3 on HPLC followed by UV detection. Alternatively, 25(OH)D_3 can be measured directly in the extract from LH 20 by a selective radioimmunoassay (RIA) (3) and the total 25(OH)D (25(OH)D_2 + 25(OH)D_3) can be measured by a competitive protein binding assay (CPBA) using vitamin D binding protein from rat serum (4).

The dihydroxylated fraction is separated by HPLC in three fractions co-eluting with 24,25$(OH)_2D_3$, 25,26$(OH)_2D_3$ and 1,25-$(OH)_2D_2$/1,25$(OH)_2D_3$, respectively.

24,25$(OH)_2$D: This fraction is known to include 24,25$(OH)_2D_2$, 24,25$(OH)_2D_3$, 25,26$(OH)_2D_2$ and 25(OH)D_3-23,26-lactone. Further purification on HPLC (1) is necessary prior to separate measurement of these metabolites. However, a selective radioimmunoassay (5) can determine 24,25$(OH)_2D_3$ in the eluate, directly.

25,26$(OH)_2$D: 25,26$(OH)_2D_3$ can be measured either by competitive protein binding assay or radioimmunoassay due to the selective collection of this D_3 metabolite in the fraction.

1,25$(OH)_2$D: In the applied HPLC system 1,25$(OH)_2D_2$ and 1,25-$(OH)_2D_3$ is almost co-eluting. By measuring either with receptor isolated from rachitic chick intestine or from calf thymus equal potency of the two metabolites results in a measurement

Vitamin D. A Chemical, Biochemical and Clinical Update

of 1,25(OH)$_2$D, including 1,25(OH)$_2$D$_2$ and 1,25(OH)$_2$D$_3$. Specific RIA's have been developed capable of measuring 1,25(OH)$_2$D$_3$ only or 1,25(OH)$_2$D$_2$ and 1,25(OH)$_2$D$_3$ together. Another HPLC system is required if 1,25(OH)$_2$D$_2$ and 1,25(OH)$_2$D$_3$ has to be separated.

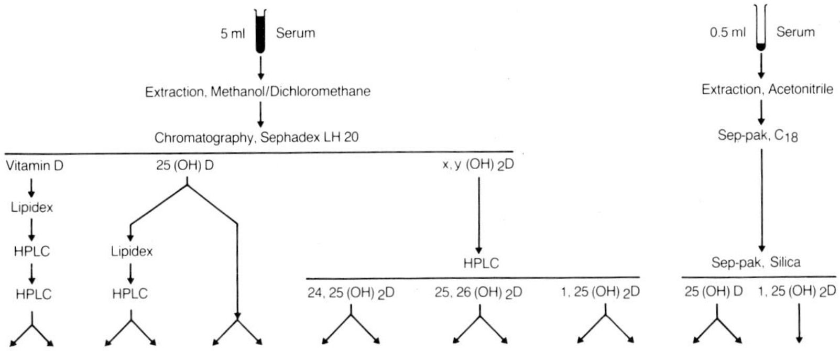

Fig. 1
Main extraction and purification steps in the two vitamin D metabolite assays.

B: "0.5 ml" VITAMIN D ASSAY

An improved isolation procedure using acetonitrile together with purification in prepacked cartridges, Sep-pak C_{18} and Sep-pak Silica has been developed. In the 25(OH)D-fraction 25(OH)D$_3$ can be measured by CPBA (rat serum), the result will include some 25,26(OH)$_2$D and 24,25(OH)$_2$D as well. In the 1,25-(OH)$_2$D fraction, the 1,25(OH)$_2$D$_2$ and 1,25(OH)$_2$D$_3$ together, can be measured by CPBA with the receptor isolated from the calf thymus.

Conclusion:

The present knowledge about vitamin D metabolism and about assay methodology stresses the need for carefully selecting the assay well suited for elucidating the clinical problem in question, taking as well specificity as sample volume, time and labor cost into consideration.

References

1. Horst RL, Littledike ET, Riley JL, Napoli JL. Anal Biochem 1981; 116: 189-203.

2. Hummer L, Riis BJ, Christiansen C, Rickers H. Scand J Clin Lab Invest 1985; in press.

3. Hummer L, Nilas L, Tjellesen L, Christiansen C. Scand J Clin Lab Invest 1984; 44: 163-167.

4. Hummer L, Tjellesen L, Rickers H, Christiansen C. Scand J Clin Lab Invest 1984; 44: 595-601.

5. Hummer L, Christiansen C. Clin Endocrinol 1984; 21: 71-79.

SECOND ANTIBODY VERSUS CHARCOAL SEPARATION IN THE RADIOIMMUNOASSAY (RIA) OF 1,25-DIHYDROXYVITAMIN D_3 (1,25(OH)$_2D_3$)

H. Schmidt-Gayk, F.-P. Armbruster, M. Schilling, S. Scharla and E. Mayer[Δ]

Chirurgische Klinik and [Δ]Abteilung für Endokrinologie, Universität, 6900 Heidelberg, FRG

The RIA for 1,25(OH)$_2D_3$ developed in this laboratory (1,2) includes a charcoal separation step to separate bound from free 1,25(OH)$_2D_3$. We have now carried out experiments to apply a second antibody separation step since in RIA of other steroid hormones this method has proven to be more specific and practicable than the charcoal separation technique.

100 µl of second antibody solution (Anti-rabbit IgG, 1:24 diluted in buffer PPPNE (see ref. above) were added to a total incubation volume of 420 µl. After a further incubation period of 2 h at 4 °C, the mixture was centrifuged for 10 min at 2000 g. The supernatants were aspirated and the precipitates dissolved in the varying washing solutions described below. Following centrifugation, the precipitate was dissolved in 10 µl 1 N NaOH and counted in 250 µl of scintillation fluid. The results are shown in table 1.

Table 1: Cpm ^{3}H-1,25(OH)$_2D_3$ obtained after washing

Washing solution	Total Bound cpm	Specific Bound cpm	Nonspecific Bound cpm
1. NaCl, 0.15 M	1250	760	490
2. NaCl + 0.001% Brij 35	1110	770	340
3. NaCl + 0.01% Brij 35	1050	980	70
4. NaCl + 0.1% Brij 35	1050	1020	30
5. Phosphate + 0.1% HSA	1250	890	360
6. Phosphate + 1% HSA	1120	860	260

Washing with solution 4 yielded high specific binding of ^{3}H-1,25(OH)$_2D_3$ in the presence of a very low nonspecific binding. Therefore solution 4 was used for all further experiments.

Applying equilibrium conditions, the sensitivity of the RIA for 1,25(OH)$_2D_3$ was higher when the second antibody was used in comparison to the charcoal method (80% B/B_o at 5 pg and 8 pg 1,25(OH)$_2D_3$/tube, resp.). With both techniques, the interference of 25-OH-D was identical (40 fold lower to 1,25-(OH)$_2D_3$.

Vitamin D. A Chemical, Biochemical and Clinical Update

Also, the influence of the saturation technique on the specificity of the second antibody RIA was assessed. Applying the sequential saturation (equilibrium method) addition of 48 pg (58 pg) of $1,25(OH)_2D_3$ and 3.6 ng (1.3 ng) of 25-OH-D were required to displace 50% of ^3H-$1,25(OH)_2D_3$ bound. Thus, the specificity for $1,25(OH)_2D_3$ vs. 25-OH-D was 75 fold (39 fold) with the sequential saturation method (equilibrium method).

Further, the specificity of the RIA for $1,25(OH)_2D_3$ was influenced by the ethanol content in the incubation mixture. With no ethanol contained already a 10 fold higher amount of 25-OH-D_3 than $1,25(OH)_2D_3$ resulted in 50% displacement of ^3H-$1,25(OH)_2D_3$, while a 28 fold higher concentration of 25-OH-D was required with 5% ethanol contained in the incubation volume.

In summary, the modification of our RIA for $1,25(OH)_2D_3$ by using a double antibody separation procedure appears to be superior to the charcoal separation, since the sensitivity for $1,25(OH)_2D_3$ is higher and nonspecific binding is lower. Further, this method is more practicable, less expensive (250 µl of scintillation fluid vs. 4 ml) and produces only a very small amount of radioactive waste.

1. Schmidt-Gayk, H., Gast, G., Jander, N., Gartner, R. and Mayer, E. (1982) in: Norman, A.W. et al. (eds.) Vitamin D: Chemical, Biochemical and Clinical Endocrinology of Calcium Metabolism, Walter de Gruyter, Berlin.

2. Scharla, S., Schmidt-Gayk, H., Reichel, H. and Mayer, E. (1984) Clin. Chim. Acta 142, 325-338.

PARATHYROID HORMONE SECRETION IN RENAL FAILURE.

E. SLATOPOLSKY, S. LOPEZ-HILKER, L. Y. CHAN, M. WEAVER, J. MORRISEY AND K. MARTIN,
Department of Medicine, Washington University, St. Louis, MO. U.S.A.

Secondary hyperparathyroidism is a universal finding in patients with renal insufficiency. Chief cell hyperplasia of the parathyroid glands and high levels of immunoreactive parathyroid hormone (iPTH) are among the earliest alterations of mineral metabolism in patients with chronic renal failure. Significant elevations in i-PTH in serum have been reported in patients with only slightly abnormal renal function (GFR 60-80 ml/min).

Although many factors are responsible for the regulation of the secretion of parathyroid hormone, it appears that in patients with renal insufficiency the most important factor for the development of secondary hyperparathyroidism is a reduction in the serum ionized calcium. The factors which may contribute to hypocalcemia and the development of secondary hyperparathyroidism in renal insufficiency include: 1) retention of phosphorus; 2) altered vitamin D metabolism; 3) skeletal resistance to the calcemic action of PTH; 4) altered set point for calcium-regulated PTH release and 5) impaired degradation of parathyroid hormone.

A number of studies have suggested that the majority of calcium-regulated parathyroid hormone that is secreted is obtained from a recently synthesized pool of protein that is not in rapid equilibrium with the bulk of the hormone stored in the cell (1,2-5). Beta-agonist stimulated hormone secretion, which is cAMP mediated, occurs from a pool of previously synthesized older protein (6). Phenomenologically, stimulation of hormone secretion by hypocalcemia, as opposed to stimulation by agents that operated through cAMP, appear to occur through different mechanisms (1,7-8).

Calcium is an inhibitor of the adenylate cyclase activity of isolated parathyroid membranes (9-13). Membranes prepared from hyperplastic glands are less susceptible to the inhibition of enzyme activity by calcium than are membranes prepared from normal human parathyroid tissue (12). This suggests that the "set point for calcium" (the calcium ion concentration causing a 50% decrease

Vitamin D. A Chemical, Biochemical and Clinical Update

in overall hormone secretion) to inhibit parathyroid adenylate cyclase is elevated above normal in hyperfunctioning human parathyroid glands. Since calcium-mediated changes in cellular cAMP cannot account for all the calcium-induced changes in hormone secretion, it is suggested that the elevated calcium set point for inhibition of adenylate cyclase is a general manifestation of the hyperplastic state.

In addition to the altered set point for the inhibition by calcium of parathyroid adenylate cyclase in membranes obtained from hyperfunctioning human glands, there is an altered set point for calcium in the inhibition of hormone secretion (14-18). Accumulated data obtained for collagenase-dispersed human parathyroid cells indicates a set point in normal cells of 0.97 ± 0.04 mM calcium ion; while in adenoma, primary, and secondary hyperplasia, the set point was found to be increased to 1.26 ± 0.13 mM, 1.09 ± 0.15 mM, and 1.17 ± 0.19 mM calcium ion respectively (18). Not only is the set point for calcium with respect to hormone secretion elevated in cells obtained from hyperplastic parathyroid tissue, but also the degree of responsiveness across the calcium sensitive range is altered. The degree of suppression of hormone secretion with increasing calcium is apparently less for cells obtained from all types of hyperplastic glands than for cells from normal glands (18).

Potential Regulation of PTH by Vitamin D Metabolites

Several investigators (19-21) have provided evidence that vitamin D metabolites directly affect regulation of PTH secretion. In 1974 Oldham et al (22) isolated a calcium-binding protein from porcine parathyroid glands with properties similar to those of the calcium-binding proteins found in mammalian intestinal mucosa. The administration of $25(OH)D_3$ to rachitic puppies increased the calcium binding protein in the parathyroid glands. Subsequently, Brumbaugh et al (23) demonstrated specific binding of $1,25(OH)_2D_3$ to cytosolic and nuclear receptors of the chick parathyroid glands *in vitro*. Chertow et al (19) subsequently performed studies *in vivo* in the rat and *in vitro* with bovine parathyroid gland slices. These investigators clearly demonstrated an inhibitory effect of $1,25(OH)_2D_3$ on PTH release. However, after these initial publications, a series of papers appeared in the literature, suggesting that $1,25(OH)_2D_3$ did not have a direct effect on the secretion of parathyroid hormone (23-24). Because of these controversial results, we studied in great detail the effect of $1,25(OH)_2D_3$ on parathyroid hormone secretion _in vitro_, using bovine parathyroid gland slices and isolated dispersed bovine parathyroid cells (26). The results failed to demonstrate an effect of $1,25(OH)_2D_3$ on PTH secretion by the isolated bovine parathyroid cells or by bovine parathyroid slices. It is critical to emphasize that the parathyroid glands used in these studies were obtained from normal cows which were not depleted of $1,25(OH)_2D_3$. Moreover, the studies were performed _in vitro_ and the incubations were conducted over a 4-hr period. The fact that the animals were not depleted of $1,25(OH)_2D_3$ may have had an effect on the outcome of the results obtained in these studies. Studies by Oldham and collaborators (27) in vitamin-D deficient dogs clearly indicated that higher concentrations of calcium were necessary to suppress the release of parathyroid hormone in these animals. When similar studies were performed in the same animals after $1,25(OH)_2D_3$ was given to the dogs, the parathyroid glands appeared to be more sensitive to mild increments in serum calcium.

The low levels of $1,25(OH)_2D_3$ observed in patients with advanced renal insufficiency (28-29) may potentially play a role in the abnormal behavior of the parathyroid glands. Thus we performed studies in dialysis patients with the use of an intravenous form of $1,25(OH)_2D_3$.

We selected 20 patients with hypocalcemia maintained on chronic hemodialysis (30). In the control part of the studies, blood was obtained before dialysis three times a week for a period of 3 weeks. In the treatment period 1,25-dihydroxy D_3 was given intravenously at the end of each dialysis for a period of 8 weeks. The starting dose was 0.5 µg and gradually was increased to a maximum of 4.0 µg per treatment. Finally, a second post-treatment control period was continued for an additional three weeks. Blood samples were obtained for total and ionized calcium, magnesium and phosphorus. PTH was measured with our chicken antibody CH9. This antibody recognizes the C terminal, middle region, and the intact PTH molecule.

The mean serum calcium increased from 8.5 mg/100 ml to 9.4 and with a peak response of 10.9 mg/100 ml during 1,25-dihyroxy D_3 administration. In the post-treatment period serum calcium decreased to a mean of 9.0 mg/100 ml. In general, there was a tendency for serum phosphorus to increase during 1,25-dihydroxy D_3 administration. Magnesium, on the other hand, remained fairly constant during the entire study in all patients. Every single patient had a substantial decrease in the levels of PTH during 1,25-dihydroxy D_3 treatment. The mean decrement in PTH was 70.1% (Fig. 1). After $1,25(OH)_2D_3$ was discontinued, PTH increased in every single patient. After three weeks of treatment, there was a gradual rise in the levels of ionized calcium. Concomitantly, there was a significant decrease in the levels of i-PTH.

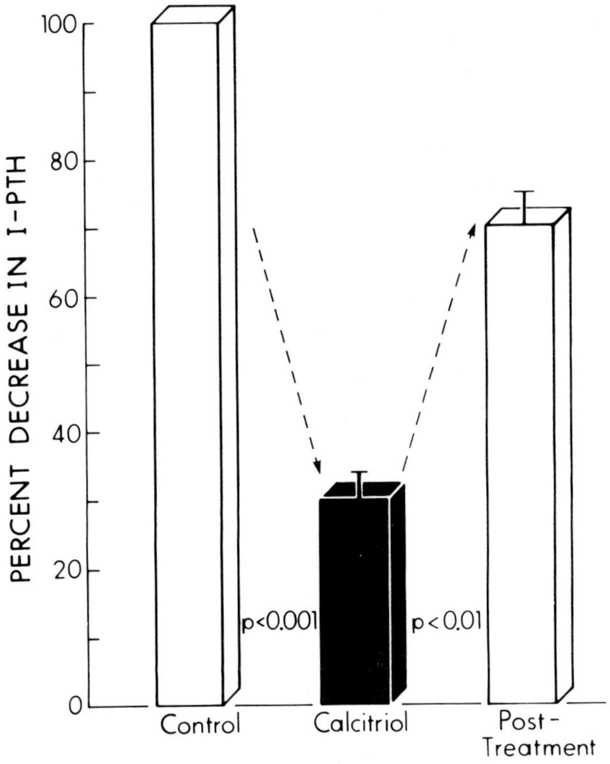

Figure 1: Changes in serum i-PTH during and after the administration of Intravenous $1,25(OH)_2D_3$ expressed as percent of pretreatment values. The mean decrement in serum i-PTH was 70.1% (Modified from Ref. 30).

However, it would seem that early during the administration of 1,25-dihydroxy D_3 before there was any significant increase in ionized calcium, already there was a decrease in the levels of i-PTH (Fig. 2).

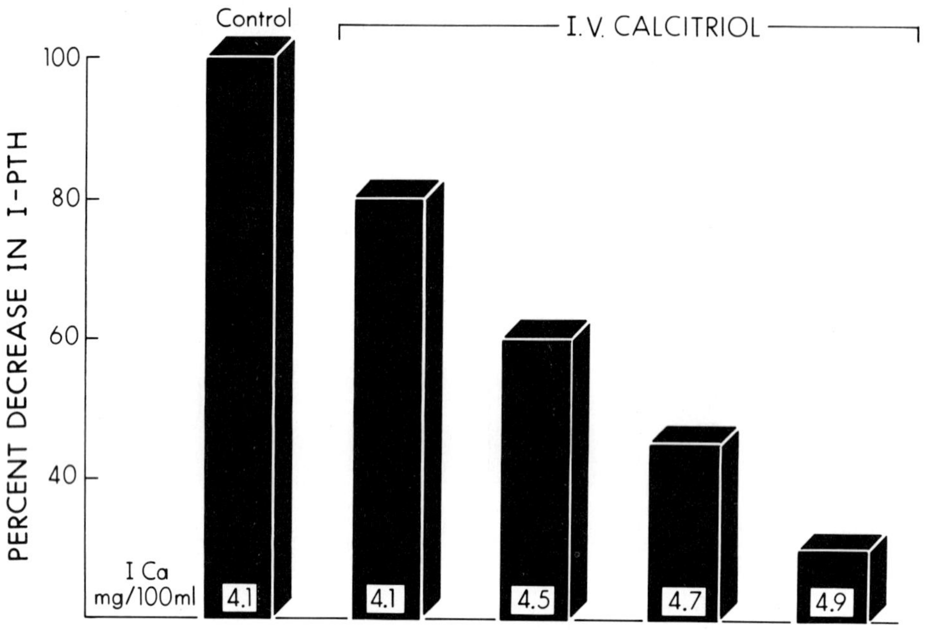

Figure 2: Temporal relationship between ionized calcium and serum i-PTH before and during intravenous $1,25(OH)_2D_3$ in all 20 patients. (Modified from Ref.30).

Thus, the present studies demonstrate that $1,25(OH)_2D_3$ has remarkable suppressive effect on the release of PTH. Likely, the effects are mainly due to elevation in serum calcium to the upper limits of normal. However, it would seem that in addition to the calcemic effect, 1,25-dihydroxy D_3 per se modified the secretion of PTH. It is known that parathyroid glands obtained from uremic patients have a shift in the set point for calcium, requiring a higher concentration of ionized calcium than normal parathyroid glands for the suppression of PTH release. These studies raise the possibility that 1, 25-dihydroxy D_3 may affect the regulation of PTH secretion by making the parathyroid gland more sensitive to calcium. Obviously, further studies are necessary to clarify this point.

In summary, the intravenous administration of $1,25(OH)_2D_3$ has a significant suppressive effect on PTH secretion in uremic patients. Although part of the changes are related to an increase in ionized calcium, it would seem that $1,25(OH)_2D_3$ per se has a direct effect on PTH release.

References

1. Morrissey, J.J., Cohn, D.V. (1979) J. Cell. Biol. 82:93-102.
2. Morrissey, J.J., Cohn, D.V. (1979) J. Cell.Biol. 83:521-528.
3. MacGregor, R.R., Chu, L.L.H., Hamilton, J.W., et al. (1973) Endocrinology 93:1387-1397.
4. MacGregor, R.R., Hamilton, J.W., Cohn, D.V. (1975) Endocrinology 97:178-188.
5. Brown, E.M., Thatcher, J.C. (1982) Endocrinology 110:1374-1380.
6. Hanley, D.A., Takatsuki, K., Birnbaumer, M.E., et al. (1980) Calcif. Tiss. Int. 32:19-27.
7. Brown, E.M. (1981) J. Clin. Endocrinol. Metab. 52:961-968.
8. Blum, J.W., Fisher, J.A., Hunziker, W.H, et al. (1978) J. Clin. Invest. 61:1113-1122.
9. Dufresne, L.R., Gitelman, H.J. in Talmade, R.V., Munson, P.L. (eds). (1972) Amsterdam, Excerpta Medica Foundation, pp 202-206.
10. Matsuzaki, S., Dumont, J.E. (1972) Biochim. Biophys. Acta. 284:227-234.
11. Rodriguez, J.H., Morrison, A., Slatopolsky, E., et al. (1978) J. Clin. Endocrinol. Metab. 47:319-325.
12. Bellorin-Font, E., Martin, K.J., Freitag, J.J., et al. (1981) J. Clin. Endocrinol. Metab. 52:499-507.
13. Ontjes, D.A., Mahaffee, D.D., Wells, S.A. (1981) Metab. 30:406-411.
14. Habener, J.F. (1978) J. Clin. Invest. 62:436-450.
15. Brown, E.M., Brennan, M.F., Hurwitz, S., et al. (1978) J. Clin. Endocrinol. Metab. 46:267-275.
16. Brown, E.M. in Cohn, D.V., Talmage, R.V., Matthews, J.L. (eds). (1981) Amsterdam, Excerpta Medica pp 35-44.
17. Brown, E.M., Wilson, R.E, Eastman, R.C., et al. (1982) J. Clin. Endocrinol. Metab 54:172-179.
18. Brown, E.M. (1983) J. Clin. Endocrinol. Metab. 56:572-581.
19. Chertow, B.S., Baylink, D.J., Wergedal, J.E., Su, M.H.H. and Norman, A.W. (1975) J. Clin. Invest. 56:668-678.
20. Au, W.Y.W. and Bukowsky, A. (1976) Fed. Proc. 35:530.
21. Dietel, M.G., Dorn, R., Montz, R. and Altenahr, G. (1979) Endocrinology 105:237-245.
22. Oldham, S.B., Fischer, J.A., Shen, L.H. and Arnaud, C.D. (1974) Biochemistry 13:4790-4796.
23. Brumbaugh, P.F., Hughes, M.R., and Haussler, M.R. (1975) Proc. Natl. Acad. Sci. USA 72:4871-4875.

24. LLach, F., Coburn, J.W., Brickman, A.S., Kurokawa, K., Norman, A.W., Canterbury, J.M. and Reiss, E. (1977) J. Clin. Endocrinol. Metab. 44:1054-1060.
25. Tanaka, Y., DeLuca, H.F., Ghazarian, J.G., Hargis, G.K. and Williams, G.A. (1979) Min. Electrolyte, Metab. 2:20-25.
26. Golden, P., Greenwalt, A., Martin, K., Bellorin-Font, E., Mazey R., Klahr, S., and Slatopolsky, E. (1980) Endocrin. 107:602-607.
27. Oldham, S.B., Smith, R., Hartenbower, D.L., Henry, H.L., Norman, A.W. and Coburn, J.W. (1979) Endocrin. 104:248-254.
28. Slatopolsky, E., Gray, R., Adams, N., Lewis, J., Hruska, K., Martin, K., Klahr, S., DeLuca, H. and Lemann, J. A. W. Norman, editor. Walter deGruyter, Publishers, Berlin-New York, 1979.
29. Christiansen, C., Christiansen, M.S., Melsen, F., Rodbro, P. and DeLuca, H.F. (1981) Clin. Nephrol. 15:18-22.
30. Slatopolsky, E., Weerts, C., Thielan, J., Horst, R., Harter, H. and Martin, K.J. (1984) J. Clin. Invest. 74:2136-2143.

ASSESSMENT OF ASSAYS OF 25-HYDROXY-VITAMIN D_3 (25-HCC), 1,25-DIHYDROXY-VITAMIN D_3 (1,25-DHCC) AND 24,25-DIHYDROXY VITAMIN D_3 (24,25-DHCC) IN HUMAN SERUM FOR USE IN LONGITUDINAL STUDIES

E.C.H. van Beresteyn, M.A. van 't Hof*, M. van Schaik, S.A. Duursma **
Netherlands Institute for Dairy Research, P.O.Box 20, 6710 BA Ede (the Netherlands)
*Department of Statistical Consultation, University of Nijmegen, Nijmegen (the Netherlands)
**Clinical Research Group for Bone Metabolism, University Hospital, Utrecht (the Netherlands)

INTRODUCTION

The reproducibility of assays of 25-HCC, 1,25-DHCC and 24,25-DHCC was studied over a short period of time. Nothing is known so far about the usefulness of these assays in longitudinal studies. Since the purpose of such studies is to measure changes in an individual with time, high-quality measurements are required, the risk being that they are jeopardized by such time-related factors as time-of-measurement effects, test effects and poor reproducibility.

Time-of-measurement effects are suspected to be caused by necessary renewal of chemicals, standards, instrumentation or change of observer. Poor reproducibility may be caused by methodological errors and by biological variability. Test effects may arise when participants become more familiar with the way in which the study is conducted (extreme sunbathing, artificial sunlight).

Within the framework of a longitudinal study, measurements of 25-HCC, 1,25-DHCC and 24,25-DHCC were taken four times at one-year intervals; the subjects were a group of pre-, peri- and post-menopausal women. From the repeated measurements and the introduction of an independent control group, it was possible to assess the longitudinal usefulness of the measurements by evaluating the confounding time-related parameters.

PARTICIPANTS

202 healthy pre-, peri- and post-menopausal women participated in the investigation. None of them was taking estrogens or drugs known to influence calcium and bone metabolism.

METHODS

Serum samples from each individual were taken at the same time of year, so as to exclude seasonal variation. They were extracted with ethylacetate/cyclohexane (1:1) and ethylacetate/cyclohexane/methanol (2,5:2,5:2). The vitamin D metabolites were separated by straight-phase HPLC on a Zorbax Sil column. The solvent was a mixture of hexane ethanol, 2-propanol and water (86:10:4:0,5). Fractions containing 25-HCC, 1,25-DHCC and 24,25-DHCC were collected and used for quantitation by competitive protein-binding assays. Dilute normal human serum was used as the binding protein in the 25-HCC and 24,25-DHCC assays. 1,25-DHCC was measured by radioimmuno-assay.

Inter-assay variations were found to be 10 %, 13 % and 15 % (n = 6) for 25-HCC, 24,25-DHCC and 1,25-DHCC respectively.

The mixed-longitudinal design of the study, the four-by-four interperiod correlation matrix, and the independent control group (measured only once) were used to evaluate time-of-measurement effects, assay reproducibility, and test effects respectively. A description of the statistical methods of evaluating the time-related parameters has been presented extensively elsewhere (1, 2).

RESULTS

The results of the estimation of the time-related parameters are given in Tables 1, 2 and 3.

Table 1. Reproducibility studied by means of the four-by-four interperiod correlation matrix analysis.

variable	reproducibility a)	waiting time b)
25-HCC	0.31	b)
1,25-DHCC	-0.08	b)
24,25-DHCC	0.23	b)

a)Estimate of test-retest correlation. > 0.9 good; 0.7 to 0.9 reasonable; < 0.7 bad.

b)Time interval (in years) during which the (variance in) individual differences in changes with time equal(s) the error of measurements: the period during which individual changes with time are observable. Waiting time could not be estimated because of poor reproducibility.

Table 2. Test effects and significance level.

variable	difference between longitudinal group and control group (%) a)	p-value ANOVA b)
25-HCC	1.0	-
1,25-DHCC	-25.3	*
24,25-DHCC	-41.0	*

a)Differences adjusted for biological age and calculated as percentages of overall level.

b)- $p > 0.05$; * $p < 0.01$

Table 3. Overall concentrations of 25-HCC, 1,25-DHCC and 24,25-DHCC in serum and estimated time-of--measurement effects and significance level.

variable	units	overall level	time of measurement							
			1980		1981		1982		1983	
			effect[a]	p-level[b]	effect[a]	p-level[b]	effect[a]	p-level[b]	effect[a]	p-level[b]
25-HCC	ng/ml	21.1	-6.2	-	5.7	-	-1.9	-	2.4	-
1,25-DHCC	pg/ml	28.4	-19.4	**	7.7	*	7.4	*	4.2	-
24,25-DHCC	ng/ml	1.92	-15.1	*	45.6	**	-8.7	*	-21.5	**

a)Calculated as percentage of overall level.

b)- $p > 0.05$; * $p < 0.05$; ** $p < 0.01$.

CONCLUSION

In spite of an inter-assay variation coefficient which is comparable to data found in the literature, the measurements of 25-HCC, 1,25-DHCC and 24,25-DHCC showed poor reproducibility on the long term. A test effect and several time-of-measurement effects were observed in the assays of 1,25-DHCC and 24,25-DHCC. The measurements of the vitamin D_3 metabolites are therefore poor variables with respect to their longitudinal usefulness, and in this study failed to give a reliable picture of changes that occur in the individual with time.

REFERENCES

1. Van 't Hof, M.A., Roede, J. and Kowalski, C.J. (1977). Human Biology 49: 165-179.
2. Van 't Hof, M.A., Kowalski, C.J. (1979). In: A mixed longitudinal interdisciplinary study of growth and development, New York, Acad. Press 161-172; 387-391.

ASSESSMENT OF THE ROLE OF VITAMIN D IN INSULIN SECRETION.

S. Ljunghall, H. Lithell and L. Lind,
Institutions of Internal Medicine and Geriatrics, UNIVERSITY OF UPPSALA, Sweden.

Insulin secretion is regulated by changes of the cytosolic calcium in the pancreatic beta cells (1, 2). The recent discovery of receptors for $1,25(OH)_2D_3$ in the endocrine pancreas, their specific localisation to the insulin-producing islets (3, 4, 5) and the demonstration of calcium-binding protein in the cells (6, 7) have led to the hypothesis that vitamin D might be involved in the regulation of insulin secretion (8). This proposed action might affect intracellular vitamin D-dependent calcium binding protein levels, $1,25(OH)_2D_3$-associated cell membrane permeability (9) mitochondrial handling of calcium (10), calcium sequestration/release cycles in organelles and/or more direct, yet unknown, effects of other calcium-sensitive biochemical processes. With respect to this latter possibility it is important to note that several studies have failed to establish any correlation between vitamin D status and calmodulin levels (11) or any consistent effects between the cellular localisation patterns of calcium-bidning protein and the ubiquitous calmodulin (12).

Several in-vitro and animal studies have been performed to corroborate these hypotheses. When pancreases from vitamin D-deficient rats were perfused with glucose and arginine, Norman et al (13) were able to demonstrate an almost 50% reduction in insulin secretion compared to the response obtained in vitamin D-deficient animals that had been replenished with vitamin D during the last few days before the experiment. The study indicated an important role for vitamin D in the endocrine functioning of the pancreas but vitamin D status had no effect on the pancreatic glucagon secretion.

Subsequent investigations have confirmed that the vitamin D-deficient animals (rats or mice) have impaired secretion of insulin in vitro upon stimulation by glucose (14, 15, 16, 17).

Repletion with vitamin D in vivo (15, 16) were also found to restore the impaired secretion towards normal, although not entirely normalising it. However, the interpretation of these data should consider the possibility that vitamin D deficiency is a complex state in which the animals eat less, have impaired growth and are hypocalcaemic. Thus, the study by Chertow and associates (14) described that vitamin D deficiency was associated by marked impairment of insulin release in vitro but that decrease in food intake might account for this impairment, at least in part, since they also found a similar defect in pair-fed normal rats. That the dietary caloric and calcium intake and the general nutritional state accounts for part of the defect insulin secretion was also reported by Kadowaki and Norman (16) and Tanaka et al. (15). Both these studies demonstrated a specific beneficial effect of $1,25(OH)_2$.

A few animal studies have also evaluated the effects of vitamin D deficiency in vivo on fasting blood glucose and insulin (15, 18). In these investigations the fasting plasma insulin levels were markedly lower in the D-deficient animals than in their D-repleted counterparts. The glucose concentrations were, however, not different (15). Collectively these studies present a picture where D-deficiency in rats and mice is associated with impaired secretion of insulin in response to glucose. This abnormality can, at least in part, be overcome by D-repletion.

There is also some evidence that glucose-stimulated insulin response in normal rats is affected by 1,25$(OH)_2D_3$ (19). In this study where an intravenous dose of the hormone was given so that the plasma levels of 1,25$(OH)_2D_3$ and calcium were elevated it was found that whereas there were no differences when isolated pancreases were perfused with low-normal calcium concentrations the response to glucose was enhanced in the presence of a high calcium perfusate.

In contrast it appeared that obese mice lost weight and displayed reduced serum levels of both glucose and insulin after four months regular treatment with active vitamin D (20). Lean mice submitted to the same treatment did not change their glucose or insulin levels compared with control animals. Also Frankel et al (21) found that islets from D-deficient obese mice had an impaired insulin release in response to glucose whereas lean littermates were less affected.

Whether these experimental findings have any relevance for the physiological regulation of insulin secretion in man is not known.

The consequences of primary hyperparathyroidism (HPT) and hypophosphataemia on glucose metabolism might, however, be relevant in this context. In primary HPT disturbances of glucose and insulin metabolism have been reported to occur (22-28). These investigations present a uniform picture where the glucose-stimulated insulin secretion is enhanced preoperatively and normalised after parathyroid surgery. A remarkable observation is that although the prevalence of diabetes is higher than expected in patients with primary HPT the glucose tolerance is significantly <u>impaired</u> when the hyperparathyroid state is reversed (26). One should rather have anticipated an improvement of glucose handling when hypercalcaemia, hypophosphataemia and high levels of parathyroid hormone were normalised. No study has measured serum levels of vitamin D and its metabolites in relation to the disturbed glucose metabolism but it is well established that in the hyperparathyroid state the levels of 1,25$(OH)_2D_3$ are elevated but that they return to normal after sucessful parathyroid surgery (29). One could speculate that impaired glucose tolerance and inadequate secretion of parathyroid hormone are only indirectly related and that the reduction of active vitamin D postoperatively has detrimental effects of glucose tolerance.

In the complex pathogenesis of diabetes and glucose intolerance is not only a reduced insulin secretion of importance but also the response to the hormone in the peripheral tissues (30). Most patients with glucose intolerance and type 2 diabetes appear to have peripheral insulin resistance as one important contributing factor. A low serum phosphate has been clearly demonstrated to cause insulin resistance in man (31). This is also reflected in an inverse relationship between fasting levels of insulin and serum phosphate (32). Obesity, another cause of insulin resistance (33), is often accompanied by lower serum phosphate values (34) but it is not known if this is a primary or secondary event. Experimentally induced phosphate depletion both in dogs (35) and man (36) also produced an enhanced insulin response to glucose.

There is no concensus regarding the possible role of vitamin D deficiency in diabetes mellitus. Experimentally induced diabetes in the rat causes an impairment in 1-alpha-hydroxylase activity (37, 38) but it has not been definitely settled whether patients with diabetes have reduced formation of $1,25(OH)_2D_3$ or other disturbances of calcium metabolism (39-42).

Reports that vitamin D might cause hypoglycaemia without affecting serum insulin levels suggest extrapancreatic effects of such treatment (43, 44).

In order to evaluate a possible role for vitamin D in the management of patients with disturbed glucose metabolism we have investigated the effects of 1α-$(OH)D_3$ in middle-aged men with glucose intolerance (45). These men, aged 59-64, were recruited from a health survey on the basis of an abnormal oral glucose tolerance test. As a group they were overweight. There were altogether 66 men in the study, 22 of them were on previous treatment with selective beta-blockade for hypertension. This was unaltered during the study period. Patients were stratified for body weight and antihypertensive treatment. Therapy was given with 0.75 µg 1α-$(OH)D_3$ for a period of 12 weeks. Before and at the end of the study period an intravenous glucose tolerance test (IVGTT) was carried out with measurements of insulin at zero, (4+6)/2 (peak) and 60 minutes. Relevant parameters for evaluation of calcium metabolism were also analysed.

During the study period there were no changes of the mean values for serum calcium or creatinine in either group. The patients on active treatment had significantly higher pretreatment values for PTH but in none of the two groups did PTH change with treatment. In the placebo group there were no changes in either fasting blood glucose, K-value (glucose elimination capacity during the IVGTT) or insulin values during the IVGTT. However, the hemoglobin A_1C values were significantly reduced, either as a consequence of the increased attention during the trial or possibly due to seasonal variation. The patients in the actively treated group displayed a similar reduction in HbA_1C without any concomitant changes of fasting blood glucose or K-value. During the IVGTT, however, the group treated with alphacalcidol had a slightly reduced peak insulin response.

Patients with low ($\leqq$0.60 mmol/l) serum levels of phosphate appeared, however, to benefit from treatment with active vitamin D. In this subgroup there was an increased peak insulin response to glucose, improvement of K-value and reduction of HbA_1C compared with patients who had high-normal serum phosphate values.

This finding suggests that prolonged studies should be carried out, perhaps also using slightly higher doses of active vitamin D, in order to further settle the important question whether such treatment can improve glucose tolerance and prevent the development of type 2 diabetes.

References

1. Grodsky, G.M. and Bennet, L.L. (1978) Diabetes 15, 910-913.
2. Wollheim, C.B. and Sharp, G.W.G. (1981) Physiol. Rev. 61, 914-???.
3. Christakos, S. and Norman, A.W. (1979) Biochem. Biophys. Res. Commun. 89, 56-63.
4. Clark, S.A., Stumpf, W.E., Sar, M., DeLuca, H.F. and Tanaka, Y. (1980) Cell Tiss. Res. 209, 515-520.
5. Christakos, S., Friedlander, E.J., Frandsen, B.R. and Norman, A.W. (1979) Endocrinology 104, 1495-1502.
6. Pike, J.W. (1981) J. Steroid Biochem. 16, 385-345.
7. Roth, J., Bonner-Weir, S., Norman A.W. and Orci, L. (1982) Endocrinology 116, 2216-2218.
8. Norman W.W., Roth, J. and Orci, L. (1982) Endocrine Reviews 3, 331-366.
9. Nemere, I. and Norman, A.W. (1982) Biochim. Biopys. Acta 694, 307-327.
10. Boquist, L., Hagström, S. and Strindlund, L. (1977) Acta Path. Microbiol. Scand. 85, 489-500.
11. Thomasset, M., Molla, A., Parkes, O. and Demaille J.G. (1981) FEBS Lett. 127, 13-16.
12. Feldman, S.C. and Christakos, S. (1982). Endocrinology 110, 688A.
13. Norman, A.W., Frankel, B.J., Heldt, A.M. and Grodsky, G.M. (1980) Science 209, 823-825.
14. Chertow, B.S., Sivitz, W.I., Baranetsky, N.G., Clark, S.A., Waite, A. and DeLuca, H.F. (1983) Endocrinology 113, 1511-1518.
15. Tanaka, Y., Seino, Y., Ishida, I., Yamaoka, K., Yabuuchi, H., Ishida, H., Seino, S., Seino, Y. and Imura, H. (1984) Acta Endocrinol. 105, 528-533.
16. Kadawaki, S. and Norman, A.W. (1984). J. Clin. Invest. 73, 759-766.
17. Frankel B.J., Sehlin, J. and Täljedal, I.-B. (1985) Acta Physiol. Scand. (in press).
18. Clark, S., Stumpf, W.E. and Sar, M. (1981) Diabetes 30, 382-386.
19. Ishida, H., Seino, Y., Seino, S., Tsuda, K., Takemura, J., Nishi, S., Ishizuka, S. and Imura, H. (1983) Life Sci. 33, 1779-1786.
20. Kawashima H. and Castro A. (1981) Res. Comm. Chem. Path. Pharm. 33, 155-161.
21. Frankel, B.J. (1985) 6th Workshop on Vitamin D (this volume).
22. Kim, H., Kalkhoff, R.K., Costrini, N.V., Carletty, N.V. and Jacobson, M. (1971) J. Clin. Invest. 50, 2596-2605.
23. Yasuda, K., Hurukawa, Y., Okuyama, M., Kikuchi, M. and Yoshinaga, K. (1975) N. Engl. J. Med. 292, 501-504.
24. Ljunghall, S., Lithell, H., Vessby, B. and Wide, L. (1978) Acta Endocrinol. 89, 580-589.
25. Hamilton, D.V., Pryor, J.S. (1981) Postgrad. Med. J. 57, 167-171.
26. Ljunghall, S., Palmér, M., Åkerström, G. and Wide, L. (1983). Eur. J. Clin. Invest. 13, 373-377.
27. Prager, R., Kovarik, J., Schernthaner, G., Woloszczuk, W. and Willvonseder, R. (1983) Metabolism 32, 800-805.
28. Prager, R., Schernthaner, G., Kovarik, J., Cichini, G., Kraushofer, K. and Willvonseder, R. (1984) Calcif. Tiss. Int. 36, 253-258.

29. Broadus, A., Horst, R.L., Lang, R., Littledike, E.T. and Rasmussen, H. (1980). N. Engl. J. Med. 302, 421-426.
30. Efendic, S., Luft, R., and Wajngot, A. (1984) Endocrine Reviews 5, 395-410.
31. DeFronzo, R.A. and Lang, R. (1980) N. Engl. J. Med. 303, 1259-1263.
32. Ljunghall, S. and Hedstrand, H. (1977). Brit. Med. J. 1, 553-554.
33. Kadowaki, T. (1984) Diabetologia 26, 44-49.
34. Ljunghall, S., Hedstrand, H. and Wide, L. (1979). Mineral Electrolyte Metab. 2, 246.
35. Harter, H.R., Santiago, J.V., Rutherford, W.E., Slatopolsky, E. and Klahr, S. (1976) J. Clin. Invest. 58, 359-367.
36. Marshall, W.P., Banasiak, M.F. and Kalkhoff, R.K. (1978) Horm. Metab. Res. 10, 369-373.
37. Schneider, L.E., Schedl, H.P., McCain, T. and Haussler, M.R. (1977) Science 196, 1452-1457.
38. Spencer, E.M., Khalil, M. and Tobiassen, O. (1980) Endocrinology 107, 300-305.
39. Fraser, T.E., White, N.H., Hough, S., Santiago, J.V., McGee, B.R., Bryce, G., Mallon, J. and Avioli, L. (1981) J. Clin. Endocrinol. Metab. 53, 1154-1159.
40. Heath III, H., Lambert, P.W., Service, F.J. and Arnaud, S.B. (1979) J. Clin. Endocrinol. Metab. 49, 462-466.
41. Storm, T.L., Sörensen, O.H., Lund, Bj., Lund, Bi., Christiansen, J.S., Andersen, A.R., Lumholz, I.B. and Parving. H.-H. (1983) Metab. Bone Dis. Rel. Res. 5, 107-110.
42. McNair, P., Fogh-Andersen, N., Madsbad, S. and Christensen, M.S. (1983). Eur. J. Clin. Invest. 13, 267-270.
43. Blahos, J., Svoboda, Z., Zarubova, V. and Justova, V. (1984) Calcif. Tiss. Int. 36, 83.
44. Boquist, L. (1980) Endokrinologie 75, 376-378.
45. Ljunghall, S., Lithell, H., Lind, L., Skarfors, E. and Selinus, I. (in manuscript).

Pancreas Diabetes
and Vitamin D
+ Metabolites

INFLUENCE OF VITAMIN D STATUS ON INSULIN SECRETION *IN VIVO* AND GLUCOSE TOLERANCE IN THE RAT.

C. CADE and A. W. NORMAN
Dept. Biochem., Univ. Calif., Riverside, CA 92521, USA.

Introduction: In light of several lines of indirect evidence including (i) the presence of pancreas-associated CaBP (1,2), (ii) demonstration of a high affinity receptor for 1,25$(OH)_2D_3$ in chick pancreas (3) and (iii) localization of $[^3H]$-1,25$(OH)_2D_3$ in the nucleus of rat β-cells (4), a role for vitamin D in pancreatic endocrine and/or exocrine function has been strongly implicated. More recently it has been demonstrated in this laboratory that vitamin D_3 is indeed essential for normal insulin (but not glucagon) secretion from the perfused rat pancreas (5,6). Accordingly the influence of vitamin D status on insulin secretion *in vivo* was investigated.

Methodology: Male weanling rats (Holtzman Co.) were raised on a synthetic D-deficient diet for 6-8 weeks after which time animals became D-depleted. These rats were then injected IP with vehicle (-D group) or 70 IU vitamin D_3 (+D groups) every other day for 10 days. During this period all animals were maintained on the -D diet. The two +D groups were either fed *ad lib* (+DAL) or pair fed to the -D rats (+DPF). In preparation for glucose tolerance tests the jugular vein was cannulated with silastic tubing the end of which was attached to a short metal elbow and pulled through the skin at the back of the neck for easy access. Glucose (2 g/kg body wt.) was subsequently infused into the vein via the cannulae and blood was withdrawn prior to and at 15, 30, 60 and 90 minutes after the glucose load. Insulin was determined by RIA. Plasma levels of glucose, calcium and phosphorus were also measured.

Results and Discussion: Vitamin D deficiency was characterized by low plasma calcium levels and depressed body weight as compared to +D AL rats (Table 1). Pair fed +D animals (included to investigate involvement of nutritional factors) were of similar weight to their -D counterparts.

TABLE 1: Effect of Vitamin D-Deficiency and Pair Feeding on Body Wt. and Various Blood Parameters.

D-Status	Body Weight (g)	Basal Plasma Concentrations (mean ±SEM for n = 7)				
		Glucose (mg%)	Insulin ($ngml^{-1}$)	Insulin/Glucose	Calcium (mg%)	P (mg%)
-D	187±12	124±3.5	0.88±0.09	0.007	4.77±28	5.20±0.4
+D PF	191±3	134±6.5	1.15±0.13	0.008	10.20±0.29	5.70±0.2
+D AL	230±8	111±3.0	0.85±0.05	0.008	10.40±0.22	6.10±0.3

Basal plasma insulin levels did not differ significantly between the three experimental groups and although basal glucose concentration was lower in the +D AL group the insulin:glucose ratio in each case was comparable.

In response to a glucose load it was demonstrated that vitamin D-deficiency impairs glucose clearance from the plasma as characterized by an elevated KG value (representing a function of the area beneath the tolerance 'curve'), as shown in Fig. 1. This increase corresponded to a significant reduction in glucose mediated insulin secretion (Fig. 2) as compared to that of the D-replete rats. The differences appeared not to be related to increased caloric intake of +D animals since the +DPF group also showed significantly higher plasma insulin levels in response to glucose. The plasma P concentration of the -D group did not at any time during the GTT differ from the values of either D-replete group and thus is unlikely to be a contributory factor in the impaired glucose tolerance.

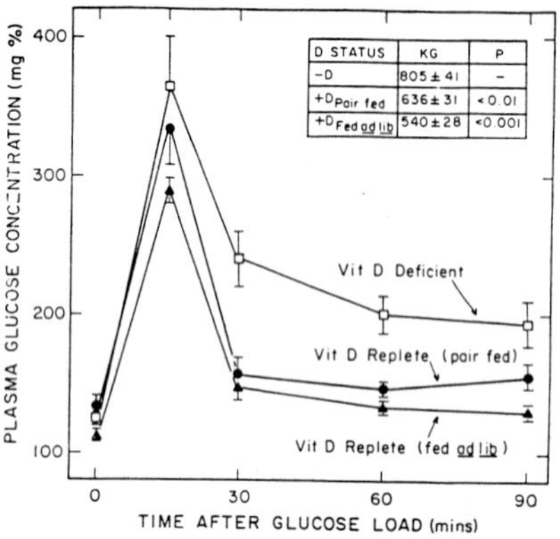

Fig. 1: Plasma glucose response to an IV glucose load

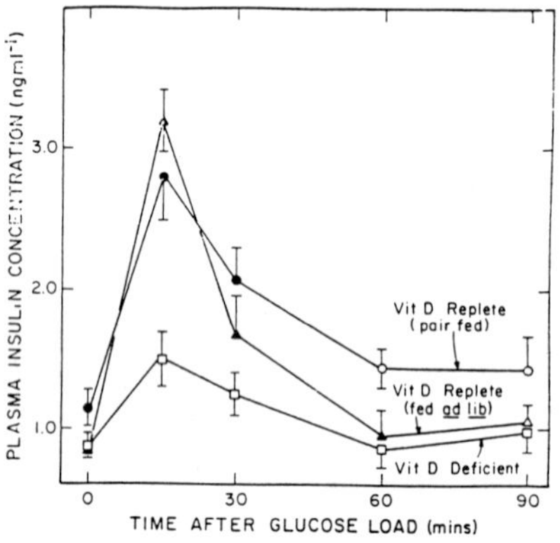

Fig. 2: Plasma insulin response to an IV glucose load

Conclusion: These results support the concept of a physiological role for vitamin D in endocrine pancreas function.

This work was supported in part by a Kroc Foundation grant.

References:

1. Roth, J., Bonner-Weir, S., Norman, A. W., and Orci, L. (1982) Endocrinology 110, 2216-2218.
2. Morrissey, R. L., Bucci, T. J., Empson, R. N., and Lufkin, E. G. (1975) Proc. Soc. Exp. Biol. Med. 149, 56-60.
3. Christakos, S., and Norman, A. W. (1979) Biochem. Biophys, Res. Commun. 89, 56-63.
4. Stumpf, W. E., Sar, M., and DeLuca, H. F. (1981) In, Hormonal Control of calcium metabolism. p.222-229. Eds. Cohn, Talmadge and Mathews.
5. Norman, A. W., Frankel, B. J., Heldt, A. M., and Grodsky, G. M. (1980) Science 209, 823-825.
6. Kadowaki, S., and Norman, A. W. (1984) J. Clin. Invest. 73, 759-766.

TIME COURSE STUDY OF INSULIN SECRETION IN THE ISOLATED, PERFUSED RAT PANCREAS AFTER 1,25-DIHYDROXYVITAMIN D_3 ADMINISTRATION.

S. Kadowaki, C. Cade, T. Fujita and A. W. Norman
Third Dept. Int. Med., Kobe Univ. Sch. Med., Kobe 650, Japan and
Dept. Biochem., Univ. Calif., Riverside, CA 92521, USA.

Introduction:

Several lines of evidence have suggested that, in addition to the classical target tissue of intestine, bone and kidney, the pancreas is also a target for $1,25(OH)_2D_3$ action and thus this metabolite may have a role in exocrine and/or endocrine pancreas function (1). We have more recently reported that, vitamin D deficiency inhibits insulin secretion and that vitamin D repletion restores it, irrespective of serum calcium concentration or dietary caloric intake (2). These data suggest a direct effect of vitamin D (or its metabolites) upon the endocrine β-cells. Such influence on insulin secretion may be mediated either as a non-genomic membrane effect or a genomic effect via production of CaBP. In this present study, a series of experiments was undertaken to investigate the time course of $1,25(OH)_2D_3$ action on arginine (20 mM) or glucose (16.7 mM)-stimulated insulin secretion in the isolated perfused rat pancreas.

Methodology:

Male weanling Holtzman rats were raised on a vitamin D-deficient diet for 7-8 weeks. After this time all of the rats were pair-fed to the vitamin D-deficient controls. A portion of these rats was subsequently treated with $1,25(OH)_2D_3$ (1.3 nmol, s.c.) at time 0 and pancreatic perfusion [employing methods previously described (2)] was performed at 0 hr, 8 hrs, 14 hrs, 24 hrs, 48 hrs or 72 hrs following this treatment. In each case serum calcium, phosphorus and glucose levels were determined from blood samples collected prior to the perfusion studies.

Results:

By 14 hrs, $1,25(OH)_2D_3$ administration was shown to significantly raise serum calcium concentrations above control levels (8.1 mg dl^{-1} vs. 4.7 ± 0.2 mg dl^{-1}, $p < 0.01$). This concentration was maintained up to 72 hrs. Insulin secretion in response to glucose (16.7 mM) exhibited a typical biphasic pattern at each time point studied (Fig. 1). Significantly enhanced insulin secretion was apparent by 8 hrs (after the $1,25(OH)_2D_3$ dose), reached a maximum at 14 hrs and then markedly decreased to control levels at 34 hrs, despite raised serum calcium concentration at this time. Likewise, arginine (20 mM)-mediated insulin secretion was significantly potentiated 8 hrs after $1,25(OH)_2D_3$ administration, peaked at 14 hrs and had gradually decreased to control values by 72 hrs (Fig. 2). Throughout both experiments the prevailing serum levels of calcium, phosphorus and glucose seemed not to be correlated to the degree of insulin secretion observed.

Vitamin D. A Chemical, Biochemical and Clinical Update

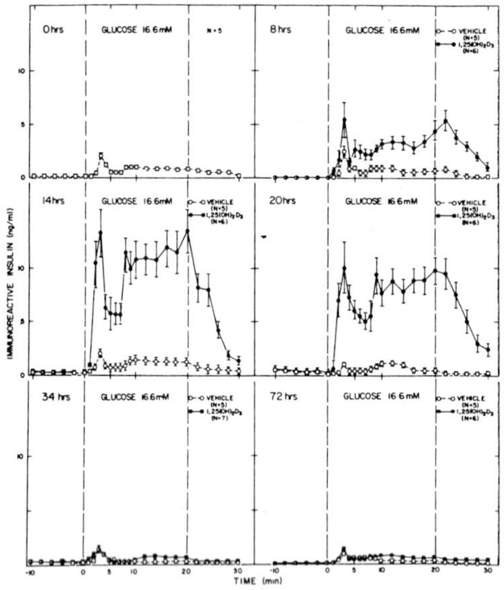

Fig. 1. Effect of a single dose of $1,25(OH)_2D_3$ (1.3 nmol) or vehicle administration in vivo on 16.6 mM glucose-induced insulin secretion by the subsequently isolated perfused rat pancreas.

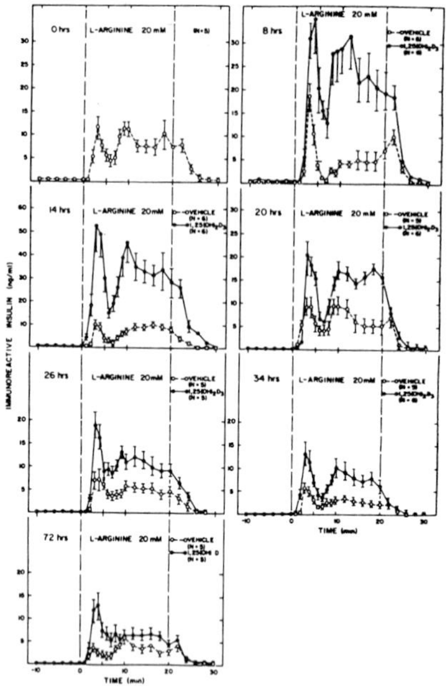

Fig. 2. Effect of a single dose of $1,25(OH)_2D_3$ (1.3 nmol) or vehicle administration in vivo on 20 mM arginine-induced insulin secretion by the subsequently isolated perfused rat pancreas.

Conclusion:

Based on these data, we can conclude:

(1) The potentiating action of $1,25(OH)_2D_3$ on glucose- or arginine-mediated insulin secretion is apparent within 8 hrs of administration of this hormone.

(2) The prevailing levels of serum calcium, phosphorus and glucose appear not to be involved in the mechanism of action.

This work was supported by grant A-82-71 from the Kroc Foundation.

References:

1. Norman, A. W. (1982) Endocrine Reviews 3, 331-366.

2. Kadowaki, S. (1983) J. Clin. Invest. 73, 759-766.

THE ROLE OF VITAMIN D FOR THE GLUCOSE STIMULATED INSULIN RELEASE FROM THE ENDOCRINE PANCREAS.

J. Harmeyer*, U. Lachenmaier-Currle and R. Kaune,
Institute of Physiology, School of Vet. Med., 3000 Hannover, FRG.

Introduction:

Nuclear 1,25-$(OH)_2D$ receptors and a vitamin D dependent calcium binding-protein have been demonstrated in B-cells of the pancreas in rats (1). The concentration of immuno-reactive insulin in plasma rises 100% in D-deficient rats after an injection of 1,25-$(OH)_2D_3$ along with a rise in plasma Ca (2). The glucose plus arginine stimulated release of insulin in perfused pancreas from D-deficient rats is significantly increased after the animals were given vitamin D_3 24 to 72 hours prior to perfusion (3). It is attempted in this study to identify the effect of long term normocalcemia on glucose stimulated release of insulin in animals which are deficient in the hormonal form of vitamin D.

Animals and Methods:

Seven to ten weeks old rachitic hypocalcemic piglets with pseudo vitamin D-deficiency rickets, type I, and normal controls were used. Glucose tolerance tests with an i.v. injection of 0.75 g glucose/kg body weight were carried out. The rachitic piglets were made normocalcemic by a two to four days lasting continuous i.v. infusion of 30 mg $CaCl_2$/h. The response of insulin was estimated from the area under the curve of insulin in plasma versus time and the disappearance rate of glucose was calculated from the slope of the semilogarithmic plot of the plasma glucose versus time curve. Glucose tolerance tests were carried out before and at the end of long term Ca infusion, three days after the end of Ca infusion and six to ten days after the end of Ca infusion.

Results:

Concentrations of Ca, glucose and immuno-reactive insulin in plasma of hypocalcemic and normal piglets are in table 1 and 2. The stimulated release of insulin and the rate constant of disappearance of glucose were significantly diminished in rachitic hypocalcemic pigs compared to normal controls (fig. 1, table 2). The turnover time of glucose in plasma was 20 min in normocalcemic piglets and 40 min in hypocalcemic piglets. Continuous three days i.v. infusion of Ca improved the glucose stimulated response of insulin and normalized the disappearance rate of glucose from plasma (fig. 1, table2). Three days after the end of the continuous infusion of Ca hypocalcemia and the diminished response of insulin release had redeveloped.

Discussion:

The diminished glucose stimulated release of insulin was partly restored by a prolonged normalization of the Ca concentration in plasma. In vitro perfusion of pancreas from vitamin D-repleted and depleted animals showed that short term normalization of Ca had no effect on glucose stimulated release of insulin in D-depleted animals (3). In other experiments with rats normocalcemia alone could also not restore physiologic B-cells

* Supported by the Deutsche Forschungsgemeinschaft, Sonderforschungsbereich 146 "Versuchstierforschung"

function (4). The experiments presented here support the assumption that vitamin D-hormon acts on B-cells function by correcting the extracellular Ca concentration. However we have also observed that the glucose induced insulin release is normalized in hypocalcemic vitamin D-repleted animals.

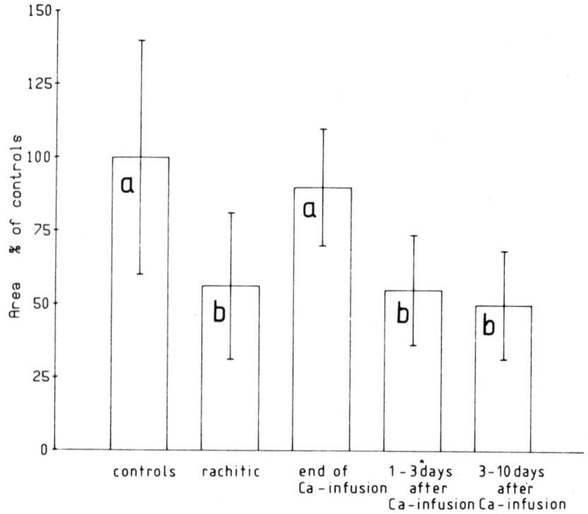

Fig. 1: Glucose stimulated increase of insulin in plasma over 6o min. Areas under the insulin versus time curves, $\bar{x} \pm$ SD, columns with different letters differ with $p < 0.05$.

Table 1: Glucose (mmol/l) and immuno-reactive insulin (mU/l) in plasma ($\bar{x} \pm$ SD)

	normal piglets	rachitic piglets
Glucose (SD)	5.5 (o.8)	5.2 (o.6)
Insulin (SD)	2o (16)	17 (12)

Table 2:
Plasma Ca concentrations (mmol/l) and rate constants of disappearance of glucose from plasma (min^{-1}) following an i.v. glucose load (*different with $p < 0.01$) (SD).

	controls	rachitic	end of Ca in-fusion	1-3 days after Ca infusion	3-1o days after Ca infusion
plasma Ca	2.7 (o.2o)	1.61* (o.24)	2.45 (o.2o)	1.97 (o.44)	1.75 (o.24)
Rate con-stant	1.5 (o.12)	o.75* (o.o6)	1.5 (o.11)	1.6 (o.o9)	1.3 (o.o9)

1.) Christakos, S., Friedlander, E.J., Frandsen, B.R., Norman, A.W. (1979) Endocrinology 1o4, 1495 - 15o2
2.) Clark, S.A., Stumpf, W.E., Sar, M. (1981), Diabetes 3o, 382 - 386
3.) Norman, A.W., Frankel, B.J., Heldt, A.M., Grodsky, G.M. (198o), Science 2o9, 823 - 825
4.) Kadowaki, S., Norman, A.W. (1984), J. Clin. Invest. 73, 759 - 766

VITAMIN D EFFECT ON INSULIN RELEASE AND NET $^{45}Ca^{2+}$ UPTAKE BY ISLETS OF LANGERHANS FROM OBESE AND LEAN MICE

B.J. Frankel, Department of Histology & Cell Biology,
University of Umeå, S-901 87 Umeå, Sweden

Introduction:

It appears (1) that insulin from the islet B cell is necessary for normal renal 25(OH)-1α-hydroxylase activity (2) and that $1,25(OH)_2D_3$, in turn, is necessary for normal insulin release (3-6) through both an indirect effect (plasma Ca) and possibly a direct effect on the B cell. Vit. D deficiency is associated with subnormal insulin release (3-6) and $^{45}Ca^{2+}$ uptake (5). ^{3}H-$1,25(OH)_2D_3$ binds to B-cell nuclei (7), and CaBP is found in islet B cells (8). Furthermore, vit. D treatment is associated with increased calcium-pyroantimonate precipitates in B-cell mitochondria (9). These data corroborate that D-deficiency suppresses insulin release, suggest that the sterol has a direct effect on the islet's Ca^{2+} handling, and show a subline difference, i.e., obese mice are more "sensitive" to the D-deficient diet than their lean littermates. (Part of these data has been presented in preliminary form; 6).

Materials and Methods:

Obese mice (Umeå-ob/ob) and lean littermates (Umeå-+/?) were fed vit.D-deficient (rat line test) diet (86% corn meal, 10% egg albumin, 3% $CaCO_3$, 1% NaCl), with only incandescent lighting. Details of culture, insulin release, and net $^{45}Ca^{2+}$ measurements previously described (6).

Results and Discussion:

Four weeks' D-deficient diet suppressed glucose-stimulated insulin release but not $^{45}Ca^{2+}$ uptake in obese-mouse islets (Fig.1, left). No significant change was seen in lean-mouse islets even after 12 weeks' D-deficient diet although there was a tendency toward suppressed glucose-stimulated $^{45}Ca^{2+}$ uptake (Fig.1, right). Thus only obese mice are susceptable to the D-deficient diet (subline difference).

Blood samples from lean mice after 0-12 weeks' D-deficient diet (Table 1), when insulin release and islet $^{45}Ca^{2+}$ uptake were not changed (data not shown), showed plasma Ca levels increased, P decreased, and $1,25(OH)_2D_3$ unchanged as compared with mice fed a normal diet. It appears that lean mice do not require a dietary source of vit.D for normal islet function or perhaps increased parathormone stimulates $1,25(OH)_2D_3$ synthesis and raises plasma Ca.

Culture of obese- and lean-mouse islets with D_3 (Fig.2) increased $^{45}Ca^{2+}$ uptake in obese-mouse islets in 3 but not 20 mM glucose, and did not affect insulin release. A similar tendency was seen in lean-mouse islets.

Conclusions:

Vitamin D_3 or one of its metabolites may have a direct effect on Ca^{2+} handling by the islet B cell in vitro, and the ob/ob islet is more sensitive than the lean-mouse islet (subline difference) to D-deficiency in vivo or culture with D_3.

Vitamin D. A Chemical, Biochemical and Clinical Update

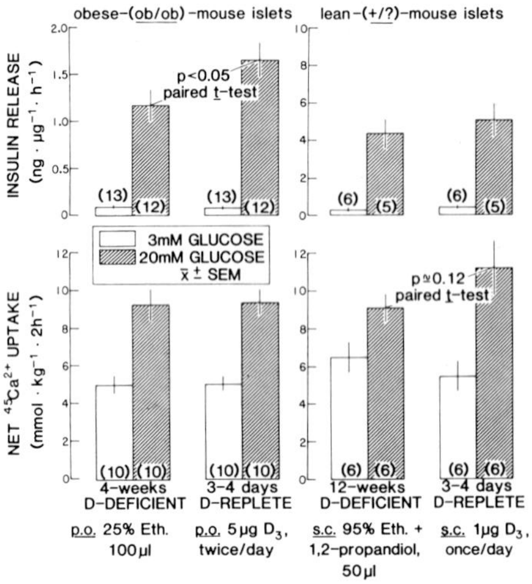

Fig.1: Effect of vit.D-deficiency in vivo on insulin release and $^{45}Ca^{2+}$ uptake by islets from obese and lean mice.

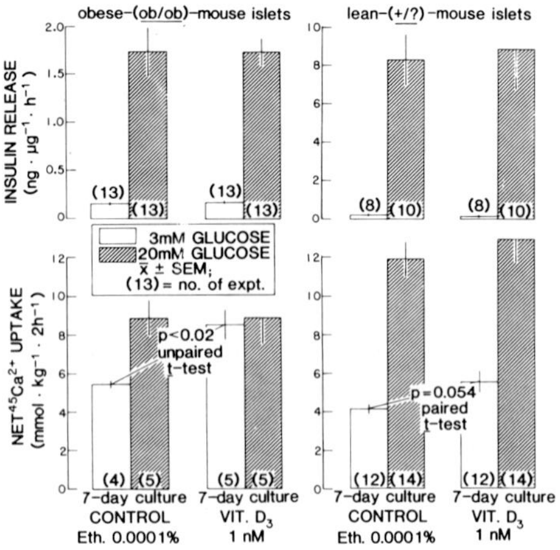

Fig.2: Effect of culture with D_3 on insulin release and $^{45}Ca^{2+}$ by islets from obese and lean mice.

Table 1: Effect of vit.D-deficient diet on lean-mouse plasma.

	D-deficient diet:	0 Weeks	4 Weeks	8 Weeks	12 Weeks
Insulin	(mU/l;n=5-7)	88±25	64±24	60±9	81±13
Calcium	(mM;n=5-7)	2.2±0.1	2.5±0.1*	2.5±0.1*	2.5±0.1*
Phosphorus	(mM;n=5-7)	1.6±0.1	0.9±0.2*	0.9±0.1*	0.9±0.1*
$1,25(OH)_2D_3$	(pg/ml;n=2)	52.5	69.2	93.8	38.2

*Mean±SE; *=P<0.05 as compared with 0 weeks (=normal diet).

References:

1. Clark, S.A., Stumpf, W.E., and Madhabananda, S. (1981) Diabetes 30, 382-386
2. Hough, S., Fausto, A., Sonn, Y., Dong, O.K., Birge, S.J., and Avioli, L.V. (1983) Endocrinology 113, 790-796
3. Norman, A.W., Frankel, B.J., Heldt, A.M., and Grodsky, G.M. (1980) Science 209, 823-825
4. Kadowaki, S., Norman, A.W. (1984) J. Clin.Invest.73,759-766
5. Chertow, B.S., Sivitz, W.I., Baranetsky, N.G., Clark, S.A., Waite, A., and DeLuca,H.F. (1983) Endocrinology 113,1511-1518
6. Frankel, B.J., Sehlin, J., and Täljedal, I.-B. (1985) Acta Physiol. Scand. 123, 61-66
7. Clark, S.A., Stumpf, W.E., Sar, M., DeLuca, H.F., and Tanaka, Y. (1980) Cell Tiss. Res. 209, 515-520
8. Roth, J., Bonner-Weir, S., Norman, A.W., and Orci, L.(1982) Endocrinology 110, 2216-2218
9. Boquist, L., Hagström, S., and Strindlund, L. (1977) Acta Path. Microbiol. Scand. Sect.A 85, 489-500

DECREASED SERUM 1,25-DIHYDROXYVITAMIN D IN DIABETES : POSSIBLE ROLE OF VITAMIN D-BINDING PROTEIN.

B.L. Nyomba, R. Bouillon and P. De Moor. Laboratorium Experimentele Geneeskunde en Endocrinologie, Gasthuisberg, B-3000 Leuven, Belgium.

The circulating 1,25-dihydroxyvitamin D [$1,25(OH)_2D_3$] level reportedly is decreased and the renal 1-hydroxylase is impaired in male rats with experimental diabetes (1). It is not known whether vitamin D metabolism is also altered in female diabetic rats or in spontaneous diabetes, and no data are available on vitamin D transport in this disease. We therefore measured vitamin D metabolites and their binding protein (DBP) in male and female rats with experimental or spontaneous diabetes.

Materials and Methods

The effects of spontaneous diabetes were studied in BB rats bred in Leuven (BB/L) from pairs provided by Dr. P. Thibert, Banting Research Centre, Ottawa, Canada. Sex- and age-matched non diabetic (N), untreated diabetic (D) and insulin-treated diabetic (I) BB/L rats were used. Carotid blood was taken at sacrifice, and urine samples were collected after a single micturition the day before the sacrifice.

Experimental diabetes was induced with streptozotocin (SZ) in 3 month-old Wistar rats 3 days after gonadectomy (Gx) or sham-operation (Shx). Diabetic rats were either untreated (D) or treated with insulin (I) from day 10 to 14 after SZ injection and were killed on day 15. Sex- and age-matched Gx or Shx rats were used as controls (N). Serum parameters were measured by established methods, and urinary DBP was determined by radioimmunoassay (2).

Results and discussion

In N rats of both strains, the serum levels of $1,25(OH)_2D_3$ (ng/l) and DBP (mg/l) were higher in males than in females (Table 1).
In male Wistar rats, $1,25(OH)_2D_3$ levels were lower in D than in N and I, but $25OHD_3$ (µg/l) levels were not significantly affected, confirming previous reports (1). In female Wistar rats, no significant difference was found. The serum DBP level was decreased in both male and female D rats, but the difference between N and D was more marked in males (2). The $1,25(OH)_2D_3$: DBP molar ratio, used as an index of "free" $1,25(OH)_2D_3$ level (ratio) was not different between N and D.
In male BB/L rats, both $1,25(OH)_2D_3$ and DBP but not $25OHD_3$ levels were decreased in D compared to N and I. In female BB/L rats, only DBP was decreased in D. The difference between N and D was also more important in males than in females. In both male and female BB/L rats, the ratio was increased in D. Urinary excretion of DBP (ng/mg creatinine) was increased in D (1,428 $\pm$ 423) compared to N (249 $\pm$ 23) and I (238 $\pm$ 37).
In view of the sex difference, Wistar rats were studied after Gx. This decreased both $1,25(OH)_2D_3$ and DBP levels in N male rats, but brought the female values up to Gx male levels. DBP concentrations in Gx diabetic rats were higher in females than in males.

Vitamin D. A Chemical, Biochemical and Clinical Update

TABLE 1 : VITAMIN D METABOLITES AND DBP IN DIABETIC RATS (Mean ± SD)

	$25OHD_3$	DBP	$1,25(OH)_2D_3$	Ratio
BB/L rats				
♂ N (35)	19 ± 6	552 ± 88	118 ± 31	2.7 ± 0.8
D (38)	15 ± 8	310 ± 124[c]	82 ± 28[c]	3.8 ± 2.4[a]
I (23)	17 ± 7	482 ± 78	109 ± 37	2.7 ± 0.8
♀ N (30)	23 ± 14	451 ± 42	63 ± 20	1.7 ± 0.5
D (18)	23 ± 16	311 ± 83[c]	69 ± 21	3.0 ± 1.5[b]
I (9)	20 ± 9	399 ± 46	80 ± 23	2.5 ± 0.9
Shx rats				
♂ N (9)	18 ± 3	608 ± 29	157 ± 29	3.2 ± 0.6
D (8)	14 ± 1[b]	434 ± 77[c]	86 ± 14[c]	2.8 ± 0.6
I (7)	15 ± 2	568 ± 99	100 ± 25	2.2 ± 0.4
♀ N (6)	32 ± 4	456 ± 13	65 ± 14	1.8 ± 0.3
D (5)	32 ± 8	365 ± 40[c]	51 ± 7	1.8 ± 0.3
Gx rats				
♂ N (8)	19 ± 2	524 ± 36[d]	113 ± 16[d]	2.7 ± 0.4
D (7)	14 ± 2[b]	361 ± 62[c,d]	78 ± 9[c]	2.6 ± 0.4
I (8)	15 ± 2	498 ± 45[d]	94 ± 26	2.4 ± 0.7
♀ N (6)	31 ± 5	523 ± 16[d]	99 ± 20[d]	2.4 ± 0.4
D (4)		428 ± 62[c,d]	63 ± 4[c]	1.7 ± 0.0
I (4)		474 ± 27	61 ± 8[c]	1.6 ± 0.2

D vs N and/or I : a : $p < 0.05$; b : $p < 0.01$; c : $p < 0.001$
Gx vs Shx : d : $p < 0.001$

The total but not the free concentrations of $1,25(OH)_2D_3$ are thus decreased in both experimental and spontaneous diabetes of the rats in parallel to DBP. This is at least partly due to increased urinary excretion. The sex difference in the concentration of the hormone and DBP is attenuated by diabetes (2) and by gonadectomy, suggesting that DBP changes induced by insulinopenia also derive from interactions with sex hormones on protein synthesis.

References

1. Schneider L.E., Schedl H.P., McCain T. and Haussler M.R. (1977) Science 196 : 1452-1454.
2. Nyomba, B.L., Bouillon, R., Lissens, W., Van Baelen, H. and De Moor, P. Endocrinology (in press).

OSTEOPOROSIS AND CALCIUM REGULATING HORMONES IN INSULIN-DEPENDENT DIABETES MELLITUS (IDDM).

G.Saggese, G.Federico, G.Cesaretti, E.Bottone, *M.F.Holick.
Dept.of Pediatrics, University of Pisa,Pisa Italy. *Vitamin D Lab.Massachusetts Institute of Technology, Boston, USA

Introduction:

In IDDM a reduction of bone mineral content (BMC) has been assessed (1). While in the experimental diabetes a derangement of calciotropic hormones regulation has been hypothized as a possible pathogenetic factor in developing osteoporosis (2), in humans the reported data do not clearly confirm this finding (3)(4)(5)(6).

Patients and Methods:

27 out patients, 18 males, 9 females aged 4.6-13 a. undertook evaluation for serum calcium (Ca), phosphate (P), alkalyne phosphatase (AP), parathyroid hormone (PTH-COOH terminal; Immunonuclear Cor.RIA kit), calcitonin (CT; Immunonuclear Cor.RIA kit), phosphaturia (PU) and calciuria (CU). 25OHD and 1.25(OH)2D were measured with a radioreceptor assay as previously described (7)(8). The control of the disease was assessed by glycaemia,glycosuria and HbAlc (nv.=4.77$\pm$0.6) determinations. BMC, Bone Width and BMC/BW for the nondominant radius were measured by photon absorptiometry (Norland 2783) and the results were mached with normal values for age and sex (unpublished data).

Results:

In all subjects we found normal or slightly elevated levels of 25OHD, normal CT, Ca, P and PU; serum AP was in the high-normal range (m$\pm$SD 870$\pm$20 U/l; nv:300-900 U/l), PTH was in the low-normal range (m$\pm$SD 0.32$\pm$0.08 ng/ml; nv:0.30-0.66 ng/ml). CU was augmented in 6 poorly controlled patients (m$\pm$SD 16.5$\pm$2.5 mEq/24h; n.v.5-12.5/24h). Serum 1.25(OH)2D levels were no significantly low in 11 patients (m$\pm$SD 26.0$\pm$2 pg/ml; nv:38$\pm$7; $p > 0.05$) and normal in the others. Bone loss was lower ($p < 0.001$) in well controlled patients (n=19; duration of disease=2.1$\pm$1.2a.; BMC=-2.1$\pm$2.8%; BMC/BW=-1.08$\pm$2.1%; HbAlc=6.5$\pm$0.6%; m$\pm$SD) than in poorly controlled ones (n=8; duration of disease=3.2$\pm$1.19; BMC=-12.8$\pm$4%; BMC/BW=-8.5$\pm$5.5%; HbAlc=10.8$\pm$1.0%; m$\pm$DS). In all subjects HbAlc values positively correlate with bone loss (BMC r=0.87; BMC/BW r=0.73).

Discussion:

Shore (1) in a trasversal as well as longitudinal study found that osteoporosis begins early in IDDM and BMC does not

Vitamin D. A Chemical, Biochemical and Clinical Update

change significantly in the next 4 years. Our data, showing that a good control of the disease is an important factor to mantain a normal bone mass, agree with Mc Nair's results (9). On the other hand our patients showed only a slight derangement of calciotropic hormones. Heath (3) found normal 1.25(OH)2D and other calciotropic hormones levels in adult diabetic patients. Christiansen (6) showed normal 1.25(OH)2D and low 24.25(OH)2D levels in adult insulin treated diabetics while Frazer (5) found low 1.25(OH)2D and elevated 24.25(OH)2D in young insulin dependent diabetics. Insulin, as showed by Henry in vitro (10), may indirectly increase calcitriol production in kidney. Recently Shavit (11) provided evidences that saccharides mediate in vitro the attachment to bone of resorptive cells and an enhanched bone resorption can be at least partially due to an abundance of these sugars on cell membran. Further studies are needed to assess the role of metabolic control and/or Vitamin D metabolites in determining osteoporosis in IDDM.

References:

1)Shore,R.M., Chesney,R.W., Mazess,R.B., Rose,P.G., Bargman,G.J. (1981) Calcif.Tissue Int. 33: 455-457.

2)Schedl,H.P., Heath,H.III, Wenger,J. (1978) Endocrinology 103: 1368-1373.

3)Heath,H.III, Lambert,P.W., Service,J.F., Arnaud,S.B. (1979) J.Clin.Endoceinol.Metab. 49: 462-466.

4)Gertner,J.M., Tamborlane,W.V., Horst, R.L., Sherwin,R.S., Felig,P., Genel,M. (1980) J.Clin.Endocrinol.Metab. 50: 862-866.

5)Frazer,T.E., Withe,N.H., Hough,S., Santiago,J.V., McGee,B.R., Bryce,G., Mallon,J., Avioli,L.V. (1981) J.Clin.Endocrinol.Metab. 53: 1154-1159.

6)Christiansen,C., Christensen,M.S., McNair,P., Nielsen,B., Madsbad,S. (1982) Scand.J.Clin.Lab.Invest. 42: 487-491.

7)Saggese,G., Bertelloni,S., Federico,G., Baroncelli,G.I., Bottone,E.(1984) Proceedings RIA '84 "Cost and Benefit of Radio Immuno Assay" Albertini A.ed., Milan,May 15-16,p.31 abs.

8)Eisman,J.A., Hamstra,A.J., Kream,B.E., De Luca,H.F.(1976) Arch.Bioch.Bioph., 176: 235-243.

9)McNair,P., Madsbad,S., Christiansen,C;, Christensen,M.S., Faber,O.K., Binder,C., Transbol,I. (1979) Diabetologia 17: 283-286.

10)Henry,H.L. (1981) Endocrinology 108: 733-735.

11)Bar-Shavit,Z., Teitelbaum,S.L., Kahn,A.J. (1983) J.Clin.Invest. 72: 516-525.

LEVELS OF 25(OH)D AND OSTEOCALCIN IN DIABETIC PREGNANCIES.

P.Catalan,M.E.Martinez,A.Lisbona*,M.Salinas,G.Balaguer,C.De Pedro,E.Sanchez Casas**,and F.Pallardo*.
Biochemistry,Endocrinology* and Obstetric** Services.C.S."LA PAZ".28046. MADRID.SPAIN.

INTRODUCTION:

There are many studies about the effects of normal pregnancy on phosphocalcium metabolism,however there are few studies which refer to the possible modifications in this metabolism in insulin-dependent diabetic pregnancies

MATERIALS AND METHODS:

Subjects studied :We studied 25(DP)belonging to the classes B&C of White .The mean age was 28±5 years,range(20-35).They were controlled weekly with divided doses of intermediate and short-acting insulin.The values of $Hb.A_1$.through the pregnancy were 8±1.5.Renal function as indicated by creatinine clearance and urinary protein excretion was normal.In parallel we evaluated 105(NP)in the three trimesters of pregnancy and also 53(NW),after the period of maximum(September-October)and minimum(March-April)solar irradiation.All the groups were of similar age and lived in the Madrid area within a radius of 50 Km and none were taking a Vit.D supplement.The(NP)and (DP)were evaluated from the 10th week and were grouped according to the time of pregnancy in trimesters:first(10-15 week)second(16-25 w)and third (26-40 w).The levels of Ca^{++},PTH,25(OH)D and Osteocalcin were evaluated in fasting conditions in the different groups.The determinations in(DP)were made every four weeks until delivery which was induced in the 35th-37th week.

Analytical methods:The $Ca^{++}$was quantified in whole blood by selective electrode(ICA 1-Radiometer-Copenhagen).The samples were placed in vacuum tubes containig sodium heparinate(Leo)and an ionic calcium concentration of 1.25 mmol/l.All handling was done under anaerobic and refrigerated conditions. The PTH(C-terminal)and the Osteocalcin were evaluated by RIA performed commercially by IRE and INC respectively.The 25(OH)D was quantified by protein-binding(Bülhman)after extraction by HPLC.

		NC	NP			DP		
			1st	2nd	3rd	1st	2nd	3rd
Ca^{++} m mol/L	n	37	27	20	31	6	14	26
	x	1.23	1.23	1.22	1.19*	1.23	1.23	1.17*
	SD	0.04	0.04	0.05	0.04	0.40	0.05	0.06
PTH m IU/ml	n	48	27	19	24	12	26	42
	x	2.4	2.2	2.3	2.77*	2.47	2.68	2.58
	SD	0.69	0.76	0.76	0.71	0.79	0.67	0.59
Ost. ng/ml	n	26	11	13	15	9	19	23
	x	2.23	1.43	0.91*	1.9	1.41	1.0*	1.25*
	SD	0.62	1.41	0.68	0.7	0.73	0.45	0.95

TABLE I:BLOOD LEVELS OF IONIC CALCIUM(Ca^{++}),PTH AND OSTEOCALCIN (Ost.)IN NORMAL WOMEN (NW),NORMAL PREGNANCIES (NP)AND DIABETIC PREGNANCIES(DP) IN THE FIRST(1st),SECOND(2nd) AND (3rd)TRIMERTERS OF PREGNANCY.VALUES MARKED WITH (*) SHOWED SIGNIFICANT DIFFERENCES AS COMPARED WITH (NC).

Vitamin D. A Chemical, Biochemical and Clinical Update

RESULTS:

We found lower levels of Ca^{++} in (NP) and (DP) in the third trimester than in (NW) (Table I). If we considered (NP) and (DP) up to the 37th week only, both groups had similar levels, but if we considered them up to the 40th week (NP) had slghtly higher levels since there was an increase after the 37th week in (NP). The levels of PTH in the first and second trimesters were slightly higher in (DP) than in (NW), but the differences were not significant (Table I). On the other hand, (NP) had increased levels of PTH in the third trimester. In the two seasonal periods studied the levels of 25(OH)D in (NP) were similar to (NW), however (DP) had lower levels than both (NW) and (NP). All groups showed higher levels of 25(OH)D in summer-autumn than in spring-winter (Fig.1). We observed no variations in the values of 25(OH)D in (DP) through the three trimesters of pregnancy (Fig. 1). The Osteocalcin was lower in (DP) than in (NW) in the last two trimesters whilst for (NP) it was only lower in the second (Table. I).

CONCLUSION:

We can assume in the group (DP) a certain hyporesponse of the PTH to the decrease on Ca^{++} in the third trimester. The levels of 25(OH)D seem to be influenced more by the season than by the trimester of pregnancy. (DP) showed lower levels of 25(OH)D than (NW) in all the seasons; this seems to be related more to diabetes than to pregnancy since (NP) have normal values. The lower levels of Osteocalcin in (DP) might be due to the low bone formation described in diabetics.

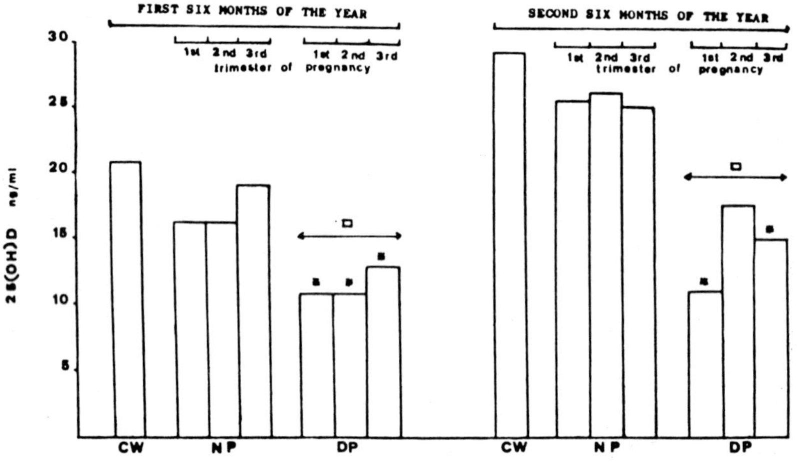

	CW	NP			DP			CW	NP			DP		
n:	24	8	11	10	7	10	15	29	23	33	23	4	11	18
mean:	21	16	16	19	11	11	13	29	25	26	25	16	22	20
± SD:	6	5	3	5	4	7	6	11	11	10	10	4	11	9

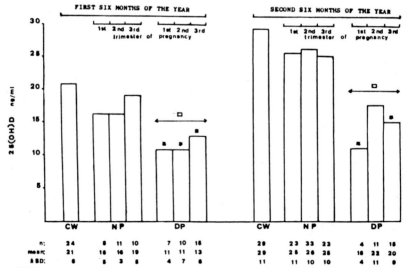

FIGURE.1. LEVELS OF 25(OH)D IN THE 1st SIX MONTHS AND 2nd SIX MONTHS OF THE YEAR IN DIABETIC PREGNANCIES (DP), NORMAL PREGNANCIES (NP) AND CONTROL WOMEN (CW) IN THE FIRST (1st), SECOND (2nd) AND THIRD (3rd) TRIMESTERS OF PREGNANCY. VALUES MARKED (*) AND (□) HAVE SIGNIFICANT DIFFERENCES AS COMPARED WITH (CW) AND (NP) RESPECTIVELY.

EFFECT OF 1α-OH-D_3 ON INSULIN SECRETION IN DIABETES MELLITUS

S. Inomata, S. Kadowaki, T. Yamatani, M. Fukase and T. Fujita
Third Division, Department of Medicine, Kobe University
School of Medicine, Kobe 650, Japan

INTRODUCTION:
Recently several investigators have reported the presence of specific cytosolic receptor protein for 1,25-dihydroxyvitamin D_3[1,25-$(OH)_2$-D_3] (1-3) and of vitamin D dependent calcium binding protein (CaBP) (4,5) in pancreatic B cells, suggesting that endocrine pancreas was one of the target tissues for vitamin D in addition to the intestine, bone and kidney et al. Subsequently, Norman et al. have reported that insulin secretion was impaired in the vitamin D-deficient rat pancreas and restored by vitamin D repletion (6). Furthermore the effectiveness of vitamin D on glucose tolerance and insulin secretion in diabetic patients has been reported (7,8), though the precise mechanism remains unknown. In this study, we have investigated the effect of vitamin D on insulin secretion, glucose tolerance along with other metabolic parameters in non-insulin dependent diabetics.

PATIENTS AND METHODS:
Seventeen non-insulin dependent diabetics (13 male and 4 female) without obesity, aged 37-78 years (mean aged 53.9 ± 3.0 years) were studied. Sixteen patients were controlled by diet therapy alone and one was treated with sulphonylurea under diet therapy. All of these patients were placed on balanced diet for 2-3 weeks, followed by daily administration of 1α-OH-D_3 (group I: 1 μg/day, N=9 or group II: 2 μg/day, N=8) for the following 3-4 weeks. The 75 g oral glucose loading test was conducted before and after the administration of 1α-OH-D_3 and plasma insulin response (single antibody immunoprecipitation techniques) was compared along with the metabolic parameters including serum calcium, phosphate and serum lipids (triglyceride, free fatty acid, β-lipoprotein and HDL-cholesterol).

RESULTS: (Table 1)
(1) The mean serum calcium level was significantly increased from 9.4 ± 0.1 mg/dl to 9.7 ± 0.15 mg/dl ($p < 0.05$) and serum free fatty acid level was decreased from 0.81 ± 0.07 mEq/L to 0.58 ± 0.08 mEq/L ($p < 0.05$) in group II, though no difference was demonstrated in group I. (2) Net insulin secretion during 120 min in response to 75 g glucose loading was significantly increased in group II (16.4 ± 3.4 μU vs. 26.0 ± 5.4 μU: $p < 0.05$), but not in group I. Insulin release in response to 75 g oral glucose load also showed no significant difference in group I at any time point. In contrast, in group II, insulin release was significantly enhanced at 30 min and 60 min respectively after treatment ($p < 0.05$). Blood glucose levels during 75 g oral glucose load showed no difference both in group I and group II. Insulinogenic index (ΔIRI/ΔBS) at 30 min also showed improvement in group II (0.04 ± 0.01 vs. 0.14 ± 0.05 : $p < 0.05$), but not in group I. (3)

There was no direct correlation between serum calcium or free fatty acid levels and insulinogenic indices.

CONCLUSIONS:

It is concluded that 1α-OH-D_3 (2 μg/day) enhances insulin secretion in non-insulin dependent diabetics and the elevation of serum calcium levels appear not to play a key role in this secretion mechanism.

REFERENCES:

1. Clark, S.A., Stumph, W.E., Sar, M., DeLuca, H.F., Tanaka, Y. (1980) Cell Tissue Res. 209: 515-520.
2. Christakos, S., Norman A.W. (1981) Endocrinology 108: 140-149.
3. Pike, J.W. (1982) J. Steroid Biochem. 16: 385-395.
4. Morrissey, R.L., Bucci, T.J., Empson, Jr. R.N., Lufkin, E.G. (1975) Proc. Soc. Exp. Biol. Med. 149: 56-60.
5. Roth, J. Bonner-Weir, S., Norman, A.W., Orci, L. (1982) Endocrinology 110: 2216-2218.
6. Norman, A.W., Frankel, B.J., Heldt, A.M., Grodsky, G.M. (1980) Science 209: 823-825.
7. Kitano, N., Tsuda, T., Kita, T., Yamamoto, Y., Taminato, T., Chiba, T., Kadowaki, S., Fujita, T. (1981) Proceeding of 18th Japanese Clinical and Metabolic Congress, Feb.
8. Blahos, J., Svoboda, Z., Zarubova, V., Justova, V. (1984) Hormone Res. 20: 83.

Table 1 Effect of 1α-OH-D_3(1 μg/day or 2 μg/day) on insulinogenic index (30 min), net blood sugar and insulin area as well as serum calcium, phosphate and serum lipids. Data are expressed as means ± SEM.

	1 μg/day		2 μg/day	
	before	after	before	after
Insulinogenic Index(30 min)	0.18±0.04	0.15±0.05	0.04±0.01	0.13±0.05*
Net insulin area (μU·120 min/ml)	25.2±5.5	25.8±3.8	16.4±3.4	26.0±5.4*
Net blood sugar area (mg·120min/dl)	224.9±23.8	217.7±22.7	263.7±17.0	236.6±22.4
Serum calcium (mg/dl)	9.3±0.17	9.4±0.23	9.4±0.10	9.7±0.15*
phosphate (mg/dl)	3.8±0.19	4.1±0.24	4.1±0.10	3.9±0.14
Serum lipids				
Triglyceride (mg/dl)	102.7±11.4	121.3±19.2	117.2±12.7	155.4±35.0
Free fatty acid (mEq/L)	0.88±0.17	0.92±0.15	0.81±0.07	0.58±0.08*
β-lipoprotein (mg/dl)	285.1±30.1	316.6±47.1	376.6±53.3	381.5±48.8
HDL-cholesterol (mg/dl)	50.0±3.5	49.3±4.6	51.6±7.8	49.2±6.1

*: Significant difference from before ($p < 0.05$)

Cancer and Vitamin D (+ Metabolites)

REGULATION OF HUMAN TARGET CELL RESPONSE TO 1,25 DIHYDROXYVITAMIN D_3

John A. Eisman
Garvan Institute of Medical Research
St. Vincent's Hospital
Darlinghurst, NSW 2010, Australia

The 1,25 dihydroxyvitamin D_3 receptor is present in a wide variety of human and animal cell lines in culture. The presence of receptors in these cells is associated with major effects of the hormone on their replication and differentiation in culture. Hence these target cells provide valuable stable in vitro models for the study of the early biochemical mechanisms of 1,25-dihydroxyvitamin D_3 action and for the regulation of the responsiveness of these target cells to the hormone's action. Such studies have previously been virtually impossible when dealing with intact animals and tissues.

Human breast cancer cell lines have been extensively studied in culture with respect to the 1,25-dihydroxyvitamin D_3 receptor and effects of the hormone on cellular function (1-11). The receptor is present in a wide variety of human cancer cell lines in culture (4) and in certain of these the active hormone regulates replication (2,5,7,12). The effect on replication is particularly interesting since low concentrations of $1,25(OH)_2D_3$ can stimulate growth (7,12) while high concentrations inhibit it (3,5,7,8). The stimulatory effect is seen in the presence of charcoal-treated but not untreated fetal calf serum (7). The replication of these breast cancer cells is also effected in a biphasic fashion by oestrogens and, in this case also, the stimulatory effect is seen in the presence of charcoal-treated but not untreated fetal calf serum (13). The mechanism for this effect has not been explained. It is not that the cells are growing at a maximal rate in the presence of untreated fetal calf serum, since the concentrations of the treated and untreated fetal calf serum can be adjusted to provide virtually identical growth rates. It seems most likely that other growth regulators are removed by charcoal-treatment. Candidates for such a role include glucocorticoids, since treatment with them can abolish the replication stimulatory respone to $1,25(OH)_2D_3$ without affecting the growth inhibitory response. This

Vitamin D. A Chemical, Biochemical and Clinical Update

area has not been investigated fully for oestrogens or $1,25(OH)_2D_3$ in any cell line.

We have been particularly interested in studying the mechanisms, by which $1,25(OH)_2D_3$ mediates its intracellular effects and possible cellular mechanisms for regulating cell responsiveness. We have concentrated on those regulatory mechanisms, which follow exposure of the cells to $1,25(OH)_2D_3$ itself rather than those mediated by other hormones. As shall be discussed below, these involve induction of metabolic enzymes for $1,25(OH)_2D_3$ and changes in receptor turnover.

METHODS

Human breast cancer cells (T47D) or human malignant melanoma cells (MM96) are grown in monolayer culture in plastic flasks or multiwell plates. The cells are cultured to near confluence in RPMI 1640 medium containing 5% fetal calf serum (FCS). Prior to experiments the cells are incubated with medium containing charcoal-treated FCS for 24-48 hours to deplete the cells of $1,25(OH)_2D_3$. For metabolism experiments, the high specific activity ^3H-$1,25(OH)_2D_3$ (90-160 Ci/mmol) is purified by HPLC immediately prior to the experiments. Cells are incubated with labelled hormone in RPMI 1640 medium containing 0.05% bovine serum albumin. Three types of studies have been performed.

In metabolism experiments, the intact cells are incubated with 0.5nM hormone (labelled either at the 23,24 or 26,27 position) in monolayer culture for periods up to 40 hours. At various times the media (or cells and media) are collected, extracted with methanol:chloroform and separated into chloroform-soluble and aqueous (methanol-water) soluble components. The chloroform-soluble material is subject to HPLC on a Waters 0.4 x 30 cm Microporasil silicic acid column in hexane:isopropanol:methanol (38:10:2) at a flow rate of 2 mL/min. Radioactivity in fractions is determined by liquid scintillation counting. At times individual radioactivity peaks are pooled and analysed further on straight phase HPLC on the same silicic acid columns in chloroform:isopropanol (90:10). Periodate sensitivity is also assessed. The aqueous phase radioactivity is further analysed by HPLC on a Waters C-18 0.4 x 40 cm Microbondapak column with a linear gradient over 45 minutes from 19 to 90% of methanol in glass-distilled water at a flow rate of 2 mL/min. As above, radioactivity in individual fractions is determined by liquid scintillation counting.

Studies on whole intact cell uptake of labelled hormone involves growth of cells in multiwell plates to near confluence. After depletion of $1,25(OH)_2D_3$ with charcoal-treated FCS containing medium, the cells are incubated in medium containing 0.05% BSA and labelled hormone at 0.5nM with or without a 100-fold excess of unlabelled hormone. At appropriate times the medium is removed and the monolayer incubated for 15 minutes at 30° with phosphate buffered saline (PBS) containing 0.5% BSA. This wash medium is removed and the monolayer gently rinsed twice with PBS. The cell monolayer is then digested with 1 mL of 1M sodium hydioxide, neutralised with acetic acid and counted in a liquid scintillation counter. Specific uptake is taken as the difference between binding of ^3H-$1,25(OH)_2D_3$ in the absence and the presence of the excess unlabelled hormone. In some experiments extra portions of labelled hormone, equivalent to 0.5nM final concentration, are added to the cell media at intervals. This is done to ensure maintenance of adequate labelled hormone level in the face of the hormone-metabolic activity of the cells. In some of the intact cell uptake studies, various cytotoxic agents are added at the initiation of the hormone incubation. These include cycloheximide (0.01mM), daunomycin (0.035mM) ethidium bromide (0.1mM) tunicamycin (0.5 mg/L), puromycin (0.5 mM), cordycepin (0.18mM), actinomycin D (0.002mM) and cytochalasin B (0.025mM). In these experiments specific uptake and hormone metabolism are studied as described above.

In the third series of experiments cytosolic receptor is studied. Cells are grown to near confluence in monolayer culture in flasks and are incubated with RPMI-1640 medium containing charcoal-treated FCS for the 24-48 hours prior to the experiments. Cells are exposed to $1,25(OH)_2D_3$ (0.5nM) in RPMI 1640 medium containing 0.05% BSA for various times up to 24 hours. The treatment medium is removed and replaced with 0.5% BSA in PBS for 15 minutes at 37°. The monolayers are then rinsed twice with PBS and the cells harvested with a rubber poleceman into homogenisation buffer A. Buffer A comprises 0.05M imidazole (pH 7.2), 0.001M EGTA, 0.002 M dithiothreitol, 0.4M potassium chloride and 1000 IU/mL of aprotinin (Trasylol). The cells are homogenised with a Teflon-glass homogeniser and the homogenate centrifuged at 189,000 g_{av} for 30 minutes at 4°. The supernatant (cytosol) is diluted with an equal volume of buffer B. Buffer B differs from buffer A by the omission of KCl and addition of 0.4% gelatin. This cytosol is then incubated with ^{3}H-1,25$(OH)_2D_3$ (0.05 - 0.2 nM) alone and with a 100 fold molar excess of unlabelled 1,25$(OH)_2D_3$ for one hour at 26°. Receptor-bound hormone is then precipated with polyethylene glycol (PEG) 4000 (26% final concentration). The pellet from the PEG precipitation is dissolved with Soluene 350 and counted with Dimilume scintillant in a liquid scintillation counter. The specific binding is taken as the difference between binding in the absence and presence of excess unlabelled hormone and is expressed as picomole per mg protein.

RESULTS AND DISCUSSION

T47D cells when incubated with labelled hormone exhibit a slow rise in specific uptake. This reaches a peak at 3-8 hours after exposure of the cells to labelled hormone. The time to peak binding has tended towards the shorter times with successive passage of the cells. The rate of rise is concentration dependent i.e. the rise is faster and the peak occurs earlier with increasing hormone concentration over the 0.05 to 1nM range tested. After the peak is reached there is a fairly rapid fall in specific binding to near zero by 12-16 hours of exposure. A similar pattern is seen with the malignant melanoma cells MM96. Investigation of the localisation of the labelled hormone in previous studies has shown a nuclear localisation (6,14). This is in direct contrast to the apparent low affinity of the unoccupied receptor for intact nuclei in our studies (6,16). It was of considerable interest to explain the slow rise and subsequent fall in specific binding. We have shown previously that oestrogen uptake is more rapid under identical conditions with the T47D cells (6,14). Also we have shown that the delay cannot be explained by a slow entry of the labelled hormone into the cells: Equilibration of labelled hormone between extra cellular and intra cellular water is complete within a matter of seconds (11). The fall in binding must reflect a disruption of the hormones receptor complex. Our further studies examined the possibilities of hormone metabolism and receptor modification, as the mechanism for this disruption.

The metabolism studies show that for at least two hours the 1,25$(OH)_2D_3$ depleted cells do not metabolise added hormone (10). However, over the following two to four hours, virtually complete metabolism of hormone occurs. This delay is not due to slow entry as pointed out earlier. The induction of the metabolism can be blocked by inhibitors of protein synthesis (puromycin, cycloheximide) or of DNA replication and transcription (e.g. actinomycin D, cordycepin). Lastly broken cell preparations from $1,25(OH)_2D_3$ depleted cells do not metabolise the hormone whereas homogenates from $1,25(OH)_2D_3$ exposed cells are extremely active in hormone metabolism. The metabolites were examined on straight phase HPLC in the two solvent systems, by double label differences and by periodate sensitivity. As we have reported previously (10), the metabolism appears to be largely the result of oxidative activity at the C-24 and C-23 carbons. Three major metabolites have been tentatively identified as $1,24,25\text{-}(OH)_3D_3$, $1,25(OH)_2\text{-}24\text{-}oxo\text{-}D_3$ and $1,23,25\text{-}(OH)_3\text{-}24\text{-}oxo\text{-}D_3$. Another chloroform-soluble metabolite and several aqueous soluble metabolites remain to be identified (10).

The metabolism studies suggest that hormone metabolism explains the loss of binding. However the repeated addition of labelled hormone was able to partially correct the loss of specific binding (Figure 1). This was completely corrected at 12-16 hours. However, even with hourly additions of fresh hormone between 3 and 6 hours, binding fell to approximately 50% of maximal at 6 and 9 hours. Examination of the media revealed that under these conditions the concentration of unaltered hormone was the same at 6 hours (with repeated addition) as it was at 3 hours, when binding was two-fold higher. In order to study the receptor changes more closely the unoccupied receptor has been measured in broken cell preparations of $1,25(OH)_2D_3$ depleted cells which had been treated with $1,25(OH)_2D_3$ (0.5nM) for appropriate periods of time. Suprisingly there is no fall in unoccupied receptor levels. In fact, as shown in Figure 1, there is a moderate increase in receptor levels. This rise appears to coincide with the fall in occupied receptor measured in the intact cells.

When the intact cells are incubated with puromycin, specific binding starts to fall immediately. It is virtually absent (less than 10% of untreated) by 9 hours. The $t\frac{1}{2}$ of receptor binding in this situation is little more than two hours. When actinomycin D is used, a similar rate of fall occurs after a delay of approximately four hours. These data indicate a rapid turnover of receptor even in the absence of hormone.

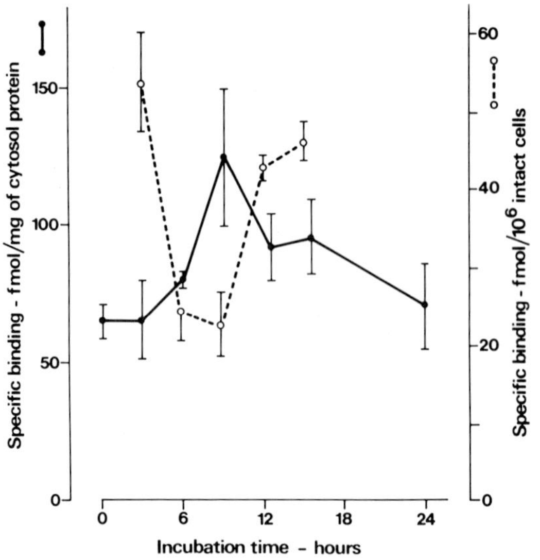

Figure 1: $1,25(OH)_2D_3$ receptor turnover in intact T47D cells and broken cell preparations.

Intact cell binding (o- - -o) was studied in monolayer culture of T47D cells which had been $1,25(OH)_2D_3$ depleted for 24-48 hours. Labelled $1,25(OH)_2D_3$ (0.5nM) was added at time zero and at hourly intervals for the three hours prior to each termination time point. For the studies of specific binding in cytosols (●——●) the cell monolayers were also $1,25(OH)_2D_3$ depleted for24-48 hours and then exposed to 0.5nM unlabelled $1,25(OH)_2D_3$ for the times indicated. Specific binding in intact cells and cytosols was determined as described in methods.

Intact cell binding declines to a nadir (approximately 50% of maximum) at 6 and 9 hours after exposure to $1,25(OH)_2D_3$. In direct contrast, cytosol binding increases to a maximum (approximately 60% above untreated) after 9 hours exposure to the hormone.

These data require careful consideration (Figure 2). In the intact cell studies, the specific binding represents the equilibrium between formation and degradation of the hormone-receptor complexes. On the other hand, the broken cell (cytosol) binding represents a "snapshot" of the unoccupied receptor at a point in time. The studies with cytotoxic agents in the intact cells clearly demonstrates the rapid turnover of receptor. The divergent data from the intact and broken cell studies could be explained by a rate-limiting step existing at the formation of hormone:receptor complexes in the intact cell. This could cause unoccupied receptor to accumulate at the expense of occupied receptor. Particularly if further reduction of the rate of hormone:receptor complex formation occurred: An alternate possibility is that there are increases in both the synthesis of receptor and the degradation of hormone:receptor complexes, while the formation of hormone:receptor complexes remain rate-limiting. This concept would fit with the transient effects of actinomycin D and cordycepin of delaying the fall in specific binding (11).

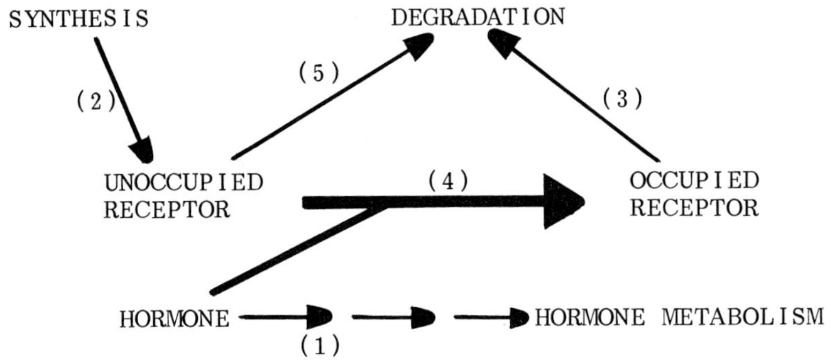

Figure 2: Scheme of regulation of cellular responsiveness to 1,25 $(OH)_2D_3$ action.

Exposure of $1,25(OH)_2D_3$ depleted cells to the hormone results in induction of hormone metabolism (1). The fall in occupied and small rise in unoccupied receptor may be due to increases in receptor synthesis (2) and occupied receptor degradation (3) particularly if formation of hormone:receptor complexes (4) is rate-limiting. Changes in degradation of unoccupied receptor (5) may also take place.

IN SUMMARY, our studies indicate that -

(a) the unoccupied $1,25(OH)_2D_3$ receptor has a short in vivo half-life,

(b) the slow rise in intact cell binding of $1,25(OH)_2D_3$ reflects an equilibrium between receptor synthesis and degradation of occupied receptor,

(c) the fall in binding would appear to be due in part to a shift in this equilibrium and in part to induction of active metabolism of the hormone by these cells.

These mechanisms likely represent pathways for the regulation of hormonal responsiveness in these human cancer cells.

1. Eisman, J.A., Martin, T.J., MacIntyre, I., and Moseley, J.M., (1979) Lancet ii, 1335-1336.

2. Eisman, J.A., Martin, T.J., MacIntyre, I., Frampton, R.J., Moseley, J.M., and Whitehead R. (1980) Biochem. Biophys. Res. Commun. 93, 9-15.

3. Findlay, D.M., Michelangeli, V.P., Eisman, J.A., Frampton, R.J., Moseley, J.M., MacIntyre, I., Whithead, R., and Martin, T.J. (1980) Cancer Res. 40, 4764-4767.

4. Frampton, R.J., Suva, J.L., Eisman, J.A., Findlay, D.M., Moore, G.E., Moseley, J.M., and Martin, T.J. (1982) Cancer Res. 42, 1116-1119.

5. Eisman, J.A., Sher, E., and Martin, T.J., (1982). In: (Norman, A.W., Schaefer, K., Van Herrath, D., Grigoleit H.G. (eds) Vitamin D: Chemical, Biochemical and Clinical Endorcinology of Calcium Metabolism. deGruyter, W. Berlin, pp.31-33.

6. Sher, E., Eisman, J.A., Moseley, J.M., and Martin, T.J. (1981) Biochem J 200, 315-320.

7. Frampton, R.J., Omond, S., and Eisman, J.A. (1983) Cancer Res. 43, 4443-4447.

8. Eisman, J.A. (1983) In: Kuman R (ed) Vitamin D Metabolism: Basic and Clinical Aspects. Martinus Nijhoff, The Hague, Boston, pp.365-382.

9. Sher, E. (1983) Ph.D. thesis, Melbourne University, Parkville, Victoria.

10. Eisman, J.A., Sher, E., Suva, L.J., Frampton, R.J., and McLean, F.C. (1984) Endorinology 114, 1225-1231.

11. Sher, E., Frampton,R.J., and Eisman J.A. (1985) Endocrinology 116 (in press).

12. Freake, H.C., Marcocci, C., Iwasaki J., and MacIntyre I. (1981) Biochem Biophys. Res. Commun. 101 1131-1138.

13. Lippman, M.E., and Bolan, D. (1975) Nature 256 592-593.

14. Sher, E. Martin, T.J., and Eisman J.A. (1985) Horm. Metabol. Res. 17 147-151.

OSTEOMALACIA ASSOCIATED WITH A MALIGNANT TUMOR OF THE UTERUS.

F.P.CANTATORE, M.D'AMORE, M.CARROZZO°, and V.PIPITONE
Department of Rheumathology, Chair of Medical Therapy°, University of Bari, Italy.

INTRODUCTION:

Osteomalacia is a metabolic bone disease characterized by bone pain, muscle weakness, and failure to calcify osteoid tissue. This type of bone disease may result from various etiologic factors that include vitamin D deficiency or alteration in vitamin D metabolism, renal disease, familial and sporadic hypophosphatemia, hypophosphatasia; fibrous dysplasia, neurofibromatosis, and osteopetrosis; neoplasms, both benign and malignant, of either bone or soft tissues.

Osteomalacia owing to neoplasia, has the unique feature of resolution after complete removal of the tumor.

In the present report one case of osteomalacia associated with an uterus adenocarcinoma is described.

CASE REPORT :

A 44-year-old woman related a 1-month history of muscle weakness, bone pain and metrorrhagie. Clinical evaluation showed a polyneuritis (confirmed by electromyography) and an uterus tumor (confirmed by computerized tomography); bone scintigraphy revealed increased uptake of ribs and ischiopubic branches symmetrically.

Serum phosphorus concentration was 2.2 mg%(n.v. 2.8-4.4 mg%), alkaline phosphatase 88 K.A. units (n.v. 50), serum 25(OH)D3 88ng/ml (n.v. 20-65), serum calcitonin 190 pg/ml (n.v. 62 ± 34), serum PTH-C terminal 50 pmol/lt (n.v. 55 ± 29).

The diagnosis of hypophosphatemic osteomalacia tumor-induced was made. Then a hysterectomy was carried out and the istological study showed a light cells adenocarcinoma of endometrium.

Postoperatively muscle weakness and bone pain dissapeared; serum phosphorus concentration, alkaline phosphatase and serum calcitonin became normal (tab.1); and after four months bone scintigraphy revealed no increased uptake.

DISCUSSION :

In our case osteomalacia is associated with an uterus' adenocarcinoma and has the feature of a complete resolution of the biochemical abnormalities of the bone disease after complete remove of the tumor.

The mechanisms proposed to explain oncogenic osteomalacia include tumor-mediated secretion of calcitonin, secretion of PTH or other phosphaturic substances, and interference with normal metabolism of vitamin D or excretion of a vitamin D antagonist by the tumor.

In our patient the levels of calcitonin were hight, serum PTH was nor-

Vitamin D. A Chemical, Biochemical and Clinical Update

mal and serum 25(OH)D3 was elevated; while other Authors described low levels of 1-25(OH)D3 in tumor-induced osteomalacia.

In this way a possible tumor-mediated disorder of vitamin D metabolism could explain our case of osteomalacia; while calcitonin is not likely to cause this sindrome because, in our experience, there is a lot of tumors with hight levels of calcitonin and without hypophosphatemic osteomalacia.

EFFECT OF SURGERY ON CALCIUM, PHOSPHORUS,VITAMIN D, CALCITONIN AND PARA=THORMONE.

	(7 days) Preoperative	Postoperative (15 days)
Phosphorus mg/dl (n.v. 3-5)	2.2	3.5
Calcium mg/dl (n.v. 9.5-10.5)	9.8	10
Alkaline phosphatase K.A.U.(n.v. 20-50)	88	45
25(OH)D3 ng/ml (n.v. 20-65)	88	68
Calcitonin pg/ml (n.v. 62 ± 34)	190	80
Parathyroid hormone pmol/lt (n.v. 55 ± 29)	50	55

TAB. 1

REFERENCES :

1. Daniels R.A.,Weisenfeld I (1979) Ann.J.Med. 67: 155-159
2. Linovitz R.J.,Resnick D.,Keissling P et al.(1976) J.Bone Joint Surg Ann 58: 419-423
3. Parker M.S.,Klein J.,Haussler M.R.,Mintz D.H. (1981) JAMA 5:492-493
4. Sweet R.A.,Males J.L., Hamstra A.J. and De Luca H.F. (1980) Ann Int Med 2: 279-280
5. Turner M.L., Dalinka M.K. (1979) AJR 133: 539-540
6. Wyman A.L., Paradinas F.J., Daly J.R. (1977) J Clin Path 30: 328-335

$1,25(OH)_2D_3$ HAS OPPOSITE REGULATING EFFECTS ON EMBRYONIC AND NON-EMBRYONIC ALKALINE PHOSPHATASES IN BREAST CANCER CELL LINES.

M.A. Mulkins and H.H. Sussman, Department of Pathology,
STANFORD UNIVERSITY, Stanford, California 94305, U.S.A.

These experiments compared the effects of treatment with $1,25(OH)_2D_3$ on the expression of alkaline phosphatase in two human breast carcinoma cell lines, MDA-MB-157 and BT20. The MDA-MB-157 cells express the alkaline phosphatase isoenzyme phenotypic to normal breast cells. The BT20 cells express the placental alkaline phosphatase isoenzyme and do not synthesize the normal breast phosphatase isoenzyme. Each cell line contains specific receptor for $1,25(OH)_2D_3$ and for hydrocortisone (HC).

MDA-MB-157 cells and BT20 cells were grown in Waymouths MB 752/1 medium, supplemented with 5% fetal calf serum and antibiotics in the presence or absence of the indicated hormone for 72 hours, and were harvested, solubilized in Triton X-100 and centrifuged (1). The concentration of alkaline phosphatase present in aliquots of the supernatant was measured by radioimmunoassay (1), using goat antiserum prepared against the breast-class phosphatase and the placental-class phosphatase isoenzymes (2), and purified phosphatase labeled with ^{125}I by a lactoperoxidase method as a tracer. All values are corrected for mg of total cellular protein per sample, and the number shown is the mean $\pm$ standard error of duplicate assays from 2-3 experiments.

Treatment	Radioimmune Assay of Alkaline Phosphatase (ng/mg/protein)	
	MDA-MB-157 Cells (Breast Class Isoenzyme)	BT20 Cells (Placental Isoenzyme)
None	297 ± 85	87 ± 9
$1,25(OH)_2D_3$ - 10^{-9} M	485 ± 60	-
- 10^{-8} M	737 ± 96	-
- 10^{-7} M	877 ± 193	44 ± 3
hydrocortisone - 10^{-6} M	636 ± 265	234 ± 21
$1,25(OH)_2D_3$ (10^{-7} M) plus hydrocortisone (10^{-6} M)	1852 ± 605	118 ± 11

As shown, the specific activity of the breast isoenzyme in the MDA-MB-157 cells can be increased 2- to 3-fold by incubating the cells for 72 hours in the presence of either $1,25(OH)_2D_3$ or hydrocortisone (HC). Simultaneous incubation of the cells with both $1,25(OH)_2D_3$ and HC resulted in an additive or synergistic increase in alkaline phosphatase activity in MDA-MB-157 cells. The increases in phosphatase activity correlated with increases in the amount of the phenotypic breast isoenzymes measured by radioimmunoassay. The increase in alkaline phosphatase activity can be inhibited by the addition of cycloheximide to the medium during the incubation with $1,25(OH)_2D_3$ and/or HC, suggesting that de novo protein synthesis is necessary for the increase in alkaline phosphatase observed after treatment with the two hormones.

Vitamin D. A Chemical, Biochemical and Clinical Update

Different and opposite results were obtained when the effects of $1,25(OH)_2D_3$ on alkaline phosphatase expression in BT20 cells was examined. Treatment of BT20 cells with 10^{-7} M $1,25(OH)_2D_3$ produced a 30% decrease in alkaline phosphatase specific activity. Furthermore, the simultaneous addition of $1,25(OH)_2D_3$ to medium containing HC effectively inhibited the 2-fold increase in alkaline phosphatase activity observed with HC alone. These changes in alkaline phosphatase activity in BT20 cells correlated with changes in the placental isoenzyme levels measured by radioimmunoassay.

Receptor Assays were conducted using untreated cells harvested during logarithmic growth and assayed for high affinity binding of $1,25(OH)_2D_3$ (3), or for hydrocortisone binding (4). The specific binding data were analyzed by the Scatchard method. Linear regression analysis was used to calculate the equilibrium dissociation constants and the maximum number of binding sites/mg of protein.

High affinity ($K_d = 3.5 \times 10^{-10}$ M) receptors for $1,25(OH)_2D_3$ were detected in MDA-MB-157 cells with maximum binding levels of 69 fmoles $1,25(OH)_2D_3$ bound per mg protein. Receptors for $1,25(OH)_2D_3$ of a much lower affinity (1.7×10^{-7} M) were measured in BT20 cells, however the cells were capable of binding at least 100 times more $1,25(OH)_2D_3$ (N_{max} = 9600 fmoles/mg protein) than were the MDA-MB-157 cells. The lower affinity is consistent with the observation that more $1,25(OH)_2D_3$ was required for those cells to elicit the response to it. Receptors for HC with similar affinities to values in the literature were measured in MDA-MB-157 ($K_d = 1.1 \times 10^{-8}$ M) and BT20 ($K_d = 0.7 \times 10^{-8}$ M) cells, with each cell line binding an approximate maximum of 200-300 fmoles HC per mg of cytosol protein.

The different effect of the $1,25(OH)_2D_3$ on the placental isoenzyme expression is of interest because it is on embryonic enzyme which is commonly expressed in malignancies (5). Its expression in neoplasms may be indicative of the de-differentiation or assumption of embryonic properties associated with neoplastic transformation. The ability of $1,25(OH)_2D_3$ to down-regulate an alkaline phosphatase isoenzyme characteristic of a more embryonic state and to up-regulate expression of a phenotypic phosphatase, associated with a more differentiated state, is important in that it is consistent with the observation in recent studies indicating that $1,25(OH)_2D_3$ is capable of inducing the differentiation of monocytes in vitro (6) and of leukemia cells in vitro (7) and in vivo (8).

1. Mulkins, M.A., Manolagas, S.C., Deftos, L.J., and Sussman, H.H. (1983) J.Biol.Chem. **258**, 6219-6225.
2. Sussman, H.H., Small, P.A., Jr., and Cotlove, E. (1968) J.Biol.Chem. **243**, 160-166.
3. Chen, T.L., and Feldman, D. (1981) J.Biol.Chem. **256**, 5561-5566.
4. Loose, D.S., Do, Y.S., Chen, T.L., and Feldman, D. (1980) Endocrinology **107**, 137-146.
5. Sussman, H.H. (1978) Scand.J.Immunol. **7**, 127-140.
6. Provvedini, D.M., Tsoukas, C.D., Deftos, L.J., and Manolagas, S.C. (1983) Science **221**, 1181-1183.
7. Miyaura, C., Abe, E., Kuribayashi, T., Tanaka, H., Konno, K., Nishii, Y., and Suda, T. (1981) Biochem.Biophys.Res.Comm. **102**, 937-943.
8. Honma, Y., Hozumi, M., Abe, E., Konno, K., Fukushima, M., Hata, S., Nishii, Y., DeLuca, H., and Suda, S. (1983) Proc.Natl.Acad.Sci.USA **80**, 201-204.

DEFECTIVE PRODUCTION OF 1,25$(OH)_2D_3$ IN MYELOMA.

P.J. LAWSON-MATTHEW, J.C. CLAYTON, D.F. GUILLAND-CUMMING, A.J.P. YATES, R.G.G RUSSELL, F.E. PRESTON and J.A. KANIS,
Department of Human Metabolism and Clinical Biochemistry, University of Sheffield Medical School, Beech Hill Road, Sheffield S10 2RX, U.K.

Myeloma is a disorder characterised by neoplastic proliferation of plasma cells within the bone marrow. Hypercalcaemia mediated by increased bone resorption is common, and might be expected to affect metabolism of vitamin D. We have investigated the effects of hypercalcaemia on vitamin D metabolism in myeloma by studying hypercalcaemic patients and healthy control subjects. In order to determine the effects of myeloma itself, we also studied a group of normocalcaemic patients without evidence of increased bone resorption.

Methods

We studied 16 patients with hypercalcaemia due to myeloma (9M, 7F; mean age 56 years), 10 normocalcaemic myeloma patients (7M, 3F; mean age 55 years) and 16 normal controls (9M, 7F; mean age 58 years) under fasting conditions. Dihydroxylated metabolites of vitamin D were extracted from 3 ml serum using hexane: butan-1-ol: propan-2-ol (93:4:3 v/v), partially purified on C_{18} Sep-Pak cartridges and separated on HPLC. 1,25$(OH)_2D_3$ was assayed using antiserum 02282 (kindly donated by Professor JLH O'Riordan) and 24,25$(OH)_2D_3$ measured by competitive protein binding assay using 1:70 000 dilution of normal human serum. 25OHD was similarly measured after protein precipitation and silica column chromatography of 200ul serum.

	HYPERCALCAEMIA	NORMOCALCAEMIA	CONTROL
SERUM CREATININE (umol/l)°	182 ± 22**	85 ± 11	81 ± 3
SERUM CALCIUM (mmol/l)	3.29 ± 0.01**	2.33 ± 0.02	2.39 ± 0.02
SERUM PHOSPHATE (mmol/l)	1.10 ± 0.06	1.06 ± 0.04	0.96 ± 0.04
ALKALINE PHOSPHATASE (IU/l)	86 ± 11	107 ± 16*	70 ± 5
URINARY CALCIUM (mol/mol creatinine)	1.24 ± 0.16++	0.19 ± 0.04	0.1 - 0.4
URINARY HYDROXYPROLINE (mmol/mol creatinine)	62.0 ± 13.0+	25.6 ± 2.5	10 30
1,25$(OH)_2D_3$ (pmol/l)	45.8 ± 7.4**	78.0 ± 7.4*	102.5 ± 7.3

Table 1 INDICES OF MINERAL METABOLISM IN PATIENTS WITH MYELOMA AND NORMAL OR RAISED SERUM CALCIUM COMPARED WITH CONTROLS (values expressed as mean ± SEM).

** $P<0.01$ vs CONTROL ++$P<0.01$ vs NORMOCALCAEMIA

* $P<0.05$ vs CONTROL + $P<0.05$ vs NORMOCALCAEMIA

° Serum creatinine in the normocalcaemic group excludes one patient with an abnormal serum creatinine. Total mean ± SEM was 116 ± 32 umol/l.

Results and Discussion

Hypercalcaemic patients had increased bone resorption as judged by fasting urinary excretion of calcium and hydroxyproline (Table 1). This was associated with low values of $1,25(OH)_2D_3$, although serum values for 25OHD were normal (data not shown). Possible mechanisms for this effect include inhibitory effects of hypercalcaemia, secondary suppression of parathyroid hormone secretion and impaired renal function. However, normocalcaemic patients, contrary to expectation, also showed significantly lower values of $1,25(OH)_2D_3$ than control subjects despite similar degrees of renal function and similar values for serum calcium, phosphate, and biochemical indices of bone turnover. An additional reason for low values for $1,25(OH)_2D_3$ in patients with myeloma includes concurrent therapy (generally intermittent melphelan and prednisolone).

Irrespective of the mechanism for this effect, these data suggest that patients with myeloma have impaired production of $1,25(OH)_2D_3$. In view of the effects of $1,25(OH)_2D_3$ on the proliferation and differentiation of bone (1) and haematological cell lines (2), the question arises whether deficient production might adversely affect tumour growth and differentiation or bone cell function in myeloma. Studies in progress suggest that administration of the bisphosphonate, clodronate, is capable of restoring values of $1,25(OH)_2D_3$ to normal at least in hypercalcaemic patients (3), but their effects on bone formation or tumour growth have not yet been studied.

Acknowlegements

We are grateful to the Leukaemia Research Fund, the MRC and to Oy Star for their support of various aspects of this work.

References

1. Dokoh, S., Donaldson, C.A. and Haussler, M.R. (1984) Cancer Res. 44, 2103-2109.
2. Manolagas, S.C. and Deftos, L.J. (1984) Ann.Intern.Med. 100, 144-146.
3. Lawson-Matthew, P.J., Clayton, J.C., Guilland-Cumming, D.F., Johnson, S.K., Vaishnav, R., Paterson, A.D., Woodhead, S., Russell, R.G.G. and Kanis, J.A. (1983) Calcif.Tissue Int. 35, 55P.

$1,25(OH)_2D_3$ RECEPTORS ARE PRESENT IN HUMAN BREAST CANCER CELL LINES (T 47 D) BUT NOT IN HYPERCALCEMIC WALKER CARCINOSARCOMA 256 OF THE RAT

J. Merke, G. Smigielsky, U. Hügel, G. Klaus, H. Minne, E. Ritz
Department Medicine, University of Heidelberg, 69 Heidelberg, FRG

The presence of $1,25(OH)_2D_3$ receptors and stimulation of calcium transport by $1,25(OH)_2D_3$ have been demonstrated in breast tissue of vitamin D_3 deficient lactating rats. Recently, $1,25(OH)_2D_3$ receptors have also been found in human breast cancer cell lines and in non-malignant breast epithelial cell lines and hypercalcemia is frequently associated with metastatic breast cancer. Therefore we examined a transplantable hypercalcemic tumor, derived from breast tissue, i.e. Walker carcinosarcoma 256 of the rat, for the presence of $1,25(OH)_2D_3$ receptor.

Material and Methods:

Non-rachitic female Sprague Dawley rats (200 g BW) raised under standard conditions. Mammary gland from rats on 17th day of gestation. Cell population (10^7 cells/ml) of Walker 256 hypercalcemic carcinosarcoma implanted (a) subcutaneously into thigh and (b) into abdominal cavity of adult rats. Solid tumor was excised after 7 days at hypercalcemic maximum. Ascites cells were collected after 3 days and purified by Percoll density gradient. Walker tumor cells and/or human breast cancer cells (T 47 D) originating from a mammary duct carcinoma were grown in RPMI 1640 (5% fetal calf serum). Before binding studies cells were incubated in serum-free medium for 24 h. Confluent cells were detached by trypsin, washed in PBS, resuspended (10^7 cells/ml) in KTEDMo (0.3 M KCl; 10 mM Tris/HCl; 1.5 mM EDTA; 1 mM DTT; 10 mM molybdate) for cytosol or TEDMo for nuclear preparations. Receptor characterisation by sucrose density gradient analysis; saturation analysis (Scatchard plot; competition with vitamin D metabolites as described (1). DNA cellulose affinity chromatography with a linear KCl gradient. Concurrent analysis of rat and chick intestinal mucosa to validate methodology.

Results:

Specific $1,25(OH)_2D_3$ receptor proteins were demonstrated by sucrose density gradient (3.2-3.5 S) in cytosolic and nuclear fractions of rat breast at 17th day of gestation and in a human breast cancer cell line (T 47 D). Receptor characterization corresponded to $1,25(OH)_2D_3$ receptor of concurrently studied intestinal mucosa of rat and chick. High affinity binding in nuclear fraction of T 47 D characterized by N_{max} = 65 fmol/mg protein and K_D of 1.08 x 10^{-10}M. Elution of receptor complex $[^3H]$-$1,25(OH)_2D_3$ from DNA cellulose column at 0.27 M KCl. In contrast, no $1,25(OH)_2D_3$ receptor could be demonstrated in cytosolic or nuclear fractions of Walker 256 (detection threshold in concurrently studied intestinal mucosa 2 fmol/mg protein). No $1,25(OH)_2D_3$ binding was seen even with postlabeling of su-

Vitamin D. A Chemical, Biochemical and Clinical Update

crose density fractions and subsequent hydroxyl-apatite assay. However, $25(OH)D_3$ was bound specifically at 5.9 S by cytosol of Walker 256. Scatchard analysis revealed low capacity (N_{max} = 514 fmol/mg protein) and high affinity ($K_D = 2{,}3 \times 10^{-9}M$). $[^3H]$ $-25(OH)D_3$ was completely displaced by 10-fold molar excess of unlabeled $25(OH)D_3$; 50% displacement by 1-fold molar excess of unlabeled $25(OH)D_3$, 200-fold for $1{,}25(OH)_2D_3$ and 5000-fold for 1-alpha-$(OH)D_3$. Protease and trypsin caused a substantial loss of binding, indicating that binding macromolecule is a protein. $25(OH)D_3$ binding protein was heat labile, could clearly be separated by sucrose density gradient from serum binding protein DBP (4.1 S) and presumably corresponded to actin/DBP 6 S complex.

Discussion:

Normal breast gland tissue of rats on day 17 of gestation and human breast cancer cell line T 47 D exhibit specific $1{,}25(OH)_2D_3$ binding. Others had speculated that hypercalcemia of mamma-derived Walker 256 carcinoma was related to $1{,}25(OH)_2D_3$. The present study fails to document $1{,}25(OH)_2D_3$ receptors (within the detection threshold) in hypercalcemic Walker carcinosarcoma 256. This contrasts with cytosolic binding of $25(OH)D_3$ by the 6 S binding complex, the function of which for biology of tumor remains to be established.

Literature:

1. Merke, J., Kreusser, W., Bier, B., Ritz, E. (1983) Europ. J. Biochem. 130: 303-308

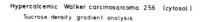

Hypercalcemic Walker carcinosarcoma 256 (cytosol)
Sucrose density gradient analysis

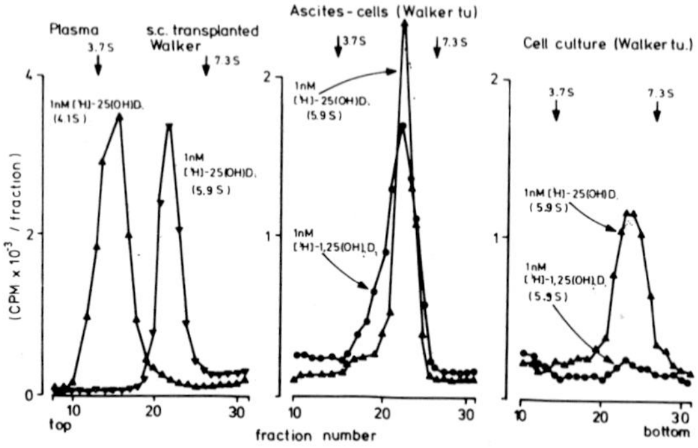

CHARACTERISATION OF 1,25 DIHYDROXYVITAMIN D_3 RECEPTORS IN RAT BREAST TUMOUR

Kay Colston and R.C. Coombes[+]
Department of Chemical Pathology, St. George's Hospital Medical School, London, and [+]Ludwig Institute for Cancer Research, Sutton, Surrey, U.K.

INTRODUCTION

Receptors for 1,25 dihydroxyvitamin D_3 (1,25$(OH)_2D_3$) have been reported to exist in several breast cancer cell lines (1) Similar receptors have also been detected in a proportion of human breast tumours (2). However, the presence of multiple binding sites and limited tissue availability have precluded complete biochemical characterisation of the receptor. A rat model of breast cancer has been reported in which tumours are induced with the carcinogen nitrosomethylurea (NMU) (3). These tumours are oestrogen receptor positive with a receptor content of greater than 10 fmols/mg cytosol protein. Growth of the tumour is oestrogen dependent and tumour incidence is low in ovariectomised rats. In this study, rat breast tumours induced by NMU were examined for the presence of 1,25$(OH)_2D_3$ receptors.

RESULTS

Female virgin Ludwig/Wistar/Olac rats (50 days old) were treated with NMU (5mg/100g body weight). Tumours became palpable at 4-5 months of age.
Sedimentation analysis on sucrose density gradients was used to examine the binding macromolecules for $[^3H]$1,25$(OH)_2D_3$ present in KTEDM extracts prepared from NMU induced rat breast tumours (4). Two binding proteins were detected: one sedimenting at 5-6S representing binding of $[^3H]$1,25$(OH)_2D_3$ to the 25OHD_3 binding protein and a second moiety sedimenting, like the rat intestinal receptor, at 3.3S. Binding of $[^3H]$1,25$(OH)_2D_3$ to the 3.3S peak was substantially reduced by a 5-fold molar excess of unlabelled 1,25$(OH)_2D_3$ (fig. 2).
Receptor content of rat breast tumours was investigated using the hydroxylapatite assay by incubating KTEDM extracts with a saturating concentration (1.3nM) of ^3H 1,25$(OH)_2D_3$ plus a 10-fold molar excess of unlabelled 25OHD_3 to eliminate binding of the hormone to the 5-6S binding species. These studies showed that $[^3H]$1,25$(OH)_2D_3$ receptor content was inversely related to tumour size. Tumours $<$0.25g consistently demonstrated higher $[^3H]$1,25$(OH)_2D_3$ binding activity than did tumours $>$1.0g when expressed on the basis of tumour weight or mg cytosolprotein.

Vitamin D. A Chemical, Biochemical and Clinical Update

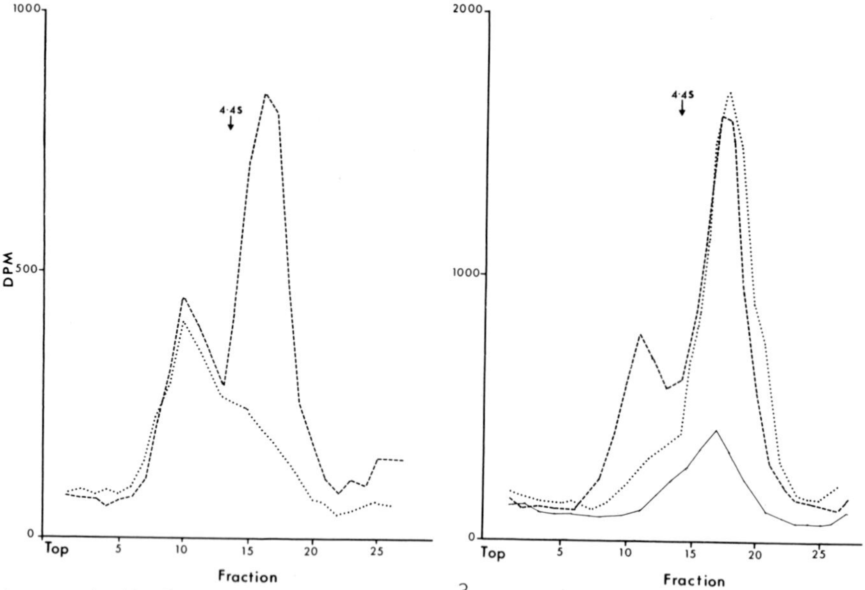

Figure 1 (left panel) ----1,3nM [^{3}H]1,25(OH)$_2$D$_3$ alone; ....plus 13nM unlabelled 25OHD$_3$
Figure 2 (right panel) -----1.3nM [^{3}H]1,25(OH)$_2$D$_3$ alone; ....plus 6.5nM unlabelled 1,25(OH)$_2$D$_3$; ——— plus 325nM unlabelled 1,25(OH)$_2$D$_3$.

Table 1
SPECIFIC [^{3}H]1,25(OH)$_2$D$_3$ BINDING IN BREAST TUMOURS

	n	[^{3}H]1,25(OH)$_2$D$_3$ bound (fmol/mg protein)
Rat breast tumours		
< 0.25 g	6	84.3
0.25-0.75g	7	35.6
Breast cancer cell lines		
T47D	-	75.3
MDA-MB-231	-	22.4
ZR-75-1	-	24.3
Human breast tumours	3	3.0

REFERENCES

1. Findlay, D.M., Michelangeli, V.P., Eisman, J.A. et.al. (1980) Cancer Res. 40, 4764-4767
2. Christakos et.al. (1983) J.Clin.Endocr.Metab. 56 686-691
3. Williams, J.C. et.al. (1981) J.Nat.Can.Inst. 66 147-155
4. Colston, K., Hirst, M. and Feldman, D. (1980) Endocrinology 107, 1916-1922.

STUDY OF 1,25-$(OH)_2D_3$ RECEPTORS IN HUMAN PRIMARY BREAST CANCERS USING POLYACRYLAMIDE GEL ELECTROPHORESIS (PAGE)

S. GUILLEMANT*, J. EURIN* and F. SPYRATOS**

Faculté de Médecine Pitié-Salpêtrière, 75013 Paris* and Centre René Huguenin, 92210 Saint Cloud**, France.

Introduction :

Breast cancer is characterized by high incidence, at least in advanced cases, of secondary bone involvement, and 1,25(OH)2D3 receptors have been described in primary breast cancers (1, 2, 3). Having previously used a PAGE technique to study 1,25(OH)2D3 receptor in chick intestinal mucosa (4), we decided to apply this technique to the detection and estimation of 1,25(OH)2D3 receptors in a series of thirty-five unselected primary breast tumors.

Materials and Methods :

Tumors : Tumors were obtained at surgery in 35 women with primary breast cancer from the Centre René Huguenin. They were immediately frozen and stored in liquid nitrogen. Estrogen and progesterone receptor analysis was carried out and tumors with specific binding site levels above 10 fmol/mg protein were considered as positive (ER+ or PR+). Histological examination was performed and tumors classed according to the histoprognostical grading of BLOOM and RICHARDSON (5).

1,25(OH)2D3 receptor assay : Tumor fragments for receptor assay, weighing 200-500 mg, were freeze-crushed after cooling in liquid nitrogen using an Autopulverizer Thermovac. The powder was taken up in 2 volumes of ice-cold Tris-HCl buffer (50 mM Tris-HCl, pH 7.4, 25 mM KCl, 5 mM MgCl2, 5 mM Dithiothreitol, 20 mM MoO4Na2, Trasylol 200 KIU/ml). Cytosols were prepared by centrifugation at 100,000 x g for 1 hr at 4°C. Fifty µl cytosol samples were incubated for 16 h at 4°C with 2 nM tritiated 1,25(OH)2D3 with or without a 200-fold excess of unlabelled 1,25(OH)2D3 (final volume 130 µl). Parallel incubations with similar excess of unlabelled 25-OHD3 were performed to ensure specificity. At the end of incubation free hormone was pelleted with Dextran-coated charcoal and to each 80 µl sample of supernatant was added a drop of Bromophenol Blue as tracking dye before layering on polyacrylamide gels.

PAGE : Electrophoresis was conducted in cyclindrical (5x130mm) separation gels without stacking gels for 2 1/2 h at 1 mA/gel and at 4°C. PAGE was performed in a multiphasic (Tris/glycine/HCl) buffer operative at pH 10.2.as previously described (6). The total concentration (T) of acrylamide monomer (Fluka A.G.) plus the cross-linking agent N,N-methylene-bisacrylamide (Sigma) was held constant at 10% and the degree of cross-linking (C) i.e. the bisacrylamide/monomer ratio maintained at 2%. When electrophoresis was completed each gel was removed and sectioned transversally into slices, 1.2 mm thick, which

Vitamin D. A Chemical, Biochemical and Clinical Update

were allowed to stand overnight with 1 ml toluene to extract the labelled steroid. The extract was mixed with 4 ml scintillation solution (Biofluor, N.E.N. C°) before radioactivity was counted. Electrophoretic relative mobility (Rf) was determined as the ratio between the distance migrated by the radioactive band and the distance migrated by the tracking dye.

Results

Specificity of the binding of 1,25(OH)2D3 by human breast tumor cytosols : Specificity of the binding was assessed by PAGE runing of breast tumor cytosol incubated with tritiated 1,25(OH)2D3 in presence of a 100-fold excess of either unlabelled 1,25(OH)2D3 (BNS) or unlabelled 25-OHD3. Specifically bound (BS) was calculated by subtracting BNS from total binding on PAGE (BT) obtained by incubation of tritiated 1,25(OH)2D3. An example is presented in Figure 1.

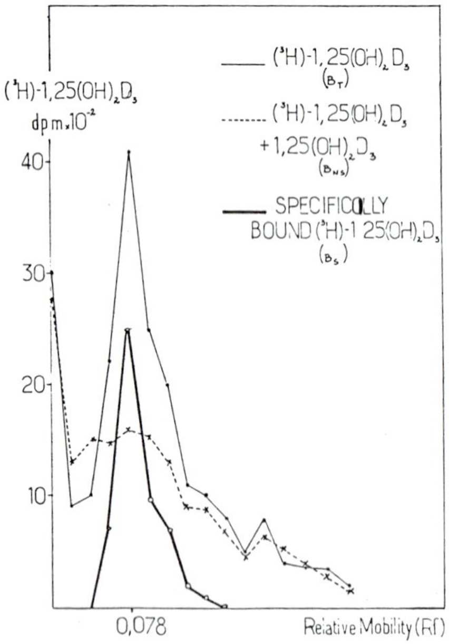

Figure 1. PAGE analysis of the binding of 1,25(OH)2D3 by human breast tumor cytosol.

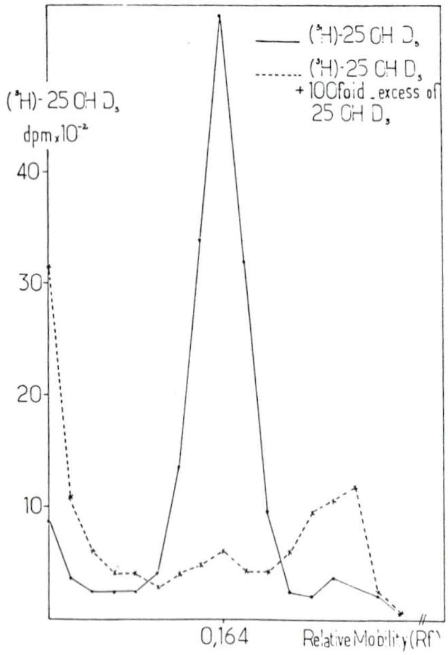

Figure 2. PAGE analysis of the binding of 25-OHD3 by human breast tumor cytosol.

Contribution of 25-OHD-binding protein (DBP): DBP contaminates any breast tumor specimen obtained at surgery as shown when PAGE runing cytosols incubated with tritiated 25-OHD3 (Figure 2). This binding protein is specific for 25-OHD3 but has a significant low affinity for 1,25(OH)2D3. It could therefore theoritically contribute to the apparent 1,25(OH)2D3 binding. Nevertheless, this possibility could be eliminated since, 1) specific 1,25(OH)2D3 binding peaks were not significantly displaced by a 100-fold excess of unlabelled 25-OHD3 and 2) Rf of DBP in that system (≃0.160) differed from that (or those) of 1,25(OH)2D3 binding activity.

Estimation of 1,25(OH)2D3 binding activity and sensitivity of the method : Estimation of specific 1,25(OH)2D3 binding activity was obtained by measuring the area, expressed as dpm, under each specific binding peak. The amount of bound 1,25(OH)2D3 was expressed on the basis of protein (fmol/mg protein). Detectable peaks (≃500 dpm) corresponded to 2-3 fmol/mg of protein. In fact only cytosols presenting specific peaks corresponding to binding activities no less than 8 fmol/mg protein were classed as receptor positive.

PAGE analysis of the binding of 1,25(OH)2D3 by human breast tumor cytosols : Some examples of PAGE analysis of breast tumor cytosols are presented in Figure 3. Receptor-positive breast tumor cytosols frequently exhibited one specific binding peak with a Rf around 0.100 in these experimental conditions. However some cytosols exhibited 2 or 3 specific binding peaks. Thirty five human primary breast cancers were studied. Nineteen (54%) of them were classed as receptor-positive according to the above defined criterions. Their levels were estimated ranging from 8 to 40 fmol/mg protein (mean±SD : 24±11 fmol/mg protein).

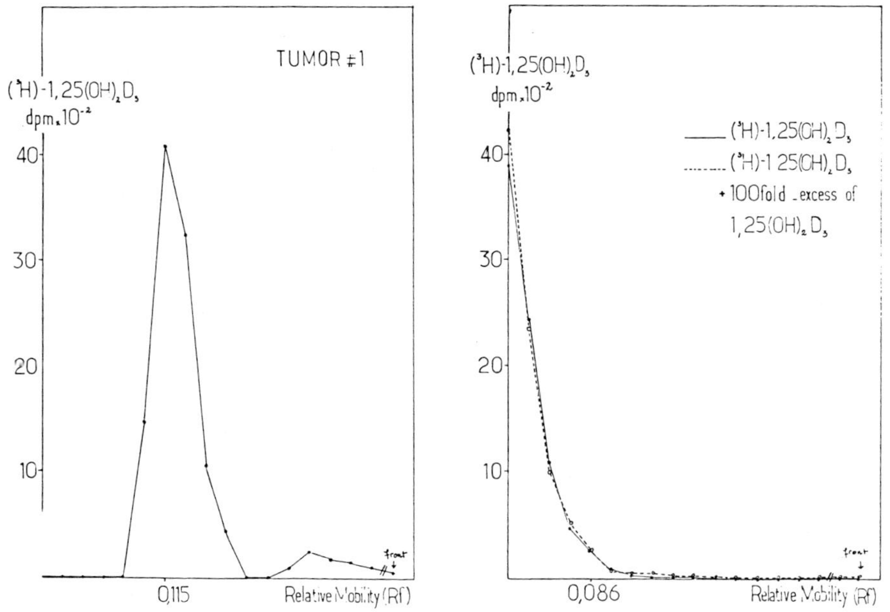

Figure 3. PAGE patterns of receptor-positive (left) and of receptor-negative (right) cytosols.

Relationship to estrogen and progesterone receptor content : 63% of the tumors examined were classed as ER+ and 49% were classed as PR+. As shown in Table 1 ER+ tumors were apparently more frequent in 1,25(OH)2D3 receptor-positive groups.

Table 1. 1,25(OH)2D3 receptor content of primary breast carcinoma in relation with the estrogen and progesterone receptor status

	1,25(OH)2D3 receptor (fmol/mg protein)	
	>8	<8
ER-	5 (26%)	8 (50%)
ER+	14 (74%)	8 (50%)
PR-	8 (42%)	10 (63%)
PR+	11 (58%)	6 (38%)

Relationship to histoprognostical grading : The results are presented in Table 2.

Table 2. 1,25(OH)2D3 receptor content of primary breast carcinoma in relation with the histoprognostical grading of BLOOM and RICHARDSON

	1,25(OH)2D3 receptor (fmol/mg protein)	
	>8	<8
Grading I	1 (5%)	1 (5%)
Grading II	12 (63%)	8 (50%)
Grading III	6 (32%)	6 (38%)
Grading not determined		1 (6%)

Our preliminary results indicate that PAGE technique is useful both for detecting and for determining 1,25(OH)2D3 receptors in small (<500 mg w.w.) of human breast cancers. The frequency (54%) and the concentrations range (<1 to 40 fmol/mg protein) are similar to those reported elsewhere (3), suggesting a good recovery of receptor although PAGE technique prohibited the use of high salt extraction buffers. Further assays are requested before establishing a relationship between the level of 1,25(OH)2D3 receptors and other prognostic indicators.

References :

(1) Eisman, J.A., Suva, L.J., Sher, E., Pearce, P.J., Funder, J.W. and Martin, T.J. (1981) Cancer Res. 41, 5121-5124.

(2) Christakos, S., Sori, A., Greenstein, S.M. and Murphy, T.F. (1983) J. Clin. Endocrinol. Metab. 56, 686-691.

(3) Freake, H.C., Abeyasekera, G., Iwasaki, J., Marcocci, C., MacIntyre, I., McClelland, R.A., Skilton, R.A., Easton, D.F. and Coombes, R.C. (1984) Cancer Res. 44, 1677-1681.

(4) Guillemant, S. and Eurin, J. (1983) Biochem. Biophys. Res. Commun. 113, 687-694.

(5) Bloom, H.J.C. and Richardson, W.W. (1957) Brit. J. Cancer 11, 359.

(6) Rodbard, D. and Chrambach, A. (1971) Anal. Biochem. 40, 95-134.

REGULATION BY 1,25-DIHYDROXYVITAMIN D_3 (1,25-$(OH)_2D_3$) OF SPECIFIC GENE EXPRESSION IN GH PITUITARY CELLS.

J.D. WARK, University of Melbourne, Department of Medicine, Royal Melbourne Hospital, 3050, Victoria, Australia.

Following the finding of a specific intracellular "receptor" for 1,25-$(OH)_2D_3$ (1,25-DR) in rat pituitary cells (1,2) the effects of vitamin D_3 metabolites on GH cells have been examined (2-5). Since serum contains vitamin D metabolites, their serum binding protein, hormones and other factors, these studies are best performed using serum-free media. Under these conditions 1,25-$(OH)_2D_3$ potently and selectively increased prolactin (PRL) gene expression in GH_4C_1 cells (ED_{50} 1-2 x 10^{-10}M; 4,5). The effects were delayed ⩾ 24h and depended on extracellular Ca^{2+}, confirming GH_4C_1 cells as a model for studying 1,25-$(OH)_2D_3$ action. In further studies the glucocorticoid hydrocortisone (HC) potently antagonized 1,25-$(OH)_2D_3$-induction of PRL gene expression.

Materials and Methods

GH_4C_1 cells in serum-supplemented Ham's F10 medium were plated (2.5 x 10^5/60mm dish) and grown for 4-5 days. Cultures were incubated in chemically-defined, hormone-free medium (4) containing 0.4mM $CaCl_2$. Added ethanol was < 0.04% and was the same in all dishes. PRL production (PRL-P) was determined by RIA of the culture medium. PRL mRNA was quantitated by cytoplasmic dot hybridization (5) followed by liquid scintillation counting.

Results and Discussion

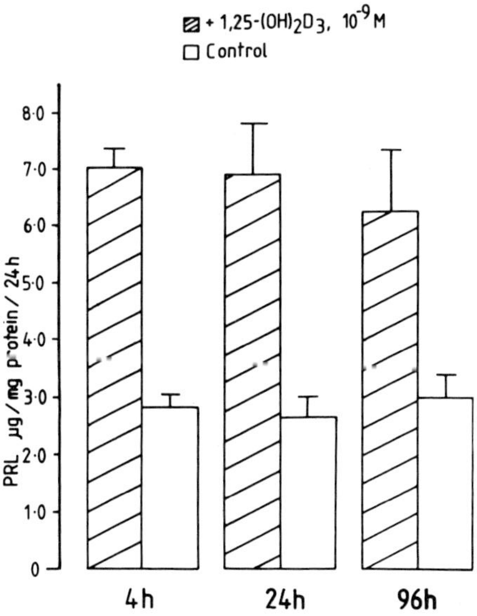

Fig. 1: Treatment with 1,25-$(OH)_2D_3$ or vehicle for 4,24 or 96h. PRL-P measured at 96h. Mean ± SEM; n=4.

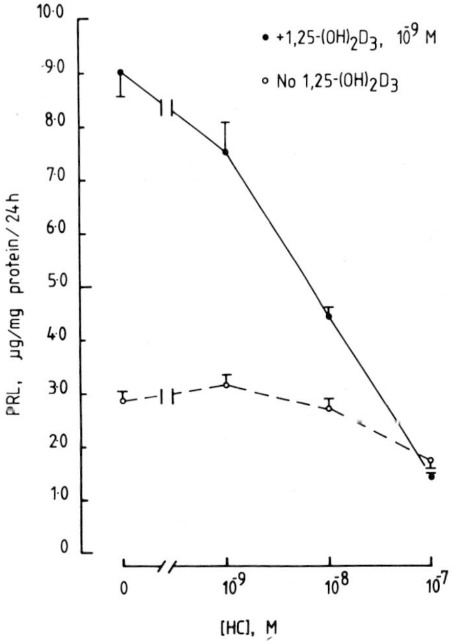

Fig. 2: Treated with 1,25-$(OH)_2D_3$ or vehicle, + HC for 96h, then PRL-P measured. Mean ± SEM; n=5,6.

Vitamin D. A Chemical, Biochemical and Clinical Update

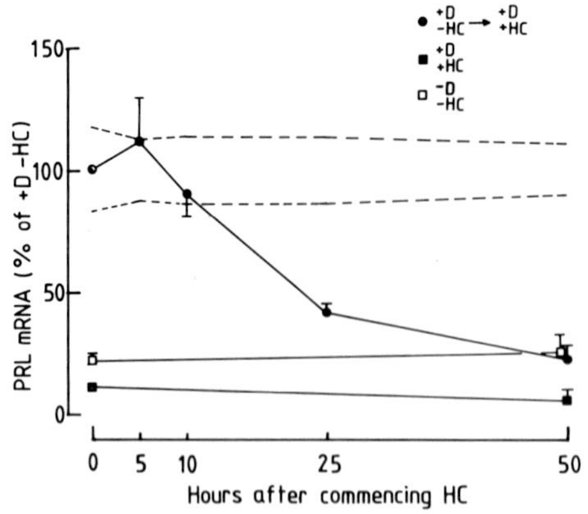

Fig. 3: Treatment for 72h prior to 0h was 10^{-9}M 1,25-$(OH)_2D_3$ (◐,●), 1,25-$(OH)_2D_3$ + 10^{-7}M HC (■), or vehicles (□). At 0h, 10^{-7} M HC added to some 1,25-$(OH)_2D_3$ treated cultures (●).
Mean ± SEM; n=4.

Removal of 1,25-$(OH)_2D_3$ did not diminish its effect on PRL-P whether it was present for 4h, 24h or 96h (fig. 1). Since < 3% of added 1,25-$(OH)_2D_3$ was recoverable after 48h (not shown), the continued presence of 1,25-$(OH)_2D_3$ was not required to maintain its biological effect. HC prevented the stimulation of PRL-P by 1,25-$(OH)_2D_3$ (ID_{50} ~5 x 10^{-9}M; fig. 2). Inhibition of basal PRL-P was modest, and did not occur at < 10^{-7}M HC. Inhibition of 1,25-$(OH)_2D_3$-induced PRL-P reflected a similar decrease in PRL-mRNA (fig. 3). HC prevented the induction of PRL mRNA; after 1,25-$(OH)_2D_3$-induction, HC decreased PRL mRNA by 59% at 25h, and to control level at 50h. In the absence of HC, PRL mRNA was maintained 50h after 1,25-$(OH)_2D_3$ withdrawal (not shown), confirming the long life of the effect of 1,25-$(OH)_2D_3$. These data support the hypothesis that 1,25-$(OH)_2D_3$ modulates PRL gene expression indirectly. HC may act directly by antagonizing a stable mediator of 1,25-$(OH)_2D_3$ action. In view of the important consequences of glucocorticoid antagonism of 1,25-$(OH)_2D_3$ action (e.g. in the intestine), it may prove valuable to study this hormonal interaction using GH cells. Endogenous glucocorticoids in serum may explain the failure of 1,25-$(OH)_2D_3$-induction of PRL gene expression in GH cells incubated in serum-supplemented medium (2-3).

This work was ably assisted by Mr. V. Gurtler and supported by the NH & MRC (Aust.). GH_4C_1 cells (Dr. A.H. Tashjian, Jr.), 1,25-$(OH)_2D_3$ (Dr. M. Uskokovic), rPRL kits (NIADDK) and plasmid pPRL-1 (Dr. D. Biswas) were generous gifts.

1. Haussler, M.R., Pike, J.W., Chandler, J.S., Manolagas, S.C. and Deftos, L.J. (1981) Ann. N.Y. Acad. Sci. 372, 502-516.
2. Murdoch, G.H. and Rosenfeld, M.G. (1981) J. Biol. Chem. 256, 4050-4055.
3. Haug, E., Pedersen, J.I. and Gautvik, K.M. (1982) Mol. Cell Endocrinol. 28, 65-79.
4. Wark, J.D. and Tashjian, A.H. Jr. (1982) Endocrinology 111, 1755-1757.
5. Wark, J.D. and Tashjian, A.H. Jr. (1983) J. Biol. Chem. 258, 12118-12121.

1-25 HYDROXYCHOLECALCIFEROL (1-25 HCC) IN THE TREATMENT OF MYELOFIBROSIS AND MYELODYSPLASIA.

Ph. Arlet, D. Adoue, E. Arlet-Suau, Y. Le Tallec.
Department of Internal Medecine, C.H.U. Rangueil, 31054 Toulouse, France

In some cases of bone diseases, especially in hyperparathyroidism and ricket, hematological abnormalities may be senn, including anemia and myelofibrosis, This is the basis of a clinical trial concerning the active metabolite of vitamin D (1-25 HCC) in the treatment of some hematological diseases particularly in myeloproliferative diseases.

PATIENTS AND METHODS

1) patients : we have studied 13 patients including : acute myelofibrosis : 2 cases, chronic myelofibrosis : 3 cases, chronic thrombocytemia : 2 cases, myelodysplasia and sideroblastic anemia, 6 cases. In all the cases, the diagnosis was well documented, particularly with bone biopsy and bone marrow aspiration.

2) therapeutic study : each patient received orally 0,25 or 0,50 µg/d of 1-25 HCC (ROCALTROL*) during 3 Months to 3 years, associated with PREDNISONE 30 mg/d, in two cases. The treatment was stopped after 3 months when it was judjed non effective. The patient's evaluation included a pre-treatment period of assessment with a survey of hematological and phosphocalcic parameters. During the 1-25 HCC treatment we performed every month a clinical and biological evaluation including C. terminal parathyroid hormone (PTH) and 25 hydroxycholecalciferol assays. We perfomed a bone biopsy six months after the beginning of this therapy.

RESULTS

. phosphocalcic abnormalities before treatment were observed in the majority of the cases : 1 case of typical hypoparathyroidism ; in other cases mild hypocalcemia or hyperphosphatemia with paradoxal low PTH plasma levels.
. a spectacular improvement of refractory anemia requiring multiple blood transfusion was observed in two cases of acute myelofibrosis (respectively 8 and 13 Months).
. in two cases of chronic myelofibrosis, dinimution of the thrombocytosis was observed with clinical amelioration. In two cases of chronic thrombocytemia, no significant result was observed.
. histolofical improvement of reticulin myelofibrosis was observed in two cases. In 6 cases of refractory anemia without myelofibrosis (myelodysplasia) no significant improvement of anemia was observed, but the clinical course of the diseases seems to be ameliorated.
The abnormalities of calcium and phosphorus plasma levels were improved in all the cases with 1-25 HCC treatment. No side effects, severe hypercalcemia, or calcinosis were observed.

COMMENTS

Clinical hematological and histological features of typical myelofibrosis were described in some cases of rickets (1) and the vitamin D supplementation cured all these features. These observations allow us to think that vitamind D is implicated in the bone marrow fonction. Recently 1-25 HCC receptors have been showed to exist on the human monocyte (2). In cultured cells (3) and in animal experimentation (4), 1-25 HCC seems to have an action on the differenciation of myeloid leukemia cell lines. MAC CARTHY (5)

Vitamin D. A Chemical, Biochemical and Clinical Update

have showed a possible inhibitory effect of 1-25 HCC on megacaryocyte capacity colony forming cells. Also 1-25 HCC seems to have an action on the differenciation of the monocyte. In our study, some hematological and histological observations seems to show that 1-25 HCC have a favorable action on the myelofibrosis with an amelioration ot the erythropoiesis in diseases were the prognosis is very bad when refractory anemia or severe thrombopenia are present (6). In these diseases, no effective treatment actually exist and an extension of the trials with 1-25 HCC may allow to prove this interesling indication of 1-25 HCC treatment. In haematological diseases, myelofibrosis, but also other myeloproliferative diseases, especially myeloid leukemia in the remission phase is probably a good indication for the future trials. Pathophysiology of these facts is not actually clear. Experimental studies allow to think that 1-25 HCC may improve myelofibrosis because 1-25 HCC enhance the macrophage formation, and the capacity colony forming cell of megacaryocyte, these two phenomenons are implicated in the degradation and the production of myelofibrosis. Thus a defect of PTH - 1-25 HCC production or an excess of consommation must be envisaged. According to this hypothesis, we find in this study a gicat number of biological abnormalities, specially phosphocalcic, and a case of typical hypoparathyroidism associated with myelofibrosis. Other investigations, with exploration of PTH-1-25 HCC axis in hematological diseases is needed to conclude.

(1) Yetgin S., Ozsoylu S., (1973) N. Engl. J. Med., 1335

(2) Bar-Shavit Z., NoffD., Edelstein S., Meyer M., Shibolet S., Goldman R. (1981) Calcif. Tissue Int., 33, 673-676

(3)Abe E., Miyaura C., Sakagami H., Takeda M., Konno K., Yamazaki T., Yosiiiki S., Suda T., (1981), Proc. Natl. Acad. Sci. USA, 79, 4990-4994

(4) Honma Y., Hozumi M., Abe E., Konno K., Fukushima M., Hata S., Nishij.Y. Deluca H.F., Suda T. (1983) Proc. Natl. Acad. Sci. Usa, 80, 201-203

(5) Mc Carthy D.M., Hibbin J.A., Goldman J.M., (1984) The Lancet, 1, 78-80

(6) Varki A., Lottenberg R., Griffith R., Reinhard E., (1983) Medicine 62, 353-371.

Renal Osteodystrophy

MORPHOLOGY OF RENAL OSTEODYSTROPHY: FACTS AND CONTROVERSIES

E. Bonucci

'La Sapienza' University, Department of Human Biopathology, Section of Pathological Anatomy, Policlinico Umberto I°, Viale Regina Elena 324, 00161 Rome, Italy

Morphological studies have yielded many definitive findings on the development and evolution of the skeletal changes which are present in patients with chronic renal failure (CRI) and are complessively indicated as Renal Osteodystrophy (RO; see 2,5,45 for review). However, several problems are still unsolved.

RO is due to development of two main pathological changes: defective calcification of bone matrix, with resultant osteomalacia (Os), and increased osteoclastic bone resorption, with consequent development of lesions, including marrow fibrosis, which are typical of hyperparathyroidism (HPT). Os and HPT are often present to a comparable degree; however, one of them can be prevalent, so that three main types of RO can result (15): RO type I, the less frequent, which is characterized by changes due to HPT with almost no Os; RO type II, which chiefly shows Os; OR type III, the most frequent, which is characterized by a variable combination of Os and HPT.

The frequence and severity of these types are rather variable and chiefly depend on duration of renal failure and dialysis, type of diet and therapy, and many other factors. Single or double iliac crest biopsies pertaining to 693 dialyzed patients, taken in 14 different nephrologic centers of north, center and south of Italy, were sent to the Section of Pathological Anatomy of the Department of Human Biopathology of Rome from 1980 to 1984. Semiquantitative evaluation of these biopsies showed that 25 (3.6%) of them had no pathological skeletal changes and 39 (5.6%) were at the upper limit of normality; RO was found in 629 patients. Of these, 24 (3.8%) had pure HPT, 49 (7.8%) HPT and initial Os, 518 (82.1%) HPT and Os of comparable degree, 29 (4.6%) Os and mild HPT, and 9 (1.4%) had pure Os. Histomorphometric evaluation carried out on bone biopsies of 94 dialyzed, unselected patients has given results (Table I) consistent with those of semiquantitative evaluation.

In the same period of time (1980-84), single or double iliac crest biopsies of 141 patients with CRI on maintenance therapy were sent to our Department. Of these biopsies, 25 (11.7%) had normal bone structure and 18 (12.8%) were at the upper normal limit. The remaining 98 patients (69.5%) had RO; 7 of them (7.1%)

Vitamin D. A Chemical, Biochemical and Clinical Update

(7.1%) had pure HPT, 6 (6.1%) HPT and initial Os, 71 (72.4%) HPT and Os of comparable degree, 12 (12.2%) Os and mild HPT, and 2 (2.0%) pure Os. Also in this case, the semiquantitative results are consistent with those obtained by histomorphometry (Table I).

Comparable bone changes develop in bone of patients with nephrotic syndrome, with or without renal failure. However, the data available on this subject are rather controversial, the reported frequency of bone changes ranging from zero (31) to 100% (34) of nephrotic patients. In a recent study (48), normal bone histology was found in 76%, Os in 17%, and Os plus HPT in 7% of 29 patients with nephrotic syndrome and normal GFR; the same parameters were respectively 35, 25 and 40% in 20 nephrotic patients with CRI (creatinine clearance 21-56 ml/min/1.73 m^2), and 53,34 and 13% in 55 patients with mild renal failure (creatinine clear. 15-58 ml/min/1.73m^2) and minimal or no proteinuria.

Table I - Histomorphometric evaluation of iliac crest biopsies of 94 dialyzed and 50 non dialyzed patients with CRI

Parameter	Normal value	Dialyzed	Non-dialyzed
OV	1.58 ± I.62	12.46 ± 8.27	5.76 ± 5.68
OS	10.27 ± 8.68	50.82 ± 26.61	30.65 ± 20.73
AOS	0.24 ± 0.61	3.85 ± 4.89	2.20 ± 2.85
TIO	13.65 ± 4.68	21.88 ± 8.18	16.16 ± 7.42
RS	1.80 ± 1.50	8.03 ± 6.82	4.01 ± 4.02
ARS	0.20 ± 0.31	2.01 ± 2.27	1.04 ± 2.47

OV: osteoid volume; OS: osteoid surface; AOS: active osteoid surface; TIO: thickness index of osteoid; RS: resorption surface; ARS: active resorption surface.

RO type I was complessively found in 31 patients (4.0%) of our two series. It showed different degrees of severity. The mildest forms were present in patients with CRI of short duration and consisted of small erosions along the trabecular borders, with occasional presence of active osteoclasts (Fig. 1a). The most severe cases showed a lot of Howship's lacunae and many osteoclasts, whose resorbing activity often produced trabecular dissection (Fig. 1b). In many of these cases intense and diffuse marrow fibrosis was present, sometimes associated with severe osteoporosis, the bone tissue consisting of few and small trabeculae of woven bone without osteoblasts (Fig. 2a).

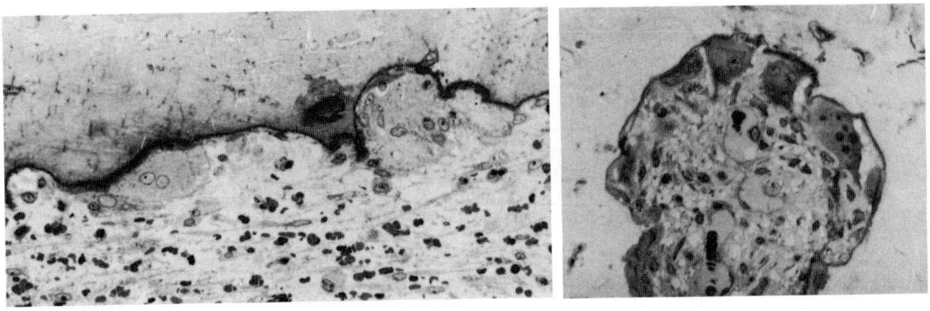

Fig. 1 - a)RO type I, early stage: active osteoclasts and Howship's lacunae along a trabecular border. b) RO type I with initial Os: group of osteoclasts in a dissecting lacuna. Undecalcified semithin sections, Azure II - Methylene blue, x 240.

RO type II seems to be the less predictable change of renal failure.In fact, it is reported to be rare and mild in some dialytic centers, very frequent and severe in others. In our series of patients, the degree and frequency of pure Os were low, with no sensible differences in different centers. Pure Os was found in 11 patients (1.51%) and Os with early HPT in 41 (5.62%).

RO type II seems to be much more frequent in other countries than in Italy. When present, it can be associated with miopathy and encephalopathy (43), a syndrome which has been related to the high aluminum levels present in dialysate water (22,43,51) and consequent Al intoxication and Al accumulation in muscle, brain and bone (1). Al presence in bone has been documented by physical (13,20,42,44) and histochemical (3,9,36) methods: they show that in RO type II Al can be localized at the boundary between the mineralized and non-mineralized matrix and along the cementing lines (Fig. 2b).

On the basis of these results, not frequently found in our cases, it has been suggested that Al presence in bone inhibits calcification and causes severe Os (8,26,42,44) either by interference with calcium phosphate formation and precipitation (45), by formation of abnormal inorganic complexes (44), or by reduction of osteoblast and osteoclast activity (10,33).

The biopsies sent to our Department were of both dialyzed and undialyzed patients: the former were dialyzed using deionized water, both were treated with aluminum hidroxide as phosphate binder. Most of these patients had high Al levels in serum and bone, confirming that aluminum hidroxide consumption alone is sufficient to induce Al intoxication (23,26). All the same, the percentage of pure Os was very low, being found in 1.4% of dia-

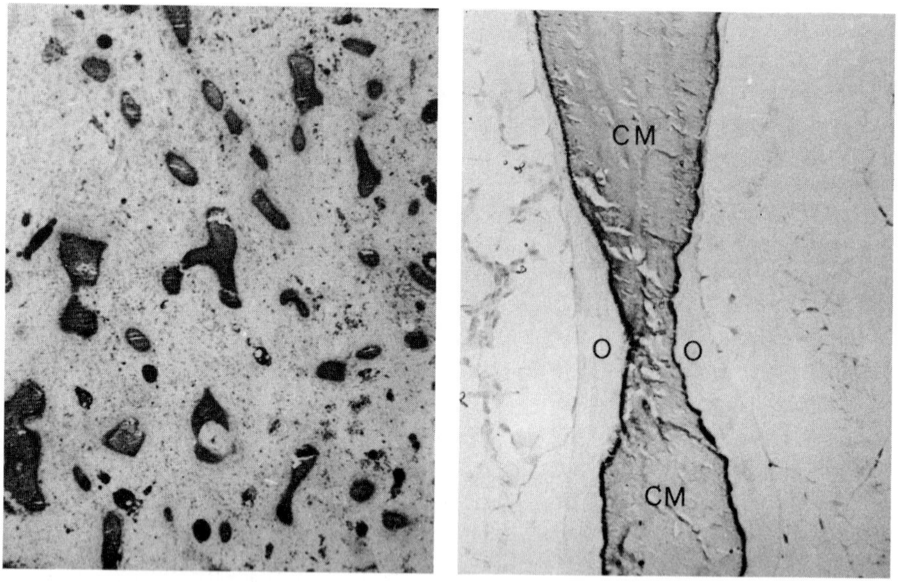

Fig. 2 - a) RO type I, advanced stage: diffuse marrow fibrosis with osteoporosis; undecalcified semithin section, Azure II - Methylene blue, x 40. b) Presence of Al between osteoid (O) and calcified matrix (CM); undecalcified semithin section, Aluminon x 300.

lyzed and 2.0% of non-dialyzed patients. In these Os cases, Al was often but not always (42% of cases) found between osteoid and calcified matrix (Fig. 2b). Moreover, Al was also present along inactive, normally calcified borders, cementing lines, and sometimes along active and inactive resorption surfaces. Al was also found in bone marrow mast cells. There was no direct relationship between Al content in bone and histomorphometric parameters, whereas there was an inverse correlation between Al and Ca concentration.

Several experimental studies have been carried out on the possible mechanism(s) of Al inhibition of the calcification process. They have given rather contradictory results. Intraperitoneal and intravenous injection of $AlCl_3$ to rats and dogs is followed by Al accumulation in bone comparable to that of dialyzed patients (3,11,20,24,25,46,50). However, defective calcification is reported only in a part of these experiments (20,25,46), the others showing persistence of normal calcification (3,11,24,50). This discrepancy might be due to different types of treatment, duration of Al injection, and other experimental conditions. Because $AlCl_3$ can induce peritonitis, we have injected aluminum lactate to normal rats and to rats treated with PTH (Ballanti et al., this volume). After 11 weeks, high Al levels were detected in bone, but Os was not present in normal rats.

These experiments seem to show that Al intoxication has no direct effects on bone calcification, and that it can induce Os when other factors, one of which could be the renal failure itself, are active. In this connection, Al administration to partially nephrectomized rats has produced Os in one experiment (46), no calcification defects in another (24); in a third experiment, Os was found in uremic animals, independently of Al treatment, but was more severe in Al treated than in untreated ones (11).

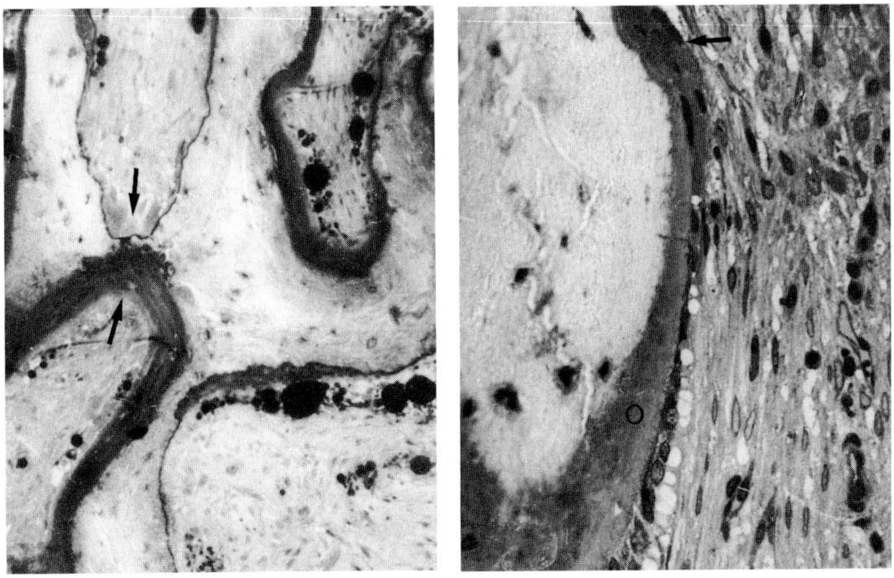

Fig. 3 - a) RO type III, advanced stage: an uncalcified osteoid border is almost in contact with a resorption area (arrows). b) RO type III, advanced stage: an osteoclast (arrow) and many vacuolized osteoblasts are in contact with an osteoid border (O); note marrow fibrosis. Undecalcified semithin sections, Azure II Methylene blue, x 100 and x 360.

It is possible that Al intoxication depresses osteoblastic activity (3,17,24,44), either by Al accumulation in mitochondria (44) or by impairment of PTH metabolism (46). PTH administration significantly enhances bone Al concentration in Al intoxicated normal rats (39, Ballanti et al., this volume) and can induce moderate increase of osteoid tissue. On the other hand, patients with RO type I or III, i.e., with HPT, have low levels of histochemically demonstrable Al, whereas those with Os and high Al concentration in bone have low PTH levels (27,41). Moreover, Al might be toxic to the parathyroid glands.

The available data are consistent with, but do not prove the hypothesis that Al intoxication plays a role in Os induction. An indirect role seems possible, cofactor(s) being probably necessary for Os development. The true mechanism of Al accumulation in bone and of inhibition of calcification remains unknown.

RO type III represents the most frequent form of bone disease induced by CRI. It consists of a combination of Os and HPT, usually of comparable degree (Fig. 3a). For this reason, the bone volume remains unchanged during the progress of the disease, although the radiological bone density decreases because of the reduced mineral content. However, uncoupling between bone resorption and formation can occur, with development of osteoporosis or, less frequently, osteosclerosis according to whether bone resorption exceedes, or is exceeded by, bone formation. Usually, OV,OS,AOS,TIO,RS and ARS are all increased in RO type III (Table I), although the available data differ to a certain extent and are sometimes contradictory (4,16,18,19,21,28,32). The variability chiefly concerns the degree of marrow fibrosis, sometimes considered a constant feature of RO type III (from which the incorrect denomination 'osteitis fibrosa'), other times infrequent or inapparent. In our 1980-84 series of 693 dialyzed patients, evidence of marrow fibrosis was found in 159 cases (22.9%). Patients with CRI have similar histomorphometric parameters (30, 32,35,40 and Table I); marrow fibrosis was present in 14 (14.3%) of our cases.

Active osteoblasts are often present in RO type III. They are roundish, basophilic cells usually forming a single row along the trabecular borders and having the ultrastructural characteristics of active synthesizing elements (6,37). They are usually similar to the osteoblasts of controls. However, in cases of severe marrow fibrosis they can have cytoplasmic vacuolization (Fig. 3b). These vacuoles probably contain lipids because are osmiophilic. Whether they are due to metabolic abnormalities induced by excessive PTH stimulation, or to the obstacle to cellular exchange due to marrow fibrosis, remains to be established. They might explain the disappearance of osteoblasts and the development of osteoporosis in cases with severe HPT.

Independently of its type, the morphology of RO depends to a large extent on several factors, chiefly duration of CRI and dialysis, associated therapies, diet, age, etc. The severity of RO increases proportionally to the duration of CRI and dialysis, although many patients with CRI are admitted to hospital with already severe skeletal changes. Both semiquantitative and quantitative data show that there is a direct correlation between Os and HPT on one side, age of renal insufficiency on the other. The degree of HPT, however, often increases to a greater extent than that of Os.

HPT development is greatly influenced by the diet, phosphate restriction preventing secondary HPT in patients with CRI, or reducing the severity of bone changes (38,47). This has been confirmed in partially nephrectomized rats: when on low phosphate intake, 80% of these animals had normal bone histology, 14% had Os and 6% Os plus HPT; when on high phosphate intake, 30% of them had normal bone, 40% Os, and 30% Os plus HPT (14).

Continuous ambulatory peritoneal dialysis (CAPD) can also improve the skeletal changes of RO. In 17 patients with end-stage renal failure treated by CAPD, the radiological and histological changes due to secondary HPT were less severe than those of hemodialyzed patients (52). These results are in agreement with those found in our Department in 35 patients treated with CAPD for 3-36 months; however, CAPD of long duration is accompanied by the development of mild RO changes.

Parathyroidectomy can greatly reduce bone resorption and is advisable, although with the utmost caution, in cases of severe HPT and when conservative therapy is ineffective. In this connection, it must be underlined that cases of Os and Al intoxication can be complicated by hypercalcemia which can be treated by reduction of Al intake and does not need parathyroidectomy, which can make worse the degree of Os (41).

Renal transplantation can greatly reduce RO skeletal changes or even completely normalize bone histology (7,19), although osteoporosis and bone necrosis can develop because of immunosuppressive therapy. In a series of 30 transplanted patients, whose bone biopsies had been sent to our Department, RO improved rapidly and bone histology remained within normal limits for about two years after transplantation, when osteoporosis was evident in almost all cases. In a few of them, who had been transplanted 8-10 years before biopsy, early RO changes were present, probably because of newly intervened renal damage.

The morphological appearance of RO can be greatly modified by therapy with vitamin D metabolites and synthetic analogues. Many papers have been recently published on the use of 25-OHD$_3$,

$1,25(OH)_2D_3$, 1α-OHD_3 and analogues, alone or in combination (see 2,5 for review). These therapies usually have beneficial effects, although the results are not satisfactory in all cases and hypercalcemia can occur. In the attempt of improving these results, and on the basis of the observation that vitamin D metabolites have different biological effects, combined therapies have been proposed. In two groups of dialyzed patients with RO, $1,25(OH)_2D_3$ and 25-OHD_3 caused marked reduction of OV,OS,AOS, TIO and ARS, whereas 25-OHD_3 alone produced significative falls only of OV, OS and TIO (12).

This concise review of the present knowledge on RO is mainly based on personal experience, chiefly concerns bone morphology, and does not claim of being complete and exhaustive. However, it points out that, despite our ever increasing knowledge of RO and its histological, histochemical and ultrastructural characteristics, several problems remain unsolved. A better knowledge of vitamin D metabolism, activity of its derivatives, and interactions with PTH is needed to reduce the residual controversial points.

References

1. Alfrey, A.C., LeGendre,G.R.,Kaehny,W.D.(1976) New Engl.J. Med.,294:184-188.
2. Avioli,L.V.(1978) in Metabolic bone disease, V.2,ed.Avioli, L.V.,Krane,S.M.,Academic Press,New York, p149-215.
3. Ballanti,P.,Mocetti,P.,DellaRocca,C.,Costantini,S.,Giordano, R.,Ioppolo,A.,Mantovani,A.,Stasolla,D.,Bonucci,E.(1983) Min. Metab.Res.Italy, 4:139-142.
4. Binswanger,U.,Sherrard,D.,Rich,C.,Curtis,F.K.(1973) Nephron, 12:1-9.
5. Bonucci,E.(1980) in Il metabolismo elettrolitico e minerale nelle malattie del rene, ed. Maschio,G.,Piccin,Padova,p162-232.
6. Bonucci,E.,Gherardi,G.,Faraggiana,T.,Mioni,G.,Cannella,G., Castellani,A.,Maiorca,R.(1976)Virchows Arch.A,371:183-198.
7. Bortolotti,G.C.,Feletti,C.,Scolari,M.P.,Bonomini,V.(1977) Calcif. Tiss. Res.,22(suppl.):486-489.
8. Boyce,B.F.,Elder,H.Y.,Elliot,H.L.,Fogelman,I.,Fell,G.S., Junor,B.J.,Nenstall,G.,Boyle,I.T.(1982)Lancet, 1009-1012.
9. Buchanan,M.R.C.,Ihle,B.U.,Dunn,C.M.(1981)J.Clin.Path., 74: 1352-1354.
10. Cann,C.E.,Prussin,S.G.,Gordan,G.S.(1979)J.Clin.Endocrinol. Metab.,49:543-545.
11. Chan,Y.L.,Alfrey,A.C.,Posen,S.,Lissner,D.,Hills,E.,Dunstan, C.R.,Evans,R.A.(1983)Calcif.Tiss.Int.,35:344-351.
12. Coen,G.,TacconeGallucci,M.,Bonucci,E.,Ballanti,P.,Bianchi,

A.R.,Bianchini,G.,Matteucci,M.C.,Mazzaferro,S.,Picca,S.,Taggi, F.,Cinotti,G.A.,Casciani,C.U.(1983)Min.Electr.Met.,9:19-27.

13.Cournot-Witmer,G.,Zingraff,J.,Plachot,J.J.,Escaig,F.,Lefèvre,R.,Boumati,P.,Bourdeau,A.,Garabédian,M.,Galle,P.,Bourdon, R.,Drüeke,T.,Balsan,S.(1981)Kidney Int.,20:375-385.

14.D'Angelo,A.,Bonucci,E.,Fabris,A.,Messa,M.,Giannini,S.,Malvasi,L.,Ferrarese,P.,Morbiato,F.,Vassanelli,P.,Maschio,G.(1982) Min.Metab.Res.Italy,3:131-134.

15.Delling,G.(1975) in Veröffentlichungen aus der Pathologie, v.98,Fischer Verlag, Stuttgart.

16.DeVernejoul,M.C., Kuntz,D.,Miravet,L.,Gueris,J.,Bielakoff, J.,Ryckewaert,A.(1981)Metab.Bone Res.Rel.Res.,3:175-179.

17.Dunstan,C.R.,Evans,R.A.,Hills,E.,Wong,S.Y.P.,Alfrey,A.C. (1984)Calcif.Tiss.Int.,36:133-138.

18.Duursma,S.A.,Visser,W.J.,Njio,L.(1972)Calcif.Tiss.Res.,9: 216-225.

19.Eastwood,J.B.(1982)J.Clin.Path.,35:125-134.

20.Ellis,H.A.,McCarthy,J.H.,Herrington,J.(1979)J.Clin.Path., 32:832-844.

21.Ellis,H.A.,Pearth,K.M.(1973)J.Clin.Path.,26:83-101.

22.Elliott,H.L.,Dryburgh,F.,Fell,G.S.,Sabet,S.,MacDougall,A.I. (1978)Brit.Med.J.,1:1101-1103.

23.Fleming,L.W.,Stewart,W.K.,Fell,G.S.,Halls,D.J.(1982)Clin. Nephrol.,17:222-227.

24.Goodman,W.G.,Gilligan,J.,Horst,R.(1984)J.Clin.Invest.,73: 171-181.

25.Goodman,W.G.,Henry,D.A.,Horst,R.,Nudelman,R.K.,Alfrey,A.C., Coburn,J.W.(1984)Kidney Int.,25:370-375.

26.Heaf,J.G.,Nielsen,L.P.(1984)Min.Electr.Met.,10:345-350.

27.Hodsman,A.B.,Sherrard,D.J.,Alfrey,A.C.,Ott,S.,Brickman,A.S., Miller,N.L.,Maloney,N.A.,Coburn,J.W.(1982)J.Clin.Endocrinol. Met.,54:539-545.

28.Huffer,W.E.,Kuzela,D.,Popovtzer,M.M.(1975)Am.J.Path.,78: 365 384.

29.Huffer,W.E.,Kuzela,D.,Popovtzer,M.M.,Starzl,T.E.(1975)Am.J. Path.,78:385-400.

30.Ingham,J.P.,Stewart,J.H.,Posen,S.(1973)Brit.Med.J.,2:745-748.

31.Korkor,J.P.,Schwartz,J.,Bergfeld,M.,Teitelbaum,S.,Avioli,L., Klahr,S.,Slatopolsky,E.(1983)J.Clin.Endocrinol.Met.,56:496-500.

32.Krempien,B.,Ritz,E.,Beck,U.,Keilbach,H.(1972)Virchows Arch. A,357:257-274.

33.Lieberherr,M.,Grosse,B.,Cournot-Witmer,G.,Thil,C.L.,Balsan, S.(1982)Calcif.Tiss.Int.,34:280-284.

34.Malluche,H.H.,Goldstein,D.A.,Massry,S.G.(1979)J.Clin.Invest. 63:494-500.

35.Malluche,H.H.,Ritz,E.,Lange,H.P.,Kutschera,J.,Hodgson,M., Seiffert,U.,Schoeppe,W.(1976)Kidney Int.,9:355-362.
36.Maloney,N.A.,Ott,S.M.,Alfrey,A.C.,Miller,N.L.,Coburn,J.W., Sherrard,D.J.(1982)J.Lab.Clin.Med.,99:206-216.
37.Maschio,G.,Bonucci,E.,Mioni,G.,D'Angelo,A.,Ossi,E.,Valvo,E., Lupo,A.(1974)Nephron,12:437-448.
38.Maschio,G.,Tessitore,N.,D'Angelo,A.,Bonucci,E.,Lupo,A.,Valvo,E.,Loschiavo,C.,Fabris,A.,Morachiello,P.,Previato,G.,Fiaschi, E.(1980)Am.J.Clin.Nutrit.,33:1546-1554.
39.Mayor,G.H.,Sprague,S.M.,Hourani,M.R.,Sanchez,T.V.(1980) Kidney Int.,17:40-44.
40.Nielsen,H.E.,Melsen,F.,Christensen,M.S.(1980)Min.Electr.Met. 4:113-122.
41.Ott,S.M.(1983)J.Artif.Organs,6:173-175.
42.Ott,S.M.,Maloney,N.A.,Coburn,J.W.,Alfrey,A.C.,Sherrard,D.J. (1982)New Engl.J.Med.,307:709-713.
43.Parkinson,I.S.,Ward,M.K.,Kerr,D.N.S.(1981)J.Clin.Path.,34: 1285-1294.
44.Plachot,J.J.,Cournot-Witmer,G.,Halpern,S.,Mendes,V.,Bourdeau A.,Fritsch,J.,Bourdon,R.,Drüeke,T.,Galle,P.,Balsan,S.(1984) Kidney Int.,25:796-803.
45.Ritz,E.,Malluche,H.H.,Krempien,B.,Mehls,O.(1977) in Calcium metabolism in renal failure and nephrolithiasis,ed.David,D.S., J.Wiley & Sons, New York, p197-233.
46.Robertson,J.A.,Felsenfeld,A.J.,Haygood,C.C.,Wilson,P.,Clarke C.,Llack,F.(1983)Kidney Int.,23:327-335.
47.Slatopolsky,E.,Caglar,S.,Gradowska,L.,Canterbury,J.,Reiss, J.,Bricker,N.S.(1972)Kidney Int.,2:147-151.
48.Tessitore,N.,Bonucci,E.,D'Angelo,A.,Lund,B.,Corgnati,A.,Lund B.,Valvo,E.,Lupo,A.,Loschiavo,C.,Fabris,A.,Maschio,G.(1984) Nephron,37:153-159.
49.Thomas,W.C.,Meyer,J.L.(1984)Am.J.Nephrol.,4:201-203.
50.Thurston,H.,Gilmore,G.R.,Swales,J.D.(1972)Lancet,881-883.
51.Ward,M.K.,Feest,T.G.,Ellis,H.A.,Parkinson,I.S.,Kerr,D.N.S., Herrington,J.,Goode,G.L.(1978)Lancet,841-845.
52.Zucchelli,P.,Catizone,L.,Casanova,S.,Fusaroli,M.,Fabbri,L., Ferrari,G.(1984)Min.Electr.Met.,10:326-332.

The personal investigations mentioned in this paper have been carried out with the financial support of CNR and MPI. The Renal Osteodystrophy Project is carried out in collaboration with:P.Ballanti,S.Berni,D.Brancaccio,G.Coen, S.Costantini,G.D'Amico,A.D'Angelo,A.DaPorto,P.Degetto,C.DellaRocca,A.Farinelli,A.Giangrande,G.Graziani,R.Maiorca,G.Maschio,G.Mioni,P.Mocetti,F.Pizzarelli,G.Schmid,G.Silvestrini,M.Surian,R.Terzigni.

THE ROLE OF $1,25(OH)_2D_3$ IN DIVALENT ION ABNORMALITIES IN EARLY RENAL FAILURE.

Francisco Llach, M.D.
Department of Medicine, Nephrology Section, University of Oklahoma Health Sciences Center and VA Medical Center, Oklahoma City, Oklahoma, U.S.A.

INTRODUCTION

A large amount of information has been accumulated in recent years which has greatly furthered our knowledge of the mechanisms that underlie the development of altered divalent ion metabolism in renal insufficiency. Nonetheless, there is uncertainty about the initial steps in the pathogenesis of either secondary hyperparathyroidism, increased bone resorption, or altered metabolism of vitamin D and the degree of interaction between various pathogenic factors. There is little doubt that parathyroid hyperplasia and high circulating levels of PTH (parathyroid hormone) are among the most consistent abnormalities of divalent ion metabolism present in patients with early renal failure.

The main factor which leads to PTH secretion and causes hyperplasia of the parathyroid glands in uremic patients is perfusion of the glands with blood containing reduced ionized calcium. However, it is likely that factors other than hypocalcemia may also be operative. This is suggested by the recent observation of Lopez et al who observed secondary hyperparathyroidism developing in dogs with 70% reduction of GFR and no apparent decrease in serum ionized calcium (1). Similar observations by Kaplan et al have demonstrated no differences in the serum calcium levels of normal dogs as compared with uremic dogs (2). Factors which may lead to hypocalcemia include: 1) phosphate retention with a rise in serum P_i and a reciprocal change in serum calcium, 2) altered vitamin D metabolism with intestinal malabsorption of calcium, 3) a decreased calcemic response to PTH, 4) an altered feedback relationship between serum calcium and secretion of PTH ("set-point" for calcium). These factors may be interrelated and it is likely that one factor may exert a more prominent role than the others at different stages of renal insufficiency.

PHOSPHATE RETENTION

The role of phosphate retention as a major factor in the pathogenesis of secondary hyperparathyroidism has been emphasized by Slatopolsky, Bricker, and their colleagues (3). As the phosphate retention theory developed, it was postulated that a transient and possibly undetectable increase in serum phosphorus occurs in early renal failure in association with a small decrement in renal function (4). The transient hyperphosphatemia was believed to temporarily decrease the blood ionized calcium which, in turn, stimulated PTH secretion. The higher levels of PTH would reduce tubular reabsorption of phosphorus, cause phosphaturia, and return both serum phosphorus and calcium toward normal but at the expense of a higher level of PTH. However, while there is considerable evidence supporting an important role of phosphate retention in producing secondary hyperparathyroidism, most of the available data refer to advanced chronic renal failure.

Vitamin D. A Chemical, Biochemical and Clinical Update

Recent data suggest that phosphate retention may not play a role in the early stages of renal insufficiency. In patients with early renal failure (ERF), low serum phosphorus levels have been reported (5-6); these observations indicate that a slight decrease in serum calcium which is sometimes noted as well in such patients (5) cannot arise as a direct consequence of hyperphosphatemia. To explain this hypophosphatemia observed by various investigators, Slatopolsky et al have suggested that post-prandial hyperphosphatemia occurs which then stimulates PTH secretion leading to low fasting serum phosphate levels (7). Thus, serum phosphorus levels could be higher in azotemic patients after a phosphate-containing meal than in normal subjects. Recent data do not support this hypothesis. Portale et al studied five children with ERF and after hourly measurements of serum phosphate and PTH, they were unable to detect any change in serum phosphate in the post-prandial period (8). Furthermore, recent studies in our laboratories in patients with ERF (GFR 40-80 ml/min) receiving an oral phosphate load have shown that rather than hyperphosphatemia and phosphate retention, these patients had an increased ability to excrete phosphate as compared with control subjects (Figure 1).

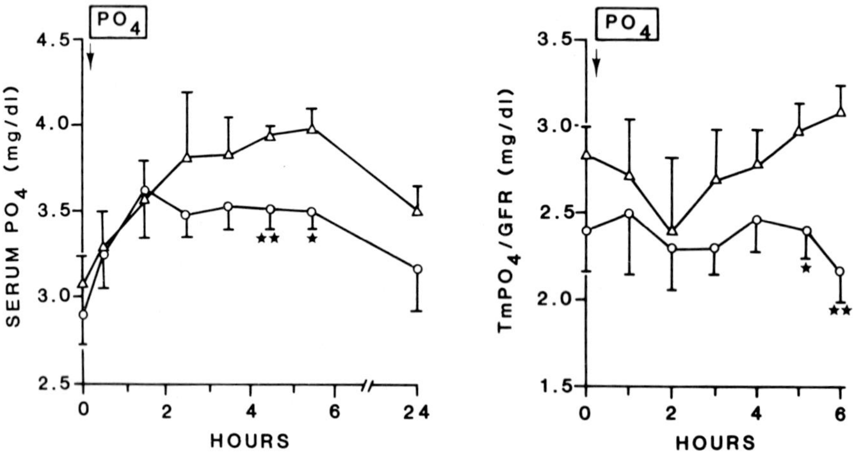

Figure 1. Mean values (±SE) of serum phosphate and $TmPO_4/GFR$ in patients with early renal failure (open circles) and normal subjects (open triangles) during the phosphate load test, prior to $1,25(OH)_2D$ therapy. *, $p < 0.05$; **, $p < 0.01$. (used with permission).

Of interest is that these patients given a phosphate load excrete phosphate in a manner similar to patients with primary hyperparathyroidism (10). With more advanced renal insufficiency, Maschio et al have demonstrated an impairment in phosphorus excretion after the same oral phosphate load and as renal disease advances and GFR falls below 25 ml/min, hyperphosphatemia usually develops (11); under such circumstances, hypocalcemia is more directly related to the level of serum phosphorus.

IMPAIRED CALCEMIC RESPONSE TO PTH

A decreased response to the calcemic action of PTH is another important cause of hypocalcemia in patients with renal insufficiency. Evanson (12) noted that the calcemic response to an infusion of parathyroid extract was significantly lower in hypocalcemic patients with renal failure than was observed in normal subjects of patients with hypoparathyroidism. Subsequently, Massry et al (14) found that the calcemic response to a standardized infusion of PTH (parathyroid extract) in patients with early renal failure (creatinine clearance of 27-87 ml/min) was significantly lower than in normals (13). This reduced calcemic response was unrelated to the initial levels of serum calcium, phosphorus, or PTH. In patients with early renal insufficiency and creatinine clearances of 34 to 93 ml/min, Llach et al (6) observed a delayed recovery from EDTA-induced hypocalcemia compared to normal subjects; this occurred despite a greater augmentation in serum iPTH levels in early renal failure patients. These observations indicate that the impaired calcemic response to PTH appears early in the course of renal insufficiency and a greater circulating PTH level may be required for the maintenance of a normal serum calcium level in patients with renal failure. Llach et al have recently observed that dietary phosphate restriction in patients with mild renal insufficiency improved the calcemic response to a standardized infusion of PTE (14).

The factors responsible for skeletal resistance to the calcemic action of PTH are, at present, uncertain. In rats with chronic renal failure (15), which have a blunted calcemic response to PTE, the administration of $1,25(OH)_2D$ resulted in a partial correction of the impaired calcemic response. Recent data in 12 patients with ERF have demonstrated a significant improvement in the impaired calcemic response to PTH after 6 weeks' administration of $1,25(OH)_2D$, 0.5 g per day (9). Such data support the possibility that altered vitamin D metabolism plays a role in the impaired calcemic response.

ALTERATIONS IN VITAMIN D METABOLISM

Abnormal conversion of vitamin D_3 to its active hormonal form probably plays a fundamental role in secondary hyperparathyroidism in early renal failure. The evidence that vitamin D metabolism is altered in renal failure is convincing. Intestinal absorption of calcium is diminished, and this defect is poorly responsive to vitamin D (16).

The consequences of reduced generation of $1,25(OH)_2D$ in ERF deserve consideration. The problems that may arise from a deficiency of this active form of vitamin D include decreased intestinal absorption of calcium and phosphorus, decreased calcemic action of PTH on the skeleton, and increased PTH secretion at any given level of serum calcium.

When in the course of progressive renal insufficiency does the abnormality of vitamin D metabolism occur? Preliminary observations reported by Slatopolsky et al in patients with serum creatinine from 1.5 to 3.5 g/dl described normal 1,25(OH)$_2$D levels (17). More recent and detailed observations by Portale et al in children with moderate renal insufficiency (creatinine clearance of 25 to 50 ml/min/1.73 m^2) have reported a 40% reduction in 1,25(OH)$_2$D levels (18). When analyzed over the range covering normal to severely impaired renal function, the PTH values in these children correlated inversely with their 1,25(OH)$_2$D levels. Chesney et al have also reported low levels of 1,25(OH)2D in ERF patients with clearances above 75-80 ml/min (19). In addition, there was a significant correlation between the creatinine clearances and the 1,25(OH)2D levels. Likewise, Juttman et al have observed subnormal levels of 1,25(OH)$_2$D in patients with creatinine clearances between 40-50 ml/min (20). Finally, Wilson et al, in our laboratory, have recently reported low levels of 1,25(OH)2D in ERF patients with GFR between 50-80 ml/min (9). Thus, the available data suggest that patients with ERF have low levels of 1,25(OH)$_2$D. Recently, we have evaluated the role of 1,25(OH)$_2$D in the pathogenesis of abnormal divalent ion metabolism in patients with ERF (9). This was accomplished by examining the calcemic response to PTH and the handling of an oral phosphate load both before and after 6 weeks of therapy with 1,25(OH)$_2$D. Twelve patients with ERF and six normal volunteers were studied. Patients with ERF as compared with normals have low serum phosphate, low urinary calcium, low serum 1,25(OH)$_2$D and high plasma PTH and urinary cyclic AMP. With EDTA infusion, an impaired calcemic response to PTH was observed in patients with ERF and not in normals. The phosphate load test showed that these patients had an increased ability to excrete phosphate. After 1,25(OH)$_2$D therapy, a significant increase in serum phosphate, urinary calcium, and a decrease in urinary cyclic AMP was observed only in ERF patients. Furthermore, the impaired calcemic response to PTH improved significantly (Figure 2), the renal handling of phosphate became normal (Figure 3), and the low baseline levels of 1,25(OH)$_2$D increased to normal after therapy with 1,25(OH)$_2$D. In addition, significant correlation between the levels of 1,25(OH)$_2$D and creatinine clearances were observed in both patients and normals. These data seem to suggest that the mild deficiency of 1,25(OH)$_2$D is present in ERF patients and that the administration of this sterol results in dramatic changes in several biochemical parameters.

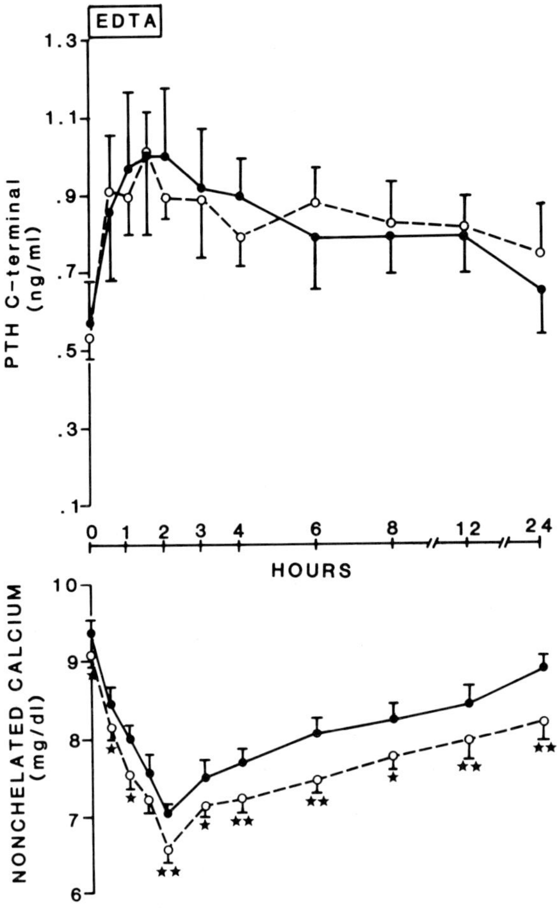

Figure 2. Mean values (±SE) of PTH and nonchelated calcium during the EDTA test in patients before (open circles) and after (closed circles) $1,25(OH)_2D_3$ therapy. Symbols are: $^*p < 0.05$; $^{**}p < 0.01$. (Used with permission).

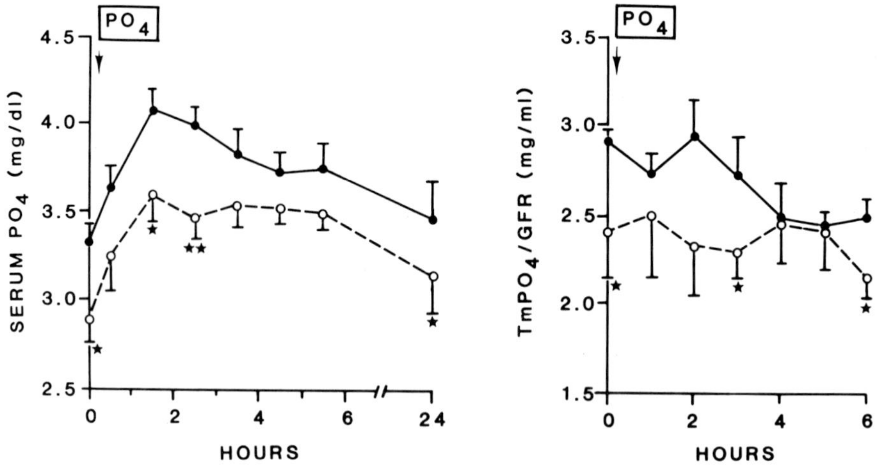

Figure 3. Mean values (±SE) of serum phosphate and $TmPO_4/GFR$ during the phosphate load test in patients with early renal failure before (open circles) and after (closed circles) $1,25(OH)_2D$ therapy. Symbols are: *, $p < 0.05$; **, $p < 0.01$. (Used with permission).

What produces a reduction in $1,25(OH)_2D_3$ synthesis is not yet defined. It is possible that $1,25(OH)_2D_3$ synthesis by the kidney is related to the functional state of the proximal renal tubules and since glomerular filtration rate reasonably reflects functional renal mass, a decrement in $1,25(OH)_2D_3$ may occur slowly and progressively as glomerular filtration declines in patients with chronic renal insufficiency. In support of such a contention are observations by Kawaguchi et al in the rat which shows progressive decrease in renal synthesis of this sterol following graded nephron mass reduction (21). Portale et al have postulated that in early renal insufficiency, an increase in the intracellular concentration of phosphorus may occur (8). This, in turn, will reduce the activity of 1, alpha hydroxylase and decrease synthesis of $1,25(OH)_2D_3$. Consistent with this hypothesis are our recent observations in four patients with ERF placed on phosphate restriction under metabolic conditions (14). A decrease in phosphate excretion, an increased intestinal absorption of phosphate as well as a decrease in PTH was observed. Most important, there was a significant increase in $1,25(OH)_2D$ following phosphate restriction. These occurred in the absence of significant changes in serum phosphorus of net external balance of phosphorus. Recent studies from Portale et al in children with ERF placed on a reduced phosphate diet have also shown an increased synthesis of 1,25(OH)$_2$D$_3$ despite a decrease in PTH (8). These findings were associated with a significant decrease in fractional excretion of phosphate. Thus, a disorder of phosphate metabolism within the renal tubular cells may lead to a decreased synthesis of 1,25(OH)$_2$D$_3$. Regardless of a cause for a decreased secretion of 1,25(OH)$_2$D$_3$, the pathophysiological consequences of such a deficiency may be important. Thus, the low levels of this sterol with ERF may impair intestinal absorption of calcium and decrease the calcemic response to PTH, leading to hypocalcemia.

A final pathophysiological consequence of a partial deficiency of 1,25(OH)2D$_3$ may be the absence of a modulating inhibitory action of this sterol on PTH secretion leading to secondary hyperparathyroidism. Recently, Booth et al have shown that under normal or near normal metabolic conditions, the prevailing circulating concentrations of 1,25(OH)$_2$D dampen an otherwise greater activity of 1, alpha hydroxylase (22). It is likely that the same may apply to PTH secretion. Silver et al have recently shown in bovine parathyroid cell cultures a significant suppression of cytoplasmic mRNA coding for pre-proparathyroid hormone by 1,25(OH)$_2$D (23). Recently, Slatopolsky et al have shown in hemodialysis patients a direct suppressive effect of intravenously administered 1,25(OH)$_2$D on PTH secretion (22). Thus, in view of these recent data, it is possible that a deficiency of 1,25(OH)$_2$D per se and not necessarily through a hypocalcemic stimulus may lead to secondary hyperparathyroidism.

ABNORMAL "SET POINT" FOR CALCIUM

The secretion of PTH appears to be regulated in a sigmoidal relationship over a narrow range of plasma calcium (25). Recently, it has been shown that isolated parathyroid cells from uremic patients requires higher extracellular calcium concentrations than normal cells in order to suppress their PTH secretion (26). Thus, the "set point" for calcium, that is the concentration of calcium required to produce a 50% decrease in PTH release, is shifted (26-27). This abnormality may be an important factor in the pathogenesis of secondary hyperparathyroidism.

An abnormal set point for calcium has been recently demonstrated by Voigts et al, in our laboratory, in patients with osteitis fibrosa (29). When dialyzed with a zero calcium bath these patients exhibited a marked increase in carboxy and amino terminal PTH even though the serum calcium was greater than 9 mg/dl. Thus, it is possible that in early renal failure, an altered "set point" for calcium may be present and this may be related to a partial deficiency of 1,25(OH)2D.

In summary, the relative roles of phosphate retention, altered vitamin D metabolism, impaired calcemic response to PTH, and altered degradation and metabolism of PTH in the pathogenesis of hypocalcemia and secondary hyperparathyroidism in renal failure are uncertain. In early renal failure, serum calcium levels and values for intestinal calcium absorption have benerally been normal, while serum phosphorus levels are either normal or low. Rather than phosphate retention, patients with early renal failure may have an increased ability to excrete phosphate not unlike patients with primary hyperparathyroidism. Observations that the restriction of dietary phosphate intake, carried out early in the course of renal failure, can greatly reduce the magnitude of secondary hyperparathyroidism and largely restore the calcemic response to PTH, indicate that phosphate per se, may be an important pathogenic factor. However, the finding of normal or low serum levels of phosphorus in early renal failure suggest that the hypocalcemia leading to secondary hyperparathyroidism may be mediated by mechanisms other than phosphate retention. It is possible that an increased intracellular concentration of phosphate in the proximal tubules may lead to a relative deficit of $1,25(OH)_2D$, which may lead to hypocalcemia; this deficit may also directly lead to increased PTH secretion by altering the "set point" for calcium.

REFERENCES

1. Lopez, S., Galceran, T., Chan, W., Rapp, N., Martin K., Slatopolsky, E. (1985) Kidney Int 27: 122.
2. Kaplan, M.A., Canterbury, J.M., Gavellas, G., Jaffee, D., Bourgoignie, J., Reiss, E., Bricker, N.S.(1978) Kidney Int 14: 207.
3. Slatopolsky, E., Caglar, S., Gradowska, L., Canterbury, J., Reiss, E., and Bricker, N.S. (1972) Kidney Int 2: 147.
4. Slatopolsky, E. and Bricker, N (1973). Kidney Int 4: 141.
5. Coburn, J.W., Koppel, M.H., Brickman, A.S., and Massry, S.G. (1973).
6. Llach, F., Massry, S.G., Singer, F.R., Kurokawa, K., Kaye, J.H., and Coburn, J.W. (1975) J. Clin. Endocrinol. Metab. 41: 338.
7. Slatopolsky, E., Rutherford, E.W., Hruska, K., Martin, K., Klahr, S. (1978) Arch. Intern. Med. 138: 848-852.
8. Portale, A.A., Booth, B.E., Halldran, B.P., Morris, R.C.(1984) J. Clin. Invest 73: 1580-1589.
9. Wilson, L., Felsenfeld, A., Drezner, M.K., and Llach, F. (In Press) Kidney Int.
10. Llach, F., Brickman, A.S., Ben-Issac, L., Coburn, J.W., Massry, S.G. (1975)Nouvelle Imprimeri Fournier, pp. 171-178.
11. Maschio, G., Tessitore, N., D'Angelo, A., Bonuci, E., Lupo, A., Valve Loschiavo, C., Fabris, A., Morachiello, P., Previato, G., and Fiashi, E. (1980) Am. J. Clin. Nutr. 33: 1546-1554.
12. Evanson, J.M. (1966). Clin. Sci. 31: 63.
13. Massry, S.G., Coburn, J.W., Lee, D.B.N., Jowsey, J., and Kleeman, C.R. (1973). Ann Intern. Med. 78: 357.
14. Llach, F., Massry, S.G. (In Press) Ann. Intern. Med.
15. Sommerville, P.J. and Kaye, M. (1978). Kidney Int. 14: 245.
16. Liu, S.H. and Chu, H.I (1943). Medicine (Baltimore) 22: 103.
17. Slatopolsky, E., Gray, R., Adams, N.D., Lewis, J., Hruska, K., Martin, K., Klahr, S., DeLuca, H., and Lemann, J. (1978). Kidney Int 14 (abstract).
18. Portale A.A., Booth, B.E., Taai, H.C., Morris, R.C., Jr. (1982). Kidney Int 21: 627-632.
19. Chesney, R.W., Hamstra, A.J., Mazess, R.B., Rose, P., DeLuca, H.F. (1982). Kidney Int 21: 65-59.
20. Juttmann, J.R., Buurman, J.C., Dekam, E., Visser, T.J., Birkenhager,

J.C. (1981). Clin. Endocrinol. 14: 225-236.
21. Kawaguchi, Y., Kimura, Y., Yakamota, M., Inamura, N., Tukwi, I., Horiwchi, N., Swada, T., Ogwra, Y., Oda, Y., Miyahara, T. (1983). Metab. Bone Dis. Rel. Res. 4: 333-336.
22. Booth, B.E., Tsai, H.C., Morris, R.C. (1985). J. Clin. Invest. 75: 155-161.
23. Silver, J., Russell, J., Lettier, I., Sherwood, L.M. (1984). Clin. Res. 32: 561A.
24. Slatopolsky E., Weerts, C., Thielan, J., Horst, R., Harter, H., Martin, K. (1984). J. Clin. Invest 74: 2136-2143.
25. Mayer, G.P. and Hurst, J.G. (1978). Endocrinology 102: 1036-1042.
26. Brown, E.M. (1983). J. Clin. Endocrinol. Metab. 56: 572.
27. Brown, E. (1981). Hormonal Control of Calcium Metabolism, (Excerpta Medica), p. 35.
28. Brown, E.M., Wilson, R.E., Eastman, R.C., Pallotta, J., Marynick, S.P. (1982). J. Clin. Endocrinol. Metab. 54: 172.
29. Voigts, A., Felsenfeld, A., Andress, D., and Llach, F. (1984). Kidney Int 25: 445-452.

RENAL OSTEOSYSTROPHY: VIEWS ON PATHOGENESIS AND MANAGEMENT - 1985.

J.W. Coburn, K.C. Norris, I.B. Salusky, D.L. Andress, P.W. Crooks, S.M. Ott, G. Hercz, H.G. Nebeker, D.A. Milliner, N.C. DiDominico, and D.J. Sherrard.

Medical & Research Services, Veterans Administration Wadsworth Medical Center and Depts of Medicine and Pediatrics, U.C.L.A. School of Medicine, Los Angeles, CA and Medical Service, Veterans Administration Medical Center and Department of Medicine, University of Washington School of Medicine, Seattle, WA, U.S.A.

In patients with end-stage renal disease, several pathogenic processes can cause alterations in calcium metabolism and bone disease. The present discussion will focus upon abnormalities encountered in patients with advanced renal failure or treated with regular dialysis. The therapeutic implications of these events will also be reviewed. Our observations have been derived from experience in the U.S., where patients undergo thrice weekly dialysis, receive diets with mild restriction of phosphate (i.e., 900-1000mg phosphorus/day), and ingest aluminum-containing phosphate binders; some but not all of the patients receive calcitriol or dihydrotachysterol.

Classification of Bone Disease: The bone diseases observed in patients with advanced renal failure comprise a spectrum of pathologic features, the classification of which has evolved with additional techniques for the evaluation of bone. Initially, features of osteitis fibrosa, osteomalacia, or a mixture of both were identified on morphologic grounds, and we followed these criteria for the initial classification (1, 2). With application of double tetracycline labelling, it was possible to identify patients with normal or even increased bone formation rates (usually variations of hyperparathyroid bone disease); other patients, particularly those with osteomalacia, demonstrated subnormal rates of bone formation (1, 2). Although a deficiency of calcitriol was initially viewed as a likely cause of impaired mineralization in renal failure, the general experience has indicated little improvement of mineralization of osteomalacia following vitamin D therapy unless substantial hyperparathyroid bone disease was also present.

The measurement of aluminum in bone by a variety of techniques (3, 4), its localization along the mineralization front in patients with refractory osteomalacia (5, 6), and the production of a low turnover bone disease in animals given parenteral aluminum (3, 7-9) provide convincing evidence of a pathogenic role of aluminum in causing osteomalacia. Also, there has been the identification of substantial numbers of symptomatic patients who do not show increased osteoid but who exhibit increased surface localization of aluminum and have markedly reduced bone formation rates; this subgroup has been termed, "aplastic" bone disease (10). Finally, there is a group of patients who exhibit no increase in osteoid nor peritrabecular fibrosis and who have a normal bone formation rate despite increased surface staining for aluminum.

Vitamin D. A Chemical, Biochemical and Clinical Update

These latter features have been largely seen in asymptomatic patients, although some may exhibit symptoms (11). The types of bone disease are noted in Table I.

Table I. CLASSIFICATION OF RENAL OSTEODYSTROPHY
Based on Morphologic Features, Bone Dynamics, and Al Staining

	Fibrosis	Osteoid	D-Response	Al Stain	Al+++ #	BFR
O.F.	>.5%	<15%	Often	low	variable	incr
MIXED	>.5%	>15%	Often	low, var.	variable	incr, var.
OM	Ø	>15%	Usually not	incr	incr.	low
MILD	Ø	<15%	? *	low	variable	normal
Apl.	Ø	<15%	Usually not	incr	incr.	low
Ind.	Ø	<15%	? *	incr	incr.	normal

Abbreviations: BFR, bone formation rate; O.F., osteitis fibrosa; OM, osteomalacia; Apl, aplastic; Ind., indeterminate; #Chemical aluminum content; *Usually asymptomatic

Secondary Hyperparathryoidism and Osteitis Fibrosa: Osteitis fibrosa, the lesion of secondary hyperparathyroidism, has received considerable attention in patients with renal failure. The high levels of serum parathyroid hormone (iPTH) have been thought to arise from hypocalcemia that occurs due to phosphate retention and a deficiency of calcitriol ($1,25(OH)_2D_3$). It is now apparent that phosphate retention and hyperphosphatemia can contribute to the reduced levels of $1,25(OH)_2D_3$ in patients with renal failure (12) However, growing evidence also indicates the existence of intrinsic alterations of the parathyroid glands, themselves, in patients with renal failure (13, 14). Through mechanisms that are poorly defined, such alterations in the parathyroid glands may contribute to both the persistence and propagation of secondary hyperparathyroidism in patients with advanced renal failure and in those undergoing dialysis.

We would like to review certain clinical observations which provide strong support for the premise that alterations in the parathyroid glands, themselves, occur commonly in patients with advanced renal failure. We carried out a prospective, double-blind trial with calcitriol for the prophylaxis of bone disease in 78 asymptomatic dialysis patients with normal skeletal radiographs (15). At the outset of the study, the mean pre-dialysis serum Ca was 9.4±0.6 mg/dl and phosphorus (P) was 4.7±0.9 mg/dl, providing evidence for good biochemical control. The patients were given $CaCO_3$ providing 1g Ca/day and either placebo capsules or calcitriol and they were followed for up to 30 months. Despite wide variations in serum iPTH with values from 44 to 3565ulEq/ml as measured with the mid-region assay (ch 9), no relationships were noted between the serum iPTH levels and either the serum P or Ca concentrations for the entire patient population. In individual patients, there were direct correlations between the serum iPTH and serum P levels in only 23% of the individual patients, while inverse correlations between serum Ca and iPTH were present in 47% of the patients. On the other hand, significant suppression of serum iPTH levels occurred in 27%

of the patients receiving $CaCO_3$ alone and in 59% of the calcitriol-treated patients, while increments of serum iPTH occurred in 39% and 11%, respectively, of patients in these two treatment groups. Thus, some factor other than a change in the serum Ca or P levels seem to account for alterations in serum iPTH levels. Indeed, a few patients actually exhibited a direct correlation between the serum Ca level and that of iPTH. Closer scrutiny of serial iPTH and Ca levels in individual subjects revealed certain interrelations and permitted the identification of a serum Ca level that was associated with a marked change in the serum iPTH. Such a serum Ca level could be identified in 83% of the patients in the study (16). We have termed this, the "apparent suppression point," although it may be analagous to the "set point," described for the regulation of PTH secretion produced by changing the calcium level in suspensions of parathyroid cells (13). In 23% of the patients in this study, the apparent suppression point for iPTH occurred with serum Ca levels above 10.4 mg/dl, and PTH suppression occurred with a serum calcium below 9.5 mg/dl in only 26% of the patients. These latter values are closer to the normal "set point" for PTH suppression. Thus, there was considerable heterogeneity from patient to patient. Also, the level of calcium leading to suppression was observed to change in a substantial number of individual subjects over the 30 month period of observation. There was a decrease in the apparent suppression point in 92% of the patients whose iPTH levels were suppressed during the study, while the apparent suppression point rose in 46% of patients who exhibited a significant rise in serum iPTH during the study. These observations raise the possibility that changes in the level of calcium that lead to suppression of PTH secretion could be related to the prolonged suppression of the parathyroid glands or account for a progressive rise in serum iPTH levels observed in other patients during the period of observation.

Further evidence that a higher serum Ca is required to reduce the serum iPTH levels came from observations in uremic children being treated with continuous ambulatory peritoneal dialysis (CAPD). In our initial observations (17), we noted that children with serum Ca levels that were slightly above normal showed improvement of secondary hyperparathyroidism, compared to worsening in those with slightly lower but normal serum Ca levels. Therefore, we carried out a prospective study utilizing larger doses of calcitriol in 17 patients undergoing CAPD to raise the serum Ca to 10.5 to 11.0 mg/dl. During this time, there was normalization of the both plasma alkaline phosphatase levels and skeletal radiographs; moreover, the serum iPTH levels fell, but only with serum Ca levels above 10.5 mg/dl (18).

These observations may provide the clinical counterpart for the in vitro observations of the increased calcium level required to reduce PTH secretion by suspensions of parathyroid cells (13). Our clinical observations suggest that some factor intrinsic to the parathyroid glands or parathyroid cells, themselves, is altered in patients with advanced renal failure.

The possibility that $1,25(OH)_2D_3$ may directly affect the secretion of PTH by the parathyroid glands has received considerable attention

(19-22). We evaluated the effect of intravenous calcitriol in a group of dialysis patients with marked secondary hyperparathyroidism; most had previously received treatment with oral calcitriol, and their pre-treatment serum Ca level was 10.3±0.16 mg/dl (23). They were given intravenous calcitriol with each hemodialysis, and there was a 27% decrease in serum iPTH levels even though the serum calcium levels did not change during the initial 4-16 weeks period of treatment. Later, when serum Ca levels rose slightly, there was further suppression of serum iPTH levels, the alkaline phosphatase levels fell and often to normal, and bone biopsy features of osteitis fibrosa improved. In another group of dialysis patients with equally elevated serum iPTH levels, treatment with oral calcitriol also lowered the serum iPTH levels before there was an increase in serum Ca levels; however, the suppression of serum iPTH was not well sustained as treatment was continued and hypercalcemia dictated a reduction of the dosage. Moreover, the patients receiving oral calcitriol had serum Ca levels of 9.3±0.14 mg/dl prior to treatment, values significantly lower than the 10.3±0.16 mg/dl in the group given parenteral calcitriol; also, the former had never received prior therapy with calcitriol. Thus, the two groups are not entirely comparable. Nonetheless, these observations and those of Slatopolsky et al (22) provide support for the view that calcitriol has a direct effect to suppress PTH secretion by the parathyroid glands; also, they may suggest a mechanism whereby a deficiency of $1,25(OH)_2D_3$ may hasten the generation of secondary hyperparathyroidism in patients with renal failure. Finally, these observations of the effectiveness of parenteral calcitriol may suggest a new therapeutic approach other than parathyroid surgery for the management of patients with overt secondary hyperparathyroidism.

Osteomalacia and defective mineralization in uremic patients. Osteomalacia is also common in patients with advanced renal failure. Its pathogenesis may vary from patient to patient. Some have observed a direct relation between the frequency of osteomalacia and the plasma levels of 25(OH)D in patients with renal failure (24, 25). such an occurrence may be limited to areas with a marginal intake of vitamin D and reduced sunlight exposure. Reduced serum phosphorus levels and hypophosphatemia may also lead to impaired mineralization (26), although hypophosphatemia is an infrequent cause of osteomalacia. Indeed, growing evidence now indicates that aluminum accumulation is the major cause of osteomalacia in dialysis patients and this disorder occurs in uremic patients who have never undergone dialysis (27).

Regarded by some as quite rare, two recent surveys in the U.S. now indicate that aluminum-related bone disease may be found in bone biopsies of 25 to 30% of dialysis patients treated in dialysis units that either have never had elevated aluminum levels in water or which employ adequate methods of water purification (28). Such observations, shown in Table II, strongly suggest that the oral intake of aluminum-containing phosphate binders that are prescribed for these patients are the source of aluminum. There is evidence for oral absorption of small amounts of aluminum in normal subjects ingesting aluminum hydroxide (29), and dialysis patients have no mechanism to excrete aluminum,so that they accumulate aluminum that is absorbed. The plasma aluminum levels have been found to correlate directly with the intake of aluminum-containing gels in uremic children treated with CAPD (30). Moreover, when oral aluminum hydroxide gels are discontinued followed by the substitution of calcium carbonate as a phosphate binder, there has been a substantial decrease in the plasma aluminum levels. It is our belief that the oral absorption of aluminum gels poses the greatest risk factor for the development of aluminum-related bone disease in patients with renal failure. Thus, the predictions that aluminum-related osteomalacia would largely disappear after the introduction of adequate water treatment systems for dialysis units have not proven to be the case.

Table II. TYPES OF BONE DISEASE ENCOUNTERED IN ASYMPTOMATIC DIALYSIS PATIENTS

LOCATION:	Seattle	Okla. City
Bone features	(Per cent of patients)	
Osteitis fibrosa	28	68
Mild	40	
Aplastic*	32	7
Osteomalacia*	8	25

*Aluminum staining

(The 27 Seattle patients were chosen for biopsy be cause they had undergone dialysis for more than 8 years; Seattle water has never had aluminum concentrations above 10 ug/L. The 142 Oklahoma City patients were enlisted to participate in a prospective study with vitamin D sterols from several large dialysis units utilizing adequate water purification methods) From Andress et al. Kidney Int. (Suppl) in press and Llach et al (28)

The two series noted above have been largely derived from asymptomatic dialysis patients. What is the incidence of aluminum-related osteomalacia in symptomatic dialysis patients? Our experience is indicated in table III, which gives the results of bone biopsies carried out in symptomatic patients who were referred for the evaluation of bone disease. The largest groups of symptomatic patients either had osteomalacia or aplastic bone disease, defined by the finding of abnormally low bone formation rate. Among the patients with osteomalacia, all demonstrated a high aluminum content in bone and intense surface staining for aluminum; none responded to therapy with calcitriol. In the group with aplastic bone disease, 90% displayed intense staining for aluminum, and many of these have shown a favorable response to treatment with desferrioxamine, a chelating agent which permits the removal of aluminum during dialysis. In the small subgroup of patients with aplastic bone but no aluminum staining, some other problem i.e., diabetes mellitus, low-turnover osteoporosis, etc., may be present to account for the low bone formation rate.

Table III. TYPES OF BONE DISEASE ENCOUNTERED IN SYMPTOMATIC DIALYSIS PATIENTS
(87 patients in Los Angeles, 1981-4)

Bone features	Per cent
Osteitis fibrosa	19
Mild	1
Mixed (OF + OM)	4.5
Aplastic	37
Osteomalacia	38

(These represent patients who were referred from several dialysis units because of symptoms indicating metabolic bone disease.)

What is the pathogenesis of aluminum-related bone disease? This remains a puzzling question without clear answers. The finding of intense deposits of aluminum along the mineralization front of bone has led to the view that aluminum may prevent the mineralization of matrix. Some in vitro support for this view is derived from observations showing that aluminum can both prevent the formation of hydroxyapatite crystals as well as inhibit their growth (31). In addition, there is the possibilty that aluminum has a direct inhibitory effect on the osteoblast. Thus, aluminum can inhibit certain enzymatic functions of the osteoblast (32); and the "aplastic" lesion, itself, suggests that osteoid synthesis is reduced to the same extent as is mineralization. The identification of patients showing a change from aplastic bone disease to classic osteomalacia raises the possiblity that both pathogenic processes may occur; thus, the inhibition of matrix synthesis by the osteoblast may be the initial process, and the subsequent accumulation of surface aluminum may block mineralization to a greater degree than it decreases matrix synthesis. Indeed, the finding of aluminum staining on the cement lines of bone indicates that new bone can form over areas with aluminum deposition.

There appear to be conditions when aluminum is not toxic; thus, patients with severe osteitis fibrosa may be protected from the effect of high aluminum levels in dialysate (33) or they may show large amounts of aluminum that is distributed diffusely throughout the bone and yet exhibit normal or increased rates of bone formation (5). Similarly, aluminum accumlation on the surface of bone in experimental animals with vitamin D-deficiency osteomalacia does not inhibit the subsequent mineralization of bone following treatment with vitamin D (34). Thus, there seems to be something about a high rate of bone turnover or high iPTH levels that may prevent the toxic manisfestations of aluminum.

There are several concerns regarding the interaction of vitamin D therapy and aluminum toxicity. There is evidence that intestinal absorption of phosphate is slightly impaired in renal failure, and calcitriol and other active vitamin D sterols can enhance the absorption of phosphate as well as that of calcium (35). Thus, therapy with a vitamin D sterol might increase the need for aluminum-containing phosphate binders and thereby increase the risk of aluminum-loading and aluminum related bone disease. There is a great need for phosphate binders that do not contain aluminum. Although far from being perfect, calcium carbonate is reasonably effectively as a phosphate binder (36). With the use of calcium carbonate, would there be increased risk of hypercalcemia when it is given with calcitriol or another active vitamin D sterol? This seems possible; however, there may be little calcium absorbed when calcium carbonate is ingested with a phosphate-containing meal. Under these circumstances, it may be safe to administer calcium carbonate in conjunction with calcitriol, although the serum calcium must be monitored closely. Finally, we have also observed clinically apparent aluminum-related bone disease that appears after secondary hyperparathyroidism has been reversed. This has been reported following parathyroidectomy (37), and our experience with anecdotal cases indicate that this can also occur after secondary hyperparathyroidism is reversed by treatment with the active vitamin D sterols. Almost certainly this has occurred when there has been pre-existent aluminum loading of bone; somehow the aluminum becomes pathogenic after correction of the hyperparathyroidism.

There are other interactions between aluminum accumulation, aluminum-related osteomalacia, vitamin D, and PTH: Thus, aluminum may inhibit PTH secretion (38), and aluminum may reduce the generation of $1,25(OH)_2D_3$ (9); also, chelation of aluminum may be associated with hypocalcemia, higher iPTH levels and an increased requirement for calcitriol. The coexistence of hyperparathyroidism may lead to greater localization of aluminum in bone; however, the presence of intact parathyroid glands may permit more rapid and complete removal of aluminum during chelation therapy with desferrioxamine (39).

SUMMARY The pathogenesis of renal osteodystrophy, once regarded as a scholarly debate about the relative roles of phosphate retention compared to reduced generation of $1,25(OH)_2D_3$, now assumes new complexity in that additional mechanisms may account for increased PTH release in response to calcium and promote the generation of hyperparathyroidism. In addition, aluminum accumulation is recognized as a clear cause of osteomalacia in chronic renal failure and dialysis patients, with the oral absorption of aluminum becoming the important route for its accumulation. This raises the problem that one disease (osteomalacia) may arise from our efforts to treat another (osteitis fibrosa). The complexity of this increases, as it seems that high PTH levels may largely protect patients form aluminum toxicity, while a lowering of PTH may predispose to aluminum bone disease, and aluminum, itself, may reduce PTH secretion. Since the therapy of hyperparathyroidism differs markedly from the treatment of aluminum bone disease, the further understanding of the pathogenic mechanisms responsible for these conditions and the identification of the best means for their management and prevention is essential.

ACKNOWLEDGEMENT Supported, in part by research funds from the Veterans Administration and by USPHS Grant AM 14750.

REFERENCES

1. Sherrard, D.J., Coburn, J. W., Brickman, A. S., Singer, F.R., and Malone, M. (1980) Contrib. Nephrol. 18:92.
2. Sherrard, D.J., Baylink, D.J., Wergedal, J.E. and Maloney, N. (1974) J. Clin. Endocrinol. 39:119.
3. Ellis, H. A., Mccarthy, J.H., and Herrington, J. (1979) J. Clin Pathol. 32:832.
4. Hodson, A.B., Sherrard, D.J., Alfrey, A.G., Brickman, A.S. (1982) J. clin. Endocrinol. Metab. 54:539
5. Gournot-Witmer, G., Zingraff, J., Pischot, J.J., Escaig, F., Lefevre, R., Boumati, P., Bourdeau, A., Garabedian, M., Galle, P., Bourdon, R., Drueke, T., and Balsan, S. (1981) Kidney Int. 20:376.
6. Maloney, N.A., Ott, S., Alfrey, A.C., Coburn, J.W., and Sherrard, D.J. (1982) J. Lab. Clin. Med. 99:206.
7. Robertson, J.A., Felsenfeld, A.J., Haygood, CC., Wilson, P., Clarke, C., and Llach, F. (1983) Kidney Int. 23:327.
8. Chan, Y., Alfrey, A.C., Posen, S., Lissner, D., Hills, E., Dunstan, C.R., and Evans, R.A. (1983) Calcif. Tiss. Internat. 35:344.
9. Goodman, W.G., Henry, D.A., Horst, R., Nudelman, R.K., Alfrey, A.C., and Coburn, J.W. (1984) Kidney Int. 25:370.
10. Sherrard, D.J., Orr, S.J., Maloney, N.A., Andress, D., and Coburn, J.W. (1984) in: Clinical Disorders of Bone and Mineral Metabolism, Ed. B. Frame & J.T. Potts, Excerpta Medica, Amsterdam, p.254.
11. Malluche, H.H., Smith, A.J., Abreo, K., and Faugere, M.C. (1984) N. Engl. J. Med. 311:140.
12. Portale, A.P., Booth, B.E., Halloran, B.P., and Morris, R.C., Jr. (1984) J. Clin. Invest. 73:1580.
13. Brown, E.M., Wilson, R.E., Estman, R.C., Pallotta, J., and Marynick, S.P. (1982) J. Clin. Endocrinol. Metab. 54:172.
14. Brown, E.M. (1983) J. Clin. Endocrinol. Metab. 56:572.
15. Coburn, J.W., N.C. DiDemonico, G.F. Bryce, L.W. Bassett, S.A. Shupien, E.G. Wong, R.B. Miller, C.M. Bennett, R.H. Gold, J.P. Mallon, O.N. Miller, and P. C. Chang. (1982) Vitamin D: Chemical, Biochemical, and Clinical Endocrinology of Calcium Metabolism. Edited by A.W. Norman et al. DeGruyter, Berlin, pp. 833.
16. Coburn, J.W., N.C. DiDomenico, G.F. Bryce, P.C. Chang, O.N. Miller. (1982) Clin. Res. 30:539.
17. Paunier, L., Salusky, I., Slatopolsky, E., Kangarloo, H., Kopple, J., Horst, R., Coburn, J., Fine, R. (1984) Pediatric Research, 18:742.
18. Salusky, I.B., L. Paunier, E. Slatapolsky, H. Kangarloo, J.W. Coburn and R.N. Fine. (1984) (1984) in: Calcitriol, A Clinical Update, Ed. J.W. Coburn, Excerpta Medica, Princeton, New Jersey, pp. 36-42.
19. Chertow, B.S., Baylink, D.J., Wergedal, J.F., Su, M.H.H., and Nornam, A.W. (1975) J. Clin. Invest. 56:668.
20. Oldham, S.G., Smith, R., Hartenbower, D.L., Henry, H.L. Norman, A.W., and Coburn, J.W. (1979) Endocrinology 104:248.
21. Madsen, S., Olgaard, K. and Ladefoged, J. (1981) J. Clin. Endocrinol. 53:823.
22. Slatopolsky, E., Weerts, C., Thielan, J., Horst, R., Harter, H. and Martin, K.J. (1984) J. Clin. Invest. 74:2136.

23. Norris, K.C,., Kraut, J.A., Andress, D.L., Koffler, A., Sherrard, D.J., and Coburn, J.W. (1985) Kidney Internat. 27:158.
24. Eastwood, J.B., Harris, E., Stamp, T.C.B., and De Wardener, H.E. (1976) Lancet 2:1209.
25. Mason, R.S., Lissner, D., Wilkinson, M., and Posen, S. (1980) Clin. Endocrinol. 13:375.
26. Kanis, J.A., Adams, N.D., Earnshaw, M., Heynen, G., Ledingham, L.G.G., Oliver, D.O., Russell, R.G.G. and Woods, C.G. (1977) in: Eds. A.W. Norman et al: Vitamin D. Biochemical, Chemical and Clinical Aspects Related to Calcium Metabolism. W. de Gruyter, Berlin, p. 671.
27. Coburn, J.W., Nebeker, H.G., Hercz, G., Milliner, D.S., Ott, S.M., Andress, D.L., Sherrard, D.J., and Alfrey, A.C. (1984) Nephrology: Proc. of IX Intl. Congress Nephrology, Ed. By R.R. Robinson, New York, Springer-Verlag, pp. 1383-1395.
28. Llach, F, Felsenfeld, A.J., Coleman, M.D., Pederson, J.A. and Rosen, R. (1984) in: Calcitriol, A Clinical Update, Ed. J.W. Coburn, Exerpta Med. Princeton, N.J., p. 11-18.
29. Kaehny, W.D., Hegg, A.P., and Alfrey, A.C. (1977) N. Engl. J. Med. 296:1389.
30. Salusky, I.B., J.W. Coburn, L. Paunier, D.J. Sherrard, and R.N. Fine. (1984) J. Pediatrics 105:717-200.
31. Blumenthal, N.C., and Posner, A.S. (1984) Calcified Tiss. Internat. 36:439.
32. Lieberherr, M., Grosse, B., Cournot-Witmer, G., Thil, C.L., and Balsan, S. (1982) Calcif. Tissue Int. 34:280.
33. Ellis, H.A. (1982) Ann. Intern. Med. 96:533.
34. Quarles, L.D., Dennis, V.W., Gitelman, H.J., Herrelson, J., and Drezner, M. (1984) Clin. Res. 32:522A.
35. Brickman, A.S., Hartenbower, D.L., Norman, A.S., and J.W. Coburn. (1977) Am. J. Clin. Nutr. 30:1064.
36. Morniere, P.H., Rousel, A., Tahiri, Y., et al. (1982) Proc. E.D.T.A. 19:784.
37. Felsenfeld, A.J., Harrelson, J.M., Gutman, R.A., Wells, S.A., Jr., and Drezner, M.K. (1984) Ann. Int. Med. 96:34.
38. Morrisey, J., M. Rothstein, G. Mayor, and E. Slatopolsky. (1983) Kidney Internat. 23:699.
29. Ott, S.M., D.L. Andress, H.G. Nebeker, D.S. Milliner, N.A. Maloney, J.W. Coburn and D.J. Sherrard. Kidney Internat. (in press)

ASSESSMENT OF $1,25(OH)_2D_3$ IN THE CORRECTION AND PREVENTION OF RENAL OSTEODYSTROPHY IN PATIENTS WITH MILD TO MODERATE RENAL FAILURE

Shaul G. Massry

Division of Nephrology and Department of Medicine, University of Southern California School of Medicine, Los Angeles, California, USA.

Introduction:

Studies in our laboratory in adults (1) and data by Portale et al. (2) in children suggest that phosphate retention, which may develop as renal insufficiency ensues, may interfere with the ability of the patients to augment the renal production of $1,25(OH)_2D$ to meet their needs. A state of absolute or relative vitamin D deficiency develops, leading to defective intestinal absorption of calcium and impaired calcium response to PTH. These two abnormalities produce hypocalcemia and, subsequently, secondary hyperparathyroidism. Vitamin D deficiency would also be associated with defective mineralization of osteoid resulting in osteomalacia.

An additional pathway through which an absolute or relative deficiency of $1,25(OH)_2D$ may mediate secondary hyperparathyroidism, and consequently hyperparathyroid bone disease, is related to the interaction between this vitamin D metabolite and the parathyroid glands. Prolonged exposure to $1,25(OH)_2D_3$ both in vivo (3) and in vitro (4) may directly suppress the parathyroid gland activity. Also, available data suggest that $1,25(OH)_2D$ may render the parathyroid glands more susceptible to the suppressive action of ionized calcium (5,6). Thus, it is possible that a deficiency of $1,25(OH)_2D$ may initiate secondary hyperparathyroidism even in the absence of overt hypocalcemia. This postulate is in agreement with recent observations by Lopez et al. (7) who found that secondary hyperparathyroidism developed in dogs with 70% decrease in glomerular filtration rate in which serum calcium was maintained normal.

The above mentioned observations assign a critical role for a relative or absolute deficiency of $1,25(OH)_2D$ in the genesis of secondary hyperparathyroidism and the other various components of renal osteodystrophy. Therefore, it is theoretically possible to prevent and/or manage the manifestations of renal osteodystrophy in patients with mild to moderate renal failure by treating them with $1,25(OH)_2D_3$.

Methods:

The present study reports the results of therapy with $1,25(OH)_2D_3$ in a large population of patients with moderate renal failure. Patients with creatinine clearance between 15 and 55 ml/min and without significant proteinuria were asked to participate in the study and only those who signed an imformed consent entered the study. The duration of the study was one year. The patients were assigned in a double-blind fashion to a placebo group and a treatment ($1,25(OH)_2D_3$) group. Thirty-three patients completed one year of study, and had iliac crest biopsy before and at the end of the study; 17 of these patients were in the treatment group and 16 patients received placebo. The dose of $1,25(OH)_2D_3$ ranged between 0.5-1.0 (0.8 ± 0.06) pg/day.

Results:

The blood levels of PTH were elevated in all but two patients with a mean value of 35 ± 4 (normal 2-6, μlEq/ml). There was a significant inverse relationship between blood levels of PTH and creatinine clearance ($r = -0.44$, $p < 0.01$). The blood levels of 25(OH)D were normal while the blood levels of $1,25(OH)_2D$ were usually low in patients with creatinine clearance below 25 ml/min; there was a significant correlation between the blood levels of $1,25(OH)_2D$ and creatinine clearance ($r = 0.43$, $p < 0.01$).

The majority of the patients showed evidence of bone disease secondary to hyperparathyroidism and/or defective mineralization. The abnormalities in bone morphometry were more frequent and severe in patients with creatinine clearance below 35 ml/min. The bone histology showed the following abnormalities: a) an increase in the number of osteoclasts (osteoclast index) and in the surface density of bone osteoclast interface; there were significant correlations between these parameters and the blood levels of PTH; b) variable degrees of endosteal fibrosis; c) increased number of osteoblasts (osteoblast index); d) increased osteoid area; and e) prolonged mineralization lag time.

After a year of placebo treatment, there were no significant changes in the blood levels of calcium, inorganic phosphorus and alkaline phosphatase. The blood levels of PTH remained elevated. There were no significant changes in creatinine clearance. The abnormalities in bone histology either worsened or remained unchanged.

Treatment with $1,25(OH)_2D_3$ for one year produced a significant rise in blood levels of calcium. Eleven of the 17 patients had one episode of mild hypercalcemia and 7 of these 11 patients had 2 episodes while only 4 of these patients had 3 episodes of hypercalcemia. Discontinuation of therapy for a few days or reduction of the dose of the vitamin D medication was adequate to reverse the hypercalcemia. The blood levels of inorganic phosphorus fell initially and rose again to baseline values. There was a gradual decline in the blood levels of alkaline phosphatase. The blood levels of PTH fell in most patients and the mean decline was $38 \pm 9\%$, $p < 0.02$; there was a significant inverse correlation between the fall in the blood levels of PTH and the rise in the blood concentrations of calcium. There were no significant changes in creatinine clearance.

Treatment with $1,25(OH)_2D_3$ resulted in either complete healing or marked improvement of all the abnormalities of bone histology including the manifestations of enhanced bone resorption and those of defective mineralization.

Conclusion:
Our data demonstrate that the prescription of small doses of $1,25(OH)_2D_3$ to patients with moderate renal failure is an effective therapeutic modality for the healing and the prevention of the progression of the derangements of divalent ion metabolism. This treatment is safe and does not cause adverse effects on glomerular filtration rate.

References:
1. Llach,F.,Massry,S.G. (Submitted for publication) J.Clin.Endocrinol. Metab.
2. Portale,A.A.,Booth,B.E.,Halldran,B.P.,Morris,R.C. (1984) J.Clin.Invest. 73:1580-1589.
3. Slatopolsky,E.,Weerts,C.,Thielan,G.,Martin,K.,Harter,H. (1983) In: Clinical Disorders of Bone and Mineral Metabolism (eds., Frame,B.,Potts,J.T., Jr., pp. 267-270).

4. Chan,W.,McKay,C.,Dye,E.,Slatopolsky,E. (1984) Proc.Amer.Soc.Nephrol. 17:
13A.
5. Oldham,S.B.,Smith,R.,Hartenbower,D.L.,Henry,H.L.,Norman,A.W.,Coburn,J.W.
(1979) Endocrinology 104:248-254.
6. Madsen,S.,Olgaard,K.,Ladenfoged,J. (1981) J.Clin.Endocrinol.Metab. 53:
823-827.
7. Lopez,S.,Galceran,T.,Chan,W.,Rapp,N.,Martin,K.,Slatopolsky,E. (1984)
Proc.Amer.Soc.Nephrol. 17:24A.

INFLUENCE OF PARATHYROID HORMONE AND 1,25-DIHYDROXYVITAMIN D_3 ON THE ORGAN DISTRIBUTION OF ALUMINIUM AND ZINC IN NORMAL AND UREMIC RATS.

R. Hirschberg, D. von Herrath, A. Pauls, K. Schaefer
Med. Abt. II, St. Joseph-Krankenhaus I, Bäumerplan 24, 1000 Berlin 42, Germany

Little is known, whether or not the organ distribution of trace elements as aluminium (AL) or zinc (ZI) is influenced by drugs or underlying metabolic disorders. Since many renal patients develop parathyroid hormone (PTH)-related disorders of calcium und phosphorus metabolism it seemed of interest to investigate not only the possible influence of PTH on the organ distribution of orally and parentally applied AL in uremia, but in addition, to evaluate the effect of PTH on the organ distribution of ZI. Furthermore, studies were performed to test whether the most potent metabolite of vitamin D_3, i.e. 1,25-Dihydroxyvitamin D_3 (1,25$(OH)_2D_3$), which is frequently given to patients suffering from renal bone disease, might exert an influence on the organ distribution of both trace elements under the above conditions.

Methods:
Studies were performed using for both investigations male Wistar rats, which were kept for 40 days on a normal diet (Altromin^R, C 1.000) but free of vitamin D, in a laboratory with UV-free artificial light. After this time, the rats (average weight now 200 g) were divided into different groups. Half of the rats were subjected to 5/6 nephrectomy carried out under ether anesthesia. The remaining rats were shamoperated. The rats participating in the AL-investigation received in order to simulate closely the human conditions, for 20 days AL i.p. and orally. All rats received except the normal and uremic controls for the same period of time a subcutaneous injection for 10 USP-U of PTH (Parathormon^R, Hormon Chemie, Munich, FRG) alone or together with 2 IU (0.05 ug i.p.) of 1,25$(OH)_2D_3$, a further group received only the vitamin D hormone. The measurement of AL and ZI was performed by atomic absorption spectrometry. The accuracy of the method was repeatedly determined and varied by 2.4 % for the different tissue samples.

Results and Conclusions:

1. With regard to the AL studies it could be demonstrated that the uremic muscle contains less AL than that of controls, whereas the uremic liver and bone reveal a higher AL incorporation than the comparable normal organs. Table 1 gives an overview on the percentage organ distribution of AL in relation to the serum. It is evident that in all rats, irrespective of the pretreatment, the liver and the bone contain the highest AL concentration.

Table 1

Rat groups	Serum	Heart	Bone	Brain	Muscle	Liver
C + AL	1.0	4.3	26.4	1.7	7.9	141.4
C + AL + D	1.0	4.2	2o.5	1.1	9.2	242.4
C + AL + D + PTH	1.0	6.4	33.1	-	8.5	200.2
C + AL + PTH	1.0	5.1	7o.7	3.1	14.5	187.3
NX + AL	1.0	4.5	76.2	1.7	3.7	177.3
NX + AL + D	1.0	12.1	62.6	1.1	11.6	2oo.6
NX + AL + D + PTH	1.0	9.9	36.2	o.8	11.3	2o5.9
NX + AL + PTH	1.0	6.2	59.8	1.7	5.4	194.6

Vitamin D. A Chemical, Biochemical and Clinical Update

The treatment with $1,25(OH)_2D_3$ and/or PTH results in higher AL concentrations in the uremic heart and muscle compared to untreated uremic rats. On the other hand, both hormones reduce the AL concentration in the uremic liver and bone.

2. The relative organ distribution of ZI in relation to the serum is depicted in Table 2.

Table 2

	Serum	Muscle	Heart	Bone	Brain	Liver
C	1	71	1o1	11o	1o8	23o
C + D	1	82	111	118	113	287
C + D + PTH	1	58	79	79	114	219
C + PTH	1	75	82	122	129	247
NX	1	83	111	122	141	416
NX + D	1	96	139	145	136	547
NX + D + PTH	1	1o8	141	144	16o	531
NX + PTH	1	116	146	17o	151	7o9

It can be seen, that under all conditions the liver contains the highest concentration of ZI. This was underlined, when uremic rats were pretreated with $1,25(OH)_2D_3$ and/or PTH, as these compounds increased further the ZI concentration of the uremic liver. An opposite pattern could be observed for the serum where a pretreatment with both compounds alone or given together resulted in a decreased ZI concentration.

The following conclusions could be drawn according to our data.

1) For physicans being involved in the care of renal patients it is important to realize, that an excess of PTH or the administration of $1,25(OH)_2D_3$ can modify the organ deposition of aluminium.

2) It should be also kept in mind, that PTH as well as $1,25(OH)_2D_3$ can augment the differences of the organ concentration of zinc, which seem to be already typical for the uremic state.

For references see

1) R. Hirschberg et al.
Organ distribution of aluminium in uremic rats: influence of parathyroid hormone and 1,25-dihydroxyvitamin D_3
Min. Electr. Metabol. (in press)

2) R. Hirschberg et al.
Parathyroid hormone and 1,25-dihydroxyvitamin D_3 affect the tissue concentration of zinc in uremic rats.
Nephron 39 (1985) 277

Al INTOXICATION IN NORMAL RATS: EFFECTS ON THE MINERALIZATION PROCESS.

P. Ballanti, P. Mocetti, C. Della Rocca, S. Costantini °, R. Giordano°, A. Ioppolo°, A. Mantovani° and E. Bonucci.

Dept. Human Biopathology, Div. Pathological Anatomy, "La Sapienza" University, 00161 Rome, Italy.

(°) Istituto Superiore di Sanità, 00161 Rome, Italy.

Introduction:

Renal Osteodystrophy (RO) with severe osteomalacia in patients on regular hemodialysis has been related to Al intoxication (1-2-3). To verify if Al has a direct role in inhibiting mineralization, normal rats were injected intraperitoneally with $AlCl_3$ (4); bone histomorphometric analysis showed slight but inconstant increase of osteoid tissue. Because $AlCl_3$ caused peritoneal irritation and organic decay, a new experiment has been carried out using Al lactate; moreover, because we have found high Al concentration in bone of RO with prevalent hyperparathyroidism changes, rats have been injected with PTH and PTH+Al to check their combined effect on bone.

Materials and Methods:

31 male Wistar rats were divided in 2 groups: part of group 1 rats (n=12) were injected intraperitoneally for 11 weeks with Al lactate (7.4 mg/week of elemental Al), and part (n=6 controls) with Na lactate; group 2 rats were partly (n=8) injected with Al lactate and, during the last week, with bovine PTH (40 USP/day), and partly (n=5 controls) with Na lactate and, during the last week, with PTH. All rats were fed a standard diet containing 1.2 % calcium, 0.8 % phosphorus and 2,500 UI/Kg Vit. D. Serum Ca and serum Al levels, and tibia Al concentration were determined by atomic absorption spectroscopy. Tibia and rib specimens were fixed in 4 % paraformaldehyde buffered at pH 7.2 and embedded in Araldite without decalcification. 1 µm thick sections were stained with Methylene blue - Azure II; histomorphometric analysis was performed on trabecular bone of tibia epiphyseal calcification center and on metaphyseal bone of tibia and rib. 2.5 µm thick sections were stained with Aluminon.

Results:

Al+PTH and PTH treated rats were hypercalcemic and had a Ca concentration significantly higher than that of Al and Na lactate treated rats. In Al+PTH treated rats, serum Ca was lower than in rats treated with PTH alone ($p < 0.001$). Al content

Table 1: Al content in Serum and Bone (ppm).

	SERUM		TIBIA	
	TREATED	CONTROLS	TREATED	CONTROLS
Group 1	0.95 ± 0.13	0.004 ± 0.002	151.08 ± 30.22	1.57 ± 0.26
Group 2	1.02 ± 0.19	0.005 ± 0.002	187.75 ± 31.14	2.59 ± 0.68
	NS*	NS*	$p < 0.02$*	$p < 0.01$*

*Student's t-test.

in serum and in bone is shown in Table 1. In Al treated rats histomorphometric measurements show a slight but not significant increase of Osteoid Volume, Osteoid Surface and Thickness Index of Osteoid. In rats of group 2 the osteoid parameters were always significantly higher in Al+PTH than in PTH treated animals. The Osteoclastic Index (ocl./mm^2) decreased to a variable extent in Al treated rats of both groups. Al Aluminon staining was positive in most of trabecular borders of Al and Al+PTH treated rats.

Discussion:

The present results confirm that Al intoxication has no direct effect on bone calcification and suggest that it can induce osteomalacia in cooperation with other factors such as increased PTH secretion. The addition of PTH resulted in increased Al content in bone. Direct Al inhibition of osteoblast and osteoclast activity seems possible.

References:

1. Cournot-Witmer G., Zingraff J., Plachot J. J., Escaig F., Lefèvre R., Boumati P., Bourdeau A., Garabédian M., Galle P., Bourdon R., Drüeke T. and Balsan S., (1981), Kidney Int., 20: 375-385.
2. Ott S. M., Maloney N. A., Coburn J. Y., Alfrey A. C., Sherrard D. J., (1982), New. Eng J. Med., 307: 709-713.
3. Boyce B. F., Elder H. Y., Elliot H. C., Fogelman I., Feel G. S., Junior B. J., Beastall G., Boyle I. T., (1982) Lancet I: 1009-1013.
4. Ballanti P., Mocetti P., Della Rocca C., Costantini S., Giordano R., Ioppolo A., Mantovani A., Stasolla D., and Bonucci E., (1983), Min. Met. Res. in IT., 4: 139-142.

Supported by grants of MPI and CNR.

VITAMIN D METABOLITES LEVELS IN RENAL OSTEODYSTROPHY.

G. Cesaretti, G. Federico, M. Massimetti and G. Saggese.
Department of Pediatrics, University of Pisa, Italy.

Introduction:

Very variable values of serum 25-OH-D have been found in renal osteodystrophy (ROD): elevated, normal or, especially in the patients with osteomalacia, often reduced. To know furtherly vitamin D metabolites levels, we investigated calcium metabolism in a group of patients with ROD.

Patients and methods:

Fourteen children aged 2.5-17.6 years with chronic renal failure (CRF) (Clcr 31.2 ± 9.2 ml/m'/mql,73) (m ± 1 SD) were examinated. None of the patients underwent to hemodialytic treatment and none received drugs acting on calcium metabolism. We effected the evaluations of serum Ca (nv: 5 ± 0.25 mEq/L), P (nv: 2.1 ± 0.35 mEq/L) and alkalyne phosphatase (nv: 600 ± 300 U/L), i-PTH (C-term) by a RIA-method (nv: 440±220 pg/ml), 25-OH-D (nv: 45 ± 12 ng/ml) and 1,25(OH)2D (38 ± 7 pg/ml) by a RRA method (1)(2) and a radiographic examination of the skeleton.

Results:

Twelve children showed radiographic signes of ROD. In all patients 1,25(OH)2D was low (15±5 pg/ml) ($p < 0.001$), while also 25-OH-levels were decreased (14.6±3.5 ng/ml) ($p < 0.001$); i-PTH were elevated (892 ± 124 pg/ml) ($p < 0.001$); furthermore alkalyne phosphatase (1054 ± 130 U/L) and phosphate (2.5 ± 0.5 mEq/L) were increased ($p < 0.001$), while calcium (4.1 ± 0.3 mEq/L) was decreased in all.

Discussion:

The findings that an impaired bone mineralization is more common in patients with low 25-OH-D (3) and that the nephrectomized patients have not often greater signes of osteomalacia than other uremic subjects (4) have suggested that a deficiency of this metabolite may contribute to the azotemic osteomalacia (5). Furthermore the bone mineralization does not always improve with calcitriol therapy (6). A decreased 25-OH-D values in children with bone demineralization could be determined by some causes:

reduced dietary intake, lacking solar exposure, nephrotic syndrome (7), hepatic diseases (8), continous dialysis. None of these conditions was present in our subjects. It is possible that the 25-OH-D deficiency could be caused by a microsomial epatic induction by the uremic toxins (8), as demonstrated by Keck (9). Elevated phosphate levels could inhibit hepatic 25-hydroxylation (10) too. Also the findings human bone cells metabolize directly 25-OH-D to 1,25(OH)2D (9) and the improvement of bone lesions induced by 25-OH-D therapy is not attributable to 1,25(OH)2D (11) indicate an autonomous action of 25-OH-D on bone, suggesting an useful therapeutic approach to ROD.

References:

1) Belsey, R.E., De Luca, H.F. and Potts, J.T. (1974) J. Clin. Endocrinol. Metab. 28: 1046-51.
2) Eisman, J.A., Hamstra, A.J., Kream, B.E., De Luca, H.F. (1976) Arch. Bioch. Bioph. 176: 235-43.
3) Eastwood, J.B., Daly, A., Carter, G.D., Alaghband-Zadeh, J. and DeWardener, H.E. (1976) Clin. Sci. 57: 473-6.
4) Favus M.J. (1978) Med. Clin. North Am. 62: 1291-327.
5) Bordier, P., Zingraff, J., Gueris, J., Jungers, P., Marie, P., Pechet, M. and Rasmussen, H. (1978) Am. J. Med. 64: 101-5.
6) Robitaille, P., Marie, P.J., Delvin, E.E., Lortie, L. and Glorieaux, F.H. (1984) 73: 315-24.
7) Goldstein, D.A., Haldimann, B., Sherman, D. and Massry, S.G. (1981) J. Clin. Endocrinol. Metab. 87: 664-9.
8) DeWardener, H.E. (1980) Rev. Pediatr. 30: 2555-62.
9) Keck, E., Dyrdel, R., West,T., Kruck,F., Meier,W., Hennes, U., Kruskemper, H.L. and Schweikert, H.U. (1983) J. Endocrinol. Invest. 6: 211-6.
10) Dominguez, J.H., Gray, R.W. and Lemann, J. (1976) 43: 1056-8.
11) Langman, C.B., Mazur, A.T., Baron, R. and Norman, M.E. (1982) 100: 815-20.

1α OH VITAMIN D3 INCREASES PLASMA ALUMINIUM IN HEMODIALYZED PATIENTS TAKING Al(OH)3.

Fournier A.[1], Demontis R.[1], Idrissi A.[1], Tahiri Y.[1], Morinière Ph.[1], Leflon A.[2] (1) Service de Néphrologie. CHU Amiens.(2) Laboratoire de Biochimie. CHU Amiens.

The vitamin D metabolites may increase plasma aluminium by increasing the need of Al(OH)3 (1), but wether or not they directly increase plasma aluminium is not known. Therefore this study was undertaken to assess the effect of 1α OH vitamin D3 on the plasma concentration of aluminium in uremic patients taking a constant dose of Al(OH)3 but not exposed to high aluminium dialysate.

PATIENTS AND METHODS :

16 patients on chronic hemodialysis for 2-108 months with a dialysate aluminium <.3 µmol/l thanks to reverse osmosis, were studied while on a constant dose of Al(OH)3 (0.5 - 4g/day). After 3 weeks of a control period, 1α OH vitamin D3 was given for 4 weeks at the dose of 6 µg per week, the drug being given at the end of each dialysis. After 1α OH vit.D3 discontinuation the followup was 2 weeks for the 16 patients and 8 weeks in 6 patients.

Before the first dialysis of each week, following plasma concentrations were measured throughout the study :

- calcium, phosphate, protein by autoanalyzer technic,
- aluminium by inductively coupled plasma emission spectrometry (normal range < 0.3 µmol/l ; detection limit 0.15 µmol/l (2),
- PTH (44-68) was measured in only 6 patients by radio immunoassay (normal range 80-220 pg/ml).

RESULTS :

Table I shows that plasma aluminium increases significantly during 1α OH D3 administration and remains significantly higher than during the control for the 2 weeks after 1α OH D3 discontinuation. During the 3 - 6th week after 1α OH D3 discontinuation mean plasma aluminium remains higher than during the control period but the significance of the difference disappears because the number of patient is only 6. During the 7-8th week after discontinuation, plasma aluminium concentrations is comparable to that of the control period. Plasma calcium concentration increases and plasma PTH concentrations decreases only during 1α OH D3.administration.

Plasma phosphate did not change significantly.The variations of plasma aluminium (versus control period)were negatively correlated with the variations of plasma PTH ($r=-0.75$, $n=6$, $p<0.05$).

DISCUSSION AND CONCLUSION :

1α OH D vitamin D3 significantly increases plasma aluminium concentration in hemodialyzed patients taking Al(OH)3. This increase may be explained either by an increase in intestinal absorption of aluminium or by a decreased tissue storage capacity for aluminium. The experimental data of DRUEKE(3)showing that uremic rats treated with 1,25 (OH)2 D acumulate less aluminium in their liver than pair fed controls when exposed to oral aluminium load but have higher plasma levels of aluminium, are consistent with the second hypothesis. To prove this hypothesis an other study is being done in patients who have been exposed to variable aluminium overload, but who are no more taking Al(OH)3 and who are taking 1α OH D3 during 4 weeks.

Vitamin D. A Chemical, Biochemical and Clinical Update

EFFECT OF 1α OH VITAMIN D3 ON PLASMA CONCENTRATIONS OF ALUMINIUM, CALCIUM, PHOSPHATE AND PTH 44 - 68 (mean + sem)

Plasma Concentrations (Numbers of patients)	Control Period	Weeks on 1 OH D3		Weeks after 1 OH vitamin D3 discontinuation			
		1 + 2	3 + 4	1 + 2	3 + 4	5 + 6	7 + 8
	(16)	(16)	(16)	(16)	(6)	(6)	(6)
Aluminium (umol/l)	1.20 ± .25	1.51 ± .3*	1.69 ± .35**	1.71 ± .3**	1.52 ± .4	1.72 ± .6	1.05 ± .5
Calcium (mmol/l)	2.28 ± .06	2.48 ± .07	2.54 ± .09*	2.38 ± .06	2.31 ± .06	2.28 ± .08	2.18 ± .06
Phosphate (mmol/l)	1.72 ± .13	1.86 ± .12	1.9 ± .11	1.81 ± .12	1.31 ± .2	1.33 ± .15	1.41 ± .10
PTH 44 - 68 (pg/ml) (only 6 pt)	1375 ± 300	--	654 ±200**	--	1173 ± 300	--	911 ±150

Comparison versus control period : * $p < .05$; ** $p < .01$

If 1α OH D3 increase significantly plasma aluminium, this increase will be explained only by aluminium redistribution. Whatever the explanation is, our observation, should lead to careful monitoring of plasma aluminium when 1α OH D3 is given to patients loaded with aluminium.

REFERENCES :

(1) FOURNIER A., MORINIERE Ph., SEBERT JL. (1984). In Nephrology. Robinson R. Editor, Springer Verlag New York 1984, Vol II, p 1357-1373.

(2) ALLAIN P., MAURAS Y. (1979). Analyt.Chem., 51, 2089-2095.

(3) DRUEKE T., LACOUR B., TOUAM M., 1985. Nephron, 39, 10-17.

EFFECTS OF DIET AND ALFACALCIDOL TREATMENT ON FEMORAL HEAD OSTEOSCLEROSIS OF LONG-TERM URAEMIC RABBITS.

E. TVEDEGAARD and O. LADEFOGED,
Medical Department P, Division of Nephrology, Rigshospitalet and Department of Animal Feeding and Nutrition, Royal Veterinary and Agricultural University, Copenhagen, Denmark.

Introduction:

Avascular necrosis of the femoral head is a rather frequent and serious complication following renal transplantation. The possible importance of pre-existing renal osteodystrophy remains to be determined. Rabbits have been used in experimental studies of femoral head necrosis (1) and previous studies have shown that chronic renal failure (CRF) in rabbits is characterized by osteomalacia and increased trabecular bone volume (2). In the present study the effects on femoral head morphology of dietary modifications regarding calcium (Ca) and phosphorus (P) as well as treatment with alfacalcidol (1α-OHD_3) in CRF rabbits were investigated.

Material and Methods:

Young, adult rabbits of the White Danish Country strain were used weighing 3-3.5 kg. CRF was induced by electrocoagulating part of the left kidney during general anaesthesia with right side nephrectomy 3 weeks later. After 3 weeks of adaptation 3 groups of CRF rabbits with comparable degrees of renal insufficiency were formed and given diets with low, medium and high contents of Ca and P (Table 1). A sham-operated group of controls with normal renal function was given the medium diet. The content of vitamin D_3 of the diets was 2ooo IU per kg. After 6 weeks on this regimen half of the rabbits within each group were given oral treatment with alfacalcidol(o.o2µg/kg/d). After 6 months the rabbits were killed and one femoral bone was analyzed chemically and the head of the other femur processed for histological examination. Undecalcified sections were stained with Goldners trichrome and histomorphometric evaluation was carried out as described by Melsen (3).

Results:

The serum concentrations are shown below in table 1.

Table 1. Serum concentrations (Means ± SEM).

Groups and Diets		Creatinine mmol/l	Calcium mmol/l	Magnesium mmol/l
Controls	+1-alfa(8)	o.11 ± o.o1	3.5 ± o.1	1.6 ± o.1
1.o%Ca,o.9%P	Placebo(6)	o.11 ± o.oo	3.5 ± o.1	1.5 ± o.1
Uraemia	+1-alfa(5)	o.35 ± o.o9	3.7 ± o.1	2.3 ± o.3
o.4%Ca,o.3%P	Placebo(5)	o.23 ± o.o3	3.5 ± o.3	1.7 ± o.1
Uraemia	+1-alfa(7)	o.25 ± o.o2	4.o ± o.1	2.2 ± o.1
1.o%Ca,o.9%P	Placebo(7)	o.24 ± o.o2	4.o ± o.1	2.1 ± o.2
Uraemia	+1-alfa(6)	o.22 ± o.o2	3.7 ± o.1	2.2 ± o.2
1.8%Ca,1.6%P	Placebo(5)	o.21 ± o.o4	3.6 ± o.1	2.1 ± o.2

A fairly uniform increase of the serum creatinine in all CRF groups was present. The serum concentrations of Ca and P tended to be increased in the CRF rabbits whereas treatment with alfacalcidol had no effect in any of the groups.
The bone mineral composition was similar in all of the groups and no effect of uraemia, diets or alfacalcidol treatment was found (Table 2).

Table 2. Bone mineral composition (Means ± SEM).

Groups and diets		Calcium (%)	Phosphorus (%)	Magnesium (%)
Controls	+1-alfa(8)	28.1 ± o.2	12.3 ± o.1	o.38 ± o.o1
1.o%Ca,o.9%P	Placebo(6)	27.9 ± o.2	12.6 ± o.1	o.4o ± o.o1
Uraemia	+1-alfa(5)	28.1 ± o.1	12.3 ± o.2	o.41 ± o.o1
o.4%Ca,o.3%P	Placebo(5)	27.8 ± o.3	12.6 ± o.2	o.42 ± o.o2
Uraemia	+1-alfa(7)	27.7 ± o.3	12.3 ± o.1	o.42 ± o.o1
1.o%Ca,o.9%P	Placebo(7)	27.7 ± o.1	12.4 ± o.1	o.43 ± o.o1
Uraemia	+1-alfa(6)	27.5 ± o.3	12.7 ± o.1	o.43 ± o.o3
1.8%Ca,1.6%P	Placebo(5)	28.3 ± o.2	12.6 ± o.1	o.43 ± o.o2

Histomorphometric analysis of the femoral head showed an increased volume of trabecular bone and increased amounts of osteoid tissue as well in all of the CRF groups. The low Ca-low P diet protected to a certain degree against these changes whereas treatment with alfacalcidol had no significant effect.

Table 3. Morphologic parameters (Means ± SEM).

Groups and diets		Trabecular bone vol(%)	Osteoid surface(%)	Osteoid volume(%)
Controls	+1-alfa(8)	46 ± 2.6	1.6 ± o.5	o.3 ± o.2
1.o%Ca,o.9%P	Placebo(6)	38 ± 5.9	2.5 ± o.6	o.6 ± o.3
Uraemia	+1-alfa(5)	53 ± 3.9	6.9 ± 3.4	o.8 ± o.4
o.4%Ca,o.3%P	Placebo(5)	43 ± 4.4	2.6 ± 1.6	o.1 ± o.1
Uraemia	+1-alfa(7)	78 ± 3.2	45 ± 11	2.6 ± o.5
1.o%Ca,o.9%P	Placebo(7)	64 ± 6.6	25 ± 1o	1.3 ± o.4
Uraemia	+1-alfa(6)	66 ± 4.4	28 ± 11	1.3 ± o.5
1.8%Ca,1.6%P	Placebo(5)	73 ± 9.6	44 ± 12	3.3 ± 1.9

Conclusions:

Osteosclerosis and osteomalacia are prominent characteristics of renal osteodystrophy in the rabbit. They may be influenced by restriction of dietary Ca and P whereas a modest dose of alfacalcidol (1α-OHD_3) has no effect.

References:

1.Rösingh,G.E., James,J. (1969) J.Bone Jt.Surg. 51B:165-174.
2.Tvedegaard,E., Nielsen,M., Kamstrup,O. (1982) Acta path. microbiol. immunol.scand.Sect.A,9o:235-239.
3.Melsen,F., Melsen,B., Mosekilde,L., Bergmann,S. (1978) Acta path. microbiol. immunol.scand.Sect.A,86:7o-81.

BONE HISTOMORPHOMETRIC EVALUATION OF THE ROLE OF BIOCHEMICAL AND HORMONAL FACTORS IN UREMIC PATIENTS.

J.L. SEBERT[1], A. FOURNIER[1], P. FOHRER[1], M.A. HERVE[1], J. GUERIS[2], A. IDRISSI[1], M. GARABEDIAN[3]
1 CHU 80030 AMIENS. 2 Laboratoire de Radio-Immunologie, Hôpital Lariboisière, PARIS. 3 Laboratoire des Tissus Calcifiés, Hôpital des Enfants Malades, PARIS, FRANCE.

The aim of the study was to evaluate the role of various simultaneously measured biochemical and hormonal factors on bone histological parameters in uremic patients.

PATIENTS AND METHODS

20 uremic patients were studied. They had been on chronic hemodialysis (12 patients) or hemofiltration (8 patients) for 28±15 months and had no symptom of bone disease. Aluminium concentration was < .3 μmol/l in the dialysate and ranged from .15 to .60 μmol/l in the substitution fluid for hemofiltration. Oral treatments consisted of aluminium hydroxide in 17 patients with a total cumulative dose of 100-6400 g, 25 OH D3 in 6 (5-30 μg/day), 1 α OH D3 in 2 (1 μg/day).
All patients had an iliac bone biopsy performed after double tetracycline labeling, for histomorphometric analysis. The bone concentration of aluminium was determined on a second bone sample taken during the same biopsy procedure. Aluminium was measured in plasma and bone by inductively coupled plasma emission spectrometry using a JOBIN YVON 38 P elemental analyzer (1). The upper limit of the normal range of plasma aluminium was .3 μmol/l. Normal values for aluminium bone concentration obtained from 7 non uremic corpses were .068 ± (SD) .036 μmol/g of fresh bone tissue. Plasma PTH was measured by radioimmunoassay using an anti serum specific of the mid region of the molecule (normal range : 80 - 220 pg/ml). Vitamin D metabolites were measured by radio competition after previous lipidic extraction of plasma and purification by chromatography on a sephadex LH 20 column followed by a second high pressure liquid chromatography. The normal range was : 6 - 30 ng/ml for 25 (OH) D, 20 - 60 pg/ml for 1.25 (OH)2 D. Statistical methods used a multidimensional analysis combining polynomial evaluation and matricial discriminant analysis (2). This multidimensional analysis leads to the determination of the D2 coefficient of MAHALANOBIS which measures the proper influence on histological parameters of each biochemical factor, independently of the others. The D2 coefficient ranges from - 1 to + 1 according to the sign of the relation.

RESULTS

Bone histology : 8 patients had pure hyperparathyroidism : they had increased active resorption surfaces (ARS) and no evidence of a mineralization defect as shown by normal to high labeled surfaces (Lab.S.) and mineral appositional rate (MAR). 8 patients had increased ARS coupled with decreased MAR. These patients had hyperparathyroidism but low bone formation rates (BFR). The remaining 4 patients had low normal bone resorption and decreased Lab. S. and MAR. Osteoid surfaces were increased in 18 patients but none had increased osteoid thickness. Osteoblastic surfaces (OBL.S.) were strongly correlated with ARS (r=.86), Lab.S. (r=.82), MAR (r=.79) and BFR (r=.79).
Biochemistry : Bone aluminium was increased in all patients with a mean value of .59 ± .44 μmol/g about 10 times higher than in non uremic controls. Plasma Al was increased in 17/20 patients with a mean value of 1.94 ± .44 μmol/l. The mean plasma level of 25 (OH) D was 14.3 ± 11.8 ng/ml and only 5/20 patients had values under the lower limit of the normal range. The 2 patients who were taking 1 α OH D3 had increased levels of 1.25 (OH)2 D. When these 2 patients were excluded, the mean plasma level of 1.25 (OH)2 D was 24.2 ± 17 pg/ml, a value located in the lower part of the normal range. Plasma PTH was increased in all but one patient.
Results of the multidimensional analysis are reported in the table below :

Vitamin D. A Chemical, Biochemical and Clinical Update

Values of the D2 coefficient of MAHALANOBIS showing the influence of biochemical and hormonal factors on bone histology.

	Aluminium		PTH	25 (OH)D	1.25 (OH)2 D	PO4
	Bone	Plasma				
OBL.S.	-.47*	-.62**	.82**	.12	.35	.73**
ARS	.27	.29	.80**	.11	.11	.23
Lab.S.	-.07	-.10	.23	.67**	.82**	.38
MAR	-.39*	-.31	.19	.53**	.80**	.49**
BFR	-.39*	-.32	.20	.29	.41*	.40

The p value of the D2 coefficient is * $p < .05$; ** $p < .01$.

PTH was positively correlated with ARS and OBL.S. which are parameters of bone turn over. In contrast there was no significant correlation between PTH and MAR or BFR. The MAR which reflects the cellular activity of osteoblasts was positively correlated with the D metabolites 25 (OH) D and 1.25 (OH)2 D and with phosphate. Negative relations were found between either plasma or bone aluminium and parameters of bone formation and mineralization.

CONCLUSIONS

These data indicate that in uremic patients on chronic hemodialysis or hemofiltration :
1) Mild aluminium intoxication mainly induced by aluminium hydroxide decreases bone formation.
2) PTH stimulates bone turn over but has no direct effect on the cellular activity of osteoblasts which is mainly dependent on vitamin D metabolites and phosphate.

REFERENCES

1 - ALLAIN P., MAURAS Y. (1979)
Analytical chemistry 51, 2089 - 2091.

2 - LEFEBVRE J. (1983)
Introduction aux analyses multidimensionnelles.
Masson, PARIS.

25-HYDROXYVITAMIN D TREATMENT IN OSTEODYSTROPHIC PATIENTS ON CONTINUOUS AMBULATORY PERITONEAL DIALYSIS (CAPD).

M.L. Bianchi, G. Valenti, L. Soldati, M. Lorenz, S. Giaretto, G. Buccianti - Clinica Medica I - Università di Milano, Italy

Introduction

The effects of CAPD on mineral metabolism are still not completely understood: early reports suggested a good control of calcium-phosphate metabolism (1), but subsequently some worsening of osteodystrophic alterations was observed (2).
The aim of our study was to evaluate the natural evolution of skeletal disease during CAPD and to investigate the results of vitamin D therapy on the main parameters of mineral metabolism in these patients.

Patients

We studied 15 patients (7 females, 8 males; mean age 53±7 yrs) for two years. In the first year, they were treated with CAPD alone; in the second year, 25-OH D_3 was added (100 µg/day). All the patients used the Travenol system for CAPD, with a dialysate calcium concentration of 3.5 mEq/l. Health conditions, diet (.8-1 g/die of calcium) and life habits were unchanged during the study.

Methods

At the beginning and every six months, the following determinations were made: plasma calcium, phosphate and alkaline phosphatase (standard laboratory methods); plasma parathyroid hormone (PTH-COOH and PTH-NH_2) and 1,25$(OH)_2D_3$ with radioimmunolocal assay and 25-OH D_3 with protein-binding assay.
At the beginning and every year, bone mineral content (BMC) was evaluated on the right forearm by direct photon absorptiometry with ^{125}I source.

Results

During the first year, we observed a general worsening on the main indexes (Table I). Calcemia decreased (from 8.7±.3 to 8.2±.3 mg/dl, NS), and both plasma alkaline phosphatase (from 73±11 to 164±42 U/l, $p<.01$) and PTH-COOH (from 1655±226 to 2568±362 pg/ml, $p<.01$) increased significanlty.
The striking decrease of plasma 25-OH D_3 determined the choice of this hormone for the second part of the study.
During the second year, we observed a general improvement of

skeletal conditions, and in particular, 25-OH D_3 reached the lower limits of normal. Plasma calcium increased significantly (to 9.4±.3 mg/dl, $p<.01$), while both alkaline phosphatase (to 46±8 U/l) and PTH-COOH (to 1435±203 pg/ml) decreased significantly ($p<.01$, for both).
Plasma phosphate remained stable throughout the study.

TABLE I

	0 *mo*	12 *mo*	24 *mo*	*p*
$PTH-NH_2$ *(pg/ml)*	347 ±53	468 ±65	302 ±49	<.01
$25(OH)D_3$ *(ng/ml)*	16 ± 2	5.6± 1	26 ± 3	<.01
$1,25(OH)_2D_3$ *(pg/ml)*	18.7± 2	11 ± 1	21.5± 2	<.01
BMC *(mg/cm^2)*	667 ±43	600 ±38	650 ±33	<.01

Conclusions

We think that CAPD alone can achieve a good control of phosphatemia; however, the high loss of protein in the dialysate should be considered at least partially responsible for the falling 25-OH D_3 levels. Our results suggest that CAPD alone seems to have both positive and negative effects on mineral metabolism, and that it cannot control the evolution of renal osteodystrophy (3). 25-OH D_3 therapy can achieve significant results on the metabolic alterations that lead to an increased bone turnover, and effectively controls the osteodystrophic lesions in these patients.

References

1. Gokal,R., Ellis, H.A., Ward, M.K., Kerr,D.N.S.(1980) in CAPD Update, Ed.Masson, New York, p249-251
2. Tielemans,C., Aubry,C., Dratwa,M.(1981) in Advances in Peritoneal Dialysis, Ed.Excerpta Medica, Amsterdam, p455-460
3. Buccianti,G., Bianchi,M.L., Valenti,G.(1984) Clinical Nephr. 22, 279-283

INFLUENCE OF VITAMIN D AND KETO ACIDS (KA) ON 1,25$(OH)_2$D LEVELS IN PATIENTS WITH CHRONIC RENAL FAILURE (rf)

P.T. Fröhling, H.Schmidt-Gayk, F.Kokot, K. Vetter, E.Mayer, K.Lindenau
St. Joseph-Hospital Potsdam, GDR, Academy of Sciences of the GDR, Central Institute of Nutrition, Research Clinic of Nutrition, Potsdam-Rehbrücke, GDR, University of Heidelberg, FRG, Silesian School of Medicine Katowice, Poland.

1,25$(OH)_2$-vitamin D-levels are reduced in advanced chronic renal failure. The results in early renal failure are different. This paper aims at investigating the influence of different therapeutic strategies on the 1,25-$(OH)_2$-D-levels in several stages of chronic renal insufficiency.

Patients and methods: 152 determinations of 1,25$(OH)_2$D levels were made in 105 patients with chronic renal failure with a radioimmunoassay which has been described in detail elsewhere (1).
Determination of c-terminal PTH, intact PTH, calcitonin, 25OHD, calcium and inorganic phosphate were performed simultaneously. Bone histology was available in all patients. In mild renal failure 14 patients were treated with pharmacological doses of vitamin D (20,000 - 80,000 u/day), 11 patients served as control group. In advanced renal failure 74 patients under low protein diet received only vitamin D (0.4 resp. 0.6 g per kg body weight), and in 39 cases a combined treatment with vitamin D and keto acids was performed, 14 patients served as control group.

Results: Figure 1 reveals the serum levels of 1,25$(OH)_2$D in several stages of chronic renal failure under different therapeutic strategies. It can be seen that 1,25$(OH)_2$D is reduced already in mild renal failure. In this stage of renal insufficiency a normalization was achieved by administration of pharmacological doses of Vitamin D. In moderate as well as in severe renal insufficiency 1,25$(OH)_2$D levels were markedly reduced in spite of vitamin D administration, but the levels were significantly lower in the control group. Additional administration of keto acids leads to a slight but significant increase of 1,25$(OH)_2$D.

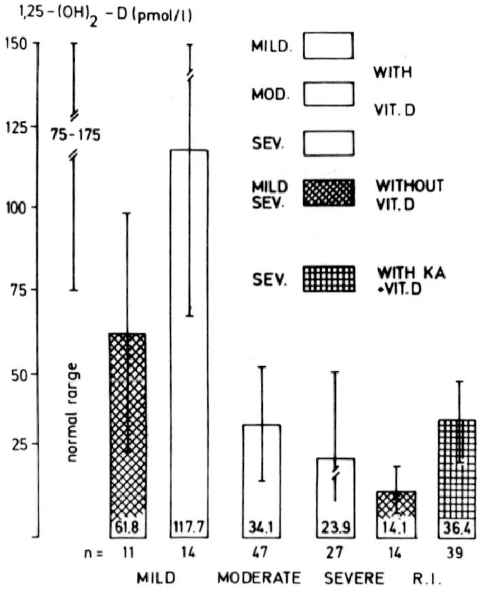

Figure 1: 1,25 $(OH)_2$- VIT.D LEVELS/SERUM IN PATIENTS WITH R.I. ON DIFFERENT THERAPEUTIC STRATEGIES

The influence of vitamin D on the 1,25 $(OH)_2D$ levels was confirmed by the pair-test in 7 cases. A significant increase of 1,25 $(OH)_2D$ was observed after 4 weeks of vitamin D treatment. The effect of keto acids in vitamin D saturated uremic patients is demonstrated by a pair-test of 12 patients. A significant increase of 1,25 $(OH)_2D$ levels could be stated 4 weeks after administration of keto acids combined with a decrease of 25OH-D.

Discussion:
The reduced level of 1,25 $(OH)_2D$ confirm the results of Llach (2). However, higher doses of vitamin D can by themselves normalize this lack combined with "therapeutic" levels of 25-OH-D increase of calcitonin and suppression of PTH (3). The effect of this prophylaxis is underlined by histological investigations (3). In spite of the increasing effect of vitamin D on the 1,25 $(OH)_2D$ levels both in moderate and in advanced renal failure, a marked lack of 1,25 $(OH)_2D$ is present in all patients. Additional administration of keto acids has a further increasing effect of 1,25 $(OH)_2D$ in advanced renal failure. These data explain the histological improvement under the combined treatment with keto acids and vitamin D (4). They also confirm Heidland's hypothesis (5) that keto acids improve the transformation of 25-OH-D to 1,25 $(OH)_2D$. In spite of the therapeutical effect of vitamin D and keto acids on the 1,25 $(OH)_2D$ levels a direct substitution of this metabolite will be necessary in a great number of patients in advanced renal failure.

References

1. Scharla, St., Schmidt-Gayk, H., Reichel, H. and Mayer, E. (1984) clinica Chimica Acata, 142, 325 - 338
2. Llach, F., Wilson, L., Felsenfeld, A. and Dreyner, S.: (1984) Intern.Congress of Nephrol. Abstr.p. 352 A
3. Lindenau, K., Kokot, F., Vetter, K., Hohmann, W.D., Werner, G., Buder, R., Großmann, I. and Fröhling, P.T. (1984) Contr. Nephrol. 37, 66 - 69
4. Fröhling, P!T, Kokot, F., Vetter, K., Hohmann, W.D., Werner, G., Großmann, I., Schmicker, R. and Linenau, K. (1984) Contr.Nephrol. 37, 62-65
5. Heidland, A., Kult, J., Röckel, A. and Hoidbreder (1978) Amer.d.Clin.Nutr. 31, 1784 - 87.

EFFECTS OF DIHYDROXYVITAMIN D3 AND DESFERRIOXAMINE THERAPY ON ALUMINIUM-RELATED OSTEOMALACIA.

P.M. CHAVASSIEUX, S.A. CHARHON and P.J. MEUNIER.
INSERM U. 234, Faculté A. Carrel, rue G. Paradin, Lyon, France.

INTRODUCTION :

Improvement in clinical symptoms and bone histology of dialysis osteomalacia (OM) probably related in several patients to aluminium (Al) overload has been reported after long term therapy with 24,25 dihydroxyvitamin D3 (24,25 D) and 1,25 dihydroxyvitamin D3 (1,25 D) (1). However, the short term effects of this therapy on bone mineralization have not been reported. We studied tetracycline labelled transiliac bone biopsies from 6 dialyzed patients with Al-related OM. Biopsies were taken before treatment and after 6 months of 24,25 D alone or in combination with 1,25 D.* In addition, the effects of desferrioxamine (DFO) therapy on bone histology were studied in two patients who showed no response to vitamin D therapy.

PATIENTS AND METHODS :

- Six hemodialyzed uremic patients (4 females, 2 males), aged 19-57, with Al-related OM were studied. All patients except one were treated in centers using low Al water. All were receiving Al hydroxide orally at daily doses ranging from 2 to 6 grams. One patient received oral calcium supplement. In each patient, a tetracycline labelled transiliac bone biopsy showed evidence of OM on the basis of an increase in the thickness index of the osteoid seams (TIOS : 31.6 ± 11.6 ; controls : 18.5 ± 4.1), a markedly decreased calcification rate and extensive bone Al deposits (Aluminon staining). Within 2 ± 1.3 months after the initial biopsies were performed, 2 patients were given 24,25 D (mean daily dose : 22 µg) and 4 patients received therapy combining 24,25 D and 1,25 D at 3.1 ± 0.7 µg and 0.31 ± 0.07 µg per day respectively. A second biopsy was realized after 6 months of therapy in each patient. Two patients who showed no improvement (one previously given 24,25 D and one given the combined therapy) received intravenous weekly DFO infusions (6 g and 3 g respectively) and combined vitamin D therapy. A third bone biopsy was performed in these 2 patients after 8 and 11 months of therapy respectively.
- The histomorphometric analysis of undecalcified trabecular bone sections was performed according to previously published methods (2,3). The following parameters were measured or calculated : the osteoid volume (OV, percent of trabecular bone volume), the osteoid surfaces (OS, percent of trabecular surfaces), the TIOS i.e. (OV/OS) x 100, the resorption surfaces, the osteoblastic osteoid surfaces (ob.OS, percent of OS covered with osteoblasts), the double labelled osteoid surfaces (DLOS, percent of OS showing tetracycline double labels), the calcification rate (CR, µm/day) and the bone formation rate at the Basic Multicellular level (BFR_{BMU} = DLOS x CR).

RESULTS (figure 1) :

- Patients receiving 24,25 D alone : one patient showed a mild increase in bone mineralization as shown by the reduction of the OV and TIOS values and the increase in the DLOS and BFR values. The other patient showed a complete clinical and histological failure of the therapy.
- Patients receiving 24,25 D + 1,25 D : an increase in DLOS and BFR values was noted in 2 patients. In one, there was a marked improvement of bone fractures. Two patients did not show any change in bone mineralization or in osteoid parameters and one of them developed new fractures.

Vitamin D. A Chemical, Biochemical and Clinical Update

In the 6 patients receiving vitamin D therapy, there was no significant change in Al covered surfaces (68.1 ± 11.7 % before, 71.1 ± 19.6 % after).
- patients given DFO therapy : relief of bone pain and healing of fractures were obtained within a few weeks. The bone biopsies taken under DFO showed a dramatic increase in bone mineralization associated with a marked reduction of OV and TIOS. The extent of the resorption surfaces and osteoblastic osteoid surfaces increased. The Al covered surfaces decreased from 95 % and 82 % before DFO to 8 % and 12 % respectively after DFO.

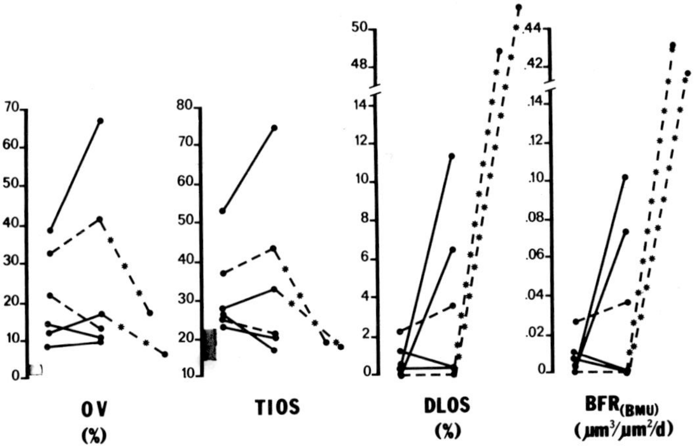

Fig. 1 : Individual values of OV, TIOS, DLOS and BFR(BMU) before and after therapy with 24,25 (•- - -•), 24,25 D + 1,25 D (•——•) or DFO (•-*-*-•).

CONCLUSIONS : 1° a mild increase in bone mineralization was observed in only 3 patients treated with 24,25 D alone or in combination with 1,25 D. 2° this contrasts with the marked improvement in clinical symptoms and bone mineralization obtained under DFO. This increase in bone formation was associated with a marked increase in the number of bone cells (osteoblasts and osteoclasts) and a dramatic reduction of stainable bone Al.

REFERENCES :

1. Hodoman, A.B., Wong, E.G.C., Sherrard, D.J., Brickman, A.S., Miller, N.G., Maloney, N.A. and Coburn, J.W. (1983) Amer. J. Med., 74, 407-414.
2. Meunier, P.J., Edouard, C., Courpron, P. and Toussaint, F. in Vitamin D and problems related to uremic bone disease. Norman A.W. et al (eds), Berlin, Walter de Gruyter, 1975, 149-155.
3. Meunier, P.J., Edouard, C. and Courpron, P. in Bone Histomorphometry, Jaworski ZFG (ed), Ottawa, University of Ottawa Press, 1976, 156-160.
4. Ackrill, P., Day, J.P., Garstang, F.M., Hodge, K.C., Metcalfe, P.J., Benzo, Z., Hill, K., Ralston, A.J., Ball, J. and Denton, J. (1982) Proc. EDTA, 19, 203-207.
5. Malluche, H.H., Smith, A.J., Abreo, K. and Faugere, M.C. (1984) New Engl. J. Med., 311, 140-144.

* 1,25 and 24,25 D were kindly provided by Hoffmann-La Roche, Nutley, USA.

CALCIUM, VITAMIN D AND BONE MINERAL METABOLISM POST-RENAL TRANSPLANTATION

S. EPSTEIN, H. TRABERG, R. McCLINTOCK, R. RAJA, and J. POSER,
Department of Medicine, Albert Einstein Medical Center, and Temple University, Philadelphia, Pennsylvania and Indiana University, Indianapolis, Indiana, and Procter and Gamble Laboratories, Cincinnati, Ohio, U.S.A.

INTRODUCTION

Renal transplantation (TP) is the treatment of choice for most cases of end stage renal failure. Despite normalization of most of the metabolic problems, bone and mineral abnormalities, such as hypercalcemia, hyperparathyroidism and bone disease may persist. We were interested to study parameters of bone metabolism especially levels of bone gla protein and the vitamin D metabolites in patients post-renal transplantation with restored renal function or near normal restored renal function.

PATIENTS AND METHODS

Twenty-three patients, who had had successful renal transplantation were studied. These patients were generally studied two years after transplantation but some were also studied immediately after transplantation at approximately one to two weeks. All the patients were on immunosuppressive therapy with glucocorticoids, immuran and cyclosporin in varying doses either singularly or in combination. No patient was on concomitant vitamin D therapy or calcium supplements. Serum levels of BUN, creatinine, calcium (Ca), phosphate (P), Parathyroid hormone (the carboxyl terminal) fragment (PTH), bone gla protein (BGP), 25(OH)D, $1,25(OH)_2D$ and alkaline phosphatase (AP) were measured from blood collected from the patients. Serum BGP was measured by radioimmunoassay using bovine anti-serum in a dilution of 1-35,000 (1). 25(OH)D and $1,25(OH)_2D$ were measured by competitive protein binding techniques after final separation by HPLC. PTH (the carboxyl terminal) was measured by radioimmunassay using a kit from Immuno Nuclear Corporation.

RESULTS

	PTH ng/ml	BGP ng/ml	25(OH)D ng/ml	$1,25(OH)_2D$ pg/ml	BUN mg/dl	CREAT mg/dl	P mg/dl
Norm.	0.43±.04 N = 20	6.6±2.2 N = 82	33.0±1.9 N = 77	31.0±11.6 N = 47	8-20 N=100	0.7-1.4 N = 100	2.5-4.5 N = 100
Patients	1.90±.31 N = 15	2.7±.34 N = 15	12.8±2.1 N = 23	19.8±3.9 N = 23	31±5 N = 23	1.8±.3 N = 23	2.9±0.3 N = 23
P Value	<.005	<.02	<.005	<.005	<.005	<.002	<.02

N = number of subjects. Mean ± SEM

In the TP patients, it was found that BUN, creatinine and PTH were significantly elevated compared to normal subjects. These figures also include the patients immediately after TP. Serum BGP, 25(OH)D, and $1,25(OH)_2D$ were significantly decreased compared to normal subjects. In the patients who had the worst renal functions (usually those immediately after TP) as judged by the elevated BUN and serum creatinine values, the lowest levels of serum $25(OH)_2D$ and the highest PTH levels were observed. In the TP patients where renal function was stable up to two years after TP, near normal serum levels of 25(OH)D and $1,25(OH)_2D$ values were found.

Vitamin D. A Chemical, Biochemical and Clinical Update

However, even in these patients PTH levels were still elevated and BGP levels were decreased as compared to normal subjects.

CONCLUSIONS

We postulate that the low 1,25 dihydroxyvitamin D levels and high serum PTH values that we observed immediately following TP, probably resulted from poor renal function. However, the results of patients who, up to two years following TP, had persistently low serum 25(OH)D and BGP levels together with elevated PTH, values, possibly reflect the effects of immunosuppressive doses of corticosteroid therapy on bone mineral metabolism (2,3).

REFERENCES

1. Epstein S, Poser J, McClintock R, Johnston Jr. CC, Bryce G, and Hui S. Differences in serum bone gla protein with age and sex. Lancet (1984) 1:307-310.

2. Hahn TJ, Halstead LR, Teitelbaum SL, Hahn BH. Altered mineral metabolism in glucocorticoid-induced osteopenia. J. Clin. Invest. (1979) 64: 655-665.

3. Beresford JN, Gallagher JA, Poser J, Gowen M, Couch M, Yates AJP, Kanis JA, and Russel RGT. Effect of the Anabolic steroid stanazolol on human bone cells in vitro. Calc. Tiss. Intnl. (1983) Calc. Tiss. Intnl. 35:25 p.

PREVENTION OF OSTEODYSTROPHY BY CALCIUM CARBONATE AND NON HYPERCALCEMIC DOSES OF 25 OH VITAMIN D 3 IN PATIENTS WITH MODERATE RENAL FAILURE.

A FOURNIER[1], A IDRISSI[1], JL SEBERT[1], A MARIE[1], J GUERIS[2], M GARABEDIAN[3] -
(1) CHU AMIENS - (2) Hôpital Lariboisière PARIS - (3) Hôpital Necker PARIS -

INTRODUCTION : It is logical to prevent osteodystrophy as soon as the first histological abnormalities occur i.e. when GFR is reduced by half(1). Whereas MASSRY et al(2)have reported promising results with 1.25(OH)2 D without phosphate binder or calcium supplement in the prevention of renal osteodystrophy because 1.25(OH)D did improve bone histology without worsening GFR, other investigators(1)have stressed the point that the efficency of 1α hydroxylated vitamin D metabolites on bone disease may be obtained at the price of a more rapid decline of GFR because of hypercalcemia and/or hyperphosphatemia. Because of these controversies, we report here an other approach of osteodystrophy prevention based on diary product restriction and an oral supplement of 3 g of $CaCO_3$ and of 25 OH vitamin D at non hypercalcemic doses(10-50 μg/d) in uremic patients with a creatinine clearance between 40-15 ml/mn.

PATIENTS AND METHODS : 21 uremic patients were included in the study. The treatment consisted in diary product restriction, a supplement of 3 g of $CaCO_3$ and a supplement of 25OH D3 at the dose of 10 μg in 13 patients(group I)in order to prevent vitamin D depletion induced by the diary product restriction or 25 μg in 6 patients and even 50 μg/d in 2 patients(with a plasma calcium below 2.25 mmol/l)(group II). None has taken $Al(OH)_3$ or other aluminium containing phosphate binder. Blood and urine phosphocalcic parameters were measured every 3 months 4 times before starting the treatment and then at least 4 times in all patients and 8 times in 17 of them. Furthermore, 12 patients had 2 successive bone biopsies at a mean interval of 15 ± 5 months after double tetracycline labeling.

RESULTS : Table I shows that plasma concentrations of 25 OH D and 24.25(OH)2 D significantly increased whereas the increase in P.I.25(OH)2 D was not significant. C Terminal PTH increased slightly after the first year whereas alkaline phosphatases decreased significantly as soon as the first year. Plasma calcium remained stable throughout the study at a low normal level. Plsma phosphate significantly increased after the first year as did plasma creatinine. However the slope of 1./PCr did not increase but rather decreased suggesting a slower decline of GFR. Plasma concentration of bicarbonate remained stable at low normal levels(25.5 mmol/l). Calciuria significantly increased whereas the rise in Tm PO4/GFR was not significant.

TABLE I : EVOLUTION OF THE BIOCHEMICAL PARAMETERS (*p < .05 versus control)

Mean ± SD	NORMAL	control (n=21)	FIRST YEAR (n=21)	SECOND YEAR (n=17)
P 25 OH D nmol/l	50±17	34±20	75±50*	
P 24.25(OH)2 D nmol/l	2.5-7.5	3.5±4	6.5±5*	
P 1.25(OH)2 D pmol/l	50-150	84±40	100±40	
P PTH pg/ml	20-45	138±60	132±60	179±60
Alk Pose IU	70-170	148±60	110±50*	112±50*
P calcium mmol/l	2.25-2.62	2.34±.01	2.34±.01	2.34±.01
P Phosphate mmol	0.64-1.3	1.13±.35	1.30±.3	1.45±.22*
P Creatinine μmol/l	71-115	300±100	370±100	440±180*
Slope of 1/PCr (1)	0	50.10-4	30.10^{-4}	30.10 4
P Bicarbonate mmol	24-29	25.5±4	25.5±5	25.5±4
U Ca/U Cr mmol/mmol		0.11±.03	0.16±.04	0.22±.06
Tm PO4/GFR mmol/l	0.8-1.3	0.6±.2	0.69±.16	0.70±.20

(1) The slope is calculated as in MITCH's paper (3) with an ordinate unit of 0.01 dl/mg and an equal abcissa unit of 1 month.

Table II shows that the initially increased osteoid volume significantly decreased. The decrease in the initially increased osteoid surface was however not significant. The osteoid seam thickness was always normal. The osteoblastic surface initially normal, decreased significantly whereas the decrease of the initially increased active resorption surface was not significant. The initially normal mineral apposition rate remained stable.

Comparison of the 2 therapeutic groups shows that they were always comparable at the exception of their alkaline phosphatase which was initially higher(180 versus 120 IU)and decreased significantly more (-20 versus -14 IU) in group II, and of their increase in P 25 OH D(+75 vs +19 nmol/l)and in P 24.25(+4.8 vs +1 nmol/l)which were greater in group II. Bone X rays were normal throughout the study. In only 1 patient with coronary heart disease did a 5 mm calcification appear on the abdominal aorta.

TABLE II : EVOLUTION OF BONE HISTOLOGY (n = 12 ; *p < .05 versus control)

Mean ± SD	NORMAL	FIRST BIOPSY	SECOND BIOPSY
Trabecular bone volume % total volume	21±5	28±8	25±5
Osteoid volume % TBV	2.5±1	5.3±3	2.8±3*
Osteoid surface % T trabecular S	13±6	39±20	23±10
Osteoid seam thickness µ	6±0.5	7±3	5±3
Osteoblastic surface % TTS	2±1	2.1±2	1±1*
Active resorption surface % TTS	0.5±0.5	2.9±2	2.1±2
Mineral apposition rate µ/day	0.5±0.1	0.48±0.1	0.45±.01

CONCLUSIONS : 1/ Restriction of diary product in association with an oral supplement of 3g of CaCO3 and of non hypercalcemic doses of 25(OH) vitamin D3 represent effective measures for the prevention of hyperparathyroidism worsening in spite of the relentless progression of renal failure. As a matter of fact, in spite of slight increase in the plasma concentration of C Terminal PTH(explained by the reduced capacity of the catabolism of these inactive fragments), the biological indices of PTH activity decreased(significant decrease in alkaline phosphatase, osteoblastic surface and osteoid volume)or did not increase(active resorption surface). 2/ These measures are safe since the speed of GFR decline is rather slowed down. 3/ These measures are able to prevent also osteomalacia since the osteoid seam thickness and mineral apposition rate remain normal.

4/ Metabolic acidosis is also prevented since the plasma concentration of bicarbonate remain normal in spite of the decrease in GFR.

5/ Comparatively to the study of MASSRY et al with 1.25(OH)2 D3, our results are less good. However our results have been obtained with a plasma calcium concentration of 2.34 mmol/l whereas a mean concentration of 2.62 was obtained in MASSRY's study. These higher plasma concentrations of calcium and the use of 1α hydroxylated vitamin D metabolites may however be hazardous for the vessels since at non hypercalcemic doses 1α OH vitamin D3 has been reported to increase the calcium content of the aorta of uremic rabbits(4)and since plasma calcium has been found to be a risk factor of vascular calcification in hemodialyzed patients (5). Furthermore according to other authors (1)it is questionable to be able to control plasma phosphate below 1.5 mmol/l when GFR decrease below 20 ml/mn without Al(OH)3 administration and its hazards of aluminium intoxication, when no CaCO3 but 1α hydroxylated D3 metabolite is given. Therefore we suggest that oral CaCO3 and 1α hydroxylated vitamin D should be compared in the prevention of renal osteodystrophy at the same level of "normal" calcemia i.e. 2.5 mmol/l.

REFERENCES :

(1) FOURNIER A, BOUDAILLIEZ B, TOLANI M, MORINIERE P, SEBERT JL - 1984 in Vitamin D et maladies des os et du métabolisme minéral - Edited by FOURNIER A, GARABEDIAN M, SEBERT JL, MEUNIER P - MASSON - PARIS - p 171-246.

(2) MASSRY WE, GRUBER H, ARIF SR, SHERMAN O, GOLDSTEIN DA, LETTERI JM - 1983 in Clinical Disorders of Bone and Mineral Metabolism - Edited by FRAME B, POTTS M, Excerpta Medica New York - p 260-265.

(3) MITCH WE, WALSER M, BUFFINGTON GA, LEMANN JJ - 1976 - LANCET - ii - 1326-1328.

(4) TVEDEGAARD E, LADEFOGED O, NIELSEN M, KRAMSTRUP O - 1983 - NEPHRON, 34, 185-191.

(5) RENAUD H, ATIK A, HERVE M, MORINIERE P, FOURNIER A - 1985 - ARCH. MAL. COEUR - (in press).

HUMAN BONE CELL METABOLISM OF 25(OH)D_3 IN CHRONIC RENAL FAILURE: EFFECT OF SURFACE BONE ALUMINUM.

D.L. Andress, G.A. Howard, D.B. Endres, D.J. Sherrard, Department of Medicine, University of Washington and Veterans Administration Medical Centers, Seattle, WA and Tacoma, WA.

Introduction

The accumulation of aluminum on the surface of mineralized bone in patients with chronic renal failure is associated with abnormally low bone formation rates (1). Many such patients also have relatively low random serum parathyroid hormone (PTH) levels (1) or PTH levels that do not respond to a hypocalcemic stimulus (2). In addition, bone-surface aluminum accumulation is increased after parathyroidectomy (3). While hypoparathyroidism seems to be an important factor in the pathogenesis of aluminum bone disease in humans, the effect of aluminum on bone cell function has not been completely evaluated. Recent studies using chick calvarial cells (4) and mouse fibroblasts (5) grown in culture have shown that aluminum affects cell mitosis in a biphasic manner; mitosis is enhanced at low levels of aluminum in the growth medium and decreased at higher concentrations. In addition, metabolism of ^{3}H-25(OH)D_3 in chick calvarial cells is inhibited at high aluminum concentrations (4). Whether aluminum has similar effects on bone cell function in humans has not been determined. The purpose of the present study was to determine if aluminum on the bone surface is associated with changes in bone cell metabolism of 1,25(OH)$_2D_3$ in humans and whether bone formation correlated with bone cell production of 1,25(OH)$_2D_3$.

Patients and Methods

Twenty patients with chronic renal failure on hemodialysis were studied. Four patients had received a prior parathyroidectomy and one patient had insulin-dependent diabetes mellitus. All were asymptomatic for bone disease at the time of the study. Each underwent an iliac crest bone biopsy after double tetracycline labeling. The bone samples were analyzed for bone-surface aluminum (as % of the total surface), osteoid area (as % of the total bone area) and bone formation rate. From a separate bone specimen, bone cells were released by enzymatic digestion with collagenase for 2 hours at 37 C. The cells were then washed and incubated with 10 nM ^{3}H-25(OH)D_3 for one hour at 37 C. The vitamin D metabolites were extracted from the aqueous phase with dichloromethane and identified using high performance liquid chromatography. The quantity of ^{3}H-1,25(OH)$_2D_3$ and ^{3}H-24,25(OH)$_2D_3$ was determined by scintillation spectrometry. Plasma was available for determination of calcium and phosphorus in all 20 patients and for intact-PTH, aluminum and 1,25(OH)$_2D_3$ in 18 of the patients.

Results

The comparisons of bone histology and bone cell production of 1,25(OH)$_2D_3$ are displayed in Table 1. Additionally, direct correlations were noted between serum PTH and bone formation ($r=.70$, $p<.01$) and between bone cell production of 1,25(OH)$_2D_3$ and 24,25(OH)$_2D_3$ ($r=.58$, $p<.01$). There were no correlations between bone cell production of 1,25(OH)$_2D_3$ and serum calcium, phosphorus, PTH, 1,25(OH)$_2D_3$ or aluminum. Bone formation was not significantly correlated with osteoid area ($r=.41$, $p<0.1$). There were no correlations of bone cell production of 24,25(OH)$_2D_3$ with any of the serum or bone histologic parameters.

Vitamin D. A Chemical, Biochemical and Clinical Update

TABLE 1. Correlation Coefficients of Comparisons of Bone Histologic Parameters and Bone Cell Production of $1,25(OH)_2D_3$

Bone Parameters		r	p value
1. Bone formation vs. bone-surface aluminum	A*	-.56	< .01
	B+	-.63	< .01
2. Bone-surface aluminum vs. bone cell production of $1,25(OH)_2D_3$	A	+.46	< .05
	B	+.52	< .05
3. Bone cell production of $1,25(OH)_2D_3$ vs. bone formation	A	-.46	< .05
	B	-.67	< .01
4. Osteoid area vs. bone cell production of $1,25(OH)_2D_3$	A	-.27	NS
	B	-.57	< .05

A* indicates all patients; B+ indicates that 5 patients have been excluded (4 with parathyroidectomy and 1 with diabetes mellitus)

Conclusions

These date suggest that bone-surface aluminum may result in increased bone cell production of $1,25(OH)_2D_3$. These findings appear to contradict studies of chick calvarial cells grown in culture in which bone cell production of $1,25(OH)_2D_3$ is decreased after incubation with high concentrations of aluminum (4). One possible explanation for the discrepant findings may relate to the absolute concentrations of aluminum. In general, the bone aluminum content in patients with aluminum bone disease (1) is lower than the concentrations used in the in vitro studies (4). Thus, it is possible that bone cell production of $1,25(OH)_2D_3$ is stimulated by low aluminum levels but inhibited at higher concentrations. It is also possible that the measurement of $1,25(OH)_2D_3$ metabolism in human biopsy specimens might still be influenced by factors within the bone microenvironment which are not encountered in tissue culture conditions. Finally, differences in species response to aluminum may also be operative. It is intriguing to suggest that the enhanced bone cell production of $1,25(OH)_2D_3$ might in part be responsible for the decreased bone formation by inhibiting osteoid synthesis. Incubation studies of $1,25(OH)_2D_3$ with cultured bone cells have shown an inhibitory effect on collagen synthesis (6). The importance of PTH in uremic bone disease (3), however, should not be ignored since bone formation directly correlates with circulating PTH. Thus, alternatively, bone cell production of $1,25(OH)_2D_3$ may be a secondary response to the PTH induced decline in bone formation. In vitro studies with cultured human bone cells may help resolve this issue.

References

1. Ott S.M., Maloney N.A., Coburn J.W., Alfrey A.C., Sherrard D.J. (1982) N. Engl. J. Med. 307:709-13.
2. Andress D.L., Felsenfeld A.J., Voigts A., Llach F. (1983) Kidney Int. 24:364-73.
3. Andress D.L., Ott S.M., Maloney N.A., Sherrard D.J. (1985) N. Engl. J. Med. 312:468-73.
4. Howard G.A. (1984) Calcif. Tiss. Int. 36:A13(abstract)
5. Smith J.B. (1984) J. Cell. Physiol. 118:298-304.
6. Raisz L.G., Maina D.M., Sworek S.C., Dietrich J.W., Canalis E.M. (1978) Endocrinology 102:731-35.

1,25-$(OH)_2D_3$ AND 24,25-$(OH)_2D_3$ IN RENAL OSTEODYSTROPHY OF THE RAT.

H.A.P.Pols, D.H.Birkenhäger-Frenkel, P.Derkx, J.J.Eygelsheim, E.E.Zijlstra, E.C.G.M.Clermonts and J.C.Birkenhäger.
Dept. of Internal Medicine III and Dept. of Pathology I, Erasmus University Rotterdam, The Netherlands.

INTRODUCTION. Previous studies (1) suggest that only the combination of 1,25-$(OH)_2D_3$ with 24,25-$(OH)_2D_3$ is adequate to restore mineralization in nutrional osteomalacia. Other studies also point to an anabolic effect of 24,25-$(OH)_2D_3$ on bone (2). In order to test the possible additive effect of 24,25-$(OH)_2D_3$ in the treatment of renal osteodystrophy, we studied the effect of both dihydroxy-D metabolites in rats with sulphacetylthiazol (SAT)-induced renal failure (3).

MATERIALS AND METHODS. Male Wistar rats (300-350 g) were maintained on normal laboratory chow (Ca: 0.8%; P: 0.4%). SAT 0.1 g/kg bodyweight (BW) was injected i.p. twice a week for 1 month. For the following 3 weeks the rats were randomly divided into 3 groups and treated with vehiculum (group I), 1,25-$(OH)_2D_3$ 10 ng/kg BW daily s.c. (group II) or 1,25-$(OH)_2D_3$ 10 ng/kg BW daily s.c. plus twice a week 24,25-$(OH)_2D_3$ 200 ng i.p. (group III). Treatment with SAT was continued twice a week 0.05g/kg BW i.p. At the end of the experimental period the animals were sacrificed. BUN and serum Ca, P, creatinine, alkaline phosphatase (Technicon-autoanalyser) and immunoreactive (i)PTH (I.N.C.) were determined. Histomorphometric measurements were done in 5 μm sections of femoral metaphyses (4). Statistics: Mann Whitney test.

RESULTS AND DISCUSSION.

Table IA: Bodyweight and serum chemistry.

Group	I (n=8)	II (n=8)	III (n=8)
serum chemistry:			
Ca (mM)	2.78± 0.04	3.53± 0.07^a	3.53± 0.06^a
P (mM)	2.27± 0.14	2.65± 0.12^b	3.01± 0.12^{a,c}
alk. phosph. (U/l)	95 ± 3.6	82 ± 8.9	76 ± 2.2^a
BUN (mM)	42.4 ± 4.2	39.0 ± 4.2	50.9 ± 6.1
creatinine (μM)	180 ±14	195 ±18	229 ±19^a
iPTH (pM)	141 ±13	144 ±22	101 ± 5^{a,c}

Table IB: Quantitative histology of metaphyseal sections.

Group	I (n=8)	II (n=8)	III (n=8)
max.metaphyseal outer diameter (mm)	4.10±0.14	4.47±0.10^a	4.91±0.09^{a,c}
cortical area (D^2-d^2)	6.6 ±0.3	7.9 ±0.7^a	8.7 ±0.6^a
osteoblast seams (%)	8.9 ±2.6	40.7 ±7.8^a	47.9 ±5.0^a
osteoid seams (%)	44.4 ±2.6	67.3 ±7.1^a	67.8 ±5.4^a
rel.osteoid vol.(%)	14.9 ±5.6	21.0 ±5.1	22.6 ±3.8
rel.osteobl.act. (%)	17.8 ±3.7	55.8 ±8.0^a	70.6 ±3.5^{a,c}
osteoclast (n/mm^2)	3.45±0.59	0.98±0.16^a	1.45±0.11^a

a) diff. from group I $p<0.01$; b) from group I $p<0.05$; c) from group II $p<0.05$.

Vitamin D. A Chemical, Biochemical and Clinical Update

The serum chemistry and histomorphometric results, obtained after 3 weeks treatment with vehiculum (group I), 1,25-(OH)$_2$D$_3$ (group II) and 1,25-(OH)$_2$D$_3$ plus 24,25-(OH)$_2$D$_3$ are summarized in Table I. In both treated groups there was a marked increase in serum Ca and P accompanied by an increase in osteoblast seams %, osteoid seams % and relative osteoblast activity. Although these observations indicate a stimulation of bone formation (at the metaphyseal endosteum), this represent not necessarily a direct effect of the D metabolite(s) on bone. The significant correlations (for the 3 groups together) between serum Ca and O.Bl% ($r=0.57$; $p<0.01$) and between serum P and O.Bl% ($r=0.62$; $p<0.01$) suggest that the improvements might be attributed to the calcemic and/or phosphatemic effects. Additional treatment with 24,25-(OH)$_2$D$_3$ led to a greater increase of the maximum metaphyseal outer diameter than treatment with 1,25-(OH)$_2$D$_3$ alone. Because we have no histomorphometric data at the periosteum it is possible, that this is due to an increase in periosteal bone formation. Further studies of a possible variability of effects of vit.D derivatives at different bone formation sites are necessary. Changes due to hyperparathyroidism (increase in osteoclast number) were only moderate in this study. Although treatment resulted in a decrease in osteoclast number, this was not related to a decrease in iPTH. We want to emphasize that in the control group we found a high serum Ca and a low serum iPTH relative to the severity of the renal insufficiency. It is possible that SAT, used to induce azotemia also has a direct effect on Ca homeostasis. Still, we found a significant decline of iPTH in the group treated with 1,25- plus 24,25-(OH)$_2$D$_3$, which was independent of the changes in serum Ca.

REFERENCES

1. Bordier,P.A., Rasmussen,H., Marie,P., Muravet,L., Gueris,J., Ryckwaert,A.(1978) J.Clin.Endocrinol.Metab. 46,284-294.
2. Kanis,J.A.,Cundy,T., Earnshaw,M., Henderson,R.G., Heynen,G., Naik,R., Russell,R.G.G., Smith,R., Woods,C.G.(1979) Quart. J.Med. 48,289-322.
3. Okano,K., Fujita,T., Oruno,H., Yoshikawa,M.(1972) Endocrinol. Japon. 19,277-283.
4. Birkenhäger-Frenkel,D.H., Clermonts,E.C.G.M., Richter,H. (1981) In: Bone histomorphometry (3rd Internat. Workshop, Sun Valley 1980), pp 453-457.

OSTEODYSTROPHY IN PATIENTS RECEIVING DIALYSIS FOR CHRONIC RENAL FAILURE: A CROSS SECTIONAL STUDY.

Y.L. Chan, T.J. Furlong, C.J. Cornish, S. Posen. Departments of Endocrinology and Renal Medicine, Royal North Shore Hospital, St. Leonards, NSW 2065, Australia.

Clinical, biochemical, radiological and histological studies were performed in 94 patients receiving dialysis for chronic renal failure in one unit over a six months' period. An attempt was made to correlate the various findings to one another and, in particular, the results of non-invasive tests to the histological lesions.

PATIENTS AND METHODS

Ninety-four (of a total of 120) patients gave informed consent for an iliac crest trephine biopsy. These patients were asked specific questions concerning pruritus, weakness and pain and they underwent a physical examination. Biochemical tests included the estimation of serum immunoreactive parathyroid hormone (iPTH) and 3 vitamin D metabolites. Radiological tests consisted of 5 standard films (chest, skull, hand, pelvis and lumbar spine). Dynamic bone histomorphometry was performed according to the method of Evans et al. (1).

RESULTS

"Skeletal" symptoms were present in 48 patients (51%) and physical signs in 21 (22%). Symptoms and signs (as well as age and sex) were of no value in predicting biochemical, radiological or histological findings. The duration of dialysis was positively correlated with total bone area, fractional osteoid area and fractional osteoid surface ($p<0.001$ for each parameter) and negatively with the mean appositional rate ($p<0.01$).

Serum alkaline phosphatase and iPTH were positively correlated with each other ($p<0.001$) and both were positively correlated with fractional osteoblastic surfaces, fractional resorption surfaces, osteoclast densities and fractional fibrous areas ($p<0.001$ for each histological parameter). The serum concentrations of 3 vitamin D metabolites (25OHD, $24,25(OH)_2D$ and $1,25(OH)_2D$) could not be correlated with any other biochemical, radiological or histological parameter. Serum 25OHD was higher in hemodialyzed than in normal subjects (Table 1) or in peritoneally dialyzed patients (see Furlong et al., this volume).

Subperiosteal erosions were predictive of severe histological parathyroid osteopathy ($p<0.001$) but this radiological sign was absent in 66% of patients with histological hyperparathyroidism. Generalized osteosclerosis was associated with an increase in fractional osteoid surfaces ($p<0.001$) but this radiological sign was absent in 87% of patients with histo-

Vitamin D. A Chemical, Biochemical and Clinical Update

logical osteomalacia. Vascular calcification showed only a weak correlation with hypercalcemia ($p<0.05$) but was not correlated with any other parameter.

Skeletal histology was abnormal in each case. Hyperparathyroidism was present as the only abnormality in 18 (19%), osteomalacia in 26 (28%) and mixed lesions in 50 (53%). There were no reliable parameters to predict the presence or severity of osteomalacia.

TABLE 1

SELECTED SERUM AND SKELETAL PARAMETERS

	Normals (n=38)	Dialysis patients (n=94)	p value
Calcium (mmol/l)	2.39±0.11	2.54±0.25	<0.001
Inorganic PO_4 (mmol/l)	1.06±0.16	1.55±0.48	<0.001
Alk. Phosphatase (U/L)	45±15	193±250	<0.001
25OHD (nmol/l)	70.0±29.6	87.5±48.0	<0.02
$24,25(OH)_2D$ (nmol/l)	7.1±3.5 (n=37)	1.5±0.98 (n=27)	<0.001
$1,25(OH)_2D$ (pmol/l)	89.3±38.0 (n=47)	17.0±12.0 (n=28)	<0.001
Immunoreactive PTH (ng/ml)	0.15±0.12	3.19±2.79	<0.001
Total trabecular area	24.6±2.8 (n=8)	33.9±10.9	<0.02
Fractional osteoid area	0.5±0.3 (n=8)	5.5±4.8	<0.01
Fractional osteoid surface	12.0±5.1 (n=8)	69.2±18.7	<0.001
Fractional resorption surface	1.7±0.5 (n=8)	5.2±4.3	<0.05
Osteoclast density	0.4±0.1 (n=8)	1.9±1.7	<0.05
Bone aluminum* (ng/mg dry weight)	<3 (n=8)	63.3±40.1	

* Performed in the laboratory of Dr. A. Alfrey

1. Evans, R.A., Dunstan, C.R., Baylink, D.J. Miner. Electrolyte Metab. 2: 179-185, 1979.

FACTORS GOVERNING CALCIUM ABSORPTION AND SERUM 1,25 DIHYDROXYVITAMIN D IN CHRONIC RENAL FAILURE

B E C Nordin* H A Morris** M Cochran+ A R Clarkson*
H Healey* T F Hartley**
* Departments of Endocrinology and Renal Medicine, Royal Adelaide Hospital, Adelaide, South Australia
** Division of Clinical Chemistry, Institute of Medical & Veterinary Science, Adelaide, South Australia
\+ Department of Renal Medicine, Flinders Medical Centre, Adelaide, South Australia

Introduction

Malabsorption of calcium is a well recognised feature of renal insufficiency usually attributed to low serum concentrations of $1,25(OH)_2D$. The latter is normally attributed to a reduction in its production by the kidney associated with renal insufficiency. In this paper, we show that hyperphosphataemia also contributes independently to calcium malabsorption in renal failure. In addition, the serum $1,25(OH)_2D$ level is determined not only by the degree of renal failure but also by the plasma phosphate and serum 25OHD levels.

Clinical Material and Methods

The series comprises 19 adult men and 27 women aged 21-82 years with varying degrees of renal insufficiency but none of them on dialysis.

Radiocalcium absorption was measured by administering 5 μC of Ca^{45} in 20 mg of calcium carrier as the chloride in 250 ml of water and taking a plasma sample 60 minutes later for the measurement of radioactivity. After correction for body weight, the result was expressed as the fraction of radiocalcium absorbed per hour by reading off a calibration curve (1). Serum $1,25(OH)_2D$ was measured by radioimmunoassay after HPLC separation (2) and serum 25OHD by competitive protein binding after LH 20 separation (3). Serum parathyroid hormone was measured by a commercial C-terminal radioimmunoassay. Plasma phosphate, creatinine and bicarbonate were measured by multichannel analyzer. All measurements were performed on fasting samples.

Results

The mean values of the measured variables are shown in the Table. Plasma phosphate and creatinine were significantly elevated, as was the serum PTH. Radiocalcium absorption (α) serum $1,25(OH)_2D$ and plasma bicarbonate were all significantly reduced. The mean serum 25OHD level was normal.

Vitamin D. A Chemical, Biochemical and Clinical Update

TABLE: MEAN VALUES OF MEASURED VARIABLES (SE)

Ca	P	Cr	HCO_3	α	25OHD	$1,25(OH)_2D$	PTH
--------- mmol/l			--------		nmol/l	pmol/l	pmol/l
2.35	1.24	.32	24.1	.41	72	49	219
(.03)	(.06)	(.03)	(.7)	(.05)	(4)	(4)	(24)

Univariate regression analysis showed that α was a significant negative function of plasma phosphate ($p<.001$), of plasma creatinine ($p<.01$) and of PTH ($p<.05$). α was significantly positively related to serum $1,25(OH)_2D$ ($p<.001$) and to plasma bicarbonate ($p<.001$). It was not related to the serum level of 25OHD. Serum $1,25(OH)_2D$ was a significant negative function of plasma phosphate ($p<.001$) and was not significantly related to the plasma PTH level. It was a significant positive function of the reciprocal of plasma creatinine ($p<.01$), of plasma bicarbonate ($p<.05$) and of plasma 25OHD ($p<.05$).

Multiple regression analysis showed that the main determinant of α was the plasma phosphate concentration to which it was negatively related ($r = .64; p<.001$). When serum $1,25(OH)_2D$ was added to the regression analysis, multiple R became 0.67, although the contribution of serum $1,25(OH)_2D$ was not in itself significant.

Multiple regression analysis to establish the determinants of the plasma $1,25(OH)_2D$ level gave the highest multiple R value when the following three independent variables were included: Reciprocal of plasma creatinine ($t = 1.4$), serum 25OHD ($t = 1.5$) and reciprocal of plasma phosphate ($t = 1.2$). Although none of these three contributions was in itself significant, the combination of the three produced a multiple R of .51 ($p<.001$).

Conclusions

The main determinant of radiocalcium absorption in renal insufficiency is the plasma phosphate concentration; the serum $1,25(OH)_2D$ level is of much less importance. The explanation may be that the calcium load is trapped in the intestine by the high digestive juice phosphate. The low serum $1,25(OH)_2D$ levels in renal insufficiency are only partly accounted for by the loss of renal tissue; hyperphosphataemia and low serum 25OHD levels in some cases are of comparable importance.

References

1. Marshall, D.H., Nordin, B.E.C. (1981) Clin. Sci. 61:477-481
2. Taylor, G.A., Peacock, M., Pelc, B., Brown, W., Holmes, A. (1980) Clin. Chim. Acta. 108:239-246
3. Edelstein, A., Charman, M., Lawson, B.E.M., Kodicek, E. (1974) Clin. Sci. Mol. Med. 46:231-240

Osteoporosis

A COMPARISON OF THE EFFECTS OF CALCITRIOL OR CALCIUM SUPPLEMENTS ON BONE IN POSTMENOPAUSAL OSTEOPOROSIS

J.C. GALLAGHER AND R.R. RECKER,
Creighton University Medical School, Omaha, NE 68131 U.S.A.

Introduction:

Although postmenopausal osteoporosis is a heterogeneous condition, two of the more common findings in osteoporotics are, first, malabsorption of calcium and second, low bone turnover as defined by bone histomorphometry and tetracycline dynamics. Whether these are related findings in the same patient or independent changes has never been established, and whether they share a common mechanism is open to speculation. One hypothesis is that reduced levels of parathyroid hormone in osteoporotics lead secondarily to decreased levels of serum 1,25 dihydroxyvitamin D (1-3) and subsequent impairment in calcium absorption (4-6). Although there is good evidence that these hormonal abnormalities are associated with impaired calcium absorption, there is little evidence that these changes are the cause of low bone turnover in osteoporosis. Circumstancial evidence suggests, however, that parathyroid hormone is important in maintaining high remodelling rates in bone. In patients with primary hyperparathyroidism, bone remodelling is higher than average, whereas in hypoparathyroidism bone remodelling is reduced. In patients with primary hyperparathyroidism both serum parathyroid hormone and 1,25 dihydroxyvitamin D levels are elevated, but it is not clear whether one or both of the elevated hormones play independent or permissive roles in bone remodelling. The evidence for a direct action on calcitriol on bone in man has not yet been established. Certainly in tissue culture systems, calcitriol can be shown to have a direct effect on bone cells. Although it is a potent agent in inducing bone resorption in cell culture lines, there is also evidence for stimulation of osteoblastic activity (7) and the formation of GLA protein (8), a possible marker of bone turnover.

Methods:

Ten patients with postmenopausal osteoporosis who had two or more vertebral fractures were treated with high doses of calcitriol, the dose ranged from 1.5 to 2 mcg/daily and was given in divided doses, twelve hours apart. In addition the calcium intake was restricted to 500 mg/day so as to avoid any possibility of the development of hypercalemia or hypercalcuria. We had shown previously that calcium absorption was positively correlated with serum 1,25 dihydroxyvitamin D levels (1). Also, in order to examine the effect of calcitriol on calcium absorption we measured urine calcium excretion and expressed it as a fraction of the calcium intake. We found a dose dependent increase in urine calcium with increasing doses of calcitriol. On a dose of calcitriol, 0.25 mcg twice daily,

Vitamin D. A Chemical, Biochemical and Clinical Update

we found that thirty percent of the calcium intake was excreted in the urine, on Ø.5 mcg twice daily, fifty percent of the calcium intake was excreted in the urine, and on 1.Ø mcg twice daily we found seventy-five percent of the calcium intake was excreted in the urine (9). Thus, on a calcium intake of 4ØØ-5ØØ mg/day one could predict that the urine calcium would not exceed 3ØØ mg. Ten patients were started on the protocol, after undergoing initial bone biopsies with Tetracycline labelling. In one patient the baseline biopsy was unsatisfactory for analysis. At the end of 4-6 months on high dose calcitriol therapy, repeat biopsies were obtained in all patients. It should be noted that the second biopsy was taken from the iliac creast on the opposite side from that of the first biopsy. Five patients were then crossed over to calcium supplements and one patient to estrogen; after three-four months on calcium or estrogen, a third bone biopsy was performed.

Results:

A summary of the initial and final biochemical changes in the patients treated with high-dose calcitriol and a restricted calcium intake is given in Table 1 below.

The results show that serum calcitriol levels doubled, urine calcium excretion increased, serum calcium rose and serum parathyroid hormone levels were suppressed, all of these changes were significant. There was no significant change in urine hydroxyproline excretion which is an independent marker of bone resorption.

Table 1:

Biochemical Changes: Pre- and Post-Calcitriol Therapy

	Baseline	4-6 Months
Serum Calcium mg.dl	9.36 ± Ø.19	1Ø.1Ø ± Ø.21*
24 Hr Urine Calcium .mg	91 ± 25	257 ± 31*
24 Hr Hydroxyproline/ Creatinine Ratio	Ø.Ø28 ± Ø. ØØ4	Ø.Ø24 ± Ø.ØØ2
Serum PTH ul.eg.ml	8.61 ± 2.14	4.Ø3 ± Ø.86*
Serum 1,25 dihydroxy D3 pg.ml	26.87 ± 4.2	68.88 ± 6.9*

* $p < Ø.Ø1$

Analysis of bone histomorphometry showed that there was a significant increase in mean double tetracycline labels in patients treated with high dose calcitriol. Seven of the patients showed a clear increase in tetracycline labels and two patients showed a small decrease. When patients were crossed over to calcium or estrogen, there was a decrease in tetracycline labels in five of the six patients. The percent of trabecular surfaces covered with osteoid generally showed a mean increase, although in one patient there was a striking decrease. (In this particular patient the percent of trabecular surface covered by osteoid was forty percent on the initial biopsy.) On crossing over to calcium or estrogen the percent of osteoid covered surfaces decreased. The percent resorption surfaces showed no significant change on calcitriol, however, on calcium supplements all patients showed a decrease in resorption activity. With regard to the dynamic measurements of bone turnover, we found that the bone formation rate, calculated either on a volume or a surface basis, increased on high dose calcitriol therapy in contrast to treatment with estrogen or calcium in which a marked decrease occurred. Sigma, which represents the length in time of a bone remodelling cycle decreased in five patients, was unchanged in two and increased in two on calcitriol, whereas on calcium or estrogen sigma was prolonged in all but one patient. In three patients on calcium sigma was prolonged beyond 1.5 years.

Discussion:

In the preliminary analysis of this study described above, we have been able to examine differences between the effect of calcitriol or calcium supplements on bone turnover. Since calcitriol increases calcium absorption it has been suggested that increasing absorption may be the only important function of calcitriol and, therefore, the use of calcium supplements in larger doses would fulfill the same objective. What our results show is that there is a distinct difference between the effect of calcitriol and calcium supplements on bone. Calcium supplements significantly slow down bone turnover, but when an equivalent or larger amount of calcium is absorbed through the action of calcitriol we do not find the same degree of depression of bone remodelling in these patients, but rather an opposite effect with activation of bone remodelling. These results argue for a direct effect of calcitriol on bone, especially since parathyroid hormone levels were suppressed on calcitriol therapy, and demonstrate subtle differences between calcium given in the form of calcium supplements and calcium absorbed through calcitriol therapy. These preliminary experiments show that calcitriol could be used in the treatment of osteoporosis in two different ways, firstly, it could be used in a small dose to increase calcium absorption and improve calcium balance as we have previously described (10). Secondly, it could be used in high doses with dietary calcium restriction as an activating agent for stimulating bone remodelling, especially in those cases where there is evidence of low-turnover osteoporosis. This opens up exciting possibilities for the use of this agent in the treatment of osteoporosis. Various experiments are now underway to look at the potential uses of calcitriol on a cyclical basis, or in combination with the use of a partial depressant of bone resorption such as low dose estrogen therapy. Of our nine patients who underwent a baseline bone biopsy, seven showed the typical histological appearances of low turn-over osteoporosis. On high-dose calcitriol most of the dynamic parameters returned to normal. After stopping calcitriol and adding calcium supplements we found that the histological picture on calcium was identical to that of the initial biopsy. What we do find perturbing is the marked depression of bone turnover which occurs in patients treated with calcium supplements .pa and in whom the histological picture is indistinguishable from that of low-turnover osteoporosis. The histological measurements performed in this study cannot address the question of whether or not there are other actions of calcitriol, calcium supplements or estrogen on bone besides the histological changes. It is quite possible for example that any of these agents could decrease the number of microfractures, which could lead to prevention of macro fractures in the vertebra. This hypothesis has some support, in so much that a decrease in vertebral fracture rates has been reported on calcitriol (10), calcium (11) and estrogen (11). It may be that histological examination of osteoporotic patients on various therapies serves mainly as a guide to the mechanisms by which therapy works, but does not ultimately answer the question of how these changes affect the outcome of osteoporosis. The final end point has to be the prevention of further vertebral fractures.

References:

1. Gallagher, J.C., Riggs, B.L., Eisman, J., Hamstra, A., Arnaud, S.B. and DeLuca, H.F. (1979) J. Clin. Invest. 64, 729-736.
2. Okano, K., Nakai, R. and Harasawa, M. (1979) Endocrinol. Jpn. Suppl. 1, 23-30.
3. Lawoyin, S., Zerwekh, J.E., Glass, K, and Pak, C.Y.C., (1980) J. Clin. Endocrinol. Metab. 50, 593-596.
4. Caniggia, A., Gennari, C., Bianchi, V. and Guideri, R. (1963) Acta. Med. Scand. 173, 613-617.
5. Gallagher, J.C., Aaron J., Horsmann, A., Marchall, D.H., Wilkinson, R. and Nordin, B.E.C. (1973) Clin. Endocrinol. Metab. 2, 293-315.
6. Nordin, B.E.C., Peacock, J.A., Crilly, R.G., Heyburn, P.J., and Horsman, A. (1980) Osteoporosis and Osteomalacia in Metabolic Bone Disease ed. L. Avioli & L. Raisz. Saunders vol. 9 no. 1.
7. Zerwekh, J.E., Sakhaee, K. and Pak, C.Y.C. (1985) J. Clin. Endocr. Met. 60, 615-617.
8. Prince, P.A. and Baukol, S.A. (1980) J. Biol. Chem. 255, 11660.

9. Gallagher, J.C. (1982) The Use of 1,25-Dihydroxyvitamin D3 in Vitamin D: Endocrinological Aspects and their Clinical Applications, ed. A. Norman et. al., W. DeGruyter, Berlin.
10. Gallagher, J.C., Jerpbak, C.M., Jee, W.S.S., Johnston, K.A., DeLuca, H.F. and Riggs, B.L. (1982) Administration of 1,25-Dihydroxyvitamin D3 to Patients with Postmenopausal Osteoporosis: Short- and Long-Term Effects on Bone and Calcium Metabolism in Proc Nat Acad Sci 79, 3325-3329.
11. Riggs, B.L., Seeman, E., Hodgson, S.F., Taves, D.R. and O'Fallon, W.M. (1982) Effect of the Fluoride/Calcium Regimen on Vertebral Fracture Occurrence in Postmenopausal Osteoporosis. N. Engl. J. Med. 306, 446-450.

Acknowledgements:
The authors wish to thank Jean Clay-Koprucki for her help in preparation of this manuscript.

ROLE OF THE VITAMIN D-ENDOCRINE SYSTEM IN PATHOGENESIS OF INVOLUTIONAL OSTEOPOROSIS

B. Lawrence Riggs
Endocrine Research Unit, Mayo Clinic and Foundation, Rochester, MN, USA

Decreased calcium absorption is a characteristic feature of involutional osteoporosis. Because the main regulator of calcium absorption is the vitamin D-endocrine system, abnormalities in the availability or metabolism of vitamin D could play a contributory role in pathogenesis.

There is growing evidence that involutional osteoporosis is a heterogeneous disorder. In this communication I summarize evidence that each of these is associated with a primary or secondary abnormality of vitamin D metabolism (Table I). Because of space limitations, I will review mainly the published work from our group. The reader is referred to the original articles for complete details of these studies and for a review of related work by others.

Table I. Abnormalities of Vitamin D Metabolism Associated with Various Types of Involutional Osteoporosis

Type	Definition	Mechanism
I	Postmenopausal osteoporosis	Sec. decrease in 25(OH)D 1α-hydroxylase activity
IIa	Senile osteoporosis	Prim. defect (mild) in 25(OH)D 1α-hydroxylase
IIb	Senile osteoporosis with nutritional vitamin D deficiency	Insufficient substrate
III	Associated with sec. hyperparathyroidism	Prim. defect (mod.) of 25(OH)D 1α-hydroxylase activity

TYPE I OSTEOPOROSIS

This classic form of the disease, which is also called postmenopausal osteoporosis, occurs mainly in women within the first two decades after menopause (1). This syndrome is characterized by an accelerated and disproportionate loss of trabecular bone (2) and is manifested by fractures of the vertebrae and distal radius, sites containing predominantly trabecular bone.

For type I osteoporosis, the predilection for women and the temporal proximity to menopause implicate estrogen deficiency as an etiologic agent. Only a relatively small subset of postmenopausal women has this form of osteoporosis, although all are estrogen deficient. In contrast to some reports, we repeatedly have found no differences in serum sex steroid

Vitamin D. A Chemical, Biochemical and Clinical Update

levels between postmenopausal women with and those without osteoporosis (3). Thus, some factor(s) must interact with menopause to determine individual susceptibility.

Virtually all investigators have found that intestinal calcium absorption and adaptation are impaired in type I osteoporosis. In 1979, our group (4) reported that, women with type I osteoporosis have a small but highly significant, decrease of about 30% in serum 1,25-dihydroxyvitamin D ($1,25(OH)_2D$) as compared with age-matched normal women. Because serum 25-hydroxyvitamin D (25-OH-D) was normal in these same patients, this suggests that osteoporotic patients have adequate vitamin D nutrition but impaired metabolism of 25-OH-D to $1,25\ (OH)_2D$. Most, but not all, subsequent investigators have confirmed these results (Table II). It is of interest that in all three studies that reported normal values, measurements were made in serum from patients who resided in northern Europe where subclinical vitamin D deficiency is common (the measurements made by Hausler et al. (14) were made on serum samples from patients who resided in Leeds, England).

Table II. Serum $1,25(OH)_2D$ Levels in Type I Osteoporosis

Results from Medical Literature			
Decreased Values		Normal Values	
Gallagher et al.	1979 (4)	Nordin et al.	1979 (12)
Lawoyin et al.	1980 (5)	Christiansen et al.	1982 (13)
Bishop et al.	1980 (6)	Hausler et al.	1984 (14)
Riggs et al.	1981 (7)		
Sorenson et al.	1982 (8)		
Lund et al.	1982 (9)		
Caniggia et al.	1984 (10)		
Nordin et al.	1984 (11)		
Aloia et al.	1985 (29)		

We have investigated the mechanisms of these abnormalities further. First, we demonstrated that there was a significant correlation between serum $1,25(OH)_2D$) levels and calcium absorption in normal subjects ($r = -0.50, p<0.01$): the correlation was maintained when values were merged with values from osteoporotic subjects (4). This suggests that the decrease in serum $1,25(OH)_2D$ levels was responsible for the decrease in calcium absorption. Second, we showed that long-term treatment with a physiological dosage of $1,25(OH)_2D_3$ corrected the impaired calcium absorption while treatment with placebo had no effect (17, and Fig.1). Third, we found that parathyroid function (assessed by PTH radioimmunoassay and by urinary cyclic

AMP excretion) was normal or decreased in most patients with type I osteoporosis (7,15,16,Table III). Moreover, the decrease in calcium absorption correlated directly (r = 0.81, p<0.005) with the decrease in parthyroid function (18). These findings are inconsistent with the primary defect in intestinal calcium transport which would produce the opposite findings.

Table III. Parathyroid Function in Postmenopausal Osteoporosis as Compared with Page-Matched Postmenopausal Women Without Osteoporosis

Method	N	Differences from controls (%)	P
Radioimmunoassay (NH_2-terminal)	32	-30.7	<0.001
Radioimmunoassay ("whole-molecule")	31	-18.8	<0.001
Urinary cAMP	12	-19.1	<0.05

Fig 1. Net calcium absorption measured by metabolic balance before and six months after treatment with either placebo or a physiologic dosage of $1,25(OH)_2D_3$.

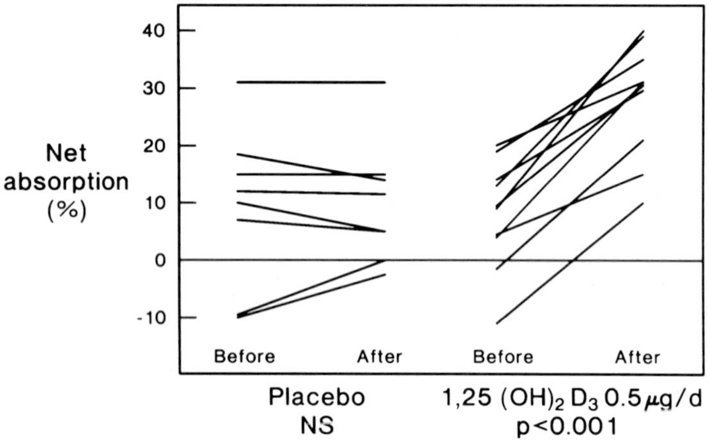

Fourth, we found a significant inverse correlation (r = -0.75,P<0.005) between parathyroid function and net bone resorption (assessed by combining results of ^{47}Ca kinetic and iliac bone biopsy studies) (18). This suggests that the decrease in parathyroid function results from rather than causes the increase in net bone resorption. Fifth, we assessed 25(OH)D 1α-hydroxylase reserve in 12 women with type I osteoporosis and in 10 age-comparable normal women (7). After administration of parathyroid extract to stimulate the enzymatic conversion of 25-OH-D to $1,25(OH)_2D$, increases in serum $1,25(OH)_2D$ were similar in both groups. This suggests that the decreased basal levels of serum $1,25(OH)_2D$ resulted from a functional rather than a structural enzymatic defect. Finally, we (19) compared findings in 21 women with osteoporosis before and after six months treatment with either placebo (9 patients) or a physiological replacement dosage of estrogen (12 patients). Both fractional calcium absorption and serum levels of total $1,25(OH)_2D$ were normalized after treatment with estrogen whereas there was no change in the placebo-treated patients. This suggests that the abnormalities of vitamin D metabolism in type I osteoporosis are a secondary consequence of estrogen deficiency. These collective findings are consistent with the model shown in Figure 2.

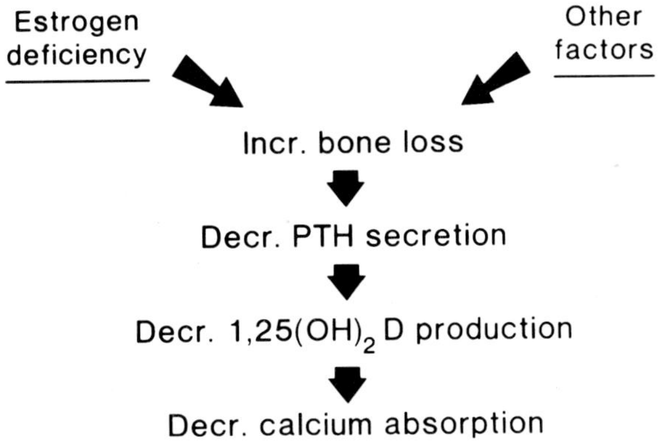

Fig. 2. Model for pathogenesis of type I (postmenopausal) osteoporosis

Although this model assumes impaired production of $1,25(OH)_2D$ is secondary, this defect could exacerbate negative calcium balance. Indeed, treatment with a small dose of $1,25(OH)_2D_3$ in 12 patients with type I osteoporosis improved calcium balance, ^{47}Ca kinetics, and bone histomorphometric findings in one study (17) and, in another two-center study, resulted in a substantial reduction in vertebral fracture rate (20).

TYPE IIa OSTEOPOROSIS

This form of osteoporosis, which is also called senile osteoporosis, occurs in a large proportion of women who are older than 75 years of age. In contrast to type I osteoporosis, bone loss is not accelerated, and there is proportionate loss of both cortical and trabecular bone. Both hip and vetebral fractures commonly occur (1).

For type IIa osteoporosis, there may be two major causes--impaired bone formation and secondary hyperparathyroidism. First, from the fourth decade of life onward less bone is formed than is resorbed at individual remodeling foci, and this imbalance increases with aging. Second, several groups including our own (16,21), have demonstrated an increase in serum iPTH and in urinary cyclic AMP excretion with aging. Our recent observation (21) that overall bone turnover among women may increase with aging (as assessed by measurement of serum bone Gla-protein and other biochemical markers) suggests that secondary hyperparathyroidism may increase the number of individual remodeling units and, thus, increase bone turnover at the tissue level. Because bone formation remains decreased at the level of individual remodeling foci, increased bone turnover would result in increased bone loss.

Aging is associated with a decrease in serum $1,25(OH)_2D$ in man (4,22,23); this is the probable cause of the well documented age-related decrease in calcium absorption which, in turn, is the cause of the increase in parathyroid function. Studies in experimental animals have shown a primary defect in 25-OH-D 1α-hydroxylase activity. We (22) studied 10 normal premenopausal women, 8 normal women within 20 years of menopause, 10 normal elderly women, and 8 elderly women with hip fracture whose ages (mean ± SE) were 37±4, 61±6, 78±4, and 78±4 years respectively. Serum 25-OH-D was similar in all groups, demonstrating nutritional adequacy of vitamin D; but basal levels of serum $1,25(OH)_2D$, the physiologically active vitamin D metabolite, decreased ($P < 0.01$) with aging (Table IV).

The stimulated levels of serum $1,25(OH)_2D$ after a 24-hr infusion of parathyroid hormone fragment 1-34, a tropic agent for the enzyme, 25-OH-D 1α-hydroxylase, correlated inversely with age (Table III) and the response was ($P < 0.001$) more blunted in elderly patients with hip fracture than in elderly controls (Table IV). These data suggest that impaired ability of the aging kidney to synthesize $1,25(OH)_2D$ could contribute to the pathogenesis of senile osteoporosis and are consistent with the model shown in Fig. 3.

Table IV. Effect of Age on Vitamin D Metabolism

	Serum $1,25(OH)_2D$, pg/ml	
	Basal	Incremental
Premenopausal normal	37±7	64±13
Postmenopausal normal	34±5	40±11
Elderly normal	20±6	25± 3
Hip fracture	21±3	13± 3

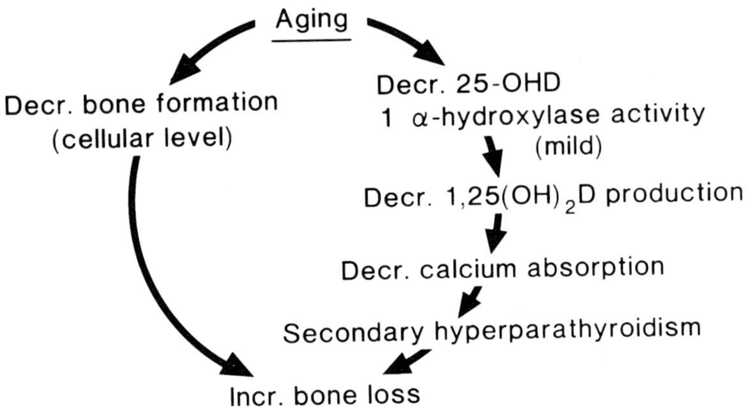

Fig 3. Model for pathogenesis of type II-A (senile) osteoporosis

TYPE IIb OSTEOPOROSIS

In northern Europe, nutritional osteomalacia may occur in the winter months, particularly in the elderly. A high proportion of elderly women in Leeds, England with fractures of the proximal femur were found to have histological osteomalacia and low serum 25(OH)D levels, with a peak incidence in the winter (25). Residents of the United States were less likely to have nutritional vitamin D deficiency because of the more southern latitude and because of the fortification of dairy products with vitamin D. In American patients with hip fractures, some investigators have found, and others have failed to find, histological evidence of osteomalacia. We, (26) have measured serum 25(OH)D levels and made bone density measurements at the mid radius and lumbar spine in 122 randomly selected, female residents of Rochester, MN, whose ages range from 33 to 94 years. Serum 25(OH)D decrease significantly with aging and levels in the elderly were almost one-half of that found in young adulthood. Bone mineral density also decreased with aging, but these decreases did not correlate with the decreases in serum 25(OH)D when age was fixed. Thus, we cannot confirm that vitamin D deficiency plays a major role in age-related bone loss in a northern American population. We believe, therefore, that type II-b osteoporosis is relatively rare in America and is most likely to be found in elderly house-bound patients, particularly in those having overall inadequate nutrition.

TYPE III OSTEOPOROSIS

Most patients presenting with the syndrome of type I osteoporosis have normal or low circulating levels of serum iPTH. In 1973, we reported that a small subgroup of patients had clearly elevated values (27), a finding that has been subsequently confirmed by others. Combined data from all re-reports suggest that about 10% of all patients with type I osteoporosis have increased levels of serum iPTH. These patients also have increased bone turnover as assessed by bone histomorphometry. Three patients that we studied (Table V) had decreased calcium absorption and inappropriately low-normal serum $1,25(OH)_2D$ levels despite high serum iPTH levels suggesting impaired 25-OH-D 1α-hydroxylase function (Figure 4).

Table V. Laboratory Values in Type III Osteoporosis

Serum	Case 1 (75,F)	Case 2 (63,F)	Case 3 (71,F)	Age-corrected normal range
Serum Ca^{++}, mg/dl	4.0	3.8	4.3	4.0-4.8
iPTH, μleq/ml	84	63	54	< 45
25(OH)D, ng/ml	26	38	21	8-30
$1,25(OH)_2D$, pg/ml	27	22	24	20-52
Ca balance				
% net absorption	-0.7	9	9	10-40

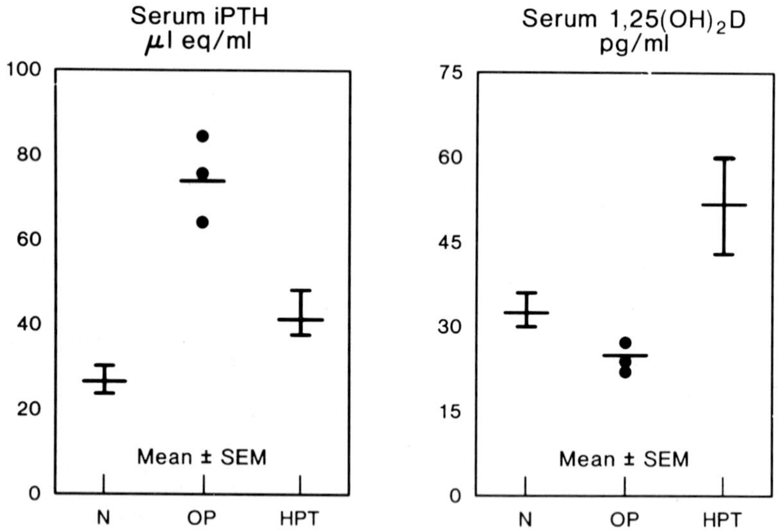

Fig. 4. Comparison of levels of serum iPTH and serum 1,25(OH)D in 20 normal women (4), 3 women with type III osteoporosis (27) and 11 women with primary hyperparathyroidism (28). Note that in type III osteoporosis serum iPTH is higher and serum $1,25(OH)_2D$ is lower than either normal or hyperparathyroid subjects. This strongly suggests impaired response of 25(OH)D 1α-hydroxylase activity in this disorder.

At present, it is unclear whether this syndrome represents a more severe form of type II-a osteoporosis occurring at an earlier age or, in fact, is a separate entity. Although less common, type III osteoporosis is important because it is potentially remediable by treatment with $1,25(OH)_2D_3$. The data are consistent with the model shown in Figure 5.

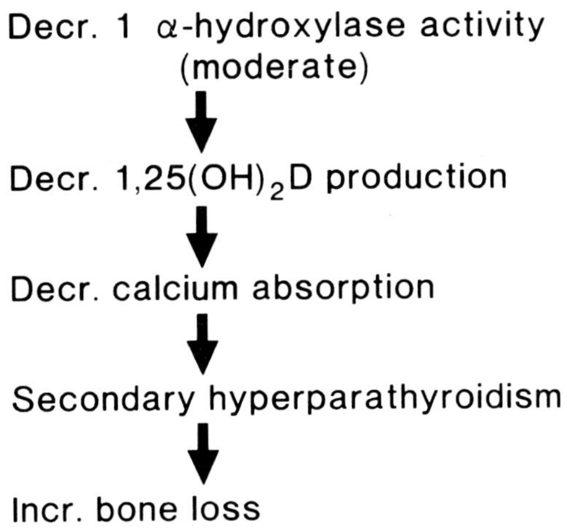

Fig. 5: Model for pathogenesis of type III osteoporosis

SUMMARY

Involutional osteoporosis is not a single age-related disorder, but consists of at least four distinct syndromes. Each syndrome is associated with a corresponding abnormality of vitamin D metabolism. In type I osteoporosis, impaired conversion of 25-OH-D to 1,25(OH)$_2$D is a secondary consequence of accelerated bone loss due to estrogen deficiency. Although this defect is secondary, it may exacerbate the bone loss caused by estrogen deficiency per se. In type II-a osteoporosis and III osteoporosis, there is evidence for a primary defect in 25-OH-D 1α-hydroxylase activity. This leads to decreased production of 1,25(OH)$_2$D to secondary hyperparathyroidism and, presumably, to increased bone loss. Nutritional vitamin D deficiency is the hallmark of type II-b osteoporosis. This seems to be relatively rare in the United States and is found mainly in elderly housebound patients.

ACKNOWLEDGEMENTS

This is a summary of almost 10 years of work which could not have been completed without the help and collaboration of Drs. C. D. Arnaud, H. Heath, III, and R. Kumar of Mayo Clinic and Foundation and Dr. H. F. DeLuca of the University of Wisconsin. Drs. P. D. Delmas, J C. Gallagher, and K.-S. Tsai made important contributions while working as postdoctoral research fellows in my laboratory.

REFERENCES

1. Riggs, B.L. and Melton, L.J. III, (1983) Am. J. Med. 75, 899-901.

2. Riggs, B.L, Wahner, H. W., Dunn, W.L., Mazess, R.B., Offord, K.P., and Melton, L. J. III, (1981) J. Clin. Invest. 67, 328-335.

3. Davidson, B.J., Riggs, B.L., Wahner, H.W., and Judd, H.L., (1983) Obstet. Gynecol. 61, 275-278.

4. Gallagher, J.C., Riggs, B.L., Eisman, J., Hamstra, A., Arnaud, S.B., and DeLuca, H.F., (1979) J. Clin. Invest. 64, 729-736.

5. Lawoyin, S., Zerwekh, J.E., Glass, K. and Pak, C.Y.C., (1980) J. Clin. Endocrinol. Metab. 50, 593-596.

6. Bishop, J.E., Norman, A.W., Coburn, J.W., Roberts, P.A., and Henry, H.L., (1980) Min. Elec. Metab. 3, 181-189.

7. Riggs, B.L., Hamstra, A., and DeLuca, H.F., (1981) J. Clin. Endocrinol. Metab. 53, 833-835.

8. Sorensen, O.H., Lumholtz, B., Lund, B., Lund, B., Hjelmstrand, I.L., Mosekilde, L., Melsen, F., Bishop, J.E., and Norman, A.W., (1982) J. Clin. Endocrinol. Metab. 54, 1258-1261.

9. Lund, B, Sorensen, O.H., Lund, B., and Agner, E., (1982) Horm. Metabol. Res. 14, 271-274.

10. Caniggia, A., Nuti, R., Lorie, F., and Vattimo, A., (1984) J. Endocrinol. Invest. 7, 373-378.

11. Nordin, B.E.C., Remarks made at the International Symposium on Osteoporosis, Copenhagen, (1984) June 3-8.

12. Nordin, B.E.C., Peacock, M., Crilly, R.G., and Marshall, D.H., IN: Vitamin D, Basic Research and Its Clinical Application, Walter deGruyter and Co., New York. (1979) pp. 99-106.

13. Christiansen, C., IN: Vitamin D, Chemical, Biochemical and Clinical Endocrinology of Calcium Metabolism, Norman A.W., Schefer, K., Herrath, D.V., Grigoleit, H-G. (Eds), Berlin, Walter de Gruyter. (1982) pp. 915-920.

14. Hausler, M.R., Donaldson, C.A., Allegretto, E.A., Marion, S.L., Mangelsdorf, J., Kelly, N.A., and Pike, J.W., IN: Osteoporosis. Proceeding of the Copenhagen International Symposium, June 3-8, 1984. Christianson, C., (Ed) Aalborg Stiftsbogtrykkeri, Copenhagen. (1984) pp. 725-736.

15. Riggs, B.L., Arnaud, C.D., Jowsey, J., Goldsmith, R.S., Kelly, P.J., (1973) J. Clin. Invest. 52, 181-184.

16. Gallagher, J.C., Riggs, B.L., Jerpbak, C.M., and Arnaud, C.D., (1980) J. Lab. Clin. Med. 95, 373-385.

17. Gallagher, J.C., Jerpbak, C.M, Jee, W.S.S., Johnson, K.A., DeLuca, H.F., and Riggs, B.L., Proc. Natl. Acad. Sci. U.S.A. (1982) 79, 3325-3329.

18. Riggs, B.L., Gallagher, J.C., DeLuca, H.F., and Zinsmeister, A.R., IN: Vitamin D, Chemical, Biochemical and Clinical Endocrinology of Calcium Metabolism. Norman, A.W., Schaefer, K., Herrath, D. V., and Grigoleit, H-G. (Eds), Walter de Gruyter, New York (1982) pp. 903-908.

19. Gallagher, J.C., Riggs, B.L, J. Clin. Endocrinol. Metab. (1980) 51, 1359-1364.

20. Gallagher, J.C., Riggs, B.L., Recker, R., and Goldgar, D., IN: Osteoporosis, National Institutes of Health Consensus Development Conference April 2-4, 1984, Program and Abstracts, (1984) pp. 52-54.

21. Delmas, P.D., Stenner, D., Wahner, H.W., Mann, K.G., and Riggs, B.L., J. Clin. Invest. (1983) 71, 1316-1321.

22. Tsai, K-S., Heath, H. III, Kumar, R., and Riggs, B.L., J. Clin. Invest. (1983) 73, 1668-1672.

23. Manolagas, S.C., Culler, F.L., Howard, J.E., Brickman, A.S., Deftos, L.J., J. Clin. Endocrinol. Metab. (1983) 56, 751-760.

24. Slovik, D.M., Adams, J.S., Neer, R.M., Holick, M.F., and Potts, J.T., Jr., N. Eng. J. Med. (1981) 305, 372-374.

25. Aaron, J.E., Gallagher, J.C., Anderson, J., Stasiak, L., Longton, E.B., Nordin, B.E.C., and Nicholson, M., Lancet (1974) I, 229-233.

26. Tsai, K-S., Wahner, H.W., Offord, K.P., Melton, L.J., III, Kumar, R., and Riggs, B.L., (1984) submitted.

27 Riggs, B.L., Gallagher, J.C., DeLuca, H.F., Edis, A.J., Lambert, P.W., and Arnaud, C.D., Mayo Clin. Proc. (1978) 53, 701-706.

28. Law, W.M., Jr., Bollman, S., Kumar, R., and Heath, H., III, J. Clin. Endocrinol. Metab. (1984) 58, 744-747.

29. Aloia, J.F., Cohn, S.H., Vasevani, A., Yeh, J.K., Yuen, K., and Ellis, K., Am. J. Med. (1985) 78, 95-100.

1,25(OH)2VITAMIN D3 IN THE LONG-TERM TREATMENT OF POST-MENOPAUSAL OSTEOPOROSIS

A. CANIGGIA, R. NUTI, F. LORE' and A. VATTIMO
Institute of Clinical Medicine, University of Siena, 53100 Siena, Italy

Postmenopausal osteoporosis is characterized by a decrease in bone mass without changes in the mineral composition of the remnant bone. There is general agreement that its primary cause is estrogen deficiency occurring after the menopause. Obviously, such a decrease in bone mass (even more than 50%) can only result from a negative calcium balance.

Albright demonstrated that negative calcium balance in postmenopausal osteoporosis was mainly due to increased fecal losses of calcium (1): evidently calcium was not absorbed enough. The mechanism of active calcium transport is impaired in postmenopausal osteoporosis, as demonstrated by the measurement of orally administered radiocalcium absorption: the circulating fraction of the administered dose is decreased and most part of radiocalcium is excreted in faeces(2). This impairment of intestinal calcium transport cannot be accounted for by the vitamin D status of the body: according to our previous results the mean serum level of 25-hydroxyvitamin D (25OHD) is higher in osteoporotic women than in age-matched controls (3); on the contrary there is increasing evidence that the serum levels of 1,25-dihydroxyvitamin D (1,25(OH)2D) are decreased (4, 5). The administration of 1,25(OH)2D3 at physiological doses (1 μg/day) to women with postmenopausal osteoporosis has been shown to restore a normal radiocalcium absorption (6); similar doses of 24,25(OH)2D3 were ineffective from this point of view. It could be suggested that the negative calcium balance of postmenopausal osteoporotic women is due to the impairment of intestinal calcium transport as a consequence of a reduced 1,25(OH)2D synthesis, resulting from an impaired activity of renal 25OHD-1α-hydroxylase (1α-OHase), which is no longer stimulated by estrogens. The findings we obtained in a double-blind study carried out in post-menopausal osteoporotic women treated with an estrogen-gestagen combination or placebo are consistent with this hypothesis: the treatment restored a normal intestinal calcium absorption whereas the placebo was ineffective (7). More recently a direct effect of estrogens on the renal synthesis of 1,25(OH)2D has been demonstrated in DeLuca's laboratory (8).

The present study was begun in 1980 (9, 10) and is still in progress. 120 women with postmenopausal osteoporosis, aged 49-78 years (mean 64 years), entered the trial. Two of them have so far been treated for more than 4 years; 9 for 3 to 4 years; 25 for 2 to 3 years; 21 for 1 to 2 years; 63 for 4 months to 1 year. The patients were given 1,25(OH)2D3 at the oral dose of 0.5 μg twice a day without calcium supplementation. There has been no interruption of the treatment since the beginning of the trial. No other drug was given (including analgesics!). The patients were

Vitamin D. A Chemical, Biochemical and Clinical Update

allowed to their usual diet. The estimated daily intake of calcium, phosphate and vitamin D was 580±120 mg, 850±190 mg, 0.5±0.2 µg, respectively.

Only women with symptomatic post-menopausal osteoporosis were admitted. They had: back pain and difficulty in walking; a radiographic finding of vertebral translucency with one or more non-traumatic vertebral fractures (edge crushes accompanied by kyphosis and/or codfishing); a decreased bone mineral content (BMC) as determined by absorptiometry at the distal end of radius and ulna, in a comparison with age-matched, non osteoporotic women; a typical histological pattern of osteoporosis as determined by microscopic inspection of bone biopsies from the iliac crest obtained by means of a Burckhardt's drill: undecalcified bone specimens were prepared in order to exclude patients with osteoid seams; normal renal function; normal values of serum calcium, phosphate and alkaline phosphatase and 24h urinary calcium, phosphate and hydroxyproline excretion; impaired intestinal radiocalcium transport, as assessed by the measurement of the circulating fraction of the administered dose. All the patients were exempt from: renal diseases; heart failure and major respiratory insufficiency; endocrine diseases; diseases of the alimentary tract, liver and biliary ducts; osteomalacia and mixed patterns of osteoporosis and osteomalacia; primary and secondary neoplastic bone disease; spondiloarthrosis, even when occurring in women with osteoporosis and decreased BMC, because in these conditions back pain is mainly dependent on the articular disease and is not relieved by 1,25(OH)2D3 treatment; long-term treatments with glucoactive corticosteroids, anticonvulsants or heparin.

Laboratory parameters were usually determined every other month.
Intestinal calcium absorption was measured by our 47Ca oral test (10

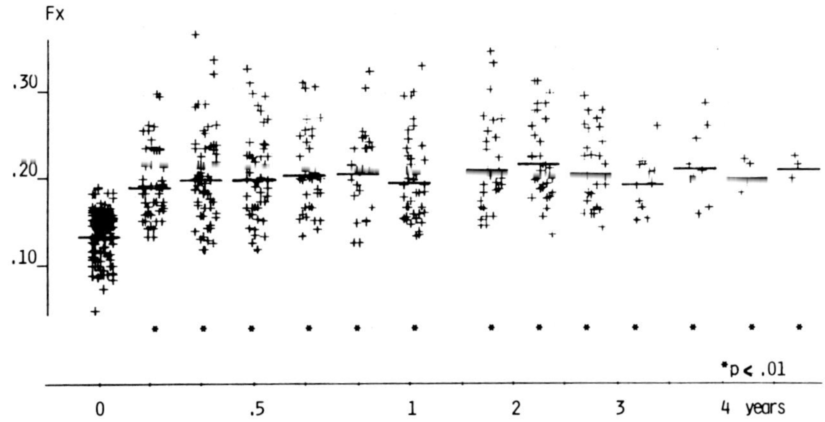

Fig. 1. Fractional intestinal radiocalcium absorption (fx) during 1,25(OH)2D3 treatment: increases were statistically significant.

uCi of 47Ca were given orally in 80 mg of CaCl as a carrier; radioactivity was measured in plasma samples obtained every 30 min for 4 h and the circulating fraction of the dose (fx) was calculated according to Marshall and Nordin (11). Basal fx values were lower than the normal range: after two months of treatment a normal fx was restored; fx remained within the normal range as long as 1,25(OH)2D3 was administered (Fig. 1).

Fasting plasma calcium during the study averaged slightly higher mean

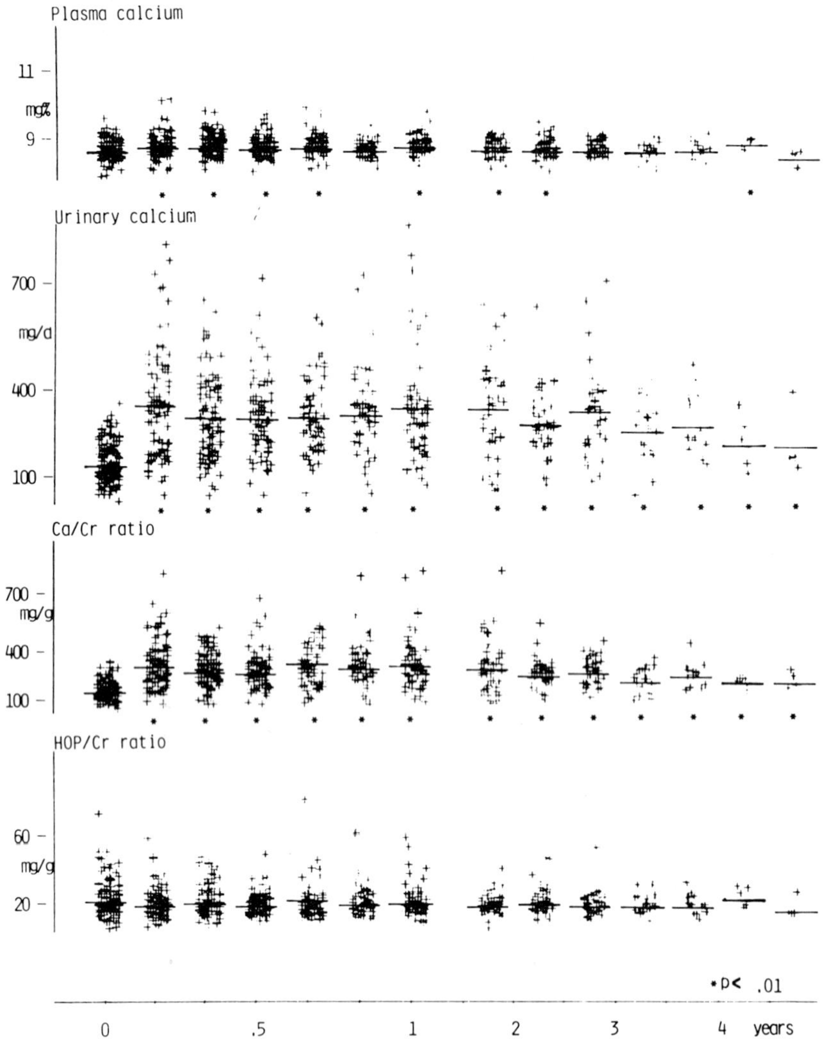

Fig. 2. Fasting plasma calcium, 24 h urinary calcium, calcium and hydroxyproline/creatinine ratios on 1,25(OH)2D3 treatment.

values as compared with the basal levels. Due to the improvement in intestinal calcium absorption increases in plasma calcium were expected, actually high plasma calcium was only exceptionally observed (Fig. 2).

The 24 h urinary calcium excretion increased remarkably in all patients so that hypercalciuria was generally observed throughout the treatment.

It has been suggested that 1,25(OH)2D3 has two indipendent target organs: the intestinal mucosa and bone, so that the improvement of calcium absorption is necessarily accompanied by an increase in bone resorption. This view is untenable according to our experience: in fact the 24h urinary excretion of hydroxyproline (HOP) did not increase during long-term treatment with 1,25(OH)2D3. This is confirmed by the urinary ratio HOP-/creatinine (determined in 24h urine) which remained unchanged, whereas the ratio Ca/creatinine increased, so that the ratio Ca/HOP (in 24 h urine) was found to increase significantly.

When each individual value of urinary calcium was plotted against the corresponding fx value a highly significant positive correlation was obtained. Fasting plasma calcium correlated significantly also with fx but not with total 24 h urinary calcium (Fig. 3).

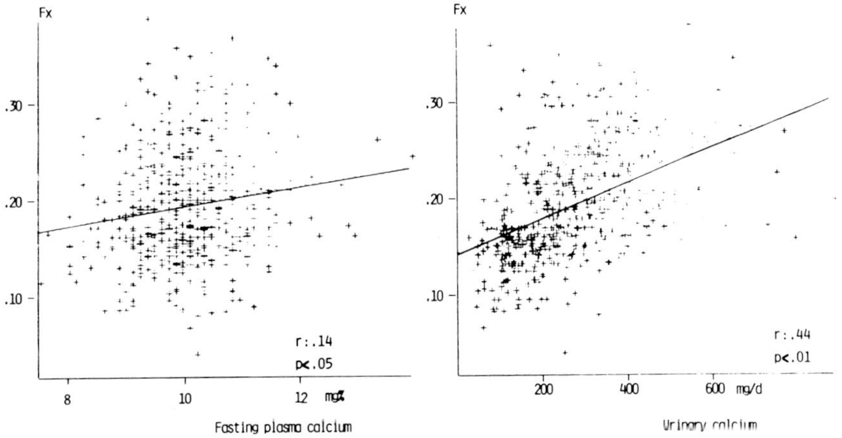

Fig. 3. Correlations between fractional radiocalcium absorption (fx) and fasting plasma calcium (left) and 24 h calcium excretion (right).

It must be concluded that in our patients hypercalciuria is exclusively the result of 1,25(OH)2D3 action on the intestinal calcium transport. Obviously this effect is mainly appreciable after the meals, rather than after an overnight fast.

Hypercalcemia and hypercalciuria are generally believed to be harmful to renal function and to increase the risk of renal stone formation. As previously stated, only patients with normal renal function and without renal stones were selected for our study. Despite the hypercalciuria (and sometimes hypercalcemia) induced by long-term 1,25(OH)2D3 administration no patient showed changes in renal function as demonstrated by urinalysis, blood urea nitrogen, creatinine levels and creatinine clearance. No renal stone developed. The conclusion can be drawn that the long-term administration of 1 µg/day of 1,25(OH)2D3 did not result in any adverse effect on renal function, in spite of a persistent hypercalciuria (Fig. 4).

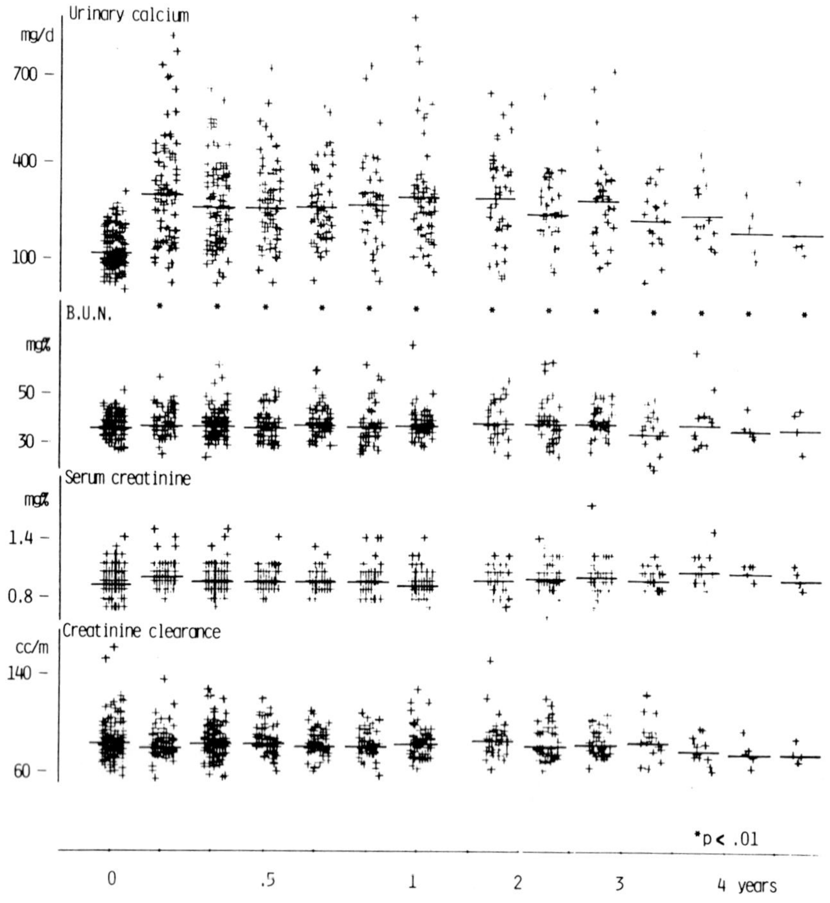

Fig. 4. Behaviour of urinary calcium and of the main parameters of renal function during 1,25(OH)2D3 treatment.

<u>Plasma phosphate</u> was not modified significantly by 1,25(OH)2D3.

The <u>24 h urinary phosphate excretion</u> increased significantly but to a lower extent as compared with calcium; it is known that 1,25(OH)2D3 is effective in promoting the intestinal absorption of phosphate (Fig. 5).

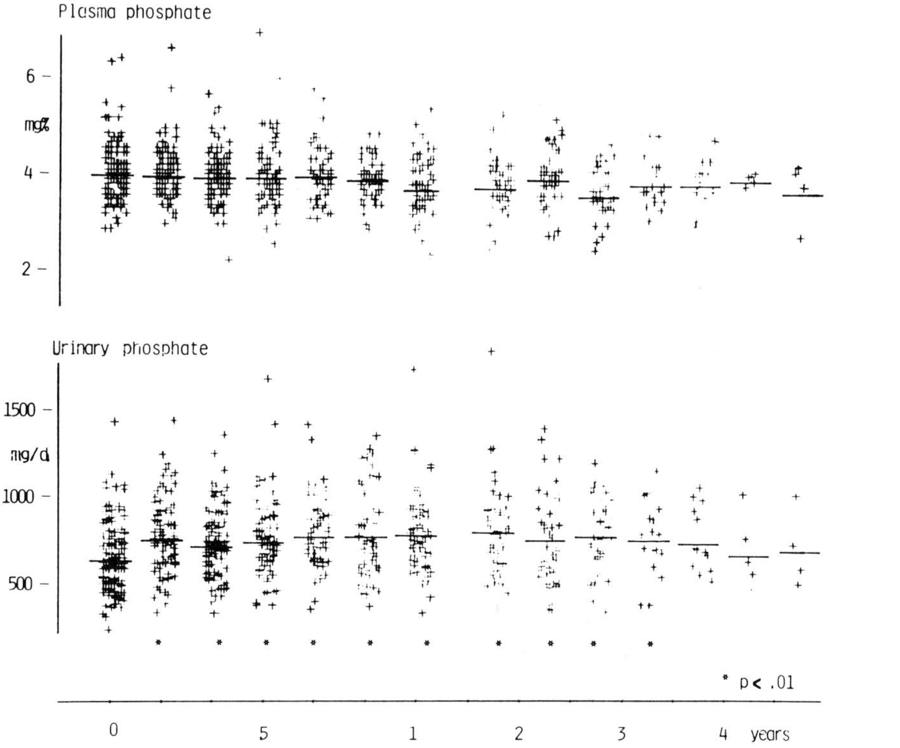

Fig. 5. Changes in fasting plasma phosphate levels and 24 h urinary phosphate excretion on treatment.

The <u>cAMP/creatinine ratio</u> on 24 h urine is recognized as a good index

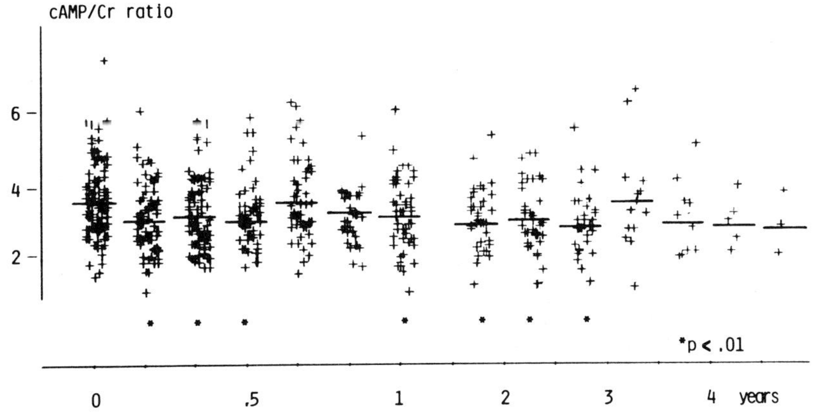

Fig. 6 Changes in 24 h urinary cAMP/creatinine ratio on treatment.

of parathyroid function. In the patients of the present study a slowly progressive, but significant decrease in this parameter was observed. This can be accounted for by parathyroid suppression and must be considered a favourable effect since it tends to reduce bone resorption rate (Fig. 6).

The serum levels of 25OHD and 1,25(OH)2D have been evaluated in a number of our patients. The basal serum concentration of 25OHD were found to be higher in our osteoporotic women, whereas 1,25(OH)2D3 levels were lower than in normal peers. These findings are probably related one to another: the low 1,25(OH)2D levels could be responsible for a reduced product-inhibition of liver vitamin D-25-hydroxylase. In fact 25OHD levels decreased significantly in our patients during 1,25(OH)2D3 treatment (12) (Fig. 7). Recent "in vitro" and "in vivo" studies have confirmed that 25OHD production is really inhibited by 1,25(OH)2D3 (13, 14).

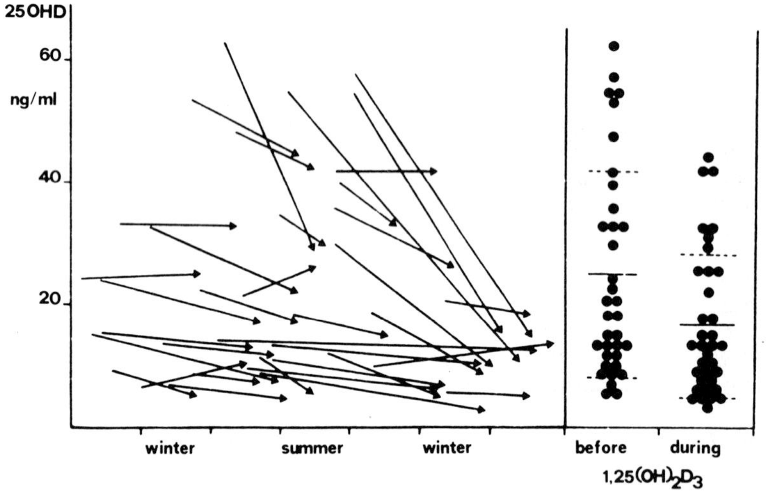

Fig. 7. Serum 25OHD levels decreased on treatment, despite the season.

Clinical results: it should be emphasized that 1,25(OH)2D3 treatment resulted in a significant and often dramatic relief from pain and improvement of motility: some of our ladies were practically bed ridden or confined to wheel-chair: after a few months of therapy they were able to walk again: significant reduction in the occurrence of new non-traumatic fractures as compared with the period preceding the initiation of therapy (respectively, 13.0 and 2.9 fractures/100 patients x year): only clinically relevant vertebral fractures were considered. These fractures were easily distinguishable on X-ray films and in most cases had manifested themselves with sudden acute pain; microfractures such as those which can only be identified on X-ray films by measuring the vertebral body heights were not taken into account, since in our hands these procedures were found to be unreliable and hardly reproducible.

Bone mineral content showed a mean increase of about 10 % as compared with the basal values, but only 10-12 months after the beginning of treatment (Fig. 8).

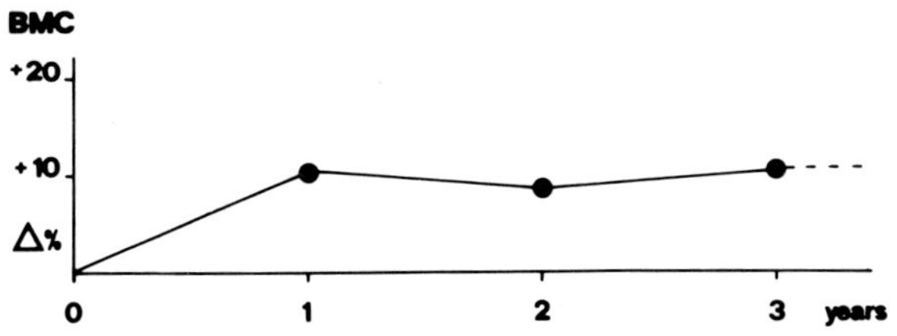

Fig. 8. Behaviour of bone mineral content (BMC) on treatment.

Patients' compliance is testified by the fact that they diligently come to our department for periodical analyses. Our study includes subjects from every part of Italy, who come regularly to Siena every other month at their own expenses. This can be considered a good measure of social compliance and is a confirmation of the beneficial effects of treatment as seen from the point of view of the patients.

The serum concentrations of osteocalcin (BGP) have been evaluated in a number of our postmenopausal osteoporotic women in basal conditions and during long-term treatment with 1,25(OH)2D3.

The behaviour of BGP in postmenopausal osteoporosis is still a matter of debate. Controversial data have been obtained in early studies, however, low BGP levels have been recently reported in osteoporotic women by Brown et al., who, on the basis of histomorphometric analyses have related this finding to the presence of low-turnover osteoporosis (15).

Prior to the initiation of treatment BGP levels averaged lower than in a group of age-matched non-osteoporotic women studied in our laboratory (16); treatment with 1,25(OH)2D3 produced significant increases in BGP levels (Fig. 9), that showed no correlation with the serum levels of alkaline phosphatase and HOP urinary excretion.

It is possible that the low BGP levels we observed in postmenopausal osteoporotic women were related to an impairment of osteoblast stimulation as a consequence of the reduced endogenous production of 1,25(OH)2D3. In any case our findings indicate that in osteoporotic women the osteoblasts had not lost their ability to respond to 1,25(OH)2D3, which is known to be a physiological stimulator of BGP synthesis (17).

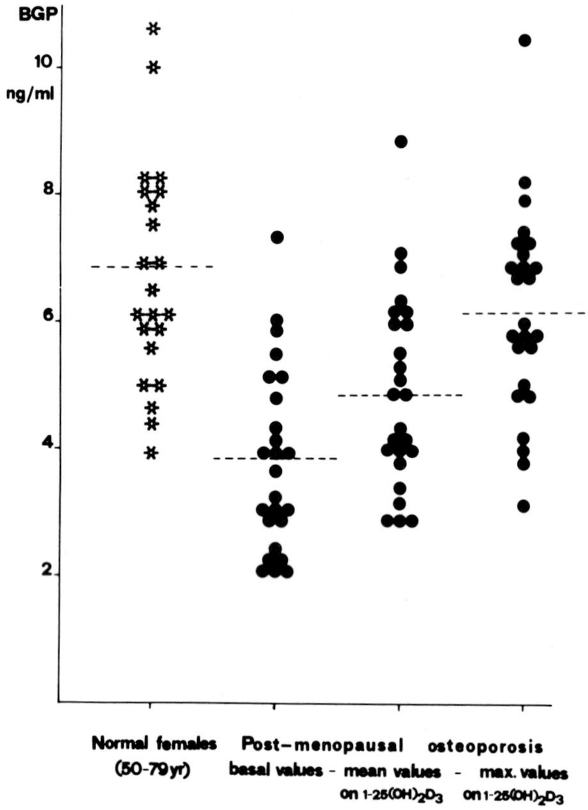

Fig. 9. Basal values of serum osteocalcin (BGP) in postmenopausal osteoporotic women as compared to age-matched normal females (left). Mean and maximum values reached during the treatment are also shown (right).

TO SUM UP:

- long-term treatment with 1 µg/day of 1,25(OH)2D3 resulted in clinical improvement in 120 women with symptomatic postmenopausal osteoporosis, with decrease in the occurrence of fractures and increase in BMC;
- this improvement was accompanied by a rapid restoration of normal values of intestinal calcium transport, i.e. the correction of what is considered the most important factor in the pathophysiology of the disease;
- no untoward effects on renal function have been observed, despite hypercalciuria;
- despite the reduced basal levels, BGP increased significantly during the treatment. The role of osteocalcin in bone physiology is still unclear, however, our findings show that osteoblasts did maintain their ability to respond to 1,25(OH)2D3 at least with an increase in BGP synthesis.

REFERENCES

1) Albright, F. and Reifenstein, B.C. (1948) The parathyroid glands and metabolic bone disease. Williams and Wilkins Co., Baltimore.
2) Caniggia, A., Gennari, C., Bianchi, V. and Guideri, R. (1963) Acta Med. Scand. 173, 613-617.
3) Loré, F., Di Cairano, G., Signorini, A.M. and Caniggia, A. (1981) Calcif. Tissue Int. 33, 467-471.
4) Gallagher, J.C., Riggs, B.L., Eisman, J., Hamstra, A., Arnaud, S.B. and DeLuca, H.F. (1979) J. Clin. Invest. 64, 729-736.
5) Loré, F., Nuti, R., Vattimo, A. and Caniggia, A. (1984) Horm. Metabol. Res. 16, 58.
6) Caniggia, A. and Vattimo, A. (1979) Clin. Endocrinol. 11, 99-103.
7) Caniggia, A., Gennari, C., Borrello, G., Bencini, M., Cesari, L., Poggi, C. and Escobar, S. (1970). Brit. Med. J. 4, 30-32.
8) Castillo, L., Tanaka, Y., De Luca, H.F. and Sunde, M.L. (1977) Arch. Biochem. Biophys. 179, 211-17.
9) Caniggia, A., Nuti, R., Lorè, F. and Vattimo, A. (1984) J. Endocrinol. Invest. 7, 373-378.
10) Caniggia, A., Nuti, R., Lorè, F. and Vattimo, A. (1984) in Steroid modulation of neuroendocrine function. Sterols, steroids and bone metabolism (Martini, L., Gordan, G.S. and Sciarra, F., eds.),pp. 231-244, Excerpta Medica, Amsterdam.
11) Marshall, D.H. and Nordin, B.E.C. (1969) Nature 222, 797.
12) Baran, D.T. and Milne, M.L. (1983) Calcif. Tissue Int. 35, 461-464.
13) Bell, N.H., Shaw, S. and Turner, R.T. (1984) J. Clin. Invest. 74, 1540-1544.
14) Lorè, F., Di Cairano, G., Periti, P. and Caniggia, A. (1982) Calcif. Tissue Int. 34, 539-541.
15) Brown, J.P., Delmas, P.D., Malaval, L., Edouard, C., Chapuy, M.C. and Meunier, P.J. (1984) Lancet 1, 1091-1093.
16) Galli, M. and Caniggia, M. (1985) Horm. Metabol. Res. 17, 165-166.
17) Price, P.A. (1983) in Bone and mineral research (Peck, W.L., ed.),pp. 157-190, Excerpta Medica, Amsterdam.

ACKNOWLEDGMENTS

This work was partly supported by C.N.R. grant n. 83.02565 (Medicina preventiva e riabilitativa).

CALCIUM ABSORPTION AND SERUM 1,25 DIHYDROXYVITAMIN D LEVELS IN NORMAL AND OSTEOPOROTIC WOMEN

H A Morris* B E C Nordin** Vicki Fraser* T F Hartley* A G Need* M Horowitz**
* Division of Clinical Chemistry, Institute of Medical and Veterinary Science, Adelaide, South Australia
** Department of Endocrinology, Royal Adelaide Hospital, Adelaide, South Australia

Introduction

Malabsorption of calcium is a well recognised feature of many forms of osteoporosis (1,2) but there is some dispute about its pathogenesis. Some workers attribute it to a reduction in serum $1,25(OH)_2D$ levels (3), whereas others suggest that it may be due in part to a gastrointestinal defect (4). In the present study, we have related radiocalcium absorption to serum $1,25(OH)_2D$ levels in 33 normal and 42 osteoporotic postmenopausal women.

Clinical Material and Methods

The clinical material comprises 33 postmenopausal women with normal spines and a mean age of 61.5 years and 42 post-menopausal women with vertebral compression fractures and a mean age of 66.4 years. Radiocalcium absorption (α) was determined by administering 5 μC of Ca^{45} in 20 mg of calcium carrier as the chloride in 250 ml of water and collecting a blood sample 60 minutes later for the measurement of plasma radioactivity. The plasma radioactivity was multiplied by 15% of body weight to yield the fraction of the dose circulating at 60 minutes and this was converted to fractional absorption by reading off a calibration curve (5). Serum $1,25(OH)_2D$ was determined by radioimmunoassay after HPLC (6). Serum 25OHD was determined by competitive protein binding assay following LH 20 chromatography (7).

Results

The osteoporotic subjects were significantly older than the normals ($p<.001$). Mean α was 0.75 ± .05 of the dose absorbed per hour in the normals and 0.57 ± .036 in the osteoporotics ($p<.01$). Mean serum $1,25(OH)_2D$ was 99 ± 8 pmol/l in the normals and 86 ± 6 pmol/l in the osteoporosis (NS). Mean 25OHD was 70 ± 4 nmol/l in the normals and 66 ± 4 nmol/l in the osteoporotics (NS).

In neither group was any of the three measured variables significantly related to age.

Serum $1,25(OH)_2D$ and α were significantly related in both groups ($p<.001$ in each group). However, in the normal group the regression equation of α on serum 1,25D was .0042 + 0.34 whereas in the osteoporotics the regression equation was

Vitamin D. A Chemical, Biochemical and Clinical Update

.0029 + .33. The difference between these slopes was highly significant ($F = 41; p<.001$).

When α was regressed on age and serum $1,25(OH)_2D$ in each group by multiple regression analysis, the contribution of age was not significant. When serum $1,25(OH)_2D$ was regressed on age and 25OHD, only the contribution of 25OHD was significant and then only in the normal group.

Discussion

Although we find serum $1,25(OH)_2D$ levels to be slightly lower in osteoporotic than normal subjects, the difference did not reach significance in this series although if the cases are classified by densitometry rather than by simple radiography, the difference in serum $1,25(OH)_2D$ between normal and osteoporotic subjects does just reach significance. However the cases are classified, the slightly reduced serum $1,25(OH)_2D$ levels in osteoporotic subjects do not explain the malabsorption of calcium which is present in many of these patients.

References

1. Saville, P.D. (1973) Clinics in Endocrinology and Metabolism, 2:177-185
2. Gallagher, J.C., Aaron, J., Horsman, A., Marshall, D.H., Wilkinson, R., Nordin, B.E.C. (1973) Clinics in Endocrinology and Metabolism, 2:293-315
3. Gallagher, J.C., Riggs, B.L., Eisman, J., Hamstra, A., Arnaud, S.B., DeLuca, H.F. (1979) J Clin. Invest. 64:729-736
4. Nordin, B.E.C., Peacock, M., Crilly, R.G., Francis, R.M. Speed, R., Barkworth, S. In: Osteoporosis: Recent Advances in Pathogenesis and Treatment, DeLuca, H.F. et al (eds) 1981, University Park Press, Baltimore, p359-367
5. Marshall, D.H., Nordin, B.E.C. (1981) Clin. Sci. 61:477-481
6. Taylor, G.A., Peacock, M., Pelc, B., Brown, W., Holmes, A. (1980) Clin. Chim. Acta. 108:239-246
7. Edelstein, A., Charman, M., Lawson, B.E.M., Kodicek, E. (1974) Clin. Sci. Mol. Med. 46:231-240

EFFECT OF THE DIPHOSPHONATE APD ON DUAL PHOTON ABSORPTIOMETRY IN INVOLUTIONAL OSTEOPOROSIS.

J.P. Huaux, J.P. Devogelaer, J.P. Brasseur, C. Nagant de Deuxchaisnes.
Department of Rheumatology, Louvain University in Brussels, St-Luc University Hospital, B-1200 Brussels.

Introduction.

(3-amino-1-hydroxypropylidène)-1,1-diphosphonate (APD) has been shown to be an effective agent in inhibiting osteolytic bone lesions (1-5). Moreover, while studying patients with Paget's disease (5 M, 9 F) given APD, 600 mg/d orally for an average period of 15.3 ± 2.2 mo., we found in this group a surprising gain of bone mineral content (0.5 % per month), as shown on single photon absorptiometry at midshaft radius (6). At distal radius, a similar increase was noted, but statistical significance was not quite reached. We therefore undertook a study of patients with involutional osteoporosis, and followed the lumbar spine (L2-L4) mineral content by means of dual photon absorptiometry.

Materiel and methods.

12 patients (4 M, 8 F), average age 56.3 ± 3.5 (SEM), received 300 mg of APD orally in 3 divided doses 30 min before meals. The treatment was discontinued every 2 months for a period of two months. The patients were followed for an average period of 8.2 ± 1.2 mo. (range : 2-14 mo.). Measurements of lumbar bone mineral (BMC/cm) content (L2-L4) were performed using dual photon absorptiometry (Novo, type-22A). Single photon absorptiometry (Norland-Cameron Bone Mineral Analyzer) was performed at distal and midshaft radius as well.
Statistical analysis was performed using Student's t test.

Results.

The results are shown in the figure and the Table. The lumbar BMC increased by 5.8 ± 1.1 %, which represents a gain of mostly trabecular bone of 0.67 % per month. This was statistically significant ($p<0.001$). Midshaft radius BMC increased, but this did not reach statistical significance.

Statistical Analysis

t test

Lumbar BMC		Signif.
Initial	Terminal (Mean±Sem)	
100%	105.8±1.1	P<0.001

Gain: 0.67% / month

Vitamin D. A Chemical, Biochemical and Clinical Update

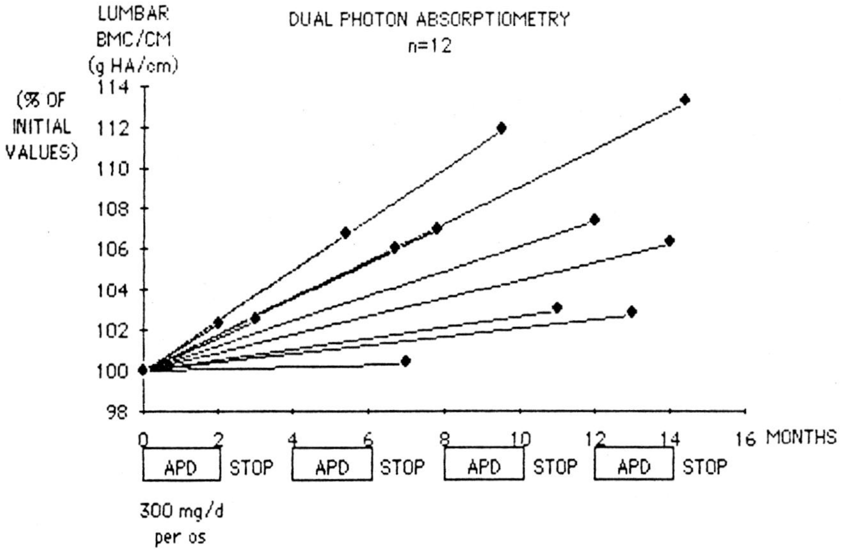

Discussion.

Our previous study (6) had shown that APD increased the cortical bone mass (0.5 % per mo.) when used in Paget's disease at the dose of 600 mg/24 h orally. This effect could not be demonstrated in this shorter study with smaller doses given intermittently. However, the present study demonstrated that APD increased the lumbar bone mass at a similar rate (0.67 %/mo.) in patients suffering from involutional osteoporosis despite the reduction of the dose to 300 mg/24 h, given only 6 mo./year. APD therefore may be the agent of choice in the treatment of involutional osteoporosis, provided in the longterm no extraskeletal side effects appear. The medication was apparently well tolerated, both clinically and biologically. More work will be needed to determine the optimal dose and mode of administration (continuously or intermittently) of APD in this indication.

References.

1) van Breukelen FJM, Bijvoet OLM, van Oosterom AT (1979). Lancet,I,803-805

2) van Breukelen FJM, Bijvoet OLM, Frijlink WB, Sleeboom HP, Mulder H, van Oosterom AT (1982). Calcif Tissue Int 34:321-327.

3) Elooma I, Blomqvist C, Gröhn P, Porkka L, Kairento AL, Selander K, Lamberg-Allardt C, Holmström T, (1983). Lancet,1,146-149.

4) Sleeboom HP, Bijvoet OLM, van Oosterom AT, Gleed JH, O'Riordan JLH (1983). Lancet,2,239-243.

5) Huaux JP, Noël H, Bastien P, Doyen C, Nagant de Deuxchaisnes C (1984). Acta Clin Belg,39,339-351.

6) Nagant de Deuxchaisnes C, Devogelaer JP, Esselinckx W, Depresseux G, Rombouts-Lindemans C, Huaux JP (1983), Brit Med J,286:1648.

DIFFERENT RESPONSES OF SERUM PARATHYROID HORMONE LEVELS IN OSTEOPOROSIS TO THE TREATMENT WITH 1 ALPHA(OH)D_3

T.NAKAMURA, K.NAKAMURA, A.NAGANO, Y.NISHII, AND T.KUROKAWA
Department of Orthopaedic Surgery, Univ. of Tokyo, Tokyo,
Chugai Pharmaceutical Laboratory, Tokyo, Japan.

Osteoporosis is a common disorder in women after menopause and has been related to several factors(3). But the precise mechanisms for the loss of bone are still uncertain and would be variable among individual patients(1). The purpose of this paper is to know the responses in patients of high parathyroid hormone(PTH) group and normal(or low) PTH group of female osteoporosis to the treatment with 1 alpha-(OH)D_3.

MATERIALS AND METHODS

Twenty three women aged 56 to 80(67.6±6.9)years were studied. All had radiological evidence of osteoporosis with vertebral fractures. They had no prior history of treatment with vitamin D, hormones, or calcium. All patients received 1 alpha(OH)D_3 at a dose of 1 microgram/day for twelve months after the initial evaluations. Serum C-PTH and vitamin D metabolites were determined every six months. Serum calcium,phosphorous, alkaline-phosphatase, and creatinine levels were measured monthly. Radiographs of hands alongside with an aluminum wedge were taken every six months for the densitometric analysis to obtain metacarpal index(MCI) and mean bone density. Serum C-PTH levels correlated with ages(r=0.55, p 0.01). High PTH(more than 1.1ng/ml) group involved seven patients and normal PTH(less than 1.1ng/ml) group involved sixteen. Significant differences between these two types of osteoporosis were found in ages(64.9±5.9 years for normal PTH group, 75.0±2.8 years for high PTH group: p 0.01), and serum creatinine levels(0.89±0.18mg/dl for normal PTH group, 1.16±0.40mg/dl for high PTH group:p 0.05).

RESULTS

Serum C-PTH levels showed the different responses to the treatment between high PTH and normal PTH groups. They were made lower significantly in the first six months. The average in normal PTH group decreased from 0.34±0.23ng/ml to 0.12±0.08ng/ml(p 0.01), and from 1.90±0.86ng/ml to 0.77±0.96ng/ml in high PTH group(p 0.01). But in the next six months they came up to the pretreatment levels of 1.79±1.14ng/ml in high PTH group, while normal PTH group maintained the reduced serum concentrations of PTH. Serum calcium levels were elevated in normal PTH group, but not in high PTH group. The average in normal PTH group was 9.7±0.12mg/dl initially, and increased to 10.0±0.34mg/dl in a year(p 0.05). But in high PTH group, 10.0±0.20mg/dl was the average initially and remained at the similar level after the treatment. Serum alkaline-phophatase levels showed the decrease in normal PTH group, but not in high PTH group. The initial mean value was 101.0±30.0IU and 76.3±13.6IU in a year(p 0.05) for normal PTH group. In high PTH group, 113.3±39.3IU was the average at the pretreatment examinations and 100.4±36.9IU in a year(N.S.).

Concerning the serum concentrations of vitamin D metabolites, no significant alterations were detected. Normal PTH group possessed the mean value of 14.5±7.7ng/ml for 25(OH)D_3 at the time of pretreatment and 14.3±5.6ng/ml in a year. On high PTH group, 10.6±5.0ng/ml was the average initially and 12.5±7.3ng/ml in a year. Results were similar in 1,25(OH)$_2$ D_3. The average concentrations of normal PTH group was 34.9±17.5pg/ml at the pretreatment period. 35.7±16.0pg/ml in six months, and 34.9±17.0 pg/ml in a year. For high PTH group, 37.7±18.1pg/ml was the initial average, 33.2±18.3pg/ml in six months and 37.9±15.1pg/ml in a year. Densitometric analysis of bone presented favourable results for normal PTH group. Normal PTH group showed the increase of MCI from the average of 0.384±0.045 to 0.403±0.051(p 0.01), while high PTH group did not indicate the significant changes on MCI, 0.374±0.061 initially and 0.387 ±0.071 in a year. No significant changes were detected with the parameter of mean bone density.

DISCUSSION

The results of the present study clearly demonstrated the different responses between high PTH group and normal PTH group to the treatment with 1 alpha(OH)D_3 at the dose of 1 microgram/day. Patients of normal PTH group responded well to the treatment, showing the steady decrease of serum C-PTH levels with the elevation of serum calcium levels. Reduced concentrations were still presented at the time of one year since the start of treatment. The increased intestinal absorption of calcium would be responsible for these changes(5). But the responses to the treatment were blunted in high PTH group. It seemed that they became less sensitive to the treatment in a year. Initial evaluations disclosed the differences between high PTH group and normal PTH group(4); age and serum creatinine level. It would be suspected that decrease of cellular function in various organs including not only ovarium but intestine, kidney and bone might be dominated in high PTH group. Serum 25(OH)D_3 levels were lower in our patients. Simple vitamin D deficiency seems unlikely and seasonal variation is not the case(2), because they were constantly decreased throught a year. We will need further investigations on the role of decreased 25(OH)D_3 levels in osteoporosis.

In conclusion, we believe we can expect the therapeutic effects on normal PTH group in postmenopausal osteoporosis with the administration of 1 alpha(OH)D . But it would not be so potent for high PTH group even with a rather high dose of 1 microgram/day.

REFERENCES

1. Davies,M.,Mawer,E.B., and Adams,H.(1977) J.Clin.Endocrinol.Metab.45, 199-208.
2. Lawoyin,S.,Zerwekh,J.E.,Glass,K., and Pak,C.Y.(1980) J.Clin.Endcrinol. Metab.50,593-596.
3. Gallagher,J.C.,Riggs,B.L.,Eisman,J.,Hamstra,A.Arnaud,S.B.,DeLuca,H.F. (1979) J.Clin.Ivest. 64,729-736.
4. Riggs,B.L.,Gallagher,J.C.,DeLuca,H.F.,Edis,A.J.,Lambert,P.W.,Arnaud, C.D.(1978) Mayo Clin. Proc.53,701.
5. Tsau,K.S.,Heath,H.,Kumar,R.,Riggs,B.L.(1984) J.Clin.Invest.73,1668-1672.

RELATION BETWEEN SERUM 1,25 DIHYDROXYVITAMIN D, CALCIUM ABSORPTION AND BONE DENSITY IN OSTEOPOROTIC POSTMENOPAUSAL WOMEN

B E C Nordin* H A Morris** Vicki Fraser** T F Hartley**
Annette Bridges* Cynthia Walker*
* Departments of Endocrinology and Radiology, Royal Adelaide Hospital, Adelaide, South Australia
** Division of Clinical Chemistry, Institute of Medical and Veterinary Science, Adelaide, South Australia

Introduction

The malabsorption of calcium which occurs in osteoporosis is only partially accounted for by reduced serum $1,25(OH)_2D$ levels. Using vertebral and forearm mineral densitometry, we have examined the relations between calcium absorption, serum $1,25(OH)_2D$ levels and vertebral and forearm density in osteoporotic postmenopausal women.

Clinical Material and Methods

The series comprises 62 postmenopausal women with varying degrees of vertebral compression and a mean age of 66.3 years. Radiocalcium absorption was measured by administering 5 μC of Ca^{45} in 20 mg of calcium carrier as the chloride in 250 ml of water and taking a plasma sample 60 minutes later for the measurement of radioactivity. After the correction for body weight, the result was expressed as the fraction of radiocalcium absorbed per hour by reading off a calibration curve (1). Serum $1,25(OH)_2D$ was measured by radioimmunoassay after HPLC separation (2). Vertebral mineral density (VMD) was measured by CAT scanning (3) and forearm mineral density (FMD) by gamma-ray absorptiometry (4).

Results

The mean radiocalcium absorption was 0.58 ± .03 of the dose absorbed per hour (NR 0.35-1.35). Mean VMD was 71 ± 4 mg/ml (NR in young adults 120-220). Mean serum $1,25(OH)_2D$ was 91 ± 6 pmol/ml (NR 50-150). Mean FMD was 290 ± 8 mg/ml (NR in young adults 420-520).

VMD was very significantly related to α ($r = .42:p<.001$) and less significantly to serum $1,25(OH)_2D$ ($r = .30:p<.02$). VMD was significantly related to age ($r = -.33:p<.01$) and serum $1,25(OH)_2D$ was also significantly related to age ($r = -.32:p<.02$). FMD was not significantly related either to α or to serum $1,25(OH)_2D$ but fell significantly with age ($r = -.32:p<.02$).

Vitamin D. A Chemical, Biochemical and Clinical Update

When VMD was regressed on α and serum $1,25(OH)_2D$ the multiple R was 0.42 ($p<.001$) but only the contribution of α was significant (Table). When VMD was regressed on age and α multiple R was 0.48 ($p<.001$) and the contributions of both age and α were significant.

Table

				t
VMD	=	45.5	α	2.47
		0.06	$1,25(OH)_2D$	0.60
		+39.0		
Multiple R	=	0.42 (59 df)	$p<0.001$	
VMD	=	-1.01	Age	2.04
		44.9	α	3.03
		+111.3		
Multiple R	=	0.48 (59 df)	$p<0.001$	

Discussion

In osteoporotic postmenopausal women, VMD is significantly related to radiocalcium absorption even after correction for age. Although there is also a correlation between VMD and serum $1,25(OH)_2D$ this is entirely accounted for by the relation between the latter and α and when both variables are considered together, the relation between serum $1,25(OH)_2D$ and VMD is lost. FMD is not related to either α or serum $1,25(OH)_2D$.

References

1. Marshall, D.H., Nordin, B.E.C. (1981) Clin. Sci. 61:477-481
2. Taylor, G.A., Peacock, M., Pelc, B., Brown, W., Holmes, A. (198) Clin. Chim. Acta 108:239-246
3. Cann, C.E., Genant, H.K. (1980) J Comput. Assist. Tomog. 4:493-500
4. Nordin, B.E.C., Robertson, A., Chatterton, B.E., Steurer, T., Bridges, A. In: Osteoporosis, C. Christiansen et al (eds) 1984, p153-156

3 YEARS TREATMENT WITH 1,25(OH)2 VITAMIN D3 DOES NOT REDUCE BONE LOSS OR FRACTURE RATE IN POSTMENOPAUSAL WOMEN WITH FRACTURE OF THE DISTAL FOREARM

J.A.Falch, O.R.Ødegaard and A.M.Finnanger.
Medical Dept.B and Dept. of Radiology, Aker Hospital, Oslo 5, Norway.

Introduction.

The incidence of fractures of the distal forearm increases rapidly in women at the age around the menopause. This is possibly due to an increased bone loss (1). In order to investigate the effect of 1,25(OH)2 Vit D on postmenopausal bone loss, females who had sustained a forearm fracture were chosen for the study.

Patients and Methods.

Postmenopausal women 50-65 years of age who had sustained a fracture of the left distal forearm during the last year were asked to participate in a single blind randomized trial. The treatment group (47 women) were given 0,25 µg 1,25(OH)2 Vit D3 twice daily. The control group were given 400 IU Vit D3 daily. There were no differences between the groups regarding age, years since menopause, bone mass or previous vertebral fractures. The treatment was given for 3 years. Changes in bone mass were evaluated by repeated photonabsorptiometry of the right distal and proximal forearm, using a double isotop equipment (Studsvik 7102). Vertebral fractures were measured from standard lateral vertebral x-rays according to Riggs (2). New long bone fractures were recorded.

Results.

In the 1,25(OH)2 Vit D3-group, 39 women (83%) completed the study. Of whom 11 (28%) had to reduce the daily dose because of slight hypercalcaemia (s-Ca above 2,65 mmol/l). No other side effects could be attributed to the treatment. In the control group 37 women (95%) completed the study. s-Ca values above 2,65 mmol/l were also occasionally seen in this group. The annual loss of bone mass of the distal forearm in the treatment group was 0,009 g/cm ± 0,047 and in the control group 0,013 g/cm ± 0,040 (Mean ∓ 1SD). For the proximal forearm the corresponding results were 0,008 g/cm ± 0,059 and 0,017 g/cm ± 0,060. The differences were not statistically significant. There was no difference in new vertebral fractures. In the treatment group 7 long bone fractures and in the control group 5 long bone fractures occured during the observation period.

Conclusion.

Treatment during 3 years with 0,5 µg 1,25(OH)2 Vit D3 did not reduce bone loss or fracture rate in postmenopausal women who had sustained a fracture of the distal forearm. Nearly 1/3 of the treated women had to reduce their daily dose because

Vitamin D. A Chemical, Biochemical and Clinical Update

of slight hypercalcaemia.

References.

1. Falch,J.A.(1983) Acta Orthop.Scand. 54, 291-295.
2. Riggs,B.L., Seeman,E., Hodgson,S.F., Taves,D.R. and O'Fallon,W.M.(1982) N.Eng.J.Med. 306, 446-450.

INSUFFICIENCY FRACTURES IN OSTEOPOROSIS CONFUSED WITH LOOSER ZONES

M.J. McKenna, M. Kleerekoper, D.S. Rao, B. Ellis, A.M. Parfitt, B. Frame,
Bone and Mineral Division, Henry Ford Hospital, Detroit, MI, U.S.A.

INTRODUCTION

Stress fractures are classified into two types, depending on whether the bone is normal (fatigue fracture) or abnormal (insufficiency fracture). A Looser zone denotes a broad lucent band perpendicular to the bone surface, symmetrically distributed at particular sites, rarely healing without specific therapy, and long considered the radiological hallmark of osteomalacia. The accuracy of this precept has been challenged since its inception (1,2) and more convincingly in recent times by reports of symmetric non-healing Looser zones in the absence of osteomalacia (3-6), raising doubts about the diagnostic utility of a Looser zone. This presentation describes six osteopenic females who presented with insufficiency fractures that were initially confused with Looser zones, until bone histologic analysis excluded a diagnosis of osteomalacia.

RESULTS

Clinical Features: All six subjects were white females and four were postmenopausal. Three of the postmenopausal females had radiologic evidence of vertebral compression, and all had low bone mass as assessed by single photon beam absorptiometry at the proximal radius site in the non-dominant forearm. Three cases had additional medical problems: alcoholism, moderate renal insufficiency, and primary hyperparathyroidism (PHPT) with iatrogenic hyperthyroidism.

Characteristics of Fractures: Twenty-six insufficiency fractures, both complete and incomplete, were recorded in the six subjects. The radiolucencies all occurred at traditional sites for Looser zones (pubic rami, medial aspect of femoral neck, lower ribs, metatarsal shafts, and lateral border of scapula). The distribution was symmetric in three cases. Fracture lines were perpendicular to the bone surface in all instances. Marginal sclerosis was an invariable finding. Various stages of healing could be seen: some had no evidence of callus, others had evidence of periosteal new bone formation, and also noted were sclerotic bands representing healed fractures. The duration of repair was protracted, and in two instances healing had not occurred after two years of observation.

Biochemical Findings: In the case with PHPT serum total calcium was mildly elevated at 10.6 mg/dl together with a raised serum parathyroid hormone at 205 ng/ml (normal <150 ng/ml) and a moderately elevated serum total alkaline phosphatase level at 225 iu/l (normal 27-83 iu/l). In the other subjects serum total calcium, ionized calcium, fasting phosphate, 25OHD, $1,25OH_2D$ values were within the respective reference ranges. In the latter five subjects the mean total alkaline phosphatase value (83±23 iu/l) was mildly elevated above the age and sex adjusted mean value (55±14 iu/l). The lady with renal insufficiency had evidence of secondary hyperparathyroidism (2^oHPT) as evidenced by an elevated serum parathyroid hormone level, a reduced $TmPO_4/GF$, and an elevated nephrogenous cyclic AMP.

Vitamin D. A Chemical, Biochemical and Clinical Update

Histologic Studies: Bone histomorphometric analysis after in vivo double tetracycline labeling excluded a diagnosis of osteomalacia, the osteoid seam width was below 15 microns in all cases. The two subjects with hyperparathyroidism (2^{O}HPT and PHPT) had an increased surface extent of osteoid and an increased bone formation rate, consistent with a high bone turnover state. In contrast the remaining subjects had low bone remodeling indices.

CONCLUSIONS

1) An insufficiency fracture may resemble the conventional radiographic description of a Looser zone, particularly if it occurs at certain sites and is slow to heal. Abnormal bone remodeling activity (both high and low bone turnover states) may retard the process of macro-fracture repair, thereby blurring the radiographic distinction between an insufficiency fracture and a true Looser zone.

2) The term Looser zone should be reserved for the following circumstances: a broad band perpendicular to the cortical surface with parallel clearly defined margins, absence of callus and of adjacent sclerosis, a minimum of three fractures preferably symmetrical and at least one appearing in either the ribs, pubis or femur. As yet such a fracture has not been described in the absence of osteomalacia (1-6). If radiological findings are equivocal, the generic term "insufficiency fracture" should be applied.

3) Previous studies have demonstrated that a true Looser zone only occurs in the presence of severe osteomalacia when clinical and biochemical features are grossly abnormal (6,7). Therefore, the following diagnostic approach is recommended both for a Looser zone (as defined above) and a suspected Looser zone or insufficiency fracture (not meeting all the above rigid criteria):

a) If compatible biochemical abnormalities are present, then this should denote severe osteomalacia; b) Conversely, normal serum chemistry should exclude osteomalacia; c) A bone biopsy is necessary to resolve cases of uncertainty.

This approach retains the customary association between a Looser zone and osteomalacia; it provides guidelines for the performance of a bone biopsy; and most importantly prevents unnecessary and potentially toxic treatment for osteomalacia.

REFERENCES

1. Dent, C.E., Hodson, C.J. (1954) Br J Radiol 27, 605-618.
2. North, K.A.K. (1966) Am J Roentgenol 97, 672-675.
3. Fulkerson, J.P., Ozonoff, M.B. (1977) Am J Roentgenol 129, 313-316.
4. Richardson, R.M.A., Rapoport, A., Oreopoulos, D.G., Meema, H.E., Rabinovich, S. (1978) Can Med J 119, 473-476.
5. Perry, H.M., Weinstein, R.S., Teitelbaum, S.L., Avioli, L.V., Fallon, M.D. (1982) Skeletal Radiol 8, 17-19.
6. McKenna, M.J., Freaney, R., Casey, O.M., Towers, R.P., Muldowney, F.P. (1983) J Clin Pathol 36, 245-252.
7. Rao, D.S., Villanueva, A., Mathews, M., et al (1983) In: Frame, B., Potts, J.T., Jr. eds. Clinical Disorders of Bone and Mineral Metabolism, Amsterdam; Excerpta Medica, 224-226.

BONE AND CORTICOSTEROIDS: THE ROLE OF ALTERED VITAMIN D METABOLISM.

G.Saggese, G.Cesaretti, S.Bertelloni, G.Federico and E.Bottone.
Department of Pediatrics, University of Pisa, Pisa, Italy.

Introduction:

A chronic treatment with corticosteroidsmay determinate a severe bone loss, so that osteopenia is one of the most important problems in these subjects. The pathogenetic pathway of steroids-induced osteopenia involves a complex alteration of bone metabolism as it demonstrated by the histologycfindings of both an increased osteoclastic activity and a decreased osteoblastic function (1)(2). Furthermore it is to be remarked steroids interfere with the bone metabolism both directly both indirectly by an alteration of vitamin D endocrine system. To clear furtherly the pathogenetic pathway of steroid-induced osteopenia we studied calcium metabolism in a group of patients treated with corticosteroids.

Patients and methods:

Thirty-one children, aged 2.1-15.2 years, treated with corticosteroids (1-2 mg/Kg/daily of prednisone) were examined. 26 were suffering from juvenil rheumatoid arthritis, 3 from dermatomysitis and 2 from systemic erythematousus lupus. All patients had radiographic findings of osteopenia. We effected the evaluations of serum Ca, P and alkalyne phosphatase, i-PTH (C-term) by a RIA-method (nv: 440 $\pm$ 220 pg/ml) (m $\pm$ 1 DS) and 25-OH-D (nv: 45 $\pm$ 12 ng/ml) and 1,25(OH)2D (38 $\pm$ 7 pg/ml) by a RRA method (3)(4).

Results:

Serum levels of Ca (4.9 $\pm$ 0.3 mEq/L), P (2.2 $\pm$ 0.3 mEq/L) and alcalyne phosphatase (624 $\pm$ 177 U/L) were in the normal range; i-PTH (760 $\pm$ 148 pg/ml) was increased ($p < 0.01$), while 25-OH-D was reduced: 27.3 $\pm$ 5.7 ng/ml ($p < 0.01$); also 1,25(OH)2D levels were decreased: 26.4 $\pm$ 7.9 pg/ml ($p < 0.01$).

Discussion:

It is known that steroids, as some other drugs, may induce hepatic enzymes. Therefore, the low 25-OH-D levels of our patients could be determin by the induction of hepatic 25-hydroxylase with the consequent formation of more polare inactive compounds (5). In fact it has been reported a negative correlation between the high steroid doses used in treatments and the serum 25-OH-D low values (6). Furthermore low 1,25(OH)2D levels, as found by Chesney (7) and in our patients too, could represent the consequence of both a reduced availability of the substratum for the kidney

Vitamin D. A Chemical, Biochemical and Clinical Update

1-alpha-hydroxylase and a stimulation of further metabolism of 1,25(OH)2D to a more polar biologically inactive intestinal metabolite (8). One of the consequences of the alteration of the vitamin D endocrine system is represented by a reduction of intestinal absorption of calcium. Moreover it has been demonstred a direct action of glucocorticosteroids on calcium transport by the intestinal mucosa (9), and moreover they would have also a calciuric effect (10). Therefore the condition of hyperparathyroidism, present also in our patients, could represent both a direct stimulation of PTH secretion by steroids (11) and the reaction to the decreased absorption of calcium, even if the levels of 1,25(OH)2D are lower than normal, in spite of the stimulation of 1-alpha-hydroxylase by the increased levels of PTH. Furthermore it is possible other endocrine alterations contribute to steroid-induced bone disease, as the reduction of serum levels of calcitonin or the ACTH-blocking effect of steroids with inhibition of adrenal synthesis of estrogen precursors. Moreover at bone levels steroids have a direct action on the activity of osteoblasts, that is inhibited, as demonstrated by some experimental studies (2). Therefore steroid-induced osteopenia represents the result of the uncoupleness between an increased bone reabsorption and a decreased bone matrix formation.

References:

1) Jowsey,J., Riggs,B.L.(1970) Acta Endocr.(Copenh) 63: 21-8.
2) Dietrich, J.W., Canalis, E.M., Maina, D.M., Raisz, L.G. (1979) Endocrinology 104: 715-21.
3) Belsey, R.E., De Luca, H.F. and Potts, J.T. (1974) J. Clin. Endocrinol. Metab. 28: 1046-51.
4) Eisman, J.A., Hamstra, A.J., Kream, B.E., De Luca, H.F. (1976) Arch. Bioch. Bioph. 176: 235-43.
5) Avioli, L.V., Birge, S.J., Sook W.L. (1968) J. Clin. Endocrinol. Metab. 28: 134-6.
6) Klein, R.G., Arnaud, S.B. and Gallagher, J.J. (1977) J. Clin. Invest. 60: 253-9.
7) Chesney, R.W., Hamstra, A.J., Mazess, R.B. and De Luca, H.F. (1978) Lancet 2: 1123-5.
8) Carre', M., Ayigbede, O., Miravet., L. and Rasmussen, H. (1974) Proc.Nat. Acad. Sci. USA 71: 2996-3000.
9) Kimberg, D.V., Baerg, R.D., Gershon, E. (1971) J. Clin. Invest. 50 :1309-21.
10) Suzuki, Y., Ichikawa, Y., Saito, E., Homma, M. (1983) Metabolism 32: 151-6.
11) Au, W.Y.W. (1976) Science 193: 1015-7.

ORAL PHOSPHATE DEPRESSES SERUM 1,25-DIHYDROXYVITAMIN-D CONCENTRATIONS IN OSTEOPOROTIC SUBJECTS

T.L. Clemens, S. Silverberg, D.W. Dempster, E. Shane, G.V. Segre, S. Williams, R. Lindsay, J.P. Bilizekian

Regional Bone Center, Helen Hayes Hospital, West Haverstraw, N.Y., Department of Medicine, Columbia University, New York, N.Y. and the Endocrine Unit, Massachusetts General Hospital, Boston, M.A., U.S.A.

Introduction:

Oral phosphate (PO_4) administration to healthy subjects acutely elevates circulating parathyroid hormone (PTH) concentrations, presumabaly by depressing serum ionized calcium (Ca^{++}) concentrations (1,2). Accordingly, it has been suggested that oral (PO_4) might be a useful "skeletal activator" in treatment regimens for low turnover osteoporosis (3). We have recently conducted experiments to evaluate the acute effects of PO_4 loading on mineral metabolism in healthy subjects and osteoporotic patients. We report here the effect of PO_4 loading on serum vitamin D metabolite concentrations.

Patients and Methods:

Five osteoporotic women (one premenopausal, aged 48 years and four postmenopausal women, aged 50 to 77) with one or more vertebral crush fractures were studied. PO_4 (as K-neutral phosphate) was given at 8:00 a.m. and 6:00 p.m. daily for 5 days. Serum PO_4, Ca^{++} (Nova 8) N-PTH (4), 25-OH-D and 1,25-$(OH)_2$-D (5) were measured at various intervals during the 4 day period. To determine the response of serum Ca^{++} to PO_4 dose we first gave doses of 0.25, 0.5, 0.75 and lg PO_4 to two healthy subjects and followed changes in serum Ca^{++} for 4 hours.

Results:

Doses of 0.75g and lg lowered serum ionized calcium at 3 to 4 hr.; lower doses were ineffective. Since lg was tolerated well in both subjects (and higher doses poorly tolerated) we used this dose to study the response in osteoporotic subjects. Oral PO_4 (lg) resulted in a rise in serum PO_4, a fall in ionized Ca^{++} and a rise in N-PTH over the first 4 hr. (Fig. 1). The fall in Ca^{++} and rise in N-PTH were variable among subjects; the greatest increment in N-PTH was 10 pg/ml (77%). These acute changes were documented in one osteoporotic subject with each of 3 successive daily doses of PO_4. In the face of increases in N-PTH, there was a 50% decrease in 1,25-$(OH)_2$-D concentrations (P 0.01) by day four in all subjects with no change in 25-OH-D levels (Fig. 2). In a separate group of 13 healthy subjects (ages 19-36 years) oral PO_4 induced changes in serum PO_4, Ca^{++} and N-PTH similar to those seen in osteoporotic subjects but the effect on 1,25-$(OH)_2$-D was collectively less impressive (mean fall 14%). However, in 4 of the healthy subjects, the magnitude of the fall in 1,25-$(OH)_2$-D was similar to that of the osteoporotic subjects. The reason for this variable response to $PO_4$is unclear at present.

Discussion:

The finding that oral PO_4 administration to osteoporotic subjects results acutely in increased PTH secretion supports previous observations in healthy subjects (1) but differs from recent findings in osteoporotic individuals (2). The major new finding from our study is the marked reduction in circulating 1,25-$(OH)_2$-D during PO_4 treatment emphasizing the importance of PO_4 in the regulation of 1-hydroxylation (6). The depressive effect of PO_4 on circulating 1,25-$(OH)_2$-D levels should be considered if PO_4 is used in treatment protocols for osteoporosis.

Vitamin D. A Chemical, Biochemical and Clinical Update

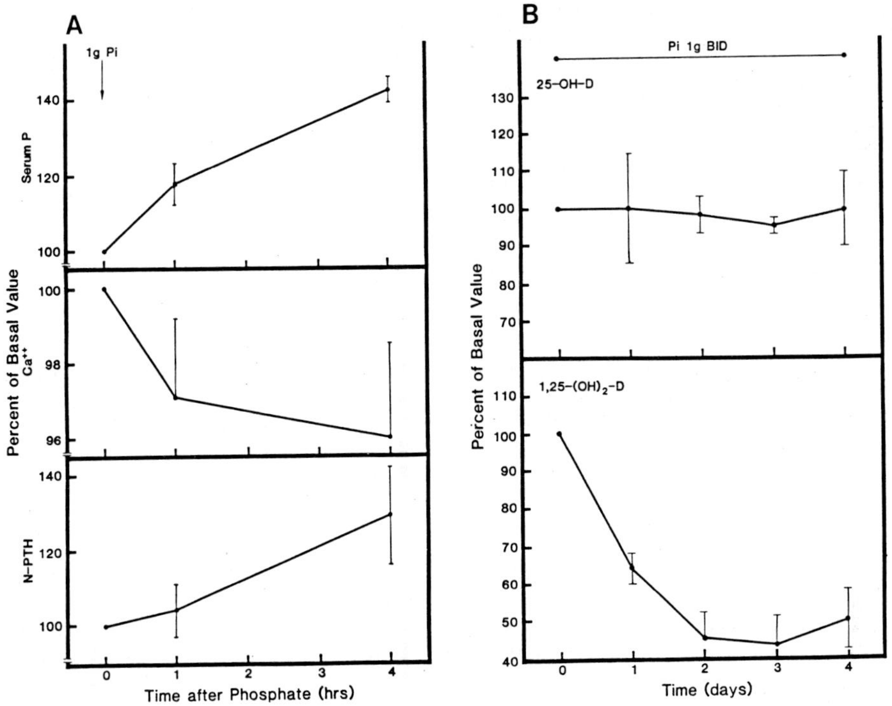

Figure 1. A. Acute changes in serum phosphorus (top), ionized calcium (middle) and N-PTH (bottom) in five osteoporotic subjects given 1 g elemental phosphorus orally. B. Changes in serum 25-OH-D (top) and 1,25-$(OH)_2$-D (bottom) concentrations in five osteoporotic subjects given 1 g phosphorus BID for five days. Data are presented as the percent of basal concentrations.

References:

1. Reiss, E., Canterbury, J.M., Kaplan, L., (1970) J. Clin. Invest. 49, 2146-2149.
2. Ittner, J., Dambacher, M.A., Ruegsegger, P., Fischer, J.A., (1984) Calc. Tiss. Intl. Program Abstract, Sixth Annual Meeting of the Society of Bone and Mineral Research, A55.
3. Anderson, C., Case, R.D.J., Crilly, R.G., Hodsman, A.B., Wolfe, B.M.J., (1984) Calc. Tiss. Intl. 36, 341-343.
4. Segre, G.V., Harris, S.J., Tully, G., Nerri, R., (1981) Proc. 63rd Annual meeting of the Endocrine Society, A585.
5. Fraher, L.J., Adams, S., Clemens, T.L., Jones, G., O'Riordan, J.L.H., (1983) 18, 151-165.
6. Maiertofer, W.J., Gray, R.W., Lemann, J., (1984) Kid. Intl. 25, 571-575.

AETIOLOGY OF OSTEOPOROSIS IN HEAVY DRINKERS

Brian Lalor, M. Davies, P.H. Adams and T.B. Counihan
Departments of Medicine, Mater Hospital Dublin, Ireland, and Manchester Royal Infirmary, England.

INTRODUCTION

There is clear evidence of a propensity to fracture and the development of osteoporosis among heavy drinkers, which suggests a causal relationship between them. The precise cause of the osteoporosis associated with chronic alcohol abuse has not been defined.

PATIENTS AND METHODS

Transilial bone biopsies (8mm) were obtained from 22 heavy drinkers with varying degrees of liver damage. Assessments were made of their nutritional status, liver function, vitamin D status and biochemical parameters of mineral metabolism, and the findings were compared with those obtained from 24 abstinent controls matched for age and sex.

RESULTS

Trabecular bone volume (TBV) tended to be reduced in the heavy drinkers, and eight had osteoporosis according to strict histological criteria. Within the drinkers, TBV was directly related to the serum albumin ($p < 0.005$), dietary calcium ($p < 0.01$) and dietary protein ($p < 0.02$). Multivariate analysis of the relevant variables showed that the major determinants of age-adjusted TBV was the serum albumin (and thus the state of liver function and the dietary protein) and the dietary calcium according to the multiple regression equation:-

TBV = 0.0197 (serum albumin) - 0.2078 (Quetelet's index) + 0.001199 (dietary calcium). $r = 0.806$, $p < 0.0001$.

The type of alcohol habitually consumed was also important. Spirit drinkers had a lower ($p < 0.007$) TBV than stout drinkers; 5 of 7 spirit drinkers and 3 of 15 stout drinkers had osteoporosis (fig 1). This effect was probably nutritional in origin and related to the nutritional value of the form of alcohol consumed. The spirit drinkers consumed less calcium and protein and fewer calories than the stout drinkers, although their basal provision (non-alcohol derived) of their nutrients was the same (Figs 2 and 3). Serum calcidiol tended to be low in the drinkers and was directly related to the state of liver function (Table 1); 4 drinkers with osteoporosis had subnormal levels of calcitriol. Six drinkers (5 with osteoporosis) had biochemical evidence of hyperparathyroidism.

All the patients with osteoporosis had a reduction in mean wall thickness, and 4 had little or no bone forming surfaces. There was no histological evidence of hyperparathyroidism or increased bone resorption.

Vitamin D. A Chemical, Biochemical and Clinical Update

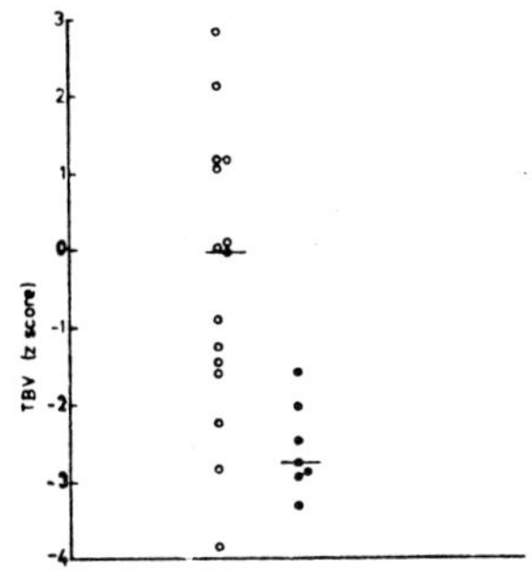

Fig.1.
Age adjusted TBV in the spirit drinkers ● and in the stout drinkers O . ——— represents the median values.

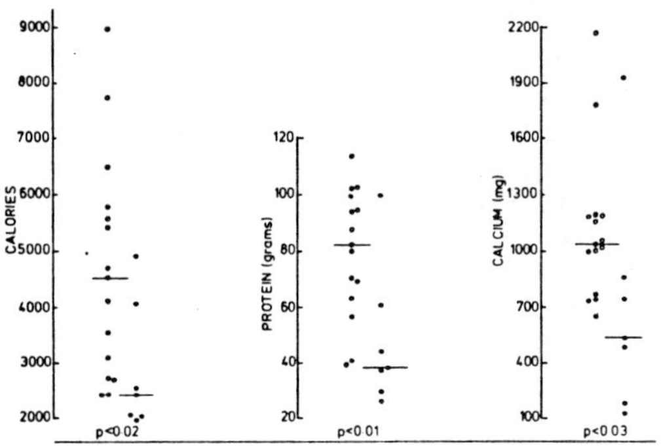

Fig.2.
Dietary intake of calories, protein and calcium in the spirit drinkers ● and in the stout drinkers O.
——— Represents the median values.

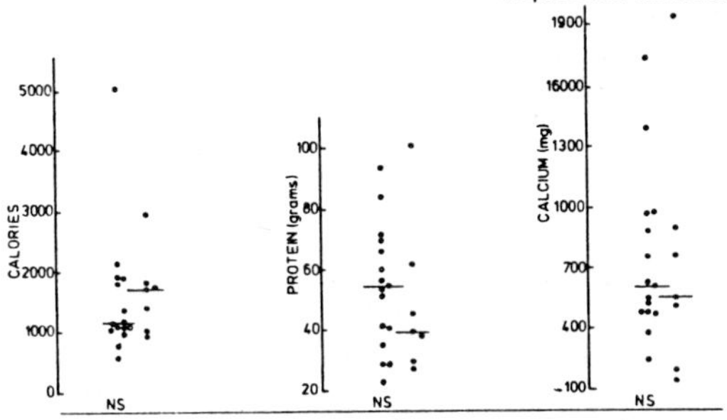

Fig.3.
Basic dietary intake (i.e. that not derived from alcoholic beverages) of calories, protein and calcium in the spirit drinkers ● and in the stout drinkers O . ——— represents the median values.

TABLE 1

ALBUMIN	rho = 0.57	$p < 0.01$
BILIRUBIN	rho = -0.621	$p < 0.005$
AST	rho = -0.552	$p < 0.01$
GGT	rho = -0.618	$p < 0.005$

Correlations between parameters of liver function and serum levels of calcidiol.

CONCLUSIONS

The development of osteoporosis among heavy drinkers is multifactorial, but seems to arise mainly through a reduction in bone formation. An important factor is protein malnutrition which is related to liver dysfunction and reduced dietary protein intake. Low vitamin D status and a reduced dietary intake of calcium are compounding factors, which might also account for secondary hyperparathyroidism and probably increased bone resorption.

PHYSIOLOGICAL INTERRELATIONS OF CALCITRIOL AND CALCITONIN

JOHN C. STEVENSON, GAMINI ABEYASEKERA, PAUL R. ALLEN[1] and MALCOLM I. WHITEHEAD[2]
Endocrine Unit, Royal Postgraduate Medical School, London W12; [1] Dept. of Orthopaedics, St. Thomas's Hospital, London SE1; [2] Academic Dept. of Gynaecology, King's College School of Medicine, London SE5.

INTRODUCTION

Certain physiological situations bring about an increased demand for calcium, particularly in women. These include growth, pregnancy and lactation. To fulfil these needs for extra calcium during such times, there is enhanced intestinal absorption of calcium and some degree of calcium retention in bone. Conversely, following the menopause there is mobilization of bone, with increased urinary calcium loss and decreased intestinal calcium absorption. In some women this postmenopausal bone loss results in an abnormally thin skeleton - osteoporosis. In all these situations there appears to be changes in the secretion of the major calcium regulating hormones, particularly calcitriol and calcitonin. We have therefore measured circulating levels of these hormones in various physiological situations to study their interrelations and possibly linked effects on bone and gut.

PATIENTS

94 healthy white women aged 16 to 75 years were studied. 39 women were pregnant (mean age 26 years, range 19-36), 15 women had normal ovarian function (mean age 33 years, range 17-44) and 40 women were without ovarian function (mean age 46 years, range 16-75). Additionally, samples were taken from 10 women with femoral neck osteoporosis (mean age 69 years, range 62-75). None of these women was taking any medication known to influence calcium metabolism. Following an overnight fast, venous blood samples were collected at midday, and the plasma was at once separated and stored at -20^0C until assayed.

METHODS (1)

Vitamin D metabolites were extracted from plasma with Extrelut columns (E. Merck) and separated by HPLC using 10% isopropynol in hexane. Calcitriol was measured using chick intestinal cytosol in a competitive protein-binding assay. Detection limit was 12.5 pmol/l with intra and inter-assay variations being <10%.

Calcitonin was extracted from plasma with Spherosil and measured in a 7 day incubation non-equilibrium radioimmunoassay. Sensitivity was 0.6 fmol/tube with intra and inter-assay variations being < 10% and <14% respectively.

Statistical analyses were performed on the $\log_{10}$ transformed values of both calcitriol and calcitonin.

Vitamin D. A Chemical, Biochemical and Clinical Update

RESULTS

The levels of calcitriol and calcitonin were elevated in the pregnant women as previously reported (2). Over the entire physiological range there was a correlation between the plasma levels of calcitriol and calcitonin ($r = 0.53$, $p < 0.001$) (Figure 1).

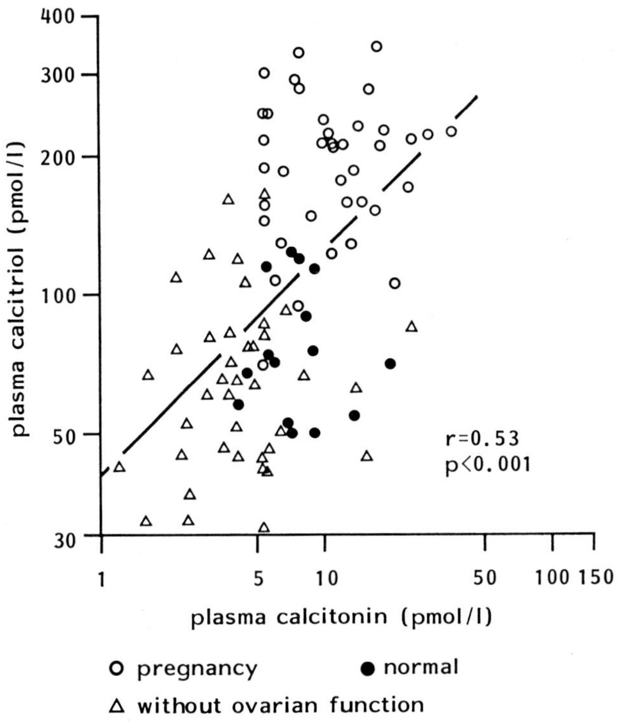

Figure 1 Correlation between plasma calcitriol and plasma calcitonin levels in normal women, pregnant women, and women without ovarian function. Expected $\log_{10}$ calcitriol (pmol/l) = 1.60 + 0.496 $\log_{10}$ calcitonin (pmol/l) (SE est = 0.24).

The $\log_{10}$ molar ratio of calcitonin:calcitriol was approximately 1:2 in premenopausal women and during pregnancy. However this ratio decreased significantly ($p < 0.002$) following the loss of ovarian function and tended to be lowest in the postmenopausal osteoporotics (Figure 2). The circulating levels of both calcitriol and calcitonin were lowest in the osteoporotics, with the mean calcitriol level being significantly lower ($p < 0.02$) than that in 10 age-matched controls. The mean plasma calcitonin level was significantly lower ($p < 0.01$) in the osteoporotics than in those controls following a 1 minute IV calcium infusion (2 mg/kg body weight).

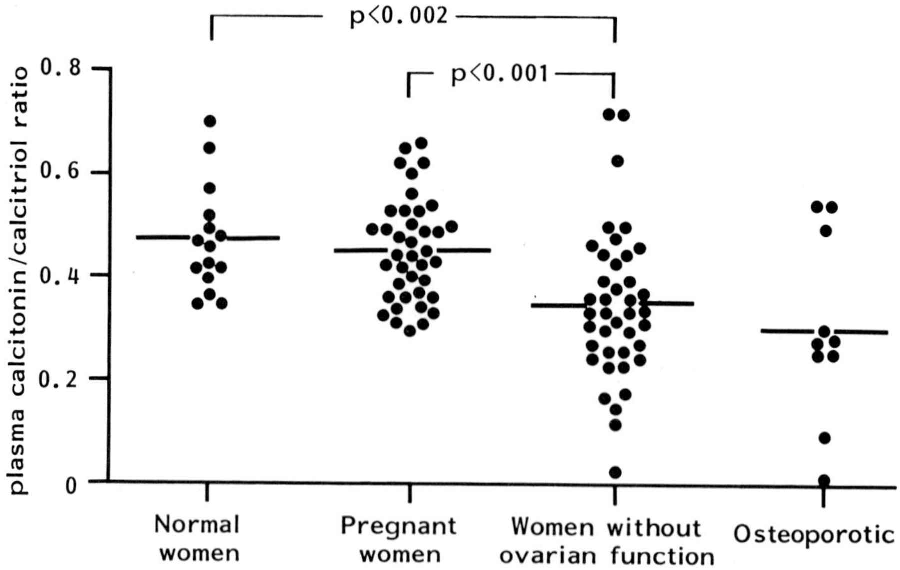

Figure 2 Plasma calcitonin/calcitriol ratios (log_{10} pmolar) in normal women, pregnant women, women without ovarian function and osteoporotic women.

DISCUSSION

The enhanced intestinal calcium absorption seen during growth, pregnancy and lactation is brought about by increased calcitriol production (2,3,4). We have previously suggested that the increase in calcitonin levels also seen at these times (5,6) prevents an unwanted increase in bone resorption. Our present finding of a correlation between the circulating levels of the two hormones supports our concept. Increased secretion of calcitriol and calcitonin may be of importance for skeletal calcium accretion, such as may occur in pregnancy (7). A number of factors may be responsible for the increased hormone secretion in these physiological situations. Calcitriol production is increased by growth hormone (8), prolactin, placental lactogen (9) and by calcitonin (10). Interestingly, calcitonin production may itself be increased by calcitriol (11,12). However, both hormones appear to be regulated by oestradiol (13,14) and hence it is of great interest to study their secretion during physiological oestrogen deficiency. There appears to be a decline in the circulating levels of both calcitriol and calcitonin following the loss of ovarian function, but the decline in calcitonin secretion is greater. Thus, following the menopause there will be an imbalance between levels of calcitriol and calcitonin which should result in an increase in bone resorption. A similar imbalance between the levels of parathyroid hormone and calcitonin could only enhance bone resorption. These alterations in the ratios of calcium regulating hormones due to loss of oestrogen may well explain the increased sensitivity of the postmenopausal skeleton to the actions of bone resorbing hormones (15). The changes in calcitriol and calcitonin secretion seem to be most marked in postmenopausal osteoporotics. Whilst factors such as declining bone formation (16) and, in very elderly women, declining renal endocrine function (17) may contribute to osteoporosis, our findings support the concept (18) that oestrogen deficiency is the single most important factor in the pathogenesis of this condition.

ACKNOWLEDGEMENTS

These studies were supported in part by Laboratoires Besins-Iscovesco and British Foundation for Age Research.

REFERENCES

1. Stevenson, J.C., Abeyasekera, G., Hillyard, C.J., Phang, K.G., MacIntyre, I., Campbell, S., Townsend, P.T., Young, O. and Whitehead, M.I. (1981) Lancet I, 693-695.
2. Whitehead, M., Lane, G., Young, O., Campbell, S., Abeyasekera, G., Hillyard, C.J., MacIntyre, I., Phang, K.G. and Stevenson, J.C. (1981) Br. Med. J. 283, 10-12.
3. Pike, J.W., Toverud, S.U., Boass, A., McCain, T.A. and Haussler, M.R., in Vitamin D. Biochemical, Chemical and Clinical Aspects Related to Calcium Metabolism, Ed. Norman, A.W. et al, Walter de Gruyter, Berlin, 1977, p.187-189.
4. Kumar, R., Cohen, W.R., Silva, P. and Epstein, F.H. (1979) J. Clin. Invest. 63, 342-344.
5. Samaan, N.A., Anderson, G.D. and Adam-Mayne, M.E. (1975) Am. J. Obstet. Gynecol. 121, 622-625.
6. Stevenson, J.C., Hillyard, C.J., MacIntyre, I., Cooper, H. and Whitehead, M.I. (1979) Lancet I, 769-770.
7. Goldsmith, N. and Johnston, J. (1975) J. Bone Joint Surg. 57, 657-668.
8. Spanos, E., Barrett, D., MacIntyre, I., Pike, J.W., Safilian, E.F. and Haussler, M.R. (1978) Nature 273, 246-247.
9. Spanos, E., Brown, D.J., Stevenson, J.C. and MacIntyre, I. (1981) Biochim. Biophys. Acta 672, 7-15.
10. Kawashima, H., Torikai, S. and Kurokawa, K. (1981) Nature 192, 327-329.
11. Juttman, J.R. and Birkenhager, J.C., in Vitamin D, Basic Research and its Clinical Application, Ed. Norman, A.W. et al, Walter de Gruyter, Berlin, 1979, p.861-865.
12. Freake, H.C. and MacIntyre, I. (1982) Biochem,. J. 206, 181-184.
13. Gallagher, J.C., Riggs, B.L. and DeLuca, H.F. (1980) J. Clin. Endocrinol. Metab. 51, 1359-1364.
14. Stevenson J.C., Abeyasekera, G. Hillyard, C.J., Phang, K.G., MacIntyre, I., Campbell, S., Lane, G., Townsend, P.T., Young, O. and Whitehead, M.I. (1983) Eur. J. Clin. Invest. 13, 481-487.
15. Heaney, R.P. (1965) Am. J. Med., 39, 877-880.
16. Lips, P., Courpon, P. and Meunier P. (1978) Calcif. Tissue Res. 26, 13-17.
17. Tsai, K.S., Heath, H., Kumar, R. and Riggs, B.L. (1984) J. Clin. Invest. 73, 1668-1672.
18. Stevenson J.C. and Whitehead, M.I. (1982) Br. Med. J. 285, 585-588.

THE RELATION BETWEEN DIETARY CALCIUM AND SERUM 1,25(OH)$_2$D LEVELS IN OSTEOPOROTIC WOMEN

Karen J Tassie* H A Morris** Vicki Fraser** M Horowitz* B E C Nordin*
* Department of Endocrinology, Royal Adelaide Hospital, Adelaide, South Australia
** Division of Clinical Chemistry, Institute of Medical and Veterinary Science, Adelaide, South Australia

Introduction

Gallagher et al (1) have reported an inverse correlation between dietary calcium intake and serum 1,25(OH)$_2$D levels in normal women below the age of 65. We have now established a similar relationship in osteoporotic postmenopausal women which is compatible with the concept that malabsorption of calcium in these cases is not due to a failure of 1,25(OH)$_2$D synthesis.

Clinical Material and Method

The subjects were 45 postmenopausal women with vertebral compression and a mean age of 67.4 years. Dietary calcium was estimated by the food frequency method (2). Serum 25OHD was measured by competitive protein binding after LH 20 separation (3). Serum 1,25(OH)$_2$D was measured by radioimmunoassay after HPLC (4). Plasma creatinine and phosphate were measured by multichannel analyzer.

Results

The mean serum 1,25(OH)$_2$D level was 88 ± 7 pmol/l (NR 50-150). The mean serum 25OHD level was 67 ± 3 nmol (NR 40-160). The mean dietary calcium intake was 827 ± 57 mg/day. The mean plasma phosphate was 1.05 ± .02 mmol/l (NR 0.7-1.25). The mean plasma creatinine was 0.79 ± .003 mmol/l (NR 0.05-0.12). In no patient was the plasma creatinine outside the normal range.

There was a significant inverse correlation between dietary calcium and serum 1,25(OH)$_2$D level ($p<.025$; Table 1). There was also a significant inverse correlation between age and serum 1,25(OH)$_2$D level (<.01; Table 1). There was no significant correlation between the serum 1,25(OH)$_2$D level and either the plasma phosphate, creatinine or 25OHD level.

When the serum 1,25(OH)$_2$D levels were regressed on age and dietary calcium simultaneously, the multiple R was 0.58 ($p<.001$) (Table 2). When 25OHD was added as a further independent variable, the multiple R rose to 0.61 ($p<.001$). When creatinine was added as a further independent variable, the multiple R rose to 0.64 ($p<.001$).

Vitamin D. A Chemical, Biochemical and Clinical Update

As seen in Table 2, the most significant determinants of the serum $1,25(OH)_2D$ were age and dietary calcium, followed by the 25OHD concentration then followed by plasma creatinine.

Table 1

$1,25(OH)_2D$	=	-0.04 Diet Ca +122
r	=	-0.35 (43 df) p<0.025
$1,25(OH)_2D$	=	-2.93 Age +286
r	=	-0.47 (43 df) p<0.01

Table 2

				t	p
$1,25(OH)_2D$	=	-0.04	Diet Ca	2.68	<0.02
		-2.89	Age	3.70	<0.001
		+317			
Multiple R	=	0.58	(42 df)	p<0.001	
$1,25(OH)_2D$	=	-0.04	Diet Ca	3.01	<0.005
		-2.80	Age	3.66	<0.001
		+0.48	25OHD	1.95	NS
		-495	Cr	1.59	NS
		+320			
Multiple R	=	0.64	(40 df)	p<0.001	

Discussion

Although malabsorption of calcium is relatively common in osteoporotic postmenopausal women, its cause has not been conclusively established to a deficiency in the production of $1,25(OH)_2D$. In our 45 osteoporotic women, there was an inverse correlation between the serum $1,25(OH)_2D$ level and the dietary calcium which was very close to the inverse correlation previously reported by Gallagher et al (1). Multiple regression analysis showed that of the other variables measured, age was a significant negative element of the serum $1,25(OH)_2D$ level. The multiple correlation coefficient was increased by introducing the serum 25OHD level which made a positive but not quite significant contribution, and the plasma creatinine concentration which made a negative but not in itself significant contribution.

References

1. Gallagher, J.C., Riggs, B.L., Eisman, J., Hamstra, A., Arnaud, S.B., DeLuca, H.F. (1979) J Clin. Invest. 64:729-736
2. Baghurst, K.I., Record, S.J. (1984) Comm. Health Studies 8:11-18
3. Edelstein, A., Charman, M., Lawson, B.E.M., Kodicek, E. (1974) Clin. Sci. Mol. Med. 46:231-240
4. Taylor, G.A., Peacock, M., Pelc, B., Brown, W., Holmes, A. (1980) Clin. Chim. Acta 108:239-246

DETERMINANTS OF VITAMIN D STATUS IN THE ELDERLY

P.Lips, M.J.M.Jongen, F.C.van Ginkel, J.C.Netelenbos, and W.J.F.van der Vijgh, Department of Internal Medicine
Academisch Ziekenhuis der Vrije Universiteit
P.B. 7057, 1007 MB Amsterdam, The Netherlands.

Introduction

Vitamin D deficiency is common in the elderly and especially in patients with hip fracture. It may lead to secondary hyperparathyroidism, high bone turnover, and cortical bone loss(1,2). The latter may be a cause of the hip fracture. We studied the determinants of vitamin D status in patients with hip fracture and aged control subjects.

Subjects and methods

The study included 125 patients with hip fracture and 74 aged control subjects (mean age±SD 75.9±11.0 yr and 75.6±4.2 yr respectively). From the patient group, 86 patients lived independently and 38 were institutionalized prior to fracture. The control subjects were healthy volunteers living independently in an apartmenthouse for aged people. Clinical and biochemical data have been published in detail(1,3). Serum levels of vitamin D metabolites (25(OH)D, 1,25$(OH)_2$D) were measured by competitive protein binding assay after gradient HPLC(4). The data were arranged according to sunshine exposure, vitamin D intake, residence, and renal function. The relative importance of the various determinants of vitamin D status was assessed by multiple regression analysis on serum 25(OH)D and serum 1,25$(OH)_2$D after correction for seasonal variation by statistical standardization.

Results

Data on vitamin D status in patients with hip fracture and aged controls are presented in Table 1. Serum 25(OH)D is lower in patients than in controls, as is sunshine exposure, whereas there is no difference in vitamin D intake. Serum 25(OH)D is higher in controls with high sunshine exposure than in those with low sunshine exposure (37.1±14.2 vs 26.3±9.3 nmol/l, $P<0.001$). A similar difference existed in the patients (24.3±11.7 vs 16.1±9.2 nmol/l, $P<0.001$). When sunshine exposure is high, there is no correlation between serum 25(OH)D and vitamin D intake. A positive correlation between serum 25(OH)D and vitamin D intake was found in patients with low sunshine exposure ($r=0.54$, $P<0.001$). According to this relationship, a vitamin D intake of about 300 IU/day is required in order to maintain serum 25(OH)D above 30 nmol/l. Patients who were institutionalized prior to fracture showed a mean serum 25(OH)D of only 14.3±6.2 nmol/l, due to negligible sunshine exposure and a very low vitamin D intake (75±39 IU/day).

The low serum 1,25$(OH)_2$D concentration in patients with hip fracture is mainly caused by a low vitamin D binding protein (DBP) concentration after the fracture. This may be inferred from the free 1,25$(OH)_2$D index, which is only little lower in patients than in controls(5). In addition, renal

Vitamin D. A Chemical, Biochemical and Clinical Update

Table 1. Vitamin D status and its determinants in patients with hip fracture and aged control subjects.

	controls	hip fractures		sign.
	mean±SD	mean±SD		
serum 25(OH)D	32.9±13.6	18.5±10.6	nmol/l	P<0.001
<30 nmol/l	46 %	87 %		
<15 nmol/l	4 %	38 %		
serum $1,25(OH)_2D$	105±31	79±46	pmol/l	P<0.001
serum creatinine	85±16	86±26	µmol/l	NS
serum DBP	371±44	315±60	mg/l	P<0.001
high/low sunshine exp.	61/39 %	32/68 %		P<0.01
vitamin D intake	114±44	116±63	IU/day	NS

functional impairment was more common in patients with hip fracture than in the control group (n=21 vs n=4). Patients with renal functional impairment (serum creatinine 111-184 µmol/l) showed a decreased serum $1,25(OH)_2D$ (52±33 pmol/l).

According to multiple regression analysis, the main determinants of serum 25(OH)D were in order of importance sunshine exposure, serum albumin and vitamin D intake in the patients with hip fracture, and sunshine exposure, serum calcium and vitamin D intake in the aged controls. Multiple regression analysis on serum $1,25(OH)_2D$ showed as most important determinants serum creatinine, serum phosphate, serum 25(OH)D and serum DBP (the latter in patients with hip fracture only).

Conclusion

Sunshine exposure is the main determinant of vitamin D status in the elderly. When sunshine exposure is low, vitamin D intake becomes important. The required intake is much higher than the observed intake. Vitamin D status is especially poor in the institutionalized. A vitamin D supplement should be considered for this group. A slight to moderate decrease of renal function causes a marked fall of serum $1,25(OH)_2D$ in the elderly.

References

1. Lips,P., Netelenbos, J.C.,Jongen,M.J.M., van Ginkel,F.C., Althuis,A.L., van Schaik,C.L., van der Vijgh,W.J.F., Vermeiden J.P.W., van der Meer,C. (1982) Metab.Bone Dis.Rel.Res.4,85-93.
2. Lips,P., Hackeng, W.H.L., Jongen,M.J.M., van Ginkel,F.C., Netelenbos,J.C.(1983) J.Clin.Endocrinol.Metab. 57, 204-206.
3. Lips,P. (1982) Metabolic causes and prevention of femoral neck fractures. Ph.D. Thesis,Vrije Universiteit,Amsterdam.
4. Jongen, M.J.M.,van der Vijgh, W.J.F., Willems,H.J.J., Netelenbos,J.C., Lips,P.(1981) Clin.Chem.27, 1757-1760.
5. Lips, P.,Bouillon,R., Jongen,M.J.M.,van Ginkel,F.C., van der Vijgh,W.J.F., Netelenbos,J.C.(1985) Metab.Bone Dis. Rel.Res. 6 (in press).

Acknowledgement

We are grateful to Dr.R. Bouillon (Rega Instituut, Leuven, Belgium) for the measurement of vitamin D binding protein.

EFFECT OF 24,25 DIHYDROXYVITAMIN D_3 ON POSTMENOPAUSAL BONE LOSS: A CONTROLLED THERAPEUTIC STUDY.

B.J. RIIS, L. HUMMER, K. THOMSEN, L. NILAS, A. GOTFREDSEN, C. CHRISTIANSEN,
Department of Clinical Chemistry, Glostrup Hospital, Denmark.

INTRODUCTION:

Postmenopausal osteoporosis have been connected with a disturbance in vitamin D metabolism (1,2). Studies have, however, demonstrated that treatment with vitamin D_3 or $1,25(OH)_2D_3$ has no beneficial effects on postmenopausal bone loss (3,4), but a recent study has postulated that $24,25(OH)_2D_3$ induce positive calcium balance in patients with osteoporosis (5). The aim of the present study was therefore to evaluate in a double blind set up, the effect of pharmacological doses of $24,25(OH)_2D_3$ on postmenopausal bone loss.

Participants and study design:

The study population comprised 53 postmenopausal women. They had passed a natural menopause 6 months to 3 years before the study. All were healthy and free of medications known to influence calcium metabolism. The participants were randomized to three groups who blindly received either $24,25(OH)_2D_3$ (10 µg/day), placebo, or estrogens/gestagens. All participants were examined before treatment and every third month for one year.

Methods:

Serum concentrations of 25(OH)D and $1,25(OH)_2D$ were determined by competitive protein binding assays with binding protein obtained from rat serum and chick intestinal cytosol, respectively (6). $24,25(OH)_2D_3$ was determined by radioimmunoassay (6). Bone mineral content in the forearms (BMC arm) was measured by single photon absorptiometry and bone mineral content in the spine (BMC spine) and in the total skeleton (TBBM) by dual photon absorptiometry (7). The serum concentrations of alkaline phosphatase and protein and urinary creatinine were measured by standard procedure. Serum and urinary calcium were determined by atomic absorptiometry. Intestinal calcium absorption was determined as the fractional absorption of an ingested dosage of ^{47}Ca (8).

RESULTS:

Table. Per cent change after 1 year study (Mean ± 1 SEM).

	$24,25(OH)_2D_3$	Placebo	Estrogens
S-$24,25(OH)_2D_3$	app. 800⇈	123 ± 27	-
S-$1,25(OH)_2D_3$	99 ± 8	92 ± 7	-
S-25(OH)D	90 ± 10	93 ± 17	-
TBBM	95⇓ ± 1	96⇓ ± 1	99 ± 1
BMD spine	96⇓ ± 1	95⇓ ± 1	101 ± 1
BMC arm	98⇓ ± 1	97⇓ ± 1	100 ± 1
S-Alkaline phos.	103 ± 5	105 ± 3	84 ⇓⇓ ± 5
S-Calcium	101 ± 1	100 ± 1	98 ± 1
24-h-urinary calcium	109 ± 14	95 ± 7	79 ⇓⇓ ± 8
Int. calcium absorp.	98 ± 8	114⇈ ± 7	130 ⇑ ± 10

Vitamin D. A Chemical, Biochemical and Clinical Update

In the $24,25(OH)_2D_3$ group the serum $24,25(OH)_2D_3$ concentration increased approximately 800 %, whereas serum 25OHD and $1,25(OH)_2D$ were unchanged. In the placebo group the serum vitamin D metabolites were unchanged. In both the $24,25(OH)_2D_3$ and the placebo groups the TBBM and BMC spine and BMC arm decreased significantly and at the same magnitude. In the estrogen treated group all three were unchanged. In both the $24,25(OH)_2D_3$ and the placebo groups serum levels af alkaline phosphatase and calcium and 24-hour-urinary calcium remained unchanged throughout the study, whereas the estrogen group showed a decrease in serum alkaline phosphatase and 24-hour-urinary calcium. The fractional intestinal calcium absorption increased significantly in the placebo group, but remained unchanged in the $24,25(OH)_2D_3$ group. In the estrogen group the calcium absorption increased significantly more than in the placebo group.

Conclusion:

10 µg daily of $24,25(OH)_2D_3$:
1) is no alternative to estrogens as prophylactic treatment of postmenopausal bone loss 2) does not improve the intestinal calcium absorption 3) does not change serum alkaline phosphatase concentration nor urinary calcium excretion rate.

References:

1. Gallagher, J.C., Riggs, B.L., Eisman, J., Hamstra, A., Arnaud, S.B., DeLuca, H.F. (1979) J. Clin. Invest. 64: 729-736.
2. Slovik, D.M., Adams, J.S., Neer, R.M., Holick, M.F., Potts, J.T. (1981) N Engl. J. Med. 305: 372-374.
3. Christiansen, C., Christensen, M.S., MaNair, P., Hagen, C., Stocklund, K-E., Transbøl, I. (1980) Eur J. Clin. Invest. 10: 273-279.
4. Christiansen, C., Christensen, M.S., Rødbro, P., Hagen, C., Transbøl, I. (1981) Eur. J. Clin. Invest. 11: 305-309.
5. Reeve, J., Tellez, M., Green, J.R., Hesp, R., Elsasser, U., Wootton, R., Hulme, P., Williams, D., Kanis, J.A., Russell, R.G.G., Mawer, E.B., Meunier, P.J. (1982) Acta Endocrinol. 101: 636-640.
6. Hummer, L., Christiansen, C. (1985) Poster, Sixth Workshop on Vitamin D, Merano, Italy, March 17-22.
7. Tjellesen, L., Gotfredsen, A., Borg, J., Christiansen, C. (1983) Clin. Phys. 3: 359-364.
8. Nilas, L., Christiansen, C., Christiansen, J. (1985) Gut 26: (in press).

CLINICAL TRIAL OF AN ADFR REGIMEN WITH CALCITRIOL AND CALCITONIN: BIOCHEMICAL OBSERVATIONS

Palummeri E., Cervellin G., Pedrazzoni M., Cucinotta D., Passeri M., Department of Medical Pathology, University of Parma, G. Stuard Hospital, 1st Medical Division (Director: Prof. M.Passeri)

INTRODUCTION

In recent years, the ADFR concempt, proposed by Frost(1)has been the subject of widespread interest both in the pathophysiological and therapeutic field, since it seems to represent an approach potentially capable of increasing the bone mass. Some clinical trials are currently in progress, to evaluate the usefulness of this regimen in the treatment of involutional osteoporosis (2). We decided to evaluate some biochemical effects of the short-term administration of calcitriol in osteopenic subjects, in view of its possible use as an activating agent in an ADFR therapeutic regimen.

SUBJECTS AND METHODS

We have studied 7 women and 1 man (mean age 68±4 years), with a reduced bone mineral content as measured by Single-Photon Absorptiometry (SPA) at the distal third of the radius. The subjects had no evidence of liver, renal and endocrine or metabolic disease on clinical and routine laboratory evaluation. After a period of normocaloric diet, each subject was given 1 microgram/day of calcitriol for seven days. Fasting blood samples were collected before treatment and at the 2nd, 4th and 7th day of the study period for the measurement of Osteocalcin (OC), Parathyroid Hormone (PTH), Calcitonin (CT), total and ionized Calcium (Ca^{2+}), Phosphate (Pi) and Alkaline Phosphatase (ALP). OC, PTH 65-84 and CT were measured by radioimmunoassay with commercial kits (Immunonuclear Corporation, USA); Ca, Pi and ALP were determined with automatized standard methods (SMA) and Ca^{2+} was directly determined by ion-selective electrode (NOVA 2). The statistical analysis of the results was performed using Student's t test for paired data and the simple regression.

RESULTS

The results are given in detail in Table 1.

	BASE	DAY 2	DAY 4	DAY 7
OC (ng/ml)	5.5 ± 1.7	5.6 ± 2.2	6.4 ± 2.2	7.1 ± 2.1*
PTH (ng/ml)	0.44 ± 0.1	0.43 ± 0.1	0.41 ± 0.1	0.37 ± 0.1
CT (pg/ml)	63 ±17	64 ±16	67 ±17	66 ±16
Ca (mg/dl)	9.3 ± 0.3	9.4 ± 0.3	9.4 ± 0.3	9.6 ± 0.2+
Ca^{2+} (mg/dl)	4.6 ± 0.3	4.7 ± 0.5	5.1 ± 0.5	4.9 ± 0.3
Pi (mg/dl)	2.7 ± 0.5	3.1 ± 0.2	3.2 ± 0.4+	2.9 ± 0.6
ALP (mU/ml)	33 ± 8.7	39 ±17.9	42 ±13.1+	43 ±16.3+

* = $p < 0.01$ + = $p < 0.05$

As shown in Figure 1, OC and ALP were significantly increased

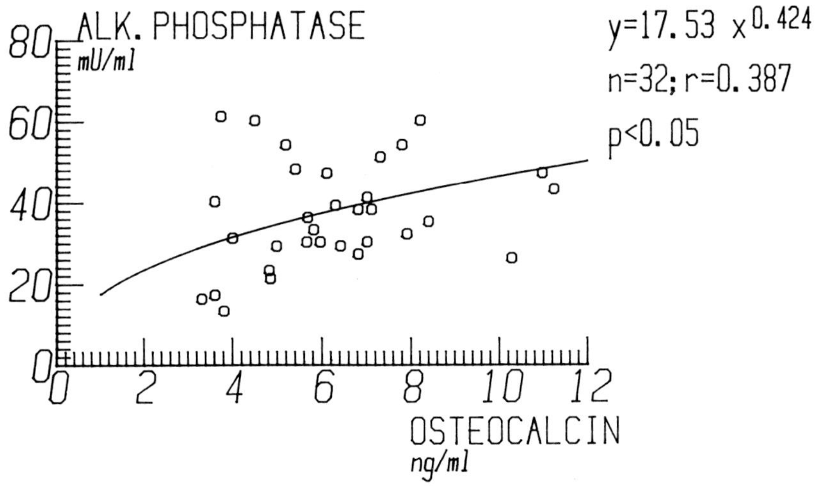

by the drug ($p<0.01$ and $p<0.05$, for OC and ALP respectively, at the 7th day). A significant correlation was found between the two parameters ($y=17.53 \cdot x^{0.424}$; $r=0.387$; $p<0.05$).

COMMENTS

The results are consistent with a calcitriol-induced activation of bone turnover and provide a rational basis for the use of calcitriol as an activating agent in an ADFR therapeutic regimen. Therefore, we have recently started a clinical trial for the treatment of postmenopausal osteoporosis. Thirty postmenopausal osteoporotic women (with at least two vertebral compression fractures on X-ray), aged between 60 and 80 years, were randomly assigned to one of the following therapeutic groups:

1) Calcium (1 gram/day PO for one year)
2) Salmon CT (100 IU every other day) and Calcium (1 gram / day PO) for one year
3) ADFR regimen as follows:
- Activation: Calcitriol (1 mcg/day for seven days)
- Depression: Salmon CT (100 IU every day) and Calcium (as above) for 21 days
- Free phase: Calcium supplementation only (as above)
- Repetition: Four such cycles every year.

The monitoring of the patients encompassed bone biopsy, Single- and Dual-Photon Absorptiometry, urinary hydroxyproline, Ca and Ca^{2+}, Pi, ALP, PTH, CT, OC. Only two patients have completed a six-month period of treatment, and no conclusion can be drawn at present.

REFERENCES

1. Frost H.M., Treatment of osteoporoses by manipulation of coherent bone cell population, Clin.Orthop. (1979) 143:227
2. Frost H.M., The ADFR concept revisited, Calcif. Tissue Int. (1984) 36:349-353

OSTEOPOROSIS IN CHILDHOOD. VITAMIN D METABOLISM IN OSTEOGENESIS IMPERFECTA.

G. Saggese, S. Bertelloni, C. Meossi, G. Cesaretti and E. Bottone.
Department of Pediatrics, University of Pisa, Pisa, Italy.

Introduction.

Osteogenesis Imperfecta (OI) is one of the most common causes of osteoporosis in childhood. An alteration of vitamin D metabolism seems to be involved in the pathogenesis of osteoporosis adults and in children (1,2). Therefore in this study we evaluated vitamin D metabolites in OI type IV in order to investigate a their possible involvment in the genesis of the OI-osteoporosis.

Case report.

A 13.11/12 years girl, born at term in normal first pregnancy, was studied. No family hystory of OI was present. She showed, at admission, short lower limbs for valgismus, dental abnormalities, multiple Wormian bones at X-ray examination of the skull, densitometric evidence of marked osteoporosis (BMC - 28 % of sex age matched control values) (3), short stature (-2.7DS). No bone fractures occurred. These data are in agreement with diagnosis of OI type IV (4). After diagnosis human calcitonin (hCT) treatment was started (25 Unit/die). The patient was periodically riexaminated in the next months.

Methods.

Serum calcium (Ca), phosphorus (P), magnesium (Mg), Alkalyne Phosphatase, urinary Ca and P were measured by standard techniques. Serum PTH and CT were detected by RIA. Serum 25-OH-D and 1,25(OH)2D were analyzed by a competitive protein assay after a preliminary HPLC-step (5,6). Assay sensitivity was 0.5 ng/ml for 25-OH-D and 2 pg/ml for 1.25(OH)2D.

Results.

Serum Ca, P, Alkalyne phosphatase, PTH, CT, urinary Ca and P were in normal range. Serum 1,25(OH)2D levels (137 pg/ml) were higher than normal values for sex and age (73.2 ± 5.1 pg/ml;n=13).25-OH-D concentrations (36.1 ng/ml) were in normal range (32.8 ± 4.0,n=25). The follow up showed a decrease in normal range of 1,25(OH)D levels after hCT therapy (Fig. 1).

Comment.

Our data, in agreement with those of Nishi (7,8), show an alterated in vitamin D metabolism in OI. The higher 1,25(OH)2D levels in presence of normal PTH, Ca, P serum levels are not known. Nishi (7) suggests that the considerable amount of uncalcified osteoid in these children might be partially responsable for the elevated 1,25(OH)2D values. Another cause might be an intrinsic augmented activity of 1alfa-hydroxylase or its hypersensivity to normal PTH values. The latter hypothesis is supported by the obsevation of a reduction of 1,25(OH)2D levels after CT therapy. CT, in fact, is able to depress 1,25(OH)2D synthesis in vitro (9). In conclusion as 1,25(OH)2D act on bone remodelling by increasing

Vitamin D. A Chemical, Biochemical and Clinical Update

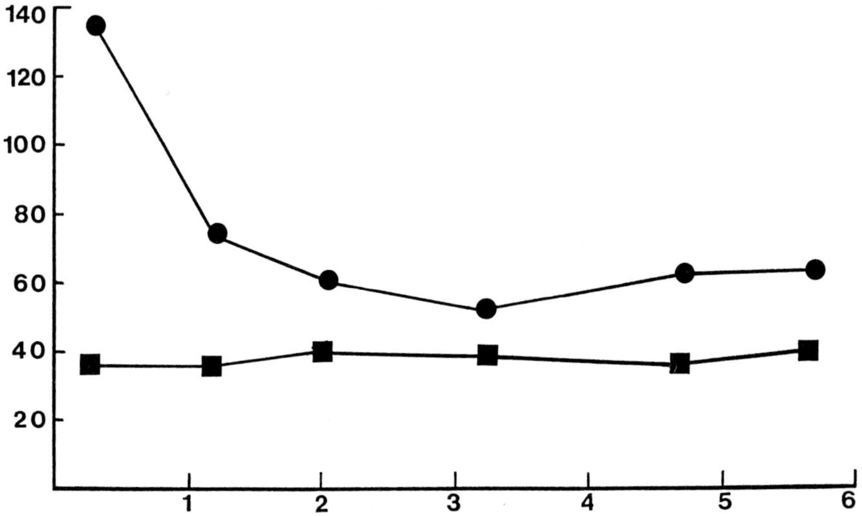

FIG.1 25-OH-D (ng/ml) (■) AND 1,25(OH)2D (pg/ml) (●) LEVELS IN OI TYPE IV DURING hCT THERAPY.

osteoblastic activity (10) osteoporosis in OI could be a consequence of excessive bone resorption induced by higher 1,25(OH)2D levels showed in this condition. At confirm the reduction of 1,25(OH)2D concentrations after hCT therapy caused an improvment of bone mineralization in our girl and in other cases (8).

References.

1) Slovik, D.M., Addams J.S., Neer, N.R., Holick M.F. (1981) N. Engl. Med. 305 :372-374.
2) Saggese, G., Federico, G., Bertelloni, S., Baroncelli, G.I., Massimetti, M., Bottone, E., Atti "IV Congresso Nazionale SIEDP", Bologna, 14-15 Ottobre, 1984,p. P8.
3) Saggese, G., Cipriani C., Federico, G., Cipriani, Y., Bertelloni, S., Baroncelli, G.I., Atti "I Incontro Nazionale Vitamina D ed omeostasi calcica in Pediatria", Pisa 25 Aprile 1985, Saggese G. ed., in press.
4) Sillence, D.O., Rimoin, D.L. (1978) Lancet I : 1041-1042.
5) Saggese, G., Bertelloni, S., Federico, G., Baroncelli, G.I., Bottone E., Proceedings "RIA '84", Albertini A. ed., Milan, May 15-16, p.31.
6) Eisman, J.A., Hamstra, A.J. (1976) Arch. Bioch.Biopn. 176: 235-43.
7) Nischi, Y., Hyodo, S., Ishida, M., Yamakoa, K., Seino, Y, Usui, T., (1983) Acta Paediatr. Scand. 72: 149-151.
8) Nischi, Y., Hyodo, S., Yoschimitsu, K., Sawano, K., Yamaoka, K., Seino, Y., Ussui, T. (1984) Pediatrics 73 : 538-542.
9) Rasmussen, H., Wong, M., Bike, D., Goodman, D.B.P. (1972) J. Clin. Invest. 51 : 2502-2509.
10) DeLuca, H.F. (1984) in "Vitamin D", Kumar R. ed., Martinus N. Pub., Boston, pp. 1-68.

CALCIUM ABSORPTION STUDIES IN NORMAL AND OSTEOPOROTIC WOMEN

B E C Nordin* H A Morris** A G Need** M Horowitz*
T F Hartley**
* Department of Endocrinology, Royal Adelaide Hospital, Adelaide, South Australia
** Division of Clinical Chemistry, Institute of Medical and Veterinary Science, Adelaide, South Australia

INTRODUCTION

There is a widespread belief that the rise in plasma calcium which occurs at the menopause leads to suppression of parathyroid hormone secretion and therefore reduced $1,25(OH)_2D$ production and malabsorption of calcium (1) and that this same mechanism is responsible for the malabsorption of calcium which is frequently found in postmenopausal women with osteoporosis. It follows from this concept that calcium malabsorption is thought to be a result rather than a cause of the osteoporotic process, that it is attributed to low serum $1,25(OH)_2D$ levels, and that it is thought to be reversible with oestrogen treatment (2). The purpose of the present paper is to show that calcium absorption and serum $1,25(OH)_2D$ levels do not normally fall at the menopause and that the malabsorption of calcium found in cases of osteoporosis is an important risk factor for osteoporosis rather than a result of the osteoporotic process.

CLINICAL MATERIAL AND METHODS

The premenopausal women included in this paper comprise young normal volunteers and women attending a menopause clinic (frequently with premenstrual tension) who were found to have premenopausal serum oestrogen and FSH levels. The normal postmenopausal women include both normal volunteers and patients attending our bone clinic who were found on investigation to have no significant degree of osteoporosis. The osteoporotic cases comprise patients with one or more compressed vertebrae or one wedged vertebra associated with a history of fracture (generally wrist fracture) since the menopause. Patients with only one wedged vertebra and no postmenopausal fracture are included in the "normal" group.

All biochemical investigations were performed after an overnight fast. Plasma calcium, phosphate and creatinine measurements were performed by routine multichannel analyzer. Calcium, phosphate, creatinine and hydroxyproline were measured in the fasting urine by methods that have been described elsewhere (3). Radiocalcium absorption was measured by administering 5 μC of Ca^{45} in 20 mg of calcium carrier as the chloride in 250 ml of water and taking a blood sample exactly 60 minutes later. The plasma

Vitamin D. A Chemical, Biochemical and Clinical Update

radioactivity was corrected for body weight and absorption expressed as an hourly fractional rate by reading off a calibration curve (4). Serum 1,25(OH)$_2$D was measured by radioimmunoassay after high pressure liquid chromotography (5).

OBSERVATIONS

The rise in plasma calcium at the menopause

Mean plasma calcium in 34 normal premenopausal women was 2.35 ± .015 mmol/l; in 52 normal postmenopausal women it was 2.38 ± .013 mmol/l; and in 53 osteoporotic women 2.45 ± .018 mmol/l. The differences between the pre- and postmenopausal women and between the normal postmenopausal and osteoporotic were both significant (Fig 1). These data confirm the rise in plasma calcium with occurs at the menopause but show that there is a further increase in plasma calcium in cases of osteoporosis. In five of the latter, the plasma calcium concentrations were just above the top of our normal range (2.55 mmol/l) but even if these cases are excluded the raised plasma calcium in the osteoporotic series remains significant. Moreover, the differences in plasma calcium between these three groups remain equally significant after correction for plasma albumin concentration.

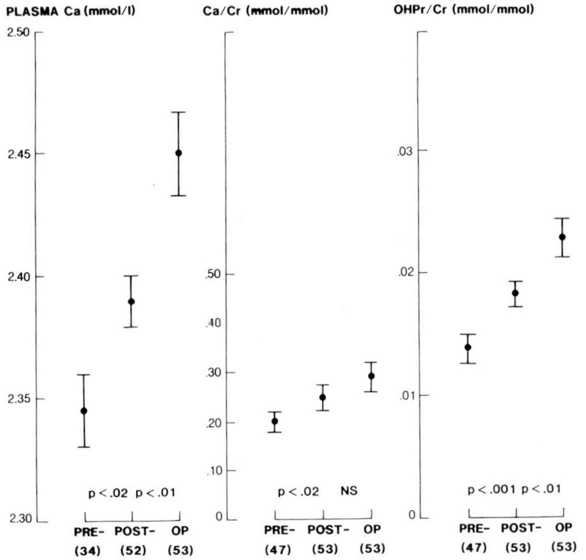

Fig 1: Fasting plasma calcium (left), urinary Ca/Cr (centre) and OHPr/Cr (right) in normal premenopausal and normal and osteoporotic postmenopausal women.

Serum 1,25(OH)$_2$D levels

We have not specifically compared the serum 1,25(OH)$_2$D levels in pre- and postmenopausal women but our normal range for serum 1,25(OH)$_2$D in young adults is 40-130 pmol/l with a mean value of 87. By comparison, the mean value in 33 normal postmenopausal women was 98 ± 8 pmol/l and in 42 osteoporotic women it was 86 ± 6 pmol/l (NS). This does not suggest any fall in serum 1,25(OH)$_2$D at the menopause but does suggest that it may be slightly reduced in osteoporotic cases though at the margin of significance. However, there was no correlation between the plasma calcium concentration and serum 1,25(OH)$_2$D in these 75 patients and no evidence whatever that those with the higher plasma calcium levels had the lower serum 1,25(OH)$_2$D levels (Table 1).

Table 1: Correlation between radiocalcium absorption, serum 1,25(OH)$_2$D and plasma calcium and phosphate in 75 normal and osteoporotic postmenopausal women

Independent Variable	Dependent Variables: Serum 1,25(OH)$_2$D	α
Serum Ca	+.10 (NS)	-.03 (NS)
Serum P	-.10 (NS)	-.07 (NS)

Calcium absorption

Radiocalcium absorption (α) in 32 pairs of age-matched pre- and postmenopausal women is shown in Fig 2. There is no significant difference in α between them. Radiocalcium absorption in 52 normal and 53 osteoporotic postmenopausal women is shown in Table 2. The difference between the two groups is highly significant ($p<.001$) and not accounted for by the difference in age.

Table 2: Radiocalcium absorption and serum 1,25(OH)$_2$D levels in 75 normal and osteoporotic women (mean ± SE)

Group	n	Age	Radiocalcium Absorption/ hour	Serum 1,25(OH)$_2$D (pmol/l)
Normal	33	61.5±1.1	.73 ± .037	98 ± 8
Osteoporotic	42	66.4±0.9	.56 ± .027	86 ± 6
p		<.001	<.001	NS

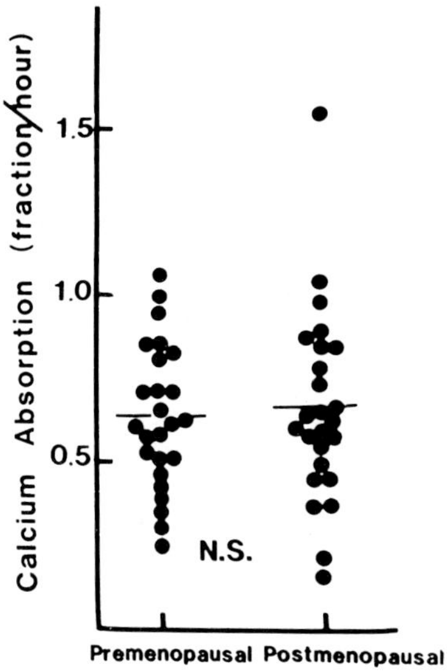

Fig 2: Radiocalcium absorption in 32 pairs of age-matched pre- and postmenopausal women (6)

The effect of oestrogen on α and serum $1,25(OH)_2D$

The effect of oestrogen administration on serum $1,25(OH)_2D$ in 15 normal postmenopausal women is shown in Fig 3. The rise in serum $1,25(OH)_2D$ is highly significant but entirely accounted for by the effect of the oestrogen on vitamin D-binding protein (7).

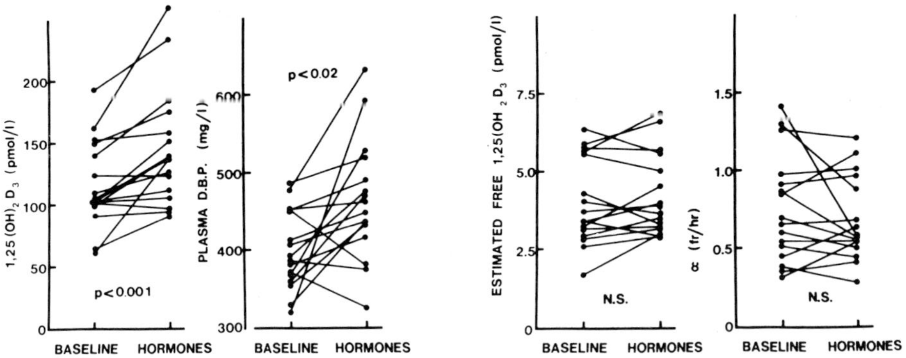

Fig 3: Serum $1,25(OH)_2D$, vitamin D-binding protein, estimated free $1,25(OH)_2D$ and radiocalcium absorption in 15 normal postmenopausal women before and during oestrogen administration (7)

The effect of oestrogen on calcium absorption in balance studies

The effect of oestrogen administration on calcium absorption as determined by balance studies is shown in Table 3 (8). There was the expected fall in urinary calcium and hydroxyproline but no effect on calcium absorption. However, it must be emphasised that these were cases whose initial calcium absorption was normal. We have as yet no data on the effect of oestrogen administration on calcium absorption in postmenopausal women with malabsorption of calcium.

Table 3: **Effect of ethinyl oestradiol on calcium absorption, excretion, balance, mineralisation and resorption rates and urine hydroxyproline in 29 postmenopausal women (mmol/day)**

	In.	Net abs.	Urine	Bal.	Min.	Res.	OHPr
Control	17.2	2.83	5.79	-2.96	6.85	9.81	0.174
Treatment	16.8	3.16	3.66	-0.50	3.07	3.57	0.106
p	NS	NS	<0.001	<0.001	<0.001	<0.001	<0.001

Urinary calcium, sodium and hydroxyproline in premenopausal, postmenopausal and osteoporotic women

Calcium/creatinine and hydroxyproline/creatinine ratios in premenopausal, postmenopausal and osteoporotic women are shown in Fig 1. The fasting urinary calcium was significantly higher in post- than premenopausal women and higher again in osteoporotic women, though this did not quite reach significance. Fasting urinary hydroxyproline was significantly higher in post- than premenopausal women and significantly higher again in osteoporotic women. Fasting urinary sodium did not differ between the three groups. Fig 1 shows that the differences in urinary calcium between the three groups reflects the differences in plasma calcium and are almost certainly the result of the latter. However, within each group there is a highly significant correlation between urinary sodium and calcium (Fig 4) and a highly significant correlation between urinary calcium and hydroxyproline (Fig 5). There are also significant correlations between urinary sodium and hydroxyproline in the two normal groups but this correlation does not quite reach significance in the osteoporotic group. The data are compatible with the concept that plasma calcium and urinary sodium are the main determinants of urinary calcium in these three groups and that the rate of calcium excretion is an important determinant of bone resorption as expressed by urinary hydroxyproline.

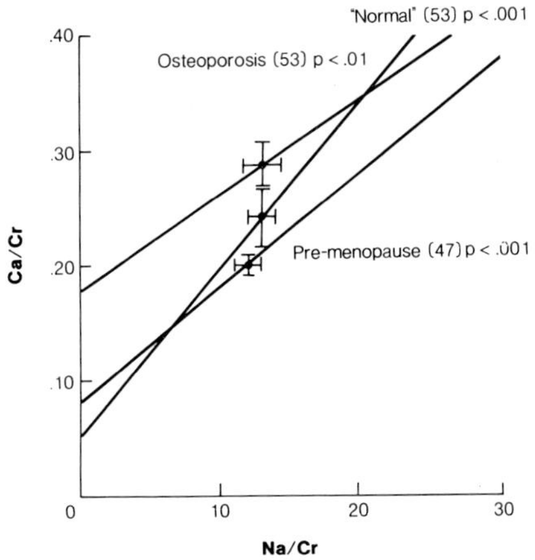

Fig 4: The relation between fasting urinary sodium and calcium in normal premenopausal, normal postmenopausal and osteoporotic women.

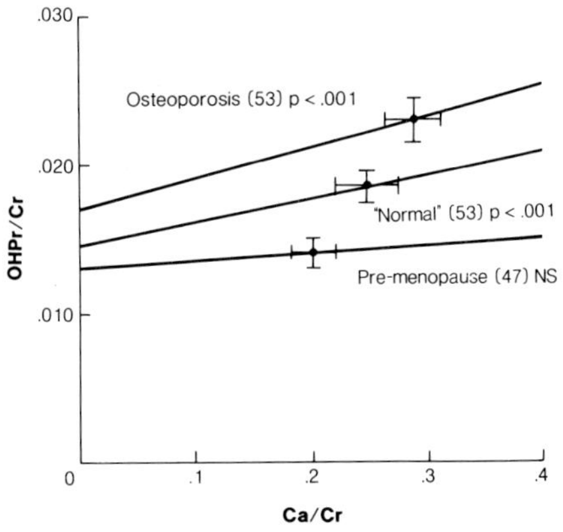

Fig 5: The relation between fasting urinary calcium and hydroxyproline in the same cases as Fig 4.

Plasma and urinary calcium, urinary hydroxyproline and serum $1,25(OH)_2D$

If increased bone resorption resulted in suppression of serum $1,25(OH)_2D$, one would expect to find an inverse correlation between the plasma and urinary calcium and urinary hydroxyproline on the one hand and the serum $1,25(OH)_2D$ on the other. This is not the case. Serum $1,25(OH)_2D$ is not related either positively or negatively to the fasting plasma or urinary calcium or the urinary hydroxyproline (Table 4).

Table 4: Correlations between serum $1,25(OH)_2D$, plasma and urine calcium and urine hydroxyproline in 75 normal and osteoporotic postmenopausal women

Variables	r	p
Ca/Cr & 1,25D	.14	NS
OHPr/Cr & 1,25D	-.10	NS
P Ca & 1,25D	+.10	NS

Calcium absorption and fasting plasma and urinary calcium and urinary hydroxyproline

If increased calcium flow from bone suppressed calcium absorption, one would expect an inverse correlation between the fasting plasma and urinary calcium and radiocalcium absorption. This is not found (Table 5). There is however an inverse correlation between radiocalcium absorption and fasting urinary hydroxyproline (Table 5). This is compatible with the suppression of absorption by increased bone resorption but is equally compatible with the concept that increased bone resorption is a response to calcium malabsorption. Since calcium absorption and fasting urinary calcium are not related, the latter explanation becomes the more probable.

Table 5: **Correlations between α and fasting urinary calcium, sodium and hydroxyproline in 105 normal and osteoporotic postmenopausal women**

Variables	r	p
α amd P Ca	+.02	NS
α and Ca/Cr	-.01	NS
α and OHPr/Cr	-.24	$<.02$
α and Na/Cr	+.08	NS

The effect of calcium and calcitriol administration

If the increased bone resorption and raised urinary hydroxyproline of osteoporotic women were the primary process, and the increased urinary calcium simply the result of this process, one would hardly expect to suppress resorption by simply administering calcium or calcitriol. If, on the other hand, the increased bone resorption were the response to the increased urinary calcium it might be expected to respond to calcium administration. Moreover, if the malabsorption of calcium (when present) was simply a response to increased bone resorption, it would be surprising if the latter could be reduced simply by administering calcitriol.

The effect on fasting urinary hydroxyproline of calcium administration (in those with normal calcium absorption) and of calcitriol (with and without calcium) in those with calcium malabsorption is shown in Figs 6 and 7. It will be seen that urinary hydroxyproline is significantly reduced by calcium administration in cases with normal calcium absorption but not in those with calcium malabsorption. Moreover, it is significantly reduced by calcitriol administration in those with calcium malabsorption and still further reduced when calcitriol is combined with calcium.

These data are compatible with the concept that the increased bone resorption is a response to urinary calcium loss and to calcium malabsorption (when present) (3,9).

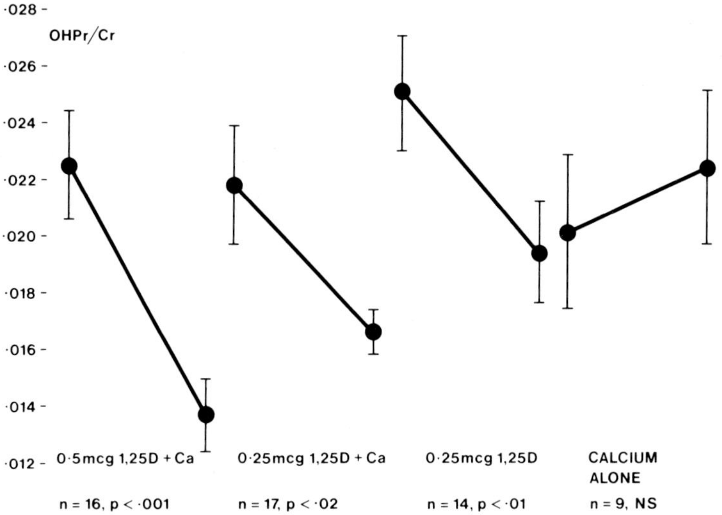

Fig 6: The effect on fasting urinary hydroxyproline of various combinations of calcitriol and calcium in osteoporotic postmenopausal women with malabsorption of calcium (9)

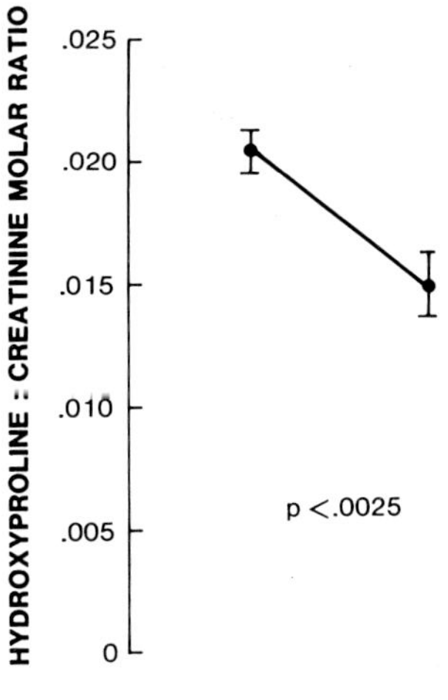

Fig 7: The effect of 1g calcium supplement given in the evening on the fasting urinary hydroxyproline in 15 osteoporotic postmenopausal women with normal absorption of calcium (3)

The effect of calcium administration on plasma ionized calcium

These data suggest that the rise in plasma (ionized) calcium which occurs at the menopause and the further rise which is associated with osteoporosis is not sufficient to suppress parathyroid hormone secretion and $1,25(OH)_2D$ production but that the rise produced by the administration of 1 g of calcium is sufficient to do so if calcium absorption is normal but not if calcium absorption is reduced. We have therefore measured the blood ionized calcium after the administration of 1 g of calcium (Sandocal) in 24 cases of postmenopausal osteoporosis with varying degrees of calcium malabsorption. The results are shown in Fig 8. It will be seen that in those with a radiocalcium absorption over 0.60/hour there is a very significant rise in the ionized calcium concentration to well above the upper limit of normal which is sustained for several hours. In those with malabsorption of calcium there is a lesser rise which is more short lived and only in some cases just exceeds the upper normal limit. The difference between the mean values in the two groups at all time intervals after calcium is significant. It is of particular interest to note, rather surprisingly perhaps, that there is a very significant difference between the basal ionized calcium concentrations in the two groups, the basal level being significantly lower in the malabsorbing group than with those with normal calcium absorption. The data are compatible with the concept that the rise in plasma calcium produced by the 1 g calcium load in patients with normal calcium absorption is sufficient to suppress serum PTH levels but in malabsorbers of calcium it is not. By implication, the rise in plasma (ionized) calcium at the menopause would not be sufficient to suppress PTH and $1,25(OH)_2D$.

It might be argued that the therapeutic value of this large dose of calcium would be counterproductive by suppressing serum $1,25(OH)_2D$ and therefore suppressing calcium absorption. We have however measured radiocalcium absorption in our patients on long term calcium supplementation and find that their good calcium absorption is maintained. We believe the explanation to be that the single calcium tablet with is routinely taken by our patients at 9 p.m. produces only a transient fall of PTH and 1,25 which is too short to cause suppression of calcium absorption because the half-time of the biological effect of $1,25(OH)_2D$ on calcium absorption is much longer (3 or 4 days at least) than the half-time of $1,25(OH)_2D$ in the blood.

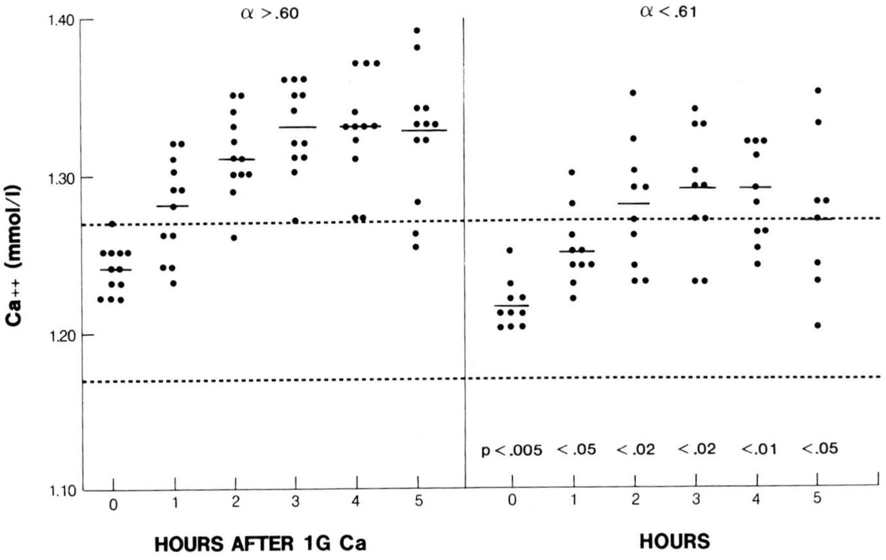

Fig 8: The effect of blood ionized calcium of a 1g calcium load in osteoporotic postmenopausal women with radiocalcium absorption over 0.60 (left) and below 0.61 (right)

CONCLUSIONS

Our data are more compatible with the concept that the malabsorption of calcium in osteoporosis is a primary event and the increased bone resorption secondary than that it is a secondary event in response to increased bone resorption. This does not of course explain the cause of the calcium malabsorption. Although serum 1,25(OH)$_2$D levels are slightly lower in osteoporotic than normal subjects, the difference is not sufficient to explain the difference in calcium absorption between these groups. Serum 1,25(OH)$_2$D and α are of course highly correlated but the slope of α on serum 1,25(OH)2D is significantly flatter in the osteoporotics than in the normals (10). This suggests a relative receptor deficiency in these cases which can be compensated for by administering extra calcitriol. Even the small dose of 0.25 mcg which we use probably produces a peak serum concentration high enough to activate the gastrointestinal receptors. However we do not exclude the possibility that this "receptor deficiency" (if such it is) is itself a response to a hormone deficiency and we do not yet know whether oestrogen administration to these cases will correct their malabsorption. We do not of course deny that a low serum 1,25$(OH)_2$D, when present, must cause calcium malabsorption but such low levels are not the main cause of calcium malabsorption in osteoporosis.

REFERENCES

1. Gallagher, J.C., Riggs, B.L., Eisman, J., Hamstra, A., Arnaud, S.B., DeLuca, H.F. (1979) J Clin. Invest. 64:729-736
2. Gallagher, J.C., Riggs, B.L., DeLuca, H.F. (1980) J Clin. Endocrinol. Metab. 51:1359-1364
3. Horowitz, M., Need, A.G., Philcox, J.C., Nordin, B.E.C. (1984) Amer J Clin. Nutrit.39:857-859
4. Marshall, D.H., Nordin, B.E.C. (1981) Clin. Sci. 61:477-481
5. Taylor, G.A., Peacock, M., Pelc, B., Brown, W., Holmes, A. (1980) Clin. Chim. Acta 108:239-246
6. Crilly, R.G., Francis, R.M., Nordin, B.E.C. (1981) Clin. Endocrinol. Metab. 10:115-139
7. Crilly, R.G., Marshall, D.H., Horsman, A., Nordin, B.E.C., Bouillon, R. In: Osteoporosis: Recent Advances in Pathogenesis and Treatment, DeLuca, H.F. et al (eds) 1981, University Park Press, Baltimore, p425-432
8. Nordin, B.E.C., Marshall, D.H., Francis, R.M., Crilly, R.G. (1981) J Ster. Biochem. 15:171-174
9. Need, A.G., Horowitz, M., Philcox, J.C., Nordin, B.E.C. (1985) Mineral Electrolyte Metab. 11:35-40
10. Morris, H.A., Nordin, B.E.C., Fraser, V., Hartley, T.F.,Need, A.G., Horowitz, M. (1985) Proceedings of 6th International Workshop on Vitamin D (this volume)

LONG TERM TREATMENT OF SENILE OSTEOPENIA WITH 1α-HYDROXYCHOLECALCIFEROL.

B. LUND, O.H. SØRENSEN, R.B. ANDERSEN, B. LUND, L. MOSEKILDE, C. EGSMOSE, T.L. STORM and S.P. NIELSEN,
Department of Rheumatology, Hvidovre Hospital, Copenhagen, Denmark.

Introduction:

The finding of reduced intestinal calcium absorption and depressed serum 1,25-$(OH)_2D$ in senile osteopenia have opened up the possibility of treating this condition with 1,25-$(OH)_2D$ and 1α-OHD.

Patients and Methods

In the present long term study, 22 patients, all with symptomatic osteopenia and at least 1 vertebral collapse were treated with 1α-OHD 1 µg per day (or less if hypercalcemia occured)for up to five years. Serum calcium, phosphorus and iPTH were not significantly different from controls at the beginning of the trial. A slight, significant increase in serum calcium was seen during the treatment.
The bone mineral content (BMC) of the forearm measured at both the 2 cm and 8 cm site increased significantly after 3 months and this increase persisted for 24 months. It was followed by a subsequent slow decline; the BMC values had returned to the starting level at the 5 year measurement (Fig. 1).
The lumbar BMC measured by dual photon absorptiometry of three lumbar vertebrae (1) confirmed the increase in the bone mass seen in the forearm. The lumbar BMC, however, was still significantly increased at the 5 year measurement. (Fig. 2).
Bone histomorphometry was performed in 22 patients on transcortical iliac biopsies after double labeling with tetracyclin (2). The measurements were carried out before and after three years of treatment.
The histomorphometric data revealed a decreased amount of trabecular bone, low turn over metabolic bone disease, increased extent of ostoid surfaces and decreased appositional rate compared with controls.

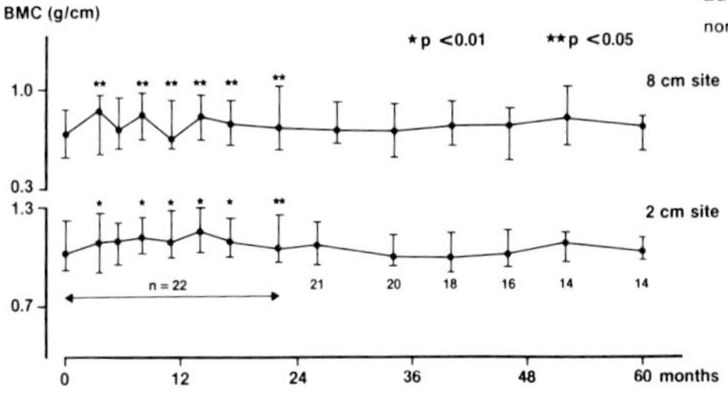

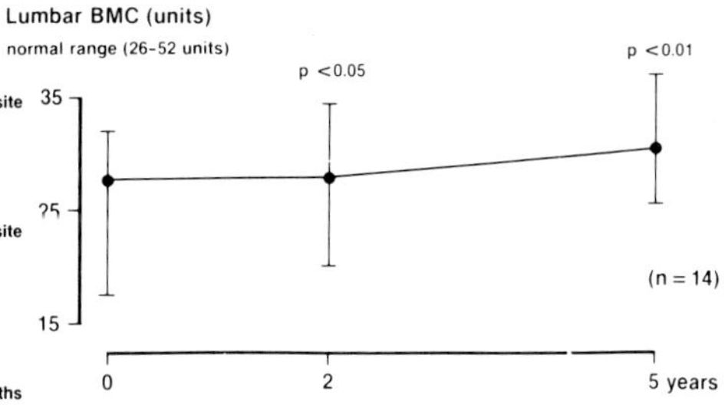

Fig. 1: BMC of the forearm measured at the 2 cm and the 8 cm site during long term treatment with 1α-OHD in osteopenic women (median and quartiles).

Fig. 2: Lumbar BMC during long term treatment with 1α-OHD in osteopenic women (median and quartiles).

Vitamin D. A Chemical, Biochemical and Clinical Update

Treatment with the active vitamin D analogue did not normalize these parametres. There was a significant decrease in the mean ostoid seam width which was normal in the first biopsies. There was no stimulation of osteoblastic activity or osteoclastic resorption (Table I).
These histological findings and the changes in the BMC are consistent with a reduction in bone remodelling rather than an influence on the coupling of the normal cycle in the structural bone unit. The changes in the BMC of the forearm during intermittent treatment with 1α -OHD support this (3).
In conclusion treatment of senile osteopenia with 1α -D_3 is followed by a temporary increase in both lumbar and forearm BMC due to a reduction of bone turn over. No stimulation of osteoblastic activity is seen.

REFERENCES

1. Krølner, B. and Nielsen, S.P. (198o) Scand. Clin. Lab. Invest. 4o: 653-663.
2. Melsen, F. and Mosekilde, L. (1978) Calcif. Tiss. Res. 26: 99-1o2.
3. Sørensen, O.H., Lund, Bj., Lund, B., Andersen, R.B., Danneskjold-Samsøe, B., Mosekilde, L., Melsen, F., Saltin, B., Friis, T. & Selnes, A.:
in Molecular Endocrinology, Eds. MacIntyre and Szelke, Elsevier/ North-Holland Biomedical Press, London 1979, p. 3o9-318.

	Osteoporosis Before	Osteoporosis 3 years treatment	Controls	
Fractional trabecular bone volume: ($V_{fract\,(b)}$, $\mu m^3/\mu m^3$)				
Median	0.13	0.12	0.18	$p < 0.05$
1. quartile	0.08	0.09	0.12	
3. quartile	0.16	0.14	0.20	
Fractional trabecular osteoid volume: ($V_{fract\,(o)}$, $\mu m^3/\mu m^3$)				
Median	0.22	0.28	0.19	$p < 0.05$
1. quartile	0.15	0.20	0.10	
3. quartile	0.29	0.36	0.23	
Fractional formation labeled surfaces: ($S_{fract\,(lab)}$, $\mu m^2/\mu m^2$)				
Median	0.13	0.11	0.11	
1. quartile	0.07	0.06	0.08	
3. quartile	0.17	0.16	0.14	
Fractional resorption surfaces: ($S_{fract\,(r)}$, $\mu m^2/\mu m^2$)				
Median	0.04	0.04	0.04	
1. quartile	0.03	0.03	0.02	
3. quartile	0.06	0.06	0.05	
Appositional rate: (${}^uM/t$, $\mu m/day$)				
Median	0.46	0.50	0.64	$p < 0.01$
1. quartile	0.42	0.28	0.59	
3. quartile	0.56	0.60	0.68	
Mean osteoid seam width: (${}^uW_f$, μm)				
Median	8.4	6.3	9.1	$p < 0.05$
1. quartile	6.7	5.4	8.2	
3. quartile	9.4	8.5	10.1	
	$p < 0.05$			
Bone formation rate, BMU level, surface referent: (${}^sV_{f\,(BMU)}$, $\mu m^3/\mu m^2/day$)				
Median	0.29	0.25	0.41	$p < 0.01$
1. quartile	0.16	0.11	0.28	
3. quartile	0.43	0.30	0.51	
Bone formation rate, tissue level, surface referent: (${}^sV_f$, $\mu m^3/\mu m^2/day$)				
Median	0.06	0.05	0.08	
1. quartile	0.03	0.02	0.06	
3. quartile	0.09	0.15	0.10	
Mineralization lag time (t_m, days)				
Median	29.3	38.3	21.2	$p < 0.01$
1. quartile	20.5	20.0	18.4	
3. quartile	43.0	101.7	23.0	

Table I: Histomorphometric data in senile osteoporosis during long term treatment with 1 -OHD.

TREATMENT OF CALCIUM DEFICIENCY OSTEOPOROSIS WITH 1α-HYDROXYCHOLE-CALCIFEROL OR 24,25-DIHYDROXYCHOLECALCIFEROL ALONE OR COMBINED.

T.S. LINDHOLM, T.C. LINDHOLM and S. ERIKSSON
From the Bone Research Group, Orthopaedic Hospital
of the Invalid Foundation, Helsinki, Finland

Experimental osteoporosis produced by feeding a low calcium diet to adult male rats can be cured by feeding an optimal calcium diet alone or combined with 1α-OHD_3 treatment. 1α-OHD_3 alone can not restore the bone mass but will produce new bone formation. (1).

In the following experiment an attempt was made to reverse the osteoporotic changes in peripheral bone of adult male rats by treating with 1α-OHD_3, 24,25$(OH)_2D_3$ only or combined.

Material

Adult male rats with a body weight of 488 g were used. The low Ca diet (0.065% Ca) was administered during 6 weeks giving significant changes of bone loss. After the treatment period of another 6 weeks with 1α-OHD_3 (0.2 µg) or 24,25$(OH)_2D_3$ (0.2 µg) or in their combination the femurs and tibiae were examined as described in the results with previously used methods (2).

Results

The bone mass could not be restored during the 6 weeks' treatment period (Fig.1). However the chemical content of bones was changed with respect to treatment with 24,25$(OH)_2D_3$ or with 24,25$(OH)_2D_3$ combined with 1α-OHD_3 in rats at low Ca intake (Fig.2).
The amounts of hydroxyproline, hexosamines, calcium and phosphorus were at the same level as in bones of rats at optimal calcium intake.
In the combined treatment group the changes were moreover significantly (< 0.001) changed which speaks for an increment of Ca and P in treated rat bones.

Conclusion

These preliminary results show that 24,25$(OH)_2D_3$ alone or combined with 1α-OHD_3 may have importance in restoring the chemical composition of calcium deficient rat bone.

Figure 1: Wet weight, dry weight, hydrated gross density and ash weight of femur in adult rats reared an optimal or low calcium diet combined with treatment with 1α-OHD_3 or 24,25$(OH)_2D_3$ or their combination.

	Optimal Ca (10)	Low Ca (10)	Low Ca 1α-OHD_3 (10)	Low Ca 24,25$(OH)_2D_3$ (10)	Low Ca 1α-OHD_3 24,25$(OH)_2D_3$ (10)
Wet weight (mg)	1.13 0.0465 -	1.08 0.0393 < 0.05	1.09 0.0304 n.s.	1.08 0.0465 n.s.	1.10 0.0368 n.s.
Dry weight (mg)	0.74 0.0345 -	0.64 0.021 < 0.001	0.65 0.015 < 0.001	0.64 0.027 < 0.001	0.66 0.206 < 0.001
Specific weight (g/cm^3)	1.57 0.0231 -	1.48 0.0115 < 0.001	1.48 0.01 < 0.001	1.48 0.0095 < 0.001	1.50 0.0111 n.s.
Ash weight (mg)	0.48 0.236 -	0.41 0.0122 < 0.001	0.41 0.0086 < 0.001	0.41 0.017 < 0.001	0.43 0.0144 < 0.001

N=10. Mean and SD. Experimental groups are compared to optimal Ca group.

Figure 2: Contents of hydroxyproline, hexosamines, calcium and phosphorus per dry weight in tibiae of adult male rats on low or optimal calcium diet treated with 1α-OHD_3 or 24,25$(OH)_2D_3$ or their combination.

	Optimal Ca (10)	Low Ca (10)	Low Ca 1α-OHD_3 (10)	Low Ca 24,25$(OH)_2D_3$ (10)	Low Ca 1α-OHD_3 24,25$(OH)_2D_3$ (10)
Hydroxy-proline (μg/mg)	21.79 1.8487 -	21.93 2.5865 n.s.	22.14 1.594 n.s.	21.12 2.205 n.s.	16.85 0.3742 < 0.001
Hexosa-mines (μg/mg)	3.38 0.4752 -	3.25 0.7148 n.s.	3.40 0.5718 n.s.	3.32 0.4146 n.s.	1.33 0.1145 < 0.001
Ca (μg/mg)	184.74 13.683 -	147.35 26.9238 < 0.001	167.93 6.4377 < 0.001	185.74 13.683 n.s.	240.24 6.8069 < 0.001
P (μg/mg)	92.26 6.2867 -	75.25 11.6224 < 0.001	83.80 3.3183 < 0.001	90.14 8.754 n.s.	124.85 2.1858 < 0.001

References:

1. Lindholm,T.S. (1979) Scand.J.Rheumat. 8:257-263.
2. Lindholm,T.S.,Nilsson,O.S.,Lindholm,T.C̄. (In press). 1-Alpha-OH-cholecalciferol (1α-OHD_3) and optimal calcium intake in calcium deficiency osteoporosis mediated by parathyroid activity. Morphologic and biochemical changes in adult male rats.

OSTEOPOROSIS IN TURNER SYNDROME. ROLE OF VITAMIN D ENDOCRINE SYSTEM.

G.Federico, S.Bertelloni, M.Massimetti, J.Cipriani and G.Saggese.
Department of Pediatrics, University of Pisa, Pisa, Italy.

Introduction:

Although osteoporosis is a common finding in Turner syndrome,its pathogenesis is still largely unknown. Brown (1) found normal parathyroid hormone (PTH) levels and concluded that bone loss was attributable to an increased sensitivity of bone to PTH.

Patients and methods:

Nine girls with Turner syndrome (aged 14.1±3.9 (m±SD) were studied; two were prepubertal, five in PH3-PH4 stage (2); two have been on estro-progestinic substitutive therapy for two years. Height was -4.3±0.8 SD (m±SD), bone age was 10.9±4.7 (m±SD). Bone Mineral Content (BMC), Bone Width (BW), BMC/BW in the non dominant radius were measured by photon absorptiometry (Norland 2783) and the results were mached with normal values for age and sex (unpublished data). We valued Calcium (Ca), phosphate (P), alkalyne phosphatase (AP), PTH (COOH-terminal), calcitonin(CT) in all patients. 25OHD and 1.25(OH)2D values were obtained by a radio receptor assay as previously described (3)(4).

Results:

All subjects showed a reduction of BMC (m±SD -20.6±4.9%) and BMC/BW (m±SD -18.9±5.4%). Bone loss resulted at a less extent in the two estro-progestinic treated girls (m±SD BMC -19.1±0.1%; BMC/BW -12.1±1.2). Serum Ca and P levels were within normal limits in all subjects. Serum AP resulted sligthly elevated (m±SD 982.3±7.5 U/l;n.v.300-900 U/l) in 3 cases. PTH was normal (n.v. 0.30-0.66 ng/ml) in the two girls on substitutive sex therapy (m±SD 0.54±0.03 ng/ml) while in the others it was at the low normal limit (4 cases) or undetectable (3 cases).Serum CT (n.v.14-44 pg/ml) was low (m±SD 11.3±2.6 pg/ml; 2 cases),undetectable (5 cases) and in the low normal limit (15.96±2.0 pg/ml m±SD) in the two sex steroid treated girls. 25OHD levels were normal in all subjects. 1.25(OH)2D values (nv:38±7 pg/ml)(m±DS) were reduced ($p < 0.05$) in 7 patients (m±SD 27.0±0.6 pg/ml), at the low limit of normal range in the two patients on sex steroid substitutive therapy (m±SD 35.1±0.1 pg/ml).

Discussion:

In our patients we found significantly low serum levels of

Vitamin D. A Chemical, Biochemical and Clinical Update

1,25(OH)2D. This finding, in the presence of normal values of 25OHD, suggests an impairment of 1-alpha-hydroxylase activity. The normal Ca and PTH levels in our subjects suggest that estrogen deficiency could affect the renal vitamin D activation. Renal receptors for estrogens have been found by Concolino (4) but other Authors (5) failed to demonstrate the estrogen stimulation of 1-alpha-hydroxylase activity in kidney cultured cells. The 1,25(OH)2D normal levels in our 2 subjects on sex substitutive therapy, as in postmenopausal osteoporotic treated women (6), support the stimulating effect of estrogens on 1-alpha-hydroxylase in vivo.

The two older girls, on estro progestinic therapy, showed the lower degree of bone loss. Unfortunately we have not data about bone ass in these patients before the therapy started; therefore the lower degree of osteoporosis could be related to the advanced age (8) rather than sex therapy. Estrogens increase CT secretion in women (9); low serum CT levels found in our patients, even if in basal condition, could represent an important adjunctive pathogenetic factor in Turner syndrome osteoporosis. Our data suggest that osteoporosis in Turner syndrome can be at least in part due to the same mechanism of the postmenopausal bone loss (7).

References:

1)Brown,D.M., Jowsey,J., Bradford,D.S.(1974) J.Pediatr. 84: 816-820.

2)Marshall,W.A., Tanner,J.M.(1969) Arch.Dis.Child. 44: 291-298.

3)Saggese,G., Bertelloni,S., Federico,G., Baroncelli,G.I., Bottone,E.(1984) Proceedings RIA '84 "Cost and Benefit of Radio Immuno Assay" Albertini A.ed., Milan May 15-16, p.31 abs.

4)Eisman,J.A., Hamstra,A.J., Kream,B.E., De Luca,H.F.(1976) Arch.Bioch.Bioph. 176: 235-243.

5)Concolino,G., Marocchi,A., Concolino,F., Sciarra,F., Di Silverio,F., Conti C.(1976) J.Steroid.Biochem. 7: 831-834.

6)Henry,H.L.(1981) Am.J.Physiol. 240: E119 abs.

7)Gallagher,J.C., Riggs,B.L., De Luca,H.F.(1980) J.Clin.Endocrinol.Metab. 51: 1359-64.

8)Shore,R.M., Chesney,R.W., Mazess,R.B., Rose,P.G., Bargman,G.J.(1982) Calcif.Tissue Int. 34: 519-522.

9)Stevenson,J.C., Abeyasekera,G., Hillyard,C.J., Phang,K.G., Mac Intyre, J., Campbell,S., Townsend,P.T., Yiung,O., Whitehed,M.I.(1981) Lancet 1: 693-695.

THE EFFECT OF CALCIUM, HORMONES AND ROCALTROL THERAPY ON FOREARM BONE LOSS IN NORMAL AND OSTEOPOROTIC POSTMENOPAUSAL WOMEN

B E C Nordin* B E Chatterton** Cynthia J Walker*
Tracy A Steurer* M Horowitz* A G Need+
* Departments of Endocrinology and **Nuclear Medicine, Royal Adelaide Hospital, Adelaide, South Australia
+ Division of Clinical Chemistry, Institute of Medical and Veterinary Science, Adelaide, South Australia

Introduction

In a previous publication (1,2) we have reported a significant fall in urinary hydroxyproline when calcium supplements are administered to cases of postmenopausal osteoporosis with normal calcium absorption and a comparable fall if calcitriol is added to the regime in cases with calcium malabsorption. We now report the effects of these therapies, alone and in combination with hormones or an anabolic steroid, on forearm mineral density.

Clinical Material and Methods

The study comprises 135 observation periods on 104 osteoporotic postmenopausal women who were separated into normal absorbers and malabsorbers of calcium by a radiocalcium absorption test (3). They were all given a 1 g calcium supplement (Sandocal) daily, to be taken in the evening, and those with malabsorption of calcium were given in addition 0.25 mcg of calcitriol (Rocaltrol). Subsets of these main groups were given in addition a hormone preparation - generally Norethisterone (Norethindrone) 5 mg daily - or Nandrolone (Deca-Durabolin) 50 mg i.m. every two weeks.

Distal forearm densitometry was performed with the Molsgaard Bone Mineral Analyzer at approximately four monthly intervals and expressed as the forearm mineral density (FMD) (mg/ml). The mean observation period was nine months.

The number of cases in each group, their mean age, and their mean initial FMD are shown in Table 1

Results

The time-weighted mean rates of change in FMD in the six groups are shown in Table 2. There was a non-significant loss of bone in the patients treated with calcium alone or with calcium and calcitriol. There was a non-significant gain of bone in the two groups who received hormones as well as calcium ± calcitriol. There was a significant increase in FMD in the 13 patients given Nandrolone plus calcium ($p<.05$) and a greater and more significant gain in the 11 patients given Nandrolone plus calcium plus calcitriol ($p<.002$).

Vitamin D. A Chemical, Biochemical and Clinical Update

Table 1

	Therapy	Number of cases	Mean Age	Initial FMD (mg/ml ± SE)
1.	Calcium	38	65.7±1.5	302 ± 8
2.	Calcium + Hormones	26	61.5±1.5	296 ± 13
3.	$1,25(OH)_2D_3$ + Ca	37	67.6±1.3	294 ± 10
4.	$1,25(OH)_2D_3$ + Ca + Horm	10	63.7±2.5	297 ± 30
5.	Nandrolone + Ca	13	64.8±2.6	265 ± 15
6.	N'lone + Ca + $1,25(OH)_2D_3$	11	69.2±3.2	364 ± 23

Table 2

	Group					
	1	2	3	4	5	6
Weighted mean rate of change in FMD	-3.3 ±2.2	+4.4 ±5.2	-1.6 ±2.5	+3.9 ±6.4	+16.0 ± 7.3	+24.6 ± 5.7
(mg/ml/yr±SE)	NS	NS	NS	NS	p<.05	p<.002

Conclusions

The data are compatible with the concept that calcium ± calcitriol, even when combined with conventional hormone therapy, do little more than hold bone status constant by inhibiting bone resorption, probably because there is secondary inhibition of bone formation. The addition of Nandrolone seems to cause an actual gain of bone, possibly due to the stimulation of bone formation.

References

1. Need, A.G., Horowitz, M., Philcox, J.C., Nordin, B.E.C. (1985) Mineral Electrolyte Metab. 11:35-40
2. Horowitz, M., Need, A.G., Philcox, J.C., Nordin, B.E.C. (1984) Am J Clin. Nutrit. 39:857-859
3. Marshall, D.H., Nordin, B.E.C. (1981) Clin. Sci. 61:477-481

EFFECT OF 1,25-DIHYDROXYVITAMIN D_3 ON BIOCHEMICAL INDICES OF BONE TURNOVER IN POSTMENOPAUSAL WOMEN

L. Tjellesen, C. Christiansen and P. Rødbro
Department of Clinical Chemistry, Glostrup Hospital; and
Department of Clinical Physiology, Aalborg Hospital, Denmark

Introduction:

Bone metabolism in postmenopausal osteoporosis is characterized by a negative calcium balance where bone resorption is more increased than bone formation (1). It has been shown that patients with postmenopausal osteoporosis have decreased serum levels of 1,25-dihydroxyvitamin D (1,25$(OH)_2$D) and decreased intestinal calcium absorption (2). Since it has been shown that 1,25$(OH)_2$D is the major regulator of intestinal calcium absorption a causal relationship between the low calcium absorption, the decreased 1,25$(OH)_2$D and development of osteoporosis has been suggested. The aim of the present study was to examine the influence of treatment with 1,25$(OH)_2D_3$ on indices of bone metabolism in postmenopausal women.

Patients and Methods:

Two groups of postmenopausal women participated in the study: group 1: 57 early postmenopausal women, and group 2: 54 70-year-old women. Informed consent was obtained from all participants. Each group were divided into 3 different treatment groups to treatment with either 1,25$(OH)_2D_3$ (0.25 ug/day, group 1, 0.50 ug/day, group 2), cyclical female hormones (Trisequens, group 1, Trisequens Forte, group 2) or placebo. Furthermore, all participants received 0.5 g calcium per day as Calcium Sandoz.

Bone metabolism was estimated by: 1) serum alkaline phosphatase (AP) (index of bone formation). 2) Fasting urinary excretion of calcium (FUCa/Cr) and hydroxyproline relative to creatinine (FUHy/Cr) (indices of bone resorption) before and after 12 months treatment.

Results:

In the female hormone treated groups the markers for bone formation and bone resorption fell significantly during the study period, whereas only small changes were seen in both the 1,25-$(OH)_2D_3$ and the placebo groups. (Table 1).

Furthermore, the statistical significance of differences between changes after 12 months treatment for each treatment group were compared with the placebo group. There was no significant difference between the 1,25$(OH)_2D_3$ subgroups and the placebo groups, whereas the mean changes in the two female hormone groups were significant for all three variables compared to the change in the placebo group (Table 2).

Vitamin D. A Chemical, Biochemical and Clinical Update

Table 1: Serum concentrations of AP and FUCa/Cr and FUHy/Cr after 12 months treatment in per cent of initial values.

	AP	FUCa/Cr	FUHy/Cr
Early postmenopausal			
1,25(OH)$_2$D$_3$	94*	139*	93
Hormones	71***	69*	67**
Placebo	99	111	100
70-year-old			
1,25(OH)$_2$D$_3$	91	113	87*
Hormones	74***	51***	78*
Placebo	89***	116	103

*$P<0.05$; **$P<0.01$; ***$P<0.001$
(Student's *t* test for paired data)

Table 2: Statistical significance of differences between changes after 12 months treatment for each treatment group compared with the placebo group.

	AP	FUCa/Cr	FUHy/Cr
Early postmenopausal			
1,25(OH)$_2$D$_3$	NS	NS	NS
Hormone	***	*	***
70-year-old			
1,25(OH)$_2$D$_3$	NS	NS	NS
Hormone	**	***	*

*$P<0.05$; **$P<0.01$; ***$P<0.001$
(Student's *t* test for unpaired data)

Conclusion:

The present study indicates that 1,25(OH)$_2$D$_3$ treatment is without significant effect on bone turnover in postmenopausal women.

References:

1. Heaney RP, Recker RR, Saville PD (1978) J Lab Clin Med 92: 964-70.

2. Gallagher JC, Riggs BL, Eisman J, Hamstra A, Arnaud SB, DeLuca HF (1979) J Clin Invest 64: 729-36.

MALABSORPTION OF CALCIUM IN ELDERLY OSTEOPOROTIC WOMEN

R.M. FRANCIS, M. PEACOCK, C.J. GIBBS and S.A. BARKWORTH
MRC Mineral Metabolism Unit, The General Infirmary, Leeds, UK.

Introduction:

Malabsorption of calcium is an important risk factor for the development of osteoporosis. We have shown that elderly women with crush fractures are "resistant" to the action of vitamin D metabolites on the bowel (1). To determine whether this "resistance" is relative or absolute, we have now performed further studies on the effect of vitamin D metabolites in elderly osteoporotic women.

Patients and Methods:

Short-term 25OHD$_3$ study: 19 women with crush fractures (age 65-86) and 21 control subjects (age 61-94) were treated with 40 µg 25OHD3 daily for 1 week (2).

Prolonged 25OHD$_3$ study: 7 women from the crush fracture group continued treatment with 40 µg 25OHD$_3$ daily for a further 3 weeks.

1,25(OH)$_2$D$_3$ study: 9 women with crush fractures (age 60-82) were treated with 1,25(OH)$_2$D$_3$ 0.25 µg twice daily (9am, 9pm) for 1 week. To avoid the effect of renal impairment (3) all women investigated had a plasma creatinine of less than 100 µmol/l. Radiocalcium absorption was measured basally and on treatment and fasting plasma was collected for determination of plasma 25OHD and 1,25(OH)$_2$D (1).

Results:

Short-term 25OHD$_3$ study: Before treatment the women with crush fractures had a mean plasma 25OHD, 1,25(OH)$_2$D and radiocalcium absorption of 20.2 nmol/l (normal 9-90), 89.7 pmol/l (normal 75-165) and 0.41 fraction of dose/hr (normal 0.3-1.3) respectively which was not significantly different from the control group values of 11.1 nmol/l, 79.3 pmol/l and 0.36. Treatment with 25OHD$_3$ increased the plasma 25OHD to 68.9 nmol/l ($p<0.001$) in the fracture group and 59.5 nmol/l ($p<0.001$) in the control group; plasma 1,25(OH)$_2$D increased to 133.3 ($p<0.01$) and 141.7 pmol/l ($p<0.001$) respectively. Despite similar increments in plasma 25OHD and 1,25(OH)$_2$D the radiocalcium absorption was unchanged in the crush fracture group (0.44) whilst it increased in the control subjects to 0.57 ($p<0.001$).

Prolonged 25OHD3 study: The 7 patients from the crush fracture group who continued treatment with 25OHD$_3$ increased their radiocalcium absorption after 3 weeks ($p<0.05$) but at supra-normal concentrations of plasma 25OHD. There was no change in plasma 1,25(OH)$_2$D (Fig. 1).

1,25(OH)$_2$D$_3$ study: Treatment with 1,25(OH)$_2$D3 produced a marked rise in radiocalcium absorption with only trivial changes in plasma 1,25(OH)$_2$D (Fig. 2).

Vitamin D. A Chemical, Biochemical and Clinical Update

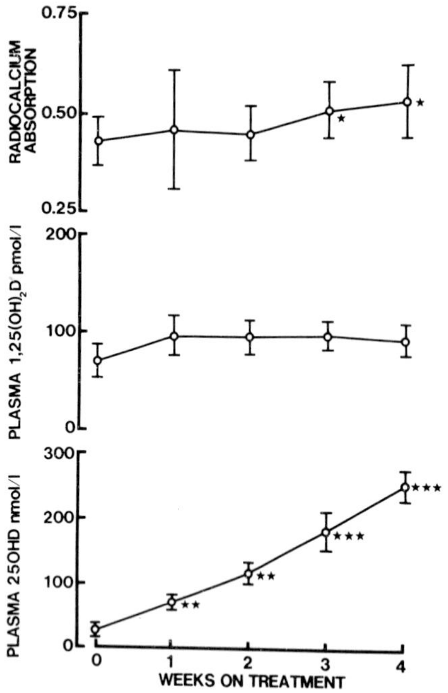

Fig. 1 Effect of treatment with 25OHD3 (40 µg/day)

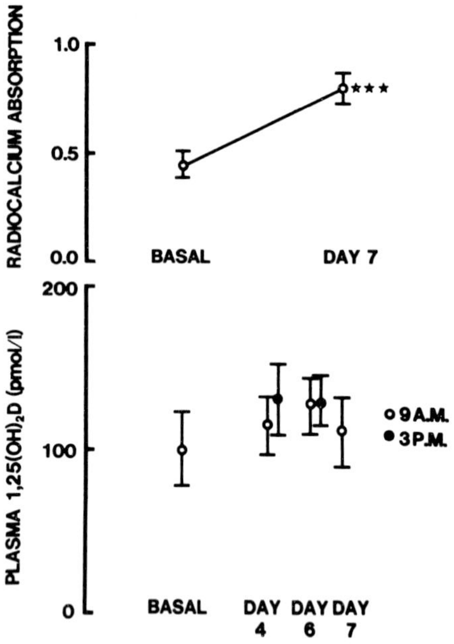

Fig. 2 Effect of treatment with $1,25(OH)_2D_3$ (0.25 µg twice daily)

Conclusions:

1. Calcium malabsorption in elderly women with crush fractures is "resistant" to increases in plasma 25OHD and $1,25(OH)_2D$ within the normal range.
2. The "resistance" is overcome at supranormal plasma 25OHD concentrations.
3. The "resistance" is also overcome by oral $1,25(OH)_2D_3$ with only small changes in plasma $1,25(OH)_2D$.
4. Low dose oral $1,25(OH)_2D_3$ acts on the bowel by a local rather than a systemic effect. This may be desirable therapeutically as the effect of $1,25(OH)_2D_3$ can be targeted on the bowel rather than the bone.

References:

1. Francis,R.M.,Peacock,M.,Taylor,G.A.,Storer,J.H.,Nordin, B.E.C.(1984) Clin.Sci.66:103-107
2. Peacock,M.,Selby,P.L.,Francis,R.M.,Brown,W.B.,Hordon,L. (1985) This volume.
3. Francis,R.M.,Peacock,M.,Barkworth,S.A.(1984) Age Ageing 13:14-20.

Sarcoidosis

PERTURBATION OF THE VITAMIN D-ENDOCRINE SYSTEM IN SARCOID AND OTHER DISEASES

N.H. BELL and P.H. STERN

Veterans Administration Medical Center and Departments of Medicine and Pharmacology, Medical University of South Carolina, Charleston, South Carolina, and Department of Pharmacology, Northwestern University Medical School, Chicago, Illinois, USA.

Introduction

The development of receptor assays, bioassays and radioimmunoassays for the vitamin D metabolites has allowed the delineation of the means by which defects in vitamin D metabolism produce hypercalcemia and abnormal metabolism of calcium in sarcoid, in chronic granulomatous diseases and in certain other diseases.

Abnormal calcium metabolism in sarcoid is characterized by increased intestinal absorption of calcium, hypercalcemia and hypercalciuria which may lead to nephrocalcinosis, renal lithiasis, renal insufficiency and even death (1-3). Increased sensitivity to vitamin D is a characteristic (1,3), and the abnormal metabolism of calcium is corrected by glucocorticoids (1,3). In sarcoid, the abnormal calcium metabolism was investigated with labeled calcium. Increased intestinal absorption (3,5) and increased turnover of radioactive calcium (4,5) were demonstrated. Glucocorticoids lowered the amount of labeled calcium absorbed as well as the rate of turnover of the isotope (3-5).

Harrell and Fisher (6) first described hypercalcemia in sarcoidosis. The similarity of abnormal calcium metabolism in sarcoid and vitamin D intoxication led to the proposal that these abnormalities resulted either from increased production of vitamin D (7) or from increased sensitivity to the vitamin (3). The observation that serum antirachitic activity from patients with sarcoid and hypercalcemia is normal (3,8) supported the idea of increased sensitivity to the vitamin in view of the fact that values for serum antirachitic activity were increased in patients with vitamin D intoxication and in individuals receiving pharmacologic doses of the vitamin (9). Further evidence that vitamin D metabolism is abnormal in sarcoid were the observations that the incidence of hypercalcemia in patients with sarcoid is seasonal, occurring during the summer months (10), that hypercalcemia and abnormal calcium metabolism often occur during the summer (7), that abnormal calcium metabolism was produced by brief exposure to ultraviolet light (11) or by small doses of vitamin D (13), and finally that the abnormal calcium metabolism is reversed by

Vitamin D. A Chemical, Biochemical and Clinical Update

omission of vitamin D from the diet and prevention of exposure to sunlight (12).

Vitamin D and its metabolites are transported in the intravascular compartment in association with an $alpha_2$-globulin, the group specific component protein or G_c protein (13). Serum concentration of vitamin D-binding protein is normal in sarcoid (14), indicating that the abnormal vitamin D metabolism in that disease does not result from an alteration in concentration of the transport protein in the peripheral circulation.

Increased Circulating $1,25(OH)_2D$ and Hypercalcemia

It is evident that hypercalcemia and abnormal calcium metabolism in a number of diseases is caused by elevated serum 1,25-dihydroxyvitamin D ($1,25(OH)_2D$). The concentration of serum $1,25(OH)_2D$ is either increased or at the upper limit of the normal range in patients with sarcoid and hypercalcemia (15-19), and in patients with hypercalcemia associated with tuberculosis (20,21), disseminated candidiasis (22), lymphomas (23,24), silicone-induced granulomas (25) or no associated disease (26,27).

In patients with sarcoid and hypercalcemia, immunoreactive parathyroid hormone (iPTH) is either suppressed or in the lower range of normal (15,17,28), and urinary cyclic adenosine 3'5'-monophosphate (cyclic AMP) is also suppressed (17). The elevated serum $1,25(OH)_2D$ is consistently lowered to values which are either within or below the normal range and hypercalcemia and abnormal calcium metabolism are corrected by treatment with glucocorticoids (15-19). The findings indicate that glucocorticoids act by reducing serum $1,25(OH)_2D$ but do not eliminate the possibility that the peripheral action of $1,25(OH)_2D$ is inhibited. With return of the serum calcium to normal, serum iPTH increases but remains within the normal range (28). Production of $1,25(OH)_2D$ in sarcoid is not regulated by PTH as it is in normal subjects. This idea is substantiated by studies in a patient with sarcoid who had developed hypoparathyroidism after subtotal thyroidectomy for non-toxic goiter and had a normal serum calcium and abnormal elevation of serum $1,25(OH)_2D$ (29).

There is evidence that the increased circulating $1,25(OH)_2D$ in sarcoid results from increased production of the metabolite. An investigation with the infusion-equilibrium method in which $[^3H]$-$1,25(OH)_2D_3$ was infused for up to 19 hours, indicated that such is the case (30). Thus, production rate and metabolic clearance rate of $1,25(OH)_2D$ were abnormally increased in two patients with sarcoid and increased circulating $1,25(OH)_2D$.

Abnormal Regulation of Circulating $1,25(OH)_2D$ in Sarcoid

Patients with sarcoidosis exhibit increased sensitivity to vitamin D (1,3). It was shown that hypercalcemia and abnormal calcium metabolism were produced by vitamin D, 10,000 units per day for 12 days, a dose which is without effect on calcium metabolism in normal subjects (3). However, in patients with sarcoid who were normocalcemic and had a history of hypercalcemia, the same dose of vitamin D produced abnormal increases in serum $1,25(OH)_2D$ but did not change the serum values for the metabolite in normal subjects (15). In larger doses, vitamin D, 100,000 units per day for 4 days, produced abnormal increases in serum $1,25(OH)_2D$ in patients with sarcoid who were normocalcemic (31). In contrast, mean serum $1,25(OH)_2D$ was not altered in normal subjects. These studies provide evidence that abnormal regulation of serum $1,25(OH)_2D$ in response to vitamin D challenge accounts for the increased sensivitity to the vitamin in sarcoid. These findings are in clear contrast to those in normal subjects in whom serum $1,25(OH)_2D$ is tightly regulated. The fact that abnormal calcium metabolism in patients with vitamin D intoxication is caused by increases in serum 25-hydroxyvitamin D (25-OHD) and not $1,25(OH)_2D$ (32) emphasizes the degree of regulation of production of $1,25(OH)_2D$. Regulation is mediated by feedback inhibition of circulating PTH by the serum ionized calcium. Thus, increases in serum calcium produced by increases in circulating $1,25(OH)_2D$ inhibit PTH secretion and the renal production of $1,25(OH)_2D$.

Ultraviolet Light and Vitamin D Synthesis

Vitamin D_3 is synthesized in the skin by the photochemical conversion from 7-dehydrocholesterol. Photons of light energy from ultraviolet light are absorbed by 7-dehydrocholesterol which then undergoes thermal conversion to previtamin D_3. Previtamin D_3, which is thermally labile, is transformed by temperature-dependent rearrangement of double bonds in the B ring to form vitamin D_3 which is thermally stable (33). Vitamin D_3 is selectively removed from the skin by vitamin D-binding protein which has a high affinity for the vitamin. Previtamin D_3 remains for eventual thermal conversion to vitamin D_3 since vitamin D-binding protein has a low affinity for this metabolite (33). The bulk of synthesis of 7-dehydrocholesterol takes place in the Malpighian and dermis layers of the skin. Very little is synthesized and therefore present in the layers stratum corneum and stratum granulosum. Synthesis of previtamin D_3 occurs primarily in the lower layer of skin which is adjacent to the capillary bed.

The production of vitamin D_3 in the skin varies with the duration of exposure to sunlight. Consequently, increases in the production of vitamin D_3 in the skin in response to exposure to sunlight is the reason for the seasonal variation of serum calcium in patients with sarcoid (10) and for the characteristic development of increases in serum $1,25(OH)_2D$ and hypercalcemia during the summer months in the northern hemisphere (15-17). It is quite clear that moderate or excessive exposure of a patient with sarcoid to sunlight or ultraviolet light can bring about an increase in the synthesis of vitamin D_3 which in turn can lead to increases in serum 25-OHD and $1,25(OH)_2D$ and to abnormal calcium metabolism. In view of the fact that sustained hypercalcemia can significantly impair renal function, the outcome in an individual patient can be tragic. As noted earlier, the abnormal calcium metabolism in sarcoid can be corrected or prevented by eliminating dietary vitamin D and preventing exposure to sunlight and ultraviolet light (12).

Extrarenal Production of $1,25(OH)_2D$

Until recently, available evidence indicated the kidney as the major if not sole source of production of $1,25(OH)_2D$. However, synthesis of $[^3H]$-$1,25(OH)_2D_3$ from $[^3H]$-25-OHD_3 was demonstrated by rat placenta (34), human decidua (35), cultured chick calvarial cells (36), and cultured human bone and osteosarcoma cells (37). The identity of $1,25(OH)_2D_3$ synthesized by rat placenta (35) and chick bone cells (38) was confirmed by mass spectral analysis. The rat appears to be unique in that no tissue other that the kidney (39,40) and placenta (34) produces $1,25(OH)_2D$. Following administration of $[^3H]$-25-OHD_3 of high specific activity, no $[^3H]$-$1,25(OH)_2D_3$ was demonstrated in serum or tissues of anephric rats (39,40).

On the other hand, low but measureable quantities of $1,25(OH)_2D$ were consistently demonstrated by both bioassay and receptor assay in the sera of anephric individuals, some of whom were on treatment with vitamin D (41). Serum 25-OHD and serum $1,25(OH)_2D$ by both assays were higher in the patients given vitamin D than in those not given the vitamin. There was a significant positive correlation between serum 25-OHD and serum $1,25(OH)_2D$, indicating that extrarenal production of $1,25(OH)_2D$ is not regulated (41). Mass spectral analysis of the hormone in the circulation of anephric subjects has not been performed, and the site of production is not known. Granulomatous inflammation of the liver and other organs as a result of spalled particles of silicone from blood-pump dialysis tubing indicates the possibility that $1,25(OH)_2D$ may be produced in the granulomatous lesions and may account for the presence of circulating $1,25(OH)_2D$ in anephric subjects (42).

The first suggestion that increased circulating $1,25(OH)_2D$ was derived from extrarenal sources, possibly granulomas, was the finding of elevated serum $1,25(OH)_2D$, hypercalcemia and suppression of PTH secretion in an anephric patient with sarcoid (18). Subsequently, synthesis of $[^3H]$-$1,25(OH)_2D_3$ was observed in 10-day-old primary cultures of pulmonary alveolar macrophages from a patient with sarcoid, elevated serum

$1,25(OH)_2D$ and hypercalcemia (43). In this patient, production of $1,25(OH)_2D$ was diminished by treatment with glucocorticoids, and little or no synthesis was seen in primary cultures of pulmonary alveolar macrophages from other patients with sarcoid who had normal calcium metabolism (43). Conversion of $[^3H]$-25-OHD_3 to $[^3H]$-$1,25(OH)_2D_3$ by the homogenate of a lymph node from a patient with sarcoid and normocalcemia was also observed (44). No conversion occurred in homogenates of lymph nodes from patients who did not have sarcoid.

Sarcoid granulomas also metabolize $[^3H]$-25-OHD_3 to two other metabolites which are biologically inactive (45). These were tentatively identified as 5(Z)-19-nor-10-oxo-25-OHD_3 and 5(E)-19-nor-10-oxo-25-OHD_3, based on their coelution with authentic standards on high pressure liquid chromatography. Neither of them bound specifically to the chick intestinal cytosol receptor. The metabolites were initially described after incubation with bovine rumen microbes and identified as 5(Z) and 5(E) isomers of 19-nor-10-keto-vitamin D_3 (46). It is proposed that these functionally inactive metabolites are in a degradative pathway of 25-OHD_3 and provide a means for regulating synthesis of $1,25(OH)_2D$ by reducing the concentration of its precursor (45).

Abnormal Vitamin D and Calcium Metabolism in other Diseases

Hypercalcemia occasionally occurs in pulmonary and miliary tuberculosis (19,20,47-52). It is associated with suppression of circulating immunoreactive PTH (47-49), and hypercalciuria (48-51), and is corrected by glucocorticoids (47,48,52). Hypercalcemia in tuberculosis results from increased circulating $1,25(OH)_2D$ (19,20). Patients with tuberculosis show increased sensitivity to vitamin D (48). This apparently results from abnormal regulation of circulating $1,25(OH)_2D$ since modest but significant increases in the serum concentration of the metabolite was produced by vitamin D, 100,000 units a day for four days, in a group of 11 patients with active pulmonary tuberculosis and a normal serum calcium (19). The production of $1,25(OH)_2D$ is probably extrarenal since hypercalcemia associated with abnormal elevation of the metabolite in the circulation occurred in a patient with end-stage renal disease who was receiving hemodialysis (20).

Although the pathogenesis of the abnormal calcium metabolism in tuberculosis and sarcoidosis is apparently similar, the presentation, clinical course and prognosis as regards mineral metabolism are usually quite different. Whereas hypercalcemia in sarcoid often occurs in the summer after exposure to sunlight and may be protracted, produce renal damage, be life threatening, and require treatment with glucocortidoids (15-18), hypercalcemia in tuberculosis usually occurs after several months of treatment with antituberculous therapy, readily is managed by hydration and seldom requires steroids (19). Thus, the prognosis for hypercalcemia is considerably better in tuberculosis than it is in sarcoidosis.

Hypercalcemia associated with abnormally elevated $1,25(OH)_2D$ was reported in a patient with disseminated candidiasis (21) and in another patient with silicone-induced granulomas in whom abnormal vitamin D and calcium metabolism were corrected by glucocorticoids (25). It is assumed but not established that the hypercalcemia reported to occur in other chronic granulomatous diseases including berylliosis (53), histoplasmosis (54) and disseminated coccidioidomycosis (55) is caused by a similar abnormality in vitamin D metabolism.

Hypercalcemia resulting from increasing circulating $1,25(OH)_2D$ was reported in six patients with lymphoma, and was associated with suppression of serum PTH and urinary cyclic AMP, impaired renal function and negative bone scans in several of them (23,24). Three of the patients had histiocytic lymphoma, one had T-cell leukemia-lymphoma, one had mixed histiocytic-lymphocytic lymphoma and one had Hodgkin's disease. The abnormal vitamin D and calcium metabolism were corrected by glucocorticoids in four of them and by surgical removal of a spleen which was infiltrated with a lymphoma in one of them (23,24). Whether the lymphoma is the site of production of $1,25(OH)_2D$ in these patients remains to be determined.

References

1. Anderson, J., Dent, C.E., Harper, C., and Philpott, G.R. (1954) Lancet 2:720-724.

2. Scholz, D.A., and Keating, R.F. (1956) Am. J. Med. 21:75-84.

3. Bell, N.H., Gill, J.R., Jr., and Bartter, F.C. (1964) Am. J. Med. 36:500-513.

4. Bell, N.H., and Bartter, F.C. (1967) Acta Endocrinol. 54:173-180.

5. Reiner, M., Sigurdsson, G., Nunziata, M.A., Milik, M.A., Poole, G.W., and Joplin, G.F. (1976) Br. Med. J. 2:1473-1476.

6. Harrell, G.T., and Fisher, S. (1939) J. Clin. Invest. 18:687-693.

7. Henneman, P.H., Dempsey, E.F., Carroll, E.L., and Albright, F. (1956) J. Clin. Invest. 35:1229-1242.

8. Thomas, W.C., Morgan, H.G., Connor, T.B., Haddock, L., Bills, C.E., and Howard, J.E. (1959) J. Clin. Invest. 38:1978-1985.

9. Warkany, J., Guest, G.M., and Graybill, F.J. (1942) J. Lab. Clin. Med. 22:557-565.

10. Taylor, R.L., Lynch, H.J., and Wysor, W.G., Jr. (1963) Am. J. Med. 34:221-227.

11. Dent, C.E. (1970) Postgrad. Med. J. 46:471-473.

12. Hendrix, J.A. (1966) Ann. Int. Med. 64:797-805.

13. Daiger, S.P., Schanfield, M.S., and Cavalli-Sforza, L.L. (1975) Proc. Natl. Acad. Sci. USA 72:2076-2080.

14. Haddad, J.G., Jr., and Walgate, J. (1976) J. Clin. Invest. 58:1217-1222.

15. Bell, N.H., Stern, P.H., Pantzer, E., Sinha, T.K., and DeLuca, H.F. (1979) J. Clin. Invest. 64:218-225.

16. Papapoulos, S.E., Clemens, T.L., Fraher, L.J., Lewin, I.G., Sandler, L.M., and O'Riordan, J.L.H. (1979) Lancet 1:627-630.

17. Koide, Y., Kugai, N., Kimura, S., Fujita, T., and Yamashita, K. (1981) J. Clin. Endocrinol. Metab. 52:494-498.

18. Barbour, G.L., Coburn, J.W., Slatopolsky, E., Norman, A.W., and Horst, R.L. (1981) N. Engl. J. Med. 305:440-443.

19. Sandler, L.M., Winearls, C.G., Fraher, L.J., Clemens, T.L., Smith, R., and O'Riordan, J.L.H. (1984) Quart. J. Med. 210:165-180.

20. Epstein, S., Stern, P.H., Bell, N.H., Dowdeswell, I., and Turner, R.T. (1984) Calcif. Tissue Int. 36:541-544.

21. Ckonos, P.J., London, R., and Hendler, E.D. (1984) N. Engl. J. Med. 311:1683-1685.

22. Kantarjian, H.M., Saad, M.F., Estey, E.H., Sellin, R.V., and Samaan, N.A. (1983) Am. J. Med. 74:721-724.

23. Breslau, N.A., McGuire, J.L., Zerwekh, J.E., Frenkel, E.P., Pak, C.Y.C. (1984) Ann. Int. Med. 100:1-7.

24. Rosenthal, N., Insogna, K.L., Ward Godsall, J., Smaldone, L., Waldone, J.A., and Stewart, A.F. (1985) J. Clin. Endocrinol. Metab. 60:29-33.

25. Kozeny, G.A., Barbato, A.L., Bansai, V.K., Vertuno, L.L., and Hano, J.E. (1984) N. Engl. J. Med. 311:1103-1105.

26. Schaefer, P.C., Fadem, S.Z., Lifschitz, M., and Goldsmith, R.S. (1978) Clin. Res. 26:533A.

27. Frame, B., and Parfitt, A.M. (1980) Ann. Int. Med. 93:449-451.

28. Cushard, W.G., Jr., Simon, A.B., Canterbury, J., and Reiss, E. (1972) N. Engl. J. Med. 286:395-398.

29. Zimmerman, J., Holick, M.F., and Silver, J. (1983) Ann. Int. Med. 98:338.

30. Insogna, I., Broadus, L., Dryer, B., and Gertner, J. (1983) Clin. Res. 31:388A.

31. Stern, P.H., De Olazabal, J., and Bell, N.H. (1980) J. Clin. Invest. 66:852-855.

32. Hughes, M.R., Baylink, D.J., Jones, P.G., and Haussler, M.R. (1976) J. Clin. Invest. 58:61-70.

33. Holick, M.F., McNeill, S.C., McLaughlin, J.A., Holick, S.A., Clark, M.B., and Potts, J.T., Jr. (1979) Trans. Assoc. Am. Phys. 92:54-63.

34. Tanaka, Y., Holloran, B., Schnoes, H.K., and DeLuca, H.F. (1979) Proc. Natl. Acad. Sci. USA 76:5033-5035.

35. Weisman, Y., Harrell, A., Edelstein, S., David, M., Spirer, Z., and Golander, A. (1979) Nature 281:317-319.

36. Turner, R.T., Puzas, E.J., Forte, M.D., Lester, G.E., Gray, T.K., Howard, G.A., and Baylink, D.J. (1980) Proc. Natl. Acad. Sci. USA 77:5720-5724.

37. Howard, G.A., Turner, R.T., Sherrard, D.J., and Baylink, D.J. (1981) J. Biol. Chem. 256:7738-7740.

38. Turner, R.T., Howard, G.A., Puzas, J.E., and Knapp, D.K. (1983) Biochemistry 22:1073-1076.

39. Reeve, L., Tanaka, Y., and DeLuca, H.F. (1983) J. Biol. Chem. 258:3615-3617.

40. Schulz, T.D., Fox, J., Heath, H., and Kumar, R. (1983) Proc. Natl. Acad. Sci. USA 80:1746-1750.

41. Lambert, P.W., Stern, P.H., Avioli, R.C., Brackett, N.C., Turner, R.C., Greene, A., Fu, I.Y., and Bell, N.H. (1982) J. Clin. Invest. 69:722-725.

42. Leong, A.S.-Y., Disney, A.P.S., and Gove, D.W. (1982) N. Engl. J. Med. 306:135-140.

43. Adams, J.S., Sharma, O.P., and Singer, F.R. (1983) J. Clin. Invest 72:1856-1860.

44. Mason, R., Frankel, T.L., Chan, Y.L., Lissner, D., and Posen, S. (1984) Ann. Int. Med. 100:59-61.

45. Okabe, T., Ishizuka, S., Fujisawa, M., Watanabe, J., and Takaku, F. (1984) Biochem. Biophys. Res. Commun. 123:822-830.

46. Napoli, J.L., Sommerfield, J.L., Pramanik, B.C., Gardner, R., Sherry, A.D., Partridge, J.J., Uskokovic, M.R., and Horst, R.L. (1983) Biochemistry 22:3636-3640.

47. Shai, F., Baker, R.K., Addrizzo, J.R., and Wallach, S. (1972) J. Clin. Endocrinol. Metab. 34:251-256.

48. Bradley, G.W., and Sterling, G.M. (1978) Thorax 33:464-467.

49. Abbasi, A.A., Chemplavil, J.K., Farah, S., Muller, B.F., and Arnstein, A.R. (1979) Ann. Int. Med. 90:324-328.

50. Need, A.G., Phillips, P.J., Chiu, F.T.S., and Prisk, H.M. (1980) Br. Med. J. 1:831.

51. Kitrou, M.P., Phytou-Pallikari, A., Tzannes, S.E., Virdidakis, K., and Mountkalakis, Th.D. (1982) Ann. Int. Med. 96:55.

52. Braman, S.S., Goldman, A.L., and Schwartz, M.I. (1975) Arch. Int. Med. 132:269-271.

53. Stoeckle, J.D., Hardy, H.L., and Weber, A.L. (1969) Am. J. Med. 46:545-561.

54. Walker, J.V., Baran, D., Yakub, Y.N., and Freeman, R.B. (1977) J. Am. Med. Assoc. 237:1350-1352.

55. Lee, J.C., Cantanzaro, A., Parthemore, J.G., Roach, R.B., and Deftos, L.J. (1977) N. Engl. J. Med. 297:431-433.

1α-HYDROXYLATION OF VITAMIN D_3 STEROLS BY CULTURED PULMONARY ALVEOLAR MACROPHAGES FROM PATIENTS WITH SARCOIDOSIS

J.S. Adams and M.A. Gacad

University of Southern California School of Medicine, Los Angeles, CA, U.S.A.

INTRODUCTION

We have previously shown that cultured pulmonary alveolar macrophages (PAM) from patients with sarcoidosis metabolize 25-hydroxyvitamin D_3 (25-OH-D_3) to 1,25-dihydroxyvitamin D_3 (1,25-$(OH)_2$-D_3). To date in our laboratory the metabolism of 25-OH-D_3 has been examined in monolayer PAM cultures established from the alveolar lavage fluid of 29 patients with pulmonary disease (19 with biopsy-proven sarcoidosis and 10 with non-sarcoidosis-related lung disease). We now report the kinetics of 1,25-$(OH)_2$-D_3 synthesis by sarcoid PAM and describe factors that alter the reaction _in vitro_ that may be important regulators of active vitamin D_3 metabolite synthesis _in vivo_.

METHODS

Seven to 17-day old PAM cultures from five patients with sarcoidosis (Table 1) were preincubated for 16 hours in serum-free medium with or without vitamin D_3 sterols, dexamethasone, or the human interferons (IFN-γ or IFN-α). This medium was replaced with serum-free BGJ_b medium containing varying amounts of $[^3H]$25-OH-D_3 solubilized in 0.2% ethanol. The cells were incubated with radiolabeled hormone for 3 hrs after which the lipid was extracted from the cells and medium. The extracts were chromatographed for purification and quantitation of metabolite yield, on normal-phase HPLC in both hexane and methylene chloride-based isocratic solvent systems.

Patient	Age (yrs)	Sex	Serum Calcium (mg/dl)	Urinary Calcium Excretion* (mg Ca/100ml GF)	Serum 1,25-$(OH)_2$-D (pg/ml)	S.A.C.E.** (I.U./L)
1	55	F	14.4	1.34	76	81
2	33	F	10.0	0.31	59	59
3	25	F	9.6	0.11	40	31
4	26	F	12.2	***	63	59
5	31	M	14.5	0.92	68	42
Normal range			8.5-10.5	<0.16	30-65	10-35

Table 1: Clinical data on patients with Sarcoidosis

RESULTS

Analysis of the kinetics of $[^3H]$1,25-$(OH)_2$-D_3 production by sarcoid PAM (Table 2) demonstrated the conversion reaction to be substrate dependent, saturable at higher substrate

Vitamin D. A Chemical, Biochemical and Clinical Update

concentrations, and greatest in PAM from patients with either hypercalcemia or hypercalciuria. The K_m of the reaction for $[^3H]25\text{-}OH\text{-}D^3$ was similar between cells from different

Patient	Substrate Range (nM)	V_{max} ($fmol \cdot 10^{-6} cells \cdot min^{-1}$)	K_m (nM)
1	3-150	5.9	52
	1-500	6.3	53
2	3-180	11.0	70
3	5-320	1.2	76
4	10-300	9.1	109
5	10-300	40.6	210

Table 2: Kinetics of $25\text{-}OH\text{-}D_3\text{-}1\alpha$-hydroxylation

patients but the V_{max} varied 40-fold. The PAM 1α-hydroxylation reaction preferred side-chain substituted sterol substrates, the yield of $[^3H]1\alpha$-hydroxyvitamin D_3 from $[^3H]$ vitamin D_3 was only 15% of that for the 1α-hydroxylated products of $[^3H]25\text{-}OH\text{-}D_3$ and $[^3H]24,25\text{-}(OH)_2\text{-}D_3$. $[^3H]1,25\text{-}(OH)_2\text{-}D_3$ synthesis by PAM was minimally resistant to inhibition by preincubation with $1,25\text{-}(OH)_2\text{-}D_3$, but was inhibited in dose-dependent fashion by dexamethasone. In PAM from three different patients $[^3H]1,25\text{-}(OH)_2\text{-}D_3$ synthesis was increased after preincubation with the human lymphokine, IFN-γ. As shown in Figure 1, this increase resulted from an increase in the V_{max} without a change in the affinity of the 1α-hydroxylation reaction for $[^3H]25\text{-}OH\text{-}D_3$.

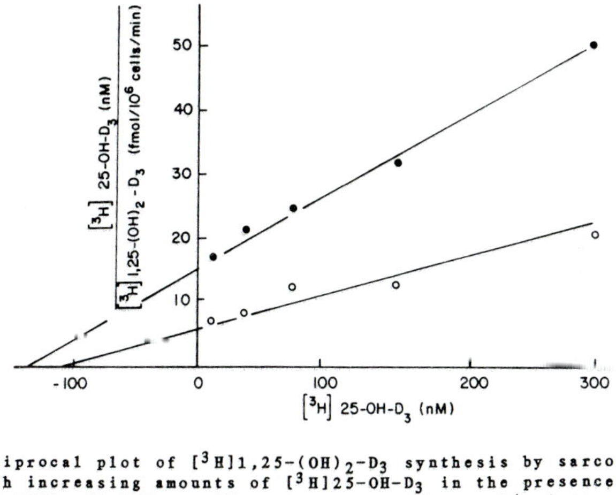

Figure 1: Reciprocal plot of $[^3H]1,25\text{-}(OH)_2\text{-}D_3$ synthesis by sarcoid PAM after incubation with increasing amounts of $[^3H]25\text{-}OH\text{-}D_3$ in the presence (o) or absence (•) of 1000 u/1 IFN-γ. (K_m=x intercept, V_{max} = 1/y intercept)

REFERENCES:

1. Adams, J.S., Sharma, O.P., Gacad, M.A., and Singer, F.R. (1983) J. Clin. Invest. 72, 1856-1860.

2. Adams, J.S., Singer, F.R., Gacad, M.A., Sharma, O.P., Hayes, M.J., Vouros, P., and Holick, M.F. (1985) J. Clin. Endocrinol. Metab. In press.

3. Adams, J.S., Gacad, M.A., Singer, F.R., and Sharma, O.P. (1985) Ann. N.Y. Acad. Sci. In press.

THE CONTROL OF PRODUCTION OF 1,25-DIHYDROXY VITAMIN D3 IN MAN: STUDIES OF VITAMIN D DEFICIENCY AND SARCOIDOSIS.

L.J. Fraher, L.M. Sandler, R. Karmali, S. Barker, K.C. Flint, B.N. Hudspith, N. McI. Johnson and J.L.H. O'Riordan.

Department of Medicine, The Middlesex Hospital, London, U.K.

INTRODUCTION

Overproduction of 1,25-(OH)2 D3 occurs during the treatment of vitamin D deficiency and can also occur in sarcoidosis. Here we describe recent studies investigating the possible pathophysiological mechanisms involved .

HUMAN VITAMIN D DEFICIENCY

The circulating concentration of 1,25-(OH)2D3 in patients with osteomalacia due to vitamin D deficiency has been an area of some controversy. In some reports (1,2) circulating 1,25-(OH)2D3 was found to be normal and in conjunction with histological studies of such patients (3), this has led to the suggestion that metabolites other than 1,25-(OH)2D3 are important in both the pathogenesis and healing of the disease. However, both our own previous findings (4) and those advanced in Manchester (5) have indicated that, in the untreated state, human vitamin D deficiency is associated with inappropriately low circulating 1,25-(OH)2D3 when considering, amongst other factors, the degree of secondary hyperparathyroidism that is typically present.

However, supranormal concentrations of 1,25-(OH)2D3 develop rapidly in these patients following administration of small doses of vitamin D3. Further to this, osteomalacia can be cured in the presence of abnormally low circulating concentrations of 25-OH D3, 24,25-(OH)2D3 and 25,26-(OH)2D3 following administration of Calcitriol alone to vitamin D deficient subjects (4). These results suggested that metabolites other than 1,25-(OH)2 D3 are not essential in the healing of osteomalacia.

In order to study the control of production of 1,25-(OH)2D3 in human vitamin D deficiency we have recently followed changes in the circulating concentrations of both 25-OH D3 and 1,25-(OH)2D3 in 29 patients with osteomalacia. To examine the circulating concentration of 1,25-(OH)2 D3 in the untreated state, we have measured serum 1,25-(OH)2 D3 in 14 patients with osteomalcia for periods of up to 4 weeks prior to therapy. In other studies the effects of differing doses of vitamin D3 on the production of 1,25-(OH)2D3 and the biochemical changes during healing were closely studied.

Vitamin D. A Chemical, Biochemical and Clinical Update

RESULTS

In 70 samples obtained from 29 different patients the range of concentrations of 25-OH D3 was from undetectable (<0.5 ng/ml) to 4.2 ng/ml, being below the lower limit of normal (3.0 ng/ml) in 67 of the samples (96%). In the same samples the concentration of 1,25-(OH)2D3 was more variable, ranging from undetectable (<4.0 pg/ml) to 41 pg/ml with a mean ±SD of 16.6 ±9.4 pg/ml. These measured concentrations were below the lower limit of normal (20 pg/ml) in 48 of the samples (69%), and within the normal range in the remaining 22 (31%). Of the 29 patients, normal concentrations of 1,25-(OH)2D3 were observed in samples from 15 individuals, but in 11 of these 15 the concentration was subnormal in other samples obtained on different days.

Sequential observations of circulating 1,25-(OH)2D3 in 14 patients studied for up to 4 weeks prior to treatment are shown in figure 1. On admission (day 0) the range of serum concentrations of 1,25-(OH)2D3 found in these patients was from undetectable to 41 pg/ml. Over the following days (or weeks) the circulating concentration decreased in 6 of the patients, increased in 5 and remained unchanged in the last 3 (in 2 of whom it was unmeasurable throughout). Sequential observations of 1,25-(OH)2D3 which were within the normal range throughout were noted in only 3 of the 14 patients.

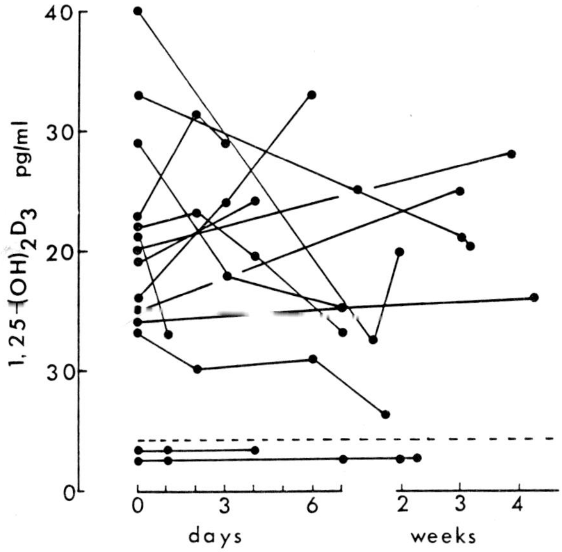

Figure 1. Sequential observations of circulating 1,25-(OH)2D3 in 14 patients with osteomalacia due to vitamin D deficiency following admission to hospital but before treatment.

EFFECT OF INCREASING DOSES OF VITAMIN D3 ON THE PRODUCTION OF 1,25-(OH)2D3

In a group of 8 Asian patients with nutritional osteomalacia the effect of treatment with increasing doses of vitamin D3 (3 were treated with 400 iu/d, 3 received 2000 iu/d and 2 received 10000 iu/d) was followed for up to 3 years. At presentation all these patients were hypocalcaemic, serum phosphate was low or near the lower limit of normal in 6 patients, and alkaline phosphatase was elevated in 6 of the 8. Amino-terminal parathyroid hormone (n-PTH) was elevated in all of them (table I).

	Ca	PO4	AlP	PTH	25- D	1,25- D
normal range	**2.2-2.55 mmol/l**	**0.6-1.3 mmol/l**	**20-85 iu/l**	**<120 pg/ml**	**3-33 ng/ml**	**20-65 pg/ml**
Patient						
1	2.11	0.55	312	750	1.4	19
2	2.17	0.96	128	620	1.8	21
3	2.14	0.53	136	270	1.8	18
4	2.15	0.51	225	160	1.6	18
5	2.19	0.51	68	380	1.2	15
6	1.67	1.20	72	870	1.0	14
7	2.12	0.66	255	425	1.9	20
8	2.11	0.60	196	388	<0.8	<4

TABLE I Biochemical details of 8 patients with osteomalacia.

Following administration of vitamin D3 the clinical and biochemical responses of all the patients were excellent. Normocalcaemia was achieved within 3 months and serum phosphate increased to such an extent that transient hyperphosphataemia was noted in all the patients. Secondary hyperparathyroidism was quickly corrected in all but one of the patients, with n-PTH falling to normal within 4 months in 7 of the 8. In the last patient, following an initial rapid decline of n-PTH from 620 pg/ml, the serum concentration plateaued at approximately 200 pg/ml for 2 years before finally reaching the normal range. In the six patients in whom it was elevated alkaline phosphatase gradually fell to normal with treatment.

In all the patients administration of vitamin D3 resulted in increases of both circulating 25-OH D3 and 1,25-(OH)2 D3. Illustrated in figure 2 are examples of the responses observed in one patient from each of the different treatment groups. Following ingestion of 400 iu/d of vitamin D3 circulating 25-OH D3 increased gradually but this was associated with the production of supranormal circulating 1,25-(OH)2 D3, which reached a peak concentration of 125 pg/ml after 4 weeks of therapy in this patient.

When 2000 iu/d was given to another patient (fig 2, middle) the increase of 25-OH D3 was again gradual, but serum 1,25-(OH)2D3 increased more rapidly to a peak concentration of 195 pg/ml within 3 weeks and, in the third example (fig 2, right), with 10000 iu/d circulating 1,25-(OH)2D3 reached 225 pg/ml within 14 days of treatment. In all these patients the concentration of 1,25-(OH)2D3 then began to decline, but the rate of fall was slower than the initial increase so that elevated serum concentrations were observed for a number of months although the other measured parameters of the disease were at, or near, normal by this time.

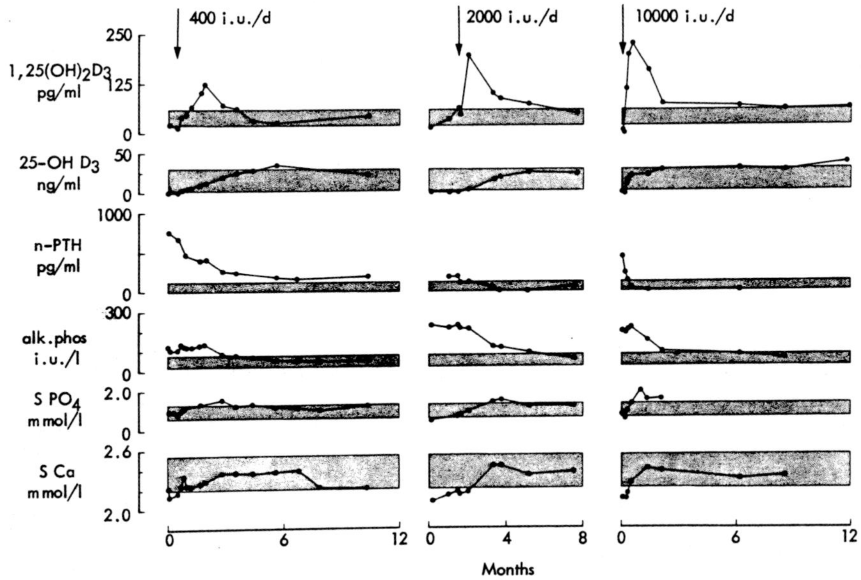

Figure 2. Sequential obervations of serum calcium, phosphate, n-PTH, alkaline phosphatase and both 25-OH D3 and 1,25-(OH)2 D3 in three patients with osteomalacia treated with vitamin D3 at a dose of either 400 iu/d (left), 2000 iu/d (middle) and 10000 iu/d (right).

In order to study the control of these phenomena all the data from the 8 patients were pooled and interdependence was tested by linear regression analysis. From this it was found that the serum concentration of 1,25-(OH)2 D3 was strongly correlated to serum 25-OH D3 during the early phase of treatment. This relationship, illustrated in figure 3, held up to the time of the peak concentration of 1,25-(OH)2 D3. However once the peak had passed, the relationship was lost and there was no evidence for a negative relationship during the prolonged decline of 1,25-(OH)2 D3 back to the normal range, even though circulating 25-OH D3 was still increasing due to continued ingestion of vitamin D3.

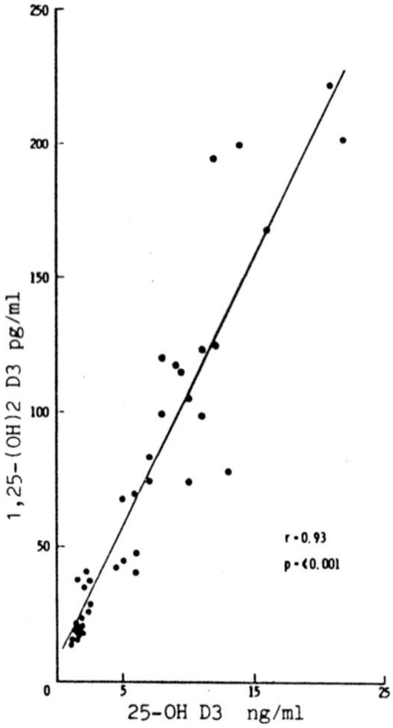

Figure 3. Relationship between circulating 25-OHD3 and 1,25-(OH)2D3 in 8 patients with osteomalacia during the early phase of treatment with vitamin D3. Analysis of data from the time of presentation to time of the peak of 1,25-(OH)2D3 in serum.

The circulating concentrations of these two vitamin D3 metabolites were not related to any other of the biochemical markers of the disease during any period of observation, neither were there any relationships between n-PTH and the other parameters. The fall of alkaline phosphatase to normal (in the 6 of 8 in whom it was elevated) was unrelated to either the dose of the vitamin given, or the circulating concentrations of the metabolites achieved, but was strongly correlated to the initial concentration. Thus, there was a positive relationship between the serum concentration of alkaline phosphatase at presentation and the time taken to fall to normal ($r=0.96$, $p<0.01$, not shown).

In summary, during the treatment of human vitamin D deficiency the production of 1,25-(OH)2 D3 is substrate dependent during the early phase until a peak concentration is reached. The magnitude and the time taken to reach this peak are affected by the dose of the vitamin given (probably through increased availability of 25-OH D3 with the larger doses), but once the peak has passed and the other parameters of the disease are normal, there is no clear biochemical explanation for the continued production of elevated circulating concentrations of 1,25-(OH)2 D3.

SARCOIDOSIS

Disordered calcium homeostasis is a frequent complication of sarcoidosis. Although hypercalcaemia has been reported in only a minority of patients, hypercalcuria can occur in up to 60 % (6) and increased intestinal absorption of calcium has also been documented (7). It is now clear that there are abnormalities of vitamin D metabolism in these patients such that when hypercalcaemia is seen, it is associated with inappropriately high circulating concentrations of 1,25-(OH)2 D3 which are produced in the face of normal concentrations of 25-OH D3 (8,9). Furthermore, the production of 1,25-(OH)2 D3 during hypercalcaemia is in a substrate dependent manner which is sensitive to glucocorticoids; the effect of steroids is to suppress elevated 1,25-(OH)2 D3 while not changing serum 25-OH D3 (10).

Following the description of an anephric patient with sarcoidosis who had spontaneous hypercalcaemia associated with supranormal circulating 1,25-(OH)2 D3 (11), putative extra-renal sites of 25-OH D3-1-hydroxylase activity have been investigated. Thus, the *in vitro* production from [3H] 25-OH D3 of tritiated material which has similar chromatographic and ligand binding characteristics to 1,25-(OH)2 D3 has been demonstrated in both cultured pulmonary alveolar macrophages (12) and lymph node homogenates (13) from patients with sarcoidosis. However, some doubts have been cast on the absolute confirmation of this material as 1,25-(OH)2 D3 following the results of animal experiments. In these latter studies (14) material produced *in vitro* from [3H] 25-OH D3 by rat peritoneal macrophages co-eluted with authentic 1,25-(OH)2 D3 on HPLC when developed in 10% isopropanol in hexane, but was shown to be dissimilar when re-chromatographed on other systems.

Here we describe studies to characterise the material assayed as 1,25-(OH)2 D3 from the circulation of patients with sarcoidosis and also give results from *in vitro* experiments investigating the ability of cultured pulmonary alveolar macrophages obtained from 28 different patients with sarcoidosis to produce putative [3H] 1,25-(OH)2 D3.

RESULTS

In order to characterise the material assayed as 1,25-(OH)2 D3 a large sample of serum was obtained from a patient with histologically proven sarcoidosis during a spontaneous episode of hypercalcaemia in the summer months. A number of 2.0 ml aliquots of this sample were extracted and fractionated by straight phase HPLC in the usual manner and the fractions corresponding to 1,25-(OH)2 D3 collected.

In radioimmunoassay using the specific antiserum S 11, the mean concentration of 1,25-(OH)2 D3 measured in 5 of these aliquots was 78 pg/ml. When a set of 3 aliquots were pooled and then serially diluted into assay, the radioligand displacement by the extract displayed parallelism to the standard curve and periodate treatment of further extracts had no effect on binding activity.

Another 5 extracts were pooled and subjected to reverse phase HPLC on a "Resolve" column eluted with 80% methanol in water at a flow rate of 1.0 ml/min. During the elution of this sample timed fractions were collected and assayed against reference 1,25-(OH)2 D3. In this separation (fig 4) the material which had been collected in the position of 1,25-(OH)2 D3 from straight phase HPLC co-eluted with reference sterol in this second system as a homogeneous peak. Thus the material assayed as 1,25-(OH)2 D3 in serum from this patient appeared to be identical to authentic 1,25-(OH)2 D3 by co-chromatography, ligand binding and periodate resistance.

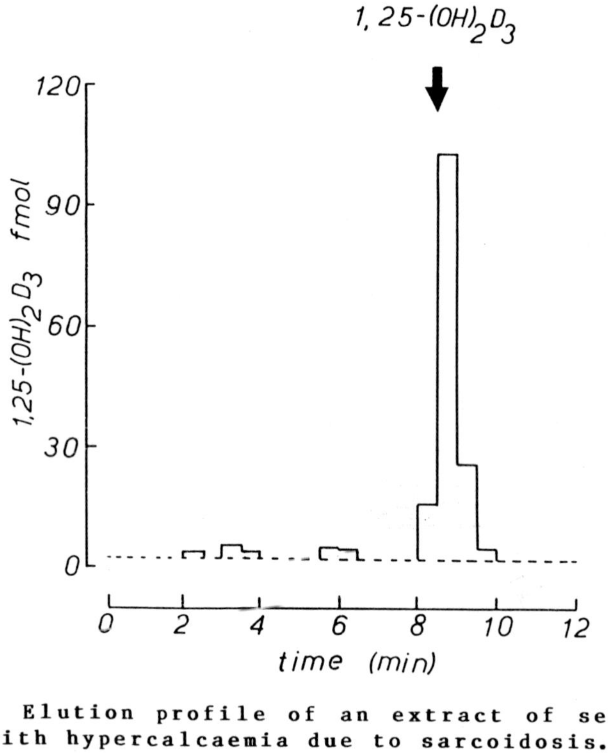

Figure 4. Elution profile of an extract of serum from a patient with hypercalcaemia due to sarcoidosis. Following initial straight phase HPLC the "1,25-(OH)2 D3" fraction was subjected to reverse phase HPLC and the column monitored by radioimmunoassay of timed fractions. The arrow indicates the elution position of reference sterol.

To study the possible ectopic genesis of 1,25-(OH)2 D3 in sarcoidosis the metabolism of [3H] 25-OH D3 was followed in cultured pulmonary alveolar macrophages (PAM) from 28 patients and 7 control subjects. In the patients serum calcium was 2.41±0.10 mmol/l (mean± SD, n=28), 25-OH D3 was 5.8±3.7 ng/ml (n=19) and 1,25-(OH)2 D3 was 59.2±16.6 pg/ml (n=19) at the time of bronchio-alveolar lavage. After 9 days of primary culture the adherent cells in duplicate wells were incubated with 5 nM 25-[26,27-3H]-OH D3 (sp act 150-180 Ci/mmol) for 3 hours. The lipid soluble material was then extracted on C18 Sep-paks and fractions corresponding to authentic 1,25-(OH)2 D3 isolated by sequential straight and reverse phase HPLC.

Tritiated material, which eluted in the position of 1,25-(OH)2 D3 from the second HPLC column was produced in cultures of cells from 14 of the 28 patients: none of this metabolite was seen in any of the control cultures. The amounts of this [3H] PAM metabolite, when produced, varied from 4.2 to 740 fmol/million adherent cells in the initial cultures/h. The metabolite co-eluted with authentic 1,25-(OH)2 D3 on Zorbax-SIL eluted with either Hex:IPA:MeOH (92:4:4) or DCM:MeOH (98:2) and on Zorbax-ODS eluted with MeOH:H20 (88:12). Furthermore, when used as the radioligand with either antiserum S 02282 or S 11 in radioimmunoassay the displacement curves by reference 1,25-(OH)2 D3 were not different from parallel assays using 1,25-[26,27-3H]-(OH)2 D3 , sp act 163 Ci/mmol, Amersham Int. PLC.

There were no relationships between the production of the [3H] PAM metabolite with either the usual biochemical features of the patients at the time of lavage or the lung involvement as assessed by either chest X-ray staging or gallium uptake. Neither was there any dependence upon the percentage of either macrophages, lymphocytes, neutrophils or eosinophils in the recovered lavage fluid. However, when the data obtained from the patients was divided into two groups according to the ability of cultured PAM's to produce the metabolite, striking differences were seen.

In the patients from whom cultured PAM produced the metabolite, there was a strong positive correlation between circulating 25-OH D3 and 1,25-(OH)2 D3. This relationship (fig 6, left) was present although serum 25-OH D3 was if anything, low (mean 5.3±2.7 ng/ml) and 1,25-(OH)2 D3 was above the upper limit of normal in only one patient. In contrast, in the group of "non producers", no such relationship could be found (fig 6, right). In this second group circulating 25-OH D3 was no different (6.2±4.6 ng/ml) yet 1,25-(OH)2 D3 was much more variable, ranging from 37 to 107 pg/ml, being elevated in 4/10 (mean 61±19 pg/ml). This latter finding is interesting since none of these patients had a history of hypercalcaemia and were both normocalcaemic and normocalcuric at the time of lavage.

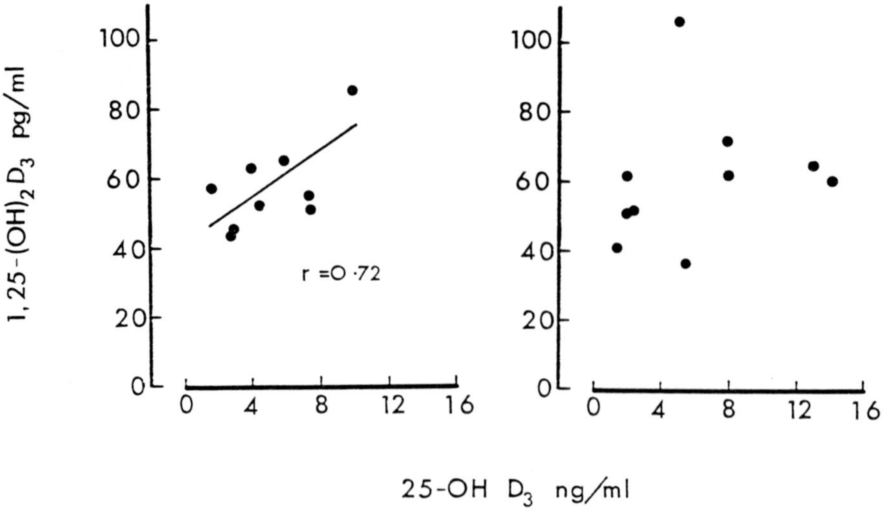

Figure 5. Relationship between circulating concentrations of 25-OH D3 and 1,25-(OH)2 D3 in two groups of patients with sarcoidosis. Left those patients in whom ectopic genesis of 1,25-(OH)2 D3 was suggested *in vitro* and Right, a group of "non-producers".

DISCUSSION

In human vitamin D deficiency the circulating concentration of 1,25-(OH)2 D3 can be variable. In the untreated state it is possible to observe "normal" serum concentrations of this metabolite. However, circulating 1,25-(OH)2 D3 can rapidly increase or decrease according to the availability of 25-OH D3, as is witnessed by the rapid, substrate dependent overproduction when treatment with vitamin D3 commences. Factors which initiate this overproduction are present when the patients are first seen, but less clear are the mechanisms which maintain elevated concentrations for many months.

In patients with sarcoidosis it is possible that ectopic genesis of 1,25-(OH)2 D3 is a major, unregulated route of metabolism of 25-OH D3. In those patients in whom it occurs, substrate dependent production of 1,25-(OH)2 D3 is suggested by the presence of a relationship between circulating 25-OH D3 and 1,25-(OH)2 D3. This relationship can be found although the concentration of both of the metabolites are within their normal ranges and the patients are normocalcaemic. Clearly an abnormality of vitamin D metabolism exists in this condition , however, sustained overproduction of 1,25-(OH)2 D3 leads to hypercalcaemia may be dependent upon the availability of substrate for the ectopic 25-OH D3-1-hydroxylase.

ACKNOWLEDGEMENTS

We would like to thank the Medical Research Council for financial support and The British Council for an award to R.K.

REFERENCES

1) Eastwood, J.B., De Wardener, H.E., Gray, R.W. and Leman, J.L.Jr. (1979) **Lancet**, i, 1377-.

2) Peacock, M., Heyburn, P.J., Aaron, J.E., Taylor, G.A., Brown, W.B. and Speed, R. (1979) in **Vitamin D: basic research and its clinical application.** eds A.W. Norman et al, Walter DeGruyter, Berlin. p 1177-.

3) Bordier, P., Rasmussen, H., Marie, P., Miravet, L, Geuris, J. and Ryckwaert, A. (1978) **J Clin Endocrinol Metab**, 46, 284-.

4) Papapoulos, S.E., Clemens, T.L., Fraher, L.J., Gleed, J. and O'Riordan, J.L.H. (1980) **Lancet**, ii, 612-.

5) Stanbury, S.W., Taylor, C.M., Lumb, G.A., Mawer, E.B., Berry, J., Hann, J. and Wallace, J. (1981) **Mineral Electrolyte Metab**, 5, 212-.

6) Studdy, P.R., Bird, R., Neville, E. and James, D.G.(1980) **J Clin Path**, 33, 528-.

7) Reiner, M., Sigurdsson, G., Nunziata, M.A., Malik, M.A., Poole, G.W. and Joplin, G.F. (1976) **Brit Med J**,2,1473.

8) Papapoulos, S.E.,Clemens,T.L.,Fraher, L.J., Lewin,I.G., Sandler,L.M. and O'Riordan,J.L.H. (1979)**Lancet**,i, 627-.

9) Bell, N.H., Stern, P.H., Pantzer, E., Sinha, T.K. and DeLuca, H. F. (1979) **J Clin Invest**, 64, 218-.

10) Sandler, L.M., Winnearls, C.G., Fraher, L.J., Clemens, T.L., Smith, R. and O'Riordan, J.L.H. (1984) **Quart J Med** 210, 165-.

11) Barbour, G.L., Coburn, J.W., Slatopolsky, E., Norman, A.W. and Horst, R.L. (1981) **New Eng J Med**, 305,440-.

12) Adams, J.S., Sharma, O.P., Mercedes, A.G. and Singer, F.R. (1983) **J Clin Invest**, 72, 1856-.

13) Mason, R.S., Frankel, T.L., Chan, Y.L., Lissner, D. and Posen, S. (1983) **Calc Tiss Int**, 35, 699-.

14) Gray, T.K., Maddux, F.W., Lester, G.E. and Williams, M.E. (1982) **Biochem Biophys Res Comm**, 109, 723-.

Other Clinical Topics

DEFECTIVE NEUTROPHIL CANDIDACIDAL ACTIVITY IN PATIENTS WITH RESISTANCE TO 1,25-$(OH)_2$-VITAMIN D_3

Y. WEISMAN, Z. HOCHBERG, S. POLLACK, T. MESHULAM, V. ZAKUT, Z. SPIRER, A. BENDERLI AND A. ETZIONI
Vitamin Research Laboratory, Ichilov Hospital, Tel Aviv and Departments of Pediatrics, Clinical Immunology and Microbiology, Rambam Medical Center, Haifa, Israel.

Introduction

Recent studies have shown that 1,25$(OH)_2D_3$ may be involved in the regulation of proliferation, differentiation and function of the immune system (1,2,3). The occurrence of the syndrome of resistance to 1,25$(OH)_2D_3$ (vitamin D dependent rickets type II) (4,5) provides an unusual opportunity of investigating the possible role of 1,25$(OH)_2D_3$ in the immune system.

Patients and Methods

Five patients, aged 2 to 11 years of 3 kindreds were the subjects of this study. Defective receptors for 1,25$(OH)_2D_3$ in cultured skin fibroblasts and in lectin-stimulated lymphocytes were demonstrated in all patients (6,7). Details of the patient's clinical and biochemical features are documented in previous reports (5,6,8). The ingestion and intraneutrophil killing of Candida albicans and Staphylococcus aureus and the endotoxin stimulated nitroblue tetrazolium (NBT) test were performed as previously described (9,10,11). Monocyte chemotaxis was measured in one patient by the response to the chemotactic peptide N-formyl-methionyl-leucyl-phenylalanine (12). Lymphoproliferative responses to phytohaemagglutinin and concanavalin A were measured by the standard method of tritiated thymidine labeling of newly synthetized DNA. T-cell subsets were quantitated by the immunofluorescent technique, using monoclonal antibodies (OKT3 for T-cells, OKT4 for helper T cells and OKT8 for suppressor T cells).

Results and Discussion

A selective defect in neutrophil candidacidal activity was found in all patients with resistance to 1,25$(OH)_2D_3$. The candidacidal activity was significantly lower (31.3 ± SEM 2.2% of ingested Candida albicans in 1h) than that of controls (82.8 ± SEM 5.1%) (Table). The bactericidal activity towards Staphylococcus aureus did not differ from that observed in controls (killing index of ingested Staph. aureus was 107.6 ± SEM 3.1% of controls). The phagocytic activity towards both microorganisms was normal. The NBT reduction test was normal in all patients. Migration of patient's 5 peripheral blood monocytes in response to N-formyl-methionyl-leucyl-phenylalanine was comparable to that of controls. Peripheral blood B and T lymphocytes and T-cell subset analysis demonstrated that the patients had normal T to B and helper (35-75%) to suppressor (13-27%) T cell ratios. Lymphocyte proliferative responses to phytohaemagglutinin and concanavalin A were comparable to those of normal controls. The mechanism that links the observed impairment of candidacidal activity to the lack of normal receptors for 1,25$(OH)_2D_3$, in patients with resistance to 1,25$(OH)_2D_3$, is unknown at present. A possible explanation is that 1,25$(OH)_2D_3$ may regulate intracellular calcium pools and intracellular free ca^{+2} level which is an important trigger of neutrophil activation. Our study also shows that lack of receptors for 1,25$(OH)_2D_3$ did not affect either helper to suppressor T-cells

Vitamin D. A Chemical, Biochemical and Clinical Update

ratio or lymphocyte proliferative response to lactins. Thus, the question whether $1,25(OH)_2D_3$ participates in the regulation of helper to suppressor T-cells ratio and mononuclear cell function, as has been shown recently in in vitro studies, is not clear yet. However, a recent study (13) shows that $1,25(OH)_2D_3$ does not suppress ^3H-thymidine incorporation into DNA in lectin stimulated lymphocytes of patients with resistance to $1,25(OH)_2D_3$, as opposed to normal subjects. This, suggests that $1,25(OH)_2D_3$ may affect some functions of mononuclear cells.

In conclusion, this study provides additional evidence for the role of $1,25(OH)_2D_3$ in the immune system including the intraneutrophil killing of microorganisms.

Table: Neutrophil phagocytic and candidacidal activities in patients with resistance to $1,25(OH)_2D_3$

Patients	Candida albicans ingested (%)	Candida albicans killed(%)	% of ingested C.albicans killed
1	31.2	9.6	30.5
2	32.3	10.8	33.4
3	72.8	18.5	25.4
4	18.7	7.2	38.2
5	45.3	12.7	28.0
mean ± SEM	40.1 ± 9.2*	11.7 ± 1.9**	31.1 ± 2.2**
controls			
mean ± SEM	53.5 ± 2.3	44.9 ± 2.9	83.8 ± 5.1

* $p > 0.05$ ** $p < 0.01$.

References

1. Editorial, Lancet (1984) 1:1105-1106.
2. Manolagas,S.C., Deftos,L.J., Ann.Intern.Med. (1984) 100:59-61.
3. Bar-Shavit ,Z., Noff,D., Edelstein,S., Meyer,M., Shibolet,S., Goldman,R. (1981) Calcif.Tissue.Int. 33:673-676.
4. Brooks,M.H., Bell,N.H., Love,L., Stern,P.H., Orfei,E., Queener,S.F., Hamstra,A.J., DeLuca,H.F. (1978) N.Engl.J.Med. 298:996-999.
5. Hochberg,Z., Benderli,A., Levy,J., Vardi,P., Weisman,Y., Chen,T., Feldman,D. (1984). Am.J.Med. 77:805-811.
6. Feldman,D., Chen,T., Cone,C., Hirst,M., Shani,A., Benderli,A., Hochberg,Z. (1982) J.Clin.Endocrinol.Metab. 55:1020-1022.
7. Liberman,U.A., Eil,C., Marx,S.J. (1983) J.Clin.Invest. 7:192-199.
8. Hochberg,Z., Borochowitz,Z., Benderli,A., Vardi,P., Oren,S., Spirer,Z., Heyman,I., Weisman,Y. (1985) J.Clin.Endocrinol.Metab. 60:57-61.
9. Lehrer,R.I., Cline,M.J. (1969) J.Bacteriol. 98:996-1004.
10. Lam,C., Mathison,G.E. (1979) J.Med.Microbiol. 12:459-469. 1970.
11. Park,H.H., Good,R.A. (1980) Lancet 2:616
12. Synderman,R., Pike,M.C. In Leukocyte chemotaxis. Gallin,J.I., Quie,P.G. ed. (1978) Raven Press, New York, p.73-78.
13. Koren,R., Ravid,A., Hochberg,Z., Weisman,Y., Novogrodsky,A., Liberman, U.A. (1985) Abstract. Sixth Workshop on vitamin D, Merano, Italy.

CLINICAL EXPERIENCES WITH HUMAN PTH (1-34).

T. J. Furlong, M.S. Seshadri, M.R. Wilkinson, C.J. Cornish, B. Luttrell, S. Posen. Department of Endocrinology, Royal North Shore Hospital, St. Leonards, NSW 2065, Australia.

Most clinical data relating to PTH infusions have been obtained with Lilly "Parathormone" which is no longer available. With the introduction of synthetic human PTH 1-34 for use in human subjects it became important to study the effect of this material in normal and abnormal subjects.

PATIENTS AND METHODS

Two hundred units of human synthetic PTH (1-34, USV, Tuckahoe, NY) were given intravenously in 2 ml normal saline over a period of 10 minutes between 10 a.m. and 10.10 a.m. There were 8 normal subjects (aged 22-59), 4 patients with surgical hypoparathyroidism, 3 patients with primary hyperparathyroidism and 6 patients with non-surgical chronic hypocalcemia not suffering from renal failure or vitamin D deficiency. The hypocalcemic patients were receiving vitamin D compounds at the time of the study. The subjects fasted overnight and remained at rest in hospital for 2 hours before the procedure and 3 hours afterwards. They drank approximately 1 liter of water during this time to ensure an adequate urine volume.

Venous blood was collected at -90, -30, +30, +90, and +150 minutes while urine collections were made at -60, 0, +60, +120 and +180 minutes. More frequent blood collections were made where indicated. Urine and plasma cyclic AMP were measured by competitive binding (Amersham kit), serum immunoreactive PTH, prolactin and osteocalcin by radioimmunoassays with commercially available reagents, serum bioactive PTH by the method of Seshadri et al. (1) and serum $1,25(OH)_2D$ by the method of Reinhardt et al. (2) Serum and urine calcium were measured by atomic absorption. Other assays were performed by standard Technicon methods.

RESULTS

There were no symptoms associated with the administration of PTH 1-34 by this method (3) and blood pressure readings remained unchanged. In the normal subjects, urine phosphate rose to a mean of approximately twice the basal value (mean basal 11.79, mean peak 21.76 µmol/100 ml glomerular filtrate). Plasma cyclic AMP rose by a factor of 3 (mean basal 12.36, mean peak 35.35 pmol/ml) while mean urinary nephrogenous cAMP rose by a factor of 38 (mean basal 1.55, mean peak 59.59 nmol/100 ml glomerular filtrate). Serum prolactin rose by 33% ($p<0.001$). Serum osteocalcin, serum immunoreactive PTH, serum calcitonin and serum vitamin D metabolites remained unaltered. Serum $1,25(OH)_2D$ concentrations were not significantly altered either at 12 hours or at 22 hours.

In 4 normal subjects multiple plasma specimens were obtained during the first 20 minutes after the termination of the infusion. Bioactive PTH in these individuals showed a mean half life of 3.8 minutes, similar to the values obtained for endogenous PTH after calcium infusions (1). No significant differences were noted between the disappearance rates of

Vitamin D. A Chemical, Biochemical and Clinical Update

bioactive PTH of normal subjects and those of patients with various forms of hypoparathyroidism.

All patients showed a rise in plasma and urine cyclic AMP except for 2 chronically hypocalcemic individuals with high basal immunoreactive PTH values (Fig 1). These 2 patients (who had no skeletal changes) presumably have one of the forms of "pseudohypoparathyroidism". Three chronically hypocalcemic individuals (members of 1 family) with elevated basal immunoreactive PTH values responded normally. No resistance to PTH was observed in the 3 hyperparathyroid individuals.

RISE IN NEPHROGENOUS cAMP IN RESPONSE TO HUMAN PTH (1-34) IN DIFFERENT DISORDERS

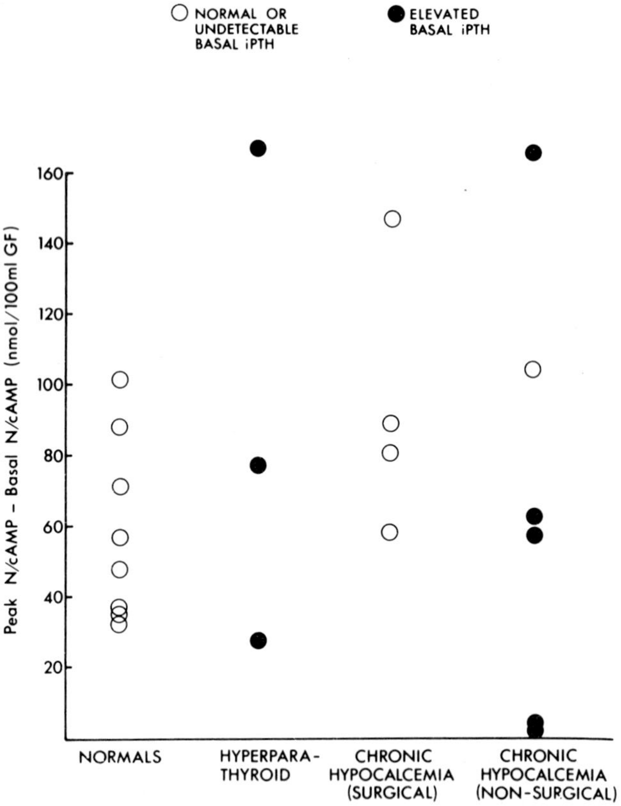

CONCLUSIONS

Synthetic human PTH (1-34) appears a safe substance if administered according to this protocol and clearly identifies some "non-responders". The current protocol is not useful for the study of vitamin D metabolites.

REFERENCES

1. Seshadri, M.S., Chan, Y.L., Wilkinson, M.R., Mason, R.S., Posen, S. Clin. 68: 321-326, 1985.

2. Reinhardt, T.A., Horst, R.L., Orf, J.W., Hollis, B.W. J. Clin. Endocrinol. Metab. 58: 91-98, 1984.

3. Slovik, D.M., Daly, M.A., Potts, J.T.Jr., Neer, R.M. Clin. Endocrinol. 20: 369-375, 1984.

125-DIHYDROXYVITAMIN D (1,25-$(OH)_2$ D) RESPONSES IN YOUNG BABOONS FED DIETS WITH VARYING CALCIUM AND PHOSPHORUS CONTENTS.

J.M. PETTIFOR, F.P. ROSS, M. CAVALEROS AND M. SLY.
Metabolic and Nutrition Research Unit, Department of Paediatrics, University of the Witwatersrand; and the National Food Research Institute, C.S.I.R., Pretoria, South Africa.

Little is known concerning the effects of dietary calcium deprivation in young primates and the resultant changes in vitamin D metabolism and bone histomorphometry. In rural vitamin D replete children on low calcium diets we have documented osteomalacia and rickets associated with elevated parathyroid hormone and 1,25-OH$)_2$D concentrations(1). In order to study the effects of dietary calcium deprivation more closely, we examined the effects of various dietary calcium and phosphorus contents on young vitamin D replete baboons over a sixteen month period.

METHODS

Four groups of seven baboons each were fed one of four diets for a period of sixteen months (Table 1). The estimated ages of the baboons on entry into the study were between six and twelve months.

	HIGH CALCIUM	MEDIUM CALCIUM	LOW CALCIUM	LOW CALCIUM LOW PHOSPHORUS
Calcium Content (mg/100 g Diet)	400	140	40	40
Phosphorus Content (mg/100 g Diet)	310	310	310	90
Vitamin D Content (IU/100g Diet)	100	100	100	100

TABLE 1: Calcium and phosphorus contents of the diets

Weights and serum calcium, phosphorus, and alkaline phosphatase were measured at approximately monthly intervals, while iliac crest bone biopsies were obtained at eight and sixteen months. 1,25-$(OH)_2$ D concentrations were assessed at 70, 180 and 410 days.

RESULTS:

Weight gain was significantly less in the low Ca group than the high Ca group for the first 200 days, thereafter weight gains were similar. Serum calcium values were similar in the four groups except for a brief period between 200 and 260 days when concentrations in the low Ca group fell sharply but then returned to normal. The low Ca group developed significant hyperphosphataemia between 200 and 400 days; this started at the time of development of hypocalcaemia. The low Ca low Phos group tended to remain hypophosphataemic for the first 300 days of the study. In all four groups alkaline phosphatase values rose significantly during the early part of the study, however values in the low Ca group rose significantly above those of the high Ca from 150 days.

1,25-$(OH)_2$ D concentrations were similar in the four groups of baboons at 70 and 180 days except for the values in the low Ca low Phos group group at 70 days, which were significantly higher at that time than in the other three groups. By 410 days however, mean concentrations had risen significantly in the low Ca and low Ca low Phos groups ($p < 0.005$ and $p < 0.025$ respectively) (Table 2).

	LOW CA	LOW CA LOW PHOS	MEDIUM CA	HIGH CA
70 days	102 + 32	187 + 21	125 + 37	139 + 58
180 days	119 + 39	91 + 21	78 + 21	98 + 40
410 days	348 + 162	262 + 130	163 + 42	122 + 59

TABLE 2: 1,25-(OH) D concentrations (pg/mℓ (mean + SD)).

Despite a lack in change in 1,25-(OH) D concentrations at 180 days, bone histomorphometry at eight months revealed a significant inverse relationship between growth plate thickness, osteoid seam thickness, volume and surface and dietary calcium content. These changes could not be correlated to serum calcium or phosphorus values. At sixteen months an increase in osteoclast numbers and resorption was associated with a concomitant rise in 1,25-$(OH)_2$ D concentrations. Despite the rise in 1,25-$(OH)_2$ D values in the low Ca low Phos group at 410 days this group did not have an increase in osteoclast numbers on bone histology at sixteen months.

It thus appears that dietary calcium deprivation in the vitamin D replete young baboons is associated with elevated 1,25-$(OH)_2$ D concentrations and features of osteomalacia and rickets on bone histology. These histological changes occur before there is a significant rise in 1,25-$(OH)_2$ D values and evidence of increased bone resorption.

References:

(1) Marie P.J., Pettifor J.M., Ross, F.P. and Glorieux F.H. (1982) N. Eng. J. Med. 307, 584-588.

DOES ALUMINUM CONTRIBUTE TO STILL ANOTHER BONE DISEASE - OSTEOPENIA OF PREMATURITY?

Gordon L. Klein, Aileen B. Sedman, Russell J. Merritt, and Allen C. Alfrey; Division of Pediatrics, City of Hope National Medical Center, Duarte, CA: Children's Hospital and USC School of Medicine, Los Angeles, CA; Departments of Pediatrics and Medicine, University of Colorado School of Medicine and VA Hospital, Denver, CO 80220, U.S.A.

Aluminum has been implicated in the pathogenesis of bone disease occurring in patients with end-stage renal disease (1) and in those receiving total parenteral nutrition (TPN) inadvertently contaminated with aluminum (2). In both groups of patients aluminum has been associated with decreased bone formation and occasional osteomalacia (1,2). Aluminum has been shown to interfere with the stimulation of acid and alkaline phosphatases by 1,25 $(OH)_2D$ in osteoblasts *in vitro* (3). It has also been shown to accumulate in the parathyroid glands (4) and to interfere with PTH secretion *in vitro* (5). Another possible effect of aluminum on calcium regulatory hormones is its interference with vitamin D metabolism. Parenteral aluminum administration to dogs (6) and to rats (7) has resulted in decreased serum levels of $1,25(OH)_2D$. The main route of aluminum excretion from the body is renal (8,9).

Sick premature infants may develop a poorly characterized 'osteopenic' bone disease, receive long-term TPN therapy, and have a lower glumerular filtration rate (10). Thus they may be at risk for aluminum loading.

To determine whether the risk of aluminum loading in these premature infants was more than theoretical, we determined plasma and urine aluminum content in 18 premature infants receiving intravenous therapy, in 8 term infants who received negligible parenteral therapy, and in 35 umbilical cord plasma samples as controls. We also analyzed autopsy samples of iliac crest from 6 premature infants who died after at least 3 weeks of parenteral therapy and for 17 infants who died acutely.

Plasma aluminum levels in the premature infants on parenteral therapy was 37 $\pm$ 45 (SD) versus 5 $\pm$ 3 ug/L in the eight term infants and the unbilical cord plasma controls ($p<.001$). Urinary aluminum/creatinine was 5.4 $\pm$ 4.6 in the premature infants versus 0.6 $\pm$ 0.8 in the control term infants ($p<.01$). Bone aluminum in the autopsied premature group was 20 $\pm$ 2 mg/kg dry weight versus 2 $\pm$ 1.4 in the infants who died acutely ($p<.0001$).

We analyzed representative intravenous solutions received by the premature infants and found that calcium and phosphate salts (5-20 mg/L), albumin (0.5-5mg/L) and heparin (0.1 - 1.5 mg/L) were highly contaminated with aluminum. Infant formulas, especially soy-based for-

Vitamin D. A Chemical, Biochemical and Clinical Update

mula (1.5 ± .1 mg/L), also was high in aluminum content. Inasmuch as the urinary aluminum/creatinine in the term infants was six times the normal adult ratio some intestinal aluminum absorption must occur.

Thus, premature infants, especially those on long-term parenteral therapy, may become aluminum loaded. It is unknown whether this amount of aluminum loading has any toxic effect on growing bones.

References

1. Ott SM, Maloney NA, Coburn JW, Alfrey AC, Sherrard DJ, (1982) N Engl J Med 307, 709-713.
2. Ott SM, Maloney NA, Klein GL, Alfrey AC, Ament ME, Coburn JW, Sherrard DJ. (1983) Ann Intern Med 98, 910-914.
3. Lieberherr M, Grosse B, Cournot-Witmer G, Thil CL, Balsan S. (1982) Calcif Tissue Int 34, 280-284.
4. Cann CE, Prussin SG, Gordan GS. (1979) J Clin Endocrinol Metab 49, 543-545.
5. Morrisey J, Rothstein M, Mayor G, Slatopolsky E (1983) Kidney Int 23, 699-704
6. Goodman WG, Henry DA, Horst R, Nudelman RK, Alfrey AC, Coburn JW (1984) Kidney Int 25, 370-375.
7. Klein GL, Vaccaro M, Jongen M, Bishop JC, Kurokawa K, Coburn JW, Norman AW (1984) Calcif Tissue Int 36, 518
8. Kovalchik MT, Kaehny WD, Jackson T, Alfrey AC (1978) J Lab Clin Med 92, 712-720.
9. Klein, GL, Ott SM, Alfrey AC, Sherrard DJ, Hazlet TK, Miller NL, Maloney NA, Berquist WE, Ament ME, Coburn JW (1982) Trans Assoc Am Phys 95, 155-164.
10. Binstadt, DH, L'Heureux PR (1978) Pediatr Radiol 7, 211-214.

PORTO-CAVAL SHUNT DECREASES SERUM CALCIUM AND CORRECTS PARTIALLY PARATHYROIDECTOMY INDUCED HYPOCALCEMIA

P.O. SCHWILLE[1], U. LINNEMANN[1], S. ISSA[2] and P. KLEIN[1]

Department of Surgery, Division of Experimental Surgery and Endocrine Research Laboratory[1], University of Erlangen; Department of Pediatrics[2], University of Bonn, West Germany

Introduction

Porto-caval shunt (PCS) has been reported as a means to restore to normal serum calcium in parathyroidectomized (PX) rats (1, 2). The existence of either a pancreatic calcium elevating peptide was assumed (3) or that the PCS mediated fall in serum phosphate would have led to stimulation of 1, 25-Dihydroxyvitamin D (1, 25$(OH)_2$D) production (2). This D metabolite might have increased intestinal calcium absorption, calcium resorption from bone or both, thereby normalizing serum calcium (2). However, during these studies animals were fed a libitum, although PCS is known to reduce food intake and weight gain thereby interfering with maintenance of normal mineral metabolism. We report data on mineral metabolism including parathyroid hormone and D metabolites, from a pair-feeding trial.

Methods

In male Sprague-Dawley rats (255-285 g; n=44) either careful PX (n=22) without damaging thyroid tissue (4) or neck sham operation (n=22) were conducted. Seven days later one moiety of PX or sham rats underwent either abdominal sham-operation (PX-Sham; Sham-Sham) or PCS (PX-PCS; Sham-PCS), respectively. All rats were pre-labelled with 45-calcium (o.1 mCi, in o.4 ml saline) at the same day, in order to monitor exchangeable bone calcium. In order to adjust the weight course of Sham to PCS rats blocks of four rats (one from each group) were fed 14 days on a normal lab chow (o.9, o.2 and o.75 per cent calcium, magnesium and elementary phosphorus, resp.) and tap water ad libitum. Thereafter, blood was drawn in Pentobarbital anaesthesia and serum stored at -3o ^{o}C. A spectrum of variables was measured (see table) using established techniques, parathyroid hormone in peripheral and portal blood and two D metabolites (5) included.

Results (table) and Comments

In the presence of statistically unchanged body weight and renal function (reflected by serum creatinine) there are a number of changed variables. Thus, PCS increases transaminase (GOT) and decreases total protein, to a lesser extent albumin, both changes long known as results of this surgical procedure. Total and 45-calcium in intact rats are lowered by PCS but are not correlated (Sham-Sham, r=o.43; Sham-PCS, r=o.o1); in PX rats, however, PCS increases total calcium and it is correlated with 45-calcium after PX-PCS (r=o.845, p< o.o1), not after PX-Sham (r=o.456, p< o.2o). Conversely, only after Sham-PCS is there a correlation between total calcium and albumin (r=o.729, p< o.o5) supporting the general view that with induction of albumin variations in blood there may result varying levels of total calcium. More important, the PCS mediated increase in total calcium of PX rats is not associated with increased albumin but rather is paralleled by a rise of 45-calcium and magnesium in the presence of lowered phosphate. However, since in these preparations 25-OHD and 1, 25$(OH)_2$D are unchanged the whole

Vitamin D. A Chemical, Biochemical and Clinical Update

spectrum of events in calcium metabolism most likely neither results from altered 1-alpha hydroxylase activity and subsequently enhanced overproduction of more polar D metabolites, what has been suggested (2), nor from elevated parathyroid hormone immunoreactivity. Although we do not dispose of bone morphometry data our data may allow to speculate that under controlled feeding conditions in the rat 1) there is no room for a splanchnic parathyroid hormone-like calcemic factor, as based on normal serum calcitonin and parathyroid hormone immunoreactivity and the portosystemic gradients (P/A) of the latter, which are not convincingly higher than unity; 2) factors other than vitamin D metabolites or the established calciotropic hormones should be considered responsible for partial restoration by PCS of PX hypocalcemia in this species. Support for independent mobilisation of bone calcium comes from other reports (6, 7).

	Parathyroid intact rats				Parathyroidectomized rats			
	SHAM-SHAM		SHAM-PCS		PX-SHAM		PX-PCS	
Postoperative weight; g	246 ± 5	(11)	233 ± 5	(8)	248 ± 6	(11)	244 ± 8	(7)
Creatinine; uMol/l	7o ± 7	(1o)	61 ± 9	(8)	84 ± 7	(11)	83 ± 7	(7)
GOT; U/l	39 ± 1	(1o)	9o ± 16[c]	(8)	43 ± 3[c]	(1o)	75 ± 9[c]	(6)
Total protein; g/l	5o ± 1	(1o)	45 ± 1[c]	(7)	51 ± 1	(11)	43 ± 1[a]	(7)
Albumin; g/l	35 ± 1	(1o)	31 ± 1	(8)	34 ± 1	(11)	27 ± 1[c]	(7)
Total calcium; mMol/l	2.26 ± o.o4	(11)	2.11 ± o.o4[a]	(7)	1.26 ± o.o7	(11)	1.71 ± o.1o[b]	(7)
^{45}Calcium; (cpm/ml).$1o^{-3}$	5.o ± o.2	(11)	4.1 ± o.3[b]	(8)	2.9 ± o.1	(11)	3.6 ± o.4[a]	(7)
Magnesium; mM/l	o.94 ± o.o2	(11)	1.o5 ± o.o4[b]	(7)	o.84 ± o.o4	(11)	1.o8 ± o.o6[b]	(7)
Phosphate; mg/dl	6.3 ± o.6	(11)	5.2 ± o.5	(7)	11.2 ± 1.o	(11)	8.2 ± o.7[a]	(7)
Alkaline phosphatase; U/l	163 ± 1o	(1o)	244 ± 12[c]	(8)	152 ± 9	(11)	289 ± 32[c]	(7)
Aortal PTH; pg-equiv/ml	382 ± 22	(11)	566 ± 58[a]	(8)	32o ± 22	(11)	352 ± 35	(7)
Portal PTH; pg-equiv/ml	381 ± 26	(11)	575 ± 1o4[a]	(6)	329 ± 27	(11)	434 ± 58	(7)
P/A; mean values	1.o		o.96		1.o		1.2	
Calcitonin; pg-equiv/ml	45 ± 7	(11)	64 ± 1o	(8)	62 ± 6	(1o)	7o ± 13	(6)
25-OHD; ng/ml	11 ± 1	(7)	15 ± 3	(6)	14 ± 2	(9)	16 ± 6	(5)
1, $25(OH)_2D$; pg/ml	17 ± 2	(7)	22 ± 3	(6)	17 ± 2	(9)	13 ± 2	(6)

( ): observations; PTH: Parathyroid hormone; [a]: $p<o.o5$, [b]: $p<o.o1$, [c]: $p<o.oo1$ vs Sham-Sham and PX-Sham, resp.

References: 1) Pfeffermann, R., Sakai, A., Kashiwabara, H., Fisch, H., Taha, M., Goldson, H., Kountz, S.O. (1977) Surgery 82, 266-27o. 2) Al-Jurf, A.S., Smith G.L. (1981) Metab. 3o, 544-548. 3) Lee, C.L., Kaplan, E.L., Sugimoto, J., Heath III, H. (198o) Ann. Surg. 192, 459-464. 4) Schwille, P.O., Steiner, H. (1975) Zschr. Versuchstierk. 17, 3o4-3o7. 5) Reinhardt, T.A., Horst, O.L., Orf, J.W., Hollis, B.W. (1984) J. Clin. Endocr. Metab. 58, 91-98. 6) Kirby, G.C., Dacke, C.G. (1983) J. Endocr. 99, 115-122. 7) Rude, R.K., Haussler, M.R., Singer, F.R. (1984) Endocr. Jap. 31, 227-233.

SERUM OSTEOCALCIN AND SERUM ALKALINE PHOSPHATASE IN PAGET'S DISEASE.

S. Posen, M.R. Wilkinson, C. Wagstaffe, L. Delbridge, J. Wiseman. Departments of Endocrinology, Nuclear Medicine and Surgery, Royal North Shore Hospital, St. Leonards, NSW 2065, Australia.

With the introduction of radioimmunoassays for serum osteocalcin (1,2) it was hoped that such assays would provide information relating to the extent of skeletal involvement in patients with metabolic bone disease. We recently measured serum osteocalcin in 49 patients with Paget's disease of bone and attempted to correlate the results with bone scintiscans and serum alkaline phosphatase.

PATIENTS AND METHODS

We investigated 49 consecutive patients (21 males, 28 females) attending the clinic because of Paget's disease of bone (3). Patients with serum creatinine values exceeding 0.12 mmol/l and patients with hypercalcemia were excluded. Eleven patients were receiving salmon calcitonin (50 U/day) at the time of the study. Bone scintiscans were scored according to the distribution of mineral in human skeletons (4). For example, involvement of an entire calvarium was scored as 15 points while each entire femur was scored as 9 points. Serum alkaline phosphatase determinations were performed on a Technicon SMAC apparatus and serum osteocalcin measurements were made by radioimmunoassay with an ImmunoNuclear kit.

RESULTS

Forty-eight of the forty-nine patients had elevated serum alkaline phosphatase values ranging from just within the upper reference limit to almost 50 times that limit. In contrast, 47% of the osteocalcin concentrations were within the reference range (2.1-8.1 ng/ml) and the highest value was 4.2 times the upper limit.

A significant positive correlation was found between bone scintiscan scores and serum alkaline phosphatase activities ($r=+0.55$, $p<0.01$). The correlation between bone scintiscan scores and serum osteocalcin concentration was closer ($r=+0.70$, $p<0.001$) than that between bone scores and osteocalcin (Fig.1).

DISCUSSION

Serum osteocalcin at present lacks sensitivity and is not useful as a screening test for Paget's disease of bone. The lack of serum osteocalcin elevation may be related to inadequate synthesis of this material by Pagetic bone or to the more rapid turnover rates of circulating osteocalcin (5) compared with those of skeletal alkaline phosphatase (6).

Vitamin D. A Chemical, Biochemical and Clinical Update

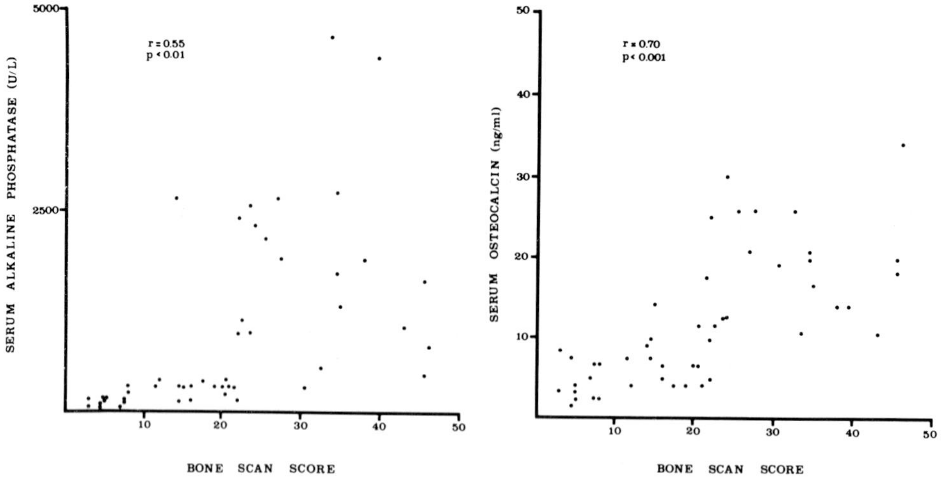

FIGURE 1

Correlation between scintiscan scores, serum alkaline phosphatase (SAP) and serum osteocalcin (OC). The p and r values were calculated by linear regression even though both SAP and OC were not normally distributed. Log transformation of the data made only minor differences to the r values and the correlation between OC and scintiscan scores remained better than that between SAP and scintiscan scores.

REFERENCES

1. Price, P.A., Parthemore, J.G., Deftos, L.J., Nishimoto, S.K. J. Clin. Invest. 66: 878-883, 1980.

2. Gundberg, C.M., Lian, J.B., Gallop, P.M. Clin. Chim. Acta 128: 1-8, 1983.

3. Steinbach, H.L. Am. J. Roengenol. 86: 950-964, 1961.

4. Bigler, R.E., Woodward, H.Q. Health Physics 31: 213-218, 1976.

5. Price, P.A., Williamson, M.K., Lothringer, J.W. J. Biol. Chem. 256: 12760-12766, 1981.

6. Posen, S., Grunstein, H.S. Clin. Chem. 28: 153-154, 1982.

REQUIREMENTS OF 1αOHD$_3$ IN VARIOUS TYPES OF RICKETS AND OSTEOMALACIA.

S. Yoshikawa, A. Ohno, T. Yoshida, H. Amagai, H. Takematsu, T. Nakamura,

Department of Orthopaedics, Institute of Clinical Medicine, University of Tsukuba, Niihari-gun, Ibaraki-ken, 305 and University of Tokyo, Tokyo, Japan

At present, 1αOHD$_3$ has been widely used in many countries, and its effectiveness in various kinds of metabolic bone diseases has been established. However, the effectiveness in each type of rickets and osteomalacia were not fully evaluated yet.

The doses that are able to attan the healing and maintain the healing may vary in different types of osteomalacia as they are intimatly related to the pathogenesis or the nature of disturbance of vitamin D metabolism in these patients.

We have reviewed our ten years' experiences of 1αOHD$_3$ treatment on 25 cases of rickets and osteomalacia to estimate the requirement or maintenance doses of 1αOHD$_3$ for healing. The cases are 10 vitamin D resistant rickets, 5 adult onset hypophosphatemic osteomalacia, 6 Fanconi syndrome, 3 anticonvulsant osteomalacia, and one vitamin D dependency. The criteria for healing was normalization of epiphyseal growth plate, maximal increase in serum phosphorus without hypercalcemia for rickets, and disapearance of Looser's zones, bone atrophy, bone pain and muscle weakness, normal levels in serum alkaine phosphatase and serum calcium, maximal increase in serum phosphatorus for osteomalacia. In some cases bone biopsy was done for histomorphometrical analysis.

Results and discussion

VITAMIN D RESISTANT RICKETS (VDRR): In ten patients with VDRR, 1αOHD$_3$ alone was able to heal the disease. Phosphorus supplementation apparently has no additional effects on healing VDRR. Maintenance doses were very large in this type of disease, varing from 0.25 to 1.9 μg/kg/day as reported previously (1). In one case it was up to 80 μg/day.

This corresponded to our previous experience with vitamin D therapy in which the maintenance doses were also as large as 200,000-800,000 units a day (2).

These results imply that 1αOHD$_3$ has rather small advantages over vitamin D for the treatment of VDRR.

ADULT ONSET HYPOPHOSPHATEMIC OSTEOMALACIA (AOHOM): In four patients with this type of disease, 6-25 μg/day, 0.07-0.49 μg/kg/day, of 1αOHD$_3$ healed the major clinical signs of osteomalacia. The amounts were less than in the case of vitamin D resistant rickets.

It was difficult in some patients to increase serum phosphate to normal levels and after discontinuation of 1αOHD$_3$ recurrences were observed in two cases. Phosphrus supplementation was not necessary. Bone or soft tissue tumors were not found during our observation period in these cases.

FANCONI SYNDROME: In five adult cases with idiopathic Fanconi syndrome, requirement of 1αOHD$_3$ was small, 1-4 μg a day, 0.04-0.13 μg/kg/day, whereas one infantile case required a larger dose, 0.5 μg/kg/day. Phosphorus supplementation was effective and indispensable in all but one patient. In this one case, 1αOHD$_3$ alone successfully managed the disease for nine years. Requirements of vitamin D in this disease was large, 10,000-20,000 units a day from our previous study (3).

ANTICONVULSANT OSTEOMALACIA (ACOM): In three ACOM cases, the requirement of 1αOHD$_3$ was relatively small, 2-4 μg/day, 0.04-0.14 μg/kg/day. Our previous experience showed that the requirement of vitamin D was also small, 20,000-50,000 units a day, in this disease.

VITAMIN D DEPENDENCY (VDD): In one patient with vitamin D dependency, the requirement of 1αOHD$_3$ was 6 μg/day, 0.143 μg/kg/day. In this case vitamin D of 250,000 units a day were required.

POTENCY RATIO OF 1αHYDROXY D$_3$ TO VITAMIN D: The potency ratio of 1αOHD$_3$ to vitamin D was evaluated from our experience with thirteen patients who had been treated with vitamin D followed with 1αOHD$_3$. The potency ratio differed among various kinds of rickets and osteomalacia. It is large, 1,000-1,700, in Fanconi syndrome and vitamin D dependency, while it is small, 200-300, in vitamin D resistant rickets and adult onset hypophosphatemic osteomalacia. Anticonvulsant osteomalacia falls between these two groupes of disease (Table 1).

This fact is considered to be the reflection of the different pathogenic mechanisms, especially various contribution of disturbed metabolism of vitamin D, in these various types of diseases.

	No. of Case	Requirement of Vitamin D/kg/day (10^3 U)	(μg)	Requirement of 1α OHD$_3$/kg/day (μg)	Potency Ratio 1α OHD$_3$/VD
VDRR					
	2	5	125	0.5	250
	3	>15	>375	1.8	> 208
	4	16	400	1.7	235
	8	15	375	1.6	234
AOHOM					
	11	4.2	105	0.38	262
	14	5.6	140	>0.49	< 285
F S					
adult	16	1.4	48	0.03	1600
	17	8.3	207	0.13	1590
	18	2.7	68	0.04	1700
	19	3.1	78	0.05	1560
infantile					
	21	6.8	170	>0.5	< 340
ACOM					
	22	1.2	31	0.07	420
VDD					
	25	5.9	147	0.14	1030

Table 1

(1) Seino, Y. et al., (1980) Arch. Dis. Child. 55,49-53.
(2) Yoshikawa, S., (1976) J. Jpn. Orthop. Ass. 50,535-549.
(3) Yoshikawa, S. et al., (1978) Bone Metabolism 11,220-231.

THE EFFECTS OF BONE OPERATION ON THE SERUM LEVELS OF VITAMIN D METABOLITES.

T. Yoshida, S. Yoshikawa, A. Ohno, H. Amagai, T. Nakamura and M. Imawari;

Department of Orthopaedics, University of Tsukuba, Niiharigun, Ibaraki-ken. 305, Japan.

Introduction:
There have been a few reports on the healing of rickets after osteotomy (1,2) and the decreased concentration of serum vitamin D metabolites in the patient sustained with femoral neck fracture (3,4). Furthermore, active contribution of bone cells to vitamin D metabolism was suggested recently by Howard et al. (5). These reports suggest the possibility of some modification of vitamin D metabolism by fracture or bone operation. Our study was undertaken to investigate on this point.
Patients and Methods:
Postoperative changes in serum vitamin D metabolites were measured in 11 patients treated with bone operation, 10 patients without metabolic bone disease and one patient with vitamin D resistant rickets. Serum levels of 25(OH)D, 24,25(OH)$_2$D and 1,25(OH)$_2$D were measured during 8 weeks after the operation using the multiple assay method described by Imawari et al. (6). The mean values ±SD (range) of 25(OH)D, 24,25(OH)$_2$D, and 1,25(OH)$_2$D were 19±5 ng/ml (10-31 ng/ml), 2.3±1.4 ng/ml (0.4-4.8 ng/ml) and 37+11 pg/ml (26-62 pg/ml)4 respectively. Other biochemical parameters (serum Ca, P, Al-P, PTH, urinary Ca, P and Ca/Cr) were measured by the standard procedure.
Results:
In the 10 patients serum 1,25(OH)$_2$D decreased significantly ($p<0.05$) from 27 11 pg/ml to 16±10 pg/ml at the 4th week and to 15±8 pg/ml at the 7th week after the operation. On the other hand, serum 25(OH)D and 24,25(OH)$_2$D did not change significantly (Fig.1). Serum phosphorus showed a continuous increase from 3.7±0.6 mg/dl to 4.2±0.6 mg/dl during 2 to 7 weeks after the operation. The increase was significant (p 0.05) at the 4th and 6th week. Serum Al-P increased slightly after from 6.4 K.A.U. to 7.8 K.A.U. In one patient with vitamin D resistant rickets, serum 1,25(OH)$_2$D was elevated slightly at the 1st and 2nd week, then falling down to the preoperative level. Changes in serum 25(OH)D, 24,25(OH)$_2$D and other parameters were similar to those of the 10 patients withozt metabolic bone disease.
Discussion:
The postoperative changes in serum Ca, P and Al-P were similar to the results reported previously (6,7). In our cases, serum levels of 1,25(OH)$_2$D significantly decreased from 3 to 8 weeks after the operation. This is supposed to be due to the increase in serum phosphorus prior to the decrease in 1,25 (OH)$_2$D. Serum 24,25(OH)$_2$D and 25(OH)D did not change

Vitamin D. A Chemical, Biochemical and Clinical Update

substantially. These results indicate that there is no major modification of vitamin D metabolism after bone operation, and hence the postoperative modification may not be the cause of the healing of rickets after bone operation. The increased serum phosphorus seems responsible for the healing as previously suggested(1,2). The pathogenesis of femoral neck fracture has been much discussed and the decrease in serum levels of $1,25(OH)_2D$ or $25(OH)_2D$ were suggested to be the cause of osteoporosis in these patients (3,4). However, it was not known whether values of vitamin D metabolites after the fracture represent those before the fracture. Our study shows that serum levels of vitamin D metabolites immediately after the fracture reflect those before the fracture, and that we should be cautious of the interpretation of serum levels of $1,25(OH)_2D$ measured from 3 to 8 weeks after the operation.

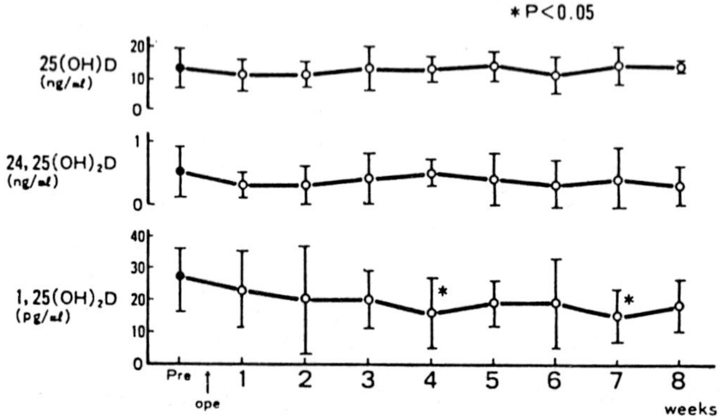

Fig.1 Changes in vitamin D metabolites of the 10 patients without metabolic bone disease

References:

1. Steendijk,R., Nielsen,H.K.L. and Kraai,A. (1968) Helv. paediat. Acta 6, 627-635.
2. Yoshikawa,S. (1976) J. Jpn. Orthop. Ass. 50, 535-549.
3. Baker,M.R.,McDonnel,H. and Nordin,B.E.C. (1979) Br. Med.J. 1, 589.
4. Lips,P., Netelenbos,J.C., Jongen,M.J., Van Ginkel,F.C., Althuis,A.L., Van Schaik,C.L., Van Der Vijigh,W.J., Vermaiden,J.P. and Van Der Meer,C. (1982) Metab. Bone Dis. Relat. Res. 4, 85-93.
5. Howard,G.A., Turner,R.T., Sherrad,D.J. and Baylink,D.J. (1981) J. Biol. Chem. 256, 773807740.
6. Imawari,M., Kozawa,K., Yoshida,T and Osuga,T (1982) Clin. Chim. Acta 124, 63-73.
7. Lal,S.K., Jacob,K.C., Nagi,O.N., Annamalai,A.L. and Nair,C.R. (1976) J. Trauma 16, 206-211.
8. Hosking,D.J. (1978) J. Bone Joint Surg. 60-B, 61-65.

VITAMIN D IN TUBERCULOUS PATIENTS

P.D.O. DAVIES,* H.A. CHURCH, R.C. BROWN and J.S. WOODHEAD,
Department of Medicine, Llandough Hospital* and Department of Biochemistry,
University Hospital of Wales, Cardiff, U.K.

Introduction

Subjects of Indian Sub-continent ethnic origin (those of Indian, Pakistani or Bangladeshi ethnic origin) resident in the U.K., form the ethnic group most at risk from Vitamin D deficient bone disease (1) and also have the highest incidence of tuberculosis (2). It has been shown that rifampicin and isoniazid reduce serum 25-hydroxycholecalciferol (25-(OH)D_3) (3). Recently it has been suggested that, in common with other granulomatous disease, tuberculosis may give rise to hypercalcaemia (4). We have measured Vitamin D metabolites, calcium and other related parameters in a group of patients with pulmonary tuberculosis and matched healthy controls prior to treatment and also throughout nine months of standard chemotherapy.

Methods

Serum 25-(OH)D_3, calcium and liver function tests were measured pre-treatment, in patients presenting with pulmonary tuberculosis to one of the Cardiff group of hospitals, and within four weeks (to avoid seasonal fluctuations) from a matched healthy control.

Blood samples for the above investigations were also taken from a smaller sample of patients and matched controls, as they presented for routine out-patient appointment during the nine months of chemotherapy.

Serum 1,25 dihydroxycholecalciferol (1,25-$(OH)_2D_3$) 24,25 dihydroxycholecalciferol (24,25-$(OH)_2D_3$), parathormone, bone and liver alkaline phosphatase were also measured pre-treatment in a random sub-group of paired samples.

Measurement of Vitamin D metabolites was by radio-immunoassay technique (5) and calcium and liver function tests by auto analyser.

Results

A total of 50 paired samples from patients pre-treatment with culture positive pulmonary tuberculosis and matched controls were available for analysis.

Serum 25-$(OH)_2D_3$ was significantly lower in patients than controls ($p<0.005$). Serum 1,25-$(OH)_2D_3$, 24,25-$(OH)_2D_3$ bone alkaline phosphatase and parathyroid hormone levels showed no significant difference. Serum calcium uncorrected for albumin was significantly lower in the patient group but was virtually the same as control values when correction was made. Other liver function tests were significantly deranged in the patient group.

Throughout chemotherapy patients' serum 25-(OH)D_3 remained significantly lower than controls' but reverted to normal within 2-4 weeks of stopping therapy. Albumin rose to control levels during chemotherapy, resulting

Vitamin D. A Chemical, Biochemical and Clinical Update

in a parallel rise in corrected calcium. Other liver function tests as evidenced by serum values of albumin, alkaline phosphatase, aspartate transaminase gradually returned to control values during chemotherapy. Gamma glutamyl transferase, however, only fell to control values after therapy was completed.

Summary

Serum 25-(OH)D_3 was significantly lower in tuberculous patients than in controls pre-treatment. Serum 25-(OH)D_3 remained significantly lower in patients throughout standard chemotherapy. Other Vitamin D metabolites, parathyroid hormone, calcium corrected for albumin and bone alkaline phosphatase showed no difference pre-treatment between patients and controls. Liver function tests showed significant derangement pre-treatment but reverted towards normal during chemotherapy.

Conclusions

Vitamin D status, as measured by 25-(OH)D_3, is lower in tuberculous patients than controls. This may be a consequence of disease but the possibility of lower Vitamin D predisposing to tuberculosis cannot be excluded. Vitamin D values remain low in patients throughout chemotherapy raising a possibility of Vitamin D deficient bone disease in patients on treatment such as those of Indian Sub-continent ethnic origin, a group known to be at risk of Vitamin D deficient bone disease. No evidence of hypercalcaemia in association with tuberculosis was found. The wide derangement of liver function tests in patients with apparent pulmonary disease only, may indicate underlying disease to be more extensive. Correction of liver function tests on treatment suggests that healing at possible extra-pulmonary sites takes place satisfactorily on standard chemotherapy.

References

1. Hunt,D.R.A.,O'Riordan,J.L.H.,Windo,J.,Truswell,A.S. (1976) Brit.Med.J. 2: 1351-1354.
2. Medical Research Council. (1980) Brit.Med.J. 281: 895-898.
3. Brodie,M.J.,Boobis,A.R.,Carmel,J.,Hillyard,C.J.,Abeyasekera,G., Stevenson,J.C.,MacIntyre,I.,Park,K.B. (1982) Clin.Pharm.&Ther. 32: 525-530.
4. Gknonas,J.P.,London,R.,Hendler,E.D. (1985) New Engl.J.Med. 311: 1683-1685.
5. Clemens,T.L.,Hendy,G.N.,Graham,F.R.,Baggiolini,E.G.,Uskokovic,M.R., O'Riordan,J.L.H. (1978) Clin.Sci.&Mol.Med. 54: 329-332.

PHYSIOLOGICAL INTERACTION BETWEEN PARATHYROID HORMONE AND ESTROGEN

James R. Buchanan, MD, Richard J.Santen, MD, Anthony Cavaliere, BA, Susanne W. Cauffman, BA, Robert B. Greer, MD, Laurence M. Demers, PhD
Divisions of Orthopaedic Surgery and Endocrinology, Hershey Medical Center, Pennsylvania State University, Hershey, Pennsylvania 17033

INTRODUCTION

Current evidence suggests that estrogen augments skeletal mass, but the underlying mechanism remains undefined. This investigation examines the hypothesis that estrogen preserves skeletal mass by blocking PTH-mediated bone resorption.

METHODS

Subjects and material: Twenty healthy caucasian women between the ages of 24 and 44 gave informed consent to participate; none were using birth control pills. Fasting serum was collected from each subject at four consecutive seven-day intervals starting within three days of menstruation. $1,25(OH)_2D$ and 25(OH)D were purified by high performance liquid chromatography and quantitated by radioreceptor assay (1) and absorbance at 254 nm respectively (2). Estrone (E_1), estradiol (E_2) and progestrone (Prog) were measured by radioimmunoassay (3,4). Immunoreactive PTH was quantitated utilizing a mid-molecular (44-68) assay (5). Interassay coefficients of variation were 15% for $1,25(OH)_2D$, 12% for 25(OH)D, 14% for E_1, 12% for E_2, 8% for Prog, and 12% for PTH.

Protocol: Based on sequential E_2 and Prog concentrations, blood samples were classified into early follicular (EF), late follicular (LF), early luteal (EL), or late luteal (LL) phase groups. Redundant phases occurred within individual subjects because of variations in menstrual cycle timing, and were deleted. Consequently, each phase group contained less than 20 samples. We tested the hypothesis that estrogen blocks PTH-mediated bone resorption by assessing the relationship between PTH and endogenous estrogen. The hypothesis predicts that PTH should vary directly with estrogen, since PTH should increase following estrogen elevation to satisfy physiologic demands for calcium.

RESULTS

Hypothesis testing: Longitudinal analysis (using ANOVA) demonstrated that PTH within individuals remained constant across menstrual cycle phases despite sharply fluctuating E_1 and E_2:

Phase	PTH pg/ml	E_1 pg/ml	E_2 pg/ml	Prog ng/ml
EF (n=17)	264 ± 39	50 ± 15	40 ± 12	0.4 ± 0.3
LF (n=19)	255 ± 65	129 ± 51	188 ± 81	0.4 ± 0.4
EL (n=17)	257 ± 77	102 ± 34	134 ± 45	13.9 ± 6.6
LL (n=14)	283 ± 70	73 ± 9	88 ± 47	7.9 ± 7.9

Cross-sectional analysis within menstrual cycle phases and across individuals (using bivariate regression) demonstrated the following

Vitamin D. A Chemical, Biochemical and Clinical Update

relationships among PTH, E_1, and E_2:

Phase	Correlation Coefficients		
	PTH vs E_1	PTH vs E_2	
EF (n=17)	-0.65^b	- 0.24	a. $p < 0.0001$
LF (n=19)	-0.84^a	- 0.29	b. $p < 0.005$
EL (n=17)	-0.39^c	- 0.17	c. $p = 0.06$
LL (n=14)	- 0.17	- 0.12	

These inverse correlations do not support the hypothesis that estrogen blocks PTH-mediated bone resorption since direct variation had been predicted.

Source of the PTH-E_1 relationship: We questioned whether the inverse relationship between E_1 and PTH during the follicular phase signified an underlying physiological link or alternatively might be artifactual. To resolve this question, we employed partial correlation to remove the effect of factors which might confound the relationship between E_1 and PTH. Controlling for 25(OH)D, phosphate and body weight had the greatest impact on the relationship between E_1 and PTH during the early follicular phase, reducing the correlation coefficient to -0.46 ($p < 0.05$). Similarly, controlling for body weight, phosphate and Prog during the late follicular phase reduced the correlation coefficient to -0.60 ($p < 0.05$). Since the correlation between E_1 and PTH persisted even after controlling for the effects of potentially confounding factors, the possibility that the PTH-E_1 relationship signified an underlying physiological link could not be excluded.

We also questioned whether the impact of E_1 on PTH might be diminished if the effect of other factors on PTH were assessed simultaneously. Stepwise regression analysis showed that only E_1, dietary calcium, and 25(OH)D each made independent significant contributions to circulating PTH (multiple $r = 0.83$, $p < 0.001$). $1,25(OH)_2D$, Prog, E_2, phosphate, and serum calcium did not contribute to PTH.

CONCLUSIONS

Our data is inconsistent with the concept that estrogen blocks PTH-mediated bone resorption, but does suggest that estrogen is associated with reduced circulating PTH. The association between E_1 and PTH may signify a physiological link, but the mechanism is unknown.

REFERENCES

1. Eisman, J.A., Hamstra, A.J., Kream, B.E., DeLuca, H.F. (1976) Arch. Biochem. Biophys. 176:235-243.
2. Shepard, R.M., Horst, R.L., Hamstra, A.J., DeLuca, H.F. (1979) Biochem. J. 182:55-69.
3. Abraham, G.E., Manlimos, F.S., Garza, R.(1977). Handbook of Radioimmunoassay, Ed. G.E. Abraham, Marcel Dekker, Inc. New York 591.
4. Kubasik, N.P., Hallaur, G.D., Brodows, R.G. (1984) Clin. Chem. 30(2):284-286.
5. Marx, S.J., Sharp, M.E., Krudy, A., Rosenblatt, M., Mallette, L. (1981) J. Clin. Endocrinol. Metab. 53:76-84.

LONG-TERM ANTICONVULSANT THERAPY DID NOT AFFECT CALCIUM OR VITAMIN D METABOLISM OR BONE MINERAL CONTENT IN CHILDREN

M. Ala-Houhala, R. Korpela, T. Koskinen, M. Koskinen and M. Koivikko
University Central Hospital of Tampere, Department of Clinical Sciences, University of Tampere, P.O. Box 607, SF-33520 Tampere, Finland

The clinical significance of the metabolic abnormalities of vitamin D due to anticonvulsant drugs has remained controversial (1,2). The purpose of the present study was to determine the effect of long-term anticonvulsant treatment on serum parameters of calcium and vitamin D metabolism and bone mineral content and their seasonal variation.

MATERIALS AND METHODS

The material consisted of 28 epileptic outpatient children and 10 normal controls. All children were ambulatory, undertook normal daily activities and nutritionally adequate diets without vitamin D supplementation during the study time from September to March. The children's general data in March is presented in Table 1:

Anticonvulsant treatment groups	Duration of therapy (years) (mean ± 1 SD)	Number of children	Sex distribution (f:m)	Age (years) (mean ± 1 SD)
Phenytoin	8.9 ± 2.7	8	3:5	14.6 ± 1.3
Carbamazepine	10.4 ± 2.1	10	4:6	14.8 ± 1.6
Combination	9.7 ± 2.2	10	4:6	14.2 ± 2.0
Controls in Sept.	-	10	4:6	14.2 ± 1.3
in March	-	10	3:7	14.4 ± 1.3

Serum 25-hydroxyvitamin D (25(OH)D) and 24,25-dihydroxyvitamin (24,25(OH)$_2$ D concentrations were measured by competitive protein binding assay and 1,25-dihydroxyvitamin D (1,25(OH)$_2$D) was analysed by the radioreceptor assay (3). Bone mineral content (BMC) was measured by single photon absorptiometry using a ^{125}I source on distal radius of each non-dominant forearm (4).

The intragroup differences between two seasons were tested by paired t-test and the intergroup differences of the same season by the Mann-Whitney -U-test.

RESULTS

Biochemical parameters (mean ± 1 SD) in serum of the anticonvulsant treatment groups and normal controls and bone mineral density in March are presented in Table 2:

Anticonvulsant treatment groups	Ca (mmol/l)	P (mmol/l)	AP (U/l)	PTH (umol/l)	BMC (% of controls)
Phenytoin	2.4±0.1	1.5±0.1	581±308	43± 8	97±16
Carpamazepine	2.5±0.1	1.4±0.1	605±338	39±11	101± 7
Combination	2.4±0.1	1.4±0.2	468±232	44±21	99±12
Controls	2.5±0.1	1.5±0.2	607±306	45± 4	100±17

Vitamin D. A Chemical, Biochemical and Clinical Update

Serum calcium (Ca), phosphorus (P), alkaline phosphatase (AP), and parathyroid hormone (PTH) levels in the epileptic patient groups did not differ significantly from the levels of the controls. The bone mineral content (BMC) of epileptic patients was also not significantly reduced in comparison to controls.

Serum vitamin D metabolites (mean ± 1 SD) of the different anticonvulsant treatment groups and the controls in two seasons are presented in Table 3:

Anticonvulsant	25(OH)D (ng(ml)		$24,25(OH)_2D$ (ng/ml)		$1,25(OH)_2D$ (pg/ml)	
treatment groups	Sept.	March	Sept.	March	Sept.	March
Phenytoin	33±17**	15± 9**	3.1±1.8*	1.6±1.6*	33±15	37±37
Carbamazepine	45±14***	17± 7***	5.7±2.9***	1.5±0.8***	41±17	42±25
Combination	33±13**	16±10**	4.5±3.9	1.8±1.6	37±12	30±13
Controls	32±10*	20± 8*	3.3±3.0	1.6±1.2	36±16	40±11

Serum 25(OH)D and $24,25(OH)_2D$ levels were consistently higher in September than in March in all groups, but no seasonal variation were found in the $1,25(OH)_2D$ levels in any group. Although the serum 25(OHO)D levels in the phenytoin group were the lowest among the anticonvulsant groups in March the difference to the control group of the same season was not significant. The $24,25(OH)_2D$ and $1,25(OH)_2D$ levels in the epileptic children groups did also not differ significantly from the controls either in September or in March.

COMMENTS

In the present study the parameters of calcium metabolism were thoroughly examined in ambulatory outpatient adolescents receiving long-term anticonvulsant drugs single or in combination. The study was carried out in two phases, in September and in March, to investigate the influence of the seasonal variation of the ultraviolet exposure at our high latitude (61°N). However, the epileptic patients with long-term anticonvulsant therapy had normal bone metabolism. The serum levels of vitamin D metabolites did not vary along the serum levels of anticonvulsants. In conclusion we can state that long-term anticonvulsant therapy did not induce the so-called "anticonvulsant rickets" in this material. This indicates that disturbances of vitamin D metabolism are not universal in children receiving long-term anticonvulsant medication and clinically significant disturbances are restricted to individual cases. Thus vitamin D supplementation does not appear to be indicated in all children on long-term anticonvulsant therapy. The data do not however allow any conclusions of the younger age groups.

References

1. Hahn, T.J., Hendin, B.A., Scharp, C.R., Bousseau, V.C., Harrad, Jr, J.G. (1975) New Engl. J. Med. 292, 550-554.
2. Keck, E., Gollnick, B., Reinhardt, D., Karch, D., Peerenboom, H. and Krüskemper, H.L. (1982) Eur. J. Pediatr. 139, 52-55.
3. Reinhardt, T.A., Horst, R.L., Littledike, E.T., Beitz, D.C. (1982) Biochem. Biophys. Res. Commun. 106, 1012-1018.
4. Karjalainen, P. (1973) Ann. Clin. Res. 5, 231-237.

MINERAL METABOLISM IN COELIAC DISEASE TREATED WITH GLUTEN-FREE DIET.

M.P. Caraceni, S. Ortolani, T. Bardella*, N. Molteni*, L. Soldati, P. Bianchi*, E.E. Polli - Clinica Medica I and Patologia Medica III* - Milan University, Milan, Italy.

Introduction

In coeliac disease a malabsorption occurs due to a lesion of small intestine mucosa caused by the gluten fraction of wheat. The osteomalacia and bone disorders, that may occur in adult coeliac patients have generally been attributed to vitamin D malabsorption accompanying steatorrhoea.
We studied peripheral bone mass and vitamin D status in patients with coeliac disease during clinical remission on gluten-free diet.

Patients and Methods

10 adult coeliac patients (ACP) (8 females and 2 males; mean age 46.2, range 23-61 yrs) were studied. Diagnosis of coeliac disease was based on physical, laboratory and histologic findings. All the patients were on gluten-free diet (mean period of diet 39, range 6-96 months) and were in clinical remission at the time of the study. One patient had laboratory signs of liver disease, none had reduced plasma proteins.
The following determinations were performed:
bone mineral content (BMC) of the distal 2/3 of the dominant forearm (^{125}I photon absorptiometry, Gambro bone densitometer connected in line to an Apple IIe computer)
plasma 25-hydroxyvitamin D (25-OHD) (protein binding assay, Buhlmann)
plasma 44-68 immunoreactive parathyroid hormone (MM-iPTH) (Immunononuclear PTH-MM RIA kit)
plasma calcium (Ca) (atomic absorption)
plasma phosphorus (P), alkaline phosphatase (AP) (standard colorimetric methods)

The BMC of treated ACP was compared to the BMC of sex- and age- matched healthy subjects.
Plasma 25-OHD of treated ACP was compared to plasma 25-OHD of 10 untreated ACP and 14 normal subjects.
The results were analyzed with appropriate Student *t* test.

Vitamin D. A Chemical, Biochemical and Clinical Update

Results

BMC was lower in the treated ACP than in the age- and sex-matched control subjects (mean±SEM: 0.53±0.04 vs 0.70±0.02 g/cm^2, $P < 0.001$)

Mean±SD of laboratory determinations were:

calcium	8.7±0.8 mg/dl
phosphorus	3.1±0.5 mg/dl
alkaline phosphatase	36.7±10.3 U/l
MM-iPTH	53.6±19 pmol/l

Plasma 25-OHD was lower in the treated ACP than in controls (mean±SEM: 26.11±4.96 vs 48.30±4.77 ng/ml, $P < 0.01$), but higher than in the untreated ACP (mean±SEM: 26.11±4.96 vs 11.24±2.60 ng/ml, $P < 0.05$)

Discussion

Our data indicate that bone and mineral disease occur in adult coeliac patients even during clinical remission, achieved with gluten withdrawal.

BMC was still low·· in the ACP after diet treatment.

Plasma 25-OHD levels were lower in the treated ACP than in normal subjects.

Vitamin D deficiency in malabsorption syndrome is caused by enteral loss of this fat-soluble vitamin. None of our patients had clinical signs of malabsorption or steatorrhoea, although complete normalization of intestinal biopsy was not observed in any patient.

It is known that responsiveness to the diet may occur with residual defects (1). Vitamin D deficiency and bone disease might be a part of this residual syndrome and careful assay of vitamin D and bone status may be useful in following these patients, to detect any persistent deficit and to determine adeguate medical treatment.

References

1 Kluge, F., Koch, H.K., Gross-Wilde, H., Lesh, R., Gerok, W., (1982) Hepato-Gastroenterol. 29, 17-23.

DIETARY CALCIUM DEFICIENCY IN BLACK CHILDREN OF TWO RURAL COMMUNITIES.

J.M. PETTIFOR, G.P. MOODLEY, AND M. SEFUBA.
Metabolic and Nutrition Research Unit, Department of Paediatrics, University of the Witwatersrand, Johannesburg, South Africa.

Over the past ten years, we have been studying the pathogenesis of rickets in rural black school-children in South Africa. Investigations have indicated that low dietary calcium intakes can lead to hypocalcaemia, elevated alkaline phosphatase levels, rickets and osteomolacia and severe bone deformities in vitamin D replete children between the ages of 5 and 18 years(1,2). This form of rickets is differentiated from that due to vitamin D deficiency by the lack of muscle weakness and the presence of normal 25-hydroxyvitamin D and elevated 1,25-dihydroxyvitamin D concentrations. further the bone disease containing adequate amounts of calcium. Although a relatively small number of children (forty) have been treated for severe bone deformities, a survey of children in a rural community in the South Eastern Transvaal (Driefontein) revealed that 13% of the children were hypocalcaemia ($<$ 2.25 mmol/ℓ) and nearly 40% had elevated alkaline phosphatase values ($>$300 IU/ℓ)(3). Those children with biochemical abnormalities had significantly lower calcium intakes than their peers with normal biochemistry. The present study aimed at assessing the prevalence of biochemical abnormalities associated with dietary calcium deprivation in a rural area in the Western Transvaal.

METHODS:

Three hundred and eighty-three randomly selected children between the ages of 6 and 16 years from two schools in Kopella were included in the study. Anthoprometric, weights and heights were measured and blood for serum total calcium, ionized calcium, phosphorus and alkaline phosphatase was obtained from each of the children. Twenty-four hour dietary recall was used to assess dietary calcium intakes in fifty-two children who participated in the study. The results obtained were compared to those obtained of the children in Driefontein.

RESULTS:

Mean weights and heights of the children calculated at yearly intervals, were similar to those previously documented in rural areas of Southern Africa, with both parameters falling below the 5th percentiles (NCHS standards) from 10 years of age. Serum calcium values were significantly higher in the Kopella children than the Driefontein children (2.43 $\pm$ 0.11 mmol/ℓ and 2.34 $\pm$ 0.12 mmol/ℓ respectively (p 0.001)). Only 2.6% of the Kopella children were hypocalcaemic (2.25 mmol/ℓ) compared to 13.2% in Driefontein. Serum phosphorus values were significantly lower in the Kopella children than in their Driefontein peers, but a similar percentage in both communities had values below 1.3 mmol/ℓ (approximately 14%). Alkaline phosphatase concentrations did not differ between the two communities, with over 25% having values greater than 300 IU/ℓ.

Calcium intakes (395 $\pm$ 167 mg/day) in the fifty-two children in Kopella in which it was assessed were approximately 50% of the recommended daily allowance. The intakes were similar to those of the normocalcaemic

Vitamin D. A Chemical, Biochemical and Clinical Update

Driefontein children (332 ± 166 mg/day), but were significantly higher than those of the hypocalcaemic Driefontein children (212 ± 149 mg/day) p < 0.001) (Table 1).

Kopella	DRIEFONTEIN	
	Serum calcium > 2.25 mmol/ℓ	Serum calcium < 2.25 mmol/ℓ
n = 52	n = 28	n = 28
395* ± 167	332 ± 166	212 ± 149

TABLE 1: Calcium Intakes (mg/day)

*p < 0.001 compared to Driefontein (< 2.25 mmol/ℓ)

CONCLUSIONS:

It appears that the prevalence of hypocalcaemia varies in different rural communities, and that this is related to the dietary calcium intake. In the Southern African context, the staple corn based diet is low in calcium and generally contains less than 300 mg/day if the diet is not supplemented with milk. Biochemical evidence of dietary calcium deficiency is uncommon in the rural community of Kopella because calcium intakes are generally higher than those in Driefontein, the calcium intakes being increased by the ingestion of milk by the majority of Kopella children.

REFERENCES:

(1) Pettifor,J.M., Ross,F.P., Moodley,G.P. and Couper-Smith,J. (1978) J. Pediatr. 92, 320-340.

(2) Pettifor,J.M., Ross,F.P., Travers,R., Glorieux,F.H. and De Luca,H.F. (1981) 2, 301-305.

(3) Pettifor,J.M., Ross,F.P., Moodley,G.P. and Shuenyane, E. (1979). Amer. J. Clin. Nutr. 32, 2477-2483.

EVIDENCE OF CIRCULATING Gc:G-ACTIN COMPLEXES IN HEALTH AND DISEASE.

PASCAL J. GOLDSCHMIDT-CLERMONT, ROBERT M. GALBRAITH, DAVID L. EMERSON, ANDRE E. NEL and WILLIAM M. LEE, Departments of Basic and Clinical Immunology and Microbiology, and Medicine, Medical University of South Carolina, Charleston, South Carolina 29425, U.S.A.

Introduction: Quantitation of Gc (Vitamin D-binding protein) by rocket immunoelectrophoresis (RIEP) (1,2) is affected by the presence of G-actin (2), and we have shown previously evidence of variable amounts of endogenous circulating G-actin complexed with Gc in serum (3,4). Since the resultant complexes (Gc:G-actin) display faster electrophoretic mobility, this may lead to overstimation of Gc using standards of purified native Gc. However, a log/linear relationship can be demonstrated between the relative amount of actin present in the sample, and the increase in rocket size related to the presence of actin (4). This allowed us to elaborate a method both for accurate measurement of total Gc in samples containing endogenous actin, and for quantitative estimation of Gc:G-actin complexes (4), which demonstrated significant variations in these parameters in health and disease (4).

Material and Method: Gc and G-actin were purified as described (2), and serum samples were obtained with informed consent from healthy subjects, and patients with fulminant hepatic necrosis (FHN). Electrophoretic procedures and mathematical analysis were carried out as previously described (2,4). Each sample was analyzed with and without addition of G-actin in amounts estimated to achieve saturation of Gc present. These were then compared with standard curves obtained respectively with native purified Gc and the same amounts of Gc saturated with G-actin. A third aliquot for each sample, containing urea (8M) to dissociate endogenous complexes (2) was also run, with extrapolation of the height obtained to the Gc only standard curve.

Results: Comparison of each sample with and without added G-actin showed the expected increase in rocket height (2,4), with the largest increases being in samples containing the smallest amount of endogeneous Gc:G-actin complexes (Fig. 1). In samples to which urea had been added to dissociate endogenous Gc:G-actin complexes, rocket heights were reduced below those of native samples, the extent of reduction being inversely related to the increase observed on addition of G-actin. Gc levels calculated from urea-containing samples corresponded in each case ($\pm$/19%) to those Gc levels obtained from appropriate analysis of rocket height in samples containing exogenous added G-actin (4). This method was then used to further compare Gc levels and endogenous Gc:G-actin complexes in normal controls and patients with FHN. This further confirmed both a significant decrease ($P<0.01$) in Gc levels in FHN patients and a significant increase ($P<0.01$) in Gc:G-actin complexes (Table I).

Discussion: Since actin is a major protein constituent of eukaryotic cells (5), release following cellular turnover into the extracellular space is to be expected. Moreover, the presence of several proteins in the circulation able to interact with actin including Gc (6,7), brevin (8), and fibrin (9), as well as the finding of increased titers of auto-

Vitamin D. A Chemical, Biochemical and Clinical Update

Table I: Serum level of Gc and precentage of Gc complexed with G-actin

	Gc (ug/ml)	Gc:G-actin (%)
Normal (n=15)	390 ± 81	29 ± 8
FHN (n=12)	101 ± 71	60 ± 16

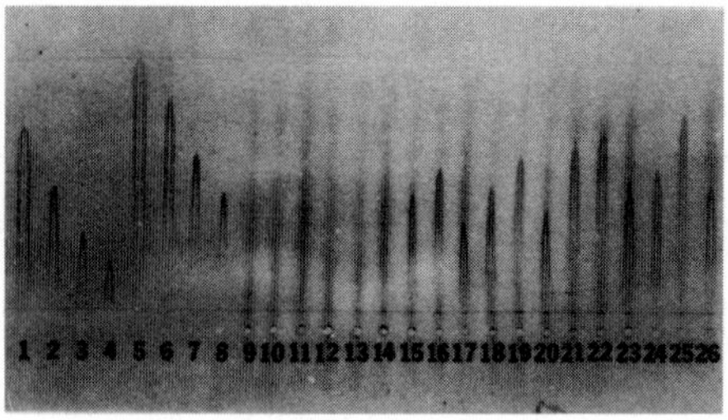

Fig. 1: Rocket immunoelectrophoresis of three samples (native, + G-actin, + 8 m urea) from each of three patients with FHN (samples 15-17, 18-20, 21-23) and a normal control (samples 24-26). Samples 9-14 correspondded to two patients with Gc level under 1 ug/ml. Levels of Gc or Gc:G-actin were calculated (4) from standard curves for Gc only (samples 1-4) and Gc:G-actin (samples 5-8).

antibodies against actin described in situations of tissue damage (10,11), provide some indirect support for this hypothesis. Recently, we have demonstrated evidence of circulating Gc:G-actin complexes (3), and other authors have reported direct evidence of actin in the extracellular space (12). Hence, the presence of actin and Gc:G-actin complexes in serum is probably not an artefact. The pathophysiological significance of these complexes remains unknown, but the availability of an apparently reliable method for their estimation in biological fluids should allow further studies in both physiological and pathological situations.

References

1. Walsh, P.G., Haddad, J.G. (1982) Clin. Chem. 28: 1781-1783.
2. Goldschmidt-Clermont, P.J., Galbraith, R.M., Emerson, D.L., Nel, A.E., Werner, P.A.M. and Lee, W.M. (1985) Electrophoresis, in press.
3. Emerson, D.L., Galbraith, R.M. and Arnaud, P. (1984) Electrophoresis 5: 22-26.
4. Goldschmidt-Clermont, P.J., Galbraith, R.M., Emerson, D.L., Werner, P.A.M., Nel, A.E. and Lee W.M. (1985) Clinica Chimica Acta, in press.
5. Korn, E.D. (1982) Phys. Rev. 62, 672-737.
6. VanBaelen, H., Bouillon, R. and DeMoor, P. (1980) J. Biol. Chem. 255, 2270-2272.
7. Haddad, J.G. (1982) Arch. Biochem. Biophys. 213: 538-544.
8. Harris, D.A. and Schwartz, J.H. (1981) Proc. Natl. Acad. Sci. U.S.A. 78, 6798-6802.
9. Laki, K. and Muszbek, L. (1974) Biochim. Biophys. Acta 371, 519-525.
10. Lidman, K., Biberfeld, G., Fragraeus, A., Norberg, R., Tortensson, R. and Utter, G. (1976) Clin. Exp. Immunol. 24: 266-276.
11. Cunningham, A.L., MacKay, I.R., Frazer, I.H., Brown, C., Pedersen, J.S., Toh, B-H., Tait, B.D. and Clarke, F.M. (1985) Clin. Immunol. Immunopathol. 34, 158-164.
12. Accinni, L., Natal, P.G., Silvestrini, M. and DeMartino, C. (1983) Connective Tissue Research 11, 69-78.

REDUCED 1α,25-DIHYDROXYVITAMIN D PLASMA LEVELS IN HUMAN FANCONI SYNDROME

G.COLUSSI, M.SURIAN°, G.ROMBOLA', E.BENAZZI, F.MALBERTI°, E.MINOLA•, P.BALLANTI*, S.ADAMI■, L.MINETTI.
Renal and Pathology• Units,E.O.Niguarda Ca'Granda,Milan; Renal Unit,Ospedale di Lodi°; Department of Human pathology,University of Rome*;Istituto di Semeiotica medica,University of Verona■, Italy .

Metabolic bone disease (MBD),either rickets in children or osteomalacia in adults,is usually,though not invariably, a most prominent clinical feature of Fanconi Syndrome (FS)(1,2). The pathogenesis of MBD in FS has not been fully elucidated: hypophosphatemia and acidosis might not be the only factors involved,since MBD may occur with normal plasma phosphate and bicarbonate levels,and can be absent despite severe hypophosphatemia (1,3); in addition, MBD often responds to treatment with pharmacological doses of vitamin D or "replacement" doses of 1α-derivatives of the vitamin, without any measurable changes in plasma phosphate levels (1).
Abnormal vitamin D metabolism in FS has been suggested by the observation that renal bioconversion of 25(OH)vitamin D (25(OH)D) is reduced both in nonazotemic children with FS (4) and in rats with maleic acid-induced FS (5).Studies "in vitro" show that the activity of the 1α-hydroxylase enzyme in renal homogenates or isolated tubules of rats with the maleic acid model of FS is markedly impaired (5).Low plasma levels of 1α,25-dihydroxy-vitamin D ($1,25(OH)_2D$) have been recently observed in 2 pediatric cases with FS (6).We have evaluated plasma levels of 25(OH)D, $1,25(OH)_2D$ and 24,25(OH) 2D in 5 patients with FS, of whom only 3 had radiographic and/or histologic evidence of MBD.

Patients and methods.

The etiologies of FS were Sjogren's disease (case 1),chronic interstitial nephritis (case 4),IgAλ mieloma (case 5) and "idiopathic"(cases 2,3)(7). The diagnosis consisted upon the presence of normoglicemic glicosuria,generalyzed aminoaciduria,type 2 RTA in all the patients;urate and phosphate reabsorption were also impaired in most patients.Only cases 1 to 3 had radiographic and/or histologic MBD.No patient was on vitamin D treatment at the time of the study;case 3 was taking alkali.Measurements of vitamin D metabolites were performed in the same blood sample using rat serum (25 (OH)D and $24,25(OH)_2D$) and specific antibody ($1,25(OH)_2D$) as receptors for HPLC fractions, as published elsewhere (8).

Results and conclusions.

The main biochemical data are shown in the table;plasma calcium (not shown) was slightly reduced only in case 2 (7.9 mg/dl;Ca++ 2.06 mEq/l,n.v. 2.1-2.55);PTH was increased only in cases 2 and 5,who had the lowest GFR values;both parameters were normal in the remaining patients.
Plasma values of $1,25(OH)_2D$ were reduced in the 3 patients with MBD in the absence of vitamin D deficiency,and were normal in the 2 patients without MBD.All the patients were acidotic,but only cases 1 and 3 were hypophosphatemic at the time of the study.Thus,low levels of $1,25(OH)_2D$ were better

correlated with the presence of MBD than acidosis and hypophosphatemia. As for the mechanism(s) responsible for the reduced levels of the metabolite, decreased GFR and the tubulo-interstitial localisation of the pathologic lesions induced by the primary disease could be a non specific explanation, though patients 4 and 5 did not differ either in renal function levels or in renal pathology, yet had normal 1,25(OH)$_2$D values.

Table I: Main metabolic parameters in the 5 patients with FS

Cases n°, sex, age	GFR°	$PHCO_3$ mEq/l	Pp mg/dl	25(OH)D ng/ml	24,25(OH)$_2$D ng/ml	1,25(OH)$_2$D pg/ml	MBD
1,♀ ,47yrs	65	18.0±1.2	2.0±0.3	12	0.22	14	+
2,♂ ,46yrs	14	15.5±0.9	3.3±0.3	15	0.27	18	+
3,♂ ,1 yr	105	17.0	2.7±0.3&	54	1.51	30	+
4,♀ ,67yrs	50	20.6±0.5	3.7±0.6	58	0.52	49	-
5,♀ ,55yrs	20	16.7±0.5	4.1±0.4	21	0.20	50	-
n.v.	>80	22-29	2.7-4.5	3-30	0.3-3	40-80	

°ml/min/1.72 mq; & n.v. in children 4-6 mg/dl

Alternatively, altered renal 1α-hydroxylase enzyme activity might be a specific component of the wide spectrum of functional abnormalities of the proximal tubule which define the FS, as suggested by animal models of FS (5). This abnormality (or reduced formation of some other(s) renal metabolite(s) of 25(OH)D), when present, might be critical for the development of MBD.

References.

1. Morris R.C., Sebastian A., in: Clinical disorders of fluid, acid-base and electrolyte metabolism, Ed. Maxwell and Kleeman (1980) p. 883-946.
2. Lee D.B.N., Drinkard J.P., Rosen V.S., Gonik H.C. (1972) Medicine, 51:107-138.
3. Rodriguez Soriano J., Houston I.B., Boichis H., Edelman C.M. (1968), J.Clin. Endocr., 28:1555-1968.
4. Brewer E.D., Tsai H.C., Morris R.C. (1976), Clin.Res. 24:154(A).
5. Brewer E.D., Tsai H.C., Szeto K.S., Morris R.C. (1977), Kidney Int. 12:244-252.
6. Kitagawa T., Akatsuka A., Owada M., Mano T. (1980), Contr.Nephrol.22:107-119
7. Colussi G., De Ferrari M.E., Surian M., Malberti F., Rombolà G., Pontoriero G., Galvanini G., Minetti L. (1985). Proc. EDTA XXI, in press.
8. Tartarotti A., Adami S., Galvanini G., Piemonte G., Lo Cascio B. (1982), J.Endocrinol.Invest. 5(suppl.1): 98-103.

HEREDITARY HYPOPHOSPHATEMIC RICKETS WITH HYPERCALCIURIA(HHRH)A NEW SYNDROME.

M.TIEDER, D.MODAI, R.SAMUEL, R.ARIE, A.HALABE, I.BAB, D.GABIZON, U.A. LIBERMAN.

Pediatric Nephrology Unit Assaf Harofeh Medical Center Zerifin, Beilinson Medical Center, Sackler Medical Faculty, Tel-Aviv University, Division of Oral Pathology Hebrew University Jerusalem, Israel.

We describe a new hereditary syndrome of hypophosphatemic rickets with hypercalciuria. Patient group consisted of 6 young subjects all belonging to a single Bedouin tribe, where intermarriage had been practiced for generations. The characteristic features consisted of low stature with disproportionally short lower limbs, bone pain, muscular weakness, deformities of lower extremities and clinical and radiological findings typical of rickets or osteomalacia.

Laboratory findings.

The salient laboratory findings were as follows: normocalcemia, severe hypophosphatemia (2-5 SD below the age related mean), significantly elevated serum alkaline phosphatase activity, increased renal phosphate (Pi) clearance (TmP/GFR = 2-4 SD below the age related mean), hypercalciuria (8.6mg/kg BW/24h), low-normal serum iPTH levels and urinary cAMP (U.cAMP) excretion and markedly elevated serum 1,25 $(OH)_2D$ concentrations (390 ± 99 vs upper normal range of 110pg/ml). No other glomerular or tubular abnormalities were observed.

Metabolic studies.

Patients were maintained on a constant diet under steady metabolic conditions. Urinary calcium/creatinine ratio (Ca/creat.) decreased to normal values following 15h fast. On oral calcium (Ca) loading test, an abnormally increased urinary Ca excretion was manifest (Δ Ca/creat=0.57 ± 0.19,vs normal values of 0.12 ± 0.02mg/mg creatinine). Simultaneously, serum Ca rose abnormally (patients=0.86 ± 0.27, vs controls=0.43 ± 0.05mg/dl) and a reciprocal further suppression of PTH activity was disclosed, expressed by a decline of U.cAMP. Oral Pi loading test demonstrated an exaggerated post load increase in serum phosphorus (S.Pi)(ΔS.Pi in patients=2.63 ± 0.59, vs controls= 1.2 ± 0.2mg/dl).200 units of PTE injected intravenously were followed by an appropriate phosphaturic response. Concomitantly U.cAMP increased abruptly 60 fold. Bone biopsy after double tetracycline labelling was consistent with osteomalacia.

Response to therapy.

Treatment consisted solely of oral neutral Pi supplementation 1.0-2.5g in 5 divided daily doses for 1-3 years. Within several weeks bone pain disappeared, muscular strength improved substantially and an accelerated linear growth rate took place. Radiological signs of rickets disappeared completely within 4-9 months. All biochemical aberrations, except for the increased renal Pi clearance, returned towards or to normal range. Bone biopsy in one patient one year after initiation of treatment showed an amelioration of osteomalacia.

Discussion.

"Resorptive" or "Renal" hypercalciuria (1,2) can be excluded in view of the low-normal values of iPTH, the decreased U.cAMP and the normalization of fasting urinary calcium (U.Ca) excretion. Intestinal hyperabsorption (1,2) is therefore strongly suggested as the etiological mechanism for hyper-

calciuria. This is further supported by the exaggerated calcemic and calciuric response to oral Ca loading test. Concerning the increased renal Pi clearance, hyperparathyroidism being excluded, the only remaining underlying mechanism would be primary renal Pi leak. We feel that this combination of primary renal Pi leak, hyperabsorptive hypercalciuria, elevated serum 1,25 $(OH)_2D$ and suppressed PTH activity unequivocally fits the framework of the "phosphate leak hypothesis"(3,4,5) as follows:The pivotal defect consists of a severe hereditary renal Pi leak resulting in hypophosphatemia and Pi depletion. This in turn stimulates renal 25$(OH)_2$D-1α hydroxylase, and the resulting enhancement of intestinal Ca and Pi absorption produces hypercalciuria. Suppression of PTH secretion further increases calciuria. Prolonged Pi depletion would generate rickets or osteomalacia(6).The favorable response to Pi supplementation lends great support to this hypothesis.
HHRH differs distinctly from the 2 types of "primary phosphopenic rickets" so far delineated;namely:familial X linked hypophosphatemia (XLH)(7) and hypophosphatemic bone disease (8). Comparing HHRH and XLH and according to currently prevailing physiological concepts two alternative pathophysiological speculations could be envisaged:1)That the affected sites for the renal tubular Pi reabsorption are different in the two syndromes. 2)That both syndromes share the same tubular locus for the defective Pi reabsorption but that in HHRH, in contrast to XLH, the integrative system for 1α hydroxylation of vitamin D is normal.
Finally, our observations support the importance of Pi as a mediator in controlling 1,25 $(OH)_2D$ production in humans.

References.

1. Coe, F. (1984) N. Engl. J. Med. 311,116-117.
2. Pak, C.Y.C., Ohata, M., Lawrence, E.C., Snyder, W. (1974) J. Clin. Invest. 54,387-400.
3. Haussler, M., Hughes, M., Baylink, D., Littledike, E.T., Cork, D., Pitt, M. (1977) Adv . Exp. Med. Biol. 81,233-255.
4. Broadus, E.E., Insogna, K.L., Lang, R., Malette, L.A., Oren, D.A., Gertner, J.M., Kliger, A.S., Ellison, A.F. (1984) J. Clin. Endocr. Metab. 54,61-69.
5. Tieder, M., Modai, D., Samuel, R., Arie, R., Halabe, A., Bab, I., Gabizon, D., Lieberman, U.A. (1985) N. Engl. J. Med. In Press.
6. Scriver, C. (1974) Am. J. Med. 57,43-49.
7. Rasmussen, H., Anast, C. (1983) In:The metabolic basis of inherited diseases. (Eds:Stanbury, J.B.,Wyngaarden, J.B.,Frederickson, D.S. pp. 1743-1773) McGraw-Hill, New York.
8. Scriver, C.R., MacDonald, W., Reade, T. (1977) Am. J. Med. Genetics. 1,101-117.

GROWTH HORMONE INDUCED CATCH–UP GROWTH AND SERUM 1,25 $(OH)_2D$ CONCENTRATIONS IN PITUITARY DWARFS. J.Łukaszkiewicz, R.Lorenc, T.Romer, M.Garabedian, S.Balsan and G.Jones.
Child's Health Center, Warsaw, Poland –Hopital des Enfants Malades, 75015 Paris, France - Sick Children Hospital, Toronto, Canada.

Introduction. Rate of renal synthesis of $1{,}25(OH)_2D$ remains under regulation of several factors including parathydroid hormone (PTH), calcium. phosphate, prolactin, $1{,}25(OH)_2D$ itself and growth hormone (GH) Because of common acceptance that $1{,}25(OH)_2D$ increases intestinal calcium absorbtion the augment of $1{,}25(OH)_2D$ production was expected in a case of rapidly growing growth hormone defficient children during GH replacement therapy, The reason of the study was to evalute the concentrations and significance of $1{,}25(OH)_2D$ in catch–up growth phase of GH deficient children during GH treatment.

Patients and methods. 23 patients with established diagnosis of pituitary dwarfism were studied before and during GH therapy. Their age was between 5,6 and 16.7 years, Diagnosis was made on the basis of clinical examination, estimation of growth rate and GH level. Patients were selected under criteria of having GH peak value below 4 ng/ml/(after stimulation with clonidyne and L'DOPA). For prolactin response curve, blood was collected at 0 , 30 , 60 , 90 and 120 minutes. Pituitary hormones were estimated by RIA double antibody method.$1{,}25(OH)_2D$ with the use of the radioreceptor assay (thymus receptor) and for PTH–RIA assay was employed.

Study protocol. 1/Before first GH injection blood sampling and hours urine collection was performed. 2/GH was applied I.M. at 9 A.M. and 9 P.M., 0,2 to 0,25IU kg of body weight per injection. 3/Next morning blood sample was taken as well as 24 hours urine collection. 4/Regular treatment of the patient twice or thrice weekly with GHI.M. injections (0.4 to 0.5 IU/kg of boody weight).No other hormonal treatment was applied, 5/Blood sampling and 24 hours urine collections were performed at 11-12 days after the commencement of the treatment.

Results. Significant increase in $1{,}25(OH)_2D$ concentration (paired t test, $0{,}01<p<0{,}02$) was observed 7–8 weeks after the therapy was instituted. No significant increase was present after 24 hours or 11–12 days of GH therapy.$1{,}25(OH)_2D$ concentrations after 7–8 weeks of GH treatment was positively correlated with growth rate and the degree of shortness given in SD scored of stature deviation from the normal mean value for age and sex. For prolactin no correlation was found between GH induced $1{,}25(OH)_2D$ levels and area under PRL stimulation curve. Alkaline phosphatase values were within normal range before, as well as during tho GH treatment.

SERUM $1{,}25(OH)_2D$ BEFORE AND DURING GH TREATMENT (MEAN±SD)

	Berofe	During treatment		
Time in days	0	1	11 - 12	49 - 56
Serum level	24.0 ± 12.8	24.4 ± 7.7	29.3 ± 13.1	32.7 ± 1.7 x
pg/ml	n=21	n=20	n=16	n=20

x Significance over time „0" /.0 1 < p <.0 2 paired t test/.

Vitamin D. A Chemical, Biochemical and Clinical Update

Discussion. Catch–up growth in growth hormone defficient children remaining on GH therapy is entirely dependent on GH.The lack of increase in 1,25$(OH)_2$D level 24 hours after substantial dose fo GH suggests that its generation is not directly related to GH.Lack of 1,25$(OH)_2$D response to overnight infusion was found also by Gertner et al (1).Significant increase of 1,25$(OH)_2$D concentration observed at the moment of considerable growth acceleration, suggests that its mechanism is related rather to catch–up growth itself than to higher concentration of growth hormone,Although the effect prolactin on 1α-hydroxylase has been reported (2) we did not find any correlation between 1,25$(OH)_2$D levels and the area under the prolactin stimulation curve,

Conclusion. Gh replacement therapy significantly increases 1,25$(OH)_2$D serum concentration.The increased serum levels of 1,25$(OH)_2$D are positively correlated with GH induced growth velocity but factors involved in this mechanism are still unknown.

Acknowledgment The work was partly supported by Wroclaw Politechnics under R,I.9.

Literature 1. Gertner, M.Tamborlane, W.V., Hinz, R.L., Horst R.L., Genel, M. (1981), J.Clin. Endocrinol. Metab. 53, 818-823 2. MacIntyre, J,Brown, D.J., and Spanos, E.(1979) In. Norman, A.W., Schaefer, K., Herrath, D.V., Grigoleit, H.-G., Coburn, J.W., Deluca, H.F., Mawer, E.B., Suda, (Eds.)Vitamin D basic research and its clinical application. Berlin, New York. pp. 523–530.

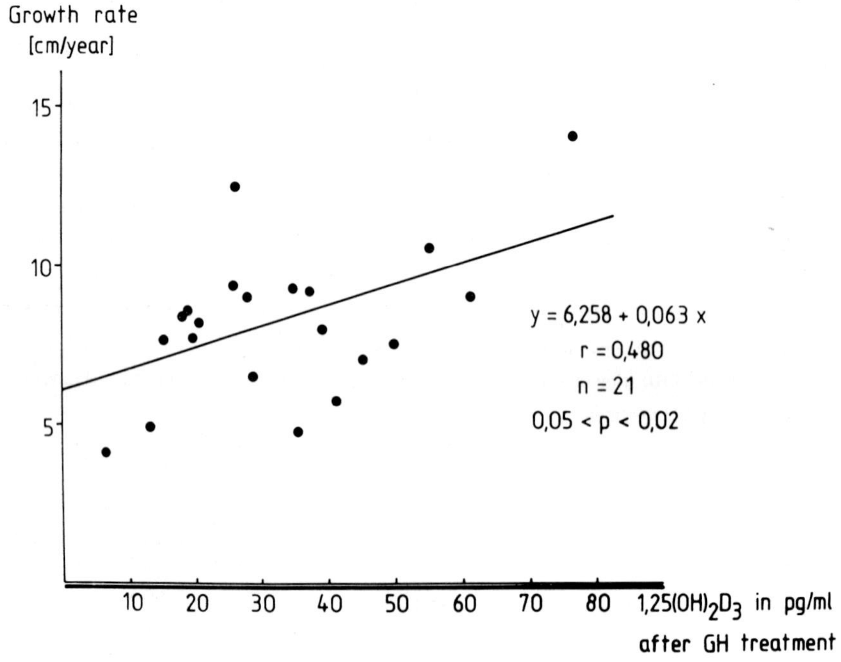

SERUM LEVELS OF VITAMIN-D METABOLITES AND OTHER CALCIOTROPIC HORMONES IN GIRLS WITH IDIOPATHIC TRUE PRECOCIOUS PUBERTY.

G. Saggese, P. Ghirri, S. Bertelloni, P. Bottone, E. Bottone and M.F. Holick*.
Department of Pediatrics, University of Pisa, Pisa, Italy.
*Vitamin D Laboratory, Massachusetts Institute of Technology, Cambridge, Boston, Massachusetts, USA.

Introduction:

The increased demands of calcium and phosphate during rapid pubertal growth are reflected by the higher serum levels of 1,25-hydroxycholecalciferol (1,25(OH)2D) during adolescence than in prepubertal and adult age (1). However an age-related increase in 25-hydroxycholecalciferol (25(OH)D) levels with no age-related differences for 1,25(OH)2D is a new finding (2). To our knowledge no data are available today on the vitamin-D endocrine system in true precocious puberty. We have studied the calciotropic hormones in girls with true precocious and normal puberty.

Patients and Methods:

We have measured the serum levels of 25-OH-D, 1,25(OH)2D, Parathyroid hormone (PTH), Calcitonin (CT), calcium (Ca) and phosphate (P) in seven girls (age 5-8 years) with idiopathic true precocious puberty. The stages of breast (B) and pubic hair (Ph) development, according to Tanner criteria (3), were BII PhII in 2 girls, BIII PhIII in 4 girls and BIV PhIII in 1 menstruated girls. We have also studied thirteen normal adolescent girls (age 11-15 years; pubertal stage P2-P3). Serum Ca and P were measured by standard techniques. Serum PTH and CT were detected by RIA-methods. Serum 25-OH-D and 1,25(OH)2D were analyzed by competitive protein-binding assay after preliminary HPLC step (4) (5).

Results:

Serum Ca, P and PTH were in the normal range in all the subjects. Serum 1,25(OH)2D levels (71.4±2.9 pg/ml) were higher than normal values for age (38.2±7.0 pg/ml n=20) but in normal range for female pubertal age (73.2±5.1 pg/ml n=13). 25-OH-D concentrations (34.5±2.2 ng/ml) were in normal range (34.6±5.4 ng/ml) with no age-related differences. Serum CT levels (83.2±6.7 pg/ml) were higher than normal values for age (46.7±19.3 pg/ml).

Discussion:

The higher 1,25(OH)2D levels in our girls with precocious puberty and in normal puberty than in prepubertal children suggest that the increased production of sex steroids in adolescence might be involved in the enhanced synthesis of

Vitamin D. A Chemical, Biochemical and Clinical Update

1,25(OH)2D. Nevertheless, sex steroids continue to rise throughout puberty while serum level of 1,25(OH)2D appears correlated to growth velocity curves and decline from stages 3-4 of puberty (6). The positive influence of puberty and gonadal steroids on serum GH responses to provocative stimuli suggest that enhanced secretion of GH induced by sex steroid may play a role in increased formation of 1,25(OH)2D. Moreover the increase of prolactin to adult levels in our girls with true precocious puberty may be involved in the enhanced formation of 1,25(OH)2D. However recent reports showed normal or only slightly elevated (7) serum levels of 1,25(OH)2D in patients with hyperprolactinemia due to pituitary adenomas. Moreover recent data suggest that prolactin could directly increase the intestinal absorption of calcium (8). The estradiol pubertal levels might be responsible also for the enhanced formation of CT in our girls. However it is possible that CT levels increase to maintain normal serum calcium in presence of rised calcium absorption induced by high 1,25(OH)2D. Our data showed that the vitamin-D endocrine system is involved in the endocrinology of true precocious and normal puberty. We have found, in agreement with Chesney (1), an increase in 1,25(OH)2D levels both in girls with true precocious and normal puberty with no differences in 25OHD levels. However more studies are needed to elucidate the regulation of vitamin D metabolites and other calciotropic hormones during puberty.

References:

1. Chesney, R.W., Rosen, J.F., Hamstra, A.J., DeLuca, H.F., (1980) Am. J. Dis. Child., 134: 135-142.
2. Taylor, A.F., Norman, M.E., (1984) Ped. Res., 18: 886-890.
3. Marshall, W.A., Tanner, J.M., (1969) Arch. Dis. Child., 44: 291-298.
4. Eisman, J.A., Hamstra, A.J., Kream, B.E., De Luca, H.F., (1976) Arch. Bioch. Bioph. 176: 235-243.
5. Saggese, G., Bertelloni, S., Federico, G., Baroncelli, G.I., Bottone, E., (1984) Proceedings RIA '84 "Cost and Benefit of Radio Immuno Assay" Albertini, A., ed., Milan, May 15-16, p.31 abs.
6. Aksnes, L., Aarskog, D., (1982) J. Clin. Endocrinol. Metab., 5 5: 94-99.
7. Brown, D.J., Spanos, E., Mac Intyre I., (1980) Br. Med. J. 1: 277-278.
8. Pahuja,D.N., De Luca,H.F. (1981) Science 214: 1038-1039.

X-LINKED HYPOPHOSPHATEMIC RICKETS. EFFECT OF 1,25(OH)2D AND PHOSPHATE ON BONE MINERALIZATION AND GROWTH RATE.

P.Ghirri, G.Cesaretti, G.I. Baroncelli, S.Bertelloni and G.Saggese.
Dept. of Pediatrics, University of Pisa, Pisa, Italy.

Introduction:

X-linked hypophosphatemic rickets (XLH) is the most commonly recognized vitamin D resistant rickets. The most tipical finding of XLH is short stature, bowing of the lower limbs, late dentition and skull deformities (1). In the pathogenesis of this disease are involved an intrinsic defect of the renal proximal tubule with decrease of phosphate reabsorption (2) and an altered 1,25-dihydroxyvitamin D (1,25(OH)2D) byosintesis too (3,4). In this study we investigate the effectiveness of 1,25(OH)2D and phosphate therapy on bone mineralization and growth rate in five children with XLH.

Patients and Methods:

Four females and one male were studied (age 6-10 yrs.). All the patients were diagnosed previously as having XLH on the basis of hypophosphatemia (0.9 ± 0.4 mEq/l)(mean±SD)(n.v. 1.4-2.8 mEq/l), hyperphosphaturia (64.3 ± 5.4 mEq/l 24h)(n.v. 20-40 mEq/l 24h), normocalcemia (4.9 ± 0.3 mEq/l) (n.v. 4.5-5.5 mEq/l), high levels of alkaline phosphatase (1220 ± 155 U/L) (n.v. 300-900 U/L), normal serum levels of immunoreactive parathyroid hormone (iPTH) (0.56 ± 0.06 ng/ml) (n.v. 0.44 ± 0.22 ng/ml) rachitic bone changes and short stature (- 3SD).Calcium, phosphate and alkaline phosphatase were measured by an autoanalyzer. Immunoreactive PTH was measured by RIA method detecting the C-terminal portion of the mulecule (Immunonuclear Kit; assay sensitivity 0.1 ng/ml).Serum 25-hydroxycholecalciferol (25-OH-D) and 1,25-dihydroxycholecalciferol (1,25(OH)2D) were analyzed by competitive protein-binding assay after preliminary HPLC step (5,6). Bone mineral content (BMC) was evaluated every six months in the nondominant forearm by the tecniques of single photon absorptiometry (Norland mod.2783, Richmond, USA). Height was measured every six months using a fixed wall stadimeter. The growth rate was evaluated by Tanner's table (7). After biochemical evaluation we started therapy with 1,25(OH)2D (Rocaltrol, Hoffman- La Roche) 2.25-3 ug/daily in three females (group A) and 0.75-1.2 ug/daily in other female and in the male (group B). All the patients received oral phosphate (2000-3000 mg/daily) every four hours for a total of five times each day. Phosphate was given as Joulie's solution.

Results:

During therapy phosphate levels rose in normal range (1.9 ± 0.4 mEq/l) in all the patients. Hypercalcemia was not found. Urinary phosphate excretion was higher (66.1 ± 4.2 mEq/l 24h) and alkaline phosphatase decreased (650 ± 93 U/L) as well as iPTH levels (0.40 ± 0.05). 25-OH-D levels were in normal range (33.1 ± 2.3 ng/ml)(n.v. 34.6 ± 5.4 ng/ml) and unchanged during therapy (35.2 ± 3.2 ng/ml). Before therapy 1,25(OH)2D

Vitamin D. A Chemical, Biochemical and Clinical Update

levels were slightly lower (29.4 ± 4.0 pg/ml) than control values (38.2 ± 7.5 pg/ml), while after therapy it increased to high normal levels (46.5 ± 4.2). Before therapy densitometric evaluation showed demineralization in all the patients (BMC -27%). After six months of treatment BMC improved in all the subjects (-13%); three females treated with higher doses of 1,25(OH)2D, in agreement with Drezner (8), showed a more marked improvement of BMC (-8%). Group A had had a more improvement of growth (-1.8 SD), while in group B stature reached -2.6 SD in male and -2.4 SD in female after 3 yrs of treatment.

Discussion:

Our data showing a more improvement both growth rate and BMC in group A than in group B suggest, in agreement with Others (9), that high 1,25(OH)2D doses may be a more appropriate therapy for XLH. Improvement of bone mineralization in patients treated with 1,25(OH)2D depends on restoration of osteoblast function which may involve the transfer of phosphate from extracellular fluid to bone matrix (10). Drezner et al.(8) found a direct correlation between mineralization front activity at the endosteal surface and the circulating levels of 1,25(OH)2D. In conclusion, the use of 1,25(OH)2D and oral phosphate supplementation is associated with improved phosphate homeostasis and improved BMC and growth rate.

References

1) Drezner M.K., in Hormonal Control of Calcium Metabolism,(1981), Ex.Med.p.243-251.
2) Mason, R.S., Rohl; P.J., Lissner, D.,Posen, S. (1982) Am.J.Dis.Child. 136: 909-913.
3) Seino, Y.,Satomura, K.,Yamaoka, K.,Tanaka, Y.,Yamamoto, T.,Ishida, M. and Yabuuchi, H.,(1984) Eur.J.Ped., 142 : 219-221.
4) Chesney, R.W.,Mazess ,R.B., Rose, P., Hamstra, A.J., DeLuca, H.F.(1980) Am.J.Dis.Child. 134: 140-143.
5) Eisman J.A., Hamstra A.J., Kream B.E. and H.F. De Luca,(1976) Arch. Bioch. Bioph., 176: , 235-243.
6) Saggese G., Bertelloni S., Federico G., Baroncelli G.I. and Bottone E.,(1984) Proceedings" RIA-84" Albertini A. ed.Milan, May 15-16.
7) Marshall W.A., Tanner J.M., (1969) Arch. Dis. Child., 44: , 291-298.
8) Drezner M.K., Lyles K.W., Haussler M., Harrelson J.M., (1980) J. Clin. Invest., 66: 1020-1032
9) Chesney, R.W., Mazess, R.B., Rose, P., Hamstra, A.J., DeLuca, H.F., Breed, A.L.(1983) Ped. 71: 559-565.
10) Meunier, P.J., Edouard, C., Arlot, M., Lejeune, E., Alexandre, C., Leroy, G., (1979) in McIntyre I., Szelke M. (eds)., Molecular Endocrinology. Elsevier, New York, p.283.

1,25 Dihydroxyvitamin D in Essential Hypertension

L.M. Resnick, J.P. Nicholson, J.H. Laragh
Cornell University Medical Center, New York, New York, U.S.A.

Introduction

We have recently described linked deviations of serum ionized calcium levels and plasma renin activity (PRA) in essential hypertensive subjects (1). We postulated that these deviations reflected altered steady-state distributions of calcium among intracellular and extracellular compartments. As calcium regulating hormones normally control the distribution of calcium between various tissue spaces, we investigated vitamin D metabolism in essential hypertension (EH).

Methods and Results

Study #1: 1,25 Dihydroxyvitamin D (1,25D) and PRA in EH.

Forty-eight EH outpatients and 10 normotensive controls had blood sampling for analysis of PRA and 1,25D. 1,25D levels were higher in low renin hypertensives (77.4±5.4 pg/ml) than in either high renin hypertensives (44.1±4.9 pg/ml, $p<0.001$) or in normotensives (57.2±5.3 pg/ml, $p<0.05$). Altogether, 1,25D and PRA were inversely related ($r=-0.64$, $p<0.001$) (Fig. 1).

Study #2: Effects of Altered Dietary Sodium Intake on BP and Calcium Metabolism.

Eleven EH outpatients were randomly allocated to both low (<50 mEq/d) and high (>200 mEq/d) salt diets, each for 3-4 weeks. Subjects on high vs. low salt whose diastolic BP (DBP) rose more vs. less than 5% had a fall in ionized calcium (Ca^{++}) ($\Delta=-0.08\pm0.04$ vs. 0.14 ± 0.15 mEq/L, $p<0.01$) and a rise in 1,25D (68.5±9.0 vs. 18.0±17.7%, $p<0.02$). The % ΔDBP was directly related to the %Δ1,25D ($r=0.74$, $p<0.01$) (Fig. 2).

Study #3: The Blood Pressure Effects of 1,25D.

1,25 D, 0.25 mcg/d. p.o, given to 15 EH inpatients on 2 Gm./day $CaCO_3$, lowered PRA (3.7±0.98 to 1.97±0.3 ng/ml/h, $p<0.01$), raised DBP in low renin subjects (ΔDBP 5.4±1.8%) but lowered DBP in higher renin subject (ΔDBP -6.5±2.4%). The BP response was predicted by the initial PRA ($r=-0.81$, $p<0.005$) and by the initial Ca^{++} ($r=-0.85$, $p<0.001$).

Discussion

PRA-linked deviations of 1,25 D levels in EH were observed in a variety of circumstances. Low renin hypertensives had higher 1,25D (Fig. 1), consistent with our earlier report of lower Ca^{++} in these subjects (1). Furthermore, increased dietary salt raised BP as 1,25D rose (Fig. 2) and Ca^{++} fell (2). Thus, we could not initially separate the potential significance of 1,25D from that of Ca^{++} itself. However, since 1,25D changed BP in a manner

Vitamin D. A Chemical, Biochemical and Clinical Update

opposite to calcium loading, despite their similar effects on Ca^{++}, the effect of calcium might depend on suppression of endogenous 1,25D (3).

Therefore, in essential hypertension, altered 1,25D, although presumed secondary to altered Ca^{++} (4), nevertheless contributes to the resultant blood pressure, especially in the low renin state. More generally, calcium regulating hormones, rather than circulating levels of Ca^{++} itself, may both reflect and/or mediate the contribution of altered calcium metabolism to hypertension.

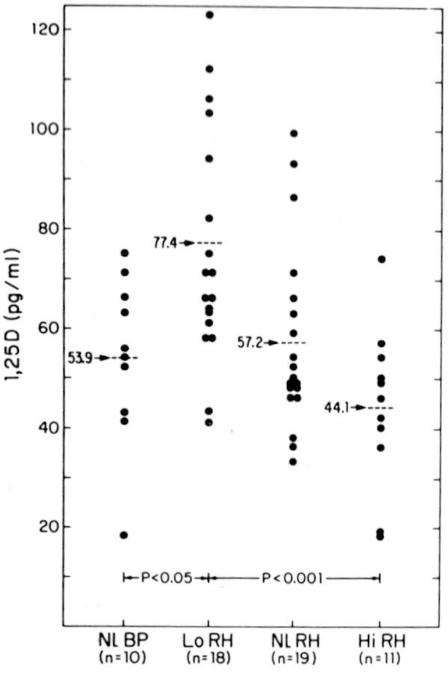

Fig. 1: Serum levels of 1,25 dihydroxyvitamin D in normotensive and renin subgroups of essential hypertension

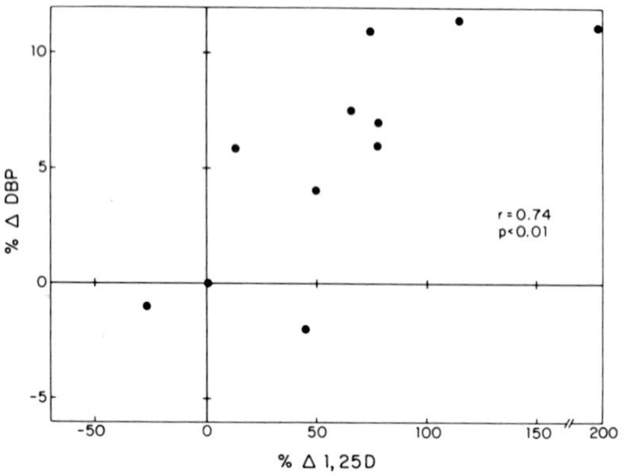

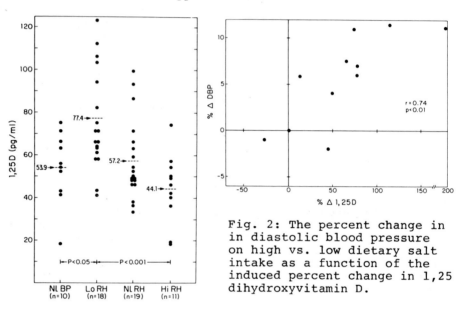

Fig. 2: The percent change in in diastolic blood pressure on high vs. low dietary salt intake as a function of the induced percent change in 1,25 dihydroxyvitamin D.

References

1. Resnick, L.M., Laragh, J.H., Sealey, J.E., Alderman, M.H. (1983). New Engl. J. Med., 309, 888-891.
2. Resnick, L.M., Nicholson, J.P., Laragh, J.H (1985). Kidney International, 27, 199.
3. Resnick, L.M., Laragh, J.H. (1984). Hypertension, 6, 792.
4. Resnick, L.M., Laragh, J.H. (1984). IX International Congress of Nephrology, Los Angeles, 224A.

CYTOSOLIC CALCIUM AS REGULATOR OF PARATHYROID HORMONE SECRETION IN CELLS OF NORMAL AND HYPERPARATHYROID GLANDS

J. Rastad, R. Larsson, C. Wallfelt, E. Gylfe, S. Ljunghall and G. Åkerström
Departments of Surgery, Medical Cell Biology and Medicine, University of Uppsala, Sweden

The calcium indicator quin2 has been used to determine the importance of the intracellular calcium activity for the abnormal release of parathyroid hormone (PTH) in hyperparathyroidism (HPT).

Bovine parathyroid glands and glands from 11 patients with primary HPT (8 adenomas, 3 familiar hyperplasias) and 3 patients with uraemic hyperplasia were enzymatically digested and purified by gradient centrifugation with Percoll (Pharmacia Fine Chemicals). After intracellular trapping of quin2 tetracetoxymethyl ester (Calbiochem-Behring), the fluorescent intensity was monitored at extracellular calcium concentrations of <0.01-6.0 mmol/l.

The PTH release was determined in duplicate incubations at an extracellular calcium concentration of <0.01-3.0 mmol/l with a radioimmunoassay employing ^{125}I-labelled bovine PTH (Inolex) and sheep antiserum (S-469) primarily recognizing the 44-68 fragment and with a somewhat lower affinity for the entire PTH molecule.

A positive sigmoidal relation was obtained between the intra- and extracellular calcium concentrations (Fig 1). The intracellular calcium activity was lower and abnormally regulated in the cells of the hyperparathyroid glands. The increase in cytosolic calcium was accompanied by a reduction of the PTH release but the abnormal cells were characterized by an increased set-point (mid-point of the curve) for both the PTH release and the cytosolic calcium activity (Fig 2). A significant correlation was attained between the set-points for the cytosolic calcium concentration and PTH release for both the normal and abnormal parathyroid cells (r = <0.92, p <0.01).

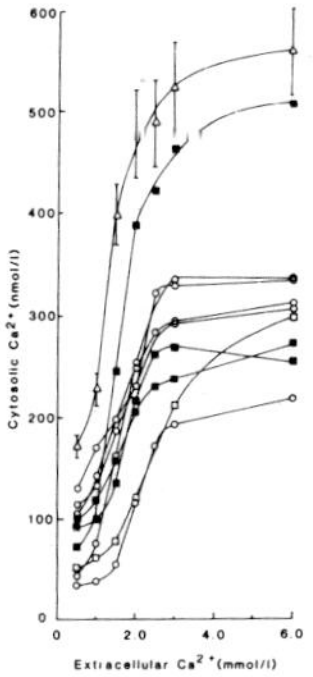

Fig 1. Intracellular and extracellular calcium concentration for 8 preparations of normal bovine parathyroid cells (▲, mean ± SEM), cells of 5 adenomas (o), 3 primary (■) and one uraemic hyperplasia (□)

Vitamin D. A Chemical, Biochemical and Clinical Update

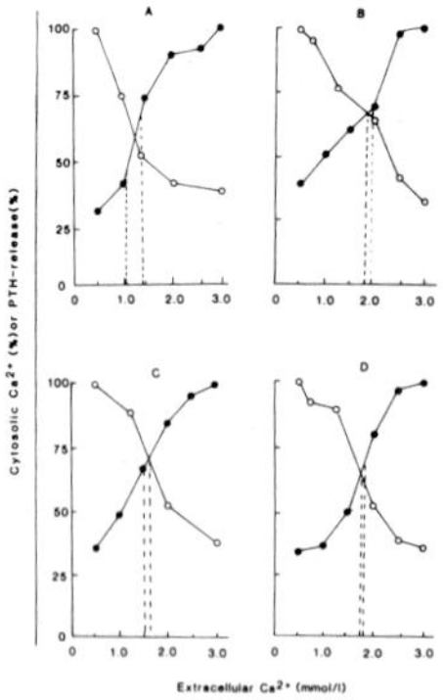

Fig 2. PTH release and the intracellular calcium activity in relation to the extracellular calcium concentration for 3 preparations of normal bovine cells (A), adenomas (B-C), and a primary hyperplasia (E).

Additions of 50 umol/l of the calcium channel blocker D-600 had no effects on the PTH release or intracellular calcium activity at extracellular calcium concentrations below 0.01 mmol/l. In the normal parathyroid cells, D-600 increased the intracellular calcium activity and inhibited PTH release at extracellular calcium concentrations of <0.01-1.5 mmol/l whereas the opposite effects were registered at higher calcium concentrations (Fig 3). In the human preparations, the transition from inhibition to stimulation of the PTH release occurred at 2.0 mmol/l Ca^{2+} and the increased set-point for the PTH release characteristically found in the abnormal cells was consequently shifted back to normal.

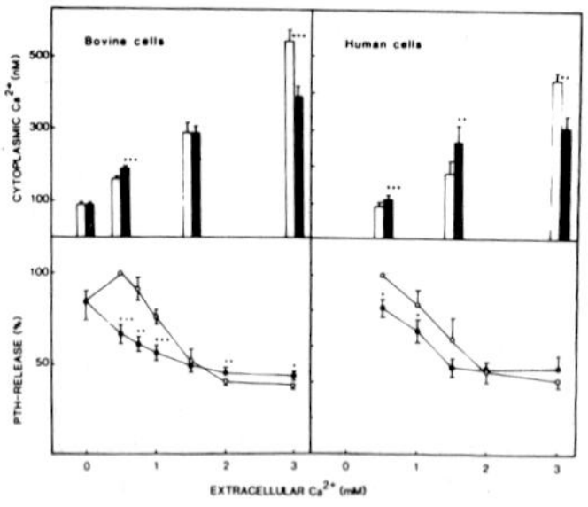

Fig 3. Effects of extracellular calcium alone (o, unfilled bars) and D-600 (•, filled bars) on PTH release (lower panels) and the intracellular calcium activity (upper panels) in normal bovine and human adenoma cells.

The results show that the intracellular calcium activity regulates the secretion of PTH in both normal and abnormal parathyroid cells. The defective release of PTH in HPT is due to an abnormal regulation of the intracellular calcium concentration. The calcium channel blocker D-600 appeared to have both calcium agonistic and antagonistic actions in facilitating and inhibiting calcium influx into the parathyroid cells at low and high concentrations of extracellular calcium, respectively. D-600 and related drugs should therefore be potentially important for the pharmacological treatment of HPT.

Acknowledgement
The study was supported by the Swedish Medical Research Council.

PSEUDOHYPOPARATHYROIDISM TYPE 1, A CASE REPORT

L. Larsson, H. Odelram, L. Aksnes, O. Eeg-Olofsson, and A. Häger,
Department of Paediatrics and Clinical Chemistry, University of Linköping, S-581 85 Linköping, Sweden and Department of Paediatrics, Haukeland Hospital, N-5016 Bergen, Norway.

The incidence of hypocalcemia due to hypoparathyroidism and pseudohypoparathyroidism is low (1). A deficient parathyroid function in children can have two reasons: first, a failure of appropriate secretion of parathyroid hormone (PTH) in response to stimuli (hypoparathyroidism) and secondly some defective end-organ responsiveness to PTH (pseudohypoparathyroidism, PHP). The latter state is a heterogenous group of disturbances with or without typical somatic anomalies of Albrights osteodystrophy (2). PHP is however a disorder which may be explained in several ways. One concept is that the end-organ resistence is due to a defect of guanine nucleotide regulatory protein (G or N unit) that links the parathyroid hormone receptor to the catalytic unit of adenylate cyclase (3). An inhibitory factor in plasma has also been suggested. This inhibition have been postulated to depend on production of PTH that lacks biological activity on the kidney (4).

The present case elucidates the special diagnostic and therapeutic problems linked to pseudohypoparathyroidism.

Our patient was a 13-year old boy referred to our hospital because of brief generalized seizures precipitated mostly by heavy physical exercise. These attacks were initially interpreted as psychomotor epilepsy and thus treatment with carbamazepine was initiated. After one months treatment routine laboratory screening revealed severe hypocalcemia. Initial clinical and laboratory values can be seen in Table 1 and 2.

Table 1

	our patient	typical PHP 1
Age of onset of hypocalcemia	13 yrs	usually > 5 yrs
Family history	not known	x-linked dominant
Somatic feature (AHO)	not present	often present
Intracranial calcification	not present	frequent
Enamel hypoplasia	not present	rare
Presence of Addison's disease, candidase etc	absent	absent

Table 2

		Reference values
S-Ionized calcium	0.66	1.20-1.35 mmol/l
S-Total calcium	1.56	2.20-2.70 mmol/l
S-Phosphate	3.10	1.00-2.00 mmol/l
S-Magnesium	0.69	0.70-1.20 mmol/l
S-Alkaline phosphatase	24.7	< 15 µkat/l
S-Parathyroid hormone	2.1	< 2.5 µg/l
S-Creatinine	53	< 115 µmol/l
S-1.25-(OH)D	90	65-180 pmol/l
S-25-OHD	57.5	30-150 nmol/l
U-Creatinine	12.3	9.7-22.0 mmol/l
U-Calcium	0.17	< 7.5 mmol/l
U-Magnesium	4.0	> 3.0 mmol/l
U-Phosphate	0.9	< 20 mmol/l

Laboratory values in our patient with PHP 1 at the time of hospital admittance. S = serum, U = urine.

It can be observed that on physical examination the boy was healthy with normal psychomotor and normal weight-height development. Routine neurological examination was normal. Thus characteristic symptoms and signs for pseudohypoparathyroidism i.e. short stature, round face, obesity, subcutaneous calcifications or mental retardation were not present.

Vitamin D. A Chemical, Biochemical and Clinical Update

Considering differential diagnostic possibilities five diagnosis were possible: 1) magnesium deficiency, 2) phosphate excess, 3) calcitonin excess, 4) vitamin D deficiency and 5) parathyroid hormone deficiency. Normal serum magnesium and urinary excretion of magnesium excludes magnesium deficiency. Basic phosphate data also indicate that phosphate excess could be excluded. A calcitonin excess was ruled out with a normal serum calcitonin level. A vitamin D deficiency could be excluded especially from a normal 25-hydroxy vitamin D level.

Intravenous infusion of PTH caused no increase in the cyclic AMP (U-c-AMP) excretion and before infusion basic PTH was normal and urinary cyclic AMP low. All laboratory findings were consistent with PHP type 1 despite the absence of typical clinical features.

Treatment with vitamin D was initiated when serum ionized calcium was very close to 0.60 mmol/l, a level described as a risk level for arrythmia development. The required dose to restore normocalcemia is shown in Figure 1.

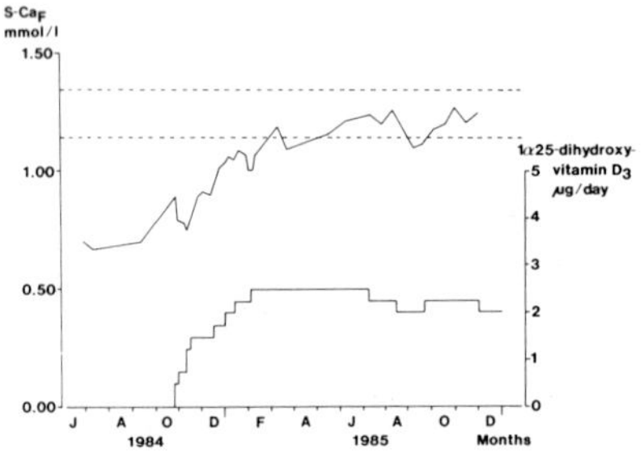

The patient soon became asymptomatic and has remained so. As PHP is a permanent condition requiring long time therapy and hypercalcemia is a danger of excessive vitamin D dosage serum ionized calcium is determined and clinical evidence of hypercalcemia is checked at each clinical visit.

In conclusion this case of PHP type 1, although an uncommon condition, stresses the diagnostic difficulties and emphasizes the importance of serum calcium determination in evaluation of different kinds of seizures.

References

1. Pseudohypoparathyroidism: continuing paradox. Editorial (1983) Lancet I, 439-440.
2. Aksnes L. and Aarskog D.: Effect of Parathyroid hormone on 1,25-dihydroxy vitamin D formation in Type I Pseudohypoparathyroidism (1980) J. Clin. Endocrinol. Metab. 51, 1223-26.
3. Spiegel A.M., Levine M.A., Marx S.J., Aurback G.D.: Pseudohypoparathyroidism: the molecular basis for hormone resistence - a retrospective. (1982) N. Engl. J. Med. 307, 679-681.
4. Loveridge N., Fischer J.A., Nagant de Deuxchaisnes C., et al.: Inhibition of cytochemical bioactivity of parathyroid hormone by plasma in pseudohypoparathyroidism type 1. (1982) J. Clin. Endocrinol. Metab. 54, 1274-75.

VITAMIN D AND OTHER PARAMETERS IN HETERTOPIC OSSIFICATIN IN SPINAL CORD INJURY IN SAUDI ARABIA.

K.M.Al-Arabi, M.W.Al-Sebai and S.H.Sedrani. College of Medicine and of Science, King Saud University, Riyadh, Saudi Arabia.

Introduction:

Heterotopic Ossification (H.O.) was originally described by Dejerine and Ceillier (1918) (1). It follows variety of central nervous system disorders and spinal cord injuries (2,3). The reported incidence varies from 16 to 49% (1-4). It commonly affects the hips, knees,shoulders and elbows in descending order of frequency. The aetiology is still unknown. The most frequently studied parameters are serum calcium, phosphorus and alkaline phosphatase activity. The results are controversial (2,4-7). An association was described with decubitus ulcers (2,4,8). There is no study of vitamin D metabolism in this condition. The purpose of this paper is to relay our experience in Saudi Arabia and to discuss its frequency, joint distribution and effect on 25(OH)D_3 and other parameters.

Subjects and Methods:

Out of 150 patients admitted to the Spinal Cord Injury Unit, Riyadh,from 1981 to 1983, 35 with H.O. were allocated as subjects and 15 with no evidence of H.O. as controls. Clinical evaluation was performed on all the joints. X-ray and Radioisotope bone scan, were performed on suspected joints. Laboratory investigations included Blood Counts, Ura and Electrolytes and serum Creatnine. Enzymes SGOT andSGPT were performed.Serum Calcium was measured using AA, Phosphorus and Alkaline Phosphatase activity by Auto-Analyzer Technique. 24 hour urine collection was measured for calcium and phosphorus content. Urine was analyzed and cultured fo micro-organisms. Blood was collected and assayed for serum 25(OH)D_3 as previously described (9) and IGG,IGA using Rate Nephelometry technique.

Results:

A. Clinical Results:

All were males with a mean age group of 30.7$\pm$10.7 years for subjects and 31.7+8.8 years for controls. The cause of injury was road traffic accident in 71% of subjects and 66.6% of controls, falls from a height in 17% subjects and 33.3% of controls and heavy objects falling on the back in 9 to 12% of subjects. Of the 35 subjects 33 were with complete cord damage (94.3%) compared to only two of the controls (13.3%) and 2 with incomplete cord damage (5.7%)compared to 13 of controls (86.7%). A total of 86 joints were involved. Their distribution is shown (Table 1). 51.4% of the subjects and 6.6% of controls had associated bed sores. 74.3% of the subjects and 60% of controls had urinery tract infection. Spasticity developed in 42.9% of subjects and 6.7% of controls. The mode of onset was artheritis like in 48.6%, DVT like in 22.8% and limitation of joint movement in 14.3%.

B. Biochemical Results:

No statistically significant difference could be detected between subjects and controls in the levels of Urea, Creatinine,Sodium,Chloride,Potassium, enzymes SGOT and SGPT and IGM. The concentration of other parameters investegated and level of significance is shown (Table 2).

Discussion and Conclusions:

Out incidence is 23.3% of admitted cases over a period of 2 years.The mode of presentation conforms to that mentioned by other authors(10,11).We found effusion in the knee joint to be an early sign in 48.6% of subjects.The knees were affected more than the hips in our experience (53.5% knees,34.8% hips). The correlation between H.O. and decubitus ulcers is high but the

Vitamin D. A Chemical, Biochemical and Clinical Update

pattern of joint involvment is different. We established a significantly higher level of alkaline phosphatase activity in subjects compared to controls. The lower level of serum calcium in subjects is worth noting. However our subjects show evidence of retention of calcium and phosphorus (Table 2). Since this is not reflected in higher levels of serum calcium and phosphorus, it could indicate their utilization in the calcification process. The level of 25(OH)D_3 in both subjects and controls is low compared to European standards. The level of this metabolite is known to be low in Saudi Arabia (9). The higher level of serum 25(OH)D_3 in our subjects compared to controls may play a role in the observed retention of calcium.

Table (1) Location and Incidence of Heterotopic Ossification in 35 Subjects wih Spinal Cord Injury and Mode of Detection.

Location	R	L	Total No.	%	X-ray	Scan
Knees	22	24	46	53.5	40	11
Hips	17	13	30	34.8	29	6
Shoulders	4	3	7	8.1	2	6
Ankles	1	-	1	1.2	-	1
Foot	-	1	1	1.2	-	1
Symphy. Pubis	-	1	1	1.2	1	1

Table (2) Concentration of Various Parameters in the Blood/or Urine of Subjects and Controls.

Parameter	Subjects		Controls		P Value
Calcium (mg/100ml)	9.4±1	(28)*	9.9±0.9	(14)	0.0394 *
Phosphorus (mg/100ml)	4.7±1.1 NS	(27)	4.6±0.6	(13)	0.3518
Alkaline Phos. (IU/l)	209.3±151	(25)*	150.6±48.4	(14)	0.0400 *
24 Hour Urine Calcium (mg/100ml)	118.2±98.6 NS	(27)	17.4±152.3	(15)	0.1305
24 Hour Urine Phosphorus (mg/100ml)	293.5±149.9	(27)*	537.1±388.3	(15)	0.0155 *
25(OH)D_3 (ng/ml)	12.3±5.6	(23)*	8.5±5.2	(12)	0.0290 *
IGG (mg/dl)	1740±485.6	(17)*	1324.9±305.2	(14)	0.0037 *
IGA (mg/dl)	276.2±81.3	(17)*	225.1±70.7	(14)	0.0342 *

* Statistically Significant

References:

1. Dejerine, Mme, Ceillier, A. and Dejerine, Mlle. Y. (1919) Rev. neurol., 26, 399-407.
2. Abramson, A.S. (1948) JBJS, 30A, 982-986.
3. Bayley, S.J. (1979) Orthop. Rev., 8, 113-120.
4. Hardy, A.G., Dickson, J.W. (1963) JBJS, 45B, 76-87.
5. Hassard, George, H. (1975) Arch Phys Med Rehabil, 56, 355-358.
6. Furman, R., Nicholas, J.J., Jivoff, L. (1970) JBJS, 52A, 1131-1137
7. Rossier, A.B., Bussat, P., Infante, F., et al (1973) Paraplegia, 11, 36-78.
8. Siver, J.R. (1969) Paraplegia, 7, 220-230.
9. Sedrani, S.H. (1984) Trop geogr Med, 36, 181-187.
10. Goldberg, M.A., Schumacher, H.R. (1977) Arch Intern Med (USA), 137(5), 619-621.
11. Hsu, J.D., Sakimura, I., Staufer, E.S. (1975) Clin Orthop (Phil.) (USA), 112, 165-169.

ISONIAZID AND VITAMIN D METABOLISM.

G.Saggese, G.Cesaretti, S.Bertelloni, E.Morganti and E.Bottone.
Department of Pediatrics, University of Pisa, Pisa, Italy.

Introduction:

Vitamin D is hydroxylated in the liver to 25-hydroxyvitamin D (25-OH-D) by a cytochrome P-450 dependent enzyme systems (1). The treatment with some drugs may induce this hepatic monoxygenase activity, reducing serum 25-OH-D serum levels. Such a finding has been described for treatments with anticonvulsants (2), antipyrine (3), cimetidyne (4) and some antitubercolar drugs, as rifampicin and isoniazid (5)(6)(7), that seem to interfere with vitamin D hepatic and renal metabolism, too. Furthermore in association to these treatments it has been described the presence of clinical signes of rickets or osteomalacia (7)(8)(9). To clear the pathogenesis of these alterations we investigated calcium metabolism in a group of patients treated with isoniazid.

Patients and Methods:

Five subjects (3 M and 2 F), aged 1.4-6.1 years, 3 with pulmonary tuberculosis and 2 with tubercular lymphadenitis, received isoniazid for 6 months (20 mg/Kg/die). At the beginning, after 3 months and 6 months of the therapy, it has been effected an evaluation of Ca, P, alkalyne phosphatase, transaminase activity, i-PTH (C-term) with a RIA method (nv: 440 ± 220 pg/ml) (m ± 1 DS), 25-OH-D with a RRA method, after a HPLC step (nv: 34.2 ± 4.5 ng/ml) (10) and 1,25(OH)2D with a RRA method (nv: 38 ± 7 pg/ml) (11). A radiographic examination of the skeleton has been effected at the beginning and after 6 months of therapy.

Results:

Ca, P, alkalyne phosphatase and transaminases always resulted in the normal range; i-PTH was normal at the beginning (415+ 59 pg/ml) and increased after 3 (528 ± 40 pg/ml) (p 0.01) and 6 months (770 ± 108 pg/ml) ($p < 0.001$); 25-OH-D resulted normal at the beginning of the study (36.6 + 2.3 pg/ml) and reduced after 3 (22.2 ± 1.9 pg/ml) ($p < 0.001$) and 6 months (19.7 ± 5.6 pg/ml) ($p < 0.001$); also 1,25(OH)2D, resulting respectively 34±6 pg/ml, 27 ± 5.2 pg/ml ($p < 0.01$) and 23±7.3pg/ml($p < 0.001$), was normal before and reduced then. No radiographic signes of bone involvement were present.

Discussion:

Mild and reversible hepatic injury is one of the most common side effects of the treatment with isoniazide. The presence of reduced levels both of 25-OH-D and 1,25(OH)2D after 3 and

6 months of therapy, in the presence of normal hepatic function is probably determinated by the effect of isoniazide on the enzymatic systems, while the consequent hyperpharathyroidism accounts for the normal calcium values. In fact, Kutt (12) showed an inhibitory effect of isoniazide on oxygenase activity in the rat and subsequently similar finding was pointed out in man (13). The decreased levels of 1,25(OH)2D could depend also by a reduced availability of 25-OH-D. Because the occurrence of osteomalacia in patients receiving antitubercular therapy has been described (8), the fall in 25-OH-D and 1,25(OH)2D serum levels could represent the earliest detectable index of the bone disease. Therefore appropriate vitamin D metabolite prophylaxis could be indicated in subjects treated with isoniazid.

References:

1) De Luca, H.F. (1979) Nutr. Rev. 37: 161-93.

2) Haussler, M.R., McCain, T.A. (1977) N. Engl. J. Med. 297: 1041-50.

3) Wilmara, P.F., Brodie, M.J., Mucklow, J.C., Fraser, H.S., Toverud, E.Z., Davies, D.S., Dollery, C.T., Hilliyard, C.J., MacIntyre, I., Park,B.K.(1979)Br.J.Clin.Pharmacol. 8: 523-8.

4) Bengoa, J.M., Bolt, M.J. and Rosenberg, I.H. (1984) J. Lab. Clin. Med. 104: 546-52.

5) Brodie, M.J., Boobis, A.R., Dollery, C.T., Hillyard, C.J., Brown, D.J., McIntyre, I. and Park, B.K. (1980) Clin. Pharmacol. Ther. 27: 810-4.

6) Brodie, M.J., Boobis, A.P., Hillyard, C.J., Abeyasekera, G., MacIntyre, I., Parh, B.K. (1981) Clin. Pharmacol. Ther. 30: 363-7.

7) Brodie, M.J., Boobis, A.R., Hillyard, C.J., Abeyasekera,G., Stevenson, I. and Park, B.K. (1982) Clin. Pharmacol. Ther. 32: 525-30.

8) Burley, D.M. in Grahame-Smith D.G., ed., Drug Interations, London, 1977, MacMillian, Press Ldt, 293-301.

9) Shan, S.C., Sharka, R.K., Chittle, H., Chittle, A.R. (1981) Tubercle 62: 207-9.

10) Saggese, G., Bertelloni, S., Federico, G., Baroncelli, G.I. and Bottone, E. (1984) In: Proceedings RIA-84: "Cost and benefit of Radio Immuno Assay", Albertini, A., ed., Milan, May 15-16, p. 31,abs.

11) Eisman, J.A., Hamstra, A.J., Kream, B.E., De Luca, H.F. (1976) Arch. Bioch. Bioph. 176: 235-43.

12)Kutt,H.,Verebely,K.,McDowell,F.(1968)Neurology 18: 706-10.

13) Kutt, H., Louis, S. (1982) 4: 256-82.

VITAMIN D METABOLITES IN CHILDREN'S CEREBROSPINAL FLUID.

S. Bertelloni, P. Ghirri, M. Massimetti, G. Saggese and M.F. Holick*.
Dept. of Pediatrics, University of Pisa, Pisa, Italy; *Massachusetts Inst. of Technology, Cambridge, USA.

Introduction:

Recent studies showed the presence of vitamin D dependent Calcium Binding Protein (CaBP)(1)(2) and of vitamin D active metabolites receptors in brain (3), suggesting a possible role of vitamin D endocrine system in the regulation of central nervous system (CNS) activity. In the present study we verified the presence of vitamin D metabolites in CNS detecting 25-hydroxy cholecalciferol (25-OH-D) and 1,25-dihydroxy cholecalciferol levels in cerebrospinal fluid of children.

Patients:

We examined 25 out-patient leukaemic children, ranging in age from 1 to 13 years (11 female and 14 males), all with satisfactory physical activity and exposure to sun-light. No one received vitamin D suplementation by mounth. All children were in maintenance chemotherapy and none showed leukaemic meningosis or any endocrine impairment. CSF samples were obtained by lumbar puncture and kept at -20°C until analyzed. No samples showed pleiocytosis. Serum samples were obtained simultaneously for each children, and stored at -20°C. All the study was performed in spring-summer.

Methods:

CSF and serum samples were used in competitive protein binding assayes for vitamin D metabolites. To assess the efficiency of extraction and subsequent chromatography step 1.500 c.p.m. of both tritiated 25(23-24-3H)-OH-D3 (98 Ci/mml; Amersham I.L., U.K.) and 1,25(23-24-3H)(OH)2D3 (85 Ci/mml; Amersham I.L., U.K.) were added to 3 ml of serum or CSF samples. After 15' at room temperature 3 ml of acetonitrile were added and than the tubes were centrifugated at 1.500g for 10 min. The upper phases were applied to a Sep-pak C18 silica cartridges (Waters Associates, Milford, Massachusetts, U.S.A.), prewashed with 2 ml of methanol and 5 ml of water. Than the Sep-pak cartridges were washed with 3.0 ml of methanol and fraction containing vitamin D metabolites was eluted with 3.0 ml of acetonitrile (4). The lipid extracts were collected, dried under a stream of nitrogen. After extraction the samples were redissolved in 50 ul of exane: isopropanolol: methanol (93: 5: 2; v: v: v); and applied to Gilson HPLC apparatus (mod 302 pump and mod Holocrome wave lenght detector fixed at 254 nm; mod 7125 Rheodyne injection valve; Spherisorb 3 u (cm 15x0.46) HPLC silica column). HPLC system was equilibrated with 93:5:2 at flow rates of 1.5 ml/min. HPLC eluition areas of vitamin D metabolites were established, before each run of samples, with both known concentrations of tritiated 25-OH-D and 1,25(OH)2D3. In HPLC step 25-OH-D eluates after 2.5' and

Vitamin D. A Chemical, Biochemical and Clinical Update

1,25(OH)2D3 after 9'. The fractions containg 25-OH-D and 1,25(OH)2D were collected, dried under nitrogen and subsequently used in competitive binding assay. 25-OH-D assay was performed in triplicate using rachitic rat serum binding protein (5); 1,25(OH)2D assay was performed in duplicate using a modified Eisman method (6).

Results:

In all children 25-OH-D and 1,25(OH)2D were detectable in CSF. 25-OH-D levels were 3.4±0.3 ng/ml (range 0.5-6.0 ng/ml). 1,25(OH)2D values were 6.4±1.8 pg/ml (range 2.3-13.5 pg/ml). Serum values were 45.3±1.5 ng/ml for 25-OH-D (n.v. 34.6±5.4 ng/ml) and 37.7±3.7 pg/ml for 1,25(OH)2D (n.v.: 38.2±7.5 pg/ml). No correlation was found between serum and CSF concentration (r= 0.311 for 25-OH-D; r= 0.142 for 1,25(OH)2D. The means of recovery were 78.1±3.2% for 25-OH-D and 64.7±5.6% for 1,25(OH)2D in liquor, and rispectively, 87.4±4.2% and 79.7±3.4% in serum. Inter- and intra-assay variations were under 10%.

Discussion:

Our data showed the presence of active vitamin D metabolites in CSF of all examined children. Serum levels of both 25-OH-D and 1,25(OH)2D were not different from normal values, and no CSF samples showed flogistic alteration in liquor. We think therefore possible that similar results may be found in CSF of non leukaemic children. The source of vitamin D metabolites in liquor is unknown. Since serum could be the source of CSF metabolites, no data are available on the passage of 25-OH-D or 1,25(OH)2D from serum into liquor and our study show none correlation between the two examined compartment. Labeled 1,25(OH)2D (3) had been showed in pituitary gland. It may be possible that pituitary can directly secrete vitamin D metabolites in CSF, as for the pituitary hormones (7). Further studies are needed to clarify the origin of 25-OH-D and 1,25(OH)2D in CSF and to elucidate their role in the regulation of brain activity.

References:

1) Feldman, S.C., Christakos, S. (1983) Endocrinology 112 : 290-301.
2) Parkes, C.O., Thomasset, M., Baimbridge, K.G., Henin, E., (1984) Eur. J. Clin. Invest. 14 : 181-183.
3) Stumpf, W.E., Sar, M., Clark, S.A., DeLuca, H.F. (1982) Science 215 : 1403-1405.
4) Fraher, L.J., Adami, S., Clemens, T.L., Jones, G., O'Riordan, J.L.H. (1983) Clin. Endocrinol. 18 : 151-165.
5) Saggese, G., Bertelloni, S., Federico, G., Baroncelli, G.I., Bottone, E., Proc. "RIA'84", Albertini A. ed., Milano, May 15-16, 1984, p.31.
6) Eisman, J.A., Hamstra, A.J., Kream, B.E., DeLuca, H.F. (1976) Arch. Bioch. Bioph. 176 : 235-243.
7) Bergland, R.M., Page, R.B. (1978) Endocrinology 102 : 1325-1338.

IS 25-HYDROXYVITAMIN D_3 OF IMPORTANCE FOR DEVELOPMENT OF HYPERCALCIURIA IN RENAL STONE FORMERS?

T. BERLIN, I. HOLMBERG and I. BJÖRKHEM,
Departments of Urology and Clinical Chemistry I, Huddinge University Hospital, S-141 86 Huddinge, Sweden.

Introduction.

The possible role of vitamin D_3 and its metabolites in hypercalciuria is a matter of controversy. In several recent studies the serum level of $1,25(OH)_2D_3$ has been reported to be increased in patients with hypercalciuria. In a previous report we showed that a group of hypercalciuric patients with urolithiasis had significantly higher serum levels of $25OHD_3$ than a group of normocalciuric stone formers (1) and similar results were reported at about the same time in a Finnish study (2). Recently, Jongen showed that a group of Dutch stone patients with hypercalciuria had significantly higher $25OHD_3$ serum levels than normocalciuric stone formers and the highest levels of $25OHD_3$ were found in a subgroup of hypercalciuric patients classified as hyperabsorbers (3). However, no elevated levels of $1,25(OH)_2D_3$ were found in different subgroups.
In the present work our previous finding that there is a relationship between serum levels of $25OHD_3$ and hypercalciuria has been confirmed and extended.

Patients and Methods.

The study was carried out in 1983. In 108 normocalcemic stone formers, all men between 31 and 51 years of age, tests were done on two occasions - in March and again in September. A 24-hour urine was collected for each of three consecutive days. Morning blood samples for determining serum $25OHD_3$, $1,25(OH)_2D$, calcium, phosphate, creatinine, urate, ALAT, albumin and PTH levels were taken after overnight fasting. Urinary excretion of cyclic AMP was determined after an overnight fast using a two-hour urine sample. The same morning a calcium load test was performed as described by Pak et al. (4). $25OHD_3$ was determined by a highly accurate method based on isotope dilution - mass spectrometry (5). $1,25(OH)_2D$ was determined by radioreceptor assay. The group of patients classified as hypercalciuric (excretion of calcium > 8.0 mmol/24 h) was subdivided according to Jongen on the basis of the fasting urinary calcium/creatinine ratio and the renal threshold phosphate concentration ($TmPO_4/GFR$) (3). The latter parameter was calculated using the nomogram described by Walton and Bijvoet (6). Hypercalciuric subjects with normal calcium/creatinine ratios (< 0.40) and normal renal threshold phosphate concentrations (> 0.80 mmol/l) were considered to be hyperabsorbers. The hypercalciuric patients were also subclassified using the oral calcium load test (4). Patients were regarded as hyperabsorbers if the ratio calcium/creatinine in urine was less than 0.31 in the fasting state and equal to or greater than 0.56 in a four-hour sample following ingestion of 1 g of calcium.

Results.

The patients were divided into three groups with respect to urinary excretion of calcium. I, hypercalciuria - excretion of calcium $\geq$ 8.1 mmol/24 hours (n=47): II, intermediate calciuria - excretion of calcium $\leq$ 8.0, $\geq$ 6.1 mmol/24 hours (n=29): III, normocalciuria - excretion of calcium

Vitamin D. A Chemical, Biochemical and Clinical Update

$\leq$ 6.0 mmol/24 hours (n=32). There was no difference between the hypercalciuric and the normocalciuric group with respect to serum calcium, phosphate, creatinine, urate, ALAT, albumin and PTH levels or fasting urinary excretion of cyclic AMP. In March the hypercalciuric stone formers had significantly higher mean level of $25OHD_3$ (30.1±1.5 ng/ml) than the normocalciuric stone formers (22.7±1.4 ng/ml) ($p < 0.0025$). Stone formers with intermediate excretion of calcium had $25OHD_3$ levels between those of the other two groups (27.5±1.7 ng/ml). With respect to $1,25(OH)_2D$ there was no difference between the hypercalciuric stone formers (29.6±1.9 pg/ml) and the normocalciuric ones (31.6±3.6 pg/ml) ($p > 0.5$). The correlation between urinary excretion of calcium and serum level of $25OHD_3$ in the individual patient was low (r=0.37), and there was no correlation to $1,25(OH)_2D$ (r=0.04) or between $25OHD_3$ and $1,25(OH)_2D$ (r=0.03). In September again the patients with high urinary excretion of calcium had significantly higher levels of $25OHD_3$ (42.0±1.3 ng/ml) than those in the group with low calcium excretion (34.0±2.0 ng/ml) ($p < 0.0025$). When the hypercalciuric patients in March were classified according to Jongen (3), the hyperabsorbers (n=18) were found to have the highest mean serum level of $25OHD_3$ (33.7±2.6 ng/ml). When the hypercalciuric patients were classfied using the calcium load test (4), the hyperabsorbers (n=7) had even higher mean serum level of $25OHD_3$ (43.3±3.9 ng/ml). This level is significantly higher than that of the hypercalciuric group as a whole ($p < 0.0025$). There was no significant difference in the serum levels of $1,25(OH)_2D$ between the hyperabsorbers and the hypercalciuric group as a whole when classified according to Jongen or Pak ($p > 0.25$).

Discussion.

In contrast to other reports but in agreement with Jongen we found no elevated levels of $1,25(OH)_2D$ in hypercalciuric stone formers. It should be emphasized that although firm evidence is presented here and in previous work (1,2,3) for a relationship between hypercalciuria and an increased level of $25OHD_3$, the correlation between calcium excretion and the level of $25OHD_3$ in the individual patient was low (r=0.37). It is evident that an abnormal vitamin D status is only one of several factors which can contribute to the development of hypercalciuria. If, however, a high $25OHD_3$ level is one of the risk factors for hypercalciuria, renal stone formers with hypercalciuria and high levels of $25OHD_3$ in the circulation may be advised to reduce their exposure to sunshine.

References.

1. Berlin, T., Björkhem, I., Collste, L., Holmberg, I., Wijkström, H. (1982) Scand. J. Urol. Nephrol. 16.269-273.
2. Elomaa, I., Karonen, S.L., Kairento, A.L., Pelkonen, R. (1982) Scand. J. Urol. Nephrol. 16.155-161.
3. Jongen, M.J.M. (1983) Thesis. Juuriaans by Amsterdam.
4. Pak, C.Y.C., Kaplan, R., Bone, H., Townsend, J., Waters, O. (1975). N. Engl. J. Med. 292.497-500.
5. Björkhem, I., Holmberg, I. (1980) Methods in Enzymology 67:385-393.
6. Walton, R.J., Bijvoet, O.L.M. (1975) Lancet 2.309-310.

VITAMIN D METABOLITES IN PAGET'S DISEASE

R.D. Devlin, J.C. Kent, D.H. Gutteridge, R.W. Retallack,
Department of Endocrinology and Diabetes, Sir Charles Gairdner Hospital, Nedlands, Western Australia.

Introduction

Severe Paget's disease has a number of features in common with osteomalacia - elevated serum alkaline phosphatase (SAP) levels, widened osteoid seams on bone biopsy and pseudofractures on radiographs. There is also a significant inverse correlation between the severity of Paget's disease (measured by SAP) and 25 hydroxy vitamin D (25OHD) ($p<0.01$; multiple linear regression) independent of age. We report here additional observations on the vitamin D status of these Paget's patients.

Subjects

25OHD, and SAP were measured in untreated Paget's patients (65 10 years) (mean ± SD) with varying severity of disease and a control group of ambulant normal volunteers (60 ± 9 years). 1,25 dihydroxyvitamin D (1,25$(OH)_2$D) and 24,25dihydroxyvitamin D (24,25$(OH)_2$D) were measured in a number of these Paget's patients and controls (Table 1).

Methods

Methods for the determination of serum 25OHD (1), SAP, and 1,25$(OH)_2$D (2) have been reported elsewhere. The 24,25$(OH)_2$D method is shown in Fig.1.

Assay characteristics of 24,25$(OH)_2$D assay

The sensitivity was 20pg per tube (0.19nmol/l in serum). Recovery of ^{3}(H)-24,25$(OH)_2D_3$ (160Ci/mmol) added to 1.0ml serum samples was 43% 13%, (n=54). Mean analytical recovery (assessed by adding 1.0ng 24,25$(OH)_2$D3 to two 1.0ml serum samples) was 99%. The interassay c.v. was 24%, and intra-assay c.v. was 12%. The normal range for 24,25$(OH)_2$D was 6.4 3.95nmol/l, n=33.

Results: see Table 1.

TABLE 1

VITAMIN D METABOLITES IN PAGET'S DISEASE

	25OHDnmol/l	1,25$(OH)_2$Dpmol/l	24,25$(OH)_2$Dnmol/l
Pagets	71 ± 25(58)*	102 ± 46(50)	2.42 ± 2.39(22)
Controls	89 ± 19(38)	110 ± 34(27)	5.46 ± 3.64(26)
	$p<0.005$	N.S.	$p<0.0025$

* Number of patients.

Discussion and Conclusions

Our solid phase extraction procedure for assay of 24,25$(OH)_2$D has yielded a sensitive and precise assay for 24,25$(OH)_2$D requiring <1.0ml serum. Although the procedure removes 25OHD3-26,23 lactone,it does not remove inhibitors of the competitive protein binding and HPLC is still required. In Paget's disease, 25OHD is significantly decreased relative to controls. 24,25$(OH)_2$D is decreased to 50% of control values, whereas 1,25$(OH)_2$D is unchanged. In Paget's disease, 25OHD and 24,25$(OH)_2$D are correlated ($r=0.44$, $p<0.05$). In contrast to 25OHD, 24,25$(OH)_2$D and 1,25$(OH)_2$D are not correlated with the severity of the disease.The profound decrease in 24,25$(OH)_2$D observed in Paget's disease is also observed in growing children who represent another high bone turnover state (3). In this situation bone formation exceeds resorption.

Acknowledgements

Professor A W Norman, Dr M Uskokovic, and Dr P Campbell who kindly provided the 25OHD3-26,23 lactone, the 24,25$(OH)_2D_3$ and the 25OHD_3 respectively.

References:

1. Kent,J.C., Devlin, R.D., Gutteridge.D.H. and Retallack,R.W. (1979)
   Biochem. Biophys. Res. Commun.89: 155-161.
2. Retallack,R.W., Kent,J.C., Nicholson,G.C., Gutteridge,D.H. (1985) Clin Endocrinol (in press).
3. Chesney.R.W., Hamstra,A.J., Deluca,H.F. (1982)
   Calcif. Tissue Int. 34: 527-530.

Fig 1. A diatomaceous earth column [Clinelut #1001] was used for extraction and 4.5mls solvent was added to silicic acid column at points 2 , 3 and 4.

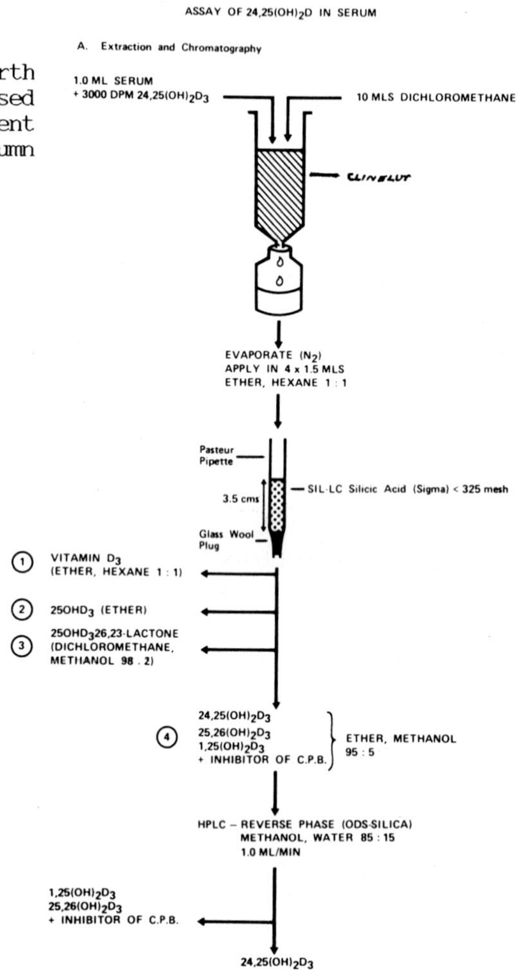

VITAMIN D ENDOCRINE SYSTEM IN LONG-TERM ANTICONVULSANT TREATED CHILDREN.

M. Massimetti, P. Ghirri, G.I. Baroncelli, A. Papini and G. Saggese. Department of Pediatrics of Pisa, Pisa, Italy.

Introduction:

Istomorphometric (1) and densitometric (2) analysis in children receiving long-term anticonvulsant therapy has shown bone demineralization in more than half of the examined subjects. The very high incidence of bone demineralization in these children has stimulated many studies on the pathogenesis of this condition in order to prevent or cure this side-effect of anticonvulsant treatment. The pathogenetic factors to consider are manifold; alterations in the metabolism of vitamin D are some of the most important.

Patients and methods:

The study comprised 35 ambulatory children aged 6-16 years receiving anticonvulsant therapy for a mean period of 4.8 years (3-11 years) and 20 normal ambulatory subjects as a control group. Serum calcium, phosphorus and alkaline phosphatase levels were determined by standard laboratory methods. Serum PTH levels were determined by radioimmunoassay using a carboxyregional antibody (Immunonuclear Corp., Stillwater, Minn. USA). Assay sensitivity was 100 pg/ml. Serum 25-OH-D was measured by a direct binding assay using the method of Belsey et al. (3) with a previous HPLC extraction. Assay sensitivity was 0.5 ng/ml. Serum 1,25(OH)2D was measured by a competitive radioreceptor assay as precedently described by Eisman (4). Assay sensitivity was 2pg/ml.

Results:

Serum calcium and phosphorus levels were lower and alkaline phosphatase levels higher in the patients receiving anticonvulsant therapy. No statistical significance (P : NS) was present. Serum PTH levels were higher in the anticonvulsant group while serum 25-OH-D levels were lower each reaching statistical significance ($P < 0.05$). No significant difference was found in 1,25(OH)2D levels between the control and the anticonvulsant treated group.

Discussion:

Our data support the presence of an impairment of the hepatic step of activation of vitamin D classically attributed to induction of hepatic microsomal enzymes (5). The low 25-OH-D circulating levels (6)(7)(8) are not related in this condition to reduced 1,25(OH)2D (9)(10), the most active metabolite of vitamin D. Evidently the presence in most of the patients of increased levels of PTH and in some of hypocalcemia represents an appropriate stimulus to induce the 1-alfa-hydroxylase activity and maintain circulating 1,25(OH)2D levels in the normal range.

On the basis of these results it seems difficult to consider the impairment of vitamin D metabolism as an important pathogenetic factor of the anticonvulsant osteomalacia. However the clinical efficacy of 25-OH-D profilactic and therapeutical administration in anticonvulsant treated children (11) shows that the impairment of the hepatic step of vitamin D activation represents an important pathogenetic aspect of bone demineralization even in the presence of normal 1,25(OH)2D circulating levels. This could mean that 25-OH-D itself might play a more important role in bone mineralization than till now thought (12).

References:

1) Mosekilde L., Melsen F. (1976) Acta Med. Scand. 199 : 349-355.

2) Hahn T.J., Henden B.A., Scharp C.R., Boisseau V.L., Haddad J.G. (1975) New Engl. J. Med. 292 :550-554.

3) Belsey R.E., De Luca H.F., Potts J.T.jr (1974) J. Clin. Endocrinol. Metab. 28 : 1946-49.

4) Eisman J.A., Hamstra A.J., Kream B.E., De Luca H.F. (1976) Science 193 : 1021-25.

5) Hahn T.J., Birge S.J., Sharp C.R., Avioli L.V. (1972) J. Clin. Invest. 51 : 741-745.

6) Stamp T.C.B., Round J.H., Rowe D.J.F., Haddad J.G. (1972) Brit. Med. J. 4 : 9-12.

7) Weisman Y., Andriola M., Reiter E., Gruskin A., Root A. (1979) South. Med. J. 72 : 400-408.

8) Saggese G., Biagioni M., Clark M.B., Bottone E. (1981) Europ. Rev. Med. Pharm. Sc. III : 145-150

9) Jubitz W., Haussler M.R., McCaine T.A., Tolman K.G. (1977) J. Clin. Endocrinol. Metab. 44 : 617-621.

10) Hahn T.J., Halstead L.R. (1979) Calcif. Tiss. Int. 27 :13-18.

11) Bottone E., Saggese G.,(1985) Terapia Pediatrica Essenziale Burgio G.R., ed. in press.

12) Bordier P., Rasmussen H., Miravet P.M.L., Gueris J.,Ryck-waert A. (1978) J. Clin. Endocrinol. Metab. 46: 284-287.

HEALING OF EHDP-INDUCED OSTEOMALACIA BY CALCITONIN.

J.P. Huaux, B. Bouchez, J.P. Devogelaer, H. Withofs, C. Nagant de Deuxchaisnes, Rheumatology Unit, Louvain University in Brussels, St-Luc University Hospital, B-1200 Brussels.

Introduction.

The CREST syndrome is sometimes complicated by severe leg ulcers. The calcinosis may interfere with the healing of the latter. Some autors have suggested that high doses of EHDP (20 mg/kg/day) may inhibit the development of calcinosis (1-2). Such a treatment was given to a patient with the CREST syndrome and severe leg ulcers.
EHDP induces mineralization defects. The healing effect of calcitonin on EHDP-induced osteomalacia has been demonstrated on clinical and radiological grounds (3). We studied whether this could be proven on histological grounds as well.

Case report.

A 72 year old woman presented the full-blown CREST syndrome (Calcinosis, Raynaud's phenomenon, Esophageal dysfunction, Sclerodactyly and Telangiectases). Calcinosis was considered as an interfering factor in the healing of the leg ulcers. Therefore EHDP (20 mg/kg/day) was given to try to inhibit the ectopic calcifications. The effect of the treatment was poor both clinically and radiologically. Neither did the ulcers heal nor did the calcinosis disappear. Osteomalacia occurred as demonstrated histologically on a bone biopsy of the iliac crest performed 2 mo. after the beginning of the treatment. Salmon calcitonin (50 U twice daily subcutaneously) was then added to EHDP. 1.5 mo. later (at time 3.5 mo.), under combined therapy, the recovery of osteomalacia took place and the healing was complete (Table) 3.5 mo. later (at time 6 mo.).

Table : Histomorphometric measurements under EHDP and combined therapy EHDP + SCT

	Normal Values	Time Zero	EHDP 20 mg/ kg/day (time 2 mo.)	EHDP + SCT 100 U/day (time 3.5 mo.)	Idem on dis-charge (time 6 mo.)
ROV* (%)	1.9 ± 1.0	1.2	12.0	7.0	3.0
ROS* (%)	11.0 ± 9.2	2.4	39.3	26.2	27.5
WOS^Δ (um)	7.7 ± 2.1	4.6	13.6	13.9	7.8
MF°° (%)	86.6 ± 8.9	99.0	55.3	81.0	89.7

ROV = relative osteoid volume; ROS = relative osteoid surface; WOS = width osteoid seams; MF = mineralization front. *Undecalcified sections stained with solochrome cyanine. °°Idem, stained with toluidine blue pH 4.6.

Vitamin D. A Chemical, Biochemical and Clinical Update

Discussion.

This case thus confirms that calcitonin indeed heals EHDP-induced osteomalacia despite the continuation of the administration of the same doses of EHDP which had produced osteomalacia. Compliance to EHDP therapy was assessed by weekly monitoring the serum phosphate level, which was consistently higher than 4.5 mg/dl. Therefore, under these circumstances, calcitonin has remineralizing properties. This is reminiscent of the findings of Boris et al. (4), who showed that calcitonin was able to correct the EHDP-induced lesions in the growth cartilage of rats. The exact mechanism of this action remains unknown.

References.

1)Rabens SF,Bethune JE (1975) Arch Dermatol,111,357-361

2)Cram RL,Bernada R,Geho WB,Ray RD (1971)N Engl J Med 285:1012-1013

3)Nagant de Deuxchaisnes C,Rombouts-Lindemans C,Huaux JP,Devogelaer JP,Malghem J,Maldague B (1979) In:MacIntyre I;Szelke M; Molecular Endocrinology. Elsevier/North-Holland Biomedical Press,Amsterdam,pp 405-433.

4)Boris A,Hurley JF,Trmal T,Mallon JP,Matuszewski DS (1979). Acta Endocrinol (Kbh.) 91,351-361

HISTOLOGIC RESPONSE IN PEDIATRIC RENAL OSTEODYSTROPHY (ROD) TO TREATMENT WITH $1,25(OH)_2D_3$ AND $24,25(OH)_2D_3$.

J.D. MAHAN[1], M.D. FALLON [2], J.E. STRIEGEL[3], Y.K. KIM[3], and R.W. CHESNEY[4], Dept of Pediatrics, The Ohio State University, Columbus, Ohio[1], Dept of Pathology, University of Pennsylvania, Phildelphia, Pennsylvania[2], Dept of Pediatrics, University of Minnesota, Minneapolis, Minnesota[3] and the University of Wisconsin, Madison, Wisconsin[4], USA.

Introduction:

Rod occurs more frequently in children with chronic renal failure (CRF) than adults (1), as manifested by short stature, bone pain, skeletal deformities and fractures. Children are prone to ROD because new bone growth is particularly sensitive to changes in mineral metabolism and bone turn-over and remodeling are more rapid than in adults. Histologic evidence of ROD develops (2) and serum levels of Vitamin D metabolites decline in children as renal function falls to <50% of normal (3). Treatment with Vitamin D metabolites can reverse many of the clinical and histologic abnormalities associated with ROD in children. Recently, $1,25(OH)_2D_3$ has been used most extensively because it has a rapid onset of action, short half life and is most potent in promoting intestinal calcium absorption. Although the benefits of $1,25(OH)_2D_3$ in the treatment of children with ROD have been well documented (4), treatment failures in some children with long-standing CRF (2) or on dialysis (6) have also been reported.

The reasons for the lack of uniform results with $1,25(OH)_2D_3$ in pediatric ROD are not well understood. Some treatment failures may represent inadequate doses of $1,25(OH)_2D_3$. Alternatively, some authors believe that "normal" circulating levels of 25-OH D_3 and/or $24,25(OH)_2D_3$ are necessary in combination with $1,25(OH)_2D_3$ to allow proper bone mineralization (2). Another factor may be the diversity of ROD histology in children. Specifically, mixed bone disease (MBD), pure osteomalacia (OM) and aplastic bone disease (ABD - with or without aluminum) may not respond as well to isolated $1,25(OH)_2D_3$ therapy as osteitis fibrosa (OF). The present study was initiated to assess the influence of pretreatment histology on results with the combination of adjusted doses of $1,25(OH)_2D_3$ and $24,25(OH)_2D_3$.

Patients and Methods:

Fourteen children with CRF (mean age 8.7 yrs, range 0.8-15.6) were studied Three children were on HD (duration 3.9 yrs, range 2.2-6.5), one on PD (duration 2.9 yrs) and the other 10 cheldren had low creatinine clearances (range 9-49 ml/min/1.73 M^2). All children were on phosphate restriction and supplemental calcium as needed. Eleven received AlOH to help keep serum phosphorous <5.5 mg/dl. Prior to this study 7 children had been on 25-OH-D_3 alone, 2 on DHT and 5 on no supplemental Vitamin D. Thirteen children had short stature, and 5 had bone pain and/or recent fractures. Pre and posttreatment, a percutaneous posterior iliac crest bone biopsy with double Tetracycline labelling was obtained. Serial sections were stained with hematoxylin and eosin, a trichome stain, and special stains for iron and aluminum and histomorphometry performed. The children were started on $24,25(OH)_2D_3$ at 100 ng/kg/day and 1-2 weeks later $1,25(OH)_2D_3$ was started at 5-10 ng/kg/day. $1,25(OH)_2D_3$ was increased until hypercalcemia occurred; at that time $1,25(OH)_2D_3$ was stopped and restarted at a slightly lower dose after an increase in $24,25(OH)_2D_3$. Dose adjustments were made every 2-4 weeks. The avg final dose $1,25(OH)_2D_3$ = 22 ng/kg/day (range 8-36) and

Vitamin D. A Chemical, Biochemical and Clinical Update

$24,25(OH)_2D_3$ = 210 ng/kg/day (range 76-577).

Serum calcium, phosphorous, creatinine, alkaline phosphatase, N-terminal parathyroid hormone (performed at Nichols Lab) and Vitamin D metabolites (25-OH D_3, $1,25(OH)_2D_3$ and $24,25(OH)_2D_3$) (7) were determined at the start and the end of therapy. Serum Ca, P and Cr were monitored every 2-4 weeks.

Results:

Three children experienced less bone pain while 2 had no improvement of their symptoms. Although some children had increased growth velocity, as a group there was no significant change during the study. Although the Alk Ptase and N-PTH tended to decline there was no significant change in Ca, P, Alk Ptase or N-PTH for the total group (see Table 1) or for specific pre-treatment sub-groups: OF, OM + MBD, OM + MBD with improved mineralization on Rx. Vitamin D metabolite levels after 6 mo of Rx revealed elevated serum $1,25(OH)_2D_3$ ($\bar{x}$ = 83 pg/ml, normal mean 43 ± 12) and $24,25(OH)_2D_3$ ($\bar{x}$ = 6.2 ng/ml, normal mean 1.7 ± 0.5) values in all subjects.

Table 1. Biochemical Response To Treatment With $1,25(OH)_2D_3$ And $24,25(OH)_2D_3$

14 Subjects	Ca (mg/dl)	P (mg/dl)	Alk Ptase (IU/L)	N-PTH (pg/ml)	(1,25 D_3)	(24,25 D_3)
before	10.3 ± 0.8	4.7 ± 8	746 ± 455	70 ± 88	41 ± 55	0.49 ± 0.44
after	10.2 ± 0.7	4.7 ± 1.0	553 ± 243	34 ± 26	83 ± 30	6.20 ± 1.0
paired T test	NS	NS	NS	NS	p <.05	p <.05

Histologic improvement was variable. In 6 children with OF, 4 improved (less bone resorption) while 1 had progression of OF and 1 developed OM. The children with pre-existing mineralization defects demonstrated improvement if there was no aluminum bone involvement. In 5 MBD children, 3 had improved mineralization; the 2 who did not improve developed Al at the mineralization front (MF). In 3 children with pure OM, 1 had improved mineralization; of the 2 who did not, 1 developed Al at the MF. The 2 children with MF Al had elevated serum Al levels (mean 78 pg/ml), were all long-term HD patients (2.2-6.5 yrs), but had no stainable bone Al on the pre-Rx biopsy.

Conclusions:

1. The combination of $1,25(OH)_2D_3$ + $24,25(OH)_2D_3$ in the Rx of pediatric ROD is well tolerated at the doses used in this study.
2. Most children with OF and those with abnormal mineralization (OM + MBD) benefit from combination Rx.
3. Aluminum associated OM can develop despite this Vitamin D metabolite Rx.
4. Although not proved to be essential in this study $24,25(OH)_2D_3$ may be a useful adjunct in the Rx of pediatric ROD.

References:

1. Ritz, E., Kremplian, B., Mehls, O., et al: Kid Int 4:116, 1973.
2. Norman, M.E.: PNCA 29:947, 1982.
3. Chesney, R.W., Hamstra, A.J., Mazees, R.B.: Kid Int 21:65, 1982.
4. Chesney, R.W., Moorthy, A.V., Eisman, J.: NEJM 298:238, 1978.
5. Chan, J.C., Kodroff, M.B., Landmehr, D.M.: Ped 68:559, 1981.
6. Mahan, J.D., Fallon, M.D., Kim Y., et al: Manuscript in preparation.
7. Shepard, R.M., Horst, R.L., Hamstra, A.J.: Biochem J 182:55, 1979.

AMYLOIDOSIS, A POSSIBLE CONTRIBUTING FACTOR TO BONE EROSIONS AND CYSTS IN AZOTEMIC RENAL OSTEODYSTROPHY ON LONGTERM HEMODIALYSIS.

J.P. Huaux*, H. Noel**, J.Malghem***, B. Maldague***, J.P. Devogelaer*, H. Van Kerckhove****, C. Nagant de Deuxchaisnes*. Departments of Rheumatology*, Pathology**, and Radiology***, Louvain University in Brussels, St-Luc University Hospital, B-1200 Brussels, Virga Jesse Ziekenhuis, B-3500 Hasselt****.

Introduction

Articular disorders may occur in patients undergoing maintenance hemodialysis for chronic renal failure. Some are related to secondary hyperparathyroidism (1) or osteomalacia, ischemic osteonecrosis or crystal-induced arthritis (4). However, some articular features still remain of unknown etiology (5). Amyloid deposits are known to produce severe carpal tunnel syndrome in dialyzed patients (6-7). We had the opportunity to observe two patients on longterm hemodialysis who developed severe articular distress with bone fractures. Their fractures were mainly due to amyloid deposits.

Case reports.

The two patients (age: 57 and 40, respectively) suffered from renal failure, unrelated to amyloidosis. Case 1 has been described elsewhere (9). They were on maintenance hemodialysis respectively over a 10 and 16 year period. Both complained of hip and shoulder pain and developed a bilateral carpal tunnel syndrome. X rays showed multiple articular erosions and bone cysts, as well as fissures of the femoral necks. Renal osteodystrophy was mainly related to secondary hyperparathyroidism in both cases, as well as to osteomalacia and aluminum toxicity in case 2. 1,25-$(OH)_2D_3$ (0.25 ug every other day) in both cases, and in addition in case 2, subtotal parathyroidectomy and 24,25-$(OH)_2D_3$ (8 ug/24 h) achieved clinical improvement, but failed to relieve all symptoms. Repeated histomorphometry of iliac crest biopsies showed in case 2 the recovery of secondary hyperparathyroidism and partial healing of osteomalacia (Table).

HISTOMORPHOMETRIC MEASUREMENTS

	NORMAL VALUES (MEAN±SD) DATE	CASE 1	CASE 2				
		10/81	3/81	6/81	7/81	1/82	5/82
TRS (%)*	2.02±0.96	4.01	5.34	0.36	0.54	0.72	0.60
ORS (%)*	1.06±0.64	2.67	4.52	0.00	0.00	0.00	0.00
OC/mm2*	0.16±0.09	2.30	1.64	0.00	0.00	0.00	0.00
ROV (%)*	1.89±0.99	9.4	35.2	16.2	20.5	19.7	15.5
AOV (%)*	0.38±0.18	1.87	8.09	6.12	3.12	3.50	2.50
ROS (%)*	11.0±9.2	44.8	76.6	64.0	74.7	72.0	48.5
TIO*	18.5±4.0	21.1	45.9	25.2	27.4	27.3	32.0
WOS (µm)*	7.72±2.08	11.3	17.4	16.6	11.9	17.7	17.4
MF (%)**	86.6±8.9	66.8	46.0	69.6	67.9	62.6	86.7
Al RS (%)***		5.0	60.0				

TRS: Total Resorption Surface. ORS: Osteoclastic Resorption Surface. OC: Osteo-clastic Count. ROV: Relative Osteoid Volume. AOV: Absolute Osteoid Volume. ROS: Relative Osteoïd Surface. TIO: Thickness Index of Osteoid. WOS: Width Oste-oïd Seams. MF: Mineralization Front. Al RS: Aluminum Relative Surface.
*: Undecalcified sections stained with Solochrome Cyanine; **: idem, stained With Toluidine Blue, pH 4.6; ***: idem, stained with Aluminon pH 5.2.

Vitamin D. A Chemical, Biochemical and Clinical Update

Femoral neck fractures occurred in both patients. Total hip replacement arthroplasty allowed us to study the bone lesions histologically. Amyloid deposits, as evidenced by staining the sections with Congo red and demonstrating typical green dichroism on polarized light, infiltrated the articular structures (synovium, tendons, ligaments), as well as the surrounding bone. The bone cysts and periarticular erosions were filled with tissue infiltrated with amyloid deposits of the AA protein type (8). The same deposits were demonstrated in the carpal tunnel tissues removed on operation as well as in the synovium of the shoulder needle biopsy in case 2.

Discussion

The two reported cases were on longterm hemodialysis. They were considered to suffer from renal osteodystrophy with bone fissures, and from lesions observed in dialyzed patients and known under the general heading of "erosive azotemic osteodystrophy" (1). However, having obtained material during three total hip replacement arthroplasties, 4 liberations of median nerve and a shoulder biopsy, we were able to ascertain that articular erosions, bone cysts as well as bone fissures and fractures were mainly due to amyloid deposits in and around the joints. The deposits seemed to play a greater role in the pathogenesis of bone lesions than the classical metabolic disturbances usually associated with renal osteodystrophy. Aluminum toxicity has repeatedly been blamed for part of these abnormalities (3-4). This may play undoubtedly an important role, but is not the determining factor in our cases, since one patient does not have more than traces of aluminum in his bone biopsy. Seven cases of amyloidosis in hemodialyzed patients have been recorded in our institution during the next year. Five of them were dialyzed in the same center and represented 20% of the patients who were hemodialyzed for at least 7 years.

References

1. Rubin LA, Fam AG, Rubenstein J, Campbell J, Saiphoo C. (1984) Arthritis Rheum 27, 1086-1094.
2. Charhon SA, Chapuy MC, Traeger J, Meunier PJ. (1984) Presse Méd 13, 1431-1434.
3. Andress DL, Ott SM, Maloney NA, Sherrard DJ. (1985) N Engl J Med 312:468-473.
4. Massry SG, Bluestone R, Klinenberg JR, Coburn JW. (1975) Semin Arthritis Rheum 4:321-349.
5. Goldstein S, Winston E, Chung TJ, Chopra S, Pariser K. (1985) Am J Med 78:82-87.
6. Assenat H, Calemard E, Charra B, Laurent G, Terrat JC, Vanel T.(1980) Nouv Presse Méd, 9,1715.
7. Allieu Y, Ascencio E, Mailhe D, Baldet P, Mion C. (1983) Rev Chir Orthop, 69: 233-238.
8. Huaux JP, Noel H, Bastien P, Malghem J, Maldague B, Devogelaer JP, Nagant de Deuxchaisnes C. (1985) Rev Rhum Mal Osteoartic : in press.
9. Wright JR, Calkins E, Humphrey R (1977) Lab Invest 36, 274-281.

CHANGES IN CALCITRIOL, AMINO-TERMINAL I-PTH, AND PHOSPHORUS IN SERA FROM GERIATRIC BEAGLES WITH UNTREATED PROGRESSIVE UREMIA

L.A. Nagode, R.S. Jaenke,* T.A. Allen,* and C.L. Steinmeyer

Department of Veterinary Pathobiology, Ohio State University, Columbus, OH 43210 and *Departments of Veterinary Pathology and Clinical Sciences, Colorado State University, Ft. Collins, CO 80523

INTRODUCTION

Human patients with advanced renal failure have very low serum calcitriol (1). With lesser degrees of renal failure, serum calcitriol correlated inversely with serum creatinine, phosphorus, parathyroid hormone (PTH) and age (2). Geriatric patients differ from younger adults and children in serum levels of calcitriol (2,3) and PTH (4).

Beagles studied are from a colony of 300 ranging from 10-13 years corresponding to human ages of 70-90. Many have progressive renal failure with degrees of uremia from mild to marked. They have renal osteodystrophy (5) and may model uremic events in geriatric human patients.

Recent reports indicate that the 1-34 amino-terminal i-PTH is superior to carboxy-terminal immunoassays in evaluating renal osteodystrophy (6,7). It is most useful for interactions between serum calcitriol and biologically active PTH (7). At the onset of hyperparathyroidism in renal failure, transitory deficits of calcitriol following excess serum phosphorus may occur. The view that such deficits help cause hyperparathyroidism (8,9) has been disputed (10).

METHODS

Serum calcium, phosphorus, creatinine and BUN were analyzed by standard methods. Amino-terminal i-PTH was assayed using the CK-67 antibody to synthetic 1-34 human PTH in the RIA (6,7). Calcitriol was assayed as previously described (11) with dextran-charcoal replacing hydroxylapatite. Creatinine and BUN were used to define uremic stages. Mildly uremic dogs were considered in two groups (Fig. 1), one with normal PTH, the second with PTH more than 2X normal.

RESULTS AND DISCUSSION

Serum creatinine values for the 5 experimental groups (Fig. 1) were 0.7 ± 0.2, 1.1 ± 0.1, 1.0 ± 0.1, 1.5 ± 0.5, and 3.4 ± 1.0 mg/dl respectively. Early hyperparathyroidism when present in mildly uremic dogs was associated with normal serum phosphorus and increased rather than decreased serum calcitriol (Fig. 1). A trade off mechanism in which both calcitriol and phosphorus return to normal at the expense of a higher level of PTH has been proposed (9) and could have been operating. Moderately uremic dogs had elevated serum phosphorus and depressed calcitriol (Fig. 1). These changes contribute to the hyperparathyroidism (8,9). In marked uremia, serum phosphorus and PTH had large increases without further change in serum calcitriol suggesting a counterbalancing of their opposing influences upon its renal synthesis (8,9). These results are similar to recent data from humans (2), supporting the view that these dogs can be useful in establishing

Vitamin D. A Chemical, Biochemical and Clinical Update

relationships among uremic factors of serum phosphorus, calcitriol and PTH in aged human patients.

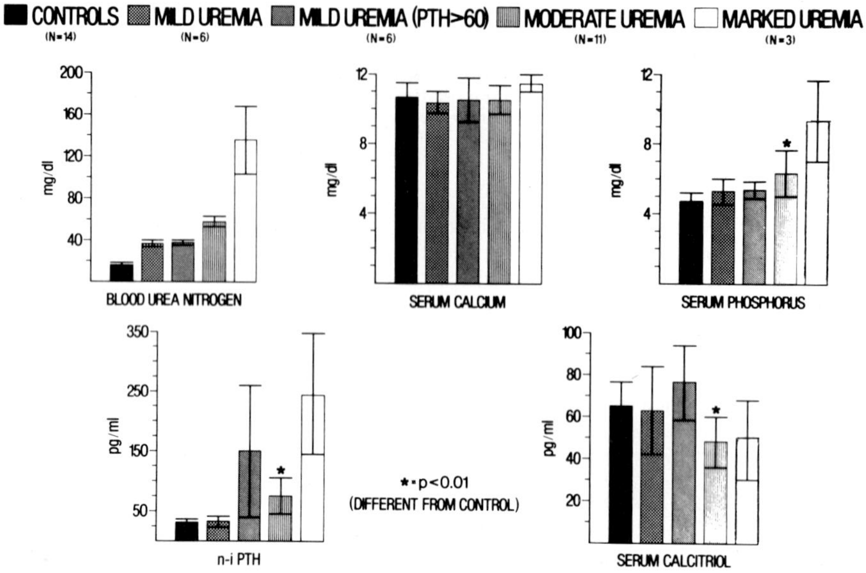

Fig. 1: Biochemical parameters of uremia in aged beagles. Data indicated are mean ±s.d. Significant differences were determined by Student t test.

Supported by a grant from the Morris Animal Foundation

REFERENCES

1. Haussler, M.R. and McCain, T.A. (1977) New Eng. J. Med. 297, 1041-1050.
2. Cheung, A.K., Manolagas, S.C., Catherwood, B.D., Mosely, C.A., Mitas, J.A., Blantz, R.C., and Deftos, L.J. (1983) Kidney Int. 24, 104-109.
3. Portale, A.A., Booth, B.E., Halloran, B.P., and Morris, R.C. (1984) J. Clin. Invest. 73, 1580-1589.
4. Marcus, R., Madvig, P., and Young, G. (1984) J. Clin. Endocrinol. Metab. 58, 223-230.
5. Norrdin, R.W., Bordier, P., and Miller, C.W. (1977) Virchows Arch. [A Pathol. Anat. Histol.] 375, 169-183.
6. Endres, D., Brickman, A., Goodman, W., Maloney, N., and Sherrard, D. (1982) Kidney Int. 21, 132.
7. Segre, G. (1983) In: Clinical Disorders of Bone and Mineral Metabolism (B. Frame and J.P. Potts, eds.) Excerpta Medica, Amsterdam, 14-17.
8. Fournier, A., Sebert, J.L., Moriniere, P. Gregoire, I., de Fremont, J.F., Tahiri, Y., and Dkhissi, H. (1984) Hormone Res. 20, 44-58.
9. Coburn, J.W. (1980) Kidney Int. 17, 677-693.
10. Slatopolsky, E., Gray, R., Adams, N.D., Lewis, J., Hruska, K., Martin, K., Klahr, S., and DeLuca, H.F. (1978) Kidney Int. 14, 733.
11. Nagode, L.A., and Steinmeyer, C.L. (1979) In: Vitamin D, Basic Research and Its Clinical Application (A.W. Norman et al., eds.) Walter de Gruyter, Berlin, 567-570.

<u>SERUM 25-HYDROXYVITAMIN D CONCENTRATIONS IN CHRONIC RENAL FAILURE</u>.

T.J. Furlong, L.S. Ibels, R.S. Mason, A. Trube, S. Posen. Departments of Endocrinology and Renal Medicine, Royal North Shore Hospital, St. Leonards, NSW 2065, Australia.

There have been conflicting reports concerning the blood levels of 25OHD in patients with chronic renal diseases (1-8). Values amongst non-dialyzed patients have been reported to be decreased (1,2,4,6-8) increased (3) or normal (5). In histological studies from this unit (6) and elsewhere (4) it was shown that the severity of osteomalacia in chronic stable renal failure was negatively correlated with serum concentrations of 25OHD while no such correlation could be established in dialysis patients (see Chan et al., this volume). We recently re-investigated this problem in 162 patients.

PATIENTS AND METHODS

There were 61 non-nephrotic patients with stable chronic renal failure (CRF) and serum creatinine values of 0.15 mmol/l or greater. Patients with serum albumin values of 30 g/l or less and patients taking vitamin D compounds were excluded from this group. There were 57 patients on hemodialysis not receiving vitamin D compounds and 25 receiving calcitriol (0.1-0.5 μg/day). There were 19 patients on regular peritoneal dialysis who were not receiving vitamin D compounds. The normal controls were apparently healthy hospital and laboratory staff. Serum and urine creatinine were measured by standard picrate methods with automated equipment, serum albumin by an automated bromocresol green method, urine protein by the benzethonium turbidometric method and serum 25OHD by a modified method of Mason and Posen (9).

RESULTS

Serum 25OHD concentrations of undialyzed patients with CRF (63.8±24.3 nmol/l) were not significantly different from those of normal subjects (69.8±29.6 nmol/l). Serum 25OHD values amongst these patients could not be correlated with serum creatinine, the reciprocal of serum creatinine, urine protein or urine protein creatinine ratios though there was a positive correlation between serum albumin and serum 25OHD (r= 0.5301, p<0.001). Patients on hemodialysis had serum 25OHD concentrations (91.7±49.2 nmol/l) significantly higher than those of normal subjects (p<0.02) or those of undialyzed patients with CRF (p<0.001). There was no significant difference between 25OHD concentrations of hemodialysis patients receiving oral calcitriol and those not receiving this medication. Patients on peritoneal dialysis had significantly lower serum 25OHD concentrations (44.2±22.8 nmol/l) than the other groups (p<0.001 in each case).

Vitamin D. A Chemical, Biochemical and Clinical Update

DISCUSSION

The 61 undialyzed patients in this study differed from those presented in previous papers in 2 important aspects: They were not referred for skeletal biopsies and they were not hypoproteinemic. While we did not question the patients specifically about skeletal symptoms we dealt with relatively "healthy" outpatients and presume that there were few individuals with gross osteomalacia of the type described by Eastwood et al. (4) and Mason et al. (6). Similarly, while we did not specifically exclude patients with gross proteinuria, the exclusion of hypoproteinemics automatically reduced the number of such individuals leaving a relatively narrow range of urinary protein values. We believe this virtual exclusion of patients with severe proteinuria may have caused the lack of correlation between serum 25OHD concentrations and urinary protein measurements which are imprecise at low values (10). The high 25OHD values amongst hemodialysis patients are presumably due to a prolonged turnover time in such subjects whilst the patients on peritoneal dialysis presumably lose various proteins (including D-binding protein) in the dialysates.

REFERENCES

1. Bayard, F., Bec, P., Thon That, H., Louve, J.P. Europ. J. Clin. Invest. 3: 447-450, 1973.

2. Offerman, G., Von Herrath, D., Schaefer, K. Nephron 13: 269-277, 1974.

3. Lund, B., Sorensen, O.H., Nielsen, S.P., Munck, O., Barenholdt, O., Petersen, K. Lancet 2: 372, 1975.

4. Eastwood, J.B., Harris, E., Stamp, T.C.B., DeWardener, H.E. Lancet 2: 1209-1211, 1976.

5. Pietrek, J., Kokot, F. Europ. J. Clin. Invest. 7: 283-287, 1977.

6. Mason, R.S., Lissner, D., Wilkinson, M., Posen, S. Clin. Endocrinol. 13: 375-385, 1980.

7. Kano, K., Nonoda, A., Yoneshima, H., Suda, T. Clin. Nephrology 14: 274-279, 1980.

8. Juttmann, J.R., Buurman, C.J., De Kam, E., Visser, T.J., Birkenhager, J.C. Clin. Endocrinol. 14: 225-236, 1981.

9. Mason, R.S., Posen, S. Clin. Chem. 23: 806-810, 1977.

10. Dilena, B.A., Penberthy, L.A., Fraser, C.G. Clin. Chem. 29: 553-557, 1983.

DOES THE SOLAR IRRADIATION COMPENSATE PERITONEAL LOSS OF 25(OH)D ON CAPD PATIENTS?

M.E. MARTINEZ*, J.L. MIGUEL, G. BALAGUER*, R. SELGAS, P. CATALAN*, A.R. CARMONA, A. PEREZ* and L. SANCHEZ SICILIA.
Biochemistry* and Nephrology Services.C.S. LA PAZ, Madrid 28046, SPAIN.

INTRODUCTION

Low levels of 25(OH)D in serum have been described in patients on continuous ambulatory peritoneal dialysis (CAPD) (1,2,3)and are attributed to a peritoneal loss of this metabolite and its transport proteins (4-5). There are also studies which show a progressive decrease in the values through the time that the patient is on CAPD (1). In previous studies we have been able to show that, in our geographic area, the levels of 25(OH)D are lower in the patients on CAPD than normal controls (3) after the period of lower solar irradiation (March, April), but there is no progressive decrease in their levels through the time on dialysis. Since in our geographic area there are important variations in the levels of 25(OH)D through the year in normal controls which are dependant on the season, the object of our study is to quantify the levels of this metabolite in patients on CAPD and find out wether solar irradiation might compensate the peritoneal loss.

MATERIALS AND METHODS

Subjects studied

We have studied 51 patients on CAPD through 2 years with a total of 167 determinations. 69% were women, the mean age was 45±15 years with an average time on dialysis of 25±16 months, range (3-60). The exchange pattern of dialysis was of three exchanges of 5 hours and 1 of 6 hours. The dialysate used contained 1.5 % glucose and 7 mg of calcium.

The patients were not restricted protein in their intake, nor did they receive treatment with either vitamin D or 25(OH)D.

The control group consisted of 73 normal subjects with a total of 80 determinations through 2 years, 57% were women and the mean age of the group was 33±9 years.

The normal subjects and the patients on CAPD were resident in the Madrid area of Spain within a radius of 50 km.

Method

The levels of 25(OH)D were quantified by protein-binding by a comercial method (Bülhman), after purification by HPLC (6).

RESULTS

In the patients on CAPD we found, as in the normal controls, significant variations in the levels of 25(OH)D through the year

In any season of the year the levels were always lower in patients on CAPD than in the normal controls

The percentage of patients with levels below the lower limit of the normal range were 72 in winter, 29 in spring, 13 in summer and 43 in autumn (Fig I .

We found no relationship between the time on dialysis and the levels of 25(OH)D.

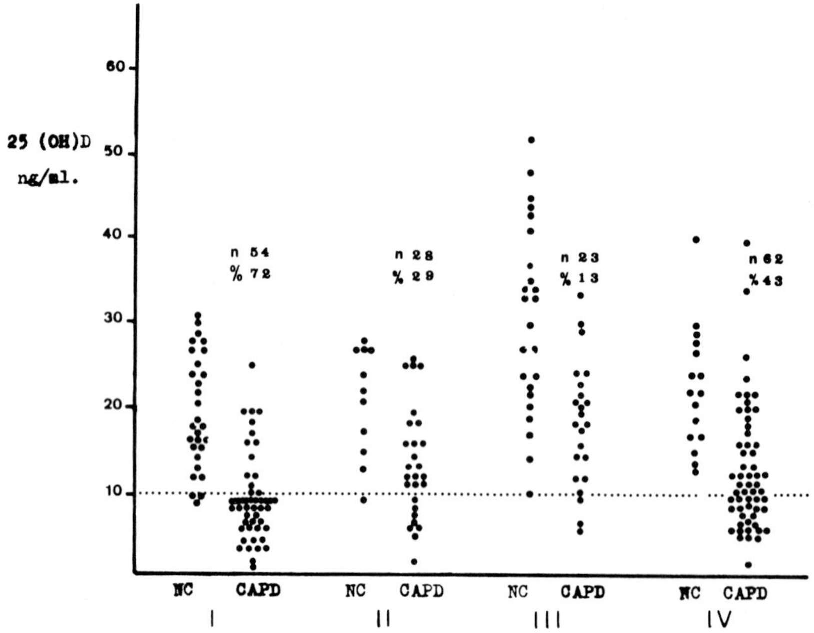

FIGURE.I

LEVELS OF 25(OH)D IN NORMAL CONTROLS(NC)AND IN PATIENTS ON CAPD IN THE FOUR SEASONS OF THE YEAR.WINTER(I),SPRING(II),SUMMER(III)AND AUTUMN(IV).DOTTED LINE SHOW THE LOWEST NORMAL RANGE.(n)INDICATE THE NUMBER OF DETERMINATIONS AND (%)THE PROPORTION OF THESE BELOW NORMAL LEVELS.

CONCLUSION

In the patients on CAPD of our geographic area, we confirmed that the levels of 25(OH)D were lower than in normal controls.

The levels seem to be influenced more by the seasons than by the time on dialysis.

If we quantify the values of 25(OH)D in the season of highest solar irradiation, it would be possible to misinterpret the results since they are within the normal range. However, during the other seasons of the year the levels are below the normal range.

REFERENCES

(1) Digenis,G., Khanna,R.,Pierratos,A.,Meema,H.E.,Rabinovich,S.,Petit,J., Oreopoulos,D.G.(1983).Perit. Dial. Bull.3(2):81-86.

(2) Aloni,Y.,Shany,S.,Chaimovitz,C.(1983).Mineral Electrolite Metab.9:82-86.

(3) Miguel,J.L.,Martinez,M.E.,Carmona,A.R.,Selgas,R., Balaguer,G., Carrasco,A.,Ibarra,M.,Martinez Ara,J.,Sanchez Sicilia,L.(1984).Kidney Int. 26:218 (Abstract).

(4) Delmez,J.A.,Slatopolsky,E.,Martin,K.J.,Gearing,B.N.,Harter,H.R.(1982). Kidney Int. 21:862-867.

(5) Guillot,M.,Lavocat,C.,Garabedian,M.,Sachs,C.,Balsan,S.,Gagnadoux,M.F., Broyer,M.(1981).Proc.EDTA.18:290-292.

(6) Traba,M.L.,Quesada,M.,Marin,A.,De La Piedra,C.,Babé,M.,Navarro,F.(1984) Rev. Esp. Fisiol. 40: 69-76.

EFFECT OF 1.25 VITAMIN D TREATMENT AND IRON STORES ON ALUMINIUM GASTROINTESTINAL ABSORPTION

JB Cannata, B Díaz-Lopez, MV Cuesta, C Rodriguez-Suarez, A Sanz-Medel.
Hospital General de Asturias. Facultad de Medicina y Ciencias Químicas. Universidad de Oviedo. Asturias, Spain.

Introduction

The risk of aluminium(Al) gastro-intestinal(GI) absorption from Al-containing phosphate(P) binders is almost worldwide accepted, nonetheless the Al-absorptive mechanism is still unknown. Since Berlyne, more than 10 years ago(1), alerted over the risk of its absorption, several factors have been blamed for enhancing Al-GI absorption
Therefore, the aim of this prospective study was to evaluate the effect of different iron stores and 1.25 vitamin D treatment on Al GI absorption in a group of patients exposed to the same dose of aluminium hydroxide($Al(OH)_3$).

Patients and Methods

We studied 29 haemodialysis(HD) patients dialysed thrice weekly with the same schedule(13.5 hours/week) using deionised water with low-Al content($< 0.3 \mu mol/l$). All patients were receiving water soluble vitamin supplements and a single fasting dose of ferrous sulphate(100-300 mg/day), they were also having $Al(OH)_3$(the necessary dose to keep serum P between 1.5-1.8 mmol/l; 4.6-5.6 mg%). In day 0 (**$Al(OH)_3$ change**) we stopped the ferrous sulphate and all patients received during the following seven days the same dose of $Al(OH)_3$(6 tablets of 475 mg=2.85 g/day). Serum Ferritin levels and parathyroid hormone (PTH) concentration were measured before introducing the 2.85 g dose (**Basal values**) using enzyme immunoanalysis(ELISA) and a human C terminal radioimmunoassay(INC) in which normal values are those lower than 1.5 ng/ml. Serum Al was measured in the Basal period and seven days after introducing the 2.85 g $Al(OH)_3$ dose (**Post-exposure**), using inductively coupled emission spectrometry.

Results

As the table I shows, patients with high iron stores (mean serum Ferritin:464 ng/ml, n=6) maintained the serum P significantly lower than the low-normal serum Ferritin group (mean serum Ferritin:91.5 ng/ml, n=23), needing significantly less $Al(OH)_3$ intake and therefore having significantly lower basal serum Al values. In all cases the 2.85 g dose meant a significant increase of $Al(OH)_3$ intake, being the highest($p < 0.005$) in the high serum Ferritin group. Nevertheless, this group was the only who did not show any change in serum Al compared with basal values. In contrast, patients with low-normal serum Ferritin levels increased their serum Al concentration almost proportionally to the $Al(OH)_3$ dose change. In this group, (serum Ferritin $<$ 250) those patients having 1.25 vitamin D treatment (n=13, mean dose:0.20 µg/day, range:0.125-0.5 µg/day)

Vitamin D. A Chemical, Biochemical and Clinical Update

had a more marked serum Al increase ($p < 0.05$) than those patients not receiving vitamin D metabolites treatment (n=10) (Figure 1). There were no differences regarding PTH levels in patients with or without 1.25 vitamin D treatment.

	Basal values		$Al(OH)_3$ change	Post-exposure	
	sFerr<250	sFerr>250		sFerr<250	sFerr>250
$Al(OH)_3$ (g/day)	1.78±1.7 *	0.77±1.1		2.8	2.8
Serum P (mmol/l)	1.68±03 *	1.31±03		---	---
Serum Al (μmol/l)	2.95±2.0 *	1.61±0.7		4.25±2.6 *	1.90±0.8
Serum PTH (ng/ml)	4.27±2.7	3.56±1.8		---	---

Table I : Basal and Post-exposure values in patients with high (* $p < 0.05$) and low-normal serum Ferritin(sFerr) levels. (± SD)

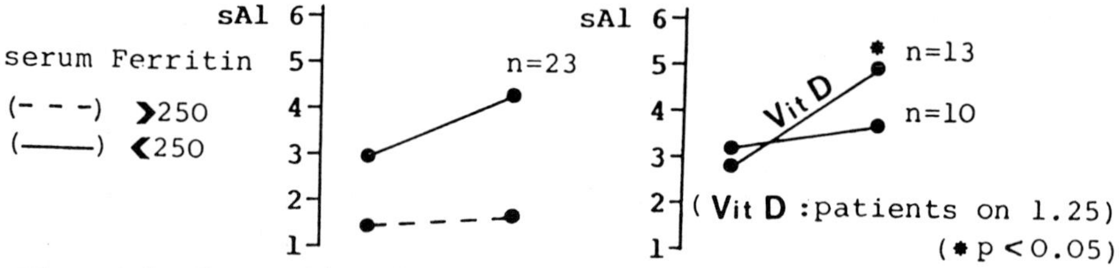

Figure 1:-Serum Al(sAl)(μmol/l). Basal and post-exposure

Discussion

In our study, patients having proportionally smaller doses of 1.25 vitamin D appeared to absorb more Al than those without vitamin D treatment, suggesting that even low-dose vitamin D metabolites could influence Al metabolism.
Although these are preliminary results with a short number of patients and further studies are needed, we suggest (2) that patients with repleted iron stores might have less chance to absorb Al and patients with low-normal iron stores would absorb Al more easily. In the latter group, 1.25 vitamin D seems to enhance Al absorption. If this is the case, serum Ferritin would be a good predictor of Al absorption and a useful index to select patients at higher risk of Al hyper-absorption while undergoing vitamin D metabolites treatment.

References

1. Berlyne GM,Ben-Ari J,Pest D,Weinberger J,Stern M,Gilmore GR,Levine R. (1970) Lancet 2,494-96.
2. Cannata JB,Suarez-Suarez C,Cuesta MV,Rodriguez-Roza R, Allende MT,Herrera J,Perez-Llanderal J. (1984) Eur Dial Transplant Assoc Proc 21, (in press).

SERUM BONE GLA PROTEIN (BGP) AND SECONDARY HYPERPARATHYROIDISM IN PREDIALYSIS CHRONIC RENAL FAILURE (CRF)

G. Coen, S. Mazzaferro, E. Bonucci, P. Ballanti, C. Massimetti, G. Donato, F. Bondatti, A. Smacchi, G.A. Cinotti and F. Taggi
Division of Nephrology and Dept. of Human Biopathology, Univ."La Sapienza"; Istituto Superiore di Sanità; Rome, Italy

The bone GLA protein (BGP) or osteocalcin, is a vit.K-dependent protein of bone produced by the osteoblasts (1). Its synthesis is stimulated by $1,25(OH)_2D_3$ (1,25D) (2). Serum levels of BGP are increased when bone turnover is accelerated (3). In spite of low levels of 1,25D in CRF serum BGP is increased (3). This finding has been mainly attributed to decreased renal disposal and consequent accumulation. The aim of this study was to correlate BGP levels with serum creatinine (Cr_s) and other humoral and bone histomorphometric parameters in order to establish whether BGP in CRF is a predictive index of osteodystrophy. The effects of long-term treatment with 1,25D on serum BGP levels have also been evaluated.

Patients and Methods:

A total of 42 patients (25 males and 17 females) with CRF with a mean age of 47.5±16.6 years were studied. Cr_s ranged from 1.5 to 9 mg/dl (4.32±1.9). 19 patients were studied within a short period,while 23 were followed with repeated biochemical controls for 17.1±8.1 months. Eleven of these patients were treated with daily doses of 1,25D, 0.25 ug, for a mean of 16.8±6.4 months. The patients were on a diet moderately restricted in proteins(0.8 g/kg b.w.) and phosphorus (12 mg/kg b.w.) and received supplements of calcium per os. In 23 patients at various stages of renal failure (Cr_s6.42 ± 2.25 mg/dl), not receiving 1,25D, a transiliac bone biopsy was performed. Serum BGP was measured by radioimmunoassay based on the method of Price et al. (4). Our normal values are 3.89±1.45 ng/ml). Serum iPTH was measured by a C-term radioimmunoassay (n.v. 0.34±0.19 ng/ml). Alkaline Phosphatase (AP) and Cr_s were measured with standard techniques. Histomorphometric evaluation was performed with the image analyzer Videoplan Kontron.

Results:

Serum BGP levels in CRF are generally higher than normal(23.5± 19 ng/ml). With progression of renal failure BGP rises strictly correlated to Cr_s.Data are fitted by a parabolic function ($p<0.001$) showing faster increments of BGP than of Cr_s in the terminal stages of CRF. Highly significant positive correlation was also found between BGP and iPTH ($p<0.001$) and BGP and AP ($p<0.001$). The correlations between bone histomorphometric parameters and BGP, AP and iPTH are reported in the table. OV correlated with BGP ($p<0.01$) and AP ($p<0.01$). OS and TIO correlated to a lesser degree ($p<0.05$) with BGP and AP. AOS% correlated with BGP, AP and iPTH equally ($p<0.01$). The same humoral parameters correlated even better and to the same degree with ARS% and OI ($p<0.001$). In this subpopulation of 23 patients BGP was more strongly correlated to bone parameters indicative of the extent of bone turnover (ARS%, OI, AOS%) than with Cr_s ($p<0.05$). The effects of treatment with 1,25D on serum BGP are shown in the figure. The D metabolite induced a decline of

Vitamin D. A Chemical, Biochemical and Clinical Update

Tab.1. Correlations between BGP, AP, iPTH and histomorphometric parameters

	BGP	AP	PTH
Total Bone Volume %	.212	.161	.130
Osteoid Volume %	.531[b]	.575[b]	.324
Osteoid Surface %	.423[a]	.473[a]	.366
Active Osteoid Surface %	.537[b]	.558[b]	.552[b]
Resorption Surface %	.649[c]	.574[b]	.618[b]
Active Resorption Surface %	.836[c]	.823[c]	.651[c]
Osteoclastic Index n°/mm^2	.835[c]	.826[c]	.657[c]
Thickness Index of Osteoid	.502[a]	.497[a]	.185

a = $p<0.05$; b = $p<0.01$; c = $p<0.001$

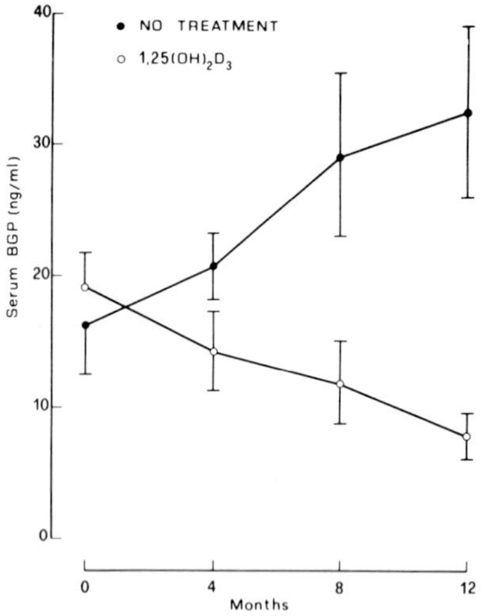

BGP while in the control patients BGP increased progressively. The difference between the slopes of treated and untreated patients was significant (Mann-Whitney U test, ($p<0.001$). The decline in BGP was parallel to the decrease in iPTH levels while no correlation was found between BGP and AP during treatment.

Discussion: The results show that with advancing renal failure serum BGP levels increase, at a faster rate in the terminal stages. However analysis of the data from the subpopulation of patients subjected to bone biopsy showed a better degree of correl-tion between BGP and iPTH ($p<0.001$) and BGP and the histomorphometric parameters indicative of bone turnover than between BGP and Cr_S. The severety of bone disease seems to be a major determinant of serum BGP levels. This conclusion agrees with the finding of the parallel decrese in BGP and iPTH during long-term treatment with 1,25D. The strong correlation between BGP and bone resorption parameters ($p<0.001$), shared also by AP, does not necessarily imply that BGP originates from the resorption of bone, since this parameter is tightly coupled to bone formation. Therefore our results should not be considered in disagreement with other published data (2) which demonstrate that BGP is produced by the osteoblasts. In conclusion serum BGP is an important index of bone turnover which can also be employed in the long-term monitoring of the effects of treatment with 1,25D os secondary hyperparathyroidism in predialysis CRF.

Aknowledgement: This study was supported by funds of Ministero della Pubblica Istruzione

References:

1. Nishimoto,S.K.,Price,P.A. (1979) J.Biol.Chem. 255,6579-6583.
2. Beresford,J.N.,Gallagher,J.A.,Poser,J.W.,Russell,R.G.G. (1984) Metab. Bone Dis. & Rel.Res. 5, 229-234.
3. Deftos,L.J.,Parthemore,J.G.,Price,P.A. (1982) Calcif.Tissue Int. 34, 121-124.
4. Price,P.A.,Nishimoto,S.K. (1980) Proc.Natl.Acad.Sci. 77,2234-2238.

EVOLUTION OF CALCIUM-PHOSPHATE METABOLISM IN CHILDHOOD CHRONIC RENAL FAILURE.

M.L.Bianchi, A.Claris-Appiani , L.Romeo , F.Ulivieri, E.Corghi
Clinica Medica I, Clinica Pediatrica II-Università di Milano

Introduction

Recent advances in the natural history of renal osteodystrophy still leave many open questions on the role of calciotropic hormones and on the evolution of the disease with respect to the degree of renal insufficiency. Most studies have been conducted in adults, and there is considerable paucity of data in the osteodystrophy of childhood renal failure (1-3).
Our study was aimed at determining the presence and evolution of renal osteodystrophy in children with renal insufficiency of different degree.

Patients

17 children, affected by tubulo-interstitial disease, were studied for one year. They were divided in 2 groups according to the levels of creatinine clearance:

GROUP 1: 10 children, mean age 7.7±1 yrs, initial GFR 47±1.4-final GFR 47.8±2.4 ml/min/1.73 m^2;

GROUP 2: 7 children, mean age 9.6±1.5 yrs, initial GFR 26.9±3.6-final GFR 26±3.2 ml/min/1.73 m^2.

Both groups followed an unrestricted diet (800 mg/day of calcium on average). During the study no variation of diet or life habits were introduced.

Methods

The following determinations were made at the beginning and every month, using standard laboratory methods: creatinine, calcium, phosphate (plasma and urine), alkaline phosphatase (plasma) and hydroxyproline (urine). At the beginning and every 6 months plasma PTH (PTH-COOH and PTH-NH_2) and 1,25(OH)$_2D_3$ and 25-OH D_3 were also checked, by RIA and protein-binding assay, respectively. At the beginning and after 1 year, bone mineral content (BMC) was evaluated at forearm midshaft by direct photon absorptiometry with a ^{125}I source.

Results

At the beginning, only 3 indexes of mineral metabolism were altered in both groups, with respect to sex/age matched controls: PTH, 1,25(OH)$_2D_3$ (Table I) and urinary hydroxyproline. Moreover, 1,25(OH)$_2D_3$ was also significantly lower in group 2 than in group 1 ($p<.01$).
A positive correlation was found between 1,25(OH)$_2D_3$ levels

Vitamin D. A Chemical, Biochemical and Clinical Update

and GFR ($r=0.73$, $p<.01$).
After one year, a different evolution of renal osteodystrophy was evident in the 2 groups. Group 1 showed an almost unchanged picture, with the exception of a 16% decrease of $1,25(OH)_2D$ (to 21$\pm$1 pg/ml, $p<.01$) and the BMC increased of 12% (controls =+13%). Group 2 showed a severe worsening of all indexes of mineral metabolism, despite a stable GFR: in particular, plasma $1,25(OH)_2D_3$ decreased of 25% (to 12$\pm$2 pg/ml, $p<.01$) and plasma $PTH-NH_2$ increased of 24% (to 289$\pm$29 pg/ml, $p<.01$). The BMC raised only 7% on average.

TABLE I - *Analysis of variance*

	CONTROLS	*GROUP 1*	*GROUP 2*	*p*
PTH-COOH *pg/ml*	397±67	723±231	955±231	<.01
$PTH-NH_2$ *pg/ml*	102±25	162±22	221±17	<.01
25-OH D_3 *ng/ml*	56±4	49±4	41±3	*N.S.*
$1,25(OH)_2D_3$ *pg/ml*	39±3	25±2	16±2	<.01

Conclusions

We think that the decreased production of endogenous $1,25(OH)_2D_3$ could be the most important factor in the progression of renal osteodystrophy. The GFR does not seem to effectively measure the decline of the endocrinologically active renal mass, so that an accelerated progression of RO can be observed even in the presence of a relatively stable GFR.

References

1. Chan,J.C.M., Kodroff,M.B. (1981) J.Pediatrics 68, 559-562
2. Portale,A.A., Booth,B.E., Tsai,H.C., Morris,R.C. (1982) Kidney Int. 21, 627-632
3. Paunier,L., Sallusky,I.B., Slatopolsky, E., Kangarloo,H., Kopple,J.D., Horst,R.L., Coburn,J.W., Fine,R.N. (1984) Pediatric Research 18, 742-747

FEMUR NECK DISEASE (FND) IN UREMIC PATIENTS UNDERGOING DIALYTIC TREATMENT: A VITAMIN D NON RELATED OSTEODYSTROPHY.

D.Brancaccio, G.Verzetti, S.Casati, M.Gallieni, S.Cantoni, G.Graziani, C.Uslenghi, F.Bellini.
Renal Units, Osp. S.Paolo, Osp. Policlinico di Milano, Osp. di Borgomanero
Departments of Radiology, Ospedale S.Paolo and ICP, Milano, Italy.

INTRODUCTION

Among the several pathological consequences of chronic renal failure, bone alterations are of primary importance. Some of them are well known in their pathogenetic mechanisms (e.g. Vit. D related osteodystrophy)(1), others are in the process of being defined (e.g. aluminum related osteodystrophy)(2), while more are probably yet to be discovered.
In uremic patients, especially those undergoing a regular dialytic treatment (RDT), the presence of bone disease is usually monitored by routine X-ray examinations, which also include a film of pelvis and upper femora. During X-ray routine examinations of our patients on RDT we observed a pattern of skeletal patholgy recently described in the literature (3) and we were struck by its remarkable frequency among the dialytic population. In order to more precisely assess the incidence of the lesion we undertook a retrospective study of pelvic X-rays of a group of patients on RDT, and results were compared to those obtained in large control groups.

THE LESION

The initial lesion may be described as multiple osteosclerosis with subsequent formation of the characteristic single cavity, whose X-ray aspect is a round radiolucency in the middle part of the femur neck approximately 1 cm in diameter (Fig. 1). However, multiple small cavities or wider single cavities, with a diameter ranging from a few millimeters to almost 2 cm, were observed; furthermore, in the large majority of patients a surrounding area of osteosclerosis was evident.

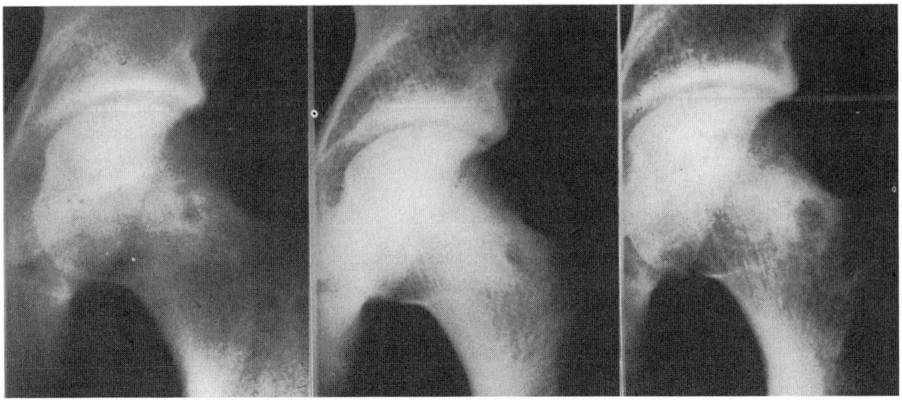

FIGURE 1. Typical evolution of the X-ray appearance of femur neck disease

Vitamin D. A Chemical, Biochemical and Clinical Update

PATIENTS AND METHODS

158 patients affected by chronic renal failure were included in this study. Patients' age spanned from 11 to 75, and some of them began dialysis treatment up to 14 years ago. For each patient we reviewed all available X-rays in order to identify the same lesions at different stages and thereby trace their course of development. All patients had X-rays taken in 1984.

The control group consisted of 483 patients divided into two groups:

a) uremic patients NOT on regular dialytic treatment (n. 60)

b) non uremic patients with random pathologies (n. 423)

RESULTS

We observed lesions of the femur neck in 45 patients on RDT, 15 of whom exhibited bilateral skeletal lesions at one time or another.

The overall frequency of femur neck disease (FND) in this study was 28.5%; the frequencies of FND at the two hospitals in which the population was studied were similar. The frequency of FND in non-uremic controls was 0.5% (2 cases); FND was not observed in the uremic control group.

We could not find any statistically valid correlation between frequency of FND in our uremic patients and both patient age and dialytic age.

The first radiological evidence of a lesion appeared as early as three months after beginning RDT. Lesions seemed to follow three possible courses: slow progression, stable state and regression; in some patients, the course changed from one type to another.

CONCLUSIONS

Considering its high frequency, femur neck disease (FND) could represent a skeletal abnormality common to patients undergoing RDT. Considering the peculiar anatomy of the terminal arterial tree supplying the proximal part of the femur and considering the appearance of the lesion on X-ray, our hypothesis is that the focal bone loss in FND could be ischemic in nature.

FND appears to behave in an unpredictable fashion: the first radiologic evidence of the lesion does not occur at any particular interval after beginning RDT and over a course of a few years, lesions may appear on X-rays, disappear and return later, suggesting that a rapidly changing, high turnover process is at work.

The discrepancy between the apparently high frequnecy of occurrence of FND and low frequency of reports of fractures of the femur neck is yet to be explained.

REFERENCES

1. Frame, B., Parfitt, A.M. (1978) Ann.Int.Med. 89:966-973

2. Ward, M.K., Feest, T.G., Ellis, H.A., Parkinson, I.S., Kerr, D.N. (1978) Lancet 1(8069):841-845

3. Pitt, M.J, Graham, A.R. SHipman, J.H., Birkby, W. (1982) Am.J.Roentg. 138: 1115-1121

CONTROVERSIES IN VITAMIN D TREATMENT FOR RENAL OSTEODYSTROPHY

E. Ritz, J. Merke and O. Mehls
Department Internal Medicine and Pediatrics, University of Heidelberg, Germany (FRG)

Until recently, the genesis of abnormal vitamin D metabolism in renal failure, and its reversal by $1,25(OH)_2D_3$ or its analogues, appear to be straightforward. The classical studies of Liu and Chu and of Stanbury and Lumb (1, 2) had established that abnormalities of Ca metabolism in uremic subjects fail to respond to physiological, but respond to pharmacological doses of vitamin D. Such vitamin D resistance found an elegant and simple explanation in the classical experiments of Kodicek who showed 1-alpha-hydroxylation of 25(OH)D in renal but not extrarenal tissue.
When $1,25(OH)_2D_3$ became available for therapy, it was soon found that administration of $1,25(OH)_2D_3$ to uremic subjects increased intestinal absorption of Ca, raised S-Ca, lowered iPTH, improved osteitis fibrosa clinically (although it falls short of normalizing bone histology), variably improved mineralisation of osteoid (resistance to the secosterol being primarily due to deposition of aluminium) and had extraskeletal effects, e.g. on muscle.
While the clinical usefulness of $1,25(OH)_2D_3$ and other vitamin D metabolites are beyond doubt, several uncertainties persist which shall be discussed in this communication.

1. Should vitamin D metabolites be administered only for treatment of symptomatic bone disease or also for prophylaxis?

While unquestionably $1,25(OH)_2D_3$ ameliorates renal osteitis fibrosa on a clinical, roentgenological and histological level, bone histology is not consistently normalized in patients with established osteitis fibrosa (4).
Apart from the failure of vitamin D or its metabolites to normalize bone histology in uremic patients, when given over prolonged periods of time in doses which normalize intestinal absorption of Ca (4), one additional argument for prophylactic administration comes from recent observations of the role of $1,25(OH)_2D_3$ in the control of PTH secretion (5). Human parathyroid cells have a characteristic receptor for $1,25(OH)_2D_3$, i.e. a 3.5 S binding macromolecule with a K_D of 4×10^{-10}M. Genomic interaction is suggested by binding of nuclear parathyroid cell $1,25(OH)_2D_3$ receptor to DNA affinity columns from which it is eluted with 0.27M KCl (fig. 1).
Despite some previous controversy, it is now established that $1,25(OH)_2D_3$ affects PTH secretion and messenger RNA for prepro-PTH. It was recently established in experimental studies that $1,25(OH)_2D_3$, but not raised ionized serum Ca levels, prevented PTH oversecretion of uremic animals (5). If these findings can be confirmed in humans, it might become necessary to give $1,25(OH)_2D_3$ prophylactically despite normal serum Ca to uremic patients in order to prevent hyperparathyroidism.

Vitamin D. A Chemical, Biochemical and Clinical Update

$1,25(OH)_2D_3$ receptor characterization in human parathyroid adenoma (nuclear fraction)

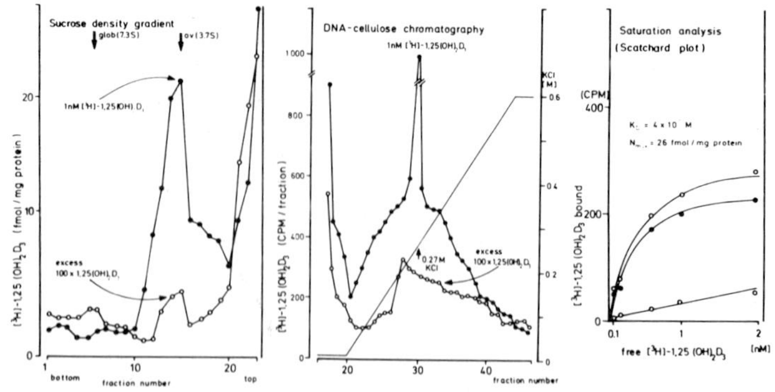

2. <u>At which stage of renal insufficiency should $1,25(OH)_2D_3$ be given prophylactically?</u>

It is currently controversial at what stage of renal failure synthesis of $1,25(OH)_2D_3$ becomes abnormal. Both in humans (6-8) and in experimental animals (9) plasma levels of $1,25(OH)_2D_3$ are normal in incipient renal failure and are not diminished until GFR is 50% normal. However, normal plasma levels by no means indicate adequate regulation of synthesis of the active secosterole. In incipient renal failure (10) the following abnormalities have been demonstrated: fasting serum Ca and Pi levels tend to be low (although this is somewhat controversial), iPTH levels are high and excessive action of PTH on target organs is reflected by increased fractional urinary excretion of cAMP (11) and increased osteoclasts (12). Obviously, in the presence of somewhat low plasma Ca and Pi and elevated PTH one should anticipate elevated $1,25(OH)_2D_3$ levels (10), as for instance in the repair phase of vitamin D deficiency osteomalacia.
One hint for abnormal regulation of $1,25(OH)_2D_3$ synthesis in the basal state has recently been given by Llach (13) who noted an increase of plasma $1,25(OH)_2D_3$ concentrations in response to Pi restriction in patients with incipient renal failure. This was accompanied by lowering of plasma iPTH and restoration of the calcemic response to PTH, indicating that even plasma $1,25(OH)_2D_3$ levels in the normal range had been unable to correct such early abnormalities of calcium metabolism.

One might conclude from these findings that $1,25(OH)_2D_3$ should be administered early in renal failure despite paradoxically normal plasma $1,25(OH)_2D_3$ levels. Indeed, recent studies show that in patients with incipient renal failure iPTH is lowered and urinary cAMP diminished by exogenous $1,25(OH)_2D_3$ (14, 15); in addition, longterm administration of $1,25(OH)_2D_3$ prevented the rise of iPTH and the development of abnormal bone histology (16), but it remains to be established that this measure is generally safe and provides worthwhile longterm benefits to the patient. In more advanced renal failure, the efficacy of routine prophylaxis with $1,25(OH)_2D_3$ in preventing uremic bone disease has been established in prospective placebo controlled trials (17-19).

Abnormal calcium metabolism despite normal plasma $1,25(OH)_2D_3$ would be compatible with an altered dose response relationship. Indeed, as shown in the table (15) in order to raise low UV_{Ca} in patients with incipient renal failure into the range noted in controls, daily administration of 1 µg/day $1,25(OH)_2D_3$ was necessary, close to the estimated endogenous daily production rate. While urinary Ca as an index of $1,25(OH)_2D_3$ action has obvious limitations, the finding is compatible with altered dose response relationship.

Table

	$1,25(OH)_2D_3$		
	0 µg/day		1 µg/day
Controls (n=13)	0.72 ± 1.26	Δ 2.59	6.31 ± 0.44
Early renal failure (n=10)	1.43 ± 0.25	Δ 1.86	3.28 ± 1.96

all data as mmol Ca/day (UV_{Ca})

We recently demonstrated (20) reduced binding capacity for $1,25(OH)_2D_3$ in basal cells of epidermis and Sertoli cells of testis of uremic rats despite low plasma $1,25(OH)_2D_3$. Obviously, the expected homologous upregulation of $1,25(OH)_2D_3$ receptors in target organs does not occur in uremia. Whether reduced binding sites for $1,25(OH)_2D_3$ also imply altered dose response relationship for exogenous $1,25(OH)_2D_3$ remains to be established in future studies.

3. Is $1,25(OH)_2D_3$ the only vitamin D metabolite required to prevent or cure renal osteodystrophy?

In humans, $1,25(OH)_2D_3$ alone was capable of completely healing the bone disease of vitamin D deficiency (21). In addition, in vitamin D deficient rats, 24,24-difluoro-25(OH)vitamin D_3 (a compound which cannot undergo 24-hydroxylation) completely normalized calcium metabolism and bony changes (22) suggesting that $1,25(OH)_2D_3$ alone is able to reverse abnormal calcium metabolism of vitamin D deficiency. Previous reports had claimed that administration of $24,25(OH)_2D_3$ to anephric patients increased intestinal Ca absorption (although this has not been confirmed by others) and reduced PTH secretion in dogs (although this again has not been confirmed by others).

One recent experimental study of Olgaard (23) showed no consistent effect of longterm administration of $24,25(OH)_2D_3$ on $S\text{-}Ca^{++}$, iPTH and bone Ca content or histology in dogs with chronic uremia, casting further doubt on a therapeutic role of this compound. On balance, there is currently lack of solid evidence that $24,25(OH)_2D_3$ is therapeutically efficacious in uremic patients.
One other problem relates to whether or not one should normalize vitamin D status in uremic patients. Low $25(OH)D_3$ levels are not rare in uremic patients (10, 24). It is controversial whether this reflects decreased cutaneous synthesis. Low $25(OH)D_3$ levels are most commonly the result of altered life style with reduced sun exposure, but low dietary intake or concomitant use of phenobarbital may occasionally play an ancillary role. Although we have previously demonstrated low plasma $25(OH)D_3$ levels in nephrotic patients (25) it is uncertain whether plasma levels of absolute free $25(OH)D_3$ are low. Vitamin D depletion, if it ever occurs, must be rare in this condition.

Low $25(OH)D_3$ levels may be important, since Bayard (26) and later Schmidt-Gayk (27) noted an inverse relation of plasma Ca and $25(OH)D_3$ in uremic patients. This may reflect substrate dependency of low residual circulating $1,25(OH)_2D_3$ levels and/or of local 1-alpha-hydroxylase in bone cells.

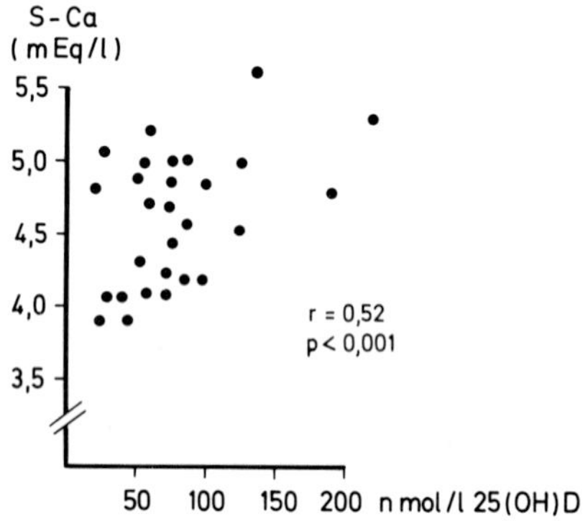

Schmidt Gayk et al, Calc. Tiss 22, 431 1977

One further consideration in this respect is the previous observation of Birge and Haddad (28) that $25(OH)D_3$ has unique actions, for instance on phosphate transport in muscle, which are not shared by $1,25(OH)_2D_3$. Although $25(OH)D_3$ levels in plasma are not regulated, $25(OH)D_3$ may generally have a permissive action on functions like phosphate flux across plasma cell membranes. These and other considerations provide a rationale to normalize low plasma 25(OH)D_3 levels, if present, in uremic patients by administration of 25(OH)D_3 or cholecalciferol, even when the patients receive adequate amounts of 1,25$(OH)_2D_3$.

4. Are 1,25$(OH)_2D_3$ or other vitamin D metabolites able to correct growth disturbance of uremia?

In previous experimental studies we could show (29, 30) that both vitamin D_3 and 1,25$(OH)_2D_3$ in equipotent eucalcemic doses improve, but fail to normalize, impaired growth in uremic rats (fig. 3).

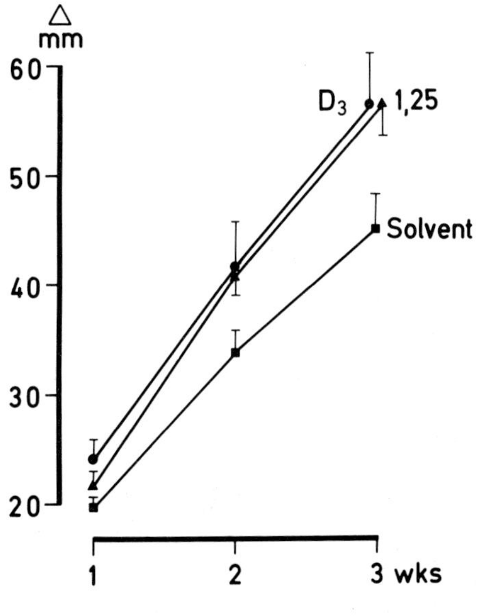

Intense interest was generated by the original communication of Chesney (31) that 1,25$(OH)_2D_3$ promoted growth in some uremic children who had failed to respond to high doses of vitamin D_3, implying a specific action of 1,25$(OH)_2D_3$ on disturbed skeletal growth in uremia. While this initial observation was supported by subsequent similar observations (32), the high hopes in this respect have been dashed by recent studies comprising larger number of subjects (33). Fig. 4 summarizes experience in children treated either with vitamin D_3; 1,25$(OH)_2D_3$ or maintenance hemodialysis. It is obvious that none of these interventions consistently corrected growth disturbance.

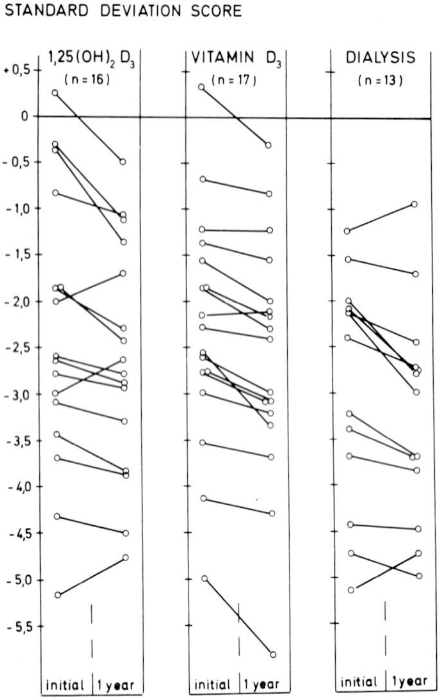

after ref. 33 (with permission)

5. Does administration of $1,25(OH)_2D_3$ to uremic patients ameliorate organ dysfunction unrelated to Ca homeostasis?

Intense interest has recently been generated by the demonstration of receptors for $1,25(OH)_2D_3$ in, and actions of $1,25(OH)_2D_3$ on, non-classical target organs for vitamin D, e.g. various endocrine systems, skeletal muscle, epidermis, macrophages and several cell species of the hematolymphatic system. Abnormalities of most of these systems have been demonstrated in uremia (34). This raises theimportant question whether some aspects of uremia are caused not by cumulation of toxins, but by deficiency of the normal renal secretory product $1,25(OH)_2D_3$. Of course one cannot predict whether lack of renal $1,25(OH)_2D_3$ is in part compensated for by local, possibly paracrine, generation of $1,25(OH)_2D_3$ in various tissues via extrarenal 1-alpha-hydroxylase or by low residual circulating $1,25(OH)_2D_3$ levels. In future it will be important, however, to examine whether exogenous administration of $1,25(OH)_2D_3$ ameliorates dysfunction of organs unrelated to calcium homeostasis. At least for skeletal muscle there is some evidence in this respect (35).

6. Does administration of $1,25(OH)_2D_3$ post longterm hazards?

The harzards of treating uremic patients with vitamin D metabolites are well known and need not be discussed in detail e.g. hypercalcemia (particularly in immobilized patients and patients with aluminium intoxication) or hyperphosphatemia (posing the hazards of raised Ca x Pi product and stimulation of PTH secretion). The pharmacokinetic properties of $1,25(OH)_2 D_3$, i.e. short elimination half life (which may be an advantage in case of intoxication) is sometimes a disadvantage if patient compliance is not impeccable and for such practical considerations metabolites which longer half life, e.g. $25(OH)D_3$ may better ensure clinical efficacy. The controversy whether $1,25(OH)_2D_3$ decreases glomerular filtration rate independent of hypercalcemia or hypercalciuria appears to be settled. The consensus today is that no such intrinsic nephrotoxicity exists for $1,25(OH)_2D_3$ (36), but this of course does not obviate the necessity to carefully avoid hypercalcemia and/or hypercalciuria in patients treated with this secosterole. However, other adverse longterm effects must be considered and looked for in the future. We have recently been able to show that $1,25(OH)_2D_3$ reversibly affects ultrastructure of aortic smooth muscle cells in tissue culture (to be published). Cholecalciferol is known to accelerate atherogenesis in non-uremic animals (37) and it is of even more concern that Tvedegaard (38) noted more severe atherosclerosis in uremic cholesterol-fed rabbits when 1-alpha-D_3 was administered. Recently, interactions between $1,25(OH)_2D_3$ and pressor systems have been recognized in hypertensive patients. The implications of this for treatment of uremic patients with $1,25(OH)_2D_3$ have not been worked out.

It is hoped that the various problems raised in this lecture will be solved in the near future.

References:

1. Liu S.H., Chu H.I. Medicine (Baltimore) 22, 103, 1943
2. Stanbury S.W., Lumb G.A. Medicine (Baltimore) 41, 1, 1962
3. Fraser D., Kodicek E. Nature 228, 764, 1970
4. Malluche H., Ritz E., Werner E., Meyer-Sabellek W. Clin. Nephrol. 10, 219, 1978
5. Lopez S. et al., 17th Ann.Meet.Am.Soc.Nephr., Washington DC, Dec. 1984, a 25
6. Slatopolsky E. et al. Kidney Intern. 14, a 177, 1978
7. Ogura Y. et al. Contr. Nephrol. 22, 18, 1980
8. Rickers H. et al. Nephron 39, 267, 1985
9. Taylor C. et al. Kidney Intern. 24, 47, 1983
10. Ritz E., Rambausek M., Kreusser W., Mehls O. Bone metabolism in renal disease; in: Recent Advances in Renal Medicine; Jones N., Peters D., Eds., Churchill Edinburgh 1982, pp 151-166
11. Kleerekoper M. et al. Adv. Exp. Med. Biol. 128, 145, 1980
12. Malluche H.H. et al. Kidney Int. 9, 355, 1976

13. Llach F., Massry SG., Koffler A., Malluche H., Singer F., Brickman A., Kurokawa K. Kidney Intern. 12, a 459, 1977
14. Wilson L.et al. Kidney Intern. 25, a 254, 1984
15. Kremer B., Lübbers E., Klooker P., Schmidt-Gayk H., Ritz, E. Min. Electr. Metab. (in press)
16. Massry S.G. Abstr. VI Workshop Vitamin D 1985, a 375
17. Sharman V.L. et al. Proc. EDTA 19, 287, 1982
18. Memmos D.E. et al. Br.Med.J. 282, 1919, 1981
19. Coburn J.W. et al. in: Vitamin D: Chemical, Biochemical and Clinical Endocrinology of Calcium Metabolism, Berlin, Walter de Gruyter, 1982
20. Merke J. et al., 22nd Congr. Eur.Dial.Transpl.Ass., Bruxelles 1985 (in press)
21. Papapoulos S.E. et al. Lancet ii, 612, 1980
22. Parfitt A.M. et al. J. Clin. Invest. 73, 576, 1984
23. Olgaard K. et al., Kidney Int. 26, 791, 1984
24. Ritz E. et al. Advances Nephrol. 9, 71, 1980
25. Schmidt-Gayk K.H. et al. Lancet ii, 105, 1977
26. Bayard F. et al. Eur.J.Clin.Invest. 3, 447, 1973
27. Schmidt-Gayk H. et al. Calc.Tiss. 22, 430, 1985
28. Birge S.J. et al. J. Clin.Invest. 56, 1100, 1975
29. Mehls O. et al. Am.J.Clin.Nutr. 31, 1927, 1978
30. Mehls O. et al. Kidney Int. 24, 53, 1983
31. Chesney R.W. et al. New Engl.J.Med. 298, 238, 1978
32. Robitaille P. et al. Acta Paed. Scand. 73, 315, 1984
33. Bulla M. et al. Klin. Wschr. 58, 511, 1980
34. Ritz E. in: Nephrology II (Proc. 9th Intern.Congr.Nephrol. Los Angeles, 1984)
35. Ritz E. et al. Am.J.Clin.Nutr. 33, 1522, 1980

VITAMIN D METABOLITES AND PARATHYROID HORMONE FRAGMENTS IN THE MILK-ALKALI SYNDROME

M. REINER, Department of Medicine, Ospedale Beata Vergine, CH-6850 Mendrisio, Switzerland.

The Milk-Alkali syndrome, due to excessive milk and calcium carbonate intake, is characterized by metabolic alkalosis, hypercalcemia, renal failure and soft tissue calcification (1). Since the introduction of non-absorbable antacids and H2-receptor blockers in peptic ulcer therapy it has become extremely rare (2).

A 50 years old man, who suffered for the past 10 years of pyloric ulcer took 10 grams calcium carbonate and 2 liters milk daily, presented during 2 weeks before admission with weakness, thirst, polyuria, burning red eyes from corneal calcification and depression. His laboratory results on admission were: Ca 4,08 mmol/l, P 1,24 mmol/l alkaline phosphatase 88 IU/l (N 170), creatinine 650 µmol/l, pH 7,50, pCO2 51,6, standard bicarbonate 38,5, PTH (C-assay) 107 ng/ml (N < 40). By rehydration and low-calcium diet the serum calcium became normal within 5 days. The possible co-existence of a primary hyperparathyroidism, masked by vitamin D deficiency in a chronic alcoholic (he also drank 2 liters of wine daily!) was ruled out by the spontaneous course of the laboratory results:

	3.6.83	14.7.83	normal values
PTH (C-assay)	107	29	(< 40 ng/ml)
PTH (N-assay)	0,35	0,19	(< 0,25 ng/ml)
Calcium	4,08	2,60	(2,1-2,60 mmol/l)
Creatinine	650	110	(44-130 µmol/l)
25 OH D3	4,3	33	(23-85 nmol/l)
1,25 (OH)2 D3	27	68	(59-170 pmol/l)

In the Milk-Alkali syndrome the decreased renal clearance of the biologically inactive C-terminal fragment of PTH results in a raised immunoreactive PTH, although the active PTH secretion is partially suppressed by hypercalcemia. This can simulate a primary hyperparathyroidism, which could hypothetically coexist as the cause of the ulcer. The Vitamin D metabolites are low because of the negative feedback by hypercalcemia.

1. Burnett, C.H., Commons, R.R., Albright, F., Howard, J.E. (1949), N.Engl.J.Med.240, 787-794.
2. Carroll, P.R., and Clark, O.H. (1983) Ann.Surg. 197, 427-433.

Addendum

$1.25(OH)_2D_3$ BINDING ALONG THE RAT NEPHRON: AUTORADIOGRAPHIC STUDY IN ISOLATED TUBULAR SEGMENTS.

N.FARMAN, C.MANILLIER, J.P.BONJOUR* and J.P.BONVALET
INSERM U246, Département de Biologie, CEN Saclay, 91191 Gif-sur-Yvette, France ; * Division de Physiopathologie, Département de Médecine, Hôpital Cantonal, Genève, Switzerland.

Introduction:

The main active metabolite of vitamin D, $1.25(OH)_2D_3$, is produced by the proximal tubule of the kidney (1). The question has arisen to know if this product could bind and act within the kidney (2). Two groups examined the existence of binding sites for $1.25(OH)_2D_3$ in defined tubular segments of the nephron of Vit.D deficient rats: Kawashima and Kurokawa (3) used biochemical methods on pools of isolated tubular segments, after in vitro incubation, whereas Stumpf et al.(4) performed autoradiographs on kidney slices, after in vivo injection of labeled hormone. They agreed to design the thick ascending limb of Henle's loop as a target segment. Binding sites were found in the proximal tubule by Kawashima (3), and not by Stumpf (4). Conflicting results also appeared concerning the cortical collecting tubules. We examined systematically the binding sites of $1.25(OH)_2D_3$ along the whole length of the nephron, at various in vitro concentrations of the hormone, by performing autoradiographs (dry film) on microdissected tubular segments (5).

Animals and methods:

Rats were injected for 7 days with the diphosphonate EHDP, which provides a selective depletion in endogenous $1.25(OH)_2D_3$. Kidney pyramids were incubated in vitro (30°C - 1 hr) in presence of collagenase, with ^3H-$1.25(OH)_2D_3$ (0.2 to 12 nM), in presence or absence of an excess unlabeled hormone. Tubular segments were microdissected and applied on a dry film, as previously described (6,7). After 1 to 4 months, the autoradiographs were developped, and tubules were fixed and stained. Silver grain counts were made over nuclear and cytoplasmic areas and over background. Specific and non specific cytoplasmic and nuclear labeling were calculated (5,6,7).

Results and discussion:

Specific, i.e. displaceable, nuclear binding sites for $1.25(OH)_2D_3$ (Fig 1) were mostly abundant in CAL and MCT. This specific nuclear binding increased between 0.2 and 1 nM concentration, and then reached a plateau, probably corresponding to saturation of receptors in these two main target segments. Specific nuclear binding sites were also observed in the distal cortical portions of the tubule: in DCT and CCT, nuclear labeling was irregular from one tubule to another and even within the same tubular segment. Particularly in the early portion of distal tubule, some groups of cells were heavily labeled, among others with no or little labeling. When DCT and CCT were considered together, their mean value of specific nuclear binding was somewhat lower than those of CAL and MCT, and appeared at higher concentrations. No specific nuclear binding was found in proximal tubule (convoluted or straight portion) and in the medullary portion of the thick ascending limb. In addition to nuclear binding sites, we also observed cytoplasmic labeling, in all nephron segments studied. It increased with steroid concentration, and was more important in medullary segments (PR, MAL and MCT). This cytoplasmic labeling was non displaceable, i.e. non specific, although it reached high values, in segments containing specific nuclear receptors, as CAL, DCT-CCT and MCT, as well as in segments lacking nuclear binding. In separate experiments, we checked that $1.25(OH)_2D_3$ was not metabolized in our incubation conditions, as determined by HPLC analysis of the radio active content of whole kidney tissue. Our observations on the localization of nuclear binding sites agree with those of Kawashima et al.(3) and

Stumpf et al.(4) to design the thick ascending limb of Henle's loop as a target site for $1.25(OH)_2D_3$. Concerning the other localizations of specific nuclear receptors, we identified the MCT (a segment not examined by the two other groups) as another main site of nuclear binding. We did not find specific binding in proximal tubule, either cytoplasmic or nuclear, in accordance with Stumpf et al.(4). These results are at variance with those of Kawashima et al.(3). We have no explanation for this discrepancy, which could partly be due to the high level of non specific cytoplasmic labeling in this segment, also noted by Kawashima et al.(3), which renders difficult a precise quantification of an eventual specific binding. The irregular, and sometimes very high, binding in DCT could correspond to the observations of Stumpf (4). In CCT, where specific binding was not described up to date, we observed a weaker, but significant, specific nuclear labeling.

The localization of binding sites described in this paper is roughly compatible with what is known on CaBP repartition along the nephron. In contrast, the establishment of a correspondance between the present observations and an eventual action of $1.25(OH)_2D_3$ along the nephron deserves further investigations.

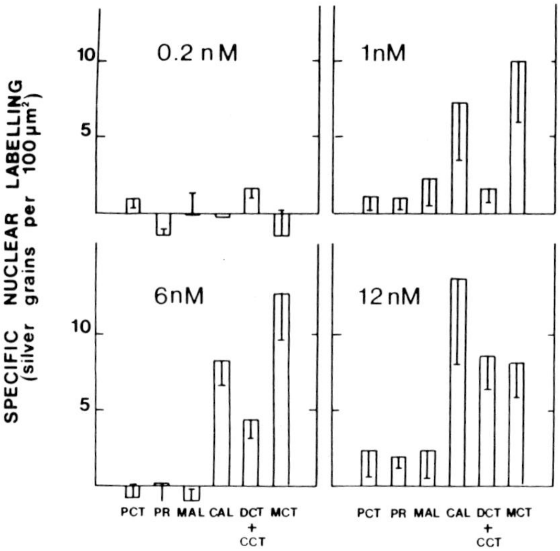

Figure 1 : Specific nuclear labeling by ^3H-$1.25(OH)_2D_3$ along the nephron, at concentrations from 0.2 to 12 nM. PCT: proximal convoluted tubule; PR: pars recta; MAL and CAL: medullary and cortical portions of the thick ascending limb of the loop of Henle; DCT: distal convoluted tubule; CCT: cortical collecting tubule; MCT: medullary collecting tubule.

References:

1. Brunette,M.G.,Chan,M.,Ferrière,C.,Roberts,K.D.(1978) Nature,276:287-289.
2. De Luca,H.F.,Schnoes,H.K.(1983) Annu.Rev.Biochem.,52:411-439.
3. Kawashima,H.,Kurokawa,K.(1982) J.Biol.Chem.257:13428-13432.
4. Stumpf,W.E.,Sar,M.,Narbaitz,R.,Reid,F.A.,DeLuca,H.F.(1980)Proc.Natl. Acad.Sci.USA 77:1149-1153.
5. Manillier,C.,Farman,N.,Bonjour,J.P.,Bonvalet,J.P.(1985) Am.J.Physiol. 248:F296-F307.
6. Farman,N.,Vandewalle,A.,Bonvalet,J.P.(1982) Am.J.Physiol.242:F69-F77.
7. Vandewalle,A.,Farman,N.,Bencsath,P.,Bonvalet,J.P.(1981) Am.J.Physiol. 240: F172-F179.

THE EFFECTS OF $1,25(OH)_2D_3$ ON THE GROWTH AND DIFFERENTIATION OF FETAL RAT "OSTEOBLAST-LIKE" CELLS AND OF A RAT OSTEOSARCOMA CELL (UMR 106).

M.P.M. Herrmann-Erlee*, C.W.G.M. Löwik*, H.A.P. Pols, J.C. Birkenhäger, C.G. Groot* and J.K. van Zeeland*. *Laboratory of Cell Biology and Histology, University of Leiden and Dept. of Internal Medicine III, Erasmus University, Rotterdam,The Netherlands.

INTRODUCTION. Previous studies have shown that $1,25(OH)_2D_3$ produces contrasting effects on growth and differentiation in osteoblast-like cells in culture. Alkaline phosphatase (ALP) activity was found to be inhibited by $1,25(OH)_2D_3$ in calvaria-derived osteoblast-like cells (1), however to be stimulated in a clonal osteoblast-like rat osteosarcoma cell line (2). A similar stimulating effects on ALP activity was found for $1,25(OH)_2D_3$ (10^{-7} - 10^{-8}M) in the Ros 17/2.8 cell line (3), when the cells were plated at low (5,000 cells/cm^2) density and show low endogenous ALP levels (immature culture). Under that condition $1,25(OH)_2D_3$ (10^{-7} - 10^{-8}M) inhibited cell growth. Lower (10^{-9} - 10^{-10}M) concentrations of 1,25 $(OH)_2D_3$ had no effects. However, these low $1,25(OH)_2D_3$ concentrations reduced ALP activity and stimulated cell growth in cultures plated at high density (25,000 cells/cm^2), a condition giving rise to cells showing higher endogenous ALP content (mature cells).

The present study was undertaken to investigate the effects of $1,25(OH)_2D_3$ on the growth (DNA) and differentiation (ALP and osteocalcin antigenicity)of fetal rat calvarium-derived osteoblast-like cells (OB). Preliminary experiments, using the osteosarcoma cell line UMR_{106} (OS) were also included in this study. In these cells DNA content and ornithine decarboxylase (ODC) activity were measured.

MATERIALS AND METHODS. Calvarium-derived osteoblast-like cells were isolated from 20-day-old rat embryos and cultured according to Boonekamp, Calcif. Tissue Int. 33, 1981, 291. They were cultured in α-MEM + 10% FCS, which has been previously treated with dextran-coated charcoal to remove endogenous Vitamin D_3 metabolites. After the first 24 h and every subsequent 24 h the medium was refreshed with α-MEM containing 2% FCS. Cells were cultured under 5% CO_2 and 95% air. ALP was measured according to the method of O.A.Bessey et al.(J. Biol. Chem., 164, 1946,321), for DNA the method of Karsten et al. (Anal. Bioch. 77, 1977, 464) was used. Ornithine decarboxylase (ODC) activity was determined according to Löwik et al. (Calcif.Tissue.Int., 35,1983,151).

Osteocalcin antigenicity was measured using a specific antiserum against rat osteocalcin raised in goat (gift from Dr. P. Hauschka).

The first antibody was visualized by rabbit-anti-goat IgG, coupled to FITC.

Table : The effect of $1,25(OH)_2D_3$ on DNA content and ALP activity in fetal osteoblast-like cells and its effect on DNA content and ODC activity in osteosarcoma cells(UMR106).

Vitamin D. A Chemical, Biochemical and Clinical Update

1,25$(OH)_2D_3$ (M)	ALP (nmoles/min/ug DNA) OB	OS	ODC (cpm/sample) OS	DNA (ug/sample) OB	OS
control	11.9 ± 0.4	n.d.	334 ± 30	7.8 ± 0.1	30.7 ± 1.1
10^{-10}	16.3 ± 0.6*	n.d.	239 ± 23**	7.4 ± 0.1	22.7 ± 1.1*
10^{-9}	n.d.	n.d.	202 ± 20**	n.d.	20.7 ± 1.4*
10^{-8}	19.8 ± 0.8*	n.d.	n.d.	7.7 ± 0.1	18.0 ± 0.9*
10^{-7}	n.d.	n.d.	n.d.	n.d.	14.7 ± 0.4*

For DNA and ALP determinations the cells were chronically treated with the hormone during 3 days, the medium was refreshed every 24 h. Plating densities for OB and OS 15,000 and 20,000 respectively. For ODC measurements OS cells were cultivated till confluency in 12 wells culture plates. The effect on ODC activity was measured 4 h after addition of the hormone. Values are mean ± SEM. Number of determinations 4 - 8. * $P < 0.01$, ** $P < 0.001$.

RESULTS. In the Table the effects of different concentrations of 1,25$(OH)_2D_3$ on the DNA content and ALP activity in fetal rat osteoblast-like cells (OB) are shown. Also included in this Table is the effect of 1,25$(OH)_2D_3$ on DNA content and ODC activity in osteosarcoma cells (OS). It follows from this table that 1,25$(OH)_2D_3$ has no effect on the DNA content of OB, however significantly reduced DNA content and ODC activity in a dose-related manner in OS. In these cells 25$(OH)D_3$ and 24,24$(OH)_2D_3$ had no effect (data not shown). In OB, ALP activity was significantly stimulated by 1,25$(OH)_2D_3$. ALP activities in OS were not yet determined.

In bone 20% of the non-collagenous matrix consists of osteocalcin. Biochemical studies (4) have shown that 1,25$(OH_2D_3$ stimulates its synthesis. In this study osteocalcin antigenicity was measured in OB cultivated to confluency (4-5 days of culture). After washing, the cells were kept for 16 hours in a Vitamin-D depleted medium (culture medium plus charcoal-treated FCS).
Subsequently, they were treated for 7 hours in a culture medium containing 2.4 x 10^{-9}M 1,25$(OH)_2D_3$ or 0.3% ethanol. After washing the cells they were frozen and thawed once to make the membranes permeable for the antibodies. The antiserum showed enhanced antigenicity in cells treated with 1,25$(OH)_2D_3$ as compared to control cells, while the preimmune serum was negative in the 1,25$(OH)_2D_3$ treated cells (data not shown).
It is concluded from this study that 1,25$(OH)_2D_3$ induces differentiation (ALP, osteocalcin) in rat osteoblast-like cells, without having effect on the DNA content. In osteosarcoma cells however, 1,25$(OH)_2D_3$ reduces ODC activity and DNA content.

REFERENCES.

1. Wong, G.L., Luben, R.A. and Cohn, D.V., (1977) Science, 197, 662-665.
2. Manolagas, S.C., Burton, D.W. and Deftos, L.J., (1981) J.Biol.Chem., 256, 7115-7117.
3. Majeska, R.J. and Rodan, G.A., (1982) J.Biol.Chem., 257, 3362-3365.
4. Price, P.A., Williamson, M.K. and Baukol, S.A., (1981) In: A.Veis (ed.) The chemistry and biology of mineralized connective tissues. 327-335, Elsevier North Holland Inc.

VISUALIZATION OF PTH BINDING SITES, CaBP AND TUBULIN IN CELL CULTURE AND INTACT TISSUE

M. DIETEL, H. ARPS AND A. NIENDORF
INSTITUTE OF PATHOLOGY, UNIVERSITY OF HAMBURG

To investigate morphologically some aspects of calcium regulating mechanisms on kidney and parathyroid glands (ptgl) the following cell culture experiments were conducted: 1) the localization of PTH binding sites and 2) of CaBP in the kidney, 3) the effect of calcium on the tubulin distribution in ptgl. Binding sites for PTH are demonstrated with a biotinylated b-PTH(1-84) and the avidin-biotin method. Immunohistological studies were performed using antisera from PROF.HESCH (Hannover) for PTH, from PROF.NORMAN (Riverside) for CaBP and from Amersham (Braunschweig) for tubulin. Tissue and cell culture were carried out as previously described (Dietel et al.1984, Biol.Cell 52:49). Tissue and cells were washed in serum free medium prior to incubation with the labeled or unlabeled hormone. Incubation was carried out for 1 to 60 minutes, followed by one wash in iced PBS and fixation in 2.5% glutaraldehyde. Binding of PTH to tubular cells is found in the majority of proximal tubular cells (Fig.1). In the distal tubule only distinct cells show positivity after incubation (Fig.2). Competition of biotinylated b-PTH(1-84) and the unlabeled hormone lead to no stain. 30 to 50% of the cultured cells expressed PTH binding, whereas CaBP was found mainly in distal parts of the nephron and in 30 to 40% of the cultured cells (Fig.3+4). Our observations show that the expression of the cytoskeleton protein tubulin is changed by different calcium levels. After 3 days of incubation a lowered calcium concentration (0,6mM) induces an increased density of tubulin filaments, whereas high calcium (2,4mM) gives opposite results (Fig.5/6). The present study is to our knowledge the first report of the visualization of PTH binding and CaBP on cultured cells. TEITELBAUM has shown the PTH dependent cAMP production on cultured kidney cells (Teitelbaum and Strewler 1984, Endocrinology 114:980). Our results can be valued as a morphological confirmation. The different distribution pattern of CaBP and PTH positive cells in tissue culture and the fact that a tenfold excess of unlabeled PTH abolished the stain completely prove the specificity of the staining. Double staining should help to solve the question in which part of the nephron PTH induces it's various functions. The preliminary result that calcium can change the density of cytoskeleton fibers possibly indicates an interrelationship between the secretory process of PTH and the cytoskeleton proteins.

The study was supported by the Deutsche Forschungsgemeinschaft, Grant Di 276 /1-1 and SFB "Rezeptoren, 232", Universität Hamburg.

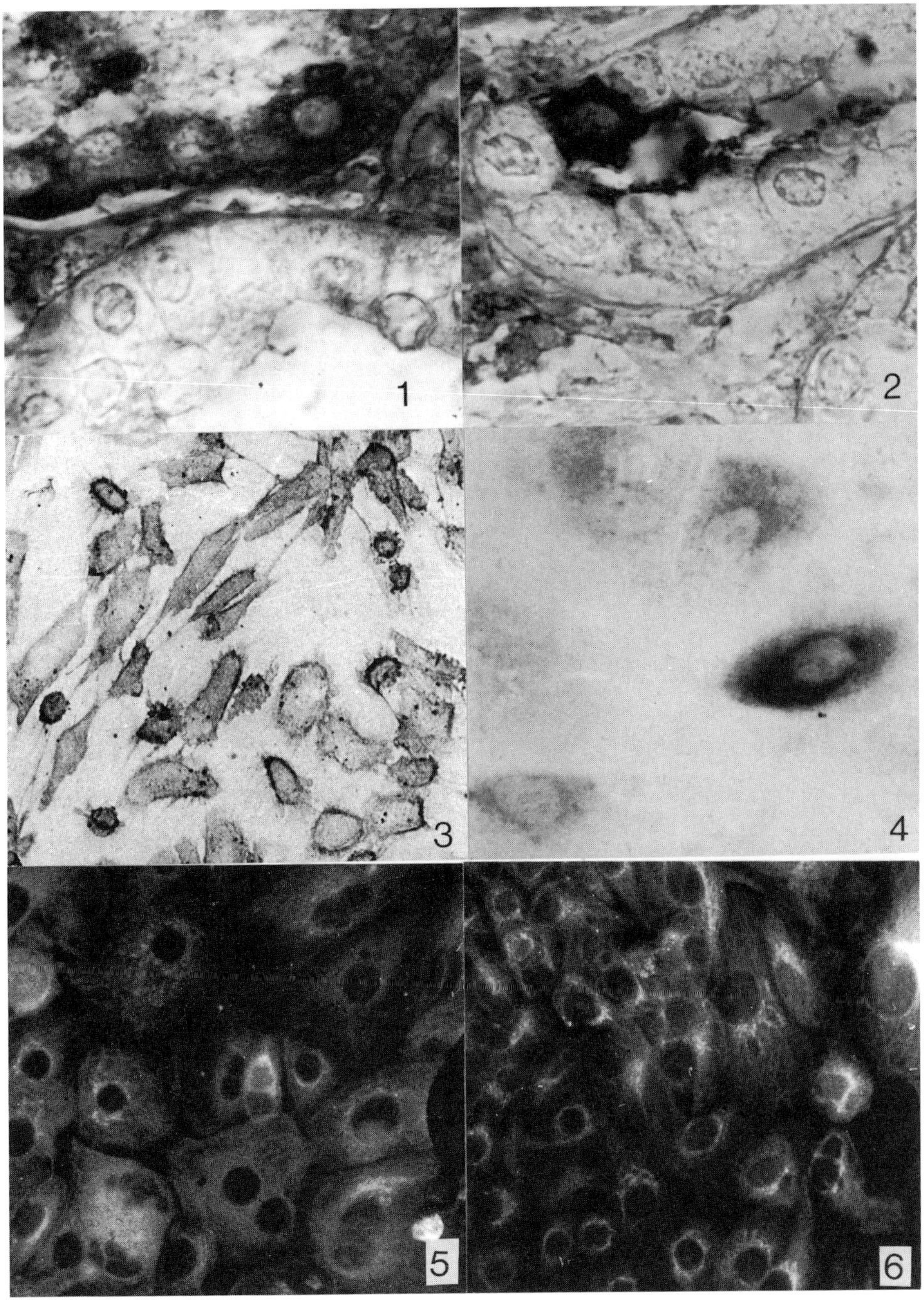

EXPLANATION OF THE FIGURES SEE TEXT

CALCITRIOL-RESISTANT LAXATIVE OSTEOMALACIA

C. Nagant de Deuxchaisnes*, C. van Ypersele de Strihou**
Departments of Rheumatology* and Nephrology**, Louvain University in Brussels, St-Luc University Hospital, B-1200 Brussels.

A woman, born in 1941, developed progressively generalized bone pain starting in the ribs (02/82), gaining the lumbar spine, the pelvis, the feet, and finally the shoulder girdle. Proximal muscular weakness was not prominent, yet a waddling gait developed probably owing to pain. A tentative diagnosis of osteomalacia was made on X rays in 07/83, because of a probable pseudofracture in one rib, and the presence of endocortical porosity in the phalanges of the fingers. Radiologic diagnosis became obvious in 09/83, when two more pseudofractures in the ribs were seen, with no tendency for the first pseudofracture to heal. The biochemistries during 1983 prior to therapy are shown in Table I. Most striking is the slight elevation of serum creatinine, the lowering of both serum Ca (total and ionized) and serum P, the elevation of both serum alkaline phosphatase and iPTH values, and the decrease in the urinary TmP/GFR. There was a mild hyperchloremic acidosis. Serum Mg, carotene and 25-OH-D levels were normal, excluding intestinal malabsorption, while the serum 1,25-$(OH)_2D$ level was lowish. In the urine (not shown in Table I), the fasting Ca /Cr ratio was low (0.02 mg/mg), whereas the fasting total hydroxyproline/Cr ratio was elevated (75 ug/mg). In the past history, there were episodes of acute gouty arthritis (onset:09/80), as well as phenacetin abuse, dating back to the year sixties. This did not continue, but was followed starting in 1972 by laxative abuse. Patient took progressively more bisacodyl (Dulcolax), a contact (stimulant) cathartic, of which she consumed 50 to 200 tablets (of 5 mg each) daily. She could never be persuaded to discontinue the medication (because she felt bloated). This habit allegedly only produced one or two watery stools daily. A bone biopsy was performed in 12/83, immediately prior to the initiation of therapy. The results of the histomorphonetric measurements (Mr. H. Withofs), performed on undecalcified sections, showed osteopenia, signs of secondary hyperparathyroidism, but above all striking osteomalacia. A that time, maximal pain was in the ribs, R. hip and L. foot. A pseudofracture had developed in the R. hip. The patient was treated with calcitriol in increasing doses, starting at 0.25 ug/day, and calcium supplements 1 g/day of elemental calcium. When on 0.50 ug/day of calcitriol, the fasting plasma level of 1.25-$(OH)_2D_3$ rose to 25.8 pg/ml. Symptomatic improvement was not achieved until the dose of calcitriol was shifted from 1.5 to 2.0 ug/day after 4 mo. of progressive increase. The fasting plasma 1,25-$(OH)_2D$ level was at that time 44.0 pg/ml. The total and ionized serum calcium were only normalized, and remained so, when the dose of calcitriol was in-

BIOCHEMISTRIES

	PATIENT VALUES	NORMAL VALUES (mean±sd)
CREATININE (mg/dl)	1.6 (7)	0.88±0.08
CALCIUM (mg/dl)	8.2 (7)	9.3±0.4
PHOSPHORUS (mg/dl)	2.3 (7)	3.1±0.5
SODIUM (meq/l)	139 (7)	140±1.6
POTASSIUM (meq/l)	4.0 (7)	3.85±0.2
CHLORIDE (meq/l)	110 (7)	104±2
TOTAL CO2 (meq/l)	19.3 (7)	24.7±2.2
PL. PROT. (g/dl)	6.7 (5)	7.1±0.3
MAGNESIUM (meq/l)	1.8 (3)	1.6±0.1
ALK. P'SE (IU/l)	105 (7)	19±7
IONIZED CALCIUM (mg/dl)	4.24 (3)	4.93±0.18
CAROTENE (µg/dl)	184 (3)	100-200
25-OH-D (ng/ml)	18.7 (2)	35.0±13.0
1,25-(OH)2D (pg/ml)	18.4 (2)	38.0±12.0
iPTH (mIU/ml)	6.7 (2)	3.5±0.9
TmP/GFR (mg/dl)	1.52 (2)	3.04±0.62

Between parentheses, number of determinations prior to therapy

Vitamin D. A Chemical, Biochemical and Clinical Update

HISTOMORPHOMETRIC ANALYSIS

	NORMAL VALUES (MEAN±SD)	PATIENT 12/83
TBV (%)*	20.9±3.60	16.9
TRS (%)*	2.02±0.96	7.01
ORS (%)*	1.06±0.64	7.01
OC/mm2*	0.15±0.09	0.88
ROV (%)*	1.89±0.99	32.3
AOV (%)*	0.38±0.18	5.45
ROS (%)*	11.0±9.20	84.9
TIO*	18.5±4.00	38
WOS (µm)*	7.72±2.08	25.5
OFS (%)*	3.50±5.13	3.93
MF (%)**	86.6±8.90	12.3

TBV: Trabecular Bone Volume TRS: Total Resorption Surface. ORS: Osteoclastic Resorption Surface. OC: Osteoclastic Count. ROV: Relative Osteoid Volume. AOV: Abosolute Osteoid Volume. ROS: Relative Osteoid Surface. TIO: Thickness Index of Osteoid. WOS: Width Osteoid Seams. OFS: Osteoblastic Formation Surface. MF: Mineralization Front

*: Undecalcified sections stained with Solochrome Cyanine; **: idem, stained with Toluidine Blue, pH 4.6.

creased to 3.0 ug/day (08/84), at which time the 24 h urinary excretion of calcium was still negligible. The pseudofractures showed incomplete signs of healing in 08/84. At that time, 3.5 ug/day of calcitriol was given, but the serum creatinine level progressively rose from 1.6 to 2.7 mg/dl, and the dose was reduced to 3.0 ug/day. Pseudofractures of ribs and R. hip had completely healed in 11/84, and all bone pain had disappeared. Serum creatinine had returned to 2.0 mg/dl. The alkaline phosphatase progressively decreased to 33 IU/l, iPTH to 4.0 mIU/ml, the total hydroxyproline/Cr ratio in the fasting urine to 26 ug/mg. Lumbar bone mineral content, as measured by dual photon absorptiometry, progressively rose from 2.85 (81 % of N) in 12/83 to 3.23 gHA/cm (92 % of N) in 11/84. In 02/85, the patient suffered an episode of "intestinal flu" and stopped taking bisacodyl for a fortnight, while continuing taking calcitriol at a reduced dose of 2.5 ug/day. Fatigue, malaise, polydipsia brought her to report at the Outpatient Clinic. The serum Ca had risen to 11.5 (ionized Ca:5.4), the serum P to 5.5, and the serum creatinine to 2.8 mg/dl. Calcitriol was discontinued, and when she was seen one week later, the serum Ca had decreased to 9.8 (ionized Ca:4.6), the serum P to 4.1, and the serum creatinine to 2.45 mg/dl. In conclusion, bisacodyl in high doses seems to produce osteomalacia, as well as a resistance to calcitriol. Interruption of bisacodyl intake soon produced clinical and biological signs of calcitriol toxicity. Our experience is that calcitriol in low doses (<1.0 ug/day) cures vitamin D-deficient osteomalacia (1), unless there is an intestinal barrier to its absorption (with among other features low serum carotene and Mg levels), as well as adult-onset hypophosphatemic vitamin D-resistant osteomalacia. In familial X-linked hypophosphatemic osteomalacia, patients seldom tolerate more than 1.5 ug/day of calcitriol when administered chronically. Laxative osteomalacia thus represents severe resistance to calcitriol. Such cases have been seldom reported, except by Frame et al. (2) in a patient taking 15 to 20 tablets daily of phenolphthalein (another stimulant cathartic) for the last 20 years. Both phenolphthalein and bisacodyl are diphenylmethane derivatives. Cure was obtained in this case when stopping the habit. This case, however, differed from ours in that the serum carotene was low and xylose absorption was impaired.

References:1.Nagant de Deuxchaisnes C, Rombouts-Lindemans C, Huaux JP, Withofs H, Meersseman F(1979).In:MacIntyre I, Szelke M. Molecular Endocrinology.Elsevier/North-Holland Biomedical Press, Amsterdam, pp 375-404. 2. Frame B, Guiang HL, Frost HM, Reynolds WA (1971). Arch Intern Med 128, 794-796.

COMPARATIVE STUDY OF 25, 1 ALPHA AND 1.25 HYDROXYLATED VITAMIN D METABOLITES USE IN LATE HYPOCALCEMIA TREATMENT

E. Mallet, B. Gügi

Department of Paediatrics, University of Rouen, 76031, France

Late neonatal hypocalcemia which occurs after the third day is associated with the presence of impaired parathyroïd secretion and additional factors such as early vitamin D deficiency. In our region, the late neonatal hypocalcemia incidence is closely correlated with the lack of sunshine and maternal vitamin D storage as demonstrated by low plasma 25-OH-D levels.

Results provided by new available vitamin D metabolites (25, 1 alpha and 1.25) were appreciated in a randomized and comparative study.

Late neonatal hypocalcemia (plasma calcium $<$ 1.90 mmol/l) was diagnosed between 3 and 10 days of life in 47 term newborns who presented symptoms of tetany with seizures in 25 p. cent of cases.

These newborns are included in a randomized therapeutic managment. They were initially treated with calcium (gluconate administrated intravenously at 1 000 mg/m^2) and hydroxylated vitamin D metabolites administrated 1-2 doses orally at a daily equivalent dosage 25-OH-D : 100 µg (n=15), 1 αOH-D : 2 µg and 1.25$(OH)_2$D : 1 µg (n=15) during the first 48 hours. Efficacy of treatment was particularly appreciated with regards to calcemic response.

There were evidence for materno-foetal vitamin D deficiency (3/4 cases with infant plasma level 25-OH-D $<$ 8 nmol/l), and hypoparathyroïd syndrome (2/3 cases with hyperphosphoremia $>$ 2.8 mmol/l and plasma immunoreactive PTH levels inappropriatly low in the presence of hypocalcemia). Before treatment, serum calcemia were not significantly different in the three groups (scheme 1).

Scheme 1

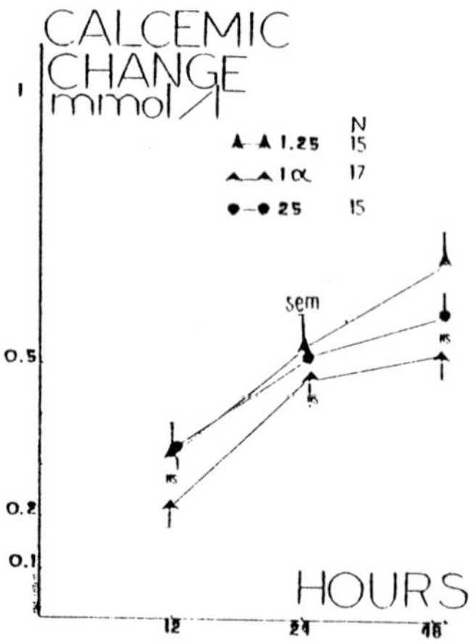

Maximal calcemic response (m ± sem mmol/l) was obtained with 1.25$(OH)_2$D (0.53 ± 0.08) as compared to 1 αOH-D (0.49 ± 0.06) and 25-OH-D (0.48 ± 0.05) at the 24th hour, but without significant difference. No hypercalcemia

Vitamin D. A Chemical, Biochemical and Clinical Update

nor any side effect were observed during treatment. No relapse of hypocalcemia occured.

There is no significant difference about calcemic response, but to explain some difference between respective metabolites effects it is possible that the explanation is the fact that 1.25 is the final and directly active metabolite. Conversely there are some delay of action probably due to kidney 1 hydroxylation for 25-OH metabolite and hepatic 25 hydroxylation for 1 αOH metabolite. Litterature provide previous studies where few cases of late neonatal hypocalcemia were treated with success by 1 αOH vitamin D metabolite (1, 2, 3).

In late symptomatic neonatal hypocalcemia which needs to be reduce shortly :

- vitamin D appears to be usefull in association with calcium, as hypercalcemic agent and because evidence of materno-foetal vitamin D deficiency especially in our region.
- 1 hydroxylated metabolites are especially indicated. Despite the fact that there is no significant advantage as regards to calcemic change during treatment, because of the therapeutic managment based on pathophysiology findings would be apply the treatment of hypoparathyroïdism 1 hydroxylated metabolites such as 1α or 1.25 may therefore be effective. Furthermore their short half life avoid hypercalcemia.

(1) David, L., Salle, B., Varenne, P., Glorieux, F. and Delvin, E. (1981) Pediatr. Res. 15, 1222
(2) Heckmatt, JZ., Peacock, M., Davies, AE., Mc Murray, J. and Isherwood, DM. (1979) Lancet 1, 546-548
(3) Doxiadis, SA. and Lapatsonis, PD. (1977) Lancet 1, 426.

COLLABORATION BETWEEN $24,25(OH)_2D_3$ AND $1,25(OH)_2D_3$ IN THE REGULATION OF ENDOCHONDRAL BONE DEVELOPMENT

A.H. Reddi and S. Wientroub
Bone Cell Biology Section, Mineralized Tissue Research Branch, National Institute of Dental Research, National Institutes of Health, Bethesda, MD 20205, U.S.A.

INTRODUCTION

The regulatory role of vitamin D metabolites on skeletal development is well known, although the precise cellular targets and the mechanism of action on endochondral bone formation is not well understood. This is in part due to the complexity of endochondral bone differentiation. The epiphyseal growth plate is a heterogeneous assemblage of different cell populations at various stages of differentiation. In view of this, it is difficult to dissect the various cellular targets in the epiphyseal growth plate. Additionally, the hormonal milieu impinging on the earliest phases of developing cartilage and bone in the fetus is complex due to contributions of fetal, maternal, and placental compartments.

The use of the matrix-induced endochondral bone differentiation system potentially circumvents these complexities and permits the study of the discrete stages of endochondral bone development, including: mesenchymal cell proliferation, chondrogenesis, cartilage calcification, bone formation, and remodelling, all resulting in the de novo formation of ossicle with hematopoietic bone marrow (1-3).

MATERIAL AND METHODS

Demineralized bone matrix was prepared from adult rat diaphyses and implanted subcutaneously over the thoracic region as previously described (1). The matrix was implanted in vitamin D-free rats, using second generation rachitic animals. These animals were obtained by depleting Long-Evans

Vitamin D. A Chemical, Biochemical and Clinical Update

female rats (8 weeks old) of vitamin D by maintaining them on a vitamin D-free diet (containing 1.0% calcium and 0.8% phosphorus), deionized water and housing them in a room free of ultraviolet light. After three weeks on the diet, serum vitamin D metabolites were not detectable and the females were mated with normal males. Male weanling rats from these litters were used at the age of 1 month for the experiments. Radiological, histological and biochemical criteria were used to confirm rickets. Vitamin D metabolites ($1,25-(OH)_2D_3$, $24,25-(OH)_2D_3$, $25-OH-D_3$) were not detectable in the serum in these rats.

Vitamin D metabolites, kindly supplied by Dr. M. Uskokovic of Hoffman-LaRoche (Nutley, N.J.), were dissolved in ethanol and then in propylene glycol to a final concentration of 100 ng/50 µl or 25 ng/50 µl. The metabolites were administered daily by i.p. injection at a dose of 100 ng or 25 ng/rat. Vitamin D deficient control animals were injected with only the vehicle.

RESULTS

Vitamin D deficiency resulted in growth retardation compared to repleted animals. It was clear that rachitic animals gained significantly less weight than the repleted animals and that the serum calcium levels in the former group (6.1 ± 0.3 mg/dl) were significantly lower than the normal range (9-10 mg/dl). $24,25-(OH)_2D_3$ appeared to be more effective in increasing the body weight but a higher dose (100 ng/day/rat) was needed for correction of serum calcium levels as compared to $1,25-(OH)_2D_3$ (25 ng/rat/day). Serum phosphate levels were decreased in the deficient animals (8.3 ± 0.4 mg/dl) and administration of various metabolites significantly increased the serum phosphate levels.

$[^3H]$ thymidine incorporation into acid precipitable DNA and ornithine decarboxylase activity (4,5) were monitored as parameters of mesenchymal cell proliferation in day 3 implants. There was a significant increase in $[^3H]$ thymidine

TABLE 1

INFLUENCE OF VITAMIN D METABOLITES ON $^{35}SO_4$ INCORPORATION IN DAY 7 PLAQUES AND PROXIMAL TIBIAL EPI-METAPHYSES

		$^{35}SO_4$ INCORPORATION			
Group	Dose (ng.)	Plaques		Epi-metaphyses	
		Acid insoluble (dpm/mg tissue)	Acid insoluble (dpm/μg DNA)	Acid insoluble (dpm/mg tissue)	Acid insoluble (dpm/μg DNA)
Vit. D. Def.		216 ± 16	45 ± 5	767 ± 52	73 ± 3
24,25-$(OH)_2D_3$	25	433 ± 58	100 ± 7	846 ± 64	135 ± 16
24,25-$(OH)_2D_3$	100	434 ± 59	97 ± 6	1244 ± 114	118 ± 12
1,25-$(OH)_2D_3$	25	207 ± 14	45 ± 3	724 ± 49	79 ± 4
1,25-$(OH)_2D_3$	100	203 ± 12	54 ± 5	747 ± 36	77 ± 4
Vit. D_3	100	380 ± 32	61 ± 7	884 ± 37	125 ± 8
25-OH-D_3	100	305 ± 11	64 ± 6	989 ± 44	122 ± 11

Values presented are the mean ± SE of 8 observations from 4 rates in each group.

TABLE 2

INFLUENCE OF VITAMIN D METABOLITES ON PHOSPHATASES AND ^{45}Ca INCORPORATION IN DAY 12 PLAQUES

Group	Dose (ng.)	Phosphatases (U/mg protein) Acid	Phosphatases (U/mg protein) Alkaline	^{45}Ca Incorporation (cpm/mg tissue)	Calcium content (µg/mg tissue)
Vit. D. Def.		0.87 ± .09	2.87 ± .22	1678 ± 176	9.0 ± 1.5
24,25-$(OH)_2D_3$	100	1.6 ± .08	1.5 ± .11	5757 ± 399	26.0 ± 1.0
1,25-$(OH)_2D_3$	100	1.6 ± .20	.90 ± .08	3643 ± 268	27.6 ± 1.8
Vit. D_3	100	1.1 ± .16	1.6 ± .31	4187 ± 265	20.8 ± 1.4
25-OH-D_3	100	1.1 ± .19	1.7 ± .19	4774 ± 571	18.2 ± 1.8
Vit. D. Def.		1.4 ± .06	2.3 ± .18	442 ± 67	1.2 ± .19
24,25-$(OH)_2D_3$	25	3.2 ± .30	1.5 ± .20	6804 ± 778	23.1 ± 1.9
1,25-$(OH)_2D_3$	25	2.0 ± .09	2.0 ± .21	3778 ± 265	13.0 ± .7

Values presented are the mean ± SE of 8 observations from 4 animals in each group.

incorporation in vitamin D deficient rats compared to controls. This increased incorporation was not changed by the administration of 24,25(OH)$_2$D$_3$ but was reduced by 1,25(OH)$_2$D$_3$ (data not shown).

Chondrogenesis was quantitated by $^{35}SO_4$ incorporation into proteoglycans on day 7. In rats treated with 24,25(OH)$_2$D$_3$ there was a significant increase in $^{35}SO_4$ incorporated (Table 1). Similar trends were observed in the proximate tibial epi-metaphyses used as an internal control (Table 1).

The alkaline and acid phosphastase activity levels reflect bone formation and resorption respectively. The ^{45}Ca incorporation represnts rate of mineralization and ^{40}Ca content as assessed by atomic absorption is an index of the extent of mineralization (5). The alkaline phosphatase levels were elevated in implants obtained from vitamin D deficient rats compared to rats treated with vitamin D metabolites (Table 2). ^{45}Ca incorporation was the lowest in rachitic rats and was stimulated by 24,25 (OH)$_2$D$_3$. However, paradoxically the calcium content appeared to be maximal in rats treated with 1, 25 (OH)$_2$D$_3$. Additional experiments revealed that in this instance the implanted matrix underwent calcification as revealed by von Kossa staining. It should be recalled that in implants in normal rats the implanted matrix does not undergo mineralization (1). At the lower doses examined (25 ng/day/rat) the implants were histologically more advanced when treated with 24, 25 (OH) $_2$D$_3$ compared to 1,25 (OH)$_2$D$_3$. Similar trends were observed with the proximal tibial epi-metaphyses (data not shown).

DISCUSSION

The present investigation was undertaken to gain better insight into the role of vitamin D metabolites in discrete stages of endochordral bone development in rachitic rats. The present experimental protocol resulted in rickets as assessed by histological, radiological and biochemical criteria. The decrease in DNA synthesis under the influence of 1,25 $(OH)_2D_3$ may suggest a regulatory role for this metabolite in proliferation of chondroprogenitor cells. The marked increase in $^{35}SO_4$ incorporation into proteoglycans by 24,25 $(OH)_2D_3$ in matrix-induced cartilage and epiphyseal cartilage is noteworthy. On the other hand 1,25 $(OH)_2D_3$ stimulated the acid phosphatase levels indicating a role in bone remodelling. The present results confirm and extend the previous work (6-10) implicating a critical role for 24,25 $(OH)_2D_3$ in cartilage and bone formation. In conclusion, the present investigation implies a temporal collaboration between 24,25 $(OH)_2D_3$ and 1,25 $(OH)_2D_3$ in the regulation of endochondral bone formation. It is likely that early chondrogenesis and bone formation is stimulated by 24,25 $(OH)_2D_3$ whereas subsequent bone remodeling and resorption is regulated by 1,25 $(OH)_2D_3$.

REFERENCES

1. Reddi, A.H. and Huggins, C.B. (1972) Proc. Nat. Acad. Sci. U.S.A. 69, 1601-1605.
2. Reddi, A.H. and Huggins, C.B. (1975) Proc. Nat. Acad. Sci. U.S.A. 72, 2212-2216.
3. Reddi, A.H. and Anderson, W.A. (1976) J. Cell Biol. 69, 557-572.
4. Rath, N.C. and Reddi, A.H. (1979) Nature, 278, 855-856.
5. Reddi, A.H. and Sullivan, N.E. (1980) Endocrinology, 107, 1291-1299.
6. Ornoy, A., Godwin, D., Nott, D. and Edelstein, C. (1978) Nature, 276, 517-519.
7. Gallagher, J.A. and Lawson, D.E.M. (1980) Calcif. Tiss. Int. 31, 215-223.
8. Corvol, M.T., Ulamann, A. and Garabedian, M. (1980) FEBS Lett. 116, 273-276.
9. Malluche, H., Henry, H., Meyer-Sabellek, W., Sherman, D., Massry, S. and Norman, A.W. (1980) Am. J. Physiol. 238, 494-498.

10. Massry, S.G., Tuma, S., Dua, S. and Golstein, D.A. (1979) J. Lab. Clin. Med. 94, 152-157.

SERUM BONE GLA-PROTEIN AND 1,25-DIHYDROXYVITAMIN D IN FULL-TERM NEWBORNS.

P.D. DELMAS[1], L. MALAVAL[1], E.E. DELVIN[3], I. MELKI[2], F.H. GLORIEUX[3], B.L. SALLE[2] and M.C. CHAPUY[1],
[1]Inserm U234 and [2]Neonatal Unit, Hopital E. Herriot, Lyon, France; [3]Genetics Unit, Shriners Hospital and McGill University, Montreal, Canada.

In newborns, the transient decrease in serum calcium characterizing the adaptation to extra-uterine life, induces a rapid increase in serum parathyroid hormone and $1,25(OH)_2D$ levels. We have previously demonstrated that this effect was particularly striking in preterm infants (1). In the present study we have looked at the same sequence of events in full term (FT) newborns by assessing during the first month of life the changes in circulating levels of several markers of bone and mineral metabolism: vitamin D metabolites, alkaline phosphatase (AP) and Bone-Gla Protein (BGP). The latter has been proposed to reflect bone formation and its synthesis to be induced by $1,25(OH)_2D$. We thus have evaluated whether in the neonatal period a rapid increase in serum $1,25(OH)_2D$ has an influence on BGP levels.

Material and Methods

Ten normal subjects were studied. Their gestational age varied from 37-40 weeks and their weight at birth from 2,700-4,500 g. Blood specimens were obtained from the cord (CB) and on day 1 and 5 on the maternity ward. Then upon check-up examination on Day 30. AP levels were measured by colorimetric assay (2) while 25-OHD and $1,25(OH)_2D$ were assessed by radioligand (3) and radioreceptor assay (4) respectively. BGP levels were measured by radioimmunoassay (5).

Results

They are summarized in Table 1. Levels of 25-OHD were low by North-American standards but comparable to other studies in the french population (1). As in preterms, $1,25(OH)_2D$ levels increased rapidly from birth to Day 5 and then decrease to reach by Day 30 values similar to those found in young children. All levels of BGP were much higher than in adult subjects (6 ± 1 ng/ml). We observed a rapid rise in BGP in the first 5 days with the value at Day 30 being not different from the one at Day 5. AP remained low during the first week and subsequently increased to high values. Levels of $1,25(OH)_2D$ and BGP were correlated in CB ($r = 0.83$, $p < 0.05$) and from birth to Day 5 ($r = 0.67$, $p < 0.001$) but not on Day 30 (Fig.1). AP levels correlated neither with $1,25(OH)_2D$ nor with BGP.

Table 1

		CB	Day 1	Day 5	Day 30
25-OHD	(ng/ml)	13 ± 2	11 ± 2	12 ± 2	17 ± 1
$1,25(OH)_2D$	(pg/ml)	38 ± 4	58 ± 10[a]	100 ± 5[c]	56 ± 6[a]
BGP	(ng/ml)	14 ± 2	17 ± 1	24 ± 2[b]	23 ± 2[b]
AP	(BU/l)	7 ± 1	7 ± 1	7 ± 1	15 ± 2

Values are mean ± s.e.m. For the significance of differences between means, all values are compared to those observed in cord blood. a) $p < 0.025$, b) $p < 0.005$, c) $p < 0.0001$.

Vitamin D. A Chemical, Biochemical and Clinical Update

Figure 1

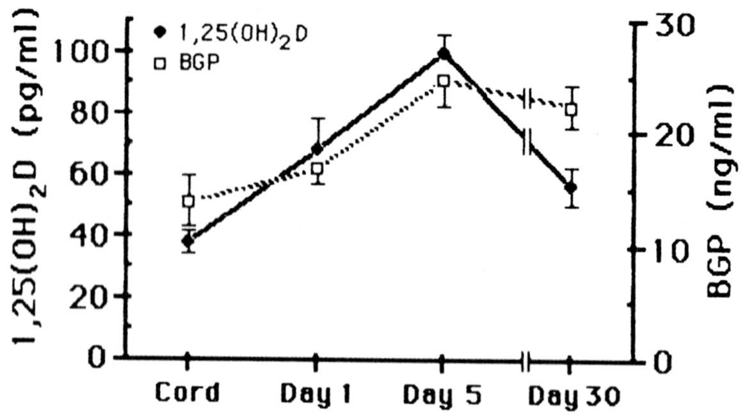

Discussion

The data support the contention that, even in the presence of low 25-OHD levels, early and significant changes in $1,25(OH)_2D$ levels reflect the perinatal equilibration of calcium homeostasis. Since the correlation between $1,25(OH)_2D$ and BGP disappeared after Day 5, BGP synthesis is not directly controlled by $1,25(OH)_2D$. Finally, since the increase in AP activity occured much later than that of BGP, it is likely that the two markers reflect different events of bone metabolism. As limitations imposed by the protocol did not allow to collect data between Days 5 and 30, further studies will be needed to elicit any possible changes in BGP and AP during that period.

References

1. Glorieux, F.H. et al. (1981) J. Pediatr. 99:640.
2. Bodansky, O. et al. (1968) Adv. Clin. Biochem. 11: 277.
3. Delvin, E.E. et al. (1980) Clin. Biochem. 13: 106.
4. Delvin, E.E. et al. (1981) Calcif. Tissue Int. 33: 173.
5. Delmas, P.D. et al. (1983) J. Clin. Invest. 71: 1316.

Supported by the Institut National de la Santé et de la Recherche Médicale and the Shriners of North America.

THE NIH PEER REVIEW PROCESS: PREPARATION OF A COMPREHENSIVE RESEARCH GRANT APPLICATION

Antonia C. Novello, MD, MPH, Executive Secretary, General Medicine B Study Section, Division of Research Grants, National Institutes of Health, Bethesda, Maryland, USA.

Obtaining Federal funds to conduct biomedical research is a lengthy, complex process, one which is becoming increasingly difficult for a variety of reasons. While it is true that research proposals which are scientifically and methodologically sound, innovative and of potential relevance to the proposed field, will always be approved by Study Section reviewers, this is not enough to insure funding. A project must also be presented in the best light, clearly written, concisely presented and prepared with a knowledge of the review process at the National Institutes of Health. In doing so, the principal investigator will submit the best possible application, and in turn will permit the study section the best evaluation of its scientific merit and prospective support. This article is written to aid the investigator in accomplishing those goals. It will attempt to summarize the pertinent points in the review process; discuss recent requirements for grant applications, make suggestions for grants improvements and finally, list the most common reasons for disapproval and poor priority scores. The main purpose, however, is to assist all investigators, experienced and non-experienced, to successfully compete in biomedical research. When preparing an application, bear in mind that you are to be reviewed by a panel of expert peers. Thus, some items to consider when writing an application are:

- Follow instructions.
- Never assume the Study Section will "know what you mean."
- Refer to the literature thoroughly and thoughtfully.
- Represent your abilities and interests honestly.
- State the goals and address the central hypothesis.
- Include well-designed and well-explained tables and figures.
- Present an organized, easy-to-comprehend set of protocols.
- Include an accurate abstract that outlines the objectives and methods of the proposed research.

Vitamin D. A Chemical, Biochemical and Clinical Update

- Use experimental systems that you are familiar with by describing the experiments, methodology and techniques, the literature, and your experience.
- Describe how you plan to analyze and interpret data.
- Address potential pitfalls and how they might be avoided.

When writing the research plan, the principal investigator must remember that the Study Section will consider the information provided as an example of the investigator's approach to a research objective and ability in the proposed area of research. In the methods section, one should not assume that the Study Section needs little information! While the Study Section might be more familiar with the methodology than the applicant, they have no way of knowing if the applicant has the same familiarity. The applicant should not leave anything to the imagination, but give details of the research plan, including descriptions of experiments or any proposed work, the kinds of data to be expected, the means by which they will be gathered and analyzed, and most importantly, why and what will be gained by this data gathering.

Likewise, when doing the biographical sketch, the PI should include a curriculum vitae for all professional personnel listed and for every collaborator. It is a good idea to include the names of mentors for the doctoral research program and for any postdoctoral research experience. Also, the PI should include any planned leave of absence as well as an updated bibliography.

Other items to consider when writing a proposal:

DO's	DON'Ts
PERSONNEL	
o describe all personnel whether professional or non-professional, by name, position, and proposed time and effort -- even if no salary is involved;	o exceed 100 percent for the collective sum of percentages of time and effort proposed for each individual.
o justify job descriptions;	o request consultants that cannot be justified -- either by lack of expertise or level of effort -- for the proposed research.

DO's -- PERSONNEL

- o list dollar amounts separately for each individual;
- o request only consultants who have agreed to participate.

EQUIPMENT AND SUPPLIES

DO's

- o request and justify all equipment necessary for the completion and performance of the proposed research;
- o request and itemize supplies needed for completion of the proposed research;
- o justify species, numbers, and cost of all animals;
- o request costs for patient care, where appropriate;
- o add subtotals.

DON'Ts

- o request to purchase equipment that appears to be duplicative (e.g., investigator in previous proposal would have had to have such equipment to conduct the research);
- o add supplies indiscriminately;
- o propose to use animal species that cannot be correlated to human data; or are not appropriate for the proposed area of research;
- o request funds for coverage of laboratory tests which are routinely provided as part of a patient's basic tests;
- o forget to check budget for errors.

DO's	DON'Ts

OTHER SUPPORT

DO's	DON'Ts
o describe for each professional -- including the investigator listed on page 2 of the application -- by time and effort all other -- active support -- applications and proposals pending review or funding; -- applications and proposals planned or being prepared for submission.	o forget to propose how priorities will be rearranged so as not to exceed 100 percent time and effort. o forget to address in detail potential overlap in scientific content between current proposal and others submitted.

TRAVEL

DO's	DON'Ts
o request travel monies and describe the purpose of the travel.	o request travel for meetings not appropriate for the proposed area of research.

The investigator can submit, up to four weeks before the Study Section meeting, any new data or manuscript that will aid the Study Section membership in accomplishing a thorough comprehensive review of the proposal. Similarly the investigator must be sure that all letters of proposed collaborators, and of recommendation, are in the hands of the Executive Secretary by the same four weeks deadline.

Other considerations when preparing an application:

1. Page Limitation

Because of the increasing volume of applications received by the National Institutes of Health (NIH) in recent years, rules on page limitation have been implemented. These rules are designed to keep applications short, concise and precise through a standard format. Page limitation is taken seriously. The applicant should adhere to the instructions summarized below:

Page Limitations

Biographical Sketch	:	2 pages
Specific Aims	:	1 page
Significance	:	3 pages
Progress Report	:	8 pages
Methods	:	No page limitation but be succinct.

If it is absolutely essential to exceed the page limitation, an explanation must be provided. In the event the above requirement is not met, the proposal will be returned with a letter requesting that the application be rewritten to comply with the page limitation requirements. If the investigator fails to respond, the application will be deferred until such time as it conforms to the rules.

2. Human Subjects

For proposals involving human subjects the applicant should:

- o describe the characteristics of the subject population;
- o describe and assess any potential risks;
- o describe the procedures followed to obtain consent, including how the procedure is designed to minimize risk and produce effectiveness;
- o assess the potential benefits to be gained by the subject and society, and
- o evaluate the risk benefit ratio.

The most recent regulations governing the protection of human subjects require the applicant to:

- o complete Form 596, assuring the protection of human subjects;
- o secure review, modification (if necessary), and approval of the proposal by the applicant's organization's local institutional review board prior to submission to the NIH.

This written documentation must be received by the NIH, attached to the application.

During the review of an application involving human subjects, if the Study Section perceives any risk (i.e., physical, psychological, or social resulting from the research), it will document its concerns, or comments and a code will be assigned. The presence of some codes prohibits issuance of an award. Only after the concerns are adequately addressed by the PI can the code be removed. Certain areas of research involving human subjects, however, are exempt from the requirments described above. These include: normal educational practices, educational tests, survey or interview procedures, observation of public behavior or collection of study of existing data (through documents, records, or specimens of information publicly available).

3. Animal Welfare

Animal welfare is of the utmost importance in the area of biomedical research. Animals must be treated in a manner to avoid unnecessary discomfort, pain, anxiety, or poor health.

When applications involving vertebrate animals in the research plan are reviewed, the applicant will have to describe

- o the appropriateness of the experimental animal species; and
- o number of animals used; and detail the maintenance;
- o care, and treatment of the animals before, during, and after experimental procedures.

As with Human Subjects, any perceived risk resulting from the research will be documented as a comment or concern, and a code will be assigned. Only after the concern is addressed will the code be removed. With animals, as with humans, when the concern is great enough, the research proposal can be disapproved.

4. Hazardous Conditions

- o Describe special facilities to protect research personnel and the environment.
- o Explain how biohazardous materials will be handled appropriately.
- o Ensure that employees will be trained adequately in safe practices.

Before final submission:

- The applicant must meet the mail deadline:

Type of Application	Receipt Dates
Competing continuation (renewals), supplemental, new program project and center, Research Career Development Award, and Fellowship applications	February 1, June 1, and October 1
New research projects	March 1, July 1, and November 1

  Although these dates are meant to be final deadlines, extensions for hardship cases may be granted, on a case-to-case basis. This is only after the application has been received by the Division of Research Grants (DRG), and after all other applications have been processed. No waiver will be considered unless a covering letter, submitted with the application, describes the extenuating circumstances that would justify special treatment.

- The applicant can provide information to facilitate the assignment and review of the proposal. This can be done in a covering letter, with the application, at the time of submission. Although the referral staff will consider these requests for specific assignments, the final decision will be based upon a number of factors. Among these are the subject matter of the application, potential conflicts of interest, timing relative to meeting date, history of the application, availability of review resources, and assigned review responsibilities of the committees as they relate to the content of the application.

- Proposals not appropriately signed by an authorized official of the applicant's institution, and by the PI properly, will be considered unacceptable, and will be returned and not reviewed.

- The applicant should contact, prior to the review, the appropriate Executive Secretary for guidance or questions. Any communication following review, however, should be addressed to the Program Director of the awarding institute.

After submission

The applicant may contact the Executive Secretary at any time before the review to:

- verify that the application received is complete and how information, if missing, can be forwarded;
- verify that the materials in the appendix are adequate and appropriate;
- provide additional information (not available at the time of submission of the application) to be included as part of the application;
- seek guidance on how corrections can be made to typographical errors discovered after submission of the application;
- determine that all assurances necessary for Form 596 (protection of human subjects) have been received.

If an investigator feels that the application has been inappropriately assigned, he or she may appeal in writing to the Referral Branch of DRG. The appeal may be made because the investigator feels that the application's main thrust is not relevant to the particular review group's expertise.

After discussions involving the Referral Officer and the appropriate Executive Secretary, a final decision is made by the Office of the Chief of the Referral Branch. Where appropriate, the Division of Research Grants Referral Branch arranges to have such an application assigned to another Study Section with similar expertise in the field or by a special Study Section.

Conflict of Interest

It is well known that members of Study Sections must leave the room when applications from their organization are being discussed and voted on. Recent policies governing conflict of interest, however, may not be generally known. These include:

- For those universities which have separate geographical campuses, e.g., the University of California, a Study Section member may not be in the room for the discussion or voting of the application from any of the campuses of that university. However, relief from this rule has been obtained for some systems, e.g., the State University of New York.

- A Study Section member must leave the room if he or she feels that there is a professional or personal conflict of interest, e.g., the application has been submitted by a recent teacher, or a recent student. In cases of close personal friends, close associates or recent number of joint publications, the application might have to go to a different Study Section.

- A Study Section may not review an application of one of its members or their spouses, parents, or children, if any one of them is listed as a principal investigator or appears on the budget page in any capacity. Such applications are reviewed by other appropriate Study Sections.

- The Initial Review Group (IRG) may review applications in which a member has no tangible involvement, e.g., the member's availability at the principal investigator's institution for discussions, being a provider of services, cell lines, reagents or other materials, or writing a letter of reference. In such cases, the member may not be in the room during the review.

All materials pertinent to the applications being reviewed are privileged communications, prepared for use only by members of Study Section and the NIH staff. Members are requested to leave all review materials with the Executive Secretary at the conclusion of the review meeting.

After the Study Section meeting, the summary statements are completed as soon as possible to allow for their timely transmission to the appropriate Councils. The summary statement and the priority score can now be obtained before Council from the program official through the Privacy Act Office of the funding Institute.

What Might Lower Your Priority Score

- Not following the prescribed instructions.

- Lack of organization, confusing aims, significance, methods.

- Absence of crucial letters of collaboration. These letters must be available during the review and explicitly include the nature and extent of collaboration.

- Poor writing, including gross typographical mistakes and grammatical errors. Suggest institutional peer review of the application prior to submission to NIH.

- o Inadequate time and level of effort proposed for the research.
- o Proposing to change direction in the middle of a project without a proper explanation, adequate expertise, or background information.
- o Unrealistic and unjustified budget.

Common Reasons for Disapproval

Although the specific reasons for disapproval vary with each application, some common faults exist.

- o Lack of new or original ideas
- o Diffuse, superficial, or unfocused research plan
- o Lack of knowledge of published relevant work
- o Lack of experience in the essential methodology
- o Uncertainty concerning the future directions
- o Questionable reasoning in experimental approach
- o Absence of an acceptable scientific rationale
- o Unrealistically large amount of work
- o Lack of sufficient experimental data
- o Uncritical approach

In addition to the above general reasons for disapproving applications, Research Career Development Awards (RCDAs) are most frequently disapproved for the following reasons:

- o Award will not enhance or be conducive to the development of an independent research career.
- o RCDA is used as a substitute for salary support.
- o Investigator has senior academic rank and is already productive.
- o The institution does not indicate proper commitment to the applicant's career development.

Additional common reasons for disapproval of renewal applications include:

- o Lack of comprehensive progress reports.

- o Lack of productivity.

- o Change in direction of the project without adequate expertise, background information or explanation.

Similarly, common reasons for disapproval of revised applications are:

- o Failure to submit documented rebuttal to the critique.

- o Failure to revise the application substantially in response to the critique.

Since the number of revised applications has increased dramatically, it is of the utmost importance to address the points previously reported in the critique. In revising an application:

- o Follow instructions in PHS-398 for Revised Applications.

- o State revised arguments based on the critique points.

- o Submit manuscripts that have been published or accepted for publication since submission of the previous proposal.

- o Be brief, clear and direct and do not exceed page limitations.

- o Remember that the members of the Study Section that reviewed the first application may have changed.

- o Be aware that if the nature of the original proposal has changed, the application might be assigned to a different Study Section.

- o Remember that for Revised Renewal Applications, the importance of the comprehensive progress report cannot be overly emphasized (as the fate of the renewal application lies almost as much with past progress as with future plans).

Rebuttal

A rebuttal is a letter and/or associated documents from a principal investigator containing information contradicting the findings and recommendations of a review group as recorded in the summary statement, project site visit report, or other related documents. A rebuttal may indicate disagreement with procedures, with details of the review, with the Bureau, Institute, or Division (BID) or IRG assignment, or with the composition of the IRG. A rebuttal may also request re-review or other special action on the application.

A letter of rebuttal is useful when it clarifies point(s), and does not vent frustration. A principal investigator should:

- o Detail the rebuttal in a letter to the appropriate Program Director.
- o Address specific points of concern.
- o Document comments with relevant literature and appropriate background information.

When a letter of rebuttal is received prior to the meeting of the appropriate National Advisory Council/Board, three options are available to program staff after appropriate consultation with review staff:

- o No intervention--if the communication is judged to provide no basis to question the efficacy or equity of the review process to date;
- o Administrative deferral for re-review by an IRG--if the communication is judged to present scientific issues, which, if considered by the IRG, may have a significant likelihood of altering the original IRG findings and recommendations; or
- o Special Council/Board consideration--if the communication is judged to present issues appropriate for resolution by the Council/Board and not requiring evaluation by an IRG.

When a letter or rebuttal is received after a Council/Board completes action, the response, in general, shall be to advise the principal investigator to submit a revised application. Theoretically an investigator has the potential to be heard and to receive additional peer review comments which should allow him or her to incorporate the new suggestions into a revised application. In the event an applicant investigator disagrees with the response to a rebuttal, that individual may make a formal appeal to the Deputy Director of NIH for Extramural Research and Training. The appeal will have to be endorsed by the signature of the responsible institutional official. The new system of appeal will soon be in place for a one-year test.

Obtaining Federal funds is influenced by a number of forces and factors, only some of which are under an investigator's control. Because of constraints in Federal funds for biomedical research over the last several years, a doubling of approved but unfunded applications in recent years, and a lowering of the cut-off point at which applications are funded, competition has become intense and obtaining funds extremely difficult. Thus this article is meant to be a guide for investigators, so that they can present their applications in the most knowledgeable and effective manner.

AUTHOR INDEX

KEY WORD INDEX